Spitz and Fisher's
MEDICOLEGAL INVESTIGATION
OF DEATH

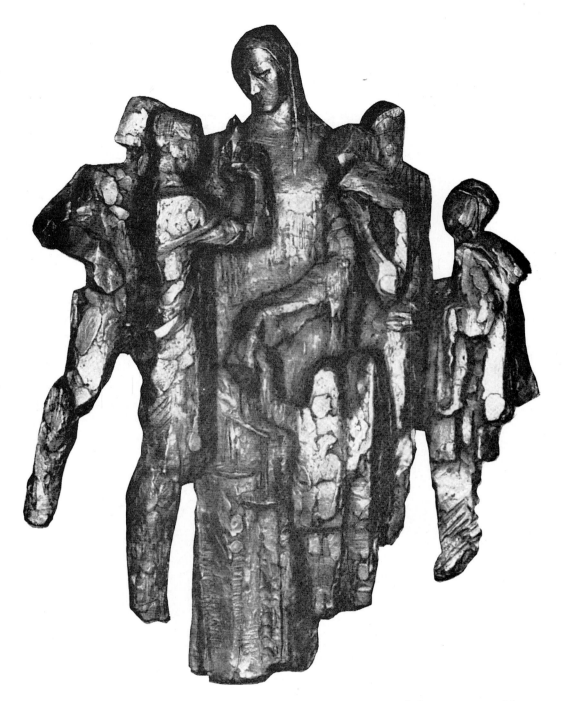

"The search for truth is the essence of forensic pathology. This truth forms an essential link between the enforcement of law and the protection of the public in the administration of justice." This illustration shows a sculpture by Una Hanbury, located in the lobby of Maryland's Medical Examiner's Building in Baltimore. The guardian figure on the left represents law. Next to it the doctor holds up the lamp of knowledge towards the symbolic figure of justice. Justice is interpreted in its aspect of love. The general public is suggested by the group of figures on the right. An inscription underneath the sculpture reads, "Wherever the art of medicine is practiced there is also a love of humanity." (Hippocrates)

Spitz and Fisher's

MEDICOLEGAL INVESTIGATION OF DEATH

Guidelines for the Application of Pathology to Crime Investigation

FOURTH EDITION

Edited by

WERNER U. SPITZ, M.D.

Consultant, Forensic Pathology and Toxicology
St. Clair Shores, Michigan
Chief Medical Examiner
Wayne and Macomb Counties (Retired)
Professor of Pathology
Wayne State University, School of Medicine, Detroit, Michigan
Adjunct Professor of Chemistry
University of Windsor
Windsor, Ontario, Canada

Co-edited by

DANIEL J. SPITZ, M.D.

Chief Medical Examiner
Macomb County, Michigan
Assistant Professor of Pathology
Wayne State University, School of Medicine
Detroit, Michigan

With a Foreword by

RAMSEY CLARK

Former Attorney General of the United States

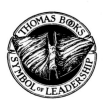

CHARLES C THOMAS • PUBLISHER, LTD.
Springfield • Illinois • U.S.A.

Published and Distributed Throughout the World by

CHARLES C THOMAS • PUBLISHER, LTD.
2600 South First Street
Springfield, Illinois 62704

©2006 by CHARLES C THOMAS • PUBLISHER, LTD.

ISBN 0-398-07544-1

Library of Congress Catalog Card Number: 2004059844

Printed in the United States of America
SR-R-3

Library of Congress Cataloging-in-Publication Data

Spitz and Fisher's medicolegal investigation of death : guidelines for the application of
    pathology to crime investigation / edited by Werner U. Spitz, co-edited by Daniel J.
    Spitz ; with a foreword by Ramsey Clark. -- 4th ed.
        p. ; cm.
    Includes bibliographical references and index.
    ISBN 0-398-07544-1
        1. Forensic pathology. 2. Death--Causes. I. Title: Medicolegal investigation of death.
    II. Spitz, Werner U., 1926- III. Spitz, Daniel J. IV. Fisher, Russell S., 1916-
    [DNLM: 1. Autopsy. 2. Forensic Medicine. 3. Pathology. W 825 S7612 2004]
    RA1063.4.S63 2004
    614'.1--dc22
                                                                              2004059844

To my father
Siegfried Spitz, M.D.
my first and foremost teacher
and to
my mother
Anna Spitz, M.D.
who relentlessly showed me the way.

CONTRIBUTORS

VERNARD I. ADAMS, M.D.

Chief Medical Examiner, Hillsborough County, Florida
Associate Professor, Department of Pathology and Laboratory Medicine
University of South Florida, Tampa

VERNON ARMBRUSTMACHER, M.D.

City Medical Examiner (Neuropathology), The City of New York,
Office of the Chief Medical Examiner
Clinical Associate Professor, Department of Forensic Medicine,
New York University School of Medicine

MICHAEL M. BADEN, M.D.

Director, Medicolegal Investigations Unit, New York State Police, Albany, New York
Former Chief Medical Examiner, City of New York

WILLIAM MARVIN BASS, III, PH.D.

Professor Emeritus
Forensic Anthropology Center, University of Tennessee
Knoxville, Tennessee

RICHARD E. BISBING, B.S.

Executive Vice President, Director of Research
McCrone Associates, Inc.
Westmont, Illinois

C. MICHAEL BOWERS, D.D.S., J.D.

Deputy Medical Examiner
Ventura, California

B. G. BROGDON, M.D.

University Distinguished Professor Emeritus of Radiology
University of South Alabama, College of Medicine
Consultant in Forensic Radiology
Office of the Medical Examiner, State of Alabama
Mobile, Alabama

HEATHER MILLER COYLE, PH.D.

Division of Scientific Services, Department of Public Safety
Connecticut State Forensic Laboratory
Meriden, Connecticut

EDMUND R. DONOGHUE, M.D.

Chief Medical Examiner, Cook County, Chicago, Illinois
Clinical Professor of Forensic Pathology
University of Illinois at Chicago College of Medicine

MARK A. FLOMENBAUM, M.D., PH.D.

First Deputy Chief Medical Examiner, City of New York
Clinical Assistant Professor of Forensic Medicine
New York University School of Medicine

RICHARD C. FROEDE, M.D.

Consultant, Forensic Pathology
Tucson, Arizona

GREGORY S. GOLDEN, D.D.S.

Chief Odontologist
County of San Bernardino, California

NEAL H. HASKELL, PH.D.

Forensic Science and Biology Professor
Saint Joseph's College, Rensselaer, Indiana
Consultant, Forensic Entomology
Rensselaer, Indiana

LYNNE M. HELTON, M.S.

Forensic Scientist
Michigan State Police
Lansing Forensic Laboratory
Biology/DNA Unit
Lansing, Michigan

JAMES M. HENRY, M.D.

Chief, Department of Neuropathology
Armed Forces Institute of Pathology
Washington, D.C.

CHARLES S. HIRSCH, M.D.

Chief Medical Examiner, City of New York, Office of the Chief Medical Examiner
Professor and Chairman, Department of Forensic Medicine, and
Professor of Pathology,
New York University School of Medicine

RAYMOND J. JOHANSEN, D.M.D.

Forensic Dental Consultant
Santa Barbara, California

STANTON C. KESSLER, M.D.

Deputy Medical Examiner, Hamilton County, Chattanooga, Tennessee
Assistant Medical Examiner, State of Tennessee
Lecturer in Pathology Harvard Medical School
Boston, Massachusetts
Chief of Staff OCME (Former)

LISA J. KOHLER, M.D.

Chief Medical Examiner
County of Summit, Ohio

CARLL LADD, PH.D.

Division of Scientific Services, Department of Public Safety
Connecticut State Forensic Laboratory
Meriden, Connecticut

HENRY C. LEE, PH.D.

Forensic Science Program, University of New Haven
West Haven, Connecticut

BARRY D. LIFSCHULTZ, M.D.

Deputy Medical Examiner, Cook County, Chicago, Illinois
Adjunct Associate Professor of Pathology
Northwestern University Medical School

HERBERT L. MACDONELL, M.S., SCD.

Director, Laboratory of Forensic Science
Corning, New York

JOSHUA A. PERPER, M.D., LL.B., M.SC.

*Chief Medical Examiner and Director of Broward County Medical Examiner and
Trauma Services Clinical Professor of Pathology, Epidemiology and
Public Health, University of Miami
Clinical Professor of Epidemiology, Novasoutheastern University*

MARVIN S. PLATT, M.D., J.D.

*Chief Medical Examiner (Retired), County of Summit, Ohio
Associate Chairman (Retired), Department of Pathology
Children's Hospital Medical Center of Akron, Akron, Ohio
Emeritus Professor of Pathology, Northeastern Ohio University College of Medicine
Rootstown, Ohio*

BARBARA A. SAMPSON, M.D., PH.D.

*Deputy Medical Examiner, City of New York
Clinical Assistant Professor of Forensic Medicine,
New York University School of Medicine*

RICHARD R. SOUVIRON, D.D.S.

*Consultant, Forensic Dentistry
Miami-Dade County Medical Examiner's Office*

DANIEL J. SPITZ, M.D.

*Medical Examiner, Macomb County, Michigan
Former Associate Medical Examiner, Hillsborough County, Florida
and Assistant Professor of Pathology and Laboratory Medicine
University of South Florida College of Medicine
Tampa, Florida*

WERNER U. SPITZ, M.D.

*Consultant, Forensic Pathology and Toxicology
St. Clair Shores, Michigan
Chief Medical Examiner, Macomb and Wayne Counties, Michigan (Retired)
Professor of Pathology, Wayne State University School of Medicine
Adjunct Professor of Chemistry, University of Windsor
Windsor, Ontario, Canada*

BOYD G. STEPHENS, M.D.

*Chief Medical Examiner, City and County of San Francisco
Clinical Professor of Pathology, University of California, San Francisco*

WILLIAM Q. STURNER, M.D.

Chief Medical Examiner
Arkansas State Crime Laboratory
Little Rock, Arkansas
Professor of Pathology, UAMS

DAVID SWEET, D.M.D., PH.D.

Associate Professor and Director
Bureau of Legal Dentistry
Vancouver, British Columbia, Canada

FRIEDRICH UNTERHARNSCHEIDT, M.D.

Chief, Department of Neuropathology (Retired)
U.S. Naval Aerospace Medical Research Laboratory, Detachment
U.S. Naval Biodynamics Laboratory, New Orleans, Louisiana

GLENN N. WAGNER, D.O.

Chief Medical Examiner, San Diego County
San Diego, California

THOMAS W. YOUNG, M.D.

Jackson County Medical Examiner
Clinical Associate Professor, University of Missouri, Kansas School of Medicine
Kansas City, Missouri

FOREWORD

"MORDRE WOL OUT," Chaucer's Prioress tells us. But those who work in homicide investigation, forensic pathology, and criminal law know better. The true manner of death which may have been murder is not determined in tens of thousands of cases annually in our violent land. The cost to the nation in truth, justice, health, and safety is enormous.

Had Hamlet put aside indecision, sentimentality, emotion, the wan grief spent on the skull of the jester of his youth "Alas, poor Yorick! I knew him, Horatio" and obtained an autopsy on his dead father, the King of Denmark, Shakespeare's play might have turned from tragical to historical. Surely, we now see how our failures can affect history itself. The violent death of a President will always cause the deepest fears and suspicions. There will always be the allegation of gunfire from a grassy knoll.

We can determine the truth, and medical science must play a major role. The coeditor of this important volume was one of four professionals I called on as Attorney General, to review the autopsy photos and x-rays of our beloved President who looked "forward to the day when America would no longer be afraid of grace and beauty." In a time of profound doubt and international concern, with the highest integrity, self-discipline, and professional skill, Dr. Fisher contributed to those most reassuring phenomena, facts linked together pointing to truth.

How many men in America can qualify for such a task? That this is the first volume in twenty-five years dealing directly and effectively with the subject of medicolegal investigation of death tells us that our neglect here is enormous. The deaths of John F. Kennedy, Medgar Evers, Malcolm X, Martin Luther King, Jr., Robert Kennedy, and Whitney Young, Jr., show how our inadequacy can alter our destiny.

About 4:45 A.M., on December 4, 1969, two young Black Panthers, Fred Hampton and Mark Clark, were killed by gunfire in the city of Chicago. The shooting occurred during the course of a police raid on Panther headquarters. There followed an official inquest, a protest inquest, three autopsies, and three grand jury investigations. Each of the autopsies was performed under conditions in a manner or reported in a way that added to speculation over the real cause of death.

A community has been left in profound doubt as to the identity of the guns from which the bullets causing death were fired, even the direction of entry and number of shots. Were the deaths accidental? Were police justified in this use of deadly force? Were the dead murdered by the police? Was Fred Hampton drugged at the time of death? That over five thousand people attended his funeral indicates the impact of our failure to establish the truth. The resulting division in the community will affect the quality of life there and, through those who live there, elsewhere, for a generation or more.

xiii

Perhaps many pathologists avoid medicolegal investigation of death because its contribution to life is not clear and the happy side of the docket is with the life savers. A study of such chapters as "Investigation of Deaths from Drug Abuse," "Forensic Aspects of Alcohol," and "Aircraft Crash Investigation" immediately demonstrates the great importance of this field in life saving and social problem solving. Indeed, few in the medical profession will be more involved in the action and passion of our times than those who seek to find and demonstrate these medical facts. We can foresee the risks of willful destruction of crowded airplanes and the meaning to mass urban technological society.

With a hundred new dangerous drugs to be created by chemical science in the next five years, with a youth culture in an age of anxiety approaching incoherence, with grossly inadequate preventive research, it often will be the autopsy that tells us of the new synthetic chemicals threatening life. With this knowledge, society can endeavor to cope with one of its most difficult problems.

There are few crueler injustices directly inflicted on an individual by government than conviction of a crime one did not commit. Important chapters such as "Sudden and Unexpected Death from Natural Causes in Adults," "Trauma and Disease," and "Injury by Gunfire" show us how easy it is to misjudge the cause of death where circumstances are suspicious. It is of the utmost importance to the individual, to society, to truth, justice, and safety that we find the facts concerning death.

Because of its pathos, we too often ignore the truths disclosed in Chapter XVIII, "Investigations of Death in Childhood—The Battered Child." How many of our most violent criminals were the subject of physical abuse as children? Forensic pathology can give us some indication. It is important that we know. The national attitude toward violent crime could be dramatically changed by this truth.

Few professionals create greater despondency about the goodness of man and the worth of life than the practice of criminal law. Not many human documents are more pessimistic than Clarence Darrow's autobiography. Few activities tend to diminish an appreciation of life more than forensic pathology as generally practiced. Neither should be. The criminal lawyer seeks justice—the forensic pathologist, truth. Noble causes. If both will abandon rhetoric, ancient dogma and fictive contentions in favor of finding and presenting fact, which is the teaching of this text, their proper purposes will be justified. Practitioners will then enjoy the satisfaction of helping people.

We must have the courage, indeed the ardent desire, to know the causes of death. We cannot let the *corpus delicti* diminish our capacity for joy. We should not faint at the photos here. They are true, and while all truth may not seem beauty, all truth can strengthen our humanity. Then, however irresolute, we will find the compassion like Hamlet to hold in our hands the skull of a beloved friend, look on it and say "Here hung those lips that I have kissed I know not how oft." The great and constant need of those who investigate homicide and practice forensic pathology or criminal law is a warm humanism. A people who will not face death cannot revere life.

But these are mere musings. Study this work.

RAMSEY CLARK
Former Attorney General
of the United States
Washington, D.C.
14 July 1972

PREFACE TO THE FOURTH EDITION

It is with great pleasure that I present this fourth edition of *Medicolegal Investigation of Death* and introduce my son Daniel as Co-editor. I am thrilled that he decided to follow in my footsteps. After working several years in Florida at the Dade and Hillsborough Counties Medical Examiner's Offices, Dan has now joined me in Michigan. His relocation enables us to exchange ideas, discuss cases and work together.

This book was first published in 1972 with Russell Fisher, then Chief Medical Examiner of Maryland. Russ was a pioneer who early on recognized the importance of teaching, research and publication in forensic pathology, if this discipline was to withstand the challenges of time. Russ died in 1987, but left an indelible mark in these pages. This is the reason why his name is and will be on the cover.

Medicolegal Investigation of Death has been applauded since its inception, primarily because of its simple style, avoidance of technical terminology and the numerous illustrations it contains. The book was meant for pathologists, pathology residents, coroners, and all those who have an interest in the recognition and interpretation of wound patterns, and mechanisms of injury, including prosecuting and criminal defense attorneys, attorneys engaged in civil litigation, detectives, investigators, forensic nurses and others.

Medicolegal Investigation of Death is a textbook in forensic pathology. It has become a tradition that this book is re-written, updated, and expanded every 10 years or so. The present version has been completely redone. Eleven new chapters and sections, an overall updated and expanded text, hundreds of new illustrations and many new contributors make this a totally new book. I want to acknowledge my profound gratitude to all contributors and welcome the new authors.

The illustrations are still in black and white and not only to reduce cost. Color evokes emotions. Black and white is more neutral. For an astute observer, the lack of color will not be significant.

The popularity of shows depicting medical legal death investigation such as, Quincy in the 1980s, and recently *CSI, Crossing Jordan,* and *Court TV,* to name but a few, have brought the world of forensic science into everyone's living room. These shows have caused the general public to become aware and intrigued, while raising expectations of what may be derived from a post-mortem examination.

Every piece of the puzzle plays a role, from the observations recorded by the police officer at the scene, EMS workers, nurses and physicians in the ER, to the forensic pathologist in the autopsy room. It is therefore important that each understand their role and the significance of their notes when reconstructing an event.

Such manpower must realize that their notes in patients records may well become evidence in later legal proceedings. Thus, what were once mere words lost in reams of paper are now subject to scrutiny and cross-examination. Diagnoses are no longer buried with the patient's demise and clinical forensic medicine where physicians are called upon as experts to testify in courts of law has grown and prospered far beyond training in the field.

This book hopes to fill the void and its' text has been adapted to a broader readership.

W.U.S.

PREFACE TO THE THIRD EDITION

Medicolegal Investigation of Death has recently celebrated its twentieth year of publication. When Russ Fisher and I were compiling the first edition, back in 1970, we were aware of a need for such a book. Ten years later, widespread demand required a second, expanded edition. Since that time, frequent queries and concerns of attorneys, investigators, pathologists and others interested in medicolegal investigation, coupled with recent developments, prompted a third edition, not only to keep abreast of the present state of the art, but perhaps, more importantly, to deal with areas not addressed in previous editions. Some of these areas are not new, but their absence in the text was obviously significant.

To those who have stimulated me by their inquiries and prompted this third, expanded edition of this book, I wish to extend my heartfelt gratitude for keeping the fire alive.

The present text is profusely illustrated, with many new photographs and added diagrams and sketches to show mechanisms of injury. Most of the old pictures have been retained because it was considered senseless to replace classic illustrations only for the purpose of novelty.

The book has largely kept its simplistic and practical approach, avoiding technical terminology where possible, in compliance with its aim of addressing not only physicians but all those who are engaged in the study of injury patterns and the practice of pathology as it relates to the law.

Unfortunately, since the last edition of this book, three prominent contributors, leaders in the field of forensic pathology and friends, are no longer with us, Doctor James T. Weston, Doctor Russell S. Fisher, and Doctor Richard Lindenberg. Their spirits live on in these pages.

A number of new contributors bring fresh ideas and expertise to this volume, and I wish to extend my sincere thanks to them for their indispensable effort.

Lastly, I wish to indicate my debt of gratitude to Diane Lucke for her tireless efforts in compiling and coordinating this entire manuscript. Without such help this book could not have been completed.

W.U.S.

PREFACE TO THE SECOND EDITION

WHEN THE FIRST EDITION of this text was published in 1973, we intended that it would fill an existing void for an up-to-date account of the current state of knowledge of death investigation. The need for a second printing three years later supported our original belief that such a publication did indeed meet a demand. Rather than continue with a third printing, we felt that it would be appropriate at this time to undertake a complete revision of the text and to include new developments, including primarily a considerable volume of material that had been previously omitted.

Consequently, many additions and alterations were made to nearly all of the chapters. New sections on sudden infant death syndrome and chemical considerations associated with postmortem changes were included. A new chapter dealing with methodology and interpretation of toxicological procedures was added. Furthermore, a shortcoming of the previous edition was corrected by devoting space to preparation of a medicolegal autopsy report and formulation of a medicolegal opinion, as have been found to be advantageous in the author's own experience.

Significantly more space was allotted to illustrations. We were almost tempted to include color, but in the interest of lower cost, photographs were again limited to black and white, although the emphasis on quality was continued.

In conformity with the first edition, an attempt was made to maintain the practical character of the book, and where possible, technical terminology was avoided in the interest of easier understanding for a wider spectrum of readers.

It is the editors' pleasure to acknowledge the assistance received from so many colleagues, pathologists, police officers and attorneys, who contributed by their questions and suggestions. As previously, a great debt of gratitude is owed to Mrs. Hannelore Russell-Wood (Schmidt-Orndorff) for assistance with the editorial work, preparation of the index and collating of the entire manuscript. Elaine Sacra, research assistant at the Wayne County Medical Examiner's Office, helped transform a raw manuscript into a coordinated text, and Nancy Whayne prepared additional drawings. Special thanks are due to our photographers, Lester Walter and Anna Faulkner, for hours of expert labor spent in providing illustrations for the new material in this edition.

W.U.S.
R.S.F.

PREFACE TO THE FIRST EDITION

WHENEVER A NEW TEXTBOOK is to be written three basic questions should be answered by the authors: Why, who needs it? Is it needed now? Why should the authors in question, rather than others, undertake the work?

In the last thirty years there has been increasing sophistication in the training of police officers assigned to homicide investigation. To a significant degree this has been due to the philosophy developed at the Harvard Medical School in the late 1940s of teaching homicide investigators the nature of the medical aspects of injuries. This has led to the development of a sizeable corps of highly expert individuals in this field. The need for this type of information has also been greatly emphasized by the fact that throughout a large part of the United States the medical investigation of death at the scene is woefully inadequate, conducted by untrained and unskilled coroners who are frequently nonphysicians. No new textbook oriented to the homicide investigator or the novice forensic pathologist has appeared in the last two and one-half decades. It is our aim to meet the need by presenting, in readable style, an authoritative text embracing all aspects of the pathology of trauma as it is witnessed daily by law enforcement officers, interpreted by pathologists of varying experience in forensic pathology and finally used by attorneys involved in the prosecution and defense in criminal cases, as well as by those engaged in civil litigation.

Since the text is addressed to a wide range of professional disciplines, some of the chapters are inevitably directed more towards readers with medical backgrounds, whereas others are suited for general understanding. Nevertheless, the large number of illustrations and diagrams will, we hope, render the text comprehensible to all who are interested in the interpretation of forensic pathologic findings.

As it has been noted above, no up-to-date textbook covering the material contained herein is currently available. While working in the Maryland Medical Examiner's Office and its partner in teaching and research, the Maryland Medical-Legal Foundation, we have accumulated a large volume of material upon which to base the text. This material and experience also serve to answer the question: Why us? We have been concerned not only with the day-to-day investigation of sudden and violent deaths in a statewide medical examiner's system but also with teaching in medical and law schools in Baltimore and elsewhere throughout the country as well as with training of young pathologists who wish to become expert in the field. Furthermore, we have been conducting the *Frances G. Lee Seminars in Homicide Investigation* for state and other police officers for many years. It is our hope that our experience and those of our coauthors will make a significant contribution to the improvement of the investigation of sudden and violent death, the prosecution and defense of those related to such events, and the protection of the public welfare.

W.U.S.
R.S.F.

ACKNOWLEDGMENTS

My sincere gratitude, as editor of this book, goes to Diane Lucke, my assistant and office manager, who has been with me 32 years. Her tireless perseverance in preparing the manuscript, often providing valuable advice, sorting the illustrations, compiling the index, proofreading and much of the work usually done by the editor, deserve special recognition. Without Diane's help, this book would not have seen the light of day.

David Woodford, Forensic Manager of the Michigan State Police Crime Laboratory in Sterling Heights merits more than just thanks for his expertise, availability to consult at all times and obtaining and confirming information on so many different topics. Indeed, Dave is not only a colleague but a dear friend. Unfortunately on March 9, 2005, while this book was in print, we lost him.

Many of the drawings and sketches were prepared by William Loechel, retired director of Medical Illustrations at Wayne State University, School of Medicine. Bill made work fun. His keen knowledge of anatomy resulted in renditions with a perfection that only Bill could have achieved. For this, my utmost gratitude to Bill.

A special thanks also, to one of the leading Evidence Photographers in the Detroit area, Edward Gostomski of the Robert J. Anderson Company for preparing a large number of the photographs in this book and his expert advise in regards to the photography chapters.

Cameron L. Marshall, Charleston, South Carolina, formerly Solicitor of the Ninth Judicial Circuit, now in private practice, provided case information and numerous hours of stimulating and delightful discussion.

Last but not least, I am deeply moved by all those unnamed individuals who provided case material, advice and encouragement in the course of preparation of the manuscript. Many thanks to them as well.

W.U.S.

ACKNOWLEDGMENTS TO THE FIRST EDITION

THE IDEA OF COMPILING a book such as this was not new to us. We had been toying with this thought many times in the past. However, by insisting on the need for such a book and by impulsively establishing contact with the publishers, Col. James T. McGuire, Superintendent of the Illinois State Police, gave us the necessary impetus to go ahead with our plan. To him goes our appreciation for his insight and understanding of the need for dissemination of experience in the pathology of trauma among law enforcement personnel to help ensure a better administration of justice.

Our thanks to all those who have contributed to this book with their knowledge and experience, and who have thereby helped us make this endeavor possible.

Finally, our sincere gratitude to Hannelore Schmidt-Orndorff for her able assistance with the editorial work. Her continuous drive and suggestions have helped immensely in the task of preparing the manuscript from its inception.

The editors also wish to acknowledge the cooperation of the photographers of the Medical Examiner's Office in Baltimore–Walter C. Carden and M. Gibson Porter–for the preparation of the illustrations of the chapters contributed by the editors as well as Chapters IV, XVII, and XXI.

W.U.S.
R.S.F.

CONTENTS

"In fine, nothing is said now
that has not been said before."

TERENCE (185–159 B.C.)

Spitz and Fisher's
MEDICOLEGAL INVESTIGATION
OF DEATH

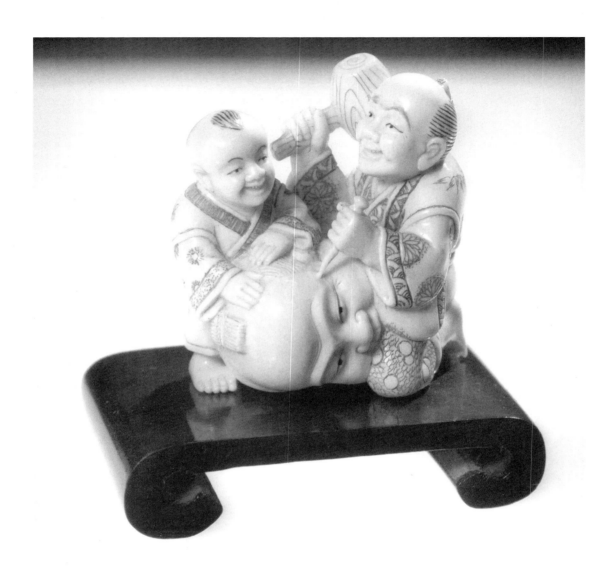

Open your mind to the wonders of forensic science.

Chapter I

HISTORY AND DEVELOPMENT OF FORENSIC MEDICINE AND PATHOLOGY

Daniel J. Spitz

EARLY DEVELOPMENT OF FORENSIC MEDICINE

THE ASSOCIATION OF LAW AND MEDICINE dates back to the Egyptian culture as early as 3000 B.C.[1] The discovery of various inscripted monuments, mummified remains and numerous papyri yields proof that the knowledge of medicine was much more scientific than first realized. Dissection of the dead gave the Egyptians and Babylonians considerable knowledge of human anatomy whereas most other cultures, which date back to these ancient times, had religious and social prejudices regarding dissection of the dead and thus were centuries behind in understanding anatomy and disease.[2]

Although evidence is lacking, some historians believe that *medical experts* were called to render opinions in ancient judicial hearings and were occasionally asked to do postmortem examinations. Imhotep was the personal physician of King Zoser and is believed to be the first man combining law and medicine. Although he was untrained in both medicine and law, Imhotep was later worshiped in Egypt as the *God of Medicine*.[1]

Clearer medicolegal associations date back to early legal systems such as The Code of Hammurabi in Babylonia in 1700 B.C. and The Code of Hittites in 1400 B.C. The Code of Hammurabi is believed to be the oldest written Code of Law. The earliest record of a murder trial was written on a clay tablet in Sumeria in 1850 B.C.[2]

In ancient Greece the work of Hippocrates was well studied and opinions based on his work were routinely used in court. Although Hippocrates studied many medical and ethical questions, he was the first to discuss forensic issues such as the relative fatality of wounds and the viability of pre-term infants. The ancient Hippocratic Oath, which is commonly referred to today, was written in 400 B.C.[1]

In ancient Roman civilizations, Roman law utilized *amicus curiae* or friends of the court to provide expert testimony and advise judges on complicated matters.[2] In general, the conclusion as to manner of death was determined by investigating the circumstances surrounding the death, however, in 44 B.C., a Roman physician named Antistius was asked to examine the slain body of Julius Caesar and render an opinion as to how he died. Antistius concluded that of the twenty-three wounds on Caesar's body, the only fatal wound was one in his chest.[3]

Developments involving medicolegal investigations continued throughout the middle ages with greater reliance on medical testimony in cases of physical injury, infanticide, rape, and bestiality. During the Middle Ages, Bologna initiated rules concerning the appointment of medical consultants to the courts which were later adopted in other Italian cities. Medicolegal autopsies were first performed in Bologna in 1302. These early autopsies were typically performed on homicide and suicide victims and criminals who were executed for their crimes.[2]

One of the first documents pertaining to postmortem examinations was a Chinese handbook published in 1250 entitled *His Yuan Lu*.[3] It contained simple autopsy techniques, proposed general postmortem guidelines, and discussed injuries caused by blunt and sharp instruments. It also offered comments on the determination of whether an individual in water had drown or died prior to submersion and whether a burned victim was alive or dead at the onset of the fire.

3

The Bamburg Code appeared in 1507 and the Constitutio criminalis Carolina enacted by Emperor Charles V appeared in 1530.[4] These early *statutes* increased the importance of legal medicine by their insistence that medical testimony was essential evidence in trials dealing with infanticide, abortion, poisoning, fatal wounds and other forms of bodily injury. At this time the statutes did not specify that autopsies were to be performed on the bodies of the victims. In 1562, a judicial autopsy was performed in Paris by a famous French surgeon, Dr. Ambroise Paré (1510–1590) and around the end of the sixteenth century performing an autopsy in medicolegal cases began to be a more frequent practice. Paré studied the lung findings in smothered children and was interested in trace evidence left during sexual assault.[5] Textbooks and scholarly writings began to appear in Western Europe at the end of the sixteenth century. These included a manuscript by Dr. Paré entitled *De rapports et des maijens d'embaumer les corps morts*, which was published in 1575.[2] Other more authoritative texts shortly followed and were critical in the further development of forensic science.

The two leading textbooks of the seventeenth century were *De Relationibus Medicorum* written by Sicilian physician Fortunatas Fidelis (1551–1630) and *Questiones Medico-Legales* written by Paulo Zacchias (1584–1659).[1] Fidelis described the findings in drowned bodies that could help distinguish homicidal and accidental drowning. The text by Zacchias was a comprehensive work that included characteristics of stab and bullet wounds, findings in asphyxial deaths, the distinction of suicide from homicide and determination of whether an infant had been born alive or dead. The influence of both men spread throughout Europe and the work by Zacchias (Fig. I-1) earned him the title, *the father of legal medicine*.[2]

The first formal lectures in the field of forensic medicine were held in Germany in the mid-seventeenth century. They were given by Professor Johann Michaelis of the University of Leipzig and later by his successor Johann Bohn.[1] During this period, Germany had the most advanced court system in Europe and it was routine for

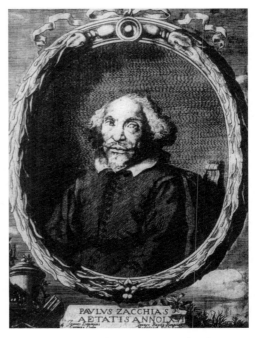

FIGURE I-1. Paulo Zacchias at age 66 (with permission, Davis Publishing Co.).

physicians to render opinions in criminal proceedings regarding injuries and cause of death. Judicial authorities all over Europe were now using forensically knowledgeable physicians in criminal and civil trials. At this time, physicians had a limited role in regard to crime scene investigation which was typically carried out by the police, however, in complicated cases police investigators occasionally consulted a physician to discuss crime scene evidence.

In 1699, an interesting medicolegal case involved the death of a young girl who was found floating in a mill dam. A lawyer named Spencer Cowper was charged with the murder. It was a common belief that if a body in water was found floating it was proof that the person was dead upon being put in the water. This was supported by two sailors who testified that when a man was killed and thrown overboard, the body would float and that if someone drowned the body would sink. During the trial interesting forensic evidence was given by Dr. Cowper (no relation) who testified that the cause of death had nothing to do with whether a body floated or sank. He stated that bodies in water always sink regardless of whether they are alive or dead. This testimony was crucial in obtaining a not guilty verdict.[1]

Throughout the nineteenth century, academic achievements in forensic and legal medicine continued to spread throughout Europe. Medicolegal lectures were now given at many European Universities and in Britain the first of such lectures were offered at the University of Edinburgh in 1791 by Sir Andrew Duncan. Andrew Duncan was a professor of the Institutes of Medicine and adopted the term *Medical Jurisprudence* for his series of lectures.[6] Continued research in forensic medicine and toxicology laid the foundation for the future of forensic pathology in Europe and the United States.

DEVELOPMENT OF FORENSIC MEDICINE IN GREAT BRITAIN

The office of the coroner originated in England as early as the eighth or ninth century, however, many historians believe that the true beginning of the British medicolegal system occurred with the election of the first county coroners in September 1194.[7] It is at this time that the office of the coroner was formally described. The office of the coroner was created by the King who laid out specific duties associated with this position. It was the job of the coroner to confiscate money and personal belongings from people who had died or from those accused of certain crimes. Until this time the collection of monies and property was done by the sheriff, however, corruption was widespread and much of the King's money was diverted into the pockets of these dishonest individuals. Creating the office of the coroner was done in an attempt to minimize the amount of money the King lost. Unfortunately, over the next century the coroners became as corrupt as the sheriffs.[7]

The term coroner originated in medieval England when everything, including the people was the property of the King. The title is derived from the Latin phrase, *Custom Plactorium Coronae* or *Supervisor of the Crown's Pleas.* When a person died the Crown sent a representative to inventory all the property and possessions of the decedent. Since everything belonged to the King, it was important to have someone secure the valuables and protect the Crown's interests. The final disposition of the property and the body of the decedent was decided by the Crown's representative. This representative became known as the *Coroner.*

Originally, the coroner was appointed by the King to represent the Crown as its magistrate in a certain district. Typically the appointed coroners were men of high rank and usually of noble blood. The office was prestigious and the coroner commanded great respect. The duty of the coroner was to ensure that the interests of the crown were maintained including keeping the peace and death investigation. When a coroner was informed of a death believed to be from felony or accident, he ordered the sheriff to bring any witnesses to him so that the truth could be determined. If the deceased had died a violent death, the coroner and selected jurors investigated the death by talking to witnesses and viewing the body to determine how and why the victim died. Following the investigation, if enough evidence was present to charge a person with the homicide, the sheriff would be instructed to seize the suspect's property and present it to the King. The coroner had the power to seize the personal belongings of those even suspected of a crime whether guilty or innocent. Likewise, people committing suicide forfeited all property and articles of value to the King.[4]

In 1272 during the rule of King Edward I, the coroner's role was described as the following:

The office and power of the coroner are similar to those of a sheriff and consists, first, in inquiring, when a person is slain or dies suddenly, or in prison, concerning the manner of his death. And this must be upon sight of the body; for if the body be not found, the coroner cannot sit. He must also sit at the very place where death happened, and the inquiry must be made by a jury from 4, 5, or 6 of the neighboring towns over which he is to preside. If any be found guilty by this inquest of murder or other homicide, the coroner is to commit them to prison for further trial and must certify the whole of his inquisition, together with the evidence thereon, to the Court of King's Bench.[8]

The use of *expert* medical testimony was often used at a coroner's inquest or at a trial involving homicide, assault, or rape. The testimony generally covered the clinical course of the victim between the injuries and death and was often given by the victim's surgeon. The injuries to the body surface were described but complete postmortem examinations were rarely conducted.[6] The first autopsy in the United Kingdom is believed to have been performed during the seventeenth century.[7] Great Britain was much slower than other European countries to adopt the practice of complete autopsies. It is believed that the first autopsy performed in Great Britain was done in 1653 by William Harvey who autopsied Thomas Parr. Mr. Parr was believed to be 152 years old when he died and the autopsy was done at the request of Charles I who was interested in aging and longevity.[7]

Over several centuries, the prestige and power of the coroner declined and with the appointment of Justices of the Peace, the coroner played a much less important role in legal proceedings. In 1791, it was decided by Lord Chief Justice Kenyon that *"inquests should only be held where marks of violence can be seen on the body."* In 1842, Lord Chief Justice Denham stated, *"The mere fact of a body lying dead does not give the coroner jurisdiction, nor even the circumstance that death was sudden; there ought to be reasonable suspicion that the party came to his death by violent or unnatural means."*[9] Needless to say, with these two rulings the coroner was left powerless in many cases and many criminal acts and other unnatural deaths went without being investigated.

The Coroners' Act of 1887 was created because of public unrest regarding the large number of overlooked homicides. It became known that homicides by poisoning and child homicide were quite rampant and that these cases often went undetected by the current methods of death investigation. The Act intended to give more authority back to the coroner which had been slowly stripped by the appointment of the Justices.[7] In addition to this Act, several influential men were instrumental in advancing death investigation by promoting postmortem examinations in certain situations.

Since the Coroners' Amendment Act of 1926, coroners in England have been responsible for both natural and unnatural death investigations and formal inquests are generally held in all unnatural deaths.[7] The coroner typically gathers information and evidence and decides if expert pathology opinions are needed. Today, the coroners are associated with and have the support of a forensic pathology department at a local university and the expertise of a trained forensic pathologist is usually sought in unnatural or complicated cases.

In more recent years Dr. Francis Camps, along with other English pathologists including Drs. Keith Simpson, Keith Mant, and Sydney Smith served as forensic pathology consultants to the coroners. As professors of pathology at prestigious medical schools in London, these men were vital in the advancement of modern day forensic pathology throughout Great Britain. In Great Britain today much of the current teaching in forensic pathology is due to the efforts of Dr. Bernard Knight, Professor of Pathology at the Wales Institute of Forensic Medicine, University of Wales College of Medicine.

In 1960, the British Academy of Forensic Sciences was founded by Dr. Camps in an attempt to unite the professions involved in medicolegal death investigations. The Academy has been successful and is associated with the respected journal appropriately called *Medicine, Science and the Law.*[10]

DEVELOPMENT OF FORENSIC MEDICINE IN THE UNITED STATES

As colonies of Englishmen began to settle in other parts of the world, the English coroner system followed. The coroners in these new lands essentially retained the same duties as they did in

Great Britain. The early colonists from England brought to America the coroner system as it existed in England during the early 1600s. Thus, there is a record of a coroner's inquest in the colony of New Plymouth, New England in 1635. The inquiry into the death of John Deacon stated:

Having searched the dead body, we finde not any blows or wounds, or any other bodily hurt. We finde that bodily weakness caused by long fasting and weariness, by going to and fro, with the extreme cold of the season were the causes of his death.[11]

The coroner's office had numerous up and down periods over the years and at the time of colonization of what is now the United States, the prestige of the office was at a low point, slightly above the status of a dog catcher.

The early American coroners, like their English counterparts, tried to use as much common sense as possible in death investigations. There were few doctors to offer professional advice and at this time pathologists did not exist. A jury was often impaneled to assist the coroner, and if there was evidence of violence or bodily injury, the jurors were authorized to render a verdict. In other cases the jurors often made hazardous guesses as to the cause of death. Certainly many of the more subtle injury cases went unnoticed and many other cases were grossly misinterpreted leading to grave injustices.

The coroner's office soon became one and the same as the sheriff's office. No additional stipend was paid for the extra death investigation duties, however, the job provided a substantial income. The sheriff was responsible for the collection of property taxes, poll taxes, and other levies of which he generally received a 10 percent commission. In 1637, the newly appointed sheriff and coroner, Thomas Baldridge gathered a jury of twelve men to hold an inquest over the body of John Bryant. Their verdict reads: *"John Bryant by the fall of a tree had his bloud bluke broken; and hath two scratches under his chinne and on the left side; and so that by means of the fall of the said tree upon him the said John Bryant came to his death."*[12] In the original colonies, autopsies were not included in the examination of the dead primarily due to religious objections. Causes of death were determined by external examination of the body

combined by statements made by witnesses. The Maryland Historical Society has record of the governor's appointment of John Robinson, high constable, as coroner for St. Mary's County. Also recorded are the coroner's duties which included the following:

Upon notice or suspicion of any body that hath or shall come to his death or her death entirely within the limits of that hundred* to warn as many inhabitants of the said hundred* as you conveniently may to view the dead body and to charge the said persons with an oath truly to inquire and true verdict to grant how the person viewed came upon his or her death according to the evidence. . . .[13]

(*the term *hundred* has a long history in England and did at one time mean an area containing a hundred able bodied men.)

Recording of vital statistics such as births, deaths, and marriages has long been practiced, but it is interesting that the Commonwealth of Massachusetts has the oldest tradition in the world of vital record keeping. It is here since 1639 that colonial laws have required that town clerks maintain such records.

Beginning around 1647, the General Court of Massachusetts Bay became concerned with the teaching of medical students and thus authorized that: *an autopsy should be made on the body of a criminal once in four years.* The first recorded application of an autopsy to ascertain medicolegal information is recorded in Maryland on March 21, 1665. This case involved the murder of Mr. Samuell Yeoungman, a servant of Mr. Francis Carpenter. Mr. Carpenter was brought before the Talbot County Court and based on the coroner's report he was vindicated. The coroner's report read:

Wee of the Jury haueing viewed the Corps of Samuell Yeoungman and finding A Depression in the Cranenum in on (one) place, and another wound where all the muscle flesh was Corrupted, and withall finding Corrupt blood betweene the Dura and Piamater, and the braine and several other bruises in the head and body therefore our verdict in that for want of Looking after the abousesaid wounds, were Cause of his death.[14]

Essentially the autopsy showed that Mr. Yeoungman died from a fractured skull and brain hemorrhage from being beaten with a club. Unfortunately, the verdict was for the defendant because it was determined that the victim died as a result of not going to a doctor. The record does not reveal whether it was Mr. Carpenter who inflicted the original wounds on the deceased's head.

A big step in the development of the law and medicine in the United States took place in 1811 when Dr. Benjamin Rush published a book entitled, *On the Study of Medical Jurisprudence*. This book was the first of its kind and served as the guideline for many medicolegal issues. Dr. Rush also gave a series of famous lectures on medical jurisprudence at the College of Medicine in Philadelphia in 1810 and spent much of his time studying and teaching forensic psychiatry.[1] Dr. Rush was a member in the Provincial Congress whereby he was one of the signers of the Declaration of Independence in 1776. Dr. Rush is now best remembered as one of the founders of medical education in this country.

In the colonies, the study of anatomy grew as the number of medical schools increased. Early on there were few bodies to autopsy until the Revolutionary War. The battlefields covered with unclaimed remains of solders provided medical students and anatomists with an unlimited supply of bodies. Unfortunately, medical students often feared for their own lives because early United States medical schools were often attacked by police and angry protestors who believed that dissection of a human body was taboo. For this reason, the University of Maryland School of Medicine had its first anatomy hall burned to the ground in 1807.[11]

Perhaps the earliest formal mention of a physician in connection with the work of the coroner was in 1860 in Maryland. It was at this time that the Code of Public General Laws authorized the coroner or his jury to require the attendance of a physician in cases of violent death. The choice of the physician was left to the coroner. Eight years later the legislature authorized the government to appoint a physician as sole coroner of the city of Baltimore. Coroners were generally an elected county official who were usually not medically trained. Until 1886 coroners were elected by popular vote and in many counties in the United States this method is still practiced. In 1877, the Commonwealth of Massachusetts initiated a statewide system requiring that the coroner be succeeded by a physician who would later be known as a *medical examiner*. At this time, the jurisdiction of the medical examiner was confined to *dead bodies of such persons only as are supposed to have come to their death by violence.*[1]

In 1883, the Medicolegal Society of New York was founded and was one of the first steps in beginning a new medicolegal investigative system in the United States. At this time the *Medico-Legal Journal* was created and was the official publication of the society. This journal was the first general periodical in the United States dealing with medicolegal issues.[2]

Although the term *medical examiner* was first designated as early as 1877, by the early 1900s the term was commonly used to refer to forensic pathologists who were involved in death investigation. In 1890, a city ordinance in Baltimore, Maryland authorized the Board of Health to appoint two physicians with the title of medical examiner and assign them the duty of performing all autopsies requested by the coroner or the state's attorney. By 1915, New York City and Massachusetts abolished the coroner system and had fully functional medical examiner departments.[2] In New York, the medical examiner was granted the authority to investigate deaths resulting from criminal violence, suicide, sudden death in an individual who appeared in good health, deaths occurring while imprisoned, or in any suspicious or unusual case. In Massachusetts, however, the law that established the medical examiner system did not initially allow the medical examiner to determine which bodies would be autopsied, but reserved this right for the district attorney. It was not until 1945 that the Massachusetts law was amended to make the performance of autopsies discretionary with the medical examiner. In 1954, Gonzales, Vance, Helpern, and Umberger wrote, *"The coroner system in practice has shown itself to be entirely inadequate for the duties it must perform. The coroner system is entirely unsuitable for the complexities of present-day civilization and needs to be replaced by a more workable type of medicolegal organization."*[4]

In 1948, Richard S. Childs who was on staff of the National Municipal League and Chairman of the League's Executive Committee joined forces with Dr. Milton Helpern and other influential people in an attempt to change the existing coroner system which was felt by some to be obsolete. At this time, most of the United States still depended on the typical elected county coroner to determine when a homicide was committed and how the responsible party should be punished. Mr. Childs gathered expert opinions and found influential allies to support his cause. In 1949, a group of authorities met at the National Conference on Government in St. Paul. Following this meeting, Dr. Richard Ford, Acting Head of the Department of Legal Medicine at Harvard University drafted what was known as *A Model State Medicolegal Investigative System*. This discussed the need for abolition of the obsolete office of the coroner and how a medical examiner system would be superior for preventing wrongdoers from *getting away with murder*. The report was endorsed by many well-respected medical and legal associations and was the primary model used to gain support for the further development of medical examiner departments across the country.

Forensic pathology in the United States essentially began in New York with Charles Norris and Thomas A. Gonzales as the two foremost figures. Dr. Norris was director of laboratories at Bellevue Hospital and was appointed the first chief medical examiner of New York City by the Civil Service Commission on February 18, 1918 (Fig. I-2). He used his own financial resources to furnish the medical examiner's office which was originally located at Bellevue Hospital in New York. Dr. Norris was a legendary figure who spent great efforts to bring the link between law and medicine closer together. He was part of numerous high profile murder trials in the early 1900s and according to a Bronx district attorney, Dr. Norris made *dead men tell more tales than live ones ever could*. Dr. Norris resigned in September 1932 and died in 1935.[15]

Through Dr. Norris' interest in toxicology, the New York office became a leader in the development of forensic toxicology. During the early years at the New York City Medical Examiner's Office, the establishment of a fully functional

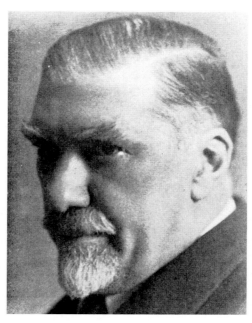

FIGURE I-2. Dr. Charles Norris, First Chief Medical Examiner, New York City from 1918–1932 (with permission, Sam Shere, TimeLife, Inc.).

forensic toxicology laboratory was developed under the direction of Alexander Gettler, who was New York's first chief forensic toxicologist (Fig. I-3). Dr. Gettler was instrumental in integrating the toxicology laboratory as a vital component of the medical examiner.

Thomas A. Gonzales began work at the New York City Medical Examiner's Office shortly after it opened in 1918 and became chief medical examiner upon the death of Dr. Norris. Dr. Gonzales taught by the philosophy that *information learned from studying the dead could be used to help the living*. He was instrumental in understanding deaths related to various drugs and poisons and worked with state government to try and decrease drug-related deaths. He left his mark on the forensic world by co-authoring one of the first comprehensive forensic textbooks entitled *Legal Medicine: Pathology and Toxicology* which was published in 1937.[15,16]

During the tenure of Drs. Norris and Gonzales, the New York office became the training ground for pathologists interested in forensic pathology. Over the years many associate medical examiners were hired at the New York office

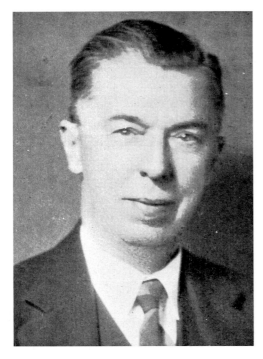

FIGURE I-3. Dr. Alexander Gettler, First Forensic Toxicology at the New York City Medical Examiner's Office.

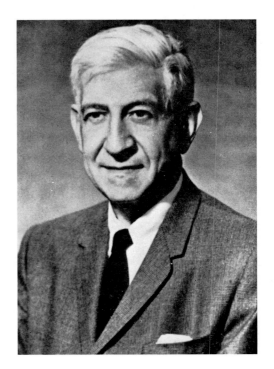

FIGURE I-4. Dr. Milton Helpern (1902–1977), Chief Medical Examiner, New York City.

including Milton Helpern, who during the tenure of Dr. Gonzales, was in charge of the main morgue in Manhattan.

Milton Helpern was the third chief medical examiner of New York City and was responsible for the construction of the medical examiner's office that is still in use today (Fig. I-4). Part of the construction included the Institute of Forensic Medicine which is the teaching arm of New York University. In 1977, the Institute was renamed in his honor.[16] Dr. Helpern founded the National Association of Medical Examiners (NAME) in 1966 and served as the association's first president. Without question, he was one of the most important figures in the development of modern day forensic pathology.

Teaching of forensic pathology as a subspecialty of pathology began in 1937 at Harvard Medical School with the establishment of the George Burgess McGrath Chair of Legal Medicine. Mrs. Frances Glessner Lee, who was responsible for obtaining the necessary funds, endowed the chair. The seminars, which were established in 1945, were initially called *The*

Frances G. Lee Seminars on Legal Medicine. Although she died in 1963, the seminars continued until 1967. From 1968 until the present the seminars have been called *The Frances G. Lee Seminars in Homicide Investigation* and have been associated with the Maryland Medical Examiner's Office and the University of Maryland. Mrs. Lee devoted much of her life to the education of homicide detectives and was extremely concerned with the development of death investigation and legal medicine in the United States. The education of police and homicide detectives with respect to the application of pathology in crime investigation were the course objectives. She continues to be remembered by her creation of miniature crime scenes which were used to recreate homicide scenes and for teaching crime investigators.[17]

Currently, many similar forensic pathology training seminars geared both toward physicians as well as police, homicide detectives, attorneys, and more recently forensic nurses are quite common. One of the most widely attended seminars is the *Medicolegal Investigation of Death* course

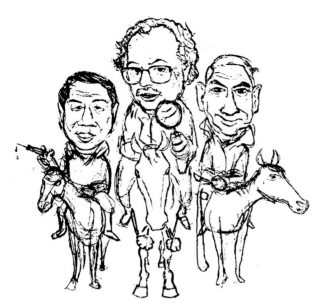

FIGURE I-5. (Right to left) Drs. Werner Spitz, Michael Baden, and Henry Lee on the verge of solving another case (by Fred Krasco).

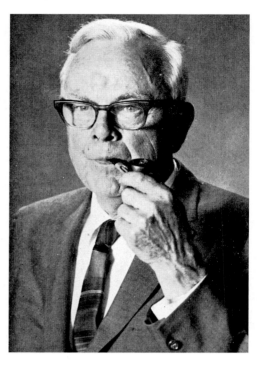

FIGURE I-6. Dr. Alan R. Moritz, Professor of Legal Medicine, Harvard University Medical School.

which had its 28th anniversary in April, 2004. The seminar is sponsored by Wayne State University School of Medicine and is directed by Dr. Werner Spitz with Drs. Michael Baden and Henry Lee on the permanent faculty (Fig. I-5).

Although forensic medicine dates back thousands of years, the development of modern day forensic pathology can be credited to a few devoted pathologists. In many ways these pathologists were our first and foremost teachers and they were instrumental in forming the current medical examiner's system that is now utilized in much of the United States.

Alan R. Moritz was one of the founders of modern day forensic pathology in the United States (Fig. I-6). Dr. Moritz organized the Department of Legal Medicine at Harvard Medical School in the late 1930s and served as its first professor. He has made long-lasting contributions through numerous academic achievements and brought respect to both forensic pathologists and the field of forensic pathology. Dr. Moritz together with R. Crawford Morris, LL.B. published the *Handbook of Legal Medicine* in 1956 and a must manuscript for all practicing forensic pathologists is Dr. Moritz's paper *Classical Mistakes in Forensic Pathology (American Journal of Clin-*

ical Pathology, 26:1383–97, 1957.) Dr. Moritz was crucial in establishing a residency training program at Harvard University for pathologists eager to train in forensic pathology and one of his best known students was Russell S. Fisher.[18]

Dr. Fisher served as the chief medical examiner of the State of Maryland from 1949–1984 (Fig. I-7). During this time, he built the Maryland office into one of the premier forensic pathology centers in the country. As a member and president of the American Board of Pathology, he was instrumental in establishing the requirements for board certification in forensic pathology. As president of the American Academy of Forensic Sciences, he oversaw continued achievements and advances in the field of forensic medicine and pathology. Dr. Fisher recognized the need for research and publication and surrounded himself with academic forensic pathologists who added vital works to the literature. Richard Lindenberg was one such scholar and a well-respected forensic neuropathologist in Germany who came to the United States shortly after World War II (Fig. I-8). Dr. Lindenberg did much of the

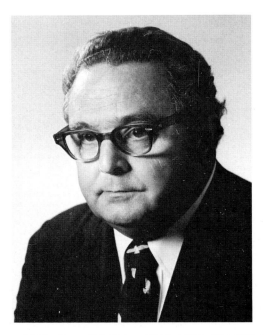

FIGURE I-7. Dr. Russell S. Fisher (1918–1984), Chief Medical Examiner of Maryland from 1949–1984.

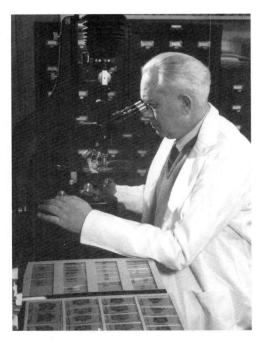

FIGURE I-8. Dr. Richard Lindenberg, Director of Neuropathology and Legal Medicine, Maryland State Department of Health and Mental Hygiene.

early work on the pathology of traumatic brain injury and is considered the father of forensic neuropathology in this country. Dr. Fisher himself was also active in scholarly work and was co-editor of the first two editions of this textbook. It was said that one of his main missions *was to use the dead to save the living.* Others stated that *"Dr. Fisher was way ahead of his time"* and that *"his goal was to help people in the future."* Homicide investigators from the United States and Canada have said that he taught them more during a five-day seminar than they could learn in 25 years on the street. Dr. Fisher inspired all those with whom he made contact and was a hands-on educator who taught by example. Over the years he trained numerous well-known forensic pathologists many of whom became chief medical examiners across the country.[19] Dr. Fisher's spirit lives on in these pages.

One of Dr. Fisher's early students was Stanley Durlacher who later moved to New Orleans to improve the forensic pathology and toxicology service of the coroner's office and to continue research and teaching at Louisiana State University School of Medicine. Joseph H. Davis

joined him as a faculty member. Dr. Durlacher was appointed the first chief medical examiner in Miami, Florida and in 1956, Dr. Davis accompanied him as assistant medical examiner. In February of 1957, Dr. Durlacher was scheduled to attend the Chicago meeting of the AAFS. As he departed, Dr. Davis joking stated *"Stan, don't have a heart attack because if you are not here I get a tight feeling in my head."* Dr. Durlacher never returned. He suffered a hemorrhagic stroke and died a short time later. Dr. Davis was appointed acting chief medical examiner and subsequently, at 31 years of age he became chief medical examiner of Dade County, recently changed to Miami-Dade County (Fig. I-9). He developed the Miami office into a world class forensic pathology center where students from around the world have come to study. Dr. Davis, together with his director of operations, Norman C. Kassoff, J.D. obtained funds to construct a three-building complex, designated by the County as *The Joseph H. Davis Center for Forensic Pathology.* It was occupied in 1988, contains approximately 89,000 square feet and houses a full service tox-

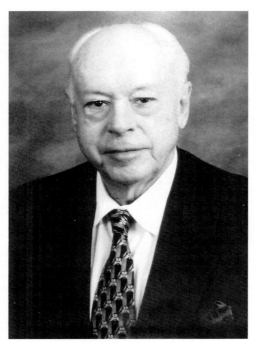

FIGURE I-9. Dr. Joseph H. Davis, Chief Medical Examiner, Dade County, Florida 1957–1996 and 2000–2001.

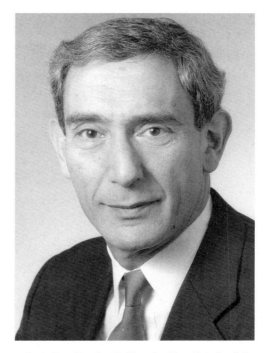

FIGURE I-10. Dr. Charles S. Hirsch, Chief Medical Examiner, New York City, New York, 1989 to present.

icology laboratory of approximately 17,000 square feet. Dr. Davis perpetuated Miami's international reputation for 39 years and 7 months prior to retiring in 1996, only to be asked to return from retirement as acting director in October 2000 until January 2001. Dr. Davis has left an everlasting impression on the world of forensic pathology and this writer is honored to have trained under him if even for a short time.

Some other well-known forensic pathologists who trained in Maryland under Dr. Fisher include Charles S. Hirsch, Charles S. Petty, and Werner U. Spitz. Following his training in Maryland, Dr. Hirsch spent several years in Cleveland, Ohio under the direction of Dr. Lester Adelson who at that time was the pathologist and chief deputy coroner for Cuyahoga County. Dr. Hirsch (Fig. I-10) was appointed the chief medical examiner of New York City, a position that he has held since January 1, 1989. After Dr. Hirsch took charge, the medical examiner office in New York City was returned to its prior status, held under Milton Helpern, as a leader in foren-

sic pathology with a training program which attracts students from all over the world.

Dr. Petty graduated from Harvard University Medical School in 1950 and studied pathology upon his graduation. In 1958, he joined Dr. Fisher's office as an assistant medical examiner and spent nine years in that position. In 1969, following two years in Indianapolis as professor of forensic pathology at Indiana University, Dr. Petty (Fig. I-11) moved to Dallas as professor of forensic sciences and pathology at University of Texas, Southwestern Medical School. Several months later he was appointed the first chief medical examiner of Dallas County. Until the development of a medical examiner system, Dallas County had ten Justices of the Peace who conducted death investigations with autopsies being performed only if they deemed necessary. Dr. Petty served as chief medical examiner and director of the Dallas County crime laboratory from 1969 until 1991 at which time he retired at age 71. Dr. Petty served as President of the American Academy of Forensic Sciences from 1967–1968 and has made countless contributions

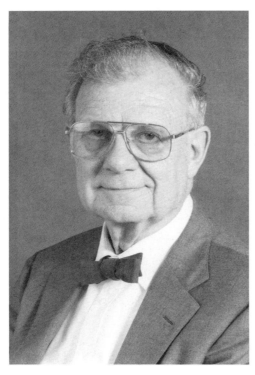

FIGURE I-11. Dr. Charles S. Petty, Director, Southwestern Institute of Forensic Sciences and Chief Medical Examiner, Dallas County, Texas 1969–1991.

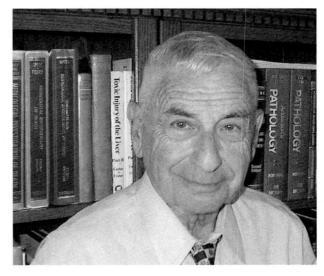

FIGURE I-12. Dr. Werner U. Spitz, Chief Medical Examiner, Wayne County, Detroit, Michigan, 1972–1988 and Macomb County, Mt. Clemens, Michigan, 1972 to present.

to the development and growth of forensic pathology. Now at age 81, he is still active and working at the University of Texas Transplant Program, which because of Dr. Petty has had a close affiliation with the medical examiner's office for many years.

After training with Dr. Fisher, Werner Spitz stayed on as the deputy medical examiner in Maryland until 1972. It was from 1967 to 1972 that Spitz and Fisher compiled and eventually published the first edition of *Medicolegal Investigation of Death*. Since it was first published in 1973, this textbook has been used worldwide and has become known as the *Bible* of forensic pathology for over 30 years. The success of this textbook can be credited to the authors of its chapters, all leaders in their respective fields. Dr. Spitz left Maryland in 1972 to serve as chief medical examiner of Wayne County, Michigan for 17 years, retiring from that position in 1988. After leaving Wayne County, he started a private consulting practice. In addition, he is also Professor

of Pathology at Wayne State University School of Medicine and medical examiner for Macomb County, Michigan. During his tenure as chief medical examiner of Wayne County, Dr. Spitz (Fig. I-12) headed an active forensic pathology training program which attracted pathology fellows and students from around the world. Many of those who trained under Dr. Spitz went on to become chief medical examiners of large offices around the country including the State of Maryland, State of New Mexico, Cook County (Chicago), IL, Philadelphia, PA, Jacksonville, FL, Harris County (Houston), TX, Tacoma, WA, and Guam.

Another distinguished figure who was important in the development of forensic pathology and a strong supporter of the medical examiner system was Geoffrey T. Mann. Dr. Mann served as the second chief medical examiner for the Commonwealth of Virginia from 1948 to 1972. After retiring from Virginia, he served as the chief medical examiner for Broward County, Florida until 1981. Dr. Mann was a founding father of NAME and part of the first group of pathologists to be certified by the American Board of Pathology in forensic pathology. He established one of the first approved training programs in forensic pathology and trained several generations of forensic pathologists including his successor David K. Wiecking. Dr. Wiecking subsequently trained the current chief medical examiner, Marcella F. Fierro. Dr. Mann died in May 2001 at the age of 86.

Growth of the Medical Examiner System in the United States

In 1939, the first statewide medical examiner system was developed in Maryland and over the next many years other states, districts, and counties followed. As of 1995, twenty-two states utilized medical examiner systems with nineteen using statewide systems, one using a district medical examiner system (Florida), and two using county medical examiners (Michigan and Arizona). A mixed medical examiner and coroner system was used in eighteen states with seven using a state medical examiner with county coroners/medical examiners and eleven using county medical examiners/coroners. The eleven remaining states solely used a coroners system of which two states used district coroners and eight states used county coroners. Puerto Rico currently uses a medical examiner system.[20]

Of the twenty-two statewide medical examiner systems, Florida is the only state using a district system which divides the state into twenty-four districts. Every district medical examiner must be a practicing pathologist and in many cases the district medical examiner is board certified in forensic pathology.[20] A medical examiner's commission representing users and providers of forensic pathology service has oversight and rule-making authority.

Of the eighteen states with a mixed medical examiner and coroner system, the qualifications of the medical examiner include a license to practice medicine and in most situations training in pathology is required. The qualifications to be a coroner are typically quite variable. In California for example, most counties utilize a coroner system or a coroner-sheriff system. In the eleven states that use a coroner system, most of the coroners are elected officials and have variable qualifications. Some states require that the coroner is a licensed physician and others states have no

specific requirements. In states or counties not utilizing a trained pathologist as a medical examiner, a death is reported to the county coroner who determines if an autopsy is needed. A trained pathologist or forensic pathologist will then typically perform the autopsy.[20]

Needless to say, death investigation in the United States varies widely from state to state, and county to county and in many ways still resembles the system implemented by the first American colonists. During the twentieth century, medical examiner systems grew quite rapidly and replaced many coroner systems, however, this trend has slowed over the past several years. As of 1997, medical examiner systems served approximately 48 percent of the national population.[21] Certainly there is room for improvement and hopefully the future will bring a more uniform approach to death investigation with more and more states utilizing a medical examiner system. Qualifications of medical examiners should also be more uniform to ensure that no death investigation is compromised. Recently proposed was formation of a National Office of Death Investigation Affairs to try to standardize the medicolegal death investigation process across the country.[28] An effort in this regard is the recently published, *Death Investigation: A Guide for the Scene Investigator* by the National Institute of Justice.[22]

A recent trend is for states or counties to outsource their medical examiner responsibilities to privately employed forensic pathologists rather than hire pathologists who are then state or county employees. The chief medical examiner is typically given a budget to run the office and is left to hire the necessary staff. Varying degrees of county interaction and support depends on the arrangement between the two parties. The hope is that money will be saved while maintaining high quality death investigations. Only time will tell if this practice will be an effective way to run a medical examiner department. A practice that is much more common today is the growth of private practice forensic pathology. These pathologists have terminated their affiliations with state or county coroner or medical examiner departments and have engaged in private consulting practices. Most of these pathologists are kept busy doing non-medical examiner autopsies and consulting in both criminal and civil lawsuits. An unfortunate trend is the decrease in the number of hospital autopsies, which is currently at an all-time low. Many hospitals are no longer doing autopsies and those that do are often charging the family up to $3,000.00 for the service. Families who want an autopsy often prefer that it is done by a pathologist who is not affiliated with the hospital where their relative died.

American Academy of Forensic Sciences

A series of informal discussions between Drs. Rutherford B.H. Gradwohl and Israel Castellanos of Cuba lead to the formation of The American Academy of Forensic Sciences in 1948. Dr. Gradwohl was an English trained pathologist who was director of the Police Research Laboratory of the Metropolitan Police Department in St. Louis, Missouri and the editor of the authoritative textbook *Legal Medicine,* published in 1954.

Both men decided that a multidisciplinary conference involving all of the forensic science disciplines was a priority and on January 19, 1948 a three-day meeting was held at the Police Academy of St. Louis for the purpose of discussing various aspects of forensic medicine. Approximately 150 persons attended the first meeting which was called the Pan American Medicolegal Congress and later called The American Medicolegal Congress. During the first meeting a steering committee was selected which met at the Hotel Pierre in New York City on October 18, 1948. At this meeting the name, The American Academy of Forensic Sciences (AAFS) was adopted.

The Academy held its second meeting in Chicago on January 26–28, 1950. During the meeting the Academy's first five officers were elected and Dr. Gradwohl was elected President. Dr. Gradwohl established seven sections within the Academy that included *Forensic Pathology, Forensic Psychiatry, Forensic Toxicology, Forensic Immunology, Jurisprudence, Police Science,* and *Questioned Documents.* Dr. Milton Helpern was appointed the first section officer for *Forensic Pathology.*

The first official publication of the Academy was a newsletter distributed at the second annual meeting in 1950. The Academy newsletter evolved from a document recording the official minutes of the Academy meetings to a more comprehensive bulletin which subsequently grew into *The Journal of Forensic Sciences.* The first copy of the *Journal* was volume 1, January to October 1956. *The Journal of Forensic Sciences* is now considered one of the premier journals in the field of forensic science.

During the 1950s (1956–1967), Alan R. Moritz, MD was the only forensic pathologist to serve as president of the Academy. In 1960, Russell S. Fisher, MD became the Academy's 11th president followed by Samuel R. Gerber, MD, JD and Milton Helpern, MD. The Academy continued to grow throughout the 60s, 70s and 80s with several forensic pathologists holding the title of president including Charles S. Petty, MD (1967–1868), James T. Weston, MD (1976–1977) and Joseph H. Davis, MD (1981–1982).[23]

National Association of Medical Examiners

The National Association of Medical Examiners (NAME) was founded in 1966 *for the purpose of fostering professional growth, education and the dissemination of professional and technical information vital to improvement of the medical investigation of violent, suspicious and unusual deaths.*

NAME was started by Dr. Milton Helpern, who filed a certificate of incorporation in New York on October 13, 1966. Dr. Helpern was the first president of NAME and its offices were located in the New York City Medical Examiner's Office. The first annual meeting was held at the Knickerbocker Hotel in Chicago, Illinois on February 21, 1968 and was held together with the annual meeting of the America Academy of Forensic Sciences. Over the years, NAME has continued to grow and currently has more than 900 members. Membership in NAME is open to all physicians, investigators, and administrators who are active in medicolegal death investigation.[24]

In 1980, NAME became the official sponsor of *The American Journal of Forensic Pathology and Med-*

icine which is sent quarterly to all members. The journal's editor-in-chief was Dr. William Eckert until 1992 at which time Dr. Vincent DiMaio took over the editorial duties. Dr. Vincent DiMaio comes from a family of physicians, in fact his father, Dominic served as chief medical examiner of New York City. Dr. DiMaio has been chief medical examiner for Bexar County, San Antonio, Texas for many years. He has written extensively in the field.

In 1988, NAME prepared accreditation standards for the purpose of improving the quality of medicolegal death investigations. Emphasis is placed on medical examiner department policies and procedures rather than on the performance of individual medical examiners. The accreditation if granted is conferred for a period of five years. Currently an inspection by NAME to receive accreditation is a voluntary process which can be arranged by sending a written request to the NAME Inspection and Accreditation Office.

Although many medical examiner offices are currently accredited by NAME, it is encouraging that each year more and more jurisdictions are requesting inspection demonstrating a strong desire to improve quality and efficiency at their offices. Unfortunately, many medical examiner offices are not accredited and the nearly 1900 coroners' offices lack a similar accreditation process.[25] Hopefully, NAME accreditation will become a mandatory process in the near future. Information regarding inspection and accreditation by NAME can be found at the NAME website (www.thename.org).

Although NAME is the leader in implementing quality assurance and quality control measures, continued efforts must be made to assure that all medical examiner departments as well as individual medical examiners are performing at acceptable standards. NAME is currently discussing ways of implementing peer reviews of autopsy and microscopic reports, autopsy photography and expert testimony. Continued efforts in quality improvement are essential to assure high quality work by all those involved in death investigation. Standardization of the death investigation protocols used throughout the Unit-

ed States is another area that needs attention and should be a priority for the near future.[25]

As of 1993 the National Association of Medical Examiners recommended that medical examiners have authority to investigate and certify any deaths that fall into the following categories:[26]

• Criminal violence
• Suicide
• Accident
• Sudden death when decedent was in apparent good health
• Death unattended by a practicing physician
• Death under suspicious or unusual circumstances
• Abortion
• Poisoning
• Diseases constituting a threat to public health
• Disease, injury, or toxic agent resulting from employment
• Death associated with diagnostic or therapeutic procedures
• Death in any prison or penal institution
• Death in any mental institution
• Death when in legal custody
• Death in which a body is to be cremated, dissected, or buried at sea
• Unclaimed bodies
• Body brought into a new medicolegal jurisdiction without proper medical certification

Forensic Pathology Training and Certification

The American Board of Pathology was organized in 1936 with the objective of providing certification of training for those who successfully completed a pathology residency in an accredited training program. Successful completion of the board examination enables the candidate to be certified in the field of anatomic and/or clinical pathology.

In the early 1950s, the board recognized the subspecialty of forensic pathology and in 1959 the first forensic pathology board examination was administered. Forty-four pathologists were certified in 1959 and joined the original 30 pathologists who received their forensic certification by a *grandfather* clause. As of January 2003,

1,144 forensic pathologists have been certified by the American Board of Pathology. Currently, there are 1,011 board certified forensic pathologists in the United States.[27,28]

It would appear that to date training programs preparing candidates for board certification have not yet reached an optimal and uniform standard for such training.

For the first time, in January 2003, the American Board of Pathology published performance results for the primary and subspecialty board examinations between 1998 and 2002. A total of 3,293 candidates took the anatomic pathology board examination, of which 2,506 were first-time takers and 787 were repeaters. The failure rate for first-time takers was 19.3%, whereas, for repeaters, the failure rate was 55.8%. For the clinical pathology board examination, a total of 2,854 candidates took the examination with 2,231 being first-time takers and 623 being repeaters. The failure rate for first-time takers was 19.5%, whereas, for repeaters, the failure rate was 61.2%. This gave an overall failure rate of 28.0% for the anatomic pathology board examination and 28.6% for the clinical pathology board examination.

During this same time period, a total of 316 candidates took the forensic pathology board examination with 235 being first-time takers and 81 being repeaters. First-time takers had a failure rate of 30.6% and repeaters had a failure rate of 60.5%, giving a failure rate of 38.2% for the total number of candidates.[29]

Forensic pathology training programs are now spread across the United States with a total of 44 accredited programs in 26 states and Puerto Rico. As of 2001–2002, the total number of accredited forensic pathology fellowship positions was 77. Forensic pathology training consists of one additional year of specialized training following successful completion of an anatomic or anatomic and clinical pathology residency. Currently, forensic pathology training requirements must be approved by the Accreditation Council for Graduate Medical Education (ACGME).

Dr. Randy Hanzlick, estimates the number of board certified forensic pathologists who are engaged in the full-time practice of forensic pathology is 300 to 400, with the greater likelihood being closer to 300.[30] A survey conducted by Dr. Brad Randall and published in the *American Journal of Forensic Medicine and Pathology* in June of 2001[31] supports Dr. Hanzlick's estimate.

Medical Examiners and the Future

Over the last ten years developments in the field of forensic pathology have led to increased knowledge regarding many previously unknown or misunderstood conditions. Recent advancements include studies related to recognition and understanding diffuse axonal injury (DAI) which has shed light on the cause and mechanism of death in many cases of blunt cerebral injuries.

Sudden cardiac death in a previously young, healthy person often creates a problem for forensic pathologists. Although, the long QT syndrome has recently been proposed as a possible explanation for some of these cases, expanding research on the genetic basis of heart disease has uncovered many genetic abnormalities associated with this and many other heart diseases. Although it is still not routinely available, more and more laboratories are now performing these complex genetic tests.

Sudden infant death syndrome (SIDS) has been a source of contention among forensic pathologists for many years. The belief that babies could asphyxiate if put down in a prone position led to a nationwide campaign to educate parents regarding this potential hazard.[32] Over the next several years, the SIDS rate dropped dramatically. This practice is now accepted by most experts and is endorsed by the American Academy of Pediatrics. The long QT syndrome has also been proposed as a possible mechanism of SIDS, but continued genetic research is necessary to define a definite association. It must be remembered that SIDS is a diagnosis of exclusion and should be made only after negative autopsy, toxicologic, microscopic and microbiologic findings and following a thorough investigation of the child's environment, sleeping arrangements, and past history.[33] Only with a diligent multidisciplinary investigation can we be certain that what we are calling SIDS is truly a natural death and not an overlooked accident or homicide. As medical examiners we must continue to work to determine the factor or factors behind this long-standing medical mystery.

The debate continues regarding child abuse and shaken baby syndrome. The term shaken impact syndrome has recently emerged and with several *high-profile* legal battles regarding injured children, several forensic and clinical experts have questioned the validity of the shaken baby syndrome. Although much is unclear regarding childhood head trauma and the mechanism of injury, what is clear is that more research is necessary before forensic pathologists and pediatricians will have a full understanding of the dynamics associated with accidental and non-accidental injuries. As of now, no one has been able to set forth a clear constellation of findings that can be used to reliably separate childhood brain injuries caused by shaking and those caused by blunt impact.

Most large medical examiner departments have in-house toxicology laboratories which are a vital resource in death investigation. Continued advances in forensic toxicology has fortunately kept up with the ever changing world of illicit drugs and drugs of abuse. As in the past ethanol is found in a large number of medical examiner cases and is commonly found in accident, homicide, and suicide victims. Cocaine and heroin are still the most common illegal drugs seen in toxicology laboratories and account for a significant percentage of deaths in large metropolitan areas. In the past several years there has been a surge in *designer drugs* including ecstasy (methylenedioxymethylamphetamine), amphetamine, methamphetamine, paramethoxyamphetamine (PMA), paramethoxymethamphetamine (PMMA), ketamine (Special K) and gamma hydroxybutarate (GHB). These drugs have primarily been found in teenagers and young adults and are particularly common among dance-club patrons. Certain prescription medications have also come into favor with teenagers and young adults with Oxycontin, Xanax, methylphenidate (Ritalin) and even Viagra being quite common.

Interesting to note is that at the time of publication of the previous edition of this book many jurisdictions were experiencing record numbers of homicides, however, over the past decade the number of homicides in the United States has steadily declined. Between 1991 and 1999 homicides in the United States dropped by 37% in steady increments.

In Miami-Dade County, the number of homicides in the year 2000 was 214, the lowest level in over 20 years and significantly less than the all-time high of 621 homicides in 1981. Since 1993, the number of homicides in Miami-Dade County has decreased by almost half from 404 to 214. Although this downward trend has not been as dramatic in every jurisdiction, many major cities in the United States have experienced similar declines. In New York City, for example the homicide rate dropped 53% between 1991 and 1996 [34] and in Baltimore the annual murder total fell below 300 (to 262) in 2000 for the first time in a decade. Overall, the number of homicides in the United States committed with a firearm fell from 18,300 in 1993 to 13,300 in 1997, a 27% decline. [34]

In the past year, however, several major metropolitan areas have experienced a re-emergence in gang violence and an increase in the homicide rate. After a decade of decline, the number of homicides committed in Los Angeles in 2000 spiked 28% to 545. Researchers and analysts have attributed the declines to a variety of factors including changes in drug markets, increased police presence, new police strategies, increased crime education and awareness programs and improved economic conditions. [35] Recent reports suggest it was inevitable that the decline in homicides would begin to slow, since crime rates are typically cyclical. Now that the downward trend may have hit a plateau, the goal will be to keep the numbers from jumping back up.

Current training guidelines for forensic pathology programs mandate that physicians training in forensic pathology be at least superficially exposed to associated forensic fields such as anthropology, odontology, and criminalistics in order to train well-rounded forensic pathologists. Most medical examiner departments have now formed close contacts with these vital forensic consultants which also include experts in firearms, serology and DNA technology, genetics, entomology, computer science, psychiatry, and electrical and mechanical engineering to name a few.

The statutory role of the medical examiner is to conduct death investigations to determine the cause and manner of death. Adelson has best defined the cause of death as: *"the injury, disease or the combination of the two responsible for initiating the train of physiological disturbances, brief or prolonged, which produced the fatal termination."*[36] Davis added that the medical examiner's expected role should go one step beyond answering *what* and attempt to answer *why* the fatal event occurred.[37] It must be remembered that medical examiners are part of a service-oriented profession with far-reaching goals and objectives. The medical examiner is typically a prominent public figure who should not only be a scientist, but also an educator. Unfortunately, monetary constraints and lack of governmental support has caused extreme difficulty for many medical examiner departments, however, other jurisdictions have been given extra resources to allow for medical examiner involvement in community educational projects related to drug and alcohol awareness and crime reduction. County and state government must be aware of the positive impact that the medical examiner can play in regards to public health, safety, and education and should provide the medical examiner with the necessary resources to become involved in these projects. Medical examiners must be effective communicators with the skill and sensitivity necessary to handle difficult issues related to police-custody deaths, religious objections to autopsy and high-profile deaths. It is essential that relations with governmental officials, law enforcement personnel, judges, attorneys, and medical colleagues remain at a professional level. It is also important to maintain close affiliations with local medical schools and hospital pathology departments. As we proceed through the twenty-first century, we must concentrate on these areas in order to guarantee the growth of our profession.

Throughout history and over the past few years several cases come to mind where the medical examiner and forensic pathology evidence played an important role. These cases, which include the assassination of President John F. Kennedy, the death of Jon Benet Ramsey and the O.J. Simpson murder trial, all served to put the field of forensic pathology on trial. We can only learn from the past and let these and other experiences prepare us for the future. It is important to understand that these cases demonstrated weaknesses in the death investigative process which includes much more than forensic pathology and the medical examiner. Forensic pathology has two components, documentation and interpretation. The interpretation of injuries relies partly on training and experience of the pathologist, but can only be accomplished accurately when evaluated in the light of the circumstances surrounding the death. If there is failure in the circumstantial investigation or failure to coordinate and correlate during the investigative phase, the chances for erroneous opinions on the part of the pathologist are enhanced. Essentially, forensic pathology service is dependent not only on the pathologist, but also on the other agencies and personnel involved in the death investigation.

The future of forensic pathology and medical examiners is bright and great discoveries lie ahead for those who are patient and inquisitive. Continued pursuit of academic achievements with emphasis on evidence-based medicine and research will continue to allow for great accomplishments. The autopsy is an incredible tool that if used correctly can speak volumes of the dead and educate the living. As medical examiners we must use all available resources and combine efforts to ensure the continued quality and success in our field. We look forward to the future with excitement and confidence that great achievements lie ahead.*

* Acknowledgment: I would like to thank Dr. Joseph H. Davis for the time he spent sharing his personal experiences and historical knowledge.

REFERENCES

1. Smith, S.: History and Development of Legal Medicine in Gradwohl, R.B.H.: *Legal Medicine.* St. Louis: C.V. Mosby, 1954.

2. Curran, W.J.: History and Development in Curran, W.J., McGarry, A.L. and Petty C.S.: *Modern Legal Medicine, Psychiatry and Forensic Science.* Philadelphia: F.A. Davis Co., 1980.

3. Camps, F.E. (Ed.): *Gradwohl's Legal Medicine,* 2nd edition. Baltimore: Williams and Wilkins, 1968.

4. Gonzalez, T.A., Vance, M., Helpern, M., and Umberger, C.J.: The Medical Examiner and the Coroner in *Legal Medicine: Pathology and Toxicology.* New York: Appleton, Century & Crofts, Inc., 1954.

5. Thorwald, J.: *The Century of the Detective.* New York: Harcourt Brace World, 1965.

6. Garland, A.N.: Forensic Medicine in Great Britain: The Beginning. *The American Journal of Forensic Medicine and Pathology, 8* (3): 269–272, 1987.

7. Mant, A.K.: Forensic Medicine in Great Britain: The Origins of the British Medicolegal System and Some Historic Cases. *The American Journal of Forensic Medicine and Pathology, 8* (4): 354–361, 1987.

8. Latrobe, J.H.B.: *Justices' Practice Under The Laws of Maryland,* 6th ed. Baltimore: Lucus, 1861.

9. Harvard, J.V.J.: *The Detection of Secret Homicide.* London: Macmillan, 39, 42–43, 1960.

10. Knight, B.: Forensic Medicine in Britain. *The American Journal of Forensic Medicine and Pathology, 1* (2): 177–180, 1980.

11. Kane County, Illinois: 1999. A Historical Perspective. http://www.co.kane.il.us/coroners.htm. 28 July 2000.

12. Browne, W.H. (Ed.): *Archives of Maryland,* Vol 4. Baltimore: Maryland Historical Society, 1887.

13. Platt, M.S.: History of Forensic Pathology and Related Laboratory Sciences. *Spitz W.U., Fisher, R.S. Medicolegal Investigation of Death,* Springfield, IL: Charles C Thomas, 1993.

14. Kornblum, R.N., and Fisher, R.S.: *A Compendium of State Medicolegal Investigative Systems.* Baltimore: Maryland Medicolegal Foundation, May 1972.

15. Eckert, W.G.: Charles Norris and Thomas A. Gonzales: New York's Forensic Pioneers. *The American Journal of Forensic Medicine and Pathology, 8* (4): 350–353, 1987.

16. Eckert, W.G.: Medicolegal Investigation in New York City: History and Activities 1918–1978. *The American Journal of Forensic Medicine and Pathology, 4* (1): 33–54, 1983.

17. Eckert, W.G.: Miniature Crime Scenes: A Novel Use in Crime Seminars. *The American Journal of Forensic Medicine and Pathology, 2* (4): 365–368, 1981.

18. Adelson, L.: Alan Richards Moritz, M.D.: An Appreciation. *The American Journal of Forensic Medicine and Pathology, 2* (4): 297–298, 1981.

19. Spitz, W.U.: A Tribute to the Late Russell S. Fisher. *The American Journal of Forensic Medicine and Pathology, 9* (4): 355–356, 1988.

20. Combs, D.L., Parrish, R.G., and Ing, R.: Death Investigation in the United States and Canada, 1995. US Department of Health and Human Services, Centers for Disease Control and Prevention, Atlanta, Georgia, August 1995.

21. Hanzlick, R., and Combs, D.: Medical Examiner and Coroner Systems: History and Trends. *Journal of the American Medical Association, 279* (11): 870–874, 1998.

22. Clark, S.C.: National Medicolegal Panel Research Report. *Death Investigation: A Guide for the Scene Investigator.* National Institute of Justice, U.S. Department of Justice, Washington, D.C., November 1999.

23. Field, K.S.: *History of the American Academy of Forensic Sciences: 50 Years of Progress.* Philadelphia: American Society for Testing and Materials, 1998.

24. Hanzlick, R.: History of the National Association of Medical Examiners and Its Meetings, 1966–93. *The American Journal of Forensic Medicine and Pathology, 16* (4): 278–313, 1995.

25. Hanzlick, R.: On the Need for More Expertise in Death Investigation (and a National Office of Death Investigation Affairs?). *Archives of Pathology and Laboratory Medicine, 120,* 329–332, 1996.

26. Hanzlick, R., Parrish, R.G., and Combs, D.: Standard Language in Death Investigation Laws. *Journal of Forensic Sciences, 39* (3): 637–643, 1994.

27. Personal Communication. The American Board of Pathology. Tampa, Florida. February, 2001.

28. Eckert, W.G.: The Forensic Pathology Specialty Certifications. *The American Journal of Forensic Medicine and Pathology, 9* (1): 85–89, 1988.

29. *The American Board of Pathology Examiner,* Vol. 25, No. 1, January, 2003.

30. Personal Communication, Randy Hanzlick, Chairman of the Board of Directors, NAME, June, 2002.

31. Randall, B.: Survey of Forensic Pathologists. *The American Journal of Forensic Medicine and Pathology, 22* (2): 123–127, 2001.

32. Sudden Infant Death Syndrome and Sleeping Position. *Pediatrics, 90:* 1158, 1992.

33. Mitchell, E., Krous, H.F., Donald, T., and Byard, R.W.: Changing Trends in the Diagnosis of Sudden Infant Death. *The American Journal of Forensic Medicine and Pathology, 21* (4): 311–314, 2000.

34. National Institute of Justice. (1997). A Study of Homicide in Eight U.S. Cities: An NIJ Intramural Research Project. http://www.ojp.usdoj.gov. February 2, 2001.

35. Zawit, M.W., and Strom, K.J.: Firearm Injury and Death from Crime, 1993–1997. US Department of Justice, Bureau of Justice Statistics. October 2000, 1–8.

36. Adelson, L.: *The Pathology of Homicide.* Springfield, IL: Charles C Thomas, 1974.

37. Davis, J.H.: The Future of the Medical Examiner System. *The American Journal of Forensic Pathology and Medicine, 16* (4): 265–269, 1995.

Chapter II

CRIME SCENE

Part 1

HERBERT LEON MACDONELL

BLOODSTAIN PATTERN INTERPRETATION

DURING THE LAST THREE DECADES, bloodstain evidence has become increasingly accepted in the forensic community as a valuable and often times essential tool for the investigation of crimes in which blood has been shed. Numerous applications of bloodstain evidence have shown that it can often be a deciding factor for apprehending a suspect and obtaining a conviction. Bloodstain evidence is frequently used to exculpate an innocent suspect or defendant. Identification or elimination of an individual by DNA has become a routine event.

Those familiar with criminal investigations are aware that eyewitness identification and other personal accounts of what they believed happened can be, and frequently are, inaccurate. The scientific reliability of physical evidence, in this case bloodstain pattern interpretation, is more accurate in reconstruction of prior events than evidence based upon the memory of an eye witness. However, bloodstain patterns, like other physical evidence, must first be detected, preserved, examined, interpreted, and properly presented in court to utilize its evidentiary value.

The study of bloodstain patterns must be directed toward the understanding of several basic pattern types and how they can be produced. These will be discussed in detail later but by way of an introduction to the significance of bloodstain patterns. The more significant considerations are listed below in a general order of significance:

- *THE SHAPE OF THE INDIVIDUAL BLOODSTAINS* which may allow their origin to be determined in three dimensions. Under certain circumstances this category can also include some transfer patterns.
- *THE SIZE OF THE INDIVIDUAL BLOODSTAINS* which suggests the kind of energy available for their production if they were the result of an impact.
- *THE DISTRIBUTION AND CONCENTRATION OF A BLOODSTAIN PATTERN* may suggest the distance between the origin of blood and the surface upon which it was deposited. This can be important in differentiating between impact spatter, expired blood, and arterial patterns.

A BRIEF HISTORY OF BLOODSTAIN PATTERN INTERPRETATION

Well over five hundred references to the subject of bloodstain pattern interpretation have been found that were published before 1975. Most are in forensic, academic, and medical libraries throughout the world.

For those who would like to read a detailed book on the early literature in this discipline, we suggest *SEGMENTS OF HISTORY, THE LITERATURE OF BLOODSTAIN PATTERN INTERPRETATION, SEGMENT 00: LITERATURE THROUGH THE 1800's.*[1] This reference includes reports of a murder case which occurred prior to 100 AD; another in London in 1514; the murder of his wife by a minister in upstate New York in

1859; and several others prior to 1900. The outstanding research of Dr. Eduard Pitrowski[2] in 1895 was undoubtedly one of the most comprehensive works of the nineteenth century. He was involved in a beating death and conducted many experiments using rabbits which he documented in great detail. His book included twenty-two color plates which illustrated his experiments.

Unfortunately, it is not possible to include the classic works of Gross, Orsos, and Balthazard in this chapter. Suffice it to say that many early forensic scientists recognized the potential value of bloodstain patterns but, for whatever reason, this subject was essentially never practiced in the United States until Dr. Paul Leland Kirk became involved with the Dr. Samuel Sheppard case in 1955. His affidavit[3] on bloodstains in that case appears to be the first in depth use of evidence of this type in the reconstruction of a homicide in recent times.

Additional information on this subject can be found which includes some five hundred and fifty references on bloodstain patterns in the inaugural issue of *QUINNIPIAC HEALTH LAW.*[4]

CHARACTERISTICS OF LIQUID BLOOD

To have a basic understanding of why blood behaves as it does, one should have some knowledge of three physical properties of human blood. These include specific gravity, surface tension, and viscosity. These properties of blood are sufficiently similar to those of water that it is unnecessary for the reader to formulate an entirely new concept to deal with blood as a liquid. Basically, it is within common experience everyone has had with water insofar as how it pours, splashes, and spatters. However, since water is colorless, it makes casual observations of this phenomenon more difficult than with blood. Bloodstains will usually have a greater contrast over their background surface.

A study of bloodstains is primarily concerned with what happens to blood once it has left the body. When blood spatters, drips, or is gushing from an artery, its behavior follows the laws of physics, specifically that of ballistics; the study of projectiles in motion. Therefore, interpretation of the significance of bloodstain evidence is best conducted by the physical scientist rather than a pathologist whose expertise is generally limited to the behavior of blood within the body. Although many pathologists may be familiar with the physical characteristics of bloodstain evidence, this subject is not normally a part of their education. They should, however, recognize the more common bloodstain patterns that are often present within a body of a deceased person. These will include petechial hemorrhages, postmortem lividity, or livor mortis, Tardieu's spots, and marbling of the skin due to hemolysis of blood in the body's superficial vessels.[5]

One of the most frequent applications of bloodstain pattern interpretation within the human body is the recognition of blanched or void patterns which appear as the result of external pressure on areas of the body, such as the back, arms, or legs. Such pressure prevents the uniform development of livor mortis in those areas and often outlines a common geometric shape which may be easily identifiable. When such patterns are observed they should be immediately photographed since such images may fade quite rapidly depending on how long it has been since livor mortis developed (Fig. II-1).

Like all liquids, blood is held together by a cohesive force that produces a skin-like surface resistant to penetration or separation. Technically, this phenomenon is known as the *surface tension of the liquid.* Surface tension produces a force across the surface of a liquid that decreases its surface area. For example, when small volumes of liquid are detached from the main body of a liquid, they assume a spherical geometry because this configuration minimizes surface area. The sphere is, in contrast to the so-called *teardrop* shape so often seen in the artist's rendition of falling raindrops. Blood drops, like all other liquids, have a spheroid or ball shape, not a *teardrop* shape.

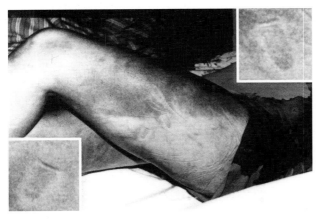

FIGURE II-1. Outlines of two 9mm cartridges are visible on the mid-thigh of the victim due to livor mortis. The inserts show detailed enlargements.

TABLE II-1
PHYSICAL PROPERTIES OF HUMAN BLOOD

Temperature (degrees centigrade	Surface Tension (Dynes/cm)	Viscosity (centipoise)
25	49–58	3.4–4.3
37	27–34	1.6–2.5

Another physical property of liquids that should be considered is that of *viscosity.* The flow of a liquid decreases as its viscosity increases. Although *blood is thicker than water,* the difference, insofar as patterns they produce, is negligible. The viscosity of blood is important when it increases greatly as a result of clotting. Seliger[6] reported the values for surface tension and viscosity as shown in Table II-1.

In a study, samples of human blood were drawn from male and female subjects ranging from two years to eighty-nine years of age. Measurements were taken on both fresh and complexed blood. The complexed blood contained EDTA, citrate, or oxalate, which are common agents used to prevent clotting. No significant differences were noted because of the subject's age or sex. Bloodstain patterns that were produced when freshly drawn blood was used were compared to those obtained when samples of complexed blood was used. No measurable differences were noted.

Law Enforcement Assistance Administration (LEAA) research confirmed that when blood drips from a dependent portion of the body, for example, after running down to the fingertips from a cut on the hand, it does so in a uniform manner. To produce a drop, blood volume increases (on a fingertip, for example) until its weight is sufficient to allow it to break away from other accumulated blood remaining behind. Therefore, before a drop can fall free, gravitational attraction for the drop must exceed the blood's surface tension. Since the surface tension of blood is quite uniform at any given temperature, each drop that falls will have a correspondingly uniform volume. The typical volume of a drop of blood has been determined to be approximately 0.05 mL or 50 micro liters (µl).[7] If the bleeding rate is rapid, blood drop volume may increase slightly, but slower bleeding does not result in drops of lower volume. Surface area of the object from which a blood drop falls may affect the size of the drop. When the object is, for example, a knife tip, drop volumes as small as 0.03 mL may be produced.

Another characteristic of blood is the terminal velocity of a drop in a free fall. This was determined to be 25.1 plus or minus 0.5 feet per second for single, typical (0.05 mL) drops in air.[7] This is a somewhat academic value. Nevertheless, it should be remembered that the smaller the droplet size the greater is its surface area and, therefore, the slower it will fall.

Contrary to popular belief, a typical drop of blood will not break up into smaller droplets as it falls through air. If a typical drop of blood is to subdivide, it must land on a rough or dirty surface or it must be acted upon by some external physical force, usually an impact, to cause it to spatter. The degree of bloodspatter that results from a single drop falling onto a surface is usually characterized as a passive drop striking a target, the surface it lands on.

TARGET SURFACE CHARACTERISTICS AND BLOODSPATTER

The degree of spatter that results when a drop of blood falls onto a surface is far more dependent upon the nature of the surface than it is on the distance the drop has fallen. In general, the harder and less porous the surface, the less spatter results. This is due to the fact that, even though the drop undergoes considerable geometric distortion upon impact by spreading out and then contracting, the surface of the drop remains intact because of blood's relatively high surface tension. Protrusions and rough texture of irregular and porous surfaces can rupture surface tension which will result in increased spatter. This condition is not unlike a rubber balloon filled with water which can be *teased about* over a smooth surface to great degrees of geometric distortion, but the same balloon will likely rupture and discharge its contents if abraded due to contact with a coarse surface such as sandpaper.

There are also distinctions which can be drawn between hard and soft porous surfaces. Raw wood and asbestos board are certainly porous, but they are also hard in contrast to newspapers or paper towels. Consequently, there will be less spatter on the raw wood and asbestos board. Likewise, irregularity of the target surface is an important factor that should not be overlooked. The two sides of a sheet of singularly corrugated cardboard may be of the same composition, but they usually differ markedly in texture.

Estimations of the distance a drop of blood has fallen from the extent of satellite spatter around the central bloodstain, or from *spines* that may also be produced, will usually be inaccurate if surface texture of the target is not considered.

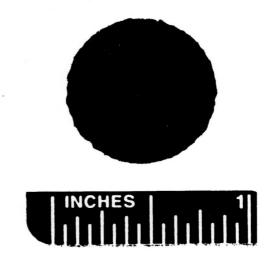

FIGURE II-2. Bloodstain produced when a typical 0.05 mL drop of human blood fell eighty feet before striking a hard, smooth, glossy cardboard surface.

Spines are the pointed streaks of blood that radiate away from the center of a bloodstain. As an example, the bloodstain shown in Figure II-2, was produced by a drop of blood that fell over eighty feet onto a hard, smooth, glossy cardboard surface producing no spatter. Surface tension of blood will prevent a drop from spattering *regardless of the height it falls before striking a smooth, hard surface*. In contrast, the bloodstain shown in Figure II-3 was produced when a drop of blood fell only eighteen inches before striking a desk blotter.

From Figures II-2 and II-3 it is obvious that correct interpretation of spattering in bloodstain patterns requires consideration of the surface texture of the target upon which it impacted.

BLOODSTAIN CHARACTERISTICS

Shape of Stain

The shape of bloodstains produced when individual drops of blood strike a surface, whether simultaneously or sequentially, will be either round or elliptical. Their directionality may often be determined from the shape of the bloodstains even when there are no edge scallops, spines, or satellite spatters. Measurements are not necessary to determine the direction of flight of a drop of blood immediately prior to an angular impact onto a flat surface because one end of the ellipse

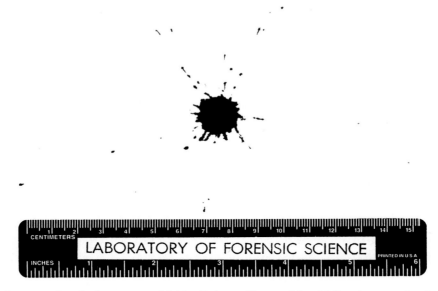

FIGURE II-3. Bloodstain produced when a typical 0.05 mL drop of human blood fell eighteen inches before it struck a soft desk blotter. Note the extensive spatter that resulted due to the blotter fibers.

is usually obvious as it will have a pointed end. This point indicates its forward direction of travel prior to impact (Fig. II-4).

A smaller droplet may sometimes be thrown from a larger parent drop upon impact to produce a *wave cast-off* (Fig. II-5).

The two-dimensional origin of a bloodstain pattern may be established by drawing straight lines through the long axis of the bloodstains. These lines represent the direction of each blood drop's horizontal travel prior to its striking the surface. The intersection of these lines represents the origin of bloodspatter in a two-dimensional configuration (Fig. II-6). The actual origin of blood spatter would have been at some point above this intersection.

Tracing bloodstain directionalities on flat surfaces to find their general area of convergence does not provide sufficient information to determine the height of the origin of bloodspatter. To achieve this, the impact angle of several individual bloodstains must be calculated and projected back above their convergence on the surface, thereby constructing a three-dimensional model.

Estimation of the height above or away from a surface may usually be established by calculation of the impact angle of each bloodstain and pro-

jecting their trajectories back to an axis that is placed 90 degrees, or normal, to the intersection of the previously established two-dimensional origin. This is discussed in greater detail later in this chapter.

Impact Angle Considerations

Blood which falls onto a flat surface that is not horizontal will produce an elliptical rather than a round bloodstain. Its degree of distortion from a circle is inversely proportional to the impact angle. That is, as the impact angle decreases from 90 degrees to 10 degrees, the bloodstain's shape becomes progressively more elongated. Figure II-7 shows nine bloodstains that resulted when single drops of blood struck a smooth surface at impact angles of 10, 20, 30, 40, 50, 60, 70, 80 and 90 degrees.

Blood drop impact angles may be determined by using the bloodstain's width-to-length ratio. This ratio has a trigonometric relationship to the angle of impact. The calculation is elementary and uses standard trigonometric tables. Simply divide the width of an elliptical bloodstain by its length. The result will always be one or less and is the sin of the impact angle. The impact angle

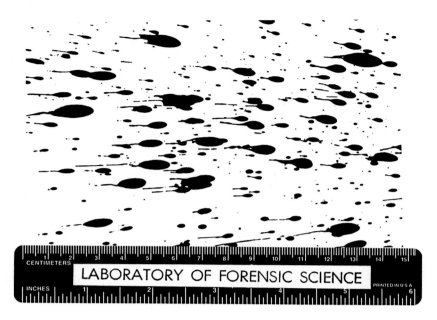

FIGURE II-4. This pattern resulted from many droplets of blood that were traveling from right to left prior to striking a flat level surface.

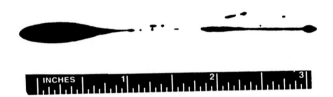

FIGURE II-5. The parent bloodstain is shown on the left and the smaller, wave cast-off is on the right. The blood drop that produced this pattern was traveling from the left to right before it struck this horizontal target at an angle of approximately sixteen degrees.

can be found from a table of trigonometric functions. Scientific calculators having trigonometric functions may also be used. In fact, this is the method of choice for both speed and accuracy. The formula to use for this calculation is:

$$\text{arc sin of} = \frac{\text{width of bloodstain}}{\text{length of bloodstain}} = \text{impact angle}$$

The accuracy in the determination of impact angle will depend upon the care that is taken in measurement of the length and width of each bloodstain. However, since the fluid nature of blood does not produce a perfect ellipse when it

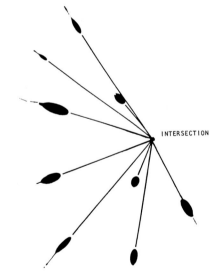

FIGURE II-6. The origin of bloodspatter on a surface can be determined by establishing a convergence of lines drawn through the long dimension of several bloodstains. This shows a two-dimensional origin.

impacts a surface at an angle other than 90 degrees, the pointed end of the bloodstain must be *rounded off* so it is symmetrical with its opposite end (Fig. II-8). The more acute the angle of

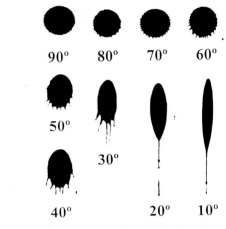

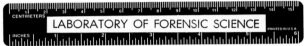

FIGURE II-7. Patterns produced when typical drops of blood fell forty-two inches onto hard, smooth, cardboard at various angles.

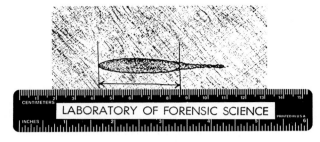

FIGURE II-8. A curved line is traced over the bloodstain to identify the length of the ellipse at its pointed end.

impact, the more pointed the forward end of the ellipse in its direction of travel prior to impact.

When evaluating bloodstains of less than five millimeters on their long dimension, measurements should be made with some type of pocket microscope that has a built-in reticle. Only bloodstains that are well defined should be measured, regardless of their size.

By determining the angles of impact for several bloodstains in conjunction with their distances from the origin, on a two-dimensional plane, it is possible to estimate the distance the origin of spatter was from the stained surface. This origin would be either the height above a floor or the distance from a wall or ceiling. A three-dimensional model may be constructed at the scene from bloodstains using string, tape, and a protractor; or it may be done back at the laboratory from measurements taken at the scene. Both the location and geometry of several bloodstains are necessary to prepare an accurate model or graph to identify the origin.

In practice, after the investigator has determined the impact angle of a bloodstain he may tape an end of elastic string, or thread, on the floor just behind the stain's pointed end. A small piece of masking tape is ideal for this. Then, with slight tension, the other end of the string should be taped well beyond where the convergence of several stains appears to be. The string is positioned so it is running parallel to the long dimension of the bloodstain. Several pieces of elastic string should be taped to the floor, wall or the ceiling in this manner. This procedure is shown in Figure II-9. After several strings have been placed, the origin on the floor should become apparent at the intersection of the strings.

Placing a vertical pole over the origin on the floor will serve as an axis from which the bloodspatter radiated. Almost any type of pole may be used. One convenient device is a discarded spring loaded pole light after its fixtures have been removed. Figure II-10 shows one that has been placed over the intersection of strings placed on the floor as previously described.

The final step in establishing the origin of spatter in space is to place a protractor beside each bloodstain and, one at a time, then have an assistant raise the other end of the string until the string reaches the previously determined angle of impact as shown in Figure II-11. The string should then be taped to the pole and the process repeated for each bloodstain. The result should show a convergence of strings on the pole in a similar manner to the intersection of the same strings when they were lying flat on the floor.

It must be emphasized that when measurements and angles are used to establish the origin or origins in space, not only will the actual origin be somewhere below the point or points of convergence, but it must be remembered that the investigator is actually determining a space and

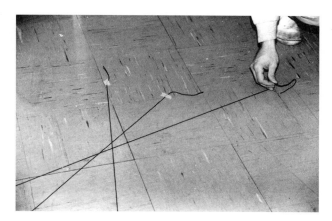

FIGURE II-9. Establishing bloodspatter origin on the floor using elastic string and masking tape. The two-dimensional origin is found at the convergence of the strings.

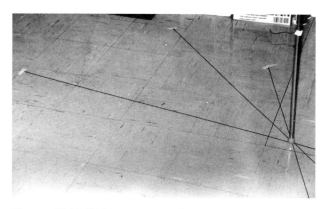

FIGURE II-10. Utilizing a spring loaded pole light to establish the vertical axis from which blood radiated as a result of an impact.

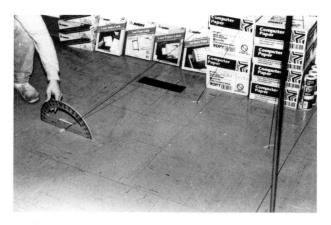

FIGURE II-11. Using a protractor to *project* the elastic strings back to the axis (pole light) at their individual angles of impact.

not a point of origin. Since the practical application of establishing this space, which is more accurately identified as a volume, it is only establishing whether the victim was standing, sitting or kneeling, on or just above the floor, in a chair or on a bed, pinpoint accuracy is not necessary.

Another technique for establishing the origin of spatter above a floor may be used. This method does not require strings and uses basic mathematics, specifically trigonometry. This method for obtaining the distance of bloodspatter away from a surface is commonly called the *Tangent Method.* This technique does not need two investigators or a protractor at the crime scene, however, it does require a scientific calculator.

All that is required to utilize the tangent method at the scene is to establish the two-dimensional point of convergence or origin on, for example, the floor, and secure a vertical axis above it as shown in Figure II-10. The next step is to calculate the angle of impact for several bloodstains using their length-to-width measurements. The only other procedure required is to measure the distance of each bloodstain away from the two-dimensional origin on the floor.

Calculation of the distance of bloodspatter origin above the floor or from a wall is a simple two-step operation. First, using a scientific calculator, enter the impact angle of a specific bloodstain, for example 37°, and press the *tangent* key. Read the value, which will be 0.753554. Second, multiply this figure by the distance the bloodstain is from the origin, for example 23 inches, and read the answer, 17.3. This is the distance in inches of the origin of spatter above or beside the surface upon which it was deposited.

The tangent method of establishing the origin of spatter is based on the simple trigonometric relationship that the side opposite an angle, in this example the height, divided by the side adjacent, in this example the distance of the bloodstain from its two-dimensional origin, is the *tangent* of that angle.

Computer programs have been developed that can calculate the exact origin of spatter from bloodstains on the walls, floor, or ceiling of crime scenes. While this is a practical application of computer technology, such precise measurements will seldom be necessary. If the origin of bloodspatter can be established within the volume of a grapefruit, or even a basketball, and that origin is either at a standing height of five to six feet above the floor, at a level consistent with sitting on the piece of furniture in question, or lying on the floor, a satisfactory reconstruction will be achieved in all but the most unusual circumstances.

Size of Stain

Information in many forensic textbooks which attempts to correlate the size of a bloodstain to the distance it had fallen is usually incomplete, inaccurate, or both. Most information on this subject frequently neglected two essential considerations in their estimation of the distance a drop of blood had fallen before it struck a surface. These are the volume of the drop of blood and the nature of the target surface.

There is a very wide range of *wetability* of surfaces. Soft porous surfaces, such as a piece of cloth, will often have a large bloodstain that results from liquid blood soaking into the fabric. Conversely, blood that falls onto glass, or some other non-porous surface, and does not *wet* the surface, will result in smaller bloodstains as it contracts before it dries because of its internal cohesive forces. The result is that a smaller bloodstain will be produced than would have been the case had the same drop of blood fallen the same distance onto a tile floor, a wooden surface, or a tight pile carpet. The cohesive proper-

ty of blood may be easily and dramatically demonstrated by simply letting drops of blood fall onto a smooth, hard surface such as the top of a coffee can. Rub a very thin layer of oil or grease onto one half of the can and leave the other half clean. Allow a drop of blood to fall three feet or so to one surface at a time. The drop that strikes the *greased surface* will immediately begin contracting until it is approximately one-half its original diameter. The drop that strikes the clean side will not contract at all because it *wets* the surface. This is an excellent way to demonstrate the terms *wetability* and *surface tension* to a lay jury. This author has found it to be a *jury friendly* exercise which helps them understand why many bloodstain patterns are produced as they are.

The resulting edge characteristics of a bloodstain are far more dependent upon the texture of the target surface upon which the drop lands than they are upon the distance it fell before impact. Therefore, conclusions as to the significance of *spines* or spatters as a function of distance fallen cannot be reliable unless texture of the target surface is considered. Bloodstains on glass will not spatter regardless of the distance they fell before impact, but bloodstains on wood or paper spatter to various degrees because they have wide variations in their surface texture.

Provided the volume of a drop of blood was known to be that of the typical 0.05 mL drop, it is possible to estimate the distance it fell prior to impact. However, in almost fifty years of study this author has yet to find a practical application for such information.

BLOOD SPATTERED FROM LOW VELOCITY IMPACT

Dripped and Splashed Blood

Blood dripping into blood produces a characteristic stain pattern. Liquid-to-liquid impact of this type results in many very small droplets being spattered upward and out away from the center of the blood pool that is being formed. This action is somewhat like a water fountain wherein small droplets are projected up and away from its center and they return to the sur-

face from whence they came at obtuse angles (Fig. II-12).

Blood acted upon by a low energy, *low velocity force,* such as when someone steps into a small pool of blood on a floor, will be splashed away from the point of impact. The drops that are produced will strike the surrounding area at very acute angles that are more streaks than ellipses. The resulting bloodstain pattern will usually have these long streaks radiating out away from the

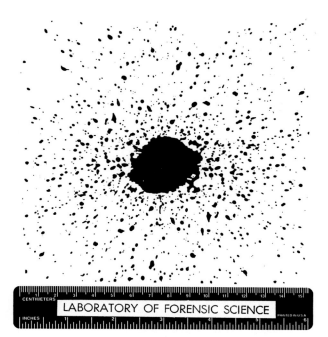

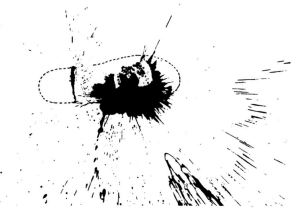

FIGURE II-13. Low velocity, surface splashing caused by stepping into a pool of blood.

FIGURE II-12. A typical drip pattern produced as blood fell into blood. Several drops of blood were released to form this low velocity impact pattern.

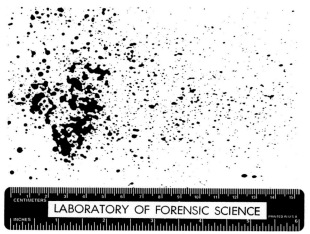

original source of blood (Fig. II-13). Blood cannot have an upward trajectory from impact by the underside surface of a flat object such as a shoe. As a result the splashed blood can only skim along the surface before the individual droplets streak to a halt. Splashed bloodstain patterns are most often formed when larger volumes of blood are available for impact of this type.

FIGURE II-14. Typical medium velocity impact spatter. Although the majority of these stains are over one millimeter in diameter, many are also much smaller.

BLOOD SPATTERED FROM MEDIUM VELOCITY IMPACT

During a beating, stabbing, or other violent act it is common for blood to be shed. As blood accumulates on the surface of the victim's clothing, or bare skin, additional blows to the same area will usually cause blood to spatter. The force of the blows, with or without a knife blade, will usually have sufficient energy to overcome blood's surface tension releasing hundreds of very small droplets. The resulting spatter pattern is identified as *medium velocity impact spatter*. It is important to understand that the velocity of the weapon is usually higher than the velocity of blood which leaves the main blood source, usually the victim's body. The preponderance of bloodstains resulting from *medium velocity impact spatter* have diameters of one millimeter or larger (Fig. II-14). It must be noted that while the diameter of most bloodstains produced by this mechanism is well over this dimension, some are also much smaller.

Homicides due to beating are usually quite characteristic because of the large amount of blood that spatters. In fact, there is usually more bloodspatter caused by a beating than a stabbing, cutting, or shooting. Exceptions, of course, do exist. If a broad axe were used as an instrument for delivering multiple blows or if a baseball bat repeatedly struck a victim's head in the same location the amount of bloodspatter would be considerable. In fact, multiple blows being struck to the head will create more bloodspatter than from any other common mechanism except gunshot wounds.

Those who administer beatings will often become spattered with blood. The absence of bloodspatter on the accused's clothing does not, however, prove non-participation as many defense lawyers would like to believe. To the contrary, it is possible to beat someone and not receive any back spatter whatsoever. This has been demonstrated and observed by over fifteen hundred participants who have attended the Bloodstain Evidence Institute.[8]

Many earlier researchers conducted beating experiments and reported that they found that blood was not always back spattered on garments worn by the perpetrator even though considerable blood was spattered elsewhere.[37] Some pointed out that assailants could also have worn outer protective garments or had simply changed their clothes after the beating. In many cases it has also been reported that the perpetrator was nude when committing the crime and afterwards simply showered and dressed so they had no blood on their body or clothing.

Scientists should concern themselves with what they *see* rather than speculate as to why they do not see something they think they should. Nevertheless, when blood spots in the medium velocity impact range are discovered on a garment, they are usually somewhat below the resolution of the average juror's eyesight. Some simple means of providing a *road map* identifying the location of these small spots of blood should be considered so a jury can understand not only their location but also their size and distribution. One convenient method is simply to place small white ring binder reinforcers around each of the bloodstains and then to photograph the garment. Reinforcers should never be glued onto the gar-

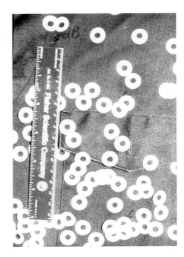

FIGURE II-15. Ring binder reinforcers used to show the locations of each small bloodstain. It is evident that the shirt pocket flap was down when it was spattered with blood during a beating.

ment but just placed around the bloodstain long enough to photograph the garment. An example of this technique is illustrated in Figure II-15.

A farm laborer beat his employer's wife to death with a hammer and wrench. His work shirt was spattered with over two hundred and fifty small bloodstains (Fig. II-15). Note the blood spots over his shirt pocket flap. Figure II-16, shows the same shirt with the flap over his shirt pocket raised up. The presence of bloodspatter beneath the flap is evidence that the flap portion of his shirt was moving up and down at the time it was spattered with blood, a movement completely consistent with raising his arm up and down as in a beating.

Another, perhaps more popular method of photographing the location of small bloodstains is to cut small, sharp triangles from masking tape and simply press them onto the garment so their most acute angle points to the individual bloodstains. The blue jeans are marked using this procedure (Fig. II-17). The triangular pieces of masking tape can be numbered for specific identification of each bloodstain, if desired. Surprisingly, masking tape adheres quite tenaciously. We have seen garments marked in this manner several years after a trial and the tape was still sticking to the garments after they had undergone considerable handling.

Impact velocity associated with beatings and stabbings has been measured at about twenty-

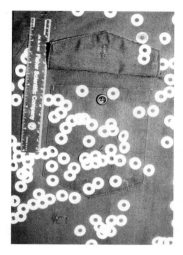

FIGURE II-16. The same shirt which was shown in Figure II-15 but the pocket flap has been raised to show blood had also spattered under the flap and onto the front of the pocket beneath it. Therefore, this flap had to be up as well as down to allow blood to spatter onto both these locations. If the person wearing this shirt were raising and lowering their arm as they were beating someone, such a motion could produce this pattern.

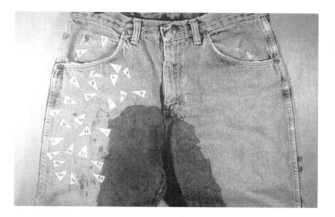

FIGURE II-17. Triangles of masking tape placed on the blue jeans to show the locations of small blood spots. Each piece of tape can be numbered so a correlation between the results of chemical tests and the stains tested can be easily established.

five feet per second. Therefore, *medium velocity impact spatter* is considered to be spatter that results from an impact to a blood source in this range. Extreme situations, of course, must always be considered. For example, a golf club may be swung at a velocity of over seventy-five feet per second. Fortunately, beatings with a golf club are rare but when such a situation is encountered, it must be given proper consideration when interpreting bloodstain patterns that result. The highest beating velocities cannot approach the velocity of the slowest projectiles fired from handguns, rifles, or shotguns. For this reason differentiation between bloodstain patterns that result from these two mechanisms is easily recognized by investigators who are familiar with evidence of this type.

Two important rules must be remembered when attempting to identify bloodstain patterns. The first is that a few bloodstains do not a pattern make! Although very small bloodstains can only be produced when some form of energy is available, there are times when the mechanism that caused bloodspatter cannot be determined. Caution is required before forming a firm conclusion as to the only manner by which a pattern could be produced. It is usually better to use the somewhat overworked cliché *consistent with* than it is to be more definite. This advice can be applied to many different bloodstain pattern types and is not restricted only to those that result from a medium velocity impact.

The second rule is in most beatings there is little, if any, bloodspatter resulting from the first blow. The first blow in a beating does not usually strike blood. If it is severe enough this blow only creates an open wound that will bleed. After blood comes to the surface of an injury any subsequent blows delivered to the same location will cause blood to spatter.

BLOOD SPATTERED FROM HIGH VELOCITY IMPACT

When considerable energy is applied to a liquid such as blood, the result is a proportionally greater disassociation of the liquid resulting in extremely small droplets. Stated quite simply, the more energy that is available, the more blood will spatter as its surface tension is ruptured by hydrostatic force. High energy allows much greater subdivision of liquids upon impact than can be accomplished during a beating. Thus, the higher the energy source, the smaller the blood drop. In almost all criminal cases wherein *high velocity impact spatter* is produced it is the result of one or more gunshots. It must be remembered, however, that almost any type of explosive force is capable of producing this type of pattern when a source of blood is available. The explosion of a hand grenade, high speed machinery, or an aircraft propeller can also produce *high velocity impact spatter*. Such cases are unusual but should caution the reader to remember that the term *high velocity impact spatter* means just that, and are not necessarily only the result of gunshot.

In the usual case of a shooting where the projectile strikes exposed skin, the energy at impact is hydrostatically transmitted throughout much of the adjoining tissue. This results in the spattering of blood in a very fine, almost *mist-like* spray. These atomized droplets of blood have a very high surface area and, therefore, cannot be projected very far in a horizontal direction. Usually, these minute droplets will be found within three or four feet of the impact point.

In addition to *mist-like* droplets, several larger droplets will be produced as well. A typical spray pattern, characterized as *high velocity impact spatter*, may be seen in Figure II-18. Note that while the vast majority of these blood spots are well under one millimeter in diameter, many larger ones are also produced. Interpreting bloodstain patterns of this type at a crime scene may be confusing when there is no body. The investigator may believe that he is seeing *medium velocity impact spatter* when he is actually looking at the larger droplet stains which were projected beyond the limits of the characteristic mist that resulted from a gunshot impact. This is an unusual situation but it has been known to occur.

The scene of a typical shooting showing extensive bloodspatter from high velocity impact is shown in Figures II-19 and II-20. The weapon was a 30-30 rifle. It is evident that void areas on the wall resulted when bloodspatter was intercepted by the brass tubing frame of the head of the bed Fig. II-20. Such well defined vertical lines demonstrate that the spatter came from a single impact and not what would likely have resulted had multiple blows been administered dur-

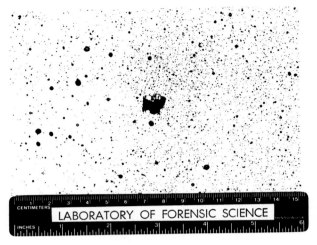

FIGURE II-18. High velocity impact pattern resulting from a gunshot. Note that the diameter of the majority of blood spots is less than one millimeter but some much larger are also produced.

ing a beating. The *mist-like* bloodstains that were on the wall cannot be resolved in these figures.

When fine bloodstains are observed in a shooting incident, they should always be considered as most likely having originated from the impact of a bullet. In more than one case the characteristic *mist-like* spray of blood was present inside the shirt cuff of a suspected suicide victim. Such evidence require the open cuff area to be facing the victim's wound indicating a posture consistent with their holding a gun to their own head.

It is necessary to examine *high velocity impact spatter* closely to be able to resolve the minute blood spots that identify this type of pattern. However, it is frequently obvious that a gunshot wound has occurred from viewing scene photographs that were taken at a distance to show an overall area. The crime scene photograph shown in Figure II-21, for example, is too distant to resolve the fine spray that can only be seen by closely examining the ceiling. Nevertheless, when blood is projected upward onto the ceiling, such as shown in this figure, it is almost always the result of a gunshot that had an upward trajectory. Such trajectory is most often associated with a suicide.

When an intense concentration of *high velocity impact spatter* is found on a floor, furniture, or

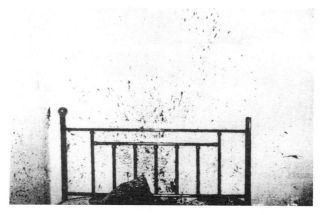

FIGURE II-19. High velocity impact spatter at the scene of a shooting. The victim was lying in bed with her head just to the right of the pillow when she was shot in the mouth with a 30-30 rifle.

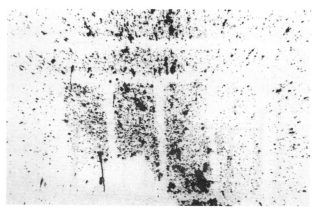

FIGURE II-20. Close-up of the bloodstain pattern on the wall behind the bed shown in Figure II-19. Void areas clearly define the outline of the brass headboard and the pillow. Such clear lines of demarcation establish the position of the victim when she was shot in the head.

other surface, it will usually be directly below the point of impact that produced it. Clothing and shoes that are stained with *high velocity impact spatter* must have been close to the victim at the time of the shooting.

A young woman found with a near-contact gunshot wound of the right temple was reported by her husband to have shot herself accidentally while cleaning a handgun. Shortly before her death, the husband had taken her to a gun range for target practice. The husband stated that he had been in the bathroom when he heard a shot, rushed out, turned his wife and claimed that he got blood on his shirt while handling the body. A bloodstain pattern interpretation of the crime scene showed that the victim had been shot on the floor.

The husband's shirt was submitted to the crime laboratory for examination. A barely visible, high velocity bloodstain mist was located on the cuff of the right sleeve. The blood penetrated the fibers, consistent with back spatter. The husband was convicted of second-degree murder.

It is important to remember that when blood is spattered as a result of a high velocity impact, the fine mist produced does not travel very far in a horizontal direction. Air resistance acts against the projected droplets slowing them down so the distance traveled is inversely proportional to their cross sections. Thus, even the extensive spatter shown in Figure II-22 did not result in any fine, mist-like droplets reaching the walls or doors as they could only travel four feet or less. An examination of the walls and door in this fig-

ure suggests that considerable energy was available to have produced such extensive spatter.

It seems appropriate to discuss an apparent difference of opinion between two schools of thought regarding terminology of impact spatter. This author prefers the term *velocity*, rather than *energy* to describe the nature of an impact that results in bloodspatter. Thus, the terms *low velocity impact spatter, medium velocity impact spatter,* and *high velocity impact spatter* are preferred over *low energy impact spatter, medium energy impact spatter,* and *high energy impact spatter*. While these two physical terms are closely related, the justification for using *velocity* rather than *energy* may be demonstrated by a comparison of the difference in bloodspatter resulting from two events of equal *energy*.

In the first example consider a bullet impacting a sponge that has been saturated with blood. The result is a very fine spray of blood, *high velocity impact spatter* which is easily recognized. In the second example an elephant steps into a large pool of blood causing very large splashes of blood to appear around the elephant's foot. The *elephant splashes* could never be mistaken as being produced by gunshot and yet the same *energy* was available in both instances. Thus, the more appropriate descriptive term *velocity* is the better choice.

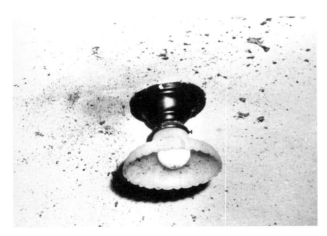

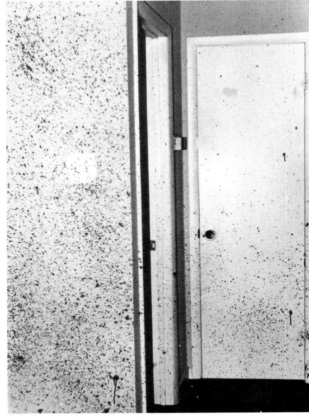

FIGURE II-21. High velocity impact blood pattern on the ceiling of a bedroom. Although the very fine individual blood spots cannot be resolved in this photograph it is easily recognized from its overall appearance.

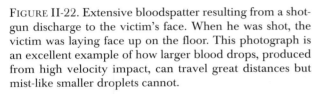

FIGURE II-22. Extensive bloodspatter resulting from a shotgun discharge to the victim's face. When he was shot, the victim was laying face up on the floor. This photograph is an excellent example of how larger blood drops, produced from high velocity impact, can travel great distances but mist-like smaller droplets cannot.

Possibly, the term *flux*, which could be used to describe the *rate of flow of energy*, ought to be considered. But how could we ever explain *flux* to a lay jury?

BLOODSTAIN PATTERNS RESULTING FROM PROJECTED BLOOD

When large volumes of blood are projected onto a surface, a somewhat unique bloodstain pattern results. The impact surface may be a wall, a floor, or any other surface. Only under unusual circumstances could it be a ceiling. The most common situation in which this occurs is when an artery, usually a major artery, has been severed or otherwise breached from gunshot or some form of blunt force injury. Systolic arterial pressure may cause blood to spurt or gush from the wound in large volume pulses. If blood is projected in this manner and strikes a surface that is relatively close to the injured victim, the resulting bloodstain pattern will fall into one of

three basic classifications each of which may be easily recognized.

- *Type I Arterial* is characterized by large bloodstains which have very elongated spines. The elongated spines indicate that an energy greater than that resulting from normal gravitational attraction was present. An example of a *Type I Arterial* projected bloodstain pattern is shown in Figure II-23.

A young girl was stabbed in the neck and her left carotid artery was severed. She fell to her knees and as she crawled away from her assailant she left a trail of large arterial splashes on a driveway. The trail of her blood

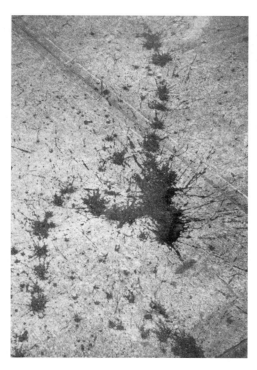

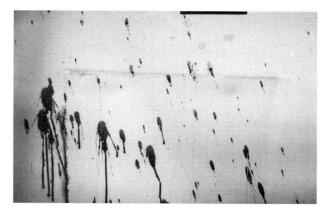

FIGURE II-24. A Type II Arterial pattern produced when blood gushed from a shotgun wound to the victim's chest. She was wearing a thin nightgown that allowed her blood to spurt from her open aorta to a nearby wall.

FIGURE II-23. A Type I Arterial pattern produced by blood which was projected from a carotid artery which had been severed by a stabbing. Well-defined pulses are evident.

extended over sixty feet from where she was stabbed to where she was found.

- *Type II Arterial* is characterized by large bloodstains which are, nevertheless, somewhat smaller than *Type I Arterial* and have well-defined borders with few, if any, spines. Bloodstains of this type have sufficient volume that blood will usually run down a wall or other vertical surface. They usually result from a wound that somewhat restricts the clean projection of blood away from the victim's body.
- *Type III Arterial* is a difficult arterial pattern to recognize because it consists of small drops rather than the large splashed blood volumes

which identifies *Types I and II Arterial*. Smaller drops of blood are produced because the artery which is breeched or severed is covered with overlaying tissue which can restrict blood from exiting in the large discrete pulses typical of *Types I and II Arterial*. Nevertheless, one characteristic of *Type III Arterial* identifies it with certainty when it is present, the appearance of a series of individual heartbeats which reflect the systolic mode of the heart. Such patterns look somewhat like one which could be produced by raising and lowering a garden hose nozzle which was set to a coarse spray while slowly moving it to one side or the other. Figure II-25 shows an excellent example of *Type III Arterial* that resulted from a self-inflicted gunshot wound to the right temporal area.

Another example of *Type III Arterial* where blood spurted from beneath crushed tissue over an anterior temporal artery may be seen in Figure II-26. These patterns resulted from spurts of blood onto a bathroom wall. Individual heartbeats are identified in this figure.

CAST-OFF BLOODSTAIN PATTERNS

During a beating, blood usually does not accumulate on the surface of the victim's wound until after the first blow. After blood covers that area, however, a *second* blow to the same area will produce spatter and often adhere to the beating instrument. As a bloody hammer is raised and

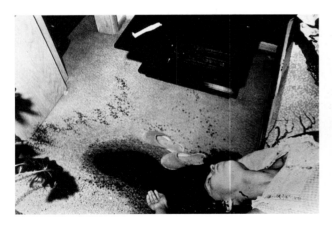

FIGURE II-25. A Type III Arterial pattern produced when blood from the victim's severed right temporal artery was projected on the carpet several feet from its origin. As her head turned slowly to her right side, blood created a zigzag pattern on the floor. This pattern is not unlike a hospital strip chart recording of a cardiogram.

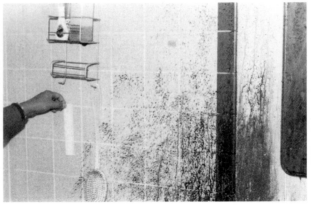

FIGURE II-26. Type III Arterial spray pattern which was produced when the victim of a beating stood in front of his bathroom sink. Blood was sprayed from his crushed temporal artery to a wall indicating that he stood in that location for several seconds. Very small droplets were produced because of his skin overlying his wound.

swung back by an assailant, the path of the hammer head is more up and back than it is in a curved motion. A study of the beating mechanism, using high speed strobe photography confirmed this rather right angle course. As a result, when the direction of the hammer head is shifted from an upward, raising motion, to a backward, swinging arc, the angular momentum of the blood adhering to the swinging hammer is usually sufficient to overcome the surface tension of blood allowing small drops to be released. These small drops usually strike the ceiling at about ninety degrees directly over the victim. A few bloodstains that were on a ceiling directly over the head of a person who was beaten on a bed are shown in Figure II-27. Direction the instrument was being swung when this pattern was made cannot be determined from blood spots that are as nearly circular as those that are shown in this figure.

As the instrument continues to be swung backward, its movement accelerates and additional blood droplets will be cast-off from its surface. If any of this blood reaches the ceiling, it will strike at ever increasing acute angles and the bloodstains will become more elongated. Figure II-28 shows the continuation of the cast-off arc pattern shown in Figure II-27, but at a distance some twenty-two inches further to the right. Direction-

ality of these bloodstains is clearly from left to right. Observing a cast-off pattern such as this on a ceiling identifies the location where the beating occurred. Although only the two ends of this pattern have been used as an illustration, the entire overhead pattern is in a *single file* straight line configuration.

Frequently, multiple *cast-off patterns* are present when a victim is struck repeatedly in the same general area so blood can accumulate on the weapon being used. If the victim did not move around the minimum number of blows may be estimated by counting the individual cast-off blood trails. One blow should be added to the total because the first blow struck will not usually allow blood to adhere to the beating instrument in a sufficient volume to produce a cast-off pattern on the backswing. If the victim moved about while being beaten ceiling cast-off patterns can appear at more than one location and do not radiate out from a single origin.

Likewise, if more than one person administers a beating, or if a single assailant moves about, more complex patterns can be produced.

If sufficient blood adheres to a beating instrument after it has been raised, cast-off patterns can also be produced on the downward, or beating stroke. If such pattern is produced it will most

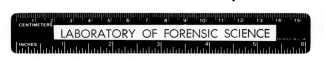

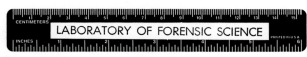

FIGURE II-27. A cast-off bloodstain pattern on a ceiling directly over the point of impact. These spots are round because they struck the ceiling at about ninety degrees.

FIGURE II-28. A continuation of the right side of the pattern shown in Figure II-27. The sharp pointed ends on the right of these bloodstains show their direction of travel, left to right.

likely consist of two or more parallel lines whose individual blood drops will show a downward directionality. The reason for the *single file* bloodstain pattern on the upswing and the *double (or triple) file* bloodstain pattern on the downswing is simply that more blood is released, or flung from the instrument nearer the end of a swing when it is at its greatest velocity. The upward swing casts blood off while the instrument is accelerating, while the downward swing has already reached its maximum velocity. This applies to walls only as these patterns reverse for cast-off bloodstains on ceilings. When there is a considerable blood volume on an instrument it may create a confusing *double file pattern* where there are bloodstains that appear to be traveling in two different directions. This only occurs when the victim is near a wall and the person doing the beating is facing that wall. Some large drops of blood are released as the instrument is raised and they do not travel upward very far before falling and they strike the wall in a downward direction. Many smaller drops are then released as the instrument continues to be swung upward and even though they are actually part of the same cast-off *single file* pattern, they were traveling in the opposite direction when they struck the wall!

Horizontal cast-off patterns are common when blows are delivered by horizontal rather than vertical movement. As a result of gravity, the end of such patterns will be seen to be falling off or downward toward the floor.

EXPIRATED BLOODSTAIN PATTERNS

If blood accumulates in the air passages of an injured person, it is frequently blown out through the mouth, the nose or a combination of both. Blood projected by such mechanism is called *expirated* blood, and not *aspirated* blood. Aspiration is the sucking in action of a chest wound, not a blowing out. Blood that is projected by expiration produces bloodstains that appear much like those which result from a medium or high velocity impact. However, droplets that are blown out of the nose or mouth can only be found in locations where such an origin is possible.

Blood spots on the fingers and hand shown in Figure II-29 appear small enough to have been produced as a result of a medium velocity impact. The actual origin of this blood, however, was the victim's mouth, as shown in Figure II-30. If there is a question as to whether or not blood could have been expirated rather than from impact photographs should be taken of the victim's face and the oral and nasal cavities should be swabbed if it is not obvious that they contain blood.

Recognition of expirated bloodstain patterns is not difficult. Common sense dictates that if the victim has no blood in the nasal or oral orifices it would have been impossible for blood to have been expirated. When air bubbles are present in

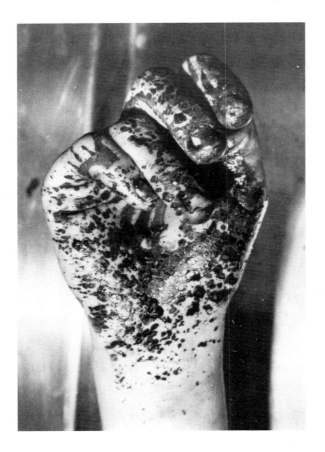

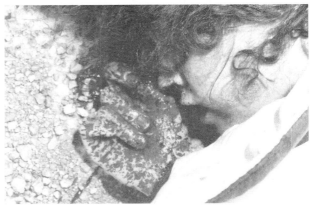

FIGURE II-29. Bloodspatter on the victim's hand suggests that it was the result of medium velocity impact, however, the actual origin of this expired bloodstain pattern was the victim's mouth.

FIGURE II-30. Actual source of the bloodstains shown in Figure II-29. Blood was expired from the mouth and/or nose onto the victim's hand.

bloodstains, this is usually evidence of expired blood. However, it should be remembered that penetrating wounds to the chest can also produce bubbles in blood. In such cases, there may not be obvious blood accumulated in the mouth or nasal passage.

TRANSFER BLOODSTAIN PATTERNS

Human blood is frequently a medium of transfer which allows geometric shapes of various kinds to be reproduced as a mirror image onto a surface. Bloody fingerprints, footprints, and footwear prints have been received in evidence countless times so an extension of this basic transfer mechanism to include fabrics, hammer heads, knives, clubs, tire irons and the like, is nothing unusual. A transfer pattern frequently encountered in homicide investigations is the hair swipe pattern. Two basic patterns of this type are quite unique in appearance and both are easily identified. The first is produced when hair that is wet with blood makes a lateral swiping of a surface and leaves characteristic fine lines and a feather edged reproduction of several individual hairs (Fig. II-31).

When hair that is wet with blood comes into contact with a surface without lateral movement the result is compression transfer rather than a swipe pattern. A young girl was killed when her assailant stomped on her head after raping her. Considerable blood had soaked into her hair and when her head came into contact with a wall and baseboard a compression transfer was produced (Fig. II-32). A study of this figure discloses several points of contact where characteristic fine, single hair replicas have been left on the baseboard and the wall above it.

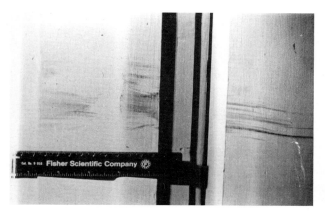

FIGURE II-31. Typical hair swipe pattern caused when bloody hair brushed laterally across a door and doorway.

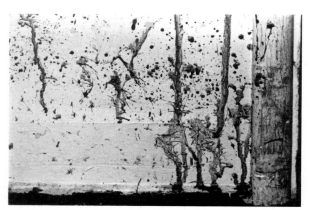

FIGURE II-32. Compression transfer pattern produced when blood soaked hair pressed against a surface without lateral motion. The fine line transfers are the impressions of individual hairs.

In most instances where a compression transfer pattern is produced, blood is deposited from a bloody object in a mirror image of the original. However, when a coarse fabric, such as corduroy, is involved, only the tops of the fabric will become stained. The presence of blood on the *ribs* or upper weave portion of a fabric will establish the staining as a transfer mechanism because had the blood been projected onto the fabric it would be equally deposited between the *ribs* as well as on top of them.

A bloodstain swipe pattern may be seen in Figure II-33 which shows how the lateral motion of a bloody finger *streaked* across the surface of a cotton shirt. This photomacrograph shows how blood was transferred only to the top of the weave pattern. Had blood been spattered onto the shirt rather than brushed over its surface, bloodstaining would have been uniform without voids. Projected blood droplets on fabric are not restricted to the top of a weave as they penetrate down into the lower portion or *valleys* as well.

Figure II-34 shows a small spot of blood which was projected onto a fabric and penetrated the weave pattern down to the base of the cloth. It is possible for a transfer pattern to appear similar to spatters when there is sufficient blood to be compressed into a fabric. However, the opposite is not possible. That is, when only the top fibers are bloodstained they could not have been stained from bloodspatter impact. This is a relatively simple observation which can be made with only a hand magnifying glass.

Some authors believe that it is possible to determine the direction of travel of the object that created a swipe transfer pattern. This may often be true with hair swipes, however, it is not possible to make this determination from fabric. Figure II-35 shows two swipe bloodstain patterns both of which were made by a right to left motion although the lower one appears to have been just the opposite. Obviously, caution must be exercised in forming a firm opinion when exceptions to general rules are known to exist.

RECOVERING AND DOCUMENTING BLOODSTAIN PATTERN EVIDENCE

Photographic Documentation

It is essential that good photographs be taken of all bloodstains at the scene of a crime. Close-up photographs should be taken of all bloodstain patterns. These should be taken normal (ninety degrees) to surface upon which the bloodstains are found. A ruler or some other scale of refer-

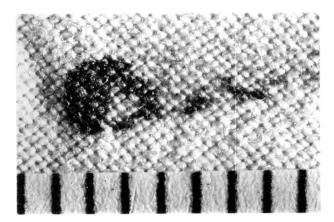

FIGURE II-33. Photomacrograph of a swipe transfer. Only the tops of several fibers are bloodstained and there is a void in the center of this stain (millimeter scale).

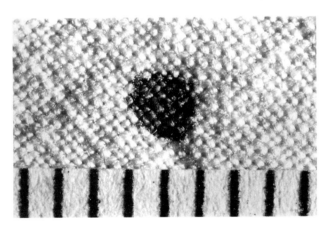

Figure II-34. Appearance of a small bloodspatter that resulted from blood which projected onto a woven fabric. Blood has uniformly penetrated the cloth in the bloodstained area (millimeter scale).

ence should be included in each photograph. It is always important to document which bloodstains are being photographed. One convenient way to achieve this is to use a felt marker to circle and number all bloodstains and/or any bloodstain patterns which are of interest. Overall photographs should be taken to show the geometric relationship of bloodstains to the general crime scene area as well as to each other.

The exact location of bloodstains which will be used for calculating angles of impact must be recorded in some systematic manner. The dis-

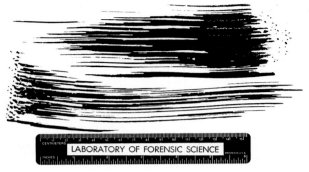

FIGURE II-35. Two lateral swipe transfer patterns. Both were produced from a lateral right to left motion.

tance of a bloodstain from the floor or ceiling and from the nearest wall should be entered on a form that provides a blank space for the width of a blood stain, its length, and its width-to-length ratio followed by space for the impact angle after it has been calculated.

Distant or overall photographs do not usually require a reference scale because furniture and/or other objects are usually present which allow the viewer a good size relationship. If the origin of bloodspatter is to be photographed, elastic string which has contrast with the background should be selected.

Lifting Bloodstain Pattern Evidence

In addition to the photographic recording of bloodstain patterns, another simpler, and perhaps even better technique should be considered; remove the bloodstain itself. This recovery method at a crime scene is apparently not often employed by investigators. Apparently they are not aware of this simple technique. The method is no more difficult than lifting a processed fingerprint and, in fact, employs the same material, transparent fingerprint tape.

After photographs have been taken, if bloodstains are on a flat, hard, smooth surface, such as major kitchen appliances, an attempt should be made to lift some of the bloodstains to preserve them as evidence. One and one-half inch wide transparent fingerprint tape, which also can serve as a scale of reference, can be used. The proce-

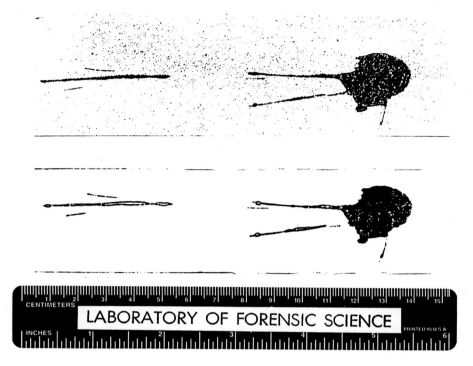

FIGURE II-36. Bloodstain lifted from a kitchen floor tile. The top stain shows how the blood appeared before it was lifted. The bottom stain is the lift that was removed from the floor with clear tape.

dure is very straightforward; one simply presses the transparent tape over the bloodstain applying considerable pressure to the stain area with a ball point pen or fingernail. The tape is then carefully peeled from the surface. The bloodstain is frequently almost completely removed. The lift should be placed on white plastic so, if for any reason, it can be lifted again in a laboratory to expose the blood. This is not to suggest that this is a method of choice for recovering blood samples for serology; *it is not*. On more than one occasion, however, blood from a lift has found its way into the serology section when, for whatever reason, no other samples were recovered at the scene. At least they could not be located if they were.

Although hard, smooth surfaces are ideal for lifting bloodstains at a crime scene, many unlikely surfaces often yield excellent results. Nothing is lost if the attempt to lift a bloodstain is unsuccessful so there is really no reason not to make the simple effort. Figure II-36 shows how effi-

ciently a bloodstain was removed from a kitchen floor tile. Bloodstain on the top of this figure as it appeared on the floor. The bottom stain is what was lifted using fingerprint-lifting tape.

Blood that remained on the floor tile consisted of very fine lines that would fill the narrow voids in the streaks of the lift. Recovery was well over ninety-nine percent effective. Many other more porous surfaces such as wallpaper often permit removal of the bloodstain, however, part of the wallpaper is frequently removed as well. In such cases, the size and shape of the bloodstain are still preserved so nothing is really lost.

Summary

Bloodstain pattern interpretation is based upon laws of physics which are well established scientific principles. When evidence of this type is properly studied and evaluated it should result in a more accurate reconstruction of events. Bloodstain pattern interpretation is rarely sufficient in and of itself for the solution of a crime. More often it will explain certain facets of a case that might have been misunderstood or misinterpreted. In conjunction with other evidence, bloodstain pattern interpretation can often be of great assistance. Frequently, bloodstain patterns will be helpful in confirming conclusions that have been established from other evidence, such as a projectile's trajectory and vice-versa.

REFERENCES

1. MacDonell, H.L.: Segments of History, the Literature of Bloodstain Pattern Interpretation, Segment 00: Literature Through the 1800's, Elmira Heights, NY, 2000, p. 47.
2. Piotrowski, E.: *Uber Entstehung, Form, Richtung und Ausbreitung der Blutspuren nach Hiebwunded des Kopfes,* Vircow, 95, Bl.1, Wein, 1895, p. 49. Note: This classic text has been republished by Herbert Leon MacDonell.
3. Kirk, P.L.: Affidavit Regarding the *State of Ohio v. Samuel Sheppard,* Court of Common Pleas, Criminal Branch, No. 64571, 26 April 1955.
4. MacDonell, H.L.: *Crime Scene Evidence—Blood Spatters and Smears and Other Physical Evidence,* Quinnipiac Health Law, v. 1, No. 1, Fall 1996, pp. 33–78.
5. Spitz, W.U., and Fisher, R.S.: *Medicolegal Investigation of Death,* 1st Ed., Springfield: Charles C Thomas, 1973, p. 17.
6. Seliger, L.: *Forensic Considerations of the Physical Properties of Human Blood,* Unpublished Independent Study Report, Elmira College, Elmira, NY, 1978, p. 105.
7. MacDonell, H.L.: *Flight Characteristics and Stain Patterns of Human Blood,* Washington, U.S. Department of Justice, L.E.A.A., N.I.L.E.C.J., 1971, p. 3.
8. Bloodstain Evidence Institute, Corning, New York, directed by Herbert Leon MacDonell, 1973–present.

Part 2

BIOLOGICAL EVIDENCE ON THE HUMAN BODY

HEATHER MILLER COYLE, CARLL LADD, AND HENRY C. LEE

INTRODUCTION

THE OBJECTIVE OF MEDICAL LEGAL DEATH investigation is not only to establish the cause and manner of death, but also to recognize, identify, collect, preserve, and examine any physical evidence associated with the death. Physical evidence can provide valuable information for determining if a questionable death is, in fact, a homicide as well as provide important leads to the solution of the case. It is crucial for medical examiners, forensic scientists, criminal investigators, crime scene technicians, and medical personnel to be aware of the many types of physical evidence that can be easily overlooked, contaminated, or destroyed. It is important to adhere to standard collection, documentation and preservation procedures and to ensure that all the evidence collected meets the scientific and legal requirements.

Physical evidence is generally either located at the crime scene or can be found on the body of a person (victim, witness or suspect). Evidence generated from both sources is equally important in death investigation. The types of physical evidence commonly found on a body can be divided into five major categories: transient evidence, conditional evidence, pattern evidence, transfer evidence and associative evidence (Table II-2).

1. ***Transient evidence*** is physical evidence that is temporary in nature and can be easily changed or altered. As time or conditions progress, the shape, form, measurements, color, consistency, or temperature of that evidence will change. Transient evidence can be altered or lost over time due to evaporation, dehydration, or a variety of other reasons. Transient evidence can be easily overlooked if crime scene processing priorities are not established properly. Commonly encountered transient evidence at a crime scene includes the color of bloodstains, color of flame, temperature of the room, and other biological or physical phenomena. Transient evidence found on a body may include body temperature (e.g. rectal temperature), body odor (e.g. alcohol on breath, almond, or decomposition odors), color of contusion, wetness of a bloodstain and body fluids and other biological phenomena (e.g. size of maggots).

2. ***Conditional evidence*** is a type of physical evidence that results from an event or action. Conditional evidence can also be easily altered or lost if it is not properly recognized and documented. The common types of conditional evidence found at a crime scene include lighting of the area or room, condition of doors and windows, condition of TV, radio and appliances, and furniture positions. Examples of conditional evidence found on a body include livor mortis and rigor mortis, condition of clothing (e.g. wet, dry, intact, torn), condition of bullet entrance and exit wounds, body condition (e.g. degree of decomposition), and stomach contents (e.g. types of food and degree of digestion).

3. ***Pattern evidence*** is generally produced by physical contact between persons, vehicles, weapons, and other objects. There are a variety of physical patterns that can be found at a crime scene.[1] Most of these patterns are in the form of imprints, indentations, striations, markings, fractures, or deposits. The recognition and identification of pattern evidence is extremely important in death investigation. It can often be used to establish the possible sequence of events, associate or disassociate the involvement of an individual, and prove or disprove a statement. The patterns most commonly found at a crime scene include fur-

TABLE II-2

TYPES OF PHYSICAL EVIDENCE

Transient:	body temperature, odors, bite marks, toolmarks, degree of decomposition
Conditional:	lividity, rigor, clothing condition, lighting, stomach contents, insects, weather
Pattern:	impressions, wound and injury markings, blood spatter, projectile trajectories
Transfer:	paint chips, hairs, soil and glass particles, fibers, botanical matter
Associative:	wallet, shoes, jewelry, money, clothing

niture damage, bloodstain distribution, glass fracture, tire marks and shoe impressions, clothing damage, and burn patterns. Pattern evidence found on a body includes tire and shoe impressions, wound and injury patterns, fabric and logo impressions, blood spatter, incendiary or burn marks, bite marks, weapon imprints, bullet trajectories, grass stains, paint smears, glass fragments, and other trace transfer patterns.

4. *Transfer evidence* is produced by physical contact between persons, objects, or both. This category of evidence encompasses many diverse types of microscopic or sub-microscopic materials as well as some examples that are easily visible to the naked eye. Because of the large number of different materials that can be included in this category, the subject is broad and diverse. Some classes of this kind of evidence are commonly encountered at a crime scene and on a body. Transfer evidence may be blood, tissue, hair, glass, soil, metal, plastics, and paint. Other types of transfer evidence; such as pollen, grass, powder, dust, fibers, and grease need experience and training to recognize and collect from a body.

5. *Associative evidence* is defined as that which can *associate* a victim or suspect with the crime scene. Examples of associative evidence include: a wallet or identification card, keys, weapons, check or notes, photographs of identifiable family members and friends, videotapes, clothing, shoes, jewelry and watches that belong to the victim or suspect.

Types of Trace Evidence Found on a Human Body

Transfer evidence, often considered as one of the largest categories of physical evidence, contains numerous categories and sub-categories of materials. For this reason, there are many examples of materials for which suitable examination methodologies have not yet been developed to an extent that would enable determination of origin. Nevertheless, there are many examples in which transfer evidence has played an important role in the investigation of homicides and serial killings.

The terms *transfer evidence* and *trace evidence* are sometimes used synonymously, although they do differ in meaning when they are carefully considered. *Trace evidence* can be thought of as evidence occurring in sizes so small that it can be transferred or exchanged between two surfaces or persons without being noticed. The examination of trace evidence generally relies on microscopic and instrumental analyses. *Transfer evidence* is exchanged between two objects or persons as the result of contact. Transfer evidence can be trace evidence or pattern evidence. Very often, it can be a combination of trace and pattern evidence such as, a bloody hand print found on victim's back, rubber residue with tire marks, gunshot residue near a bullet entrance wound or on a decedent's hand, fiber residue with a ligature mark, or metal fragments with a handcuff mark.

Trace evidence is often a result of direct contact, but may be encountered without direct contact. Such contact-less exchanges are less common and include the entrapment of airborne particles or situations in which small amounts of material are projected or fall onto another surface. The deposit of blood spatter on a victim's body or projection of glass fragments are two of the more common examples of transfer without direct contact. Just as trace evidence is not always transferred, all examples of transfer evidence are not trace evidence. Most examples of transfer evidence represent small amounts of finely divided material, but sometimes the amount or color of the material transferred

TABLE II-3

COMMON TYPES OF TRANSFER EVIDENCE FOUND ON THE HUMAN BODY

Animal and Insect Parts	Asphalt and Tar
Blood and Body Fluids	Bone and Tissues
Concrete and Road Construction Material	Chemicals
Dust and Mineral Particles	Glass and Debris
Explosive and Gunpowder Residues	Gasoline and Accelerants
Grass and Vegetative Matter	Grease and Lubricants
Hair and Fibers	Glass and Plastic Lenses
Fungi and Algae	Seeds and Wood Fragments
Paint and Auto Body Repair Bonders	Plaster and Insulation
Rubber Tire Smears and Debris	Metal Parts and Fragments
Soil and Dirt	Oil and Debris

makes it clearly visible and the term *trace* seems inappropriate. An obvious long paint smear transferred from a vehicle to a hit-and-run victim's body or a bloody shoe print deposited on a person's face are two commonly encountered examples.

The diversity of transfer evidence is indicated by the many different varieties listed in Table II-3. Although this list is extensive, there are countless other items that could be found on a human body during death investigation.

There are many different classification schemes that have been used to characterize commonly encountered trace and transfer evidence. Each classification is useful for offering a different conceptual perspective for physical evidence. Some of these categories are based on the type of material that is transferred, others are based on the nature of the evidence or the type of question to be resolved. Although they are all useful for the examination of trace evidence, none of these classification methods can account for all of the different investigation perspectives. For forensic death investigation, the following is a simple and practical classification method:

1. Biological Evidence
   a. Blood and Bloodstains
   b. Semen and Seminal stains
   c. Urine and Urine stains
   d. Tissue and Organs
   e. Hairs and Feathers
   f. Bones and Teeth
   g. Vomit and Fecal Material
   h. Tears, Milk and Other Body Fluids
   i. Meats, Fat and Food Residues
   j. Insect and Animal Matter

2. Chemical Evidence
   a. Drugs, Poisons and Narcotics
   b. Paints, Dyes and Inks
   c. Grease and Lubricants
   d. Oil, Gasoline and Accelerants
   e. Explosive and Gunshot Residues
   f. Rubber and Abrading
   g. Cosmetics, Lipsticks, Eyeliners
   h. Acids, Caustic Powder and Cleaning Materials

3. Mineralogical and Metallic Trace Evidence
   a. Glass and Porcelain
   b. Soil and Dirt
   c. Dust, Powder, and Plaster
   d. Rocks, Concrete and Construction Materials
   e. Asphalt and Tar
   f. Bullet Fragments
   g. Weapon Parts
   h. Metallic Materials
   i. Minerals and Crystals

4. Polymeric Material Evidence
   a. Fibers and Fabric
   b. Yarn and Threads
   c. Twines and Ropes
   d. Film and Plastics

5. Pattern Transfer Evidence
   a. Fingerprints and Handprints
   b. Tire Prints
   c. Footprints and Shoeprints
   d. Bite marks
   e. Weapon Impressions
   f. Toolmarks
   g. Ligature Marks
   h. Tape, Cuff, and Rope Marks
   i. Injury Patterns

TABLE II-4

TYPES OF BIOLOGICAL EVIDENCE

Body Fluids:	blood and bloodstains, semen, saliva, urine, tears, bile, perspiration
Soft Body Tissues:	skin, internal organs, hair and hair fragments, fingernails
Structural Tissues:	teeth, bone and bone fragments, skull
Other:	fecal matter, vomit

   j. Cloth and Fabric Patterns
   k. Jewelry and Watch Patterns
   l. Gunshot Residue Patterns
6. Vegetative Matter Evidence
   a. Grass and Grass Stains
   b. Plant Leaves and Roots
   c. Wood and Saw Dust
   d. Flowers and Pollen
   e. Fruits and Seeds
   f. Food Residues
   g. Fungi and Algae

Recognition, Collection, and Preservation of Biological Evidence

The importance of transfer evidence such as hair and fibers found in fingernail scrapings, seminal material found on a vaginal swab, gunpowder and soot found in bullet wound tracks and a knife tip found in a stab wound have long been recognized. However, the value of other types of trace evidence in death investigations has just been realized. Sometimes, due to its nature and size, it is extremely difficult to locate such evidence. In addition, some medical examiners lack sufficient experience to collect or examine such evidence and thus the full potential of trace and transfer evidence is not realized. It is extremely important for a forensic investigator to conduct a detailed examination of the crime scene, the decedent's clothing and the body. The body surface of a victim, witness or suspect also needs to be searched for physical evidence.[2-4] All trace evidence including biological stains, DNA, latent prints, accelerants, pollen, gunshot residue, soil, hair and fibers should be photographed in place, collected, and packaged. All body orifices should be examined for semen,

blood, hair, fibers, and drugs. Physical evidence on and in bodies should be collected expeditiously to prevent alteration and deterioration. Physical evidence is often lost during transfer of the body to the morgue or during washing prior to autopsy.

Trace amounts of biological evidence can be difficult to collect since it may take diligent observation and significant time to recognize such evidence and document it at a crime scene (Table II-4). Biological evidence is present in many forms, shapes and sizes and may not be conclusively identifiable at the scene. For these reasons, investigators should use the standard collection procedures for trace evidence. Several different methods are available for collecting transfer evidence. Each of these methods has its advantages and limitations. Most common types of biological evidence can be collected by swabbing, picking, tape lifts, scraping, and seizure of articles (e.g. weapons, clothing) that may have associated trace evidence. In order to meet the scientific and legal requirements of collection and preservation of evidence, a combination of several methods should be used to ensure that the evidence is accurately documented, collected, and stored.

Hair and fiber evidence should be collected using forceps or tape lifts. Hairs and fibers from the same area can be packaged together but hairs and fibers recovered from different locations of the body should be packaged separately. Microscopic examination of hair and comparison to known reference hair samples can aid in identifying the species, somatic and racial origin of the hair. If the hair root is still attached, DNA typing can be performed to identify the genetic profile of the person who contributed the hair to the crime scene.[5] A specialized form of DNA testing using mitochondrial DNA can be used to obtain a DNA profile from the hair shaft when the hair root is not present. Twenty-five to fifty pulled hairs from a victim or suspect should be collected as known reference samples.

Blood evidence requires special precautions during collection and preservation. Blood and bloodstains need to be photographed and documented for later pattern interpretation prior to collection. Investigators also need to be properly protected from biological hazards such as, hepatitis and HIV, by wearing disposable latex gloves and eye protection. Evidence collection team members should wear gloves not only for their own protection against pathogens but also to prevent contamination of the DNA sample. If the collector sheds a few skin cells into the biological sample, that profile may be detectable during the DNA analysis process.[6] Blood is usually found as a liquid or dried stain. Wet bloody clothing should be air-dried prior to packaging for transport to the laboratory. Bloodstains can be lifted from objects and collected on sterile cotton swabs. If a bloodstain is on a small, removable object then the object should be collected, packaged, and transported to the laboratory. Dried bloodstains on walls, for example, can be scraped into a druggist fold and packaged in an outer container or transferred to a swab. Known blood samples should be collected from the victim and suspect for later comparison with evidentiary DNA profiles.

DNA profiles can be obtained from blood, semen, tissues, organs, bones, teeth, hair, fingernails, toenails, saliva, urine, and perspiration stains. Although one nanogram of DNA is typically sufficient for polymerase chain reaction (PCR)-based testing, some biological fluids are more likely to yield complete profiles.[7] The success of generating a DNA profile from saliva, urine and perspiration stains is dependent on the number of shed epithelial cells present in a sample. Therefore, success rates with saliva, urine, and perspiration stains are more variable than with whole blood samples.

Other factors affect the ability to obtain a complete DNA profile including sample quantity, sample quality, and sample purity. Different DNA testing methods require different amounts of DNA template in order to generate a complete profile. For restriction fragment length analysis (RFLP), approximately fifty nanograms of DNA are required. For PCR-based testing, as little as one nanogram is necessary for generating an individual's DNA profile.[8,9] Table II-5 shows the amount of DNA present in each type of biological evidence. Sample quality can significant-

TABLE II-5

AVERAGE AMOUNTS OF DNA IN
BIOLOGICAL SAMPLES

Bloodstain (1 cm²)	250–500 ng*
Semen (postcoital vaginal swab)	10–3,000 ng
Hair (with root)	pulled 1–750 ng
	shed 1–12 ng
Saliva (oral swab)	1,000–1,500 ng
Urine	1–20 ng/mL
Bone	3–10 ng/mg of bone

* ng = nanogram, mL = milliliter, mg = milligram

ly affect DNA testing. If a sample has been degraded by environmental factors, only a partial profile may be generated. A final factor in DNA testing is sample purity. High quality DNA of sufficient quantity may be present in a sample, but an inhibitory substance may prevent the laboratory from being able to generate a DNA profile. Some inhibitory substances include textile dyes, grease, soil, phytochemicals (resins and tannins) and chemical solvents. Inhibited samples can become an issue when biological samples are collected from carpets (due to dyes or chemical cleaning treatments), some fabrics, wood chips or leather.[10,11] Various purification techniques have been proposed, however, they are not always successful. Therefore, the collection and preservation of a DNA sample are extremely important.

Most physical evidence should be collected in a primary container and placed into an outer container. The primary container can be a small jar or paper druggist's fold. The outer container can be an envelope, paper bag, canister, or cardboard box. The outer containers should be sealed with evidence tape and labeled with the following information: description of the item, initials of the collector, time, date and location evidence was collected, and the agency case identification number. Inappropriate documentation can prevent evidence from being introduced in court.[12] For special types of evidence like volatile liquids, leak-proof and airtight containers should be used. Biological evidence such as wet bloodstains should be air-dried prior to packaging and placed in sealed paper bags, never in airtight plastic containers. Each evidence item should be collected and packaged separately to avoid cross-contamination.

Field and Laboratory Tests of Biological Evidence

Tests for biological evidence are classified into two groups: chemical screening (*presumptive*) tests and confirmatory tests. Presumptive tests are valuable for a quick screening of large quantities of evidence for the presence of biological stains. They do not replace the need for more definitive confirmatory serological and DNA tests. Chemical screening tests should be used with caution, however, so as not to interfere with subsequent testing. Whenever possible, a portion of the stain should be retained for the confirmatory tests. Some blood enhancement reagents may inhibit DNA testing. This problem can be addressed by collecting a portion of the stain prior to using the enhancement reagent. There is a variety of tests for the presence of blood. These tests include: phenolphthalin (Kastle-Meyer), ortho-tolidine, luminol, leucomalachite green (LMG), tetramethylbenzidine (TMB) and fluorescin. Tests for the presence of other types of body fluids include: acid phosphatase (semen), creatinine (urine), amylase (saliva), and gastric acid (gastric contents). After a biological fluid has been identified, confirmatory, serological and DNA tests are performed.

Chemical Screening (Presumptive) Tests

This chapter is not intended to be a comprehensive review of all possible types of presumptive tests but will focus on the most commonly used tests in forensic laboratories. Several excellent reviews have been published on chemical screening methods.[13,14]

1. **Blood**: Presumptive tests for blood are based on the detection of heme (a component of hemoglobin in red blood cells) or heme derivatives. These tests work on the principle of converting a colorless reagent to a colored or fluorescent product. A positive color change test result suggests the substance could be blood but does not confirm blood since occasional false positive reactions can be obtained. Plant material and cleaning agents are known to yield false positives. For this reason, anti-human hemoglobin tests to determine species of origin or DNA tests are performed as confirmatory/identification tests. The Kastle-Meyer test is a common color change test used to presumptively identify blood. A positive test result is bright pink. The change from colorless to pink for a positive reaction occurs in seconds. Many other chemical reagents and sprays are used to enhance bloody patterns (e.g. bloody fingerprints, handprints). Any pattern should be photographed, documented and measured prior to spraying with a chemical enhancement reagent. In addition, a portion of the sample without the pattern should be tested prior to spraying the reagent.

2. **Semen:** Many standard sexual assault evidence kits have been developed that are used to collect trace and biological evidence transferred to the victim during an assault. Vaginal, oral, anal and genital swabs are collected from the victim and samples from the swabs are microscopically examined at the forensic laboratory for the presence of spermatozoa. If no spermatozoa are identified, several presumptive tests can be used to determine the presence of semen.

   A common screening test for the presence of semen is the acid phosphatase (AP) test. Acid phosphatase is present in high levels in semen but also in low levels of other biological samples, such as vaginal secretions, saliva, or fecal matter. Plant material can also give a positive AP test result. A confirmatory test for semen is the immunological human seminal fluid protein (p30) test. The human seminal fluid protein test is useful for identification of semen especially in cases of aspermic males. After semen or sperm has been identified, samples are typically collected for further DNA analysis.

3. **Saliva:** Amylase is a starch-digesting enzyme found in saliva and in other body fluids. The concentration of amylase is much higher in

saliva, however, than in other body fluids. One presumptive test for saliva involves the release of a blue dye that has been attached to a substrate. In the absence of amylase, the dye-substrate complex remains as a precipitate. In the presence of amylase, the dye is released from the substrate and the solution turns blue. Since other body fluids contain amylase, a positive reaction is not definitive confirmation for the presence of saliva. However, the color change will occur more quickly with saliva stains since the amylase concentration is greater in that body fluid.

4. *Urine:* The presence of urine can be determined by the presence of creatinine or urea. The Jaffe test is a presumptive test for urine that detects creatinine. A negative result is bright yellow and a positive result is reddish-orange, respectively. Some substances such as Mountain Dew soda and certain brands of lemonade can give a false positive result.

5. *Gastric contents:* Pepsin is a digestive enzyme found in stomach contents. Stomach contents, especially vegetable matter, can also be identified under the microscope. Plant cells have a cellulose wall that resists acid digestion in the stomach. In addition, different plant species have characteristic cellulose wall shapes that can aid in the identification of stomach contents.[15]

Species Determination of Blood

An immunological Ouchterlony test can be performed to determine if blood at a crime scene or on a body is from a human source. The Ouchterlony test is a double diffusion test that is based on the principle of antibody-antigen recognition. Anti-human hemoglobin antibody is placed in a central well of an agarose plate. Liquid extracts from potential bloodstains are placed in wells around the perimeter of the plate. The antibody and antigens in each sample each diffuse into the agarose plate. If the antibody recognizes the antigen as being human, a white line of precipitation will form where the two samples meet. This is a specific test for the presence of human blood.

A quantitation step during the DNA process can also determine if the DNA sample is of human origin. In many body fluids, bacteria or yeast may be present in addition to human cells. The Quantiblot system (Applied Biosystems Inc.; Foster City, CA) is used to estimate DNA yield from an evidentiary sample, a human-specific probe is used to distinguish between human DNA and bacterial or yeast DNA.

Genetic Typing of Human Blood and Other Biological Evidence

Genetic polymorphisms or differences between individuals based on protein or DNA variation have been used in forensics since the early 1900s.[16] Early antibody-antigen based tests (ABO blood grouping system, Rh-typing, or HLA histocompatability system) were used to group individuals.[17,18] Elimination of a suspect based on blood grouping was conclusive, however, inclusion in a particular blood group was not equivalent to an identity statement. This is because up to 40% of the general population could share a particular blood type. Other systems (e.g. isoenzymes, serum proteins, hemoglobin variants) have been used to detect variation between individuals in forensic tests but none have the discriminating power of DNA testing.

Deoxyribonucleic acid (DNA) is a macromolecule found in all living cells and contains an individual's unique genetic information. Genomic DNA is in the cell nucleus and is organized into long threads called chromosomes (Fig. II-37).[19] In all human cells (except sperm and egg reproductive cells) there are twenty-three pairs of chromosomes. One of each chromosome pair is maternally inherited and the other is paternally inherited. This pattern of inheritance provides the genetic basis for paternity testing. If a chromosome is unwound from its associated proteins, the *threads* are comprised of two strands of linked nucleotides. A DNA nucleotide has three parts: a deoxyribose sugar, a nitrogenous base and a phosphate group. The nucleotide bases always pair in a specific arrangement: adenine (A) bonds with thymine (T) and cytosine (C) bonds with guanine (G) in a process called complementary

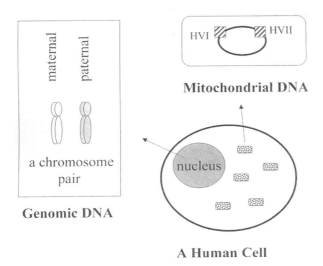

Mitochondrial DNA

nucleus

Genomic DNA

a chromosome pair

maternal paternal

A Human Cell

FIGURE II-37.

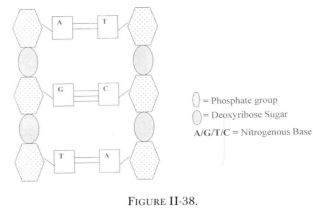

= Phosphate group
= Deoxyribose Sugar
A/G/T/C = Nitrogenous Base

FIGURE II-38.

base pairing (Fig. II-38). The order of the linked nucleotide bases provides the critical identifying information that is called the genetic code.

Another form of DNA, mitochondrial DNA, exists in subcellular organelles and can be used in human identity testing (Fig. II-37).[20-22] The mitochondrial DNA (mtDNA) molecule is a circular chromosome of 16,569 nucleotides and is maternally inherited. Mitochondrial DNA analysis is used when sample quantity is extremely limited, sources are ancient, or if the source does not contain nucleated cells (e.g. hair shaft). Mitochondrial DNA analysis is not as discriminating as genomic DNA analysis but has the advantage of requiring even less DNA than many PCR-based tests. This feature is due to differences in the mtDNA copy number per cell. For every cell, one nucleus is present that contains the genomic DNA. However, hundreds or thousands of mitochondria per cell are present depending on the cell type. Since mitochondrial DNA is inherited from mother to daughter/son, this form of DNA is useful for identification of human remains even if only a distant maternal relative is alive to provide a reference sample for comparison.

Several basic scientific concepts are important for understanding human identity test methods.

On chromosomes, many different defined segments (loci) of DNA can be tested for variation. Two types of variation are exploited in forensic testing: sequence and length variation (Fig. II-39).[23] Sequence variation refers to differences in a single nucleotide at a specific location on a chromosome. Length variation refers to differences in the number of repeating units that an individual possesses. The specific combination of sequence and length variation patterns (alleles) that an individual possesses is what is used to identify that person at the DNA level. A DNA profile is typically expressed as a string of numbers, letters, or a combination of the two depending on the type of DNA test performed.

A single individual's DNA is the same in all of the different cell types found throughout the body. This allows DNA comparisons to be made between DNA profiles from two different cell types (e.g. blood and semen) from the same individual. Environmental insults will not change one DNA profile into another profile. Exposure of DNA to harsh environmental conditions, however, can degrade the DNA to a point where it is difficult for a laboratory to obtain a complete DNA profile. Although it is preferable for tissue samples not to be fixed in formalin and paraffin-embedded, it is sometimes possible to obtain DNA profiles from these treated samples. Typically, the best results are obtained if the tissue was not soaked in formalin for an extended period of time. Many stains (e.g. Coomassie Blue) do not appear to negatively affect the ability to

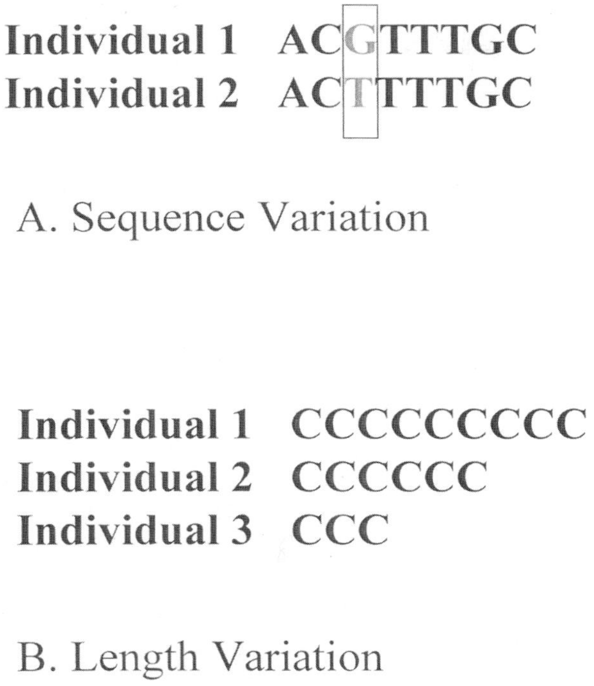

Individual 1   ACGTTTGC
Individual 2   ACTTTTGC

A. Sequence Variation

Individual 1   CCCCCCCC
Individual 2   CCCCCC
Individual 3   CCC

B. Length Variation

FIGURE II-39.

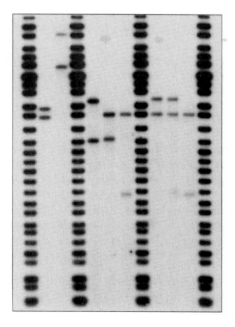

Lane #

1 2   3 4 5   6 7 8

Lane Key: 1 = K562   5 = brother A
             2 = KJL   6 = sister A
             3 = victim   7 = sister B
             4 = father   8 = brother B

FIGURE II-40. RFLP results from an accident reconstruction where the driver of the vehicle could not be identified using fingerprints or dental records. Reverse-paternity testing was performed by DNA testing of the father and siblings. In this case, the mother's body was not available for exhumation, so the siblings were typed in order to determine what the mother's profile must have been. K562 and KJL are laboratory positive controls and this photo shows the results of DNA testing with the D1S7 probe.

obtain a DNA profile from cells adhered to a slide.

A Brief History of DNA Typing Methods

Genomic DNA: Most DNA typing methods use genomic DNA, the DNA found in the cell nucleus. The first type of DNA testing was a form of restriction fragment length polymorphism (RFLP) analysis that used a multilocus system that generated a highly discriminating but very complex banding pattern called a *DNA fingerprint*.[24] This RFLP system was effective on single source samples but mixed biological sample profiles were difficult to interpret. The second-generation RFLP system used single-locus probes to generate the banding patterns and was more suitable for forensic work.[25,26] Four or five single-locus probes are used to achieve the level of discrimination necessary to distinguish between individuals (Fig. II-40).

With the development of polymerase chain reaction (PCR) technology, the ability to amplify minute quantities (1–10 nanograms) of sample for testing became a practicality.[27] The first forensic PCR tests were the reverse dot blot Ampi-Type PM and DQA1 and AmpliFLP D1S80 assays.[28-34] The PM and DQA1 tests detect sequence variation at six loci. Amplified DNA is denatured, incubated with nylon strips containing allele-specific probes and detected by a col-

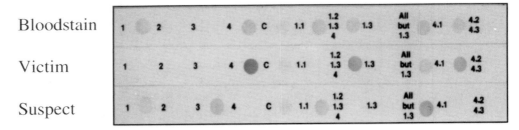

FIGURE II-41. DQA1 test results showing that the bloodstain collected from a crime scene could not have come from either the victim or the suspect.

orimetric assay (Fig. II-41). The D1S80 test detects length variation in tandem repeats. The D1S80 alleles are separated by size on acrylamide gels after PCR amplification and visualized by silver staining. Although PCR tests are faster and require less DNA than RFLP analysis, they are not as discriminatory.

A PCR test called short tandem repeat (STR) analysis uses a four base repeat form of length variation to generate an identification pattern for distinguishing between individuals.[35-39] STR testing combines the advantages of PCR with the high discrimination power of RFLP analysis and is rapidly replacing older forms of forensic DNA testing.[40] Most laboratories use fluorescent dye incorporation to visualize the DNA results. The fluorescent dye is incorporated during the PCR amplification step so that the amplified products will fluoresce when excited by a laser. PCR products are separated on a gel polymer matrix either in capillary tubes or between gel plates.[41] As the DNA fragment passes by the laser, the dye is excited and a camera records the color (Fig. II-42). The colored band pattern images are subsequently analyzed with software programs to assign numeric values to each band for the DNA profile (Fig. II-43).

Mitochondrial DNA: Mitochondrial DNA analysis detects sequence variation in polymorphic regions of the mtDNA molecule called hypervariable regions (HVI and HVII). To detect sequence variation in HVI and HVII, mtDNA is PCR amplified and DNA sequenced.[42,43] The order of the nucleotide bases is determined in each of the HV regions and varies from person to person in a random population. Some unrelated individuals in a population may share the same DNA sequence at HVI and HVII.[44] This makes mtDNA analysis less discriminating than STR testing. However, mtDNA analysis is highly effective on skeletal remains and is important for establishing familial relationships. Mitochondrial DNA is maternally inherited, therefore, individuals in the same maternal lineage share the same mtDNA profile.

Y-STR Typing: A specialized DNA typing method, Y-STR typing, is used to separate male and female components in a mixed biological sample. The most common example of this type of mixture is when vaginal swabs are processed for DNA from a sexual assault. During the DNA processing, a differential extraction is performed to separate the female epithelial cells from the male spermatozoa. Due to the acidic vaginal environment, cells begin to degrade prior to sample collection and often a complete separation of the male and female cells is not possible during DNA extraction. Y-STR typing is useful for looking at the DNA profile from only the male component (the Y chromosome) of the mixture. This method of DNA typing effectively allows for a comparison between the Y chromosome variation from a sperm source and a known reference sample from a male suspect. Y-STR typing is more sensitive than the thirteen loci STR typing method because it avoids PCR primer competition with female DNA. Less variation exists in the male Y chromosome population, however, so it is a less discriminating method. Y-STR typing is also useful for determining if more than one male is a contributor to the semen sample. This is important for establishing if the DNA profile

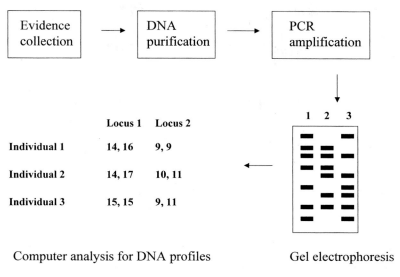

Computer analysis for DNA profiles   Gel electrophoresis

FIGURE II-42.

Electropherogram for green fluorescently-labeled STR loci

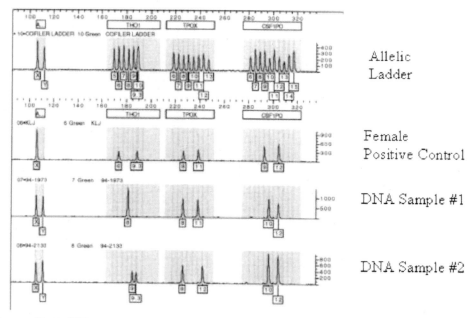

FIGURE II-43. STR test results for the DNA fragments (loci) labeled with a green fluorescent dye. An allelic ladder is electrophoresed on the same gel to aid in sizing of the DNA fragments in the DNA samples. The first green locus determines the sex of the individual that deposited the biological sample. The other three loci (THO1, TPOX, CSF1PO) aid in individualizing the sample to determine whom may have been the depositor of the sample. DNA sample #1 is a known blood sample from a suspect and does not match to DNA sample #2, a semen sample from a sexual assault.

might be a combination of DNA from a consensual partner and a suspect. Y-STR typing can be used to determine the number of male contributors in a gang rape situation as well. In addition, since Y-chromosomes are paternally inherited, Y-STR typing can establish relatedness in paternity casework.

DNA Casework Examples

Several landmark cases illustrate the importance of evidence collection and the power of DNA testing in homicide investigation.[45]

In August of 1993, Jim Peng visited the home of his mistress Jennifer Ji in Orange County, California. He found her dead in a pool of blood and their infant son, Kevin, suffocated in his crib. Jennifer Ji's body had multiple stab wounds and a bite mark on her left arm. Swabs were collected from the bite mark for DNA testing. Investigators learned that Peng's wife was visiting him from Taiwan and that she was angry when she discovered Peng had been living in the United States with another woman. Peng's wife, Lisa, immediately became a suspect and an odontologist was called in to make a wax impression of Lisa's teeth for comparison with the bite mark. The wax impression was a match to the bite mark but was not sufficient for an arrest. Lisa Peng had returned to Taiwan before police had obtained a blood sample for comparison to the DNA profile from swabs of the bite mark. However, sufficient saliva had been transferred to the wax impression for a known reference DNA profile to be obtained. The DNA from Lisa Peng's wax impression and the swabs from the bite mark matched. In January of 1994, Lisa Peng was arrested and charged with Jennifer Ji's murder.

DNA evidence was critical to the identification of a rapist and murderer of three women in New York City in 1990. Each victim was raped and manually strangled within a twenty-three day time span. DNA profiles had been obtained from the first two rapes and indicated the same person committed the crimes. Unfortunately, a DNA profile could not be obtained from semen on the third victim. Investigators collected rubbish from the crime scene and discovered a crumpled handkerchief with nasal mucous on it. The DNA profile matched the rapist from the first two crime scenes and linked him to the third attack. Through intensive police investigation, Dudley Friar was identified as the murderer, confessed, and served three life sentences for his crimes.

In January of 1998, a twelve-year-old girl was found floating in a pond in Bavaria. She lived for five days after she had been attacked and sexually assaulted but never regained consciousness. DNA samples once more provided critical forensic evidence to link a thirty-one-year-old window installer to the crime. Several cigarette butts were collected from the crime scene and the saliva from the cigarettes yielded a DNA profile that matched semen collected from the young girl's body. A blood sample confirmed the identity of her attacker and he was sentenced to life in prison.

In March of 1997, an elderly female was sexually assaulted in her apartment by an unknown male in the state of Connecticut. Seminal evidence was collected and processed to obtain a DNA profile. A suspect was developed in this case and a known blood sample was obtained from him to determine if it matched the DNA profile from the semen. This first suspect was excluded as the source of the semen and was released. In July of 1997, the profile from the semen source was entered into the Connecticut State DNA Database and a *cold hit* (matching profile) was identified. A confirmatory blood sample was drawn from this individual and DNA tests showed that he was, with a high degree of certainty, the depositor of semen in the March assault. The frequency of his profile in the general population was less than one person in five million individuals.

Re-testing of DNA evidence has exonerated more than seventy people in the United States since the late 1980s according to the Manhattan-based Innocence Project. In October of 2000, a mentally retarded man was pardoned for a 1982 rape and homicide in Virginia after DNA testing showed he did not commit the crime. In Oklahoma, two men who were convicted of a 1982 rape and homicide based on hair comparison evidence, were released in 1997 after DNA testing exonerated them. Those same DNA tests point to a witness that testified against them at their trials as being the real rapist and killer. These are just a few examples of homicides and sexual assaults where DNA evidence was appropriately collected and played a major role in obtaining convictions or exonerating a wrongly accused individual.

Non-human DNA Sources

On occasion, DNA from unusual sources has been used to solve criminal cases. Canine DNA has helped convict two suspects of a 1996 murder in Seattle, Washington:

The victim's dog was shot during the attack and investigators wanted to know if blood from the dog matched the blood found on one defendant's clothing. DNA testing confirmed a match. Genetic testing on dogs is performed by the American Kennel Club to verify parentage in canines and has now been successfully used for forensic tests. DNA data-bases have been constructed of many different canine breeds to examine their genetic diversity.[46]

Feline DNA has also been used as evidence in a criminal trial in Canada.[47]

A mother of five disappeared from her home and her body was discovered in a shallow grave several months later. A bag containing a man's leather jacket covered with the missing woman's blood and several white cat hairs was discovered near the woman's home. The genomic DNA recovered from the roots of the cat hairs was used to link the jacket to a suspect through his pet cat. He was later convicted of murder.

Even plant DNA has been used as evidence in a homicide.[48]

In 1992, a female body was discovered in the Arizona desert under a Palo verde tree. Palo verde seed pods were collected from a suspect's vehicle and DNA matched the tree under which the victim was found. These case examples emphasize the importance of using non-human DNA to effectively link criminal evidence to a suspect. The use of non-human DNA is a new but potentially powerful area of forensic science.

DNA Databases

The Federal Bureau of Investigation (FBI)[49] has established a uniform set of thirteen STR loci that are used to generate DNA profiles for both state and national DNA databases of convicted sex offenders.[50,51] The national DNA database is called CODIS for COmbined DNA Index System. Standardizing the number and type of loci to be tested in biological evidence enables investigators to search DNA profiles from state to state. DNA databases are a highly effective investigative tool due to the high rate of recidivism observed in sex offenders.[52] Many states are expanding their DNA sex offender databases to include other types of criminal convictions (all felons, violent crimes, burglary) that have a positive correlation with *cold hits* in the database.

Over two million DNA samples have been collected nationwide but only a fraction of those DNA samples have been analyzed due to limitations in laboratory resources.[53] Even so, DNA databases have generated more than 2,100 *cold hits* or investigative leads leading to numerous convictions. As more DNA samples are processed, it is expected that the *hit* rate in the database will increase substantially. Recently, many states have dramatically expanded the number of qualifying offenses for their DNA databases. All states collect samples for sexual assaults, 39 states collect for homicides, 29 states collect for assault and battery, and 27 states collect for kidnaping.

The DNA database is particularly useful for providing investigative leads for *no-suspect* sexual assault cases. Frequently, victims do not recognize the attacker or are so traumatized that they cannot give a good physical description to law enforcement officials. In these cases, the sperm-rich fraction of the vaginal swabs collected from the victim can be processed for DNA and the profile searched against the database of previously convicted sex offenders. If a match is discovered, law enforcement officials further investigate the suspect. It is important to remember that DNA evidence from intimate samples will substantiate sexual contact between two individuals but cannot determine if that contact was consensual.

Some interesting legal circumstances have arisen due to the implementation of DNA databases. In England, where the legal system is substantially different from the one in the United States, *DNA dragnets* have been used to screen the male population of an entire town to identify a sexual predator and killer. In the United States, *John Doe* warrants have been issued in many states (e.g. Wisconsin) based on using a DNA profile as the sole identifier. The purpose of the *John Doe* warrants was to provide a means of identifying a suspect before the statute of limitations expired. Many states have since extended the statute of limitations on sexual assault cases from 5 to 20 years.

Identification of Human Remains

Dental, anthropological, and fingerprint identification methods are used primarily in the identification of human remains. In many circumstances, such as in war crimes, aircraft accidents, terrorist bombings, natural disasters, and dismemberment of bodies, the identification of the victim is of utmost importance for criminal and civil investigations.[54] However, individuals with incomplete or nonexistent dental records or fingerprint records may require DNA to confirm identity. In addition, dismembered, badly burned, and decomposed bodies may require DNA for the positive identification of remains. In these cases, reverse paternity testing is performed to show a biological relationship between parent and child. If parents are living, they are asked to submit a blood sample as a reference for DNA testing. Since one half of a person's DNA is inherited from the mother and the other half from the father, a child's DNA profile can be reconstructed and compared to the parent types to establish a genetic relationship.[55] If reference samples are not available from the parents, DNA testing can be performed on the remains and compared to another relative (sibling) to determine the genetic relationship. However, as the family relationship becomes more distant, the genetic test comparison becomes less definitive. If there are no surviving parents, a *known* reference sample can be used from the victim's residence or workplace (hairs from a hairbrush or saliva from a toothbrush). It is preferable to find a living relative, however, since hairbrushes and toothbrushes may be shared by more than one person.

The Armed Forces DNA Identification Laboratory (AFDIL) was established in 1991 to aid in the identification of missing persons from the Korean War, the Vietnam War, and World War II. There are estimates of more than 75,000 men still missing from World War II, more than 8,000 missing from the Korean conflict, and approximately 2000 missing individuals from the Vietnam War. Anthropological data and dental records are primarily used for identification of war remains, but often DNA testing is the only method for conclusive identification.[56-58] One of the most famous cases has been the identification of one set of remains from the Tomb of the Vietnam Unknowns.

In 1998, the casket carrying the remains of suspected Air Force pilot 1st Lt. Michael Blassie was disinterred and the remains tested using mitochondrial DNA. Two families were identified as possible relatives based on historical evidence. The mitochondrial DNA test results from the remains were compared to those of the two families and only the Blassie family matched.

Summary

Since 1984 when *DNA fingerprinting* was first established as a scientific technique, DNA has steadily gained ground as an important tool in crime scene investigations. Primarily, this is a result of advancing technology that allows a DNA profile to be obtained from only a few cells from an individual. In comparison, identification by fingerprints requires a substantial portion of a complete print with significant detail. Forensic evidence, however, is only as good as the investigators who recognize, collect, package, and preserve it. Improper collection and documentation can impede the ability of the forensic scientist to interpret the crime scene evidence. Poor packaging and preservation may destroy critical DNA evidence by encouraging bacterial and fungal growth. Exposure to environmental insults can degrade the DNA molecule so that complete DNA profiles are impossible to obtain. As DNA technology advances, it is imperative that investigators and scientists continue with their education to keep abreast of the latest techniques for collecting, preserving, and testing biological evidence. As forensic science and DNA testing becomes more powerful, it must be handled with greater care if the guilty are to be convicted and the innocent exonerated.

DNA, in the form of databases, is also an effective tool for providing investigative leads in many crimes including homicides. In the United States, all fifty states have a DNA database of convicted sex offenders. Due to the high rate of recidivism in sex offenders, the DNA databases are very successful in providing investigative leads for *no-suspect* sexual assault cases. In addition, *no-suspect* burglary, arson and homicide cases frequently match to someone in the convicted sex offender database. Some states are expanding their DNA databases to include these additional offenses because of the positive correlation of *cold-hits* in the sex offender database. Missing person databases are also being established to aid in the identification of skeletal remains. Thousands of unclaimed dead are awaiting identification in morgues across the country. Establishing a missing person DNA database as a reference source will assist many families in finding closure to tragic situations.

REFERENCES

1. Lee, H.C., Ed.: *Physical evidence.* Enfield, CT: Magnani and McCormic, 1995.
2. Lee, H.C., Gaensslen, R.E., Bigbee, P.D., and Kearney, J.J.: Guidelines for the collection and preservation of DNA evidence. *J. Forensic Ident. 41:* 344–356, 1991.
3. Lee, H.C., Ed.: *Crime scene investigation.* Taoyuan, Taiwan: Central Police University Press, 1994.
4. Lee, H.C., Palmbach, T., and Miller, M.: *Henry Lee's Crime Scene Handbook.* New York: Academic Press (in Press), 2001.
5. Lee, H.C., Ladd, C., Scherczinger, C.A., and Bourke, M.T.: Forensic applications of DNA typing: Collection and preservation of DNA evidence. *Am. J. Forensic Med. Path., 19:* 10–18, 1998.
6. Scherczinger, C.A., Ladd, C., Bourke, M.T., and Lee, H.C.: A systematic approach to PCR contamination. *J. Forensic Sci., 44:* 1042–1045, 1999.
7. Lee, H.C., Ladd, C., Bourke, M.T., Pagliaro, E.M., and Tirnady, F.: DNA typing in forensic science I: Theory and background. *Am. J. Forensic Med. Path., 15* (4): 269–282, 1994.
8. Herrin, G., and Gaensslen, R.E.: DNA Typing: Criminal and civil applications. Cyril Wecht (Ed.). *Forensic Sciences,* Vol 3, Chapter 37. Matthew Bender & Co., Inc., 1996.
9. Inman, K., and Rudin, N.: *An introduction to forensic DNA analysis.* Boca Raton, FL: CRC Press, 1997.
10. Adams, D.E., Presley, L.A., Baumstark, A.L., Hensley, K.W., Hill, A.L., Anoe, K.S., Campbell, P.A., McLaughlin, C.M., Budowle, B., Guisti, A.M., Smerick, J.B., and Baechtel, F.S.: DNA analysis by restriction fragment length polymorphisms of blood and other body fluid stains subjected to contamination and environmental insults. *J. Forensic Sci., 36:* 1284–1298, 1991.
11. Boles, T., Snow, C., and Stover, E.: Forensic DNA testing on skeletal remains from mass graves: A pilot project in Guatemala. *J. Forensic Sci., 40* (3): 349–355, 1995.
12. Lee, H.C., and Ladd, C.: Criminal justice: An unraveling of trust? *The Public Perspective, 8:* 6–7, 1997.
13. Gaensslen, R.E.: *Sourcebook in forensic serology, immunology, and biochemistry.* Washington, DC: US Government Printing Office, 1983.
14. Lee, H.C., and Gaensslen, R.E., eds.: *Advances in forensic science.* Foster City, CA: Biomedical Press, 1985.
15. Bock, J., and Norris, D.: Forensic botany: An underutilized resource. *J. Forensic Sci. 42:*364–367, 1997.
16. Gaensslen, R.E., Berka, K.M., Pagliaro, E.M., Ruano, G., Messina, D.A., and Lee, H.C.: Studies on DNA polymorphisms in human bone and soft tissue. *Analytica Chimica Acta, 288:* 3–16, 1994.
17. Gaensslen, R.E., and Lee, H.C.: Procedures and evaluation of an antisera for the typing of antigens in bloodstains: Blood group antigens ABH, RH, MNSs, Kell, Duffy, Kidd, Serum group antigens Gm/Km. Washington, D.C.: National Institute of Justice, U.S. Government Printing Office, 1984.
18. Lee, H.C. Identification and grouping of bloodstains. *Forensic Science Review.* Saferstein, R. (Ed). Englewood Cliffs, N.J.: Prentice Hall, 267–337, 1982.
19. Kahn, R. An introduction to DNA structure and genome organization. Farley, M.A., and Harrington, J.J. (Eds) *Forensic DNA Technology,* 25–38. Boca Raton: CRC Press, 1991.
20. Budowle, B., Adams, D.E., Comey, C.C., and Meril, C.R.: Mitochondrial DNA: A possible genetic material suitable for forensic analysis. Lee, H.C., and Gaensslen, R.E. (Eds.). *Advances in Forensic Sciences: DNA and Other Polymorphisms,* 3: 76–97. Chicago: Mosby Year Book, 1990.
21. Davis, C.L.: Mitochondrial DNA: *State of Tennessee v. Paul Ware. Profiles in DNA 1*(3): 6–7, 1998.
22. Fourney, R.M.: Mitochondrial DNA and forensic analysis: A primer for law enforcement. *Can. Soc. Forensic Sci. J., 31:* 45–53, 1998.
23. Bieber, F.: Overview of human identity testing and forensic genetics. *Current Protocols in Human Genetics,* Suppl. 15, 1997.
24. Jeffreys, A.J., Wilson, V., and Thein, S.L.: Individual-specific "fingerprints" of human DNA. *Nature 318* (6046): 577–579, 1985.
25. Budowle, B.: The RFLP technique. *FBI Crime Laboratory Dig., 15* (4): 97–98, 1988.
26. Gill, P., Jeffreys, A.J., and Werrett, D.J.: Forensic application of DNA "fingerprints." *Nature, 316* (6023): 76–77, 1985.
27. Fildes, N., and Reynolds, R.: Consistency and reproducibility of ampliType PM results between seven laboratories: Field trial result. *J. Forensic Sci., 40:* 279–286, 1995.
28. Budowle, B., Smerick, J.B., Keys, K.M., and Moretti, T.R.: United States population data on the Multiplex Short Tandem Repeat Loci HUMTHO1, TPOX, and CSF1PO-and the VNTR locus D1S80. *J. Forensic Sci., 42* (5): 846–849, 1997.
29. Budowle, B., Lindsey, J.A., DeCou, J.A., Koons, B.W., Giusti, A.M., and Comey, C.T.: Validation and population studies of the Loci LDLR, GYPA, HBGG, D7S8, and GC (PM Loci) and HLA-DQα Using a

Multiplex Amplification and Typing Procedure. *J. Forensic Sci. 40:*45–50, 1995.

30. Comey, C.T., and Budowle, B.: Validation studies on the analysis of the HLA-DQα Locus Using the Polymerase Chain Reaction. *J. Forensic Sci., 36:* 1633–1648, 1991.

31. Fregeau, C.J., Bowen, K.L., and Fourney, R.M.: Validation of highly polymorphic fluorescent multiplex short tandem repeat systems using two generations of DNA sequencers. *J. Forensic Sci., 44* (1): 133–166, 1999.

32. Saiki, R.K., Bugawan, T.L., Horn, G.T., Mullis, K.B., and Erlich, H.A.: Analysis of enzymatically amplified B-Globin and HLA-DQ alpha DNA with Allele-specific Oligonucleotide Probes. *Nature 324:* 163–166, 1986.

33. Tahir, M., Balraj, E., Luke, L., Gilbert, T., Hamby, J., and Amjad, M.: DNA typing of samples for Polymarker, DQA1, and nine STR loci from a human body exhumed after 27 years. *J. Forensic Sci., 45* (4): 902–907, 2000.

34. Word, C.J., Sawosik, T.M., and Bing, D.H.: Summary of validation studies from twenty-six laboratories in the United States and Canada on the use of the AmpliType PM PCR. *J. Forensic Sci., 42:* 39–48, 1997.

35. AmpFlSTR Profiler PCR Amplification Kit User's Manual. Perkin Elmer Corporation, 1997.

36. Hochmeister, M., Budowle, B., Borer, U., Rudin, O., Bohnert, M., and Dirnhofer, R.: Confirmation of the identity of human skeletal remains using Multiplex PCR Amplification and Typing Kits. *J. Forensic Sci., 40* (4):701–705, 1995.

37. van Oorschot, R.A., Gutowski, S.J., Robinson, S.L., Hedley, J.A., and Andrew, I.R.: HUMTHO1 validation studies: Effects of substrate, environment, and mixtures. *J. Forensic Sci., 40:* 142–145, 1996.

38. Whitaker, J.P.,Clayton, T.M., Urquhart, A.J., Millican, E.S., Downes, T.J., Kimpton, C.P., and Gill, P.: Short Tandem Repeat Typing of bodies from a mass disaster: High success rate and characteristic amplification patterns in highly degraded samples, *BioTech., 18* (4): 670–676, 1995.

39. Word, C.J.: STR Data goes to court. *Profiles in DNA 2*(1): 7–8, 1998.

40. Lleonart, R., Riego, E., Sainz de la Pena, M., Bacallao, K., Amaro, F., Santiesteban, M., Blanco, M., Currenti, H., Puentes, A., Rolo, F., Herrera, L., and de la Fuenta, J.: Forensic identification of skeletal remains from members of Ernesto Che Guevaras Guerillas in Bolivia based on DNA typing. *International Journal of Legal Medicine, 113* (2): 98–101, 2000.

41. Butler, J.M.: The use of capillary electrophoresis in genotyping STR Loci. *Methods in Molecular Biology, 98:* 279–289, 1998.

42. Parsons, T.J., Muniec, D.S., Sullivan, K., Woodyatt, N., Alliston-Greiner, R., Wilson, M.R., Berry, D.L., Holland, K.A., Weedn, V.W., Gill, P., and Holland, M.M.: A high observed substitution rate in human Mitochondrial DNA Control Region. *Nature Genetics, 15:* 363–368, 1997.

43. Ryan, J.H., Wadkins, M.J., Yang, N., Barritt, S.M., Wilson, R.E., Huffine, E.F., Parsons, T.J., and Holland, M.M.: Improvements in Mitochondrial DNA amplification and sequencing through the use of "Mini-Primer Sets" for highly degraded forensic specimens. *Proc. Am. Acad. For. Sci., 5:* 74–75, 1999.

44. Budowle, B., Wilson, M.R., DiZinno, J.A., Stauffer, C., Fasano, M.A., Holland, M.M., and Monson, K.L.: Mitochondrial DNA Regions HVI and HVII Population Data. *Forensic Sci. Internat., 103:* 23–35, 1999.

45. Innes, B.: *Bodies of evidence.* Reader's Digest Association, 2000.

46. Basten, C.J.: Implications of canine population structure for DNA forensics. Proceedings of Cambridge Healthtech Institute's 3rd Annual DNA Forensics Meeting. June 13–15, McLean, VA, 1999, pp. 1–13.

47. Menotti-Raymond, M.A., David, V.A., and O'Brien, S.J.: Pet cat hair implicates murder suspect. *Nature 386:* 774, 1997.

48. Yoon, C.K.: Botanical witness for the prosecution. *Science 260:* 894–895, 1993.

49. Bromwich, M.R.: Justice Department Investigation of the FBI Laboratory: Executive Summary, Department of Justice Office of the Inspector General. *The Criminal Law Reporter, 61:* 2017–2039, 1997.

50. McEwen, J.E.: Forensic DNA Data Banking by state crime laboratories. *Am. J. Hum. Genet., 56* (6): 1487–1492, 1995.

51. McEwen, J.E., and Reilly, P.R.: A review of state legislature on DNA Forensic Data Banking. *Am. J. Hum. Genet. 54* (6): 941–958, 1994.

52. Uniform Crime Reports. U.S. Department of Justice, Federal Bureau of Investigation, 2000.

53. CODIS Statistics. U.S. Department of Justice, Federal Bureau of Investigation, 2000.

54. Brannon, R., and Kessler, H.: Problems in mass-disaster dental identification: A retrospective review. *J. Forensic Sci. 44* (1): 123–127, 1999.

55. Sozer, A., Kelly, C., and Demers, D.: *Molecular analysis of paternity. Current protocols in human genetics.* New York: John Wiley, 1998.

56. Corach, D., Sala, A., Penacino, G., Iannucci, N., Bernardi, P., Doretti, M., Fondebrider, L., Ginarte, A., Inchaurregui, A., Somigliana, C., Turner, S., and Hagelberg, E.: Additional Approaches to DNA typing of skeletal remains: The search for "missing" persons killed during the last Dictatorship in Argentina. *Electrophoresis, 18* (9): 1608–1612, 1997.

57. Holland, M., Fisher, D., Mitchell, L., Rodriquez, W., Canik, J., Merril, C., and Weedn, V.: Mitochondrial DNA sequence analysis of human skeletal remains: Identification of remains from the Vietnam war. *J. Forensic Sci., 38* (3): 542–553, 1993.

58. Raskin, J.S., Cayea, C.A., Ernst, C.M., Parsons, T.J., Ryan, J.H., Smigielski, K.B., Steighner, R.J., Yang, N., and Huffine, E.F.: Looking Beyond HV1 and HV2: The Application of VR1/VR2 Testing of Mitochondrial DNA to further discriminate ancient skeletal remains of American war casualties. *Proc. Am. Acad. For. Sci., 5:* 68, 1999.

Part 3

TRACE EVIDENCE

RICHARD E. BISBING

This chapter is intended as an introduction to the potential value of trace evidence, to the general methods of recognition and collection of trace evidence, and to the use of trace evidence by medicolegal investigators to determine the identity of the deceased, the time of death, the cause and manner of death, and the identity of the perpetrator in the case of homicide. This chapter is not intended to train medicolegal specialists in the nuances of the analysis, identification and comparison of trace evidence; there are other sources.[1-3]

What is Trace Evidence?

Trace evidence might be anything that can be described as small bits of solid material used as associative evidence in a forensic investigation, like particles of dust creating a footwear impression, torn scraps of paper from a threatening note, crusts of blood, gunshot residue particles, clothing fibers, paint chips, pubic hairs, or diatoms. Trace evidence associates people with places, objects with people, objects with places and objects with objects and provides evidence to help understand the behavior of parties to accidents, crime, and death.

Often, trace evidence will be microscopic in size and initially invisible to the unaided eye. Therefore, the trace evidence examiner is necessarily skilled in microscopy in order to handle and analyze the small motes and usually has the knowledge, skills and means to analyze all kinds of materials. Likewise, the collector of trace evidence must think small and must be capable of recognizing a wide variety of materials as evidence.

Clues in the Dust

Dust, as an example, is the microscopic debris that covers our clothes and covers our floors, accumulates everywhere from the disintegration of the various components of our environment. Dust has three distinguishing characteristics that make it useful as trace evidence: (1) it is found as small particles in a pulverized state created by the disintegration of other materials into smaller bits, (2) its compositional and morphological features derive from its origin, and (3) its microscopic size facilitates its transfer and makes it relatively difficult to detect by either the criminal party or the investigator.[4] The French microscopist, Edmond Locard, explained to criminalists: "The microscopic debris that covers our clothing and bodies are the mute witnesses, sure and faithful, of all our movements and all our encounters."[5]

Notwithstanding, trace evidence is more than dust; it includes many other types of associative evidence. The term associative evidence was defined by James Osterburg[6] and signifies that some connection or association has been established between crime scene and criminal. Traces can be any mark or material left at a scene. Some associative evidence is so specialized that it is not often thought of as trace evidence; some examples are fingerprints, bullets, and blood. Nevertheless, they are associative evidence, they often involve transfers of microscopic-size bits of materials, and they are traces left behind as evidence. Although they vary greatly with regard to how they are analyzed, in a medicolegal investigation they are all used to track the movements, encounters, or identity of both the deceased and the perpetrator.

Locard Exchange Principle

Trace evidence usually results from the transfer of material from one object to another. As explained by Locard and the Exchange Principle attributed to him, whenever two objects come in contact, material from one object will transfer to

TABLE II-6
GENERIC TRACE EVIDENCE

- Impressions and Marks
- Fractured Fragments
- Genetic Markers
- Somatic Samples
- Manufactured Portions
- Natural Samples

the other. Oftentimes, material transfers from both objects to the other in a cross transfer, providing even more evidence of contact. The transferred material may in itself be important, like blood transferring to the blade of a knife or hair to the claw of a hammer. Additionally, in many instances the material transfers in a pattern, like a shoe print on a child's clothing, fingerprints, the striations on a bullet where the bullet material transferred to the barrel and the marks from the barrel left a pattern on the bullet, or a fabric impression left on a dashboard from the crash victim's clothing.

Trace Evidence Types

One way to recognize trace evidence is to consider the possibilities in generic groups rather than trying to remember every possibility individually, which might be applicable to every imaginable case scenario. Trace evidence will originate from any of the following groups: impressions like from shoes or tools; fractured fragments like torn paper; genetic markers found in blood and semen; somatic samples from the body like hairs; manufactured materials such as fibers, paint, and glass; or soil and other natural samples from the ecological environment [Table II-6].

Successful criminalists understand that if an object or person left a mark which appears to be an impression of a surface, it is very likely that the object can be associated with the mark through comparison of class and accidental characteristics caused by biological variability, earprints, etc. (Fig. II-44) or by normal use and wear, shovel marks, etc. (Figure II-45 and Table II-7). The fingerprint or firearms specialist will probably be able to assist best with these types of

evidence. Footwear impressions are one of the most often overlooked clues (Fig. II-46).[7,8]

Likewise, if something is torn or broken, like a broken tooth or a torn fingernail, if the broken counterpart can be found, the two pieces can be physically placed back together to show they were once one whole piece. Before a valid association can be claimed, the fractured pieces must be realigned; the pieces must interfit along an irregular edge-to-edge border verified by surface markings or verified by a three-dimensional fit; and the pieces must possess accidental characteristics or a unique design. The types of fracture matches include: (1) fractures in a plane along a two dimensional irregular edge or cuts through unique arrays, like tape or paper; (2) fractured solids which are aligned either over two contiguous surfaces or two noncontiguous surfaces, like plastic vehicle parts such as taillight lens or piece of a grille. Along with fingerprints and other impressions, fracture matches are some of the best kinds of associative evidence and should never be overlooked (Table II-8).

Other groups of trace evidence (genera) include: genetic markers such as DNA which will always be available to associate animal specimens such as, blood, sperm, and skin cells, or even a plant with its origin; somatic samples from the body such as hairs, handwriting and voice prints; any portion of a manufactured material for example, textile fibers, paint, plastic, and glass can be identified by its morphology and composition and compared with other possible portions from questioned and known sources; and a wide variety of natural samples such as soil and diatoms can be used as associative evidence with varying degrees of success (Tables II-9 and II-10).

Trace Evidence Analysis

There are excellent descriptions elsewhere of methods of analysis for impressions, genetic markers and somatic samples.[1,2] The analysis of the important group of microtraces from manufactured portions is relatively straightforward. The microtraces are first identified by microscopic or chemical analysis, that is, put into pre-

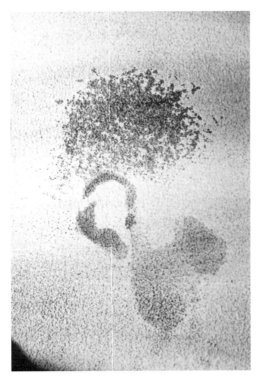

FIGURE II-44. Latent earprint, with hair and cheek impressions, developed on wall with black powder.

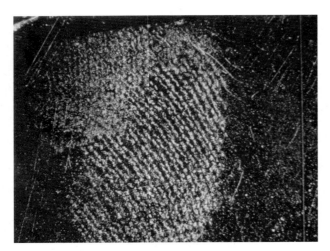

FIGURE II-45. Latent glove finger fabric impression developed on glass with silver powder.

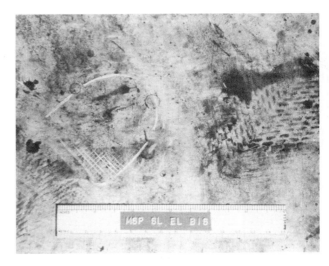

FIGURE II-46. Latent footwear impressions developed on tile floor with black powder.

TABLE II-7

IMPRESSIONS

• Fingerprints	• Rubber stamps
• Palmprints	• Tire tracks
• Footprints	• Ear prints
• Footwear impressions	• Lip prints
• Bitemarks	• Fabric impressions
• Bullets	• Toolmarks
• Cartridge Casings	• Typewriting and printing

TABLE II-8

FRACTURED FRAGMENTS

• Torn Paper	• Torn tape
• Paper pads	• Torn skin
• Paper matches	• Broken bones
• Broken tools	• Torn fabric
• Fingernails	• Broken glass

defined classes such as trilobal nylon carpet fiber or acrylic paint. The second phase is usually an attempt to use more individualizing characteristics such as color, optical properties, morphology, structure, additives and trace constituents to compare the questioned microtrace with exemplars from known sources relevant to the medicolegal investigation. For example, after identifying a particle as glass, it is then compared with the potential source by measuring a combination of refractive index and dispersion of the refractive index, density, and the quantity of trace elements in the questioned and known glass (Table II-11).

In most every instance, microtraces of these types are found and manipulated using micro-

TABLE II-9

GENETIC MARKERS

- Blood
- Semen
- Sweat
- Skin
- Hair

TABLE II-10

SOMATIC SAMPLES

- Hair
- Handwriting
- Voice prints

TABLE II-11

MANUFACTURED PORTIONS

• Fabric	• Safe insulation
• Fibers	• Road dust
• Paint	• Building materials
• Plastic	• Tape
• Metal	• Pellets, Wads, shot collars
• Gunshot residues	• Rubber
• Glass	• Ink
• Cosmetics	• Powders

scopic techniques. The particles are small and a great deal of analysis must be conducted on each particle while attempting to preserve a portion for someone else to analyze. Therefore, the techniques applicable to trace evidence analysis include those methods that can be conducted on a micro-scale. The microtraces are best analyzed by the particle approach, where the particles are isolated, characterized, and identified using microscopic techniques.

The alternative to the particle approach is a bulk specimen trace analysis in which the analytical chemist prepares the samples by dilution, mixing, dissolving or grinding, and thereby generates a homogeneous sample which is analyzed for its trace constituents. These trace analyses, if not applied appropriately, are often difficult and conclusions are often misleading. The usual methods of chemical analysis in the trace evidence laboratory include: polarized light microscopy (PLM) with microchemical tests, infrared microspectroscopy (FTIR), Raman spectroscopy, scanning electron microscopy (SEM) with energy dispersive x-ray spectrometry (EDS), pyrolysis gas chromatography (Py-GC) and mass spectrometry (GC/MS), visible and ultraviolet microspectrophotometry (MSP), thin layer chromatography (TLC), and some means for trace element analysis such as atomic absorption spectroscopy (AA) or inductively coupled plasma mass spectrometry (ICP/MS). Each of these techniques can produce data on microscopic size fragments of almost any material, which assist in first identifying the material and secondly comparing the questioned and known samples. If the materials are indistinguishable, an association can be asserted.

The relative certainty of a trace evidence association depends to some extent on the generic class from which the evidence comes and in other ways upon the context in which the evidence is used. Obviously, a fingerprint match is positive, unequivocal evidence that a person touched an object. Likewise, bullets and footwear impressions can be positively associated with the gun and boot, respectively. Torn and broken fragments can be proven beyond doubt to have once been one and the same, thereby providing a certain association between the fragment found at the crime scene and the fragment found in the suspect's pocket, if that were the case. Modern DNA technology can determine from whom the blood or semen originated with near certainty. In contrast, hairs cannot be associated with one particular person to the exclusion of all others and manufactured portions like clothing fibers, window glass or automobile paint could always have originated from another similar item fashioned from the same batch of raw material.

Soil is different than most types of associative evidence. The assumption is that soil from a spot of ground is probably unique. The accepted method for forensic soil analysis involves comparison of soil color and separation of sand grains for mineral identification using polarized light microscopy. The identification of anthropogenic artifacts in the soil is, of course, possible and other natural microscopic constituents, like pollen, phytoliths, etc, may on occasion be useful

TABLE II-12

NATURAL SAMPLES

• Soil	• Grass
• Pollen	• Insects
• Diatoms	• Mold
• Feathers	• Algae
• Seeds	• Lichens
• Feces	• Wood

for comparison. On the other hand, soil comparisons are problematic usually because of the lack of good exemplars and, in practicality, rarely lead to an unequivocal association (Table II-12).

Each type of trace evidence may play a role in any medicolegal investigation. If the case circumstances are right, none of the evidence types should be ignored or unused solely because of lesser amount of certainty of the association. Consider two more examples. In fatal vehicle accidents, determining who was driving is often important. If two friends who often drive the same car die in a vehicle accident, the presence of a fingerprint on the rearview mirror is of little value for determining who was driving at the time of the accident, even if the fingerprint can unequivocally be identified with one person to the exclusion of all others. On the other hand, the likelihood is very low that the hairs imbedded in the head strike in the windshield, which exhibit the same microscopic characteristics as occupant A but different than occupant B, came from anyone other than occupant A, regardless of how certain the association. In this context, the trace evidence can be very useful for identifying the driver and passenger, after considering occupant kinematics, and the value of the somatic sample to the medicolegal investigation is not measured by whether the match was absolutely positive or not. A second example illustrates the same point but with opposite consequences. If a questioned hair was found on a bank floor after a robbery, the likelihood that the hair originated from an unknown third party seems more likely and the somatic sample now might be of little value to the investigation.

As expected, if more than one type of evidence can be used in combination to associate objects, the relative certainty of the association should be greater. In other words, considering all the degrees of freedom with regard to types of trace evidence and types of cases, these generic classes of associative trace evidence produce a plethora of potential trace evidence available for use by the medicolegal investigator, especially when used in combinations. The combination of evidence types available for the comparison of a strip of duct tape used to bind the deceased with a tape roll found in the suspect's trunk is a good example. The tape might support fingerprints, bloodstains, or soil from the owner's locale. The torn end can be fracture matched with the roll from which it originated using the irregular edge and surface extrusion striae. Fibers or paint chips in the adhesive can be associated with the owner's environment. The material from which the questioned strip was made (polymer film, reinforcing fiber, adhesive polymer, pigments and fillers) can be compared with the composition of the tape on the roll. If the tape from the body is compared with the roll from which it originated, there is little excuse for why there should not be credible evidence of an association considering all the possible types of trace evidence it likely supports.

HOW IS TRACE EVIDENCE USED?

Trace evidence can assist on occasion in each of the areas of a medicolegal investigation of death. Although its analysis and interpretation is often left to other specialists, the importance of trace evidence to the pathologist's responsibilities should not be minimized. In every case, trace evidence is collected and studied to first determine the identity and potential source of the questioned unknown material and secondly to use the findings to help in the reconstruction of a human behavioral event.

In his autobiography, *Mostly Murder*, Sir Sydney Smith describes the role of the forensic pathologist a half century ago and gives some sage advice that applies today with regard to trace evidence. The medicolegal expert is not responsible necessarily for the trace evidence. Nevertheless, he may be expected to use his knowledge and intelligence to help the police or accident investigator use trace evidence to help solve the crime. Basically his role is simply to furnish the police with specific information on matters of which he has specialized knowledge and not necessarily only medical information. He may be the only scientific person who sees the case as a whole. He is often asked to observe, infer, and even speculate about the case, particularly about medical aspects, but oftentimes about other scientific matters. It is likely that because of his special knowledge, a non-medical clue may have a significance that even an astute police officer has not grasped. His peculiar experience and talents may enable him alone to deduce the correct interpretations of the facts. The police will want to know who the dead person is, or they will want to be told of any detail that may help identification, if the dead person's identity is not readily evident. They will want to know the cause and manner of death, whether due to natural causes or to violence; and if the latter, whether it is a case of accident, suicide, or homicide. How did the person die? When did death take place? Where did death take place? Why did it happen? A better understanding of the whole field of trace evidence by this central figure in the medicolegal investigation of death can only benefit the whole investigation.[9]

More today than in the twentieth century, the forensic specialties within trace evidence are dividing and increasing in numbers. There are fingerprint specialists and footwear specialists; firearms examiners and gunshot residue analysts; serologists and DNA specialists; hair examiners and fiber specialists; paint and glass specialists; fire debris chemists and drug chemists; and, forensic microscopists with skills in the analysis of soil, pollen, diatoms, wood, and feces. The fields of forensic science, criminalistics, microscopy, chemistry, and the academic sciences produce all the necessary experts to handle every conceivable type of trace evidence that might be encountered and used in the medicolegal investigation of

death; but it might remain an important responsibility of the forensic pathologist to find these people and encourage them to cooperate in order to accomplish a successful scientific investigation.

Identification of Human Remains

The trace evidence types described in this chapter are often thought of as a means to associate the perpetrator with the crime; nevertheless, trace evidence can be used in other equally important aspects of the investigation. For example, identification of otherwise visually unidentifiable human remains, normally the province of the medical examiner with assistance from a forensic anthropologist or odontologist, is often assisted by fingerprint technologies and genetic markers (DNA) where possible. The identification can also be assisted by the comparison of trace evidence from the body with antemortem materials. For example, the wrappings, whether clothing or something like a blanket can be identified and its origin determined either by tracing the items to the missing person via manufacturing and retail sources or by comparison with fibers collected from the antemortem environment of the deceased. Blankets and carpets usually support an abundance of stray fibers from locations where they were used and the microtraces can be collected for comparison. In other instances, hair remaining on the skull or fingernail polish on the nails of the skeletonized remains can be used to assist the anthropologist with the biological profile. Furthermore, the trace evidence examiner can compare the hair with antemortem hair collected from the missing person's brush or compare the polish with bottles of polish from the missing person's residence.

Identification of Weapons

The identification of weapons causing injury is obviously of value to first assist in determining the manner of death as well as for associating the weapon with the perpetrator. The trace evidence associated with bite marks can likewise assist in confirming the identity of the assailant. In fact,

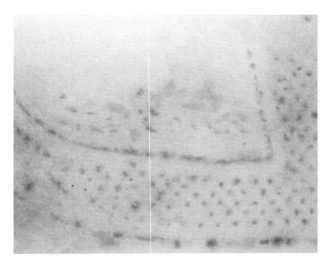

Figure II-47. Heel impression in bruised area of child's chest.

bite marks are a good example of dual associative evidence, impressions and genetic markers, that is, tooth impressions and saliva. The forensic odontologist will compare the marks with known impressions and the saliva likely found around the impression can be compared with the suspected assailant by the DNA laboratory.

Blunt force injuries, those that cause contusion or abrasion, usually involve a Locard exchange and should result in a transfer of trace evidence from the body to the weapon. Sometimes the transfer results in a patterned impression such as an imprint of the front license plate from a hit and run vehicle or a heel print on the chest of a child (Fig. II-47). If there is laceration, there will likely be a transfer of blood, tissue or hair to the weapon. If there is any cutting, particularly of bone, such as might occur from a sharp force injury, there is always the possibility of toolmarks (impressions) from the instrument or a transfer of paint to the cut surface.

Gunshot Wounds

With gunshot wounds, the direction and distance between shooter and victim is determined partly by determining the concentrations and patterns of gunshot residues, identification of any intervening materials on the projectiles, and by identification of microtraces on the gun from blowback and backsplash. Gunshot residues can be found on vehicles, upholstery, clothing, hair, skin, in nostrils, surrounding entrance and exit wounds and along the wound track.

Vehicle Crashes

The force and violence resulting from crashes of planes, trains, and automobiles produce trace evidence to help reconstruct what occurred. In few cases is the trace evidence more abundant or a better illustration of the Locard Exchange Principle. For example, in fatal hit and run crashes, the pedestrian is struck, trace evidence from the vehicle transfers to the victim and trace evidence from the victim transfers to the vehicle. Hair, blood, tissue and clothing fibers will likely be transferred to the vehicle. Glass, paint, plastic and metal will likely be transferred to the victim. Fabric impressions on the vehicle prove beyond a doubt that the vehicle struck someone with force. Blood, tissue, hair, and fabric impressions on interior surfaces will help determine the kinematics of the occupants.

Litigation over vehicle crash worthiness has fostered the use of trace evidence to determine occupant location and occupant kinematics. The seat belt and the trace evidence it supports can also be a witness to a vehicle crash. Fortunately, a limited number of common questions are presented to the trace evidence examiner during the investigation of vehicle crashes. *"Who was driving and where were the riders?"* or *"Which way did they go and what did they hit?"* are the most common questions.

Criminalists understand how to identify and associate hairs, fibers, and blood and the methods are well known; although, the relevance of the associations depends on whether the hairs, fibers, or blood are a result of the impact. Therefore, it is sometimes necessary to determine whether a hair was broken or cut. Likewise, fabric impressions prove that fibers are present due to impact, and blood spatter analysis can serve the same purpose.

If use of the belt is questioned, loading is evidenced by partial separations and forceful

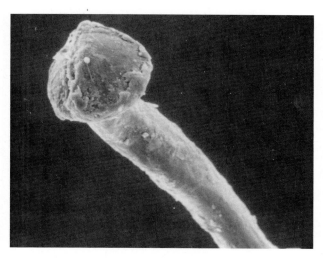

FIGURE II-48. Bulbous end of seatbelt fiber broken by tensile forces as the belt separated during a high-speed crash.

gerprints, the tape lift can keep the microtraces in context.

Once in the laboratory, samples can be examined in situ for morphological features using a stereomicroscope or a low vacuum scanning electron microscope (LV SEM); or, analyzed for chemical composition by attenuated total reflectance (ATR) infrared microspectroscopy (IR) or energy dispersive x-ray spectrometry (EDS) in a low vacuum scanning electron microscope (LV SEM). Particles can be transferred to microscopic slides for analysis by analytical light microscopy (ALM) techniques including polarized light microscopy (PLM), to a thin polished salt plate for IR, or to a beryllium plate for EDS.[10-14]

Identification of Foreign Bodies

Finally, the trace evidence examiner can assist the pathologist with the identification of foreign bodies found in organs, tissues, and body fluids. Sometimes materials identified in the stomach contents (foodstuffs, pharmaceuticals and bezoars) can help determine the time, cause, and manner of death. Hair in a hairball (trichobezoar) as sometimes found in the mentally diseased can be analyzed segmentally to determine the presence of certain drugs (Fig. II-49). Fragments of bullets or gunpowder residues in tissues can help determine range of fire or even the nature of the ammunition. The true identity of crystalline deposits in tissues can help determine the etiology of disease. For example, in individuals suffering from silicosis, are the crystalline deposits in their lungs crystalline silica, asbestos, remnants of cigarette smoke, or something else? Using ultramicroanalysis techniques, the crystalline materials can be positively identified and therefore correctly evaluated by the pathologist (Fig. II-50).

exchanges of material; and if the belt breaks, the separation mechanism is determined by a microscopic examination of the separated fiber ends looking for characteristic tensile breaks and cuts (Fig. II-48).

Applying the Locard Exchange Principle, identification, comparison, and association of microtraces will assist in determining impact points. The interiors of vehicles are covered primarily with fabric and plastic; therefore, the types of materials requiring analysis are relatively limited. If samples can be collected at all, usually only microscopic-sized samples are allowed. Alternatively, some analyses must be conducted without disturbing the samples. Microscopic examination is mandatory, documentation (photomacrography, photomicrography, and video recording) is necessary, and preservation of samples is usually required. Particles can be collected most easily in the field with sticky tape, like a latent print lift; furthermore, as with fin-

WHERE IS TRACE EVIDENCE FOUND?

Once the investigator knows what types of trace evidence are useful, he needs to know where to look. It seems logical that one would begin from the outside and work inward. The search for trace evidence in a medicolegal investigation is remarkably like the search for evidence in a house burglary. Evidence such as tire tracks, footwear impressions, and discarded cigarettes are collected from the approach (distal space) to the house; fingerprints and earprints

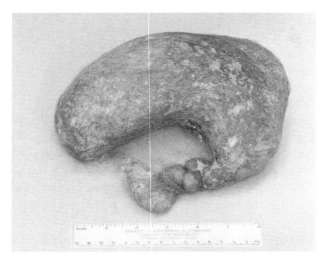

FIGURE II-49. Hairball, measuring seven inches across. The hairball is in the exact shape of the stomach and small segment beyond pylorus.

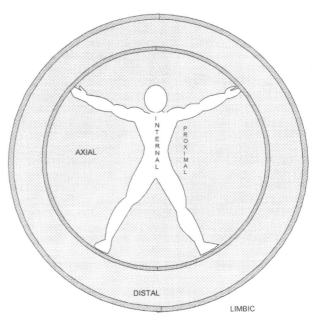

FIGURE II-51. Diagram of areas within and outside of the body as described in somatotactics (Table II-9).

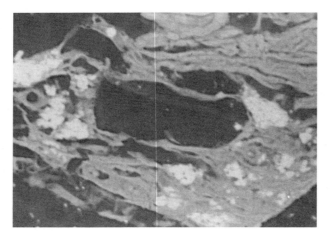

FIGURE II-50. Backscattered electron SEM image of talc particles in histological section. The bright areas are due to the higher atomic number of the silicon and magnesium in talc compared with the carbon, oxygen, and nitrogen in the tissue.

Trace Evidence Somatotactics

Somatotactics is a way to describe movements and relative distances from the central core of the body. Although esoteric, these descriptions can be used to suggest where types of trace evidence might be found on and near the body. The *internal space* is obvious and is most often thought of as the province of the pathologist. Although some trace evidence like bullet fragments and diatoms will be found in the internal spaces, trace evidence is more often associated with each of the following spaces (Fig. II-51).

Proximal space consists of the area between the body and its coverings (clothing, hair or ornament), including primarily the skin surface. Just as internal space can be entered through the natural orifices of the body (sexual penetration) or invaded through injury at unnatural sites (wounds), so too proximal space can be entered in several ways: by secretions from internal space or assailant (saliva in a bite mark), by movements from axial space which glide beneath the clothing (struggling), puncture through the clothing (stab or bullet wounds), or by stripping away the coverings (torn clothing)

from the point of entry (axial space), glass and clothing fibers from the broken entry and exit (proximal space), and many things from the interior where all types of trace evidence has been admixed inside or taken away from inside the house (internal space).

TABLE II-13
TRACE EVIDENCE SOMATOTACTICS

Distance Category	*Location*	*Item*	*Examples*
Internal	Fluids Tissues Organs	Blood, Urine, Saliva, Semen, Skin	Semen, Bullets
Proximal Axial-Proximal	Surface Coverings	Skin Clothing	Impressions, Saliva, Semen Hairs, Fibers, Paint, Gunshot residues
Axial	Reach Contacts	Hands, Feet, Fingernails	Hair, Fingerprints
Distal	Approach Leaving	Floors, Ground	Footwear impressions, Tire tracks, Weapons
Limbic	Intent Secret	Messages, Hiding places	Voice, Paper, Computers, Weapons, Vehicles

such as might occur during a physical assault. To the pathologist, the wounds at the internal-proximal boundary are often the most meaningful. To the criminalist, the evidence on the skin and clothing at the proximal-axial boundary is usually the most valuable.

The *axial space* extends from the external boundary of proximal space to the limit of the areas controlled by the extended arms and legs, that is, within the individual's reach. Defense wounds occur at the axial-distal boundary, as do footwear impressions, fingerprints, and fingernail debris. *Distal space* embraces the knowable world at any one moment in time. Cell phones and guns amplify the range of contact within the distal space and thus enormously extend certain parts of the distal-limbic boundary. The *limbic space* is beyond ordinary sensory contact and the evidence there will be derived from investigation away from the focus of the crime scene or corpse. Evidence in limbic space might include notepads with threats readable in impressed writing or a tool used to crimp wires of a homemade bomb secreted away in a favorite hiding spot (Table II-13).[15]

In summary, if the investigator considers the possible genera of trace evidence, the places near and on the body where trace evidence might be found, the possible questions before the investigator, and some simple guidelines regarding the collection of microtraces; the whole process can be reduced to a single stimulus: ***Aha, there is something!*** Once recognized and once the decision is made to recover the evidence, the stimulus is reduced to a process of finding a way to collect and preserve the trace evidence so that it is unaltered and identifiable later by the appropriate specialist.

CRIME SCENE INVESTIGATION

Investigations start at the site of the death. Therefore, the forensic pathologist has a role at the crime scene or accident site; and, in some jurisdictions, the medical examiner or representative must be there at some point in time to initiate the medicolegal portion of the investigation. Part of the pathologist's role is to assist in the collection of trace evidence. Trace evidence includes the most fragile and smallest items present, and the most likely items to be lost. Latent footwear impressions on tile and wood floors are the best examples of trace evidence that is too often overlooked and thereby too often destroyed inadvertently during the crime scene search. Just as the perpetrator had to walk across the floor to enter and exit the crime scene, so too the crime scene investigators must walk across that same floor to enter and exit. If the crime scene has not been processed for trace evidence, the medicolegal investigators need to wait, ask first, and proceed with caution so that valuable trace evidence is not lost.

Protecting Trace Evidence at the Crime Scene

All crime scenes are protected in the same general way until the evidence can be collected. The scene must be left like a frozen section in space, time, form, and context. The action needs to be stopped so that nothing foreign is introduced to contaminate the scene, nothing is destroyed, and nothing inadvertently removed. Ideally, the first police officer arriving at the scene will take control of protecting it from the usual intruders: police commanders, prosecutors, the press, and unnecessary medical personnel.

Contamination is prevented by taking measures against the five major contaminators: weather, relatives, friends and associates, the curious and collectors, and officials. Only the weather is uncontrollable. When the scene is adequately protected, the trace evidence will be observed or discovered in place, photographed, measured and mapped, and expertly collected with a short chain of custody and with very much less chance of contamination or loss. There is usually only one chance to recognize and recover all the evidence; therefore, the success or failure of the crime scene search will depend first and foremost upon crime scene protection.

Likewise, the autopsy begins when the pathologist first sees the body, whether at the scene where the deceased was first discovered or in the morgue. In either venue, the process is the same with regard to trace evidence. There should be a careful, slow, and thorough inspection of the clothing and skin surfaces. There is no better way to search than to get close to the surfaces, with a bright light, and look from short range.

The nude body of a white female was found in a field. During the search of the body at the crime scene, a tire impression and three small chips of paint were discovered on her leg. The impression matched the tread of the spare tire in the trunk of the suspect's car and the paint chips were simi-

lar to the flaking paint on the jack post in the same trunk. If the body had not been searched up close and personal at the crime scene, there is no doubt that the trace evidence would have been lost forever.

The forensic pathologist has a special expertise in the interpretation of injury and by affording him the opportunity to assist in the crime scene or accident scene investigation, that expertise can be put to good use. Relating injury with the circumstances and the items at the scene are invaluable contributions to the investigation.

One clear example of this involved the death of a teenage girl found on a wooded pathway. Postmortem findings suggested a heavy but broad blunt force injury to the head. The pathologist thought the injury was consistent with a fall, which seemed inconsistent with the wooded pathway, the physical evidence at the scene, and the story told by the boyfriend. Upon his own initiative, the forensic pathologist visited the crime scene and wandered down the path. Lo and behold, he looked up and saw a tree house. Later questioning confirmed that the deceased had been pushed from the tree house and subsequently carried to where she was found a short distance down the path.

Crime Scene Search

When the crime scene search begins, it must be conducted thoroughly and with an open mind. Hypotheses and preconceived opinions are developed early in most death investigations, so it is important for the forensic scientists participating in the investigation, whether criminalist or pathologist, to provide the needed objectivity and not immediately exclude alternate hypotheses that might be supported by the physical and medical evidence. The search must be systematic and well-planned. The search needs to start on the periphery of the scene and progress toward a focal point in a way that ensures that nothing is overlooked and nothing is destroyed before it can be collected. In the case of a death investigation, the deceased will be a logical focal point and a path giving access to the body needs to be searched. Evidence in the pathway should be recorded, collected and preserved before the body and the immediate vicinity are searched.

Obviously, the body is important and the trace evidence it supports may be crucial to determining the cause and manner of death. The position of the body needs to be documented and trace evidence should be collected from the surfaces and surrounding area before the body is even rolled over. Hairs and fibers can be collected using forceps or lifting tape. Loose hairs should be picked from the surface and placed in individual labeled paper packets. The scalp and pubic hair can be combed for foreign hairs and fibers. Sometimes, if the tines of the comb are partially filled with previously unused (new) cotton batting, the foreign hairs and fibers are secured a little better during the combing. Stains can be collected from the skin either by scraping with a clean scalpel or by swabbing with a moistened cotton swab. The wet swab should be dried before it is repackaged and sealed. Microtraces on the clothing and skin can be collected with sticky tape.

Gunshot Residues

Gunshot residue can be collected from the hands and face. In the past, a cotton swab moistened with five percent nitric acid was used to collect gunshot residues from hands for analysis by atomic absorption spectroscopy (AA). Today, a better method is to use a specially designed sticky stub, which is analyzed in a scanning electron microscope (SEM/EDS). The sticky surface is dabbed over the area where gunshot residues are suspected.

The analysis of gunshot residues (GSR) using SEM/EDS has proven to be a valuable addition to the trace evidence arsenal. The basic principle upon which the technique depends is that small particles characteristically left as a residue after a weapon is fired can be collected using adhesive-coated SEM stubs. Opaque conductive carbon-filled double-sided tape disks are used on the stubs (Fig. II-52). Subsequent analysis is performed by SEM directly on the adhesive surface and particles unique to GSR are identified by their morphology and chemical composition. Particles containing lead, antimony and barium are considered unique to gunshot residues (Figs. II-53, II-54, and Table II-14).

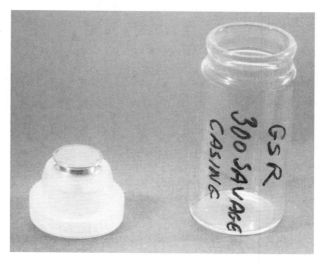

FIGURE II-52. SEM sticky stub used to collect gunshot residue particles from hands, face, hair, and clothing.

Moving the Body and Clothing

Most trace evidence can be collected before the body is removed from the scene. When the body is removed from the scene, it should first be wrapped in a new clean, white bed sheet, paper blanket, or body bag for transport. The wrappings need to be marked for identification and carefully removed at the time of autopsy and preserved for trace evidence examination. Not only do new and clean wrappings protect the body from contamination and subsequent loss of trace evidence, but the wrappings themselves are effective collectors of the tiny motes that will likely transfer from the victim's clothing or body while being moved.

Normally, the clothing should not be removed until the forensic pathologist has had an opportunity to inspect the body. Clothing should be unbuttoned, unzipped and pulled off, never torn. Each garment should be placed in a separate clean paper bag. If the clothes cannot be removed without cutting, care must be taken to avoid bullet holes and stabs. Some fabrics will display the pattern of a blunt weapon, such evidence must be preserved.

After the body has been removed, the crime scene search can continue. There will likely be

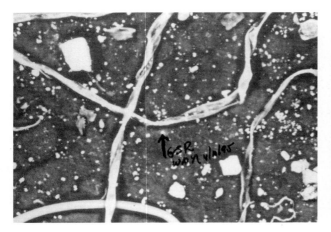

FIGURE II-53. Backscatter electron SEM image of gunshot residue and other particles on sticky stub.

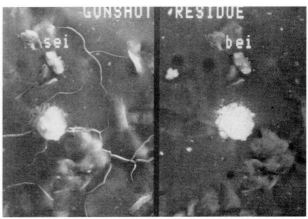

FIGURE II-54. Gunshot residue spheres on sticky stub.

TABLE II-14

GUNSHOT RESIDUE SEM KITS

• Sealed Kit Container • Instruction Sheet • Analysis Request Form • Disposable Gloves	• Vials with 10–15mm aluminum SEM stubs covered with a carbon filled adhesive which fits into the vial cap for: – "Right Back" – "Right Palm" – "Left Back" – "Left Palm"

other physical evidence at the scene. Obviously a bullet through a clock face stopping the clock is of value.

In one case, the conclusion that the multiple stab wounds were self-inflicted was assisted by the presence of an empty aspirin bottle supporting the victim's fingerprints found in the wastebasket at the crime scene, a bloody fingerprint of the victim in a nearby public restroom, and undissolved tablets in the stomach contents. The toxicolo-gist reported lethal concentrations of aspirin in the blood. The stab wounds were superficial in an initial attempt to commit suicide, ultimately accomplished by an overdose of aspirin.

In the final analysis, there will be a great deal of useful evidence at the scene that will assist the pathologist in answering the important questions. The medicolegal investigation cannot occur solely on the autopsy table.

COLLECTING TRACE EVIDENCE

When evidence is collected, the source and disposition of that evidence must be documented in a complete chain of custody. There needs to be a clear record as to whom the items were given or where they were stored. Forms and containers designed for all of the varied types of trace evi-dence are not usually readily available, although commercial sexual assault evidence collection kits provide much of what is needed. These kits usually contain instructions and chain of custody forms, labeled envelopes for each of the types of evidence to be collected, such as combed and

TABLE II-15
SEXUAL ASSAULT EVIDENCE

- Hospital Report Forms
- Paper containers for clothing items
- Miscellaneous trace evidence container
- Fingernail scrapings kit and container
- Head hair collection kit and container
- Pubic hair combings collection kit and container
- Saliva sample kit and container
- Oral, anal, and vaginal swab kit with swabs, slides, and containers
- Blood tube

pulled head and pubic hairs, and swabs and slides for semen. A tube for a known blood sample is also included (Table II-15).

Documenting Trace Evidence

Regardless of how the evidence is collected or the types of containers used, each container must be marked so that the pathologist can identify with certainty the specific item in court. Furthermore, each piece of trace evidence needs to be described in notes and reports including the date and time of collection, name of person(s) collecting the evidence, the description of the evidence, a unique identifier-like case number and item number, the location from which each item was recovered, how it was detected, how it was collected, and how it was preserved, supplemented by sketches, measurements and photographs whenever possible. Any impressions must be photographed to ensure that the image of interest (impression) fills the frame of the viewfinder while the film plane is parallel with the surface on which the impression is found, so that the imaging does not distort the evidence. If chemical enhancements are attempted, the impressions should be photographed before and after the treatment. A scale should be included in each photograph so the photographic print can be made to actual size.

Collecting Trace Evidence

The most common way to collect trace evidence is direct picking using gloved fingers or clean forceps. To protect the collected item from loss or contamination, it is immediately placed in a clean container such as a new Petri dish, plastic bag, envelope, or folded paper packet. Adhesive tape is also frequently used to pick up evidence and the collected lifts are typically placed adhesive side down on a transparent backing such as a clear plastic sheet protector, glass slide or Petri dish. Additionally, a clean spatula, scalpel or pocketknife can be used to scrape and dislodge trace evidence from an item onto a clean piece of paper. The paper with the collected debris, blood crusts, or paint chips is usually folded like a pharmacy fold in order to securely contain the small bits of trace evidence. The folded paper can be marked for identification and secured in another container such as a plastic bag or sealed envelope.

Adhesive tape is especially valuable for lifting otherwise invisible microscopic-size materials. Most often, tape is used by the trace evidence examiner for collecting fibers. The same technique that is used for lifting fingerprints can be used to collect trace evidence, whether lifting a footwear impression, a fabric impression or an accumulation of hairs and fibers. After the impression or debris is discovered, an identification tag for the lift is prepared upon which is written: (1) case number, (2) date, (3) time, (4) name of person collecting lift, (5) object from which material is being lifted, and (6) location on object, including distances from landmarks and orientation directions (up and down or compass direction). The tag can be shown in its correct orientation (right side up) in any close-up photographs of the evidence and then incorporated in the lift as an identification tag.

To lift something like a fabric impression, use one and a half inch wide transparent tape (wider if for a shoeprint or a widespread 1:1 replication lift or lay strips parallel to each other to cover the area of interest), strip off a length of tape and attach the loose end to the surface near the impression so that the tape can be positioned over the fabric impression or debris of interest. Press down firmly, starting at the end attached to the surface and apply even pressure across the length and width of the tape. After the impression or area of interest is completely covered by the tape, lift it off with a smooth, even movement, holding the still attached roll. The powder, fibers and other particles will adhere to the tape. Stick the loose end to a clean surface like a clipboard, slide a clear plastic backer under the tape, and again starting at the affixed end apply pressure toward the other end still attached to the roll. Place the identification tag, which might already have been used in a photograph, between the tape and the backer in a position where it does not interfere with the microtraces, just before the remaining tape is pressed onto the backer. If need be, the tape can be further pressed onto the backer using a pencil eraser.[16,17] Gelatin lifters can also be used in a similar way for lifting footwear impressions from floors.

It is sometimes valuable to replicate the location and patterns of the microtraces over wider areas on clothing, vehicle interiors and furniture upholstery, so that there is one-to-one correspondence between the particles recovered with the tape and the exact location from where they originated. The entire surface of interest is covered with strips of tape and each piece is numbered, photographed, and mapped in order to allow the exact location of each tape to be documented (Fig. II-55). When the tapes are pulled from the surface, the 1:1 taping method records the precise original location of all the microtraces. Ideally, the method should be used right at the crime scene before anything is moved. In cases of homicide, bodies and the area surrounding the body are good candidates for replication taping.[18]

Less commonly, a vacuum cleaner equipped with a specially designed disposable filter trap can be used to recover trace evidence from larger areas such as carpets and vehicles. The filter and its contents should be immediately packaged to avoid loss of the dust. The nearby vacuum parts, hose, etc. must be rigorously cleaned between each vacuuming to avoid cross-contamination with the next sample. Vacuuming should only be considered after other techniques have been attempted, as the sweeping is relatively non-discriminating and usually results in the collection of a large amount of out-of-context extraneous dust.

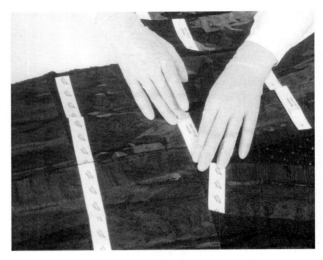

Figure II-55. A 1:1 replication taping of a sweater. Each strip of tape is labeled and the location photographed or diagramed.

A clean comb or brush can be used to recover microtraces in hair. The comb and collected debris from the hair can be packaged together. Finally, material can be clipped. Trace evidence can be recovered from fingernails by nail clipping or scraping. Fingernails can be clipped with clean scissors or clippers and packaged in clean paper packets. Alternatively, fingernails can be scraped with a clean toothpick to collect debris from under the nails. Clipping is also appropriate for collecting debris and crusted material in hair or from the pile of carpets. The clippings and debris are folded into a paper packet (Table II-16).

Regardless of the collection technique, the principles are the same. The trace evidence needs to be collected in sufficient quantity to be representative of its source and to allow for a full analysis. It needs to be protected from contamination, deterioration or loss and it needs to be identifiable when the collector is asked at a later date whether the item is the same item claimed to have been collected previously. If the item is wet, it generally needs to be dried. If it is liquid, it needs to be kept cold (refrigerated or frozen) to minimize bacterial growth that might alter the material. If it was discovered in water, it needs to be initially kept in the water until it can be pre-

TABLE II-16

TRACE EVIDENCE COLLECTION

• Picking	• Sweeping
• Lifting	• Combing
• Scraping	• Clipping

served in the laboratory. If it is volatile, it needs to be sealed in an inert airtight container so the material of interest does not evaporate.

Exemplars

To complete the trace evidence comparison process, the pathologist often assists with the collection of exemplars such as, hair and blood from the deceased. The identification and comparison of trace evidence requires quality exemplars which adequately represent the tissues sampled. For DNA analysis, a sample of blood should be placed in a tube which has been charged with EDTA, like a purple top Vacutainer®. On occasion, bone, usually best the femur, or thigh muscle can be used when whole blood is not available.

In addition to the combed *hair samples* collected primarily for the purpose of locating foreign hairs, known pulled hairs should be collected from each of the hairy regions of the body. Between 50 and 100 pulled head hairs and more than 25 pulled pubic hairs should be collected for comparisons. Although normally scalp and pubic hairs are collected, if the deceased has a beard or large amount of chest hair, samples from these regions should also be obtained. If there is a blunt force wound near the eyebrow, samples of eyebrow hairs should be obtained for comparison with hairs on the weapon. No hair comparison can be made without obtaining an exemplar from the homologous somatic region unless the hairs are to be compared by DNA alone. Scalp hairs must be compared with scalp hairs, beard hair with beard hair, and pubic hair with pubic hair. There is usually only one chance to obtain the necessary exemplars. Exhumation has been required on too many occasions because the appropriate exemplars were not obtained at the time of autopsy.

Glass is often valuable trace evidence. For example, small microscopic size glass fragments from broken windows are often trapped on burglars' clothing. The trace evidence laboratory can recover these fragments. The investigator must collect known samples for comparison. Normally, the known sample will come from a broken window at the crime scene. It must be remembered that glass still remaining in the window is required as an exemplar. Before the glass is removed from the window, it should be marked *outside* and *inside*. Sometimes it is important to know from which direction the window was broken and the properly identified pieces from the window can be used for that determination. In addition to the exemplar from the window itself, all of the broken glass lying below the window needs to be collected and preserved. The loose glass will be searched for finger and footprints and used to reconstruct how the window was broken. In the case of multiple gunshots through the window, the reconstructed glass can show which trajectory was first. If a relatively large piece of broken glass is found associated with the burglar, it can be fracture matched with a piece from the broken window.

Sometimes questioned paint samples from the scene of a hit and run accident will be sufficient in size that they can be fracture matched with the remaining chips at the scene or on a hit and run vehicle (Fig. II-56). More commonly, the finish and primer coat sequences can be determined even from very small chips of paint. From this information, it is sometimes possible to determine the possible make and model of automobile even before a suspect vehicle is found. When a suspected source is located, it is mandatory that the known paint, whether scraped from a door jam or from a car, include all layers. The chips collected must be scraped all the way to the substrate (wood, plastic or metal), using a gouge. It is also likely that similar appearing paint from different locations on a vehicle will actually be different paint; therefore, exemplars should be collected from all the various parts of a vehicle

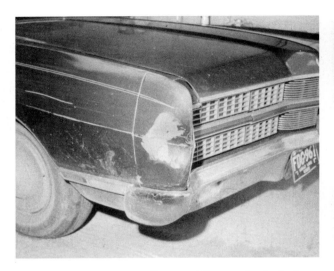

FIGURE II-56. Figure 13: Corner of damaged vehicle from which large fragments of paint have fractured.

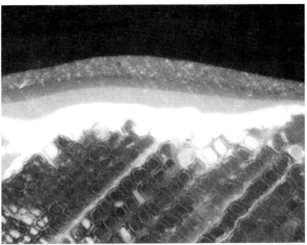

FIGURE II-57. Layers of paint on wooden hull of damaged ship.

and different parts of a door or cabinet (Fig. II-57).

Soil seems relatively simple to collect from vehicles, clothing and bodies. In general, the soil needs to be picked from the surface or scraped into a folded paper or foil packet, plastic film canister, Petri dish, or plastic bag. If it appears that the questioned soil differs in color or texture from place to place, the different appearing crumbs need to be collected separately and packaged in separate containers.

Unfortunately, experience and anecdotal evidence continue to suggest that difficulties with forensic soil analysis revolve mainly around problems of sample collection. Without good exemplars, soil comparisons are often useless. The main question in forensic soil cases is: Could a questioned soil sample have originated from the scene of the crime? In order to answer that question properly, it must be probable that if the questioned soil came from the scene, that the same soil is found at the scene and collected as a known sample. There is nothing else in criminalistics where the proper choice of an exemplar is more difficult than with soil. The reason for the difficulty is because soil is a dynamic accumulation of particles constantly changing and usually changing over very short distances affected by both natural processes and man. There is local

spatial heterogeneity in both profile depth and landscape area. There are also distinct regional or geographic differences affected primarily by the geology and terrain of the region.

Four distinct types of soil samples might need to be collected in a single case. (1) Questioned samples may be either unconsolidated dust, crumbs, stratified, or bulk accumulations of soil. They are samples about which we ask, what is their origin? (2) Primary comparison samples are of known origin from the locus or spot from which it is thought the questioned sample originated, (3) Alibi samples are used as elimination samples. The source of these samples is dictated by the accused as an excuse for the soil associated to them. Alibi samples are of paramount importance because criminalistics is essentially an exclusionary process where exclusions enhance the associated evidence, and (4) Delineating samples constitutes a site survey. These samples are either prescribed by a previously agreed upon collection pattern, like the so-called *grid*, or selected at the site. These samples help measure the variability of soil in the region and across the site and thereby help establish the probative value of the soil evidence.

In order to select the proper sample, soil samples should be thought of as a sampling volume rather than as the sampling area. Although soil is an accumulation of heterogeneous particles, the sample must reflect a coherent consolidated volume of soil. Samples are chosen either from the exact location (locus) from which the questioned soil was apparently transferred as suggested by a footwear impression in the soil, for example; or geomorphologic features of the site, such as (1) relief, drainage, erosion; (2) color and mottling; (3) texture, structure (crumb, granular, blocky, prismatic, columnar and platy) and consistency (dry–hard or soft; moist–firm or friable; wet–sticky or plastic); and (4) vegetation are used to detect the various soils present from which samples are collected at random with the hopes that one might match the questioned soil (Fig. II-58). Particularly in burials, differences can also occur due to digging through the surface, which is detected by slump, compaction, vegetation changes, disturbed soil profiles, and impressions. Mixed soil from burials is often mottled in color and texture. Of all these characteristics, probably color is the most useful and can be relied on to identify different soils in the field. The investigator will need a little empathy with the criminal activity and empathy with environmental factors, which might account for the transfer of soil to the participants, in order to be lucky enough to find the right exemplar. Soils do not vary in the field by equal invariable distances, units or increments like a grid; the different soils will occur more like a mosaic with fractal dimensions rather than a grid. The more that is known about the crime and about the questioned soil sample, the more likely that the location from where the soil originated will be found.

The collection technique is not trivial either. Surface samples are most commonly needed and should be collected with a sharpened 3–5 inch pointed trowel (archaeologist's trowel) from the surface to a depth of no more than 1/4 inch,

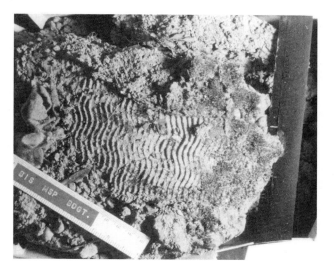

FIGURE II-58. Clod of soil with footwear impression.

although a spoon will work. Samples from soil profiles are often necessary, particularly for comparison of soil on tools used to bury evidence. A test excavation or pit is dug and the best-lighted face is troweled clean and vertical revealing the entire soil profile. Blocks of soil from each profile of interest are then cut with the trowel and kept intact as much as possible. The blocks are wrapped in aluminum foil in order to preserve the orientation and structure of the coherent volume. In the laboratory, the samples can be dried in place by opening the foil. If thin layers of soil are represented in the profile, then micro-monoliths can be collected from the profile; each sample then represents a volume with intact layers. Either a stainless steel pocket box or a plastic Petri dish, used like a cookie cutter, can be used to collect the layered samples. The micro-monoliths can then be impregnated with resin while still in the box to serve as a permanent exhibit of the layering or small samples of each layer can be excised for analysis in the laboratory.

EXAMPLES OF USING TRACE EVIDENCE

There are too many types of trace evidence and too many case situations where trace evidence can be useful to list them all effectively or to illustrate them all in detail within a chapter's length. Continuing a well-intentioned discussion about more trace evidence might only momentarily teach the investigator what to look for and where. Crime scene investigators cannot be expected to rely upon memory alone to recognize trace evidence; therefore the goal is to help them to think more divergently, thereby becoming more attuned to using all types of trace evidence to solve cases.

Hence, this chapter culminates in a series of homely stories that illustrate how trace evidence is collected and used to resolve death investigations. They are entitled with reference to their place in the **somatotactsis**. The stories are parabolic in some ways and are intended to arrest the attention of the readers, encourage them to compare features of each story to their own experiences, and excite curiosity about how trace evidence could be used during their career. In most of the stories, the actual findings from the trace evidence examination are not described in detail in order to leave the story stuck in the reader's psychic craw and force the reader to think through the possibilities illustrated. In that way, the investigator may be better prepared to make the necessary choices to resolve dilemmas and unanticipated circumstances and to make better use of previously unrecognized trace evidence.

The characters are: Victoria Timm, the female victim who is raped, murdered and run over by a car; Dominick Guy, the suspect who never commits a crime without leaving a clue; Inspector C. S. I. Wright, the trace evidence specialist and crime scene investigator, who seems to understand the value of trace evidence more than anyone; and Dr. Florence P. Whydoc, the board certified forensic pathologist, who often plays a central role in the medicolegal investigation of death.

Limbic Intent

Victoria Timm lay dead in the morgue and an autopsy was about to be conducted by Dr. Florence P. Whydoc. Timm had been found dead of an apparent gunshot wound to the side of her head. It was obvious to Dr. Whydoc that the weapon had not been in close contact with the head, but otherwise, the initial observations did not indicate whether Timm had died from a self-inflicted wound or whether from the hand of another.

Inspector C.S.I. Wright found the gun at the scene where Timm had been discovered along with a handwritten suicide note signed "Victoria." The rain the night before seemed to preclude the discovery of fingerprints on the gun and likewise, gunshot residues were not evident on Timm's hands. The gun was unregistered. Bad blood between Timm and an ex-boyfriend, Dominick Guy, caused some suspicion, nonetheless. Wright collected the note and gun as evidence and proceeded to look into the whereabouts of Guy.

Wright contacted Guy and asked for a sample of his handwriting for comparison with the suicide note. He noticed a pad of paper on the coffee table which seemed to be similar to the paper on which the suicide note had been written, so he asked if he could have it. He would later ask the laboratory to determine if the suicide note could have originated from the pad and to see if there was any impressed writing on the pad. Wright also noticed that there was a makeshift target range behind Guy's house, even though Guy said he did not own a gun. Behind the target, Wright removed fired bullets from a tree. The handwriting samples and bullets were compared with the handwriting on the note and the bullet recovered from Timm's brain. They both matched. Guy had written the note and had at one time owned or used the gun used to shoot Timm.

Distal Approach

Inspector C.S. I. Wright faced a daunting task as he was confronted with three fire victims who could not escape an apparent arson fire. Initial evidence at the fire scene indicated that someone had broken through a rear door of the two-flat apartment building and thrown a Molotov cocktail into the first floor hallway igniting an inferno from which no one escaped. The only hope of determining who may have started the fire would have to come from trace evidence collected outside of the building. Inspector Wright knew that the arsonist must have approached the building from the alley behind; therefore, that is where he began his search.

The ground was soft next to the garage across the alley from the fire scene. Wright located tire impressions from a vehicle that had pulled into the space next to the garage and backed out and continued down the alley. The width of the vehicle stance and wheelbase were measured; the tire impressions were photographed and plaster-casted. In the location where the driver must have stepped out of the vehicle, footwear impressions were photographed and casted. As is often the case where old cars are used in crimes, debris had fallen from the interior as the door was opened. The debris included tuffs of carpet and a paper matchbook. The carpet fibers were collected and packaged and the matchbook was protected for fingerprints. A paper match found outside the back door of the burned building was subsequently physically matched with the matchbook, thereby demonstrating the connection between the arson and the vehicle. As the vehicle backed out of the space and sped down the alley, it bumped over a parking block and left behind a clod of dirt that apparently fell from the undercarriage. The dirt proved to have an interesting assortment of minerals, grass and weed seeds that could be compared with dirt remaining attached to the undercarriage.

Axial Reach

As Dr. Florence P. Whydoc and Inspector C.S.I. Wright viewed the scene of another murder together, they pondered how they might find trace evidence to connect the suspect, Dominick Guy, with the shooting death of a total stranger, Victoria Timm. There was no evidence of forced entry into Timm's apartment, but there was evidence of a brief struggle before Timm had been shot three times. Drawers and cabinets in the apartment had been opened and rummaged. Guy was arrested on a tip from a confidential informant. He denied responsibility and denied he knew Timm or knew where the apartment was located. He claimed to have never been in the apartment, "wherever it was." Dr. Whydoc headed back to the hospital to await delivery of

the body. If the gun could be located, Dr. Whydoc knew she would be able to recover bullets from the body for comparison. Otherwise, the evidence at the scene was likely more valuable for identifying the perpetrator.

Wright had the foresight to ask that gunshot residue samples be collected from the hands and face of the suspect. As he had nothing to hide, Guy agreed to the procedure and samples were collected in accordance with the procedures outlined in the kit. Inspector Wright confirmed that the samples had been collected along with controls from the officers collecting the samples. Guy's clothing had also been collected and packaged in new paper bags.

The crime scene was processed for fingerprints. Finger and palm impressions were recorded and lifted where possible. A number of items were collected from the scene and sent to the laboratory for processing using superglue and other enhancement techniques available. Three loose dark brown head hairs were collected from the rummaged cupboards and a broken fingernail was recovered from inside an open drawer. Timm's nails seemed to be intact. A call to the police station confirmed immediately that the suspect's right thumbnail appeared to have been recently broken off. Guy remarked to the detective, "Yeah, that thumbnail seems to grow faster and it is always breaking off."

Axial-proximal Clothing

Sexual homicide is one of the most heinous crimes and as the medicolegal investigative team stood around the autopsy table which held Victoria Timm, the victim of the most recent brutal attack, Inspector C.S. I. Wright was asked for his advice on how to best preserve evidence that might still be on the clothing. Wright explained that the clothing itself is a potential source of all types of trace evidence but the search should have begun at the scene of the crime before Timm was even moved to the morgue. Nevertheless, the clothing was searched using a strong light and by concentrating on small areas over her entire body, front and back. After each item of interest was photographed and its location indicated on an appropriate diagram, it was placed in a separate container (paper packet or envelope), marked for identification, and described in the notes. Direct inspection of Timm's clothing revealed a faint impression, possibly footwear, on the back of her jacket. Fragments of glass, paint, and metal were found scattered over the back of her pants.

The second step was to use transparent tape as a lifter to collect the microscopic size microtraces. The tape can be used as a roller device, but in this case Wright chose to use individual strips and laid them over the entire surface of the clothing. After each piece was numbered, photographed and mapped, the individual pieces were removed and placed sticky-side down on transparent plastic sheet protectors.

Finally, the clothing was removed, one item at a time, without cutting or damaging the item in any preventable way. As each item of clothing was removed, it was immediately spread out onto a clean piece of paper to allow the garment to dry as much as possible before it was folded together with the paper on which it was laid and placed in a clean paper bag in order to preserve any trace evidence that might have fallen off the clothing onto the paper. The bag was then marked for identification and the contents described in the investigator's notes.

A variety of trace materials were ultimately identified on Timm's clothing including blood, semen, and saliva from the assailant, foreign pubic hairs, fibers from the assailant's sweater, soil from where she had been initially assaulted, and her own feces. Feces were found at the scene of the assault as well.

Proximal Surface

The bruised and battered body of Victoria Timm lay on the autopsy table. She had been found lying nude along side the highway. Dr. Florence P. Whydoc noted some marks on Timm's body and showed them to Inspector C.S. I. Wright. Wright photographed a number of marks which were either footwear impressions or impressions from a fabric or floor mat. There were also marks that could be a transfer of ink

from a label or some other type of printing. Each mark was photographed so that the image filled the viewfinder of the camera and the film plane was parallel with the surface on which the impression was found. A scale (ruler) was included in each photograph along with a label that identified the case number, location, time, date and person collecting the evidence. The exact source of the impressions would not be known until comparison sources were submitted.

A bright light and alternate light source (ALS) were also used by Wright to search for stains on the body. Suspected blood, semen, and saliva stains were collected with a cotton swab moistened with deionized water. The swab was allowed to dry naturally, that is, without extra heat, and packaged in a paper envelope for safekeeping. The location of each sample was documented. No other trace evidence was found. The deceased was then ready for autopsy.

Proximal Entrance

In most cases, the cause and manner of death are obvious, the external wounds are apparent and often account for death. Victoria Timm's autopsy was such an example. Timm had been assaulted in her bedroom by an intruder. As Dr. Florence P. Whydoc viewed the body, she knew that her responsibility would be to assist the police in demonstrating the manner and cause of death, but, more importantly, assist the police in identifying the killer. Therefore, in addition to anatomical findings, physical evidence from the body would need to be collected. As Dr. Whydoc proceeded with the autopsy, the trace evidence became apparent. Timm had been assaulted in three distinct ways.

One, she had been struck with a blunt object on the head which left a surface mark that seemed to represent the size and shape of a hammer head. The mark was photographed using a scale and keeping the film plane parallel to the surface. In another area of the scalp, a depressed fracture of the frontal bone was found under a deep laceration. Marks from two tines of a claw hammer were evident. After careful photography, the portions of bone which included the fractures were excised with a bone saw to permit the laboratory to have a good look at the cut and fractured surfaces in the event that tool marks or paint left on the bone might be compared with the claw hammer recovered at the scene.

Two, she had been shot with a single shotgun blast to her chest. The shot was from relatively close range. The pathologist was able to recover wads, shot collar, and steel shot from the entrance wound in addition to pieces of clothing and apparent intervening paper and glass of unknown origin. The fragments of paper and glass turned out to be from a family picture normally sitting on Timm's bedside stand.

Three, Timm had been sexually assaulted. A broken wooden table leg had been inserted into her vagina, penetrating through her uterus into her abdomen. The broken and splintered table leg was found at the crime scene and Dr. Whydoc recovered wood splinters and semen from Timm's vagina.

Internal Organs

Victoria Timm lay on the autopsy table, the victim of a drive-by shooting. Dr. Florence P. Whydoc was all too familiar with these cases. The autopsy was routine and the only real physical evidence were the bullets and bullet fragments to be recovered. X-rays documented the locations of the bullets. The bullets were never touched with a metal tool and care was always taken to preserve the markings which could allow the bullets to be associated with the gun. As each was recovered, where possible the base of the bullet was inscribed with initials and identifying number, being careful not to mark anywhere near the rifling marks. In those instances where the bullet was too small or damaged to permit initialing, the bullet itself was not marked, but simply placed in a small box or envelope, which was immediately labeled with the case number, a description of where the bullet was recovered, the date, time and initials of the person recovering and sealing the evidence. None of the bullets were rinsed or washed before they were packaged. Dr. Whydoc knew that the forensic microscopist might want to inspect the

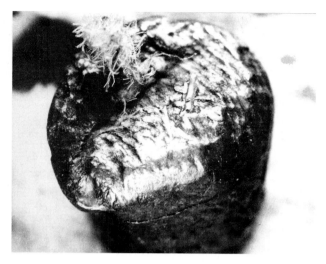

FIGURE II-59. Fibers from clothing trapped in the soft lead of a .38 caliber bullet.

bullets for evidence of intervening materials such as paint, glass, or fibers (Fig. II-59). The presence of these trace evidence materials sometimes assists with determining the trajectory of ricocheted bullets and thereby assists with determining the location of the shooter. The wound track and trajectory of one bullet was of particular interest and Dr. Whydoc noted in the x-ray images the presence of opaque fragments. The larger fragments were recovered directly, using just the fingers, and placed in separate envelopes. Smaller fragments were left in excised tissue, either to be recovered in the trace evidence laboratory or by sectioning in the histology laboratory.

Internal Tissues

Dr. Florence P. Whydoc sat at her microscope and pondered a case she had received from a colleague. The colleague was assisting an attorney who was investigating a case of possible medical malpractice. Although Dr. Whydoc did not have many details, she knew the case involved a 35-year-old woman on TPN following bowel resection. Dr. Whydoc was asked to look at the histological slides to help determine the origin of what seemed to be foreign material in the lung tissue sections. She identified the material as being consistent with magnesium silicate (talc) but instead of speculating on the origin of the material based solely on its morphology and reaction to histological stains, she decided to send the unstained microscopic slides together with photographs of areas which contained the crystalline materials on these slides to the laboratory. At the laboratory the foreign material was identified by a combination of polarized light microscopy (PLM) and electron microscopy (SEM and TEM) as talc.

Internal Fluids

No sooner had Dr. Florence P. Whydoc entered the autopsy suite, that Inspector C.S.I. Wright blurted out, "Doc, we need to know when she died." After several minutes of explanation of how difficult it was and after learning more about the circumstances surrounding Victoria Timm's demise, Dr. Whydoc began the autopsy. During the course of the autopsy, Dr. Whydoc recovered all the stomach contents and transferred them to a clean jar. She directed Wright to take them to the trace evidence laboratory and ask that they identify the contents. Fortunately, Wright called ahead, because the laboratory told him they did not do this type of analysis and directed him to a more specialized laboratory which had experience in the microscopic identification of all sorts of materials, including foodstuffs. The laboratory wanted to know from Wright what types of food were reportedly consumed by Timm and when. While Wright collected the information, he kept the stomach contents refrigerated.

Proximal Exit

Victoria Timm had obviously been shot from long range. The fatal shot was to the head and the trajectory was reasonably clear to Dr. Florence P. Whydoc. On the other hand, a second through and through wound to her left thigh was more problematic. The entrance and exit were similar in appearance and the only difference was a thin black ring on one of the wounds. Realizing that this black discoloration may represent soot, in which case the wound in question would

be an entrance bullet wound of a shot fired at contact range, she decided to collect a sample from the injury and submit it to the laboratory for gunshot residue (GSR) analysis. At the same time, Dr. Whydoc did microscopic examination of another portion of the wound with the expectation of gunpowder in the deeper tissues.

Proximal Surface

Dr. Florence P. Whydoc knew from the livor mortis on Victoria Timm's back that she had been moved at least once since she was shot. The police were obviously interested in learning where she died. Dr. Whydoc noted mud smeared on Timm's buttocks. She carefully scraped the mud from the skin surface using a new scalpel and transferred the material to a clean, folded paper packet. The mud was marked for identification and given to Inspector C.S.I. Wright for transfer to the forensic microscopy laboratory to be compared with the environment in which Timm had been found and to determine whether any trace evidence might suggest a possible locale from where she had been moved.

The laboratory had explained to Wright sometime before that the dust particles are identified by optical microscopy using a polarizing microscope. After some delay, Inspector Wright received a telephone call with the report from the microscopy laboratory. Timm had been found nude in a plowed field along side a paved highway. The mud from her body included at least four types of materials that seemed to be from mutually exclusive environments: quartz and limestone dust particles, clay, feldspar mineral grains and pollen from soil; yellow paint particles, reflective glass beads, asphalt particles and tire wear particles from the highway; and degraded carpet tufts and trunk lining fibers, apparently from the trunk of the suspects car; and paper fibers, plaster dust, wood fragments, and paint chips.

Proximal-axial Clothing

Sadly, on New Year's Eve a speeding motorist struck Victoria Timm when she was crossing the street. The police were in search of a hit-and-run driver. Fortunately, Timm's clothing was immediately sent to the laboratory for analysis. The trace evidence recovered from the clothing included an impression of a license plate on the inside of the right pant leg and small chips of green paint on the left elbow of her fleece jacket.

Axial Contact

Inspector C.S. I. Wright entered Dominick Guy's house for the first time early Saturday morning. He had a search warrant and a problem. Victoria Timm's body had been found slumped in the passenger side seat of her car. A bullet had ripped through her left external carotid artery and fourth cervical vertebra, killing her. The bullet had exited and Inspector Wright suspected he might find it in a wall of Guy's house. He was also looking for blood spatters. Timm had been in Guy's house often before, therefore the mere presence of fingerprints or even some blood stains were of no use.

Sure enough, there was a small hole in the drywall just under a picture on a bedroom wall. There also appeared to be a fine mist-like spatter pattern on the headboard of the bed. A search of the room behind the wall did not reveal an exit hole; therefore the bullet must either be lodged in the wall or have fallen where it would be found on the baseplate between the studs. A small hand saw was used to cut away the drywall surrounding the hole and when the bullet was not located, a portion of the drywall at the base of the wall was similarly removed. The bullet, which lay on the baseplate, was secured in a sealed box and transferred to the trace evidence laboratory for inspection.

In the meantime, the fine spatter was photographed to demonstrate its presence and a specialist in blood spatter analysis was called for assistance. After investigating and documenting the spatter, the small crusts were scraped from the headboard and placed in a folded paper packet. Additional material was collected with a moistened swab. The evidence were submitted to the DNA laboratory.

Soon thereafter, Dominick Guy protested that the bullet was from his gun, which he had accidentally discharged a month or so earlier. He produced the gun and proclaimed his innocence. Microscopic examination of the bullet revealed small pieces of a gold necklace worn by Timm and pieces of bone embedded in the lead.

Distal Leaving

After a short struggle, an exchange of gunfire between a dry cleaning establishment owner and a would-be robber left the owner dead. Soon thereafter, Dominick Guy was apprehended not too far away by a responding police officer. Unfortunately, the clerk who witnessed the shooting could not identify Guy as the shooter. She did describe the clothing worn by the robber and produced a pile of clothing left by the robber for dry-cleaning.

Inspector C.S.I. Wright obtained the clothing left at the cleaners and found a stocking cap just outside the door, which seemed to match the description given by the clerk.

The laboratory told Wright that there were numerous short reddish-colored dog hairs on the clothing and several head hairs in the stocking cap. Wright contacted the prosecuting attorney and obtained search warrants for Guy's residence and head hair exemplars. Guy's dog was not located, but the couch was covered with abundant short reddish animal hairs which were recovered and placed in a paper envelope. Guy's head hair was vigorously combed to collect hairs that might more likely fall naturally and accumulate in the stocking cap. Additional hairs totaling more than 50, were pulled from all the separate regions of Guy's scalp. The combed and pulled hairs were packaged and marked separately. These exemplars were submitted to the laboratory for comparison and an additional request was made to search the combed hairs for stocking cap fibers.

Limbic Secreted

As Inspector C.S.I. Wright and Dr. Florence P. Whydoc entered the bank, they immediately saw the bank manager lying face down in the middle of the lobby, dead. Bank tellers reported to the police that the manager, in his sixties, had tried to restrain an elderly woman who had attempted to hold up the bank. Instead the woman fought him off and shot him. As the robber left the bank, the tellers were convinced that it was a man disguised as an elderly woman.

Inspector Wright's colleagues soon learned through an informant the probable identity of the bank robber. The informant led Wright to a place where part of the disguise was secreted away and to another place where the gun was hidden. The gun was in a box that included pieces of a wig. The disguise had included a shaggy wool coat with a dark green acrylic pile lining. Based on the information and discovery of the disguise, a search of Dominick Guy's apartment revealed associative evidence that would ultimately link him, in a trace evidence chain, with the bank manager. Fibers stuck to the bank manager's shirt buttons matched the shaggy outer wool fibers of the coat. Wig fibers on the coat matched the fibers comprising the wig pieces found with the gun. Pieces of the wig were also found in Guy's apartment. Head hairs similar to Guy's were recovered from the pieces of wig from the apartment. Dark green acrylic fibers similar to the coat's lining fibers were found on a black polyester pantsuit found in Guy's apartment.

REFERENCES

1. Siegel, J.A. (Ed.): *Encyclopedia of forensic sciences* (3 volumes). London: Academic Press, 2000.
2. Saferstein, R. (Ed.): *Forensic science handbook* (4 volumes). Englewood Cliffs, N.J.: Prentice Hall, 1982-2001.
3. Houck, M.M. (Ed.): *Mute-witnesses: Trace evidence analysis.* London: Academic Press, 2001.
4. Bisbing, R.E.: Clues in the dust. *American Laboratory,* November 1989.
5. Locard, E.: The analysis of dust traces. *The American Journal of Police Science, 1:* 276, 1930.
6. Osterburg, J.W.: *The crime laboratory.* New York: Clark Boardman Company, 1982.
7. Hilderbrand, D.S.: *Footwear, the missed evidence.* Temecula, CA: Staggs Publishing, 1999.
8. Bodziak, W.J.: *Footwear impression evidence detection, recovery and examination,* 2nd edition. Cleveland: CRC Press, 1999
9. Smith, S.: *Mostly murder.* New York: David McKay Company, Inc., 1959.
10. Humecki, H.J. (Ed.): *Practical guide to infrared microspectroscopy.* New York: Marcel Dekker, Inc., 1995.
11. McCrone, W.C., McCrone, L.B., and Delly, J.G.: *Polarized light microscopy.* Chicago: McCrone Research Institute, 1995.
12. Messerschmidt, R.G., and Harthcock, M.A. (Eds.): *Infrared microspectroscopy.* New York: Marcell Dekker, Inc., 1968.
13. Pelton, W.R.: Distinguishing the cause of textile fiber damage using the scanning electron microscope (SEM). *Journal of Forensic Sciences, 40:* 874–882, 1995.
14. Postek, M.T., Howard, K.S., Johnson, A.H., and McMichael, K.L.: *Scanning electron microscopy.* Burlington, VT: Ladd Research Industries, 1980.
15. Spiegel, J., and Machotka, P.: *Messages of the body.* New York: The Free Press, 1974.
16. Bridges, B.C.: *Practical fingerprinting.* New York: Funk & Wagnalls Company, 1942.
17. Myre, D.C.: *Death investigation.* Alexandria, VA: International Association of Chiefs of Police, 1974.
18. Robertson, J., and Grieve, M.: *Forensic examination of fibers,* 2nd edition. Sydney: Taylor & Francis, 1999.

Chapter III

TIME OF DEATH AND CHANGES AFTER DEATH

Part 1

ANATOMICAL CONSIDERATIONS

JOSHUA A. PERPER

DEFINITION OF DEATH

THE DEFINITION OF DEATH is important to both the medical and legal professions. While it is true that for the clinician the demise of a patient signals the unfortunate end to the medical effort, the very determination of death may carry secondary therapeutic implications regarding transplantation of organs. Death is often the starting point for involvement of the forensic pathologist. Similarly for attorneys, the death of an individual may generate a great number of legal challenges related to inheritance rights, estate management, criminal liability and tortious injuries.

Until the 1960s, the *cessation of circulation and respiration* was the unchallenged definition of death. For example, the 1968 edition of *Black's Law Dictionary* defined death as: *the cessation of life; the ceasing to exist; defined by physicians as the total stoppage of the circulation of the blood, and a cessation of vital functions consequent thereon, such as respiration, pulsation, etc.*

As a matter of fact, even today in most deaths, particularly in those which occur outside hospitals or are unwitnessed, the criteria used are still the cessation of circulation and respiration.

However, the classical definition of death has been challenged in recent times by two medical advances:

1. Advanced resuscitation techniques (cardiopulmonary resuscitation [CPR], mouth-to-mouth, heart massage, electric shock) capable of effectively reviving many of the *clinically dead.*
2. Advanced life-sustaining equipment capable of maintaining blood pressure, circulation, and respiration in individuals with severe brain injury.

Though the first instance of mouth-to-mouth resuscitation was recorded long ago in the biblical story of the Prophet Elijah resuscitating a child (II Kings 4: 32–36), modern cardiac massage, electric shock, and routine CPR came into use only three decades ago.

These developments necessitated, in many cases, the obvious revision of the definition of death from just *cessation* to *irreversible cessation* of respiratory and heart activity following modern resuscitation attempts. The reversibility of the death process is dependent on the capability of tissues to recover from the effects of ischemia/anoxia occurring between the advent of clinical death to the initiation of effective resuscitation. The resistance of various organs to ischemia/anoxia is variable, with the central nervous system displaying a particularly high sensitivity. The classic literature indicates that a four to six minute period of cerebral anoxia from a delay in effective resuscitation will commonly result in irreversible and extensive brain damage. However, more recent experimental and clinical evidence points to instances where the reversible interval may be as long as fifteen to sixteen minutes.[1]

Young children and hypothermic individuals are known to resist cerebral hypoxia for thirty minutes or more with no ill effects. In a case reported by Kvittingen and Naess,[2] a five-year old boy fell into a partly frozen river and recovered fully following a presumed submersion time of twenty-two minutes.

The development of life-sustaining equipment has also changed the definition of death by permitting a dissociation between a severely hypoxic or dead brain (incapable of sustaining spontaneous respiration and circulation) and the peripheral organs which can be kept alive artificially. Therefore, the definition of death in a person with severe and irreversible brain injury, incapable of sustaining spontaneous respiration and/or circulation, had to be revised to include what is now defined as *brain death.*

The clinical definition of *brain death* was first advanced in 1968 by the *Ad Hoc* Committee of the Harvard Medical School.[3] The committee, which consisted of physicians, a theologian and a lawyer, defined the following conditions for determining irreversible brain death:

1. *Unreceptivity and unresponsitivity,* including a total lack of response to the most intense painful stimuli.
2. No movement or spontaneous respiration, defined as no effort to breathe for three minutes off the respirator with the patient's carbon dioxide tension normal and room air being breathed for ten minutes prior to the trial.
3. No reflexes fixed, non-reactive pupils, and a lack of cranial nerve reflexes (corneal, pharyngeal, ocular movements in response to head turning and irrigation of ears with ice water, etc.).
4. Isoelectric electroencephalogram.

The committee suggested that all tests be repeated in twenty-four hours and emphasized that the determination of the irreversibility of cerebral damage should be made only after the exclusion of potentially reversible conditions, such as hypothermia (temperature below 90° F [32.2° C]) and central nervous system depressants such as barbiturates.

In subsequent years, the list of reversible causes of coma has been expanded to include metabolic neuromuscular blockade, shock and young age (less than five years of age).

Also, additional objective tests besides electroencephalogram were added to the determination of brain death, such as cerebral angiograph and radionuclide studies, in order to confirm the absence of cerebral blood flow.

In 1977, the National Institute of Neurological Diseases and Stroke conducted a collaborative study which somewhat refined the Harvard criteria. The criteria of brain death proposed by the collaborative study were as follows:

1. Coma and cerebral unresponsiveness.
2. Apnea.
3. Dilated pupils.
4. Absent cephalic (brainstem) reflexes.
5. Electrocerebral silence.

These criteria were to be present for thirty minutes at least six hours after the onset of coma and apnea, and all appropriate diagnostic therapeutic procedures were to be performed. Confirmatory tests of cerebral blood flow were necessary if one of the standards was doubtful or could not be tested.

Starting with Kansas in 1968, increasing numbers of states have adopted the definition of brain death. In 1980, representatives of the American Bar Association and the National Conference of Commissioners of Uniform State Laws agreed upon a model legislative definition of death: *An individual who has sustained either, (1) irreversible cessation of circulatory and respiratory functions or, (2) irreversible cessation of all functions of the entire brain, including the brainstem, is dead. A determination of death shall be made in accordance with accepted medical standards.*

It has been pointed out that in spite of some differences between the legal definitions of brain death in various states, *physicians can meet the requirements of all of them by:*

1. Using the commonly accepted criteria of brain death.
2. Having two physicians, one of whom is a neurologist, make the brain death determination.
3. Avoiding a conflict of interest in having physicians separate from the transplant team, certifying the brain death of a potential donor.
4. Determining brain death before removing any organs or disconnecting life-support systems.[4]

As a matter of fact, a number of states have formally incorporated such provisions into their laws.

The Pathology of Brain Death and Persistent Vegetative State (PVS)

The brain findings of *brain death* or so-called *respirator brain* are characteristic on gross examination. The brain has a dusky, grayish appearance, with marked swelling and evidence of transtentorial hippocampal and tonsillar herniation. A musty odor may be present. Depending on survival time, the cerebral parenchyma shows a variable spectrum of anoxic/ischemic damage from minimal changes to severe encephalomalacia and liquefaction, and generally cannot be satisfactorily examined prior to fixation.

Microscopic findings in *respirator brains* are variable, non-specific, non-diagnostic and correlate poorly with gross findings.

Brain death changes generally become apparent approximately twelve to sixteen hours after cessation of the cerebral circulation. In some cases, changes may be evident after only six hours, and in others they may be delayed for twenty-four hours or longer.

Rapid *respirator brain* changes may be observed in cases with acute onset, such as severe head trauma or sudden cardiac arrest with delayed resuscitation. Delayed manifestations of brain death are seen in chronically ill persons with brain tumors or metabolic problems.[5]

Sometimes identification of true ante mortem hemorrhages or contusions may be substantially obscured or hampered by *respirator brain*-related hemorrhages.

Agonal changes in the microcirculation, such as petechiae in leptomeninges and cerebral parenchyma, may be dramatically accentuated in cases of brain death. Stagnant or stasis thrombi in veins and arteries may also be present and should be distinguished whenever possible from non-agonal clots.

It is important to distinguish between *brain death* and the irreversible brain injury known as *Persistent Vegetative State (PVS)*. Patients with either condition are clinically, irreversibly comatose and show severe brain injury with neuronal death. However, the diagnosis of *brain death* is based on *brainstem death* determination, while

PVS involves only permanent and total destruction of frontal lobe function.

In persistent vegetative state, vegetative functions such as respiration, anatomic functions and sleep-wake cycles occur, but there is no response to external stimuli and awareness is absent.

Autopsies of patients with persistent vegetative state reveal, in the majority of cases, diffuse axonal injury changes. Other findings may include secondary thalamic degeneration and atrophy, skull fractures, ischemic encephalopathy, contusions and intracranial bleeding.

Disconnection of life-support equipment is permissible following a determination of brain death, while it is much more problematic in cases of PVS, where a *living will* or specific court approval is required.

One should emphasize that premature or illegal discontinuation of life-supporting systems for an irreversibly unconscious but not *brain dead* patient may result not only in civil liability but also in criminal charges.

The Medicolegal Implications of the Determination of Death

The practical major medicolegal implications related to the new definition of death are:
1. The earliest determination of death for prompt *harvesting* of organs for transplantation purposes.
2. The legality of discontinuation of life-supporting equipment.
3. The determination of the time of death in criminal and civil litigation.

In medicolegal cases the transplantation procedures require not only a prior authorizing donation by the deceased and/or his family but also the specific consent of the medical examiner or coroner.

Medicolegal offices are a major source of organs for transplantation purposes, and their standing policies may substantially advance or impede the transplantation program of a particular community. The humanitarian value of transplantation procedures notwithstanding is incumbent on the forensic authority to insure not only that the harvesting of organs is duly authorized, but also that it does not substantially interfere with the medicolegal autopsy.

We have recently seen two cases of *shaken baby syndrome* with no external injuries in which the abusing parents authorized tissue donation. It is unclear whether the motivation of the parents was purely altruistic or an attempt to cover up possible homicide. Regardless of the motive, when the cause and manner of death are unclear, postmortem *harvesting* of organs may substantially interfere with the medicolegal autopsy.

If one wishes to approve the harvesting of organs under such circumstances, it is strongly recommended that a forensic pathologist be present during the procedure. Such presence is required to insure proper documentation and interpretation of findings of medicolegal significance and to avoid the interference of confusing artifacts.

The Determination of Death and Survivorship

When two individuals who previously designate each other as mutual heirs die together in a single incident, the legal question of whether they died at the same time is of paramount importance in determining who will be the ultimate inheritor.

This question, known as *survivorship,* is often posed to the forensic pathologist who will have to weigh the specific circumstances of each case, including the age of the deceased, the state of health, the extent of injuries and the corresponding reactive changes, the level of alcohol and toxic substances, and the nature and state of postmortem changes.

One should critically evaluate the various parameters in order to ensure that they are comparable under similar conditions. For example, two individuals showing marked differences in the development of postmortem changes may still have died simultaneously if one was more prone to accelerated death (e.g. excessively obese, septicemic or close to a hot radiator).

The Death Certificate and the Determination of the Cause and Manner of Death

Though the laws of many states are unclear in regard to who should make the actual determi-

nation of death, all legislatures require that every deceased be issued a certificate which is to be signed by the last attending physician or by the coroner/medical examiner.

The central medicolegal requirement of the death certificate is the determination of the cause and manner of death. The cause of death is the medical finding or findings responsible for the death, and the manner of death is the legal classification of death, whether it be natural, suicide, homicide, accident or undeterminable.

The death certificate has two major groupings for the cause of death: the primary or immediate cause of death and the secondary cause of death. The primary cause of death is subdivided into a three-link sequential chain, for example:
1. Primary cause of death:
   - Hypoxemic necrosis of brain *(brain death)*
   due to
   - Exsanguination
   due to
   - Gunshot wound (GSW) of abdomen

The secondary cause of death includes conditions which are not related to the primary cause of death but are substantially contributory to the individual's demise (e.g. emphysema of lungs, hypothermia, arteriosclerotic cardiovascular disease).

In cases of sudden unexpected death, suspicious death or unnatural death (suicide, accident or homicide) the coroner/medical examiner is the exclusive authority who has the jurisdiction to issue the death certificate. When the death follows shortly after a catastrophic event (e.g. traffic accident, suicide attempt, accidental drug intoxication, homicidal gunshot wound) the reporting is generally accurate and prompt.

Problems arise when the injured individual survives a longer period of time and dies of either predictable or unexpected complications or when death is a result of a combination of preexisting natural disease and the initial injury. It is not uncommon that the last physician to treat the patient is unaware of, or forgets, the initial traumatic or toxic event which triggered the chain of complications. Furthermore, many physicians are unaware of the medicolegal approach to the determination of the manner of death when both natural and unnatural causes of death coexist. A simple rule of thumb states that if an unnatural cause of death (trauma, drug overdose, electrocution, drowning, etc.) plays a contributory role in the death, then the manner of death is unnatural (i.e. accidental, suicidal or homicidal), and, therefore, the case falls under the jurisdiction of the coroner/medical examiner.

It is immaterial, whether the unnatural factor (i.e. trauma) was a direct, indirect, complicating or aggravating element, or whether it was a major or minor factor in the causation of death. The same is true for the unnatural physical or chemical injury which occurs long before the patient's demise, providing that the death can be traced back to the initial physical or chemical injury. A continuous chain of symptoms and/or findings must be demonstrated, however, in order to link the initial injury to its later complications and the death.

For example, the case of a seventy-year-old woman who dies of pneumonia or pulmonary embolism after being confined to bed for several weeks following a hip fracture sustained in a fall is clearly a case to be reported to the coroner/ medical examiner. The accidental hip fracture and the subsequent immobilization can be viewed as the triggering elements of the bronchopneumonia or embolism. This obviously colors the manner of death as accidental and implicitly makes it a reportable *forensic case.*

The lack of clinical continuity of symptoms between an injury (e.g. trauma) and a subsequent, apparently natural death does not necessarily classify the death as *purely natural* and unrelated to the trauma. A physical or chemical injury may trigger subclinical but nevertheless potentially fatal complications which may be substantiated only at autopsy.

A fifty-five-year-old man who dies four to five days following a symptom-free interval from the time of a physical assault is to considered a *forensic case* if the autopsy demonstrates a recent infarction, subclinical cardiac contusions, or other fatal complications related to the incident.

Difficulties also occur when the death is intraoperative, peri-operative or related to the patient's care, and the question arises whether this is or is not a reportable case. When a substantial

active medical misadventure occurs, the case is clearly a *prima facie* coroner/medical examiner case.

Such active misadventures include both physical and chemical injuries, such as perforation and/or laceration of blood vessels or other organs, disconnection of anesthetic equipment causing asphyxia, administration of the wrong type of blood, burns or electrocution by the medical equipment, overdose of anesthetics or other medications, administration of mistaken medication, and anaphylactic reactions.

The jurisdiction of the coroner/medical examiner in *unexplained* deaths may be exercised only when the *manner of death is unexplained.* If a diagnostic determination was reliably made that the death is natural, no jurisdiction exists. The precise cause or mechanism of death, in a natural death, may be medically tantalizing and may have public health significance, but its mystery cannot prompt the forensic jurisdiction unless specific authority is granted under state law. Therefore, the failure to know the precise cause or mechanism of death in an otherwise natural death does not activate the coroner/medical examiner's jurisdiction.

The same approach applies to *suspicious deaths.* It is only when reasonable and reliable information indicates that the death is *suspicious* that the forensic jurisdiction may be assumed. In such situations, the presence of a potentially fatal natural cause of death is not incompatible with the coroner's assumption of jurisdiction, as the natural condition may well be only the background on which a subtle unnatural fatal injury occurred. Obviously, only a forensic autopsy may confirm or exclude, in such cases, the possibility of poisoning or other unnatural causes of death.

Embalmment and Exhumation

Postmortem embalming is a widespread custom on the North American continent of which most religious denominations approve. The embalming procedure usually includes the application of cosmetic cream to the face and hands of the deceased, covering of the eyes under the eyelids with plastic cups, fixation or wiring of jaws, injection of embalming fluids in the neck

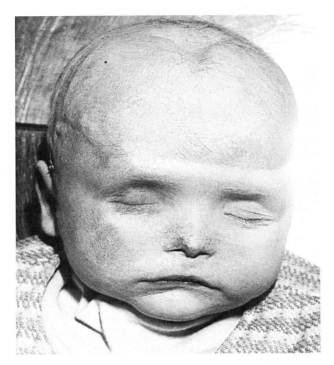 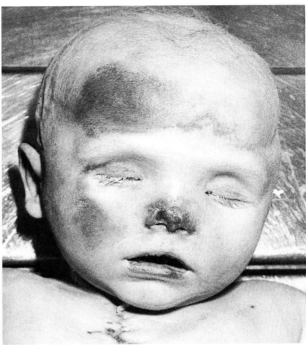

FIGURE III-1. Embalmed five-month-old child. (a) Cosmetic cream covering the face, successfully concealing extensive bruising. (b) Face after removal of cream.

(carotid), axilla (axillary) and groin (iliac and femoral) arteries, and injection through trocar of cavity fluid into the abdomen and thorax.

Autopsies performed after embalming and/or exhumation require special techniques. Embalming artifacts may conceal or mimic real injuries.

The sticky embalming cosmetics placed on the face and hands of the deceased may effectively mask substantial bruises and abrasions of the skin and, therefore, should be carefully removed with an alcoholic solution or scraped away (Fig. III-1). The injection of embalming fluids into the body cavities will obviously affect the composition, appearance and amount of any previously present fluid. Perforations of the internal organs by the embalmer's trocar may be difficult or impossible to differentiate from genuine lacerations.

Perhaps the most intrusive artifactual complication of embalming is the chemical alteration of the blood and tissues by the injected embalming fluid. Embalming fluids contain various mixtures of formaldehyde, glutaraldehyde, alcohols and other preservatives (e.g. hexylresorcinol, phenol, methylsalicylate, sodium benzoate, sodi-

um and calcium oxalates, quaternary ammonium compounds, EDTA).[6] The use of metallic salts (e.g. arsenic, mercury, lead, copper, silver, etc.) in embalming fluid is now prohibited to prevent concealing of heavy metal poisoning. However, embalming still interferes with the chemical analysis of many compounds. Some compounds, such as ethanol, opiates, carbon monoxide and cyanide, are destroyed or cannot be reliably tested.

Other chemicals (such as barbiturates, tricyclic compounds and benzodiazepines) can be qualitatively tested if only a few weeks or months have elapsed since embalming. However, a quantitative evaluation of these compounds is largely unreliable because of dilution and other factors. In some cases, analysis of more protected biological fluids (such as vitreous of the eye and cerebrospinal fluid) may give a fairly good quantitative estimate.

Metallic compounds and metalloids (e.g. arsenic) may be recovered from the embalmed body after many years. However, their elution into the environment or diffusion from the environment if the soil has a higher concentration, makes one doubt the reliability of their quantitation.

When testing embalmed tissues for metals and metalloids, it is recommended that the embalming fluid be analyzed as well in order to exclude the possibility that it contains related contaminants.

The situation becomes more complex when there is a need to examine an embalmed body after exhumation. In cases where the death is due to trauma, it is advantageous that a forensic pathologist be present during the exhumation to ensure that the coffin did not collapse, and that the body was not otherwise physically damaged in the process.

Similarly, if poisoning is suspected, the forensic pathologist should collect samples of the soil around the coffin (above, below and sides) as well as any water which may have leaked into the coffin which may contain increased amount of the chemical suspected in the poisoning. A typical poison which may be present in increased amounts in the soil is arsenic, but obviously, other toxic substances and metals may be present as well.

Following exhumation, most bodies show significant fungal growth on the face and exposed skin areas which may severely disfigure the deceased and practically obliterate bruised or abraded areas. Areas of bruising are especially difficult to evaluate because of the black, gray or greenish discoloration due to the combination of fungus and decompositional changes. Usually, fungal growth is maximal in areas of premortem injury and bleeding. *Aspergillus nigrans,* which is black, and flaky white mildew, is especially common on the body surface (Fig. III-2). Interestingly, decomposition is usually reduced in areas with fungal growth because of the bacteriostatic effect of most strains of fungi.

Furthermore, if fluid is present in the coffin, the skin may become very soggy and slippery and develop adipocere. The preservation of the internal organs varies considerably with the quality of embalming. In some cases, we have seen excellent preservation after ten or more years, in others we observed advanced internal decomposition a few weeks following burial.

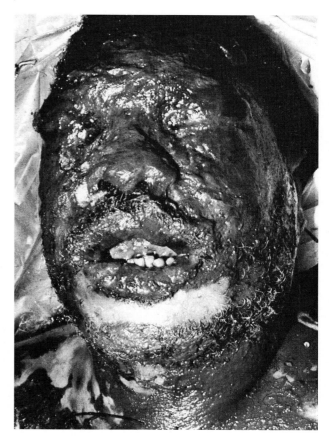

FIGURE III-2. Mildew on the face and chin. A leak in the roof had caused water to accumulate on the floor and soak the furniture. Death was due to alcoholism.

Incineration and Cremation

Close to seventy percent of the human body consists of water, twenty-five to twenty-six percent of combustible organic tissue and less that five percent of *fireproof* inorganic compounds. Most of the latter are present in the bones in the form of calcium salts, mainly as crystalline hydroxyapatite and partly as amorphous calcium phosphate. Upon exposure to temperatures in excess of 1000°C, the soft tissues of the body and the organic components of the bone literally go up in smoke leaving only a relatively small amount of ash.

In most fires, temperatures do not reach such levels, and variable amounts of soft tissue in different stages of carbonization are still present. In rare instances where temperatures are so high that the bones burn extensively, incinerated bones which may remain, appear as white or white-gray, porous, friable, calcinated fragments of various size.

Careful sifting through incinerated bones reveals, in most cases, fragments which are large enough to be recognized as human by an experienced examiner, particularly an anthropologist.

The funeral disposition of human remains by fire is known as cremation. In some parts of the world, such as India, this is the common funeral method. In the United States, the incidence of cremations has increased considerably in recent years.

In the past, most cremations involved paupers and unclaimed bodies, fetuses and body parts. Recently, larger numbers of upper-middle class professionals are opting for this method of postmortem disposal. In most states, cremation requires a special permit by the local health department and/or the coroner/medical examiner, and a mandatory twenty-four hour postmortem waiting period.

Cremation is by open flame or oven heating (calcination) at temperatures between 1600° F and 2200° F. Cremation at these temperatures and subsequent grinding of the cremated bones results in a mixture of small calcinated fragments of various color (brown, light-brown, gray and blackish) which cannot be diagnosed by current methods as being specifically human. The total volume of these cremated remains depends not necessarily on the weight of the individual but on the mass of skeletal bones, as most soft tissues incinerate with very little trace.

In a personal study of the cremated remains of two hundred and forty-six males and one hundred forty-eight females, the weight generally varied between 1,500 and 5,510 grams, with a mean in men of 3,035 grams and in women of 2,508.3 grams, and a standard deviation of 538.6 grams and 598.4 grams, respectively. If the total weight exceeds 6,000 grams, it is likely that the cremated remains consist of more than one person. A few legal suits have indeed alleged that negligent funeral directors have, on occasion, mixed the ashes of several people and sometimes animals.

POSTMORTEM CHANGES AND THE DETERMINATION OF THE TIME OF DEATH

Following death, numerous physicochemical changes occur which ultimately lead to the dissolution of all soft tissues. The medicolegal importance of these postmortem changes is related primarily to their sequential nature which can be utilized in the determination of the time of death and the related destructive and/or artifactual changes which may simulate premortem injuries or modify toxicological findings.

The determination of the time of death is generally based on the principle of using sequential changes as a *postmortem clock*. The evaluation may include:
1. Physicochemical changes evident upon direct examination of the body, such as changes in body temperature, livor, rigor and decomposition. These changes are routinely reported in protocols and are most commonly used in postmortem timing.
2. Changes in the chemical composition of body fluids or tissues (e.g. postmortem potassium concentration of vitreous fluid). These changes are not routinely evaluated and many claim their lack of reliability.
3. Postmortem residual reactivity of muscles to electrical or chemical stimuli (e.g. electrical stimulation of the masseter muscle and reaction of the iris to chemicals.) The recording of these changes, primarily popular in European medicolegal centers, is exceedingly uncommon, if practiced at all, in the United States.
4. Evaluation of physiological processes with established starting time or progress rate and cessation at death (e.g. presence of gastric contents as affected by time of digestion and the gastric emptying time). Recording of the amount, nature and appearance of gastric contents is routine in any adequate autopsy.
5. Survival time after injuries, particularly when the time of infliction is known. The nature, extent and severity of injuries as well as the quantitation of associated complications (e.g.

the amount of bleeding, early tissue reaction to injury) are often useful in determining the time of death.

The major problem encountered when relying upon the results of these methods is the variation in the environmental and individual factors on magnitude and kinetics of postmortem phenomena.

For example, the physicochemical changes following death are greatly dependent on environmental conditions and the metabolic status of the individual prior to death. Therefore, the deceased must be considered in view of environmental factors (temperature, ventilation, humidity) and his characteristics (body build, premortem exercise, state of health). Because of significant variation of kinetics of postmortem phenomena, the time of death cannot be pinpointed exactly but is estimated within a variable time frame. Furthermore, the longer the time interval since death, the wider the estimated range.

Because of inherent inaccuracies in timing of individual postmortem changes, the following approach is usually effective:

1. An initial determination of a wide *window of death* which is subsequently narrowed and refined by using variable parameters. The *window of death* is defined as the time interval prior to which one may assert with confidence that the individual was alive. The *window of death* should be established according to the most reliable testimony or evidence as to when the individual was last alive (e.g. witnesses, verified signed documents, last time newspapers were brought into the house, last time of withdrawal on bank accounts).
2. Conservative determinations of time of death as a range utilizing individual postmortem changes.
3. An algebraic integration of all postmortem timing changes.

Postmortem Cooling (Algor Mortis)

Postmortem body temperature declines progressively until it reaches the ambient temperature. Under average conditions, the body cools at a rate of 2.0° F to 2.5° F per hour during the first hours and slower thereafter, with an average loss

of 1.5° F to 2° F during the first twelve hours, and 1° F for the next twelve to eighteen hours. The final slowing of the rate of cooling is attributed to the reduced gradient between body temperature and ambient temperature. Careful studies under controlled conditions have shown that the decrease in the postmortem body temperature is not rectilinear but sigmoid in shape with a *plateau* at the beginning and at the end of the cooling process.[7]

The initial plateau, which rarely lasts more than three to four hours, is generally explained on the basis of heat generated by the residual metabolic process of dying tissues and by the metabolic activity of intestinal bacteria. A study by Hutchins[8] reports elevations of the temperature rather than a plateau within the first hours following death, with a return to base line within four hours. Whereas, the average postmortem temperature increment in Hutchins' series is minimal, it is significant that during the first few hours following death, the temperature did not decline as would have been expected under the above rule of thumb. It is also significant that all of Hutchins' cases were patients in a hospital setting who had died from natural causes with a possibility of an acute occult infection in progress.

The skin, as the closest organ to the environmental air, cools quite rapidly and is not useful for sequential temperature measurements. Temperature changes of the *inner core* are preferred, because the decline is slower and more regular.[9] Many sites have been tried for taking body temperatures. The most convenient and commonly used procedure involves hourly measurements of the deep rectal temperature (8" depth). Some prefer the liver and brain as more representative sites of *inner core* temperatures.

The postmortem rate of cooling may be used for estimating the time interval since death. As a matter of fact, literature surveys indicate that more than a hundred and fifty years ago postmortem cooling was used for this purpose in medicolegal cases. Since then, numerous studies by forensic scientists have attempted to refine the use of the cooling rate as a reliable postmortem clock. A thorough historical review of various methods of estimating the time of death from body temperature by Bernard Knight[10] conclud-

TABLE III-1

BODY COOLING:
IMPORTANT FACTORS

Clothing
State of nutrition
Environmental temperature and wind
Relative humidity
Contact of body with hot and cold objects
Temperature of body at death

ed that *in spite of the extensive application of physical theory and a great deal of direct experimentation, the level of accuracy remains low, even in the artificial venue of a controlled experiment.* This does not mean that measurements of postmortem temperatures are worthless in determining the postmortem interval, but that the data should be cautiously interpreted in view of variables affecting postmortem cooling (Table III-1).

Postmortem cooling of the human body at the skin surface (i.e., loss of heat to the environment) takes place by three major mechanisms:

1. **Conduction:** transferal of heat by direct contact to another object.
2. **Radiation:** transfer of heat to the surrounding air by infrared rays.
3. **Convection:** transfer of heat through moving air currents adjacent to the body.

Internal organs cool primarily by conduction. It follows that factors which affect these mechanisms are bound to affect the rate of cooling as well.

For example, body insulators such as clothing and increased body fat will decrease the rate of heat loss and, therefore, decrease the rate of cooling. Active air currents increase heat loss by convection and, therefore, accelerate the rate of cooling. Similarly, immersion in cold water will increase the heat loss by conduction and accelerate rate of cooling.

The rate of body cooling in water, such as in a warm swimming pool at air temperature, may be double that on dry land. Under these circumstances it would be possible to estimate the time since death in a body recovered from a pool.

A larger body surface ratio to body mass, such as is in children, will increase relative heat loss and therefore increase the rate of cooling. Furthermore, the rate of cooling is dependent on the temperature gradient between the body and the environment, and its calculation assumes that the environment is cooler than the body temperature; the higher the gradient, the faster is the loss of heat.

However, if the environment is warmer than the body temperature, the postmortem body temperature will be increased. In calculating back to the time of death, one should not necessarily assume that the body temperature at the time of death was normal (36.5°C to 37°C, or 98.6°F). People may die with hyperthermia at much higher than normal body temperature because of a variety of factors including sepsis, hyperthyroidism, physical exercise, heat stroke, seizures or drugs (cocaine, amphetamines, anticholinergic drugs, phenylcyclidine). Head injury, with damage of the hypothalamic area of the brain, may cause a terminal body temperature of 105°F or higher. Obviously, postmortem cooling would be significantly affected in such cases. On the other hand, individuals may die in a state of hypothermia caused by shock, environmental exposure or drugs (alcohol, sedative-hypnotics, opiates, phenothiazine).

Early Postmortem Ocular Changes

The eyes often exhibit some of the earliest postmortem changes. An immediate sign of death in the fundi of the eyes is the arrest of capillary circulation with settling of red blood cells, in a *rouleaux* or *boxcar* pattern.

When the eyes remain open, a thin film may be observed within minutes on the corneal surface, and within two to three hours corneal cloudiness develops. If the eyes are closed, the appearance of the corneal film may be delayed by hours and that of corneal cloudiness by twenty-four hours or longer.

If the eyes are partly open in a dry environment, the exposed areas between the lids may develop a blackish-brown discoloration known as *tâche noire* (black spot) (Fig. III-3). This phenomenon has been mistakenly interpreted as bruising. Absence of intraocular fluid suggests a time of death of at least four days. (Even in the absence of fluid within the eyeballs, the interior of the globes

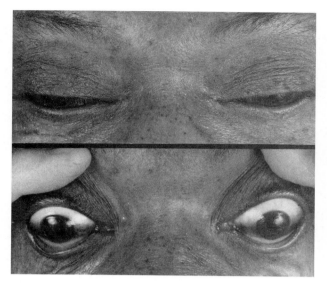

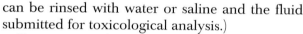

FIGURE III-3. Postmortem dark discoloration of sclera (tâche noire) due to drying, along the exposed area between the lids. The sclera covered by the lids retains moisture.

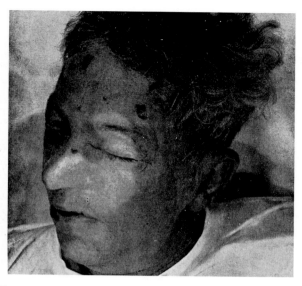

FIGURE III-4. Livor mortis. Blanched area where face was pressed against the floor. Death was due to heart disease. The abrasions on the forehead were sustained when he collapsed.

can be rinsed with water or saline and the fluid submitted for toxicological analysis.)

Postmortem changes of the pupils, consist of dilatation of the pupils and central positioning, resulting from relaxation of the iris muscle. The iris muscle, like all muscles in the body, abides by the rules governing rigor mortis.

In life, constricted pupils occur as a result of certain drugs, such as heroin and morphine, and differences in the size of the pupils may have neurological significance, such as, stroke or brain tumor. However, postmortem differences in pupillary size are variable and unreliable for such determination.

The miosis (constriction) of the pupils may persist in some narcotic deaths, while it may disappear in others. Similarly, differences in the shape of the pupil are equally variable and unreliable. Postmortem changes may affect the shape of the iris and create artefactual irregularities.

Postmortem Lividity (Livor Mortis)

Postmortem lividity (livor mortis) or postmortem hypostasis is a purplish-blue discoloration due to the settling of blood by gravitational forces within dilated, toneless capillaries of the deceased's skin.

Accordingly, livor is seen in the dependent areas, i.e., on the back if the body was in a supine position, and on the face and front if the body remained prone. A body which remained hanging for several hours, as after suicide, will have livor mortis from the elbows to the fingertips and from the mid-abdominal level down to the toes. Within the circumscribed sites of livor, one may see pale areas where the skin was pressed against a hard surface or object preventing postmortem sedimentation (Fig. III-4). Postmortem lividity may be evident as early as twenty minutes after death or may become apparent after several hours. The development of lividity is a gradual process which progressively becomes more pronounced. However, even after a number of hours postmortem lividity may be difficult to discern in cases of severe anemia or following extensive blood loss. In a case of a ruptured aortic aneurysm or severed aorta, postmortem lividity may be so faint as to be practically indiscernible. At all times, evaluation of the presence of livor mortis requires good lighting conditions: daylight is best.

In individuals with dark skin pigmentation, lividity in the skin can go unnoticed. At autopsy,

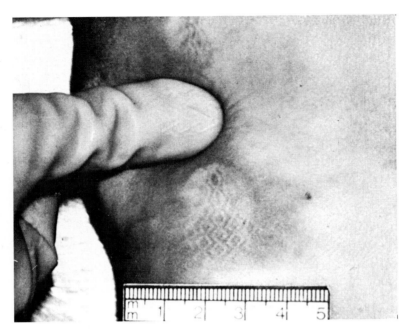

FIGURE III-5. Livor is blanched by the patterned glove compression seven and one-half hours after death.

finding congestion of internal organs may assist in determining the presence of lividity.

In the early stages, livor can be blanched by compression (Fig. III-5) and may shift if the position of the body is changed. Depending on temperature, but usually after eight to twelve hours, the blood congeals in the capillaries or diffuses into the extravascular tissues and does not usually permit blanching or displacement. In advanced stages of livor, skin capillaries in livorous areas often burst and cause pinpoint hemorrhages known as *Tardieu spots* (Figs. III-6 and III-7 a-c).

Unusual discoloration of postmortem lividity may serve as a diagnostic clue regarding the cause of death. The pathological mechanism responsible for the abnormal discoloration is usually the presence of an abnormal hemoglobin compound (e.g. carboxyhemoglobin, methemoglobin). In some instances cherry-red discoloration may be caused by the poisoning of cellular respiration (inhibition of cytochrome oxidase) resulting in excessive oxygen in the venous blood, as in cyanide and fluoroacetate poisoning (see Table III-2).

Cherry-pink livor is also seen in bodies recovered from water, wearing or covered with wet clothes, or lying on wet metal trays. Moisture on the body surface prevents the escape of oxygen, causing retention of an excess of bright red oxyhemoglobin in the skin. Some say that the bright red zone on the back is the result of reoxygenation by room air (ambient oxygen). However, in view of the fact that the red zone is usually below the purple area, i.e., the red zone involves an area the body is lying on, this theory does not seem likely.

The change in color of livor mortis in refrigerated bodies is a result of oxidation by air of reduced hemoglobin to oxyhemoglobin. The factors affecting this reaction are unknown. In cases of methemoglobinuria, livor mortis may be brown-red and in cases of hydrogen sulfide poisoning, livor mortis is often green.

A peculiar type of livor mortis may be seen in infants dying with fulminant sepsis and Waterhouse-Friederichsen Syndrome. In such cases the livor may be associated with a hemorrhagic rash, but in others the hemorrhagic rash is not clear and a diffuse skin discoloration of a slightly red-

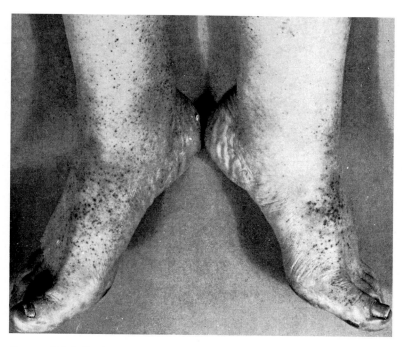

FIGURE III-6. Tardieu spots on the feet of a hanging victim. Swelling of the ankles resulted from settling of fluid due to several hours of hanging.

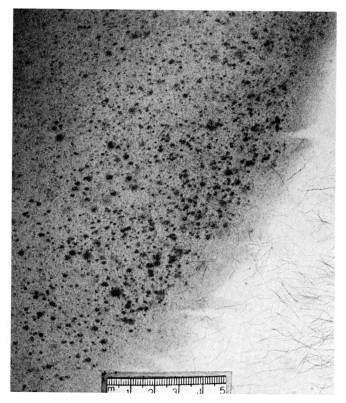

FIGURE III-7a. Close-up of Tardieu spots over the abdomen in an area of intense livor. Absolute confinement of spots to the area of livor.

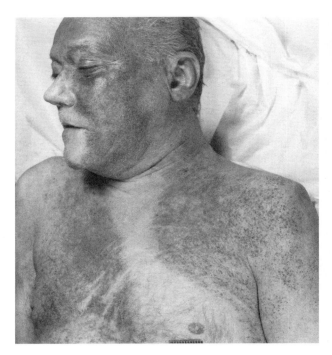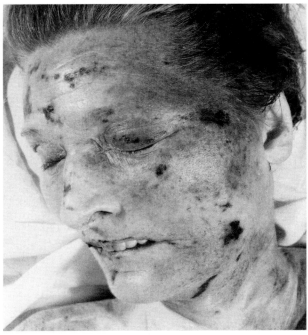

FIGURE III-7b–c. Only areas blanched by contact with the floor in the center of the face and chest show absence of Tardieu spots. The presence of Tardieu spots is a postmortem occurrence and indicates early stages of decomposition. When Tardieu spots are dense the entire area resembles bruising and care must be taken to identify the individual spots at the periphery. The use of a magnifying glass is usually of assistance. The examination may be further compounded if ants or roaches fed on the remains as well (c). (See Fig. III-40.)

TABLE III-2
POSTMORTEM LIVIDITY DISCOLORATION

Etiology	Color of Livor	Mechanism
Normal	Blue-purplish	Venous blood
Carbon Monoxide	Pink, cherry-red	Carboxyhemoglobin
Cyanide	Pink, cherry-red	Excessive oxygenated blood because of inhibition of cytochrome oxidase
Fluoroacetate (insecticide/rodenticide)	Pink, cherry-red	Inhibition of oxidative cellular metabolism
Refrigeration/hypothermia/ immersion in water	Pink, cherry-red	Oxygen retention in cutaneous blood by cold air
Sodium chlorate and inorganic nitrite	Brown	Methemoglobin
Hydrogen sulfide	Green	Sulfhemoglobin

dish-violaceus color is present on both dependent and non-dependent areas of the body with a superimposed pattern of the worn clothing. This phenomenon of diffuse livor discoloration is probably caused by increased perimortem capillary permeability.

Some researchers have claimed that changes in the color of livor mortis may be used to determine the postmortem interval, as with passage of time livor becomes darker and more purple. While this is true, the practical application of this information is of little relative value.

In certain cases it may be difficult to distinguish between postmortem livor and antemortem bruises. Incision of the skin may be required. Livor mortis is entirely intravascular and in its early stages can be drained. In a bruise, blood diffusely infiltrates the interstitial tissue and cannot be removed by drainage. With the onset of decomposition blood vessels become permeable and permit the escape of livor blood into the interstitial tissues. Differentiation of such areas from true bruises may be difficult or impossible. Massive postmortem hemorrhage may be seen from wounds in areas of livor mortis when the injured individual had been taking Coumadin or other blood thinners, including aspirin.

Since scars are devoid of blood vessels, livor mortis does not affect scarred areas. Thus, a scar in an area of lividity is usually easily noticeable. Also, the absence of blood retards decomposition of a scarred area (Fig. III-8). A cirrhotic liver, for instance, is likely to decompose at a slower rate than a normal liver.

A similar process to the gravitational movement of blood in capillaries as seen in livor discoloration of skin, occurs in the internal organs and is known as postmortem internal hypostasis. Its importance is not in determining the length of the postmortem interval, but in differentiating it from a vital process. For example, hypostasis seen in the posterior parts of the lungs in bodies lying in a supine position may be misinterpreted for severe congestion or pneumonia and the dark hypostatic area in the posterior wall of the left ventricle of the heart may be mistaken for an acute myocardial infarction.

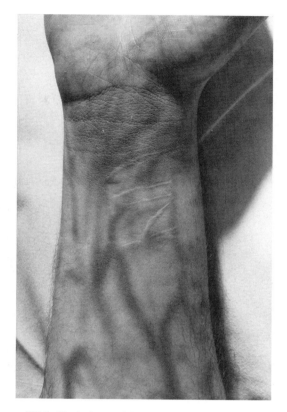

FIGURE III-8. Healed suicidal scars on the wrist of a decomposing body with evidence of marbling. Scars become more noticeable due to their white color and dark discoloration caused by decomposition. Scars contain no blood vessels, hence decomposition of a scar is delayed.

Postmortem Rigidity (Rigor Mortis)

Following death, the muscles become flaccid (flabby), and the lower jaw and extremities can be passively moved. Flaccidity is followed by increasing stiffness or rigidity of the muscular mass, which *freezes* the joints and is known as postmortem rigidity or rigor mortis. Rigidity then gradually subsides, and the body becomes flaccid again.

In temperate climates, under average conditions, rigor becomes apparent within half an hour to an hour, increases progressively to a maximum within twelve hours, remains for about ten or twelve hours and then progressively disappears within the following twelve hours (Fig. III-9). In an unconscious individual with no

vital signs, where intubation is difficult, consideration should be given to the possibility that rigor mortis is setting in.

Rigor mortis develops and disappears at a similar rate in all muscles. However, because of a lesser volume, small muscles (e.g. masseters, hands) become rigid before the large volume muscles (e.g. thigh muscles), a phenomenon which formerly led to the misleading belief that rigor progresses from the head downwards. Once fully established, the breaking of rigor in joints is irreversible, and it will not reappear. However, if the rigor is broken before it is fully developed, a variable extent of rigidity will reappear.

The occurrence of postmortem rigor is a physicochemical process following somatic death where the muscles continue their metabolic activity of glycolysis for a short time. During

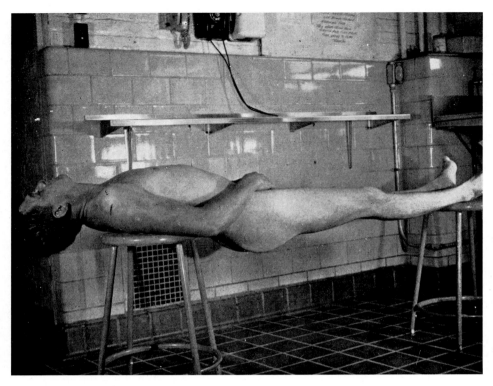

FIGURE III-9. Rigor mortis, intense enough to support the body. Death had occurred eighteen hours before the photograph was taken.

this process, ATP is hydrolyzed to ADP, and lactic acid is produced, lowering the cellular pH. The lack of ATP regeneration after death and the increased acidity result in the formation of *locking chemical bridges* between the two major muscle proteins, actin and myosin. This interlocking connection is fixed and produces rigor, without shortening of the muscle. In physiologic contraction, in contrast, the actin molecules slide inwards over the myosin, and the muscle shortens. Animal experiments indicate that in addition to the declining postmortem levels of ATP, a certain concentration of free calcium ions is also required for the development of rigor mortis, and that rigor is inhibited by calcium binding agents.[11]

With decomposition of body proteins, the chemical bridges between actin and myosin of the muscles in rigor break down, and the muscles becomes flaccid again.

As with other sequential postmortem changes, rigor mortis can assist in estimating the postmortem interval. However, one should remember that the progression of rigor may be substantially modified by a variety of factors which affect the underlying chemical process. Rigor mortis appearance and disappearance is accelerated by prior exercise, convulsions, electrocution, hyperpyrexia or hot environmental temperature. In a hot environment, for example, rigor mortis may come and go in only nine to twelve hours. Similarly, metabolic states associated with acidosis and uremia hasten the process. Hypothermia and cold environmental temperatures slow the chemical reactions and, therefore, delay the rigor process. Rigor mortis development is also affected by total body muscle mass and has been shown to develop poorly in young children, the elderly and the debilitated. Drugs affect postmortem rigor according to their physiological actions. Strychnine poisoning, which is associated with strong tetanic convulsions, accelerates rigor while carbon monoxide poisoning, associated with shock or hypothermia, delays it.

Drugs or poisons associated with tetanic convulsions can also result in excessive postmortem rigidity. For example, Hemlock Dropwort (Denanthe Crocata) a very poisonous plant belonging to the Umbelliferae family may result in accidental death when its root is mistaken for parsnip or when its leaves are used in salads or soups. The plant can cause severe tetanic convulsions and rapid death. In such cases severe postmortem rigidity is observed, often with the fist strongly clenched and thumbs applied to palm, as in cadaveric spasm (Fig. III-13).

The variability of postmortem rigor makes its use as a postmortem clock tenuous, to be considered only in conjunction with other timing indices. When the appearance of rigid limbs is inconsistent with gravitational forces, rigor is a reliable indicator of a postmortem shift in the position of the body. For example, an individual who is found in rigor with arms raised, defying gravity, was obviously moved from his original position after rigor was established (Figs. III-10 and III-11).

Rigor Mortis of Involuntary Muscles

Rigor mortis affects not only the voluntary muscles but the involuntary muscles and the heart muscle as well, producing misleading artifacts. Rigor mortis, for example, may, to a different extent, affect the iris of each eye and produce an artifactual difference between pupil diameter which may simulate a significant premortem pupillary disparity. The arrectores pilorum, the tiny muscles of the hair follicles in the skin, may be strikingly affected by rigor, resulting in cutis anserina or *gooseflesh* (Fig. III-12). Some believe erroneously that *gooseflesh* is somehow associated with drowning or death in water. Some believe mistakenly that hair grows after death because rigidity of the arrectores pilorum muscles causes hair to erect and appear longer.

Rigidity of facial arrectores pilorum may suggest early beard growth, as in 5 o'clock shadow, but, must be recognized as artifactual and not considered in estimating time of death.

Another manifestation of postmortem rigidity is the finding of semen at or near the tip of the

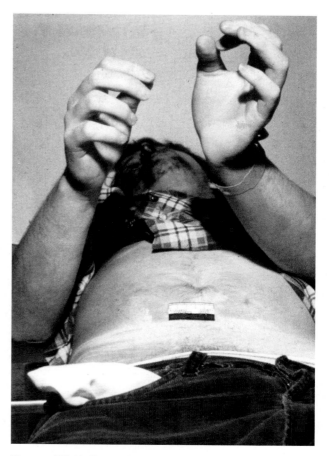

FIGURE III-10. Supine body with rigid forearms and hands in air, defying gravity. The body has been displaced from a prone position while holding a rifle.

penis. This expulsion of semen is the result of contraction due to postmortem rigidity of the layer of muscle in the wall of the seminal vesicles, which function as semen reservoirs (Fig. XXIV-7).

Muscle layers in the wall of the stomach churn the gastric contents, then pass them on into the small bowels for absorption of nutrients and the large bowel for elimination of waste. These muscle layers also obey the rules of flaccidity and rigidity associated with the dying process. During the period of flaccidity, i.e., the period where tone has been lost but rigidity has not yet developed, the pylorus opens and stomach contents leak into the duodenum or vice versa. Duodenal contents in the stomach causes bile staining of the gastric lining and contributes to autodigestion of the

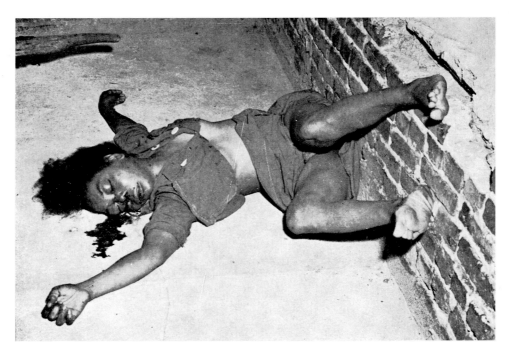

FIGURE III-11. Rigidity maintaining the legs against the brick wall. The flexed position of the legs led to the immediate conclusion that she had died elsewhere and had been moved after being dead at least six hours. Search of the area disclosed bloodstains in the home where she had been beaten. Her male friend confessed to having moved her body from the house hours later during darkness, concealing it in the yard of an adjacent house.

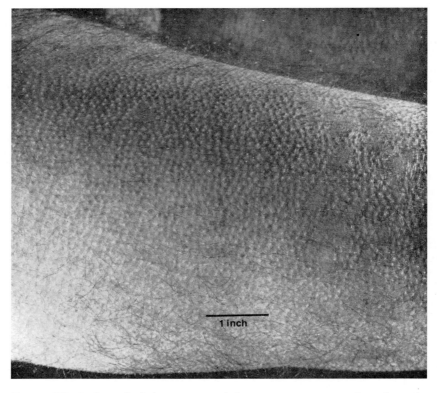

1 inch

FIGURE III-12. Gooseflesh (cutis anserina) due to postmortem rigidity of muscle fibers of the hair follicles (arrectores pilorum).

stomach wall and perforation. The change in the gastric wall is known as gastromalacia. The anal sphincter also relaxes in the same way as does the pylorus, only here rectal contents spill by gravity. Usually, fecal matter situated higher up in the large bowel, as in the sigmoid or descending colon, does not spill due to the more convoluted anatomical route to reach the opening.

We have had a case where the expelled feces were of a composition different from that in the remainder of the colon. Prompting the prosector to conclude that it was not from the deceased. Suffice it to say that the composition, and consistency of feces throughout the bowels differs depending on the diet consumed at different times.

Leakage of urine, again by gravity, is the result of relaxation of the bladder sphincter. Clothes stained with urine may be used for toxicological analysis.

The heart in rigor mortis may simulate hypertrophy, while secondary flaccidity may mimic pathologic dilatation. It is interesting to note that following open heart surgery cardiac patients may develop an ischemia-related, irreversible contraction of the heart, resembling rigor, which has been graphically described as stone heart.[12-14]

Frozen Bodies

As mentioned above, cooling delays the onset of postmortem rigidity. However, sufficient exposure of dead bodies to freezing temperatures results in rock-hard bodies that cannot be autopsied until defrosted. Such bodies should be externally examined and photographed as soon as possible, because once defrosted, decomposition progresses rapidly.

A closeup photograph of the face, unusual tattoo or an unusually shaped scar can be shown to relatives or friends for the purpose of identification, although a frozen body may be so well preserved that the body itself can be shown. Under such circumstances, photographs are advantageous as a permanent record.

Cadaveric Spasm

In rare instances, a forceful agonal contraction or seizure is converted almost immediately to

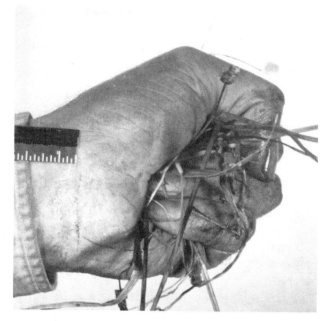

FIGURE III-13. Cadaveric spasm in a case of drowning.

tight rigor without preceding flaccidity. In such cases, labeled as cadaveric spasm, the clenched fist may be seen tightly holding a cigarette, blades of grass, clothing or some other object. Cadaveric spasm usually occurs in deaths preceded by great excitement, fear or tension. It is sometimes seen in cases of drowning, with the deceased grasping weeds or other aquatic vegetation (Fig. III-13), and in cases of homicide where the victim may be clutching some of the assailants hair or clothing.

Stomach Contents

The presence, appearance and amount of stomach contents may be helpful in estimating the time of death. This estimate is based on the assumption that the stomach empties at a known rate. However, the rate of emptying may only be approximated, because it changes depending on various factors, including the amount and type of food, drug or medication intake, prior medical and emotional condition of the deceased and other individual variables.

An ideal postmortem evaluation protocol of the rate of gastric emptying should include:

1. A description of the nature, amount, size and condition of the stomach contents.
2. A microscopic examination of the contents, if the contents are difficult to identify or are partially liquefied by the digestive process.
3. An examination of the small intestine for undigestible markers (e.g. corn kernels, tomato peels) to see how far ahead certain digested foods traveled.
4. A toxicological examination of both blood and stomach contents for drugs and alcohol.
5. An evaluation of the prior medical and psychological status and related medications and drugs.

Gastric emptying is a complex process which depends on signals originating not only in the stomach, but in the intestines and brain as well.[15] The stomach's distention by the meal affects the emptying process through reflex relaxation of the gastric fundus. Additionally, the meal's presence stimulates the gastric mucosa to secrete hormonal substances of a peptide nature (e.g. gastrin) which delay gastric emptying. Osmotic and calcium binding receptors in the duodenal mucosa respond to the composition of the incoming food and trigger the release of additional hormonal peptides (e.g. cholecystokinin) which have both a direct and indirect neural effect on post-prandial gastric emptying. Furthermore, additional chemical receptors in the distal small intestines and colon trigger the release of additional factors, such as peptide VV, which also affect the rate of gastric emptying. Finally, the central nervous system also exerts a substantial control over gastric emptying.

This complicated array of monitoring stations is affected by many factors. The rate of emptying, for example, is substantially influenced by the physical state of the food. Solid foods empty slower than ground foods and liquids.

While the half-emptying time for one hundred and fifty grams of orange juice is reported to average about half an hour, the amount of time required to digest and empty fifty grams of solid food may require two hours.[16,17] This, however, depends on the type of food and its nutritive density (isocaloric value). The greater the nutritive density and osmolarity of a meal, the slower the

meal is transferred from the stomach into the duodenum. Starchy and fatty foods may delay both the digestive process and emptying of the stomach. Light meals are usually present in the stomach for up to one and a half to two hours, medium meals up to three to four hours and heavy meals four to six hours or more.[18,19] The *head* of the meal usually reaches the cecum within six to eight hours. Gastric emptying and bowel motility are reduced at night and during sleep. An evening meal may be expected to be evacuated the next morning.

The stomach does not empty instantaneously; neither are large amounts of food expelled periodically. Only a small amount of food (a few grams) is expelled per minute, after having been ground to small particles. Therefore, the size of food particles and the extent of mastication also affects the rate of gastric emptying. Individuals who gulp their food without adequate mastication, whether because of lack of dentition or poor eating habits, have prolonged gastric retention.

Drugs and alcohol also affect the rate of gastric passage. The presence of concentrated alcoholic beverages (more than 80 proof) in the stomach causes constriction of the pyloric sphincter, which delays gastric emptying. A variety of compounds, including narcotics (heroin, meperidine, etc.), phenothiazines, atropine, beta-adrenergic drugs, potassium salts and synthetic progestins also substantially inhibit gastric emptying, while others such as diazepam (Valium®), metoclopramide and bulk laxatives accelerate it.

Natural diseases may also affect the rate of gastric emptying. For example, diabetes, bulimia and pyloric diseases (e.g. pyloric stenosis or peptic ulcers) are associated with delayed gastric emptying. The final emptying time for an idiopathic functional dyspeptic patient, for example, was found to be delayed by more than forty percent as compared to normal.[20]

Emotional stress (fear, excitement, etc.) also affects the time of gastric emptying by delaying it for many hours. Similarly, individuals in shock may retain gastric contents for days. Age and body build also affect the rate of gastric emptying. The elderly and the obese have a slower emptying gastric rate. Finally, environmental factors such as extreme cold or very hot weather may also retard gastric emptying.

Subtotal gastrectomy with gastroenterostomy and certain types of moderate exercise, such as running, have been shown to accelerate the gastric emptying rate. On the other hand, exhaustive exercise, such as a marathonic run, substantially slows the rate of gastric emptying.

In conclusion, the emptying of the stomach is a complex, multifactorial process, and its evaluation for determining time of death requires caution and careful review of all limiting factors. Consideration must also be given to the possibility of one or more close consecutive meals.

It has been found that under normal circumstances stomach contents which are readily identifiable by naked eye inspection were usually ingested within a two-hour period, and maintenance on life support may delay gastric emptying to the point where the stomach may contain undigested food for several days.

The question of the true nature of certain elements within gastric contents is sometimes raised when attempting to establish whether the particular contents match a known meal consumed at a known time. Microscopic examination of stomach contents, whether in the stomach or airway, may help identify the material. Biologists and botanists may be able to assist the pathologist in this identification process.

Decomposition

The disintegration of body tissues after death is known as decomposition. Decomposition follows the arrest of the biochemical processes which preserve the integrity of the cellular and subcellular membranes and organelles. During decomposition, the tissue components leak and break up, hydrolytic enzymes are released from the intracellular lysosomal sacs, and bacteria and other microorganisms thrive on the unprotected organic components of the body.

Accordingly, two parallel processes of decomposition have been distinguished:
1. *Autolysis:* self-dissolution by body enzymes released from disintegrating cells.

2. *Putrefaction:* decomposition changes produced by the action of bacteria and other microorganisms.

A third kind of postmortem destruction of the body occurs as a result of anthropophagy (i.e. attacks by various types of predators) from small insects to larger animals, particularly rodents.

Autolytic Changes

Early autolytic changes occur in organs rich in enzymes such as the pancreas, the gastric wall and the liver. Focal autolytic changes of the pancreas are frequently seen at autopsy.

Gastromalacia is the autodigestion of the gastric wall, often with perforation. It has been described as occurring during the late stages of coma or shortly before or after death. We have observed gastromalacia in cases of closed head injury, possibly related to stimulation of the heat regulatory centers in the brain and a terminal surge of body temperature, promoting autolysis. It usually occurs in the area of the gastric fundus and is devoid of vital reaction. In the recumbent body, acid and enzyme rich stomach contents flow up into the esophagus, causing digestion of the esophageal wall, known as esophagomalacia and spillage into the left chest cavity. When this happens the fluid in the left chest cavity should not be mistaken for hemorrhage. The lower lobe of the left lung and the chest wall, in contact with the digestive fluids undergo chemical change, turning dark gray, even black and become firm and rubbery as a result of interaction with tissue proteins.

Putrefaction

Putrefactive changes are dependent primarily on environmental temperatures and the prior state of health of the individual. Changes which in temperate climates take days to develop may develop within hours in a warm environment.

Furthermore, several individuals dying in the same area may show very different stages of decomposition, according to their individual degree of exposure to the sun or proximity to a source of heat (stove, radiator, etc.) (Fig. III-14).

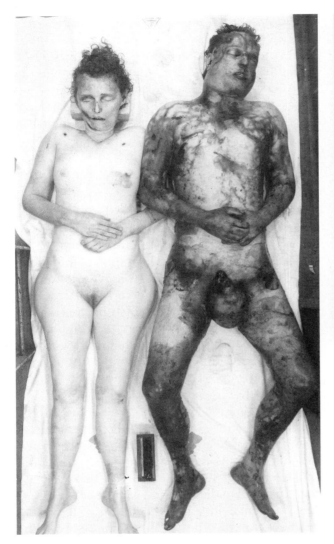

FIGURE III-14. The effect of environmental temperature on postmortem decomposition. This couple was killed within a few minutes of each other by a mentally deranged son. The body of the mother was found in the cool basement, while the body of the father was discovered in a warm upstairs room. Outside temperature was 90° F, postmortem interval about forty-eight hours.

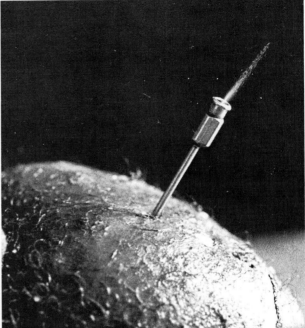

FIGURE III-15. Jet of ignited putrefaction gas (methane) at the end of a 13-gauge autopsy needle inserted into distended scrotum of a decomposed body.

Individuals with sepsis usually undergo rapid decomposition with putrefaction. In some cases of gas-producing *Clostridia* sepsis, one may witness an amazingly rapid progression of putrefactive changes in the liver, from a seemingly normal appearance at the beginning of the autopsy, to a mushy, decomposing mass an hour or so later. The putrefactive gases include methane, carbon dioxide, hydrogen and particularly malodorous ammonia, hydrogen sulfide and mercaptans. This gas burns readily when ignited (Fig. III-15).

Fever prior to death, such as encountered in sepsis, rhabdomyolysis and cocaine intoxication, also substantially accelerates decomposition and putrefaction. In such cases advanced putrefaction may be observed in less than twelve hours. Putrefaction is also more rapid in obese individuals and diabetics. The faster tissue breakdown in diabetics seems to be related to their greater sugar content. The putrefactive process is accelerated in edematous or exudative areas of the body and delayed in dehydrated tissues or following massive blood loss. On the other hand, in infants and thin individuals, putrefaction proceeds at a significantly slower pace.

The rate of putrefaction also depends on the physical environment in which the body lies. It is generally accepted that putrefaction in air is more rapid than in water, which is more rapid than in soil (Table III-3).

TABLE III-3

PUTREFACTION

One week in air equals
Two weeks in water or
Eight weeks in soil.

Exposure to cold also substantially delays the decomposition process. When evaluating post-mortem changes, it is, therefore, important to consider any intermittent period of exposure to cold, refrigeration or freezing. A further consideration is postmortem rewarming or thawing of the body. Experiments have shown that previously frozen and thawed animal tissues decompose significantly faster than freshly-killed animals. Tissues which are damaged by trauma show accelerated rates of decomposition.[21]

Decomposition gases may cause tissue artifacts mimicking softening cysts in the brain (encephalomalacia) and elsewhere, although the *Swiss cheese* pattern of the cavities easily indicates their postmortem character (Fig. XXV-14).

Similarly, decomposition gases may make difficult the diagnosis of air and fat embolism and cause the lungs of stillborns to float, which may lead to an erroneous determination of spontaneous breathing at birth.

Under conditions that promote putrefaction, especially in hot and humid environments, one may occasionally see a peculiar red discoloration of the teeth (pink teeth). The red discoloration is due to diffusion of hemoglobin from hemolyzed red blood cells into dentin canaliculi. Some studies have reported a frequency as high as twenty percent of pink teeth in sequential autopsies.[22]

A rare change caused by decomposition is the presence of white-gray, pinpoint foci, called *miliaria,* which are scattered below the endocardium and below the capsules of the liver, kidneys and spleen. The miliaria are easily distinguished from granulomas, fungi or fatty necrosis and are presumably due to autolytic changes resulting from precipitation of calcium crystals and other salts.

In temperate climates, early decomposition becomes manifest within twenty-four to thirty hours with greenish discoloration of the abdomen, due to denaturation by colonic bacte-

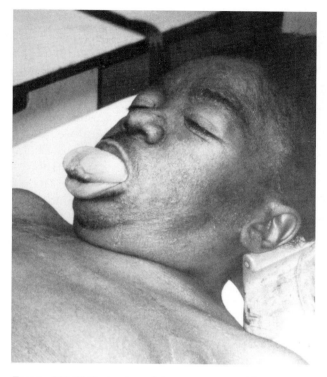

FIGURE III-16. Protrusion of the tongue caused by putrefactive gas buildup in the neck and chest, pushing the tongue up and out of the mouth.

ria, of hemoglobin to biliverdin and its reaction with hydrogen sulfide. Such discoloration is more prominent in the right lower abdominal area because of the close proximity of the cecum to the anterior abdominal wall.

This is followed by gaseous bloating, dark greenish to purple discoloration of the face and *purging* of bloody decomposition fluids from the nose, mouth and ruptured blisters. The blood-like purge does not clot. The tongue swells and progressively protrudes from the mouth (Fig. III-16), and the eyes bulge because of accumulating retrobulbar decomposition gases.

If putrefaction is advanced, the entire body and, of course, the neck may be considerably swollen by decomposition gases. A scarf or other piece of clothing around the neck may become very tight as a result of such swelling and be mistaken for a ligature. To avoid any misinterpretation, the length of the ligature may be compared with the collar size of the shirt of the deceased.

The greenish and purplish discoloration rapidly spreads within thirty-six to forty-eight hours to the chest and extremities, displaying a *marbling* pattern which delineates the decomposition of the blood and formation of sulfhemoglobin and hematin within dilated subcutaneous blood vessels (Fig. III-17a–b).

Decomposition of the internal organs progresses at different rates. The abdominal organs and especially the bowels decompose at an accelerated rate due to their high bacterial content. The brain liquifies into a gray creamy substance and eventually disappears (Fig. III-18) except for less than an ounce of inorganic crystals resembling dried mud and precipitated to one area by gravity.

Postmortem discoloration of the skin may be so dark that white individuals may be mistaken for black (Fig. III-19).

As decomposition progresses, the skin becomes slippery with blisters and slippage of the epidermis (Fig. III-20a–b), and generally, after three days, the entire body becomes markedly bloated. Swelling is particularly dramatic in areas of loose skin (eyelids, scrotum and penis). The skin of the hands often sheds, together with the fingernails, in *glove*-like fashion, and the skin of the legs and feet in a *stocking*-like pattern, a phenomenon which is also seen following prolonged immersion in water and in cases of second degree burns (Figs. III-21 and III-22).

In a body which remained *hogtied* for a period of eight hours before it was discovered, skin slippage of the medial surfaces of the knees resulted from extended pressure of one knee against the other and preservation of heat in the area (Fig. III-23).

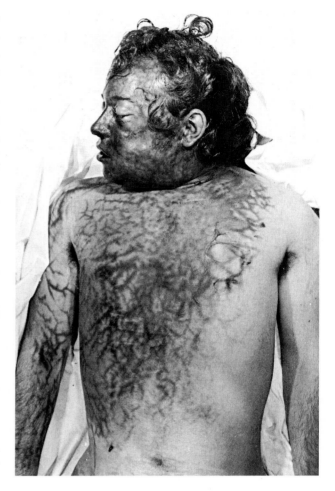

FIGURE III-17a. The cutaneous network of veins shows up due to decomposition of blood within. The phenomenon is called marbling and in this case occurred two days after death. The discoloration of the face is the result of more enhanced decomposition due to greater abundance of bacteria. Marbling is limited to areas of livor mortis.

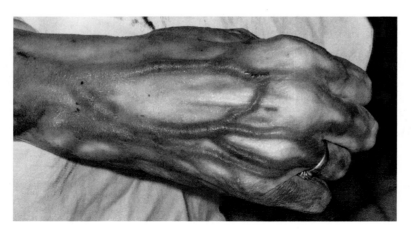

FIGURE III-17b. Bulging skin veins due to marbling with gas formation.

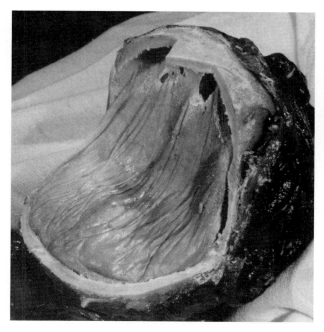

FIGURE III-18. Advanced decomposition caused liquifaction of the brain which caused the dura to separate from the skull and droop into the cranial cavity.

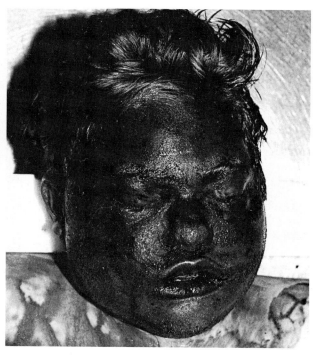

FIGURE III-19. Postmortem discoloration of the face and swelling, mimicking black racial features in a white man with straight, light-brown hair.

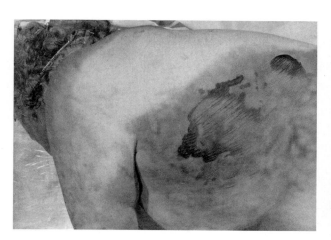

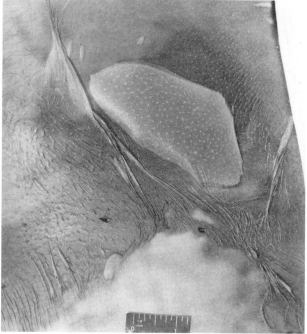

Figure III-20. (a) Epidermal blisters, resembling second degree burns, in areas of more pronounced decomposition. (b) The blisters will eventually rupture leaking decomposition fluid.

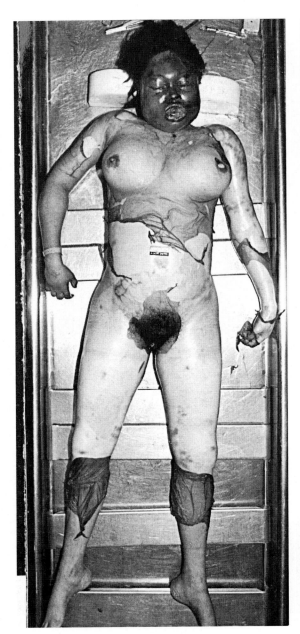

FIGURE III-21. Epidermal *stockings* and left *glove*. Bloating of body, especially of the breasts and marked discoloration of the face (three and a half days after death).

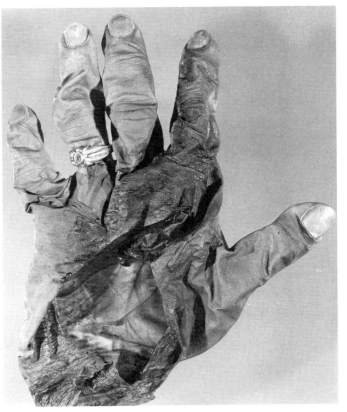

FIGURE III-22. Postmortem detachment of the epidermis in glove form. Note that the nails stay with the epidermis. These gloves often yield a full set of fingerprints and should be retained until identification is confirmed.

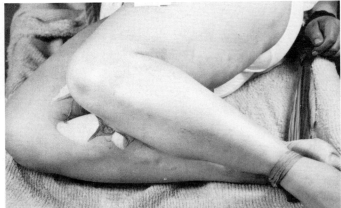

FIGURE III-23. *Hogtied* body found after 8 hours. The skin slippage between the medial surfaces of the knees was caused by body heat and extended pressure of one knee against the other.

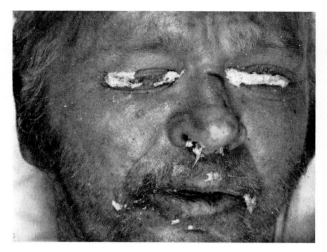

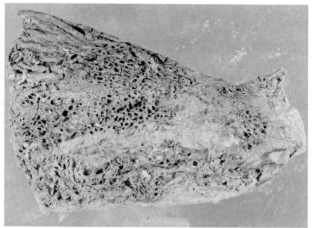

FIGURE III-24. Eggs laid by flies in the moist areas between the eyelids, nares and angles of the mouth.

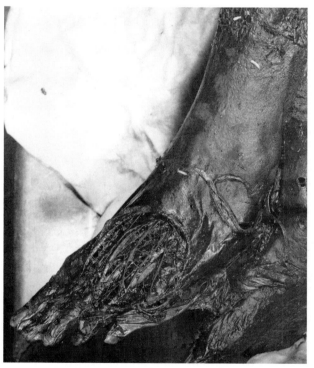

Additional destruction of the body is caused by maggots. Fly eggs initially deposited at the corners of the eyes, mouth and other mucocutaneous junctions (Fig. III-24) develop into innumerable crawling maggots which rapidly destroy soft tissues (Fig. III-25a–b). The maggots concentrate primarily in areas of body openings and perforations where they seek shelter and feed on blood and tissues. Clusters of fly eggs often resemble grated cheese (Fig. III-26).

Anytime a decomposed body is found with an unusually large concentration of maggots in a particular area, it is probable that a wound pre-existed in that location. In the case of a close range gunshot wound, maggots may remove tissue at the edges of the wound but leave soot deposited on the bone and gunpowder undisturbed.

Ultimately, decomposition ends in complete skeletanization. In temperate areas, under average conditions, the minimum period for full skeletanization is about one-and-a-half years.

The rate of putrefaction is significantly faster in arid environments. Galloway et al., in reviewing the earliest time of postmortem change in the hot, dry climate of Arizona, reported bloating of bodies as early as two days, gases at three days, advanced sagging of tissue and advanced intrathoracic and intra-abdominal activity of maggots at four days, partial mummification with leath-

Figure III-25a–b. (a) Lace-like skin caused by feeding maggots. (b) Decomposition of the foot with large undermined area from maggots feeding and intricate network of nerves, tendons and blood vessels remains.

ery change of skin at four days, and skeletanization after six to nine months.[23]

Under most *favorable* conditions, particularly with necrophagous insect activity, skeletanization may occur even earlier. Stewart[24] reports the case of a thirteen year old Mississippi girl, victim

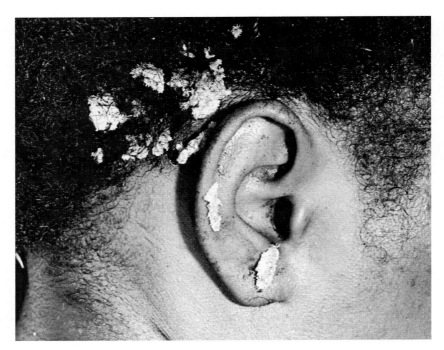

FIGURE III-26. Blowfly eggs resembling grated cheese.

of a homicide, whose body became almost completely skeletonized within ten days during late summer.

Post-Skeletanization Weathering Changes and the Time of Death

Once the body is fully skeletonized, the bones undergo a slow process of weathering and breaking down, lasting decades or centuries. Typical weathering of bones includes bleaching, exfoliation (desquamation) of cortical bone and demineralization. The rate and severity of these changes depends on environmental conditions, whether the bones were buried or exposed, the acidity of the soil and extent of humidity. Soil staining, which is a brown or sometimes tan discoloration of the bone surface, is variable, but may occur in as little as one to two years after complete skeletanization. Green discoloration of the bone surface is often caused by contact with copper or brass and may be seen as early as six months after exposure.

In hot, arid climates such as Arizona, bleaching of bones has been reported to occur as early as two months and exfoliation as early as four months, though usually the former takes six months and the latter as long as twelve to eighteen months. Demineralization is a late process, commonly seen in old bones or those found in archaeological excavations. It results in very light, porous and friable bones. Such bones may turn to dust on touching. Contact with certain roots may significantly accelerate bone demineralization.

Mummification and Adipocere

Two types of postmortem changes, mummification and adipocere, may counter substantially the process of tissue destruction by decomposition. Mummification results from drying of tissues under conditions of high environmental temperature, low humidity and good ventilation.

The conjunctivae of the eyes dry along the opening between the lids, causing a dark-brown horizontal band across the corneal surface sometimes referred to as *tâche noire* (Fig. III-3). The scrotum dries at the sides where exposed and not in contact with the moist skin of the thighs (Fig.

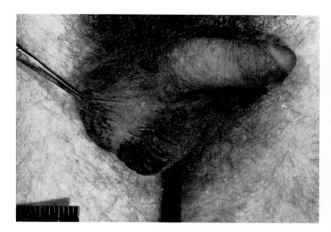

FIGURE III-27. Drying of the scrotal skin, sometimes mistaken for bruising. Where the scrotum is in contact with the thigh and along the cleavage, moisture is maintained.

III-27). Tight mummified skin displays a brownish discoloration and a parchment-like appearance and consistency. This transformation preserves facial contour (Fig. III-28). Bent knees and elbows are especially prone to this type of change. Similar drying may be observed in fingers and toes exposed to hot, dry air. Mummified fingers and toes are shriveled with wrinkled, firm, brown skin (Fig. III-29). The process begins at the finger tips which become spindly. Fingers in this condition are unsuitable for fingerprinting unless first soaked in warm water to stretch and unfold the skin for the return of its natural texture. Shrinkage of the nail beds has occasionally misled investigators and mystery book writers to conclude that fingernails and toenails grow after death.

The skin around the fingernails and toenails shrinks as a result of drying and may give the erroneous impression that the nails have grown after death. Drying of certain parts of the body may cause shrinkage of the skin to the extent of causing large splits that resemble actual injury. Such splits are especially common in the groins, neck and armpits.

In mummified bodies in temperate areas, the internal organs are usually poorly preserved or may have totally disappeared due to decomposition. Once mummification is fully developed, the body remains preserved as a shell for long

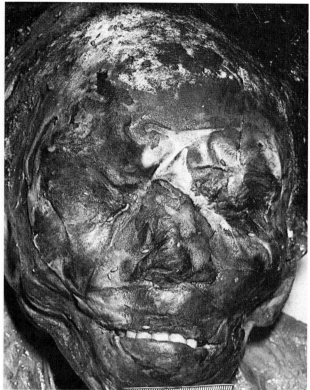

FIGURE III-28. Leathery, shrunken face of mummified body two months after death. The body was found covered by clothing in a basement.

periods of time, even years (Fig. III-30). The rate of mummification and its extent depend on the humidity of the air and the intensity of the environmental heat, and its full development in temperate areas generally requires at least three months of postmortem interval.

Adipocere (waxy fat) (Fig. III-31a–b) develops under conditions of high humidity and high environmental temperature and especially involves the subcutaneous tissue of face, extremities, buttocks and female breasts. The chemical process underlying adipocere consists of hydration and dehydrogenation of body fats, a process which imparts a grayish-white color and soft, greasy, clay-like, plastic consistency to the soft tissues of the body.

Recent research has demonstrated that bacterial enzymes of both intestinal and environmental sources, particularly *Clostridia,* are primarily responsible for adipocere, by converting unsatu-

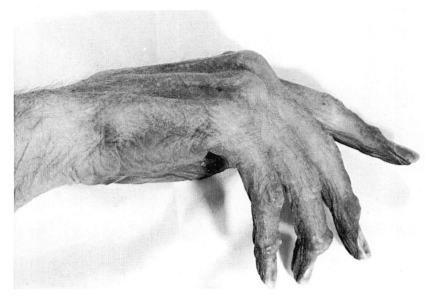

FIGURE III-29. Mummification of fingers showing shriveling and discoloration due to drying, one week after death.

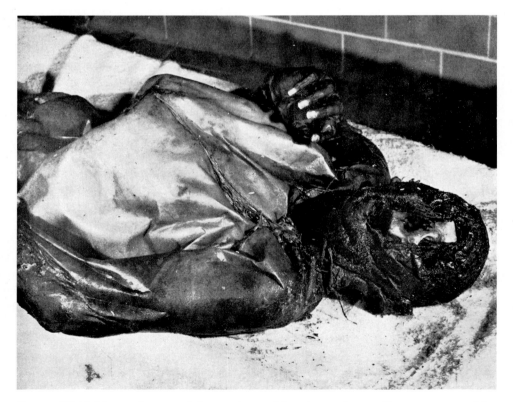

FIGURE III-30. Mummification of chest and arms. Note the parchment-like appearance of the skin in these areas. The skull is partly exposed by maggots, the surrounding tissues decomposed and blackened. The body was found in an apartment in the middle of July.

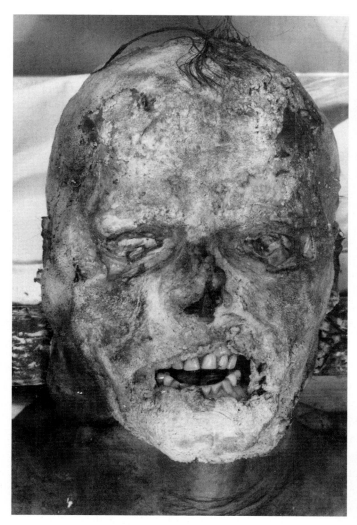

Figure III-31a. Adipocere formation in the face and head of a sea-man who had drowned six months before recovery of his body in April in the Chesapeake Bay. During winter the bay was covered with ice for two or three weeks. Water temperature when body was recovered was near 60° F. A key with the Norwegian word for cook was found in the pocket of the seaman and helped to establish identification.

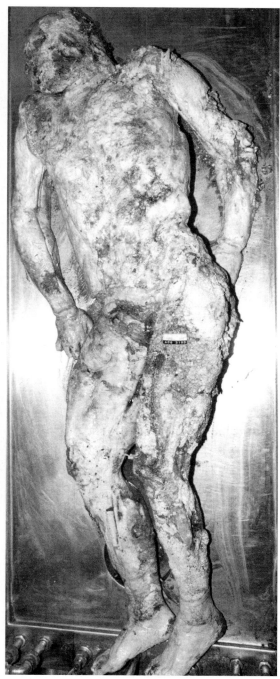

FIGURE III-31b. Adipocere involving the entire body.

rated liquid fats (oleic acid) to saturated solid fats (hydroxystearic acid and oxostearic acid).[25]

The time for the development of adipocere is estimated to be at least three months, and usually is not observed before six months.

Stillbirths

A stillbirth is the delivery of a viable fetus which is not breathing and shows no sign of life (Apgar score zero).

In such cases, the questions which the forensic pathologist must address are:

1. What is the gestational age of the fetus (by weight and dimensions)?
2. Was the fetus viable by estimated age, weight and size, and alive at birth? (Did the child breathe air?)
3. Were there traumatic injuries present in the fetus, and what was their significance?
4. What was the cause and manner of death?

The examination of the umbilical cord of the stillborn may reveal significant abnormalities such as true knots, torsion, arterial agenesis, thrombosis and funisitis. Common histological abnormalities of the placenta in stillbirth cases include placental infarcts, hemorrhagic endovasculitis, retroplacental hematomas, acute chorioamnionitis and hydrops.[26]

When intrauterine death has occurred days or months prior to delivery, the body of the fetus shows postmortem changes defined as maceration. Maceration is an autolytic process, i.e. a decomposition due to self-disintegration of the body by released cellular enzymes. The fetus and the bathing amniotic fluid are sterile and, therefore, will not undergo putrefaction if the membranes are intact. The macerated fetus initially shows a reddish, dusky discoloration and an easily peeling skin with fluid accumulation beneath the epidermis and formation of large bullae (blisters). The reddish discoloration is due to diffuse hemolysis and involves both the skin and the internal organs. Easy separation of the epidermis

does not occur until the last trimester of pregnancy. Before this period, the epidermis is less differentiated and is tightly adherent to the dermis.

This is followed, within one to three days, by further darkening of the skin, flaccidity, separation and overlapping of the cranial bones, dislocation of the temporomandibular joints and accumulation of hemolyzed blood and fluid in the body cavities. Rigor is almost never observed in macerated fetuses. In fetuses which are retained for more than seven to ten days, the reddish dark color starts to change into a light greenish-brown. Within a few days, the brain liquifies and the abdominal tissues decompose, often with disintegration of the intestinal wall, releasing meconium into the abdominal cavity. In cases where pregnancy continues, the dead fetus may be gradually resorbed or mummified (papyraceous appearance). In rare cases, usually associated with ectopic pregnancy, the dead fetus may calcify (lithopedion).

It is important to realize that some body measurements, including weight of a macerated fetus, may be altered by postmortem changes, and be unsuitable for estimating the gestational age. This makes it difficult, from the pathologist's point of view, to correlate the gestational age of the fetus to a dire traumatic event to the mother.

Decomposition certainly complicates the autopsy of a macerated fetus, although major developmental anomalies can still be detected. One should be careful not to interpret as traumatic, the subarachnoid or intraventricular hemorrhages often observed in stillborns as a result of hypoxemia.

Microscopic examination of lungs of stillborns frequently reveals some evidence of amniotic fluid aspiration with keratin squames in the alveoli, a finding which has been related to fetal distress. Other histological findings seen in fetal distress are tubulocystic change in the adult cortex of the adrenal gland, involution *(starry sky appearance)* of the thymus and meconium staining of the skin and placental membranes.

POSTMORTEM ARTIFACTS

Distinction of antemortem injuries from postmortem artifacts is of obvious importance. Problems in differential diagnosis may occur as a result of faulty autopsy technique, distorting post-

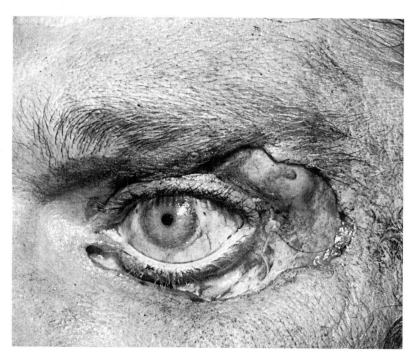

FIGURE III-32a. Anthropophagy: Irregular, bloodless defect under the eye, caused by postmortem nibbling.

mortem changes, and destructive environmental factors such as high environmental temperatures, postmortem mechanical trauma and anthropophagy, i.e. destructive changes by scavengers.[27]

Dogs and cats and other carnivorous animals will feed on a dead body when no other food is available, for example, in a closed house (Fig. III-32a–b). Occasionally, outdoors limbs, even the head are removed from the body, taken some distance away and chewed clean.

Even examination of fresh bodies may give rise to diagnostic difficulties when fatal injuries are accompanied by minimal hemorrhage or when immediate postmortem trauma opens blood vessels and causes artifactual bleeding.

I. Faulty Autopsy Technique

Faulty autopsy techniques can create confusing postmortem artifacts. For example, careless removal of congested neck organs before extracting the chest and abdominal organs may produce artifactual hemorrhages in the strap muscles of

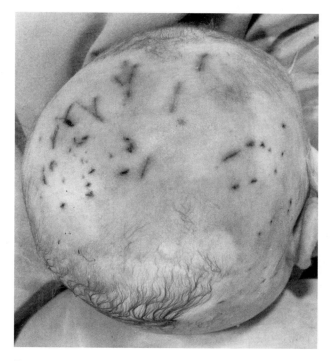

FIGURE III-32b. Typical cat scratches on the head of an infant.

the neck or laryngeal fractures, mimicking strangulation. Similarly, prying the skull with a chisel to break any remaining bridge of bone missed by sawing, may produce linear basilar fractures simulating fractures sustained during life. Removing the chest plate at the autopsy involves tearing large arteries and veins and may result not only in *bleeding* within the chest and abdominal cavities, but also in drawing air into blood vessels, mimicking air embolism. Inspection of the conjunctivae utilizing forceps to turn and lift the eyelids cause pinch marks and tears sometimes misinterpreted as the result of actual trauma.

II. Errors in Interpretation of Decomposition Changes

The following is a non-inclusive list of common situations in which distortions due to postmortem changes may be subject to misinterpretation:

1. Postmortem bloating of the body may create a misleading appearance of obesity.
2. Bloody decomposition fluid purging from the mouth and nose may be misinterpreted as premortem bleeding due to trauma.
3. The presence of decomposed bloody fluid in the chest cavity may be misconstrued as hemothorax.
4. Agonal or postmortem autolysis and perforation of the stomach may be misinterpreted as a perforated ulcer.
5. Postmortem dilatation and flaccidity of the vagina and anus may produce the appearance of a sexual attack or sodomy.
6. Pinpoint foci of extravasated blood from burst capillaries in areas of intense livor may simulate premortem petechial hemorrhages.
7. Diffusion of hemolyzed blood into tissues in areas of livor may be difficult to distinguish from genuine bruising in cases of moderately advanced decomposition.
8. Focal autolytic changes in the pancreas may be misinterpreted as focal necrosis or focal hemorrhagic pancreatitis.

Failure to carefully examine areas where decomposition is particularly advanced may result in missing of significant trauma, particularly since premortem injuries undergo more rapid decomposition.

Examination of a decomposed, charred or otherwise mutilated body can be a challenge for the examiner. These types of cases are best handled by an experienced forensic pathologist.

Alterations in blood and tissue levels of premortem toxic substances as a result of postmortem hydrolysis or decomposition may make a diagnosis of poisoning or overdose difficult if not impossible. For example, cocaine disappears rapidly from postmortem blood and tissue as a result of hydrolysis while postmortem levels of alcohol can substantially increase or decrease due to tissue decomposition.

A less known toxicological artifact results from postmortem redistribution of drugs. Postmortem diffusion of certain drugs, such as pentodiazepines, barbiturates and digoxin, has been reported to occur from areas of high tissue concentration into the blood.[28]

III. Destructive Environmental Factors

Exposure of the body to environmental forces may result in pathological changes which may obscure, modify or mimic genuine premortem injuries.

Some of the artifactual injuries clearly point to their etiology, while others are less specific and more questionable. Postmortem thermal artifacts often seen in fire victims include fractures of the skull and epidural hemorrhage due to intracranially generated steam, fractures of the extremities due to thermal contractions of tendons, and wide splitting of skin and muscles, simulating lacerations, cuts and stab wounds. However, subdural and subarachnoid hemorrhages are not artifactually produced in conflagrations.

Frozen bodies of infants may show artifactual folding of the skin of the neck, simulating ligature strangulation. Drowning fatalities recovered from larger bodies of water (rivers, lakes, oceans) may show extensive postmortem mutilation due to boat propellers, simulating injuries sustained during life.

Similarly, postmortem injuries caused by various scavengers (such as flies, ants, beetles, roaches, dogs, rodents, aquatic animals) may cause injuries (anthropophagy) simulating premortem trauma (Figs. III-33 to III-42). Superficial (epidermal) skin defects produced by insect feeding,

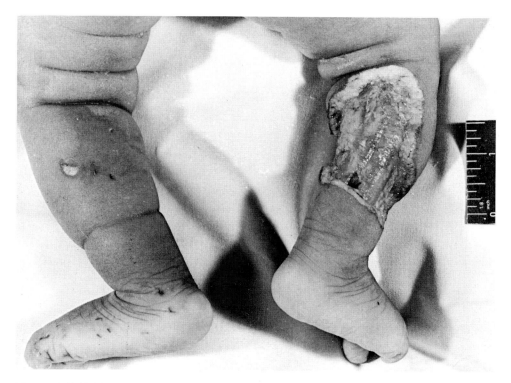

FIGURE III-33. Postmortem feeding by rats. There is complete absence of hemorrhage in the wound edges.

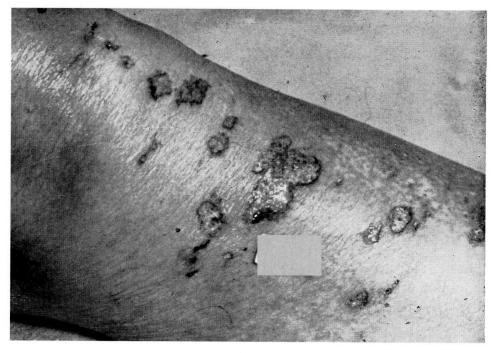

FIGURE III-34. Postmortem injury by mice. The scene suggested violence with a pool of nearly a pint of blood which had drained from these lesions onto the floor. Cause of death was chronic heart failure with marked venous hypertension.

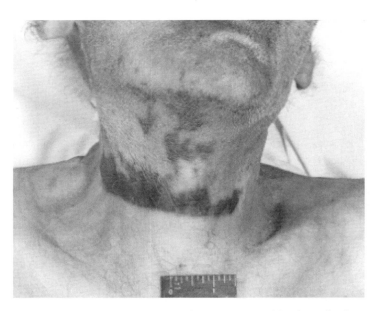

FIGURE III-35. Postmortem injury by ants restricted by the collar line could suggest strangulation.

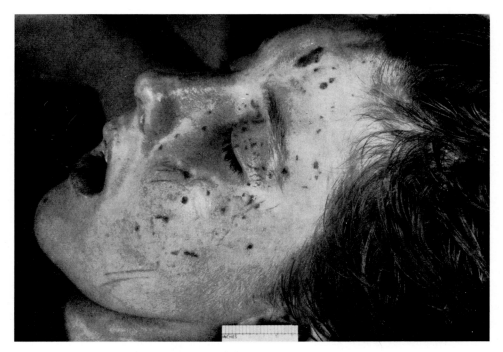

FIGURE III-36. Postmortem artifacts produced by ants. The girl was dumped face-down in a wooded area after being raped and strangled. The injuries of the face were first mistaken for fingernail marks. The fine linear scratches are due to twigs and undergrowth.

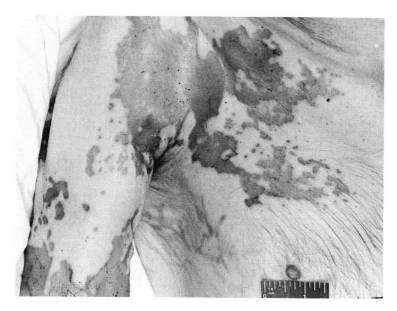

FIGURE III-37. Postmortem artifacts. Skin lesions of arm and chest by roaches. These are often misinterpreted as antemortem abrasions if roaches are not observed when the body is discovered. Note the similarity with postmortem injuries produced by ants. The latter are smaller and more discreet.

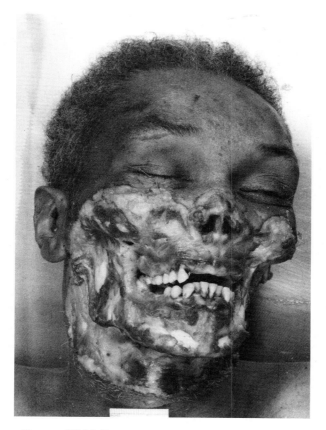

FIGURE III-38. Postmortem gnawing by small pet dog.

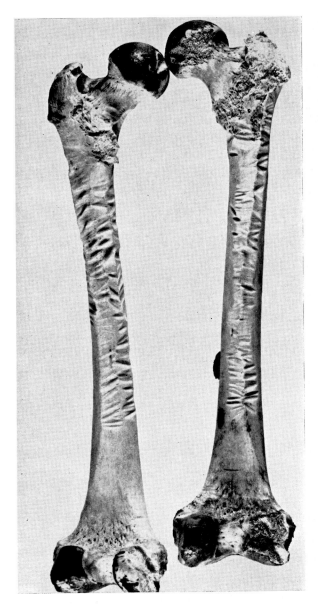

FIGURE III-39. Postmortem gnawing of human femurs, which were exposed for some months in a wooded area. The teeth marks are likely from dogs, but smaller animals, such as opossums or skunks, may leave similar marks.

especially when situated in the webs between fingers and toes may be mistaken for cigarette burns. When in doubt, microscopic examination of such areas readily reveals the true nature of such lesions. We have seen cases where dogs removed the head from a decomposing body and gnawed it at some distance away. Outdoors,

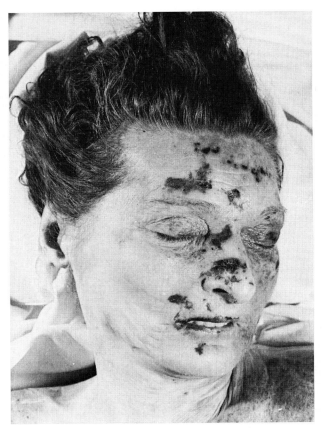

FIGURE III-40. Superficial confluent skin injuries produced after death by ants and roaches. Injuries resemble abrasions and possibly assault.

animals often take body parts and sometimes such parts are never recovered. It is often possible to determine the size of an animal by examining the edges of the injuries on the body. Areas on bone that have been gnawed are especially helpful.

Anthropophagy and Postmortem Vegetal Growth

Anthropophagy (Greek: eating of man) is the assault of the human body by prey animals and/ or scavengers.

Postmortem anthropophagy has to be differentiated from animal attacks on the body which occurred during life. Important forensic questions which are often raised regarding cadavers, showing evidence of animal attacks, is what animal caused the attack, whether the individual

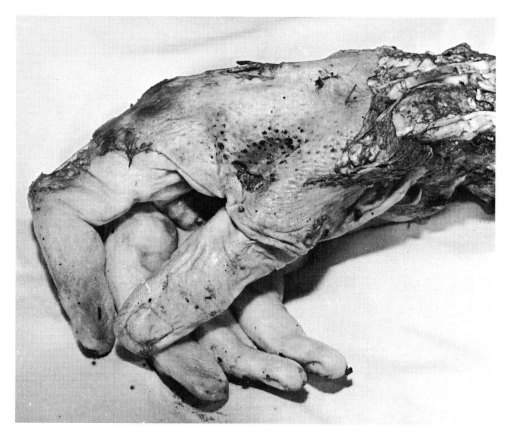

FIGURE III-41. Body recovered from water after several months during the winter. The head was above the water level when the body was found. The small defects near the web of the thumb were caused by fly maggots which burrow in and out while feeding. (See also Fig. III-25a.)

was alive at the time of the attack, whether he or she was conscious at the time of the attack, and what, if any, was the contribution of the animal related injuries to the victim's death.

The identification of the animal that caused the injuries is made on the basis of the pattern of the injuries, their location, and on the information of the fauna prevalent in the area where the body was found. Such injuries can be caused by both land-based animals, such as insects, ants, dogs and cats and aquatic animals, such as crabs, sharks, fish and alligators. Ants usually produce typical punctiform, discrete injuries, which occasionally may coalesce into larger injuries, mimicking abrasions. Crabs usually attack the areas adjacent to the eyes and mouth. The bite marks of dogs or large carnivorous aquatic animals, such as sharks, alligators and crocodiles, can be recognized by the patterned injuries caused by

their teeth on soft tissues and bones. The determination of whether the anthropophagy occurred during life is made on the basis of associated soft tissue hemorrhage. Bloodless injuries are usually indicative of postmortem injuries, except when advanced decomposition makes such determination questionable or impossible. Also, animals often lick the area, especially when blood is oozing out from a wound, which may complicate the distinction of anti and postmortem infliction.

Identification of a specific scavenger and the stage of its development may assist in estimating the minimal period of time which elapsed since death. For example, identification of maggots as being those of a particular fly (e.g. the bluebottle fly) permits determination of the minimum time which elapsed from the deposition of the eggs to the hatching of larvae. Most flies require at least

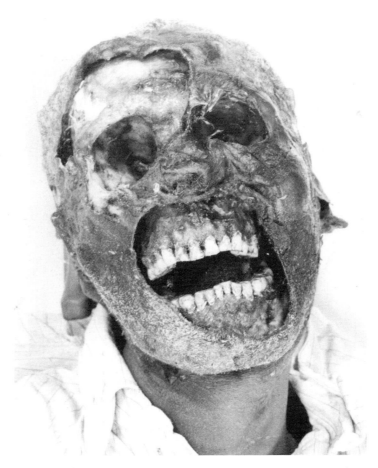

FIGURE III-42. Undermined skin defects by feeding maggots. (See also Fig. III-25b.)

twenty-four hours for hatching, but knowledge of the life cycle of a particular fly permits a more precise determination of the hatching time.[29]

Maggot size (length) may permit further evaluation of the time which elapsed from hatching to the time of recovery of the larvae. Pupae, the next stage of larval development, will obviously indicate an even longer postmortem interval. It is recommended that larvae be measured, preserved in a fixative (70% alcohol or 4% formalin solution) and submitted for examination by an entomologist. Similarly, botanists may be helpful in determining the minimal time interval since death by identifying the type and stage of postmortem growth of fungi and vegetation on bodies which were buried or left exposed to soil.[30]

Recent Developments for Determination of the Time of Death

In recent years a number of new methods have been suggested for determining the time of death. Some of the methods are based on progressive postmortem increases in levels of 3 methoxytyramine (3MT) in the basal ganglia of the brain and on the circadian variations in the levels of betareceptors and melatonin in the pineal gland.

Unfortunately, these methods involve intricate and time-consuming chemical or radioimmune techniques and dedicated expertise, and are as yet insufficiently confirmed and largely in early experimental stages.

CONCLUSION

In conclusion, none of the methods used in establishing the time of death are totally reliable and mathematically precise. Dogmatic and pinpoint accuracy in this matter is clearly not achievable.

However, careful consideration of environmental and individual influences, and the concomitant use of as many postmortem *clocking* devices as possible, frequently permit determination of a realistic range of the postmortem interval.

REFERENCES

1. Safar, P., Breivik, H., Abramson, N., and Detre, K.: Reversibility of clinical death in patients: The myth of the 5-minute limit. *Ann Emer Med, 16:*495, 1987.
2. Kvittingen, T.D., and Naess, A.: Recovery from drowning in fresh water. *Br Med J, 5341:*1315, 1963.
3. Ad Hoc Committee, Harvard Medical School: A definition of irreversible coma. *JAMA, 205:* 85, 1968.
4. Compos-Outcalt, D.: Brain death—Medical and legal issues. *J Fam Pract, 19:* 349, 1987.
5. Leestma, J.E.: *Forensic neuropathology.* New York: Raven Press, 1988.
6. Strub, E.G., and Frederick, L.G.D.: *The principles of embalming.* Professional Training Schools, Inc., 5th ed., 1989.
7. Shapiro, H.A.: Medicolegal mythology—Some popular forensic fallacies. *J Forensic Med, 1:* 144, 1953.
8. Hutchins, G.M.: Body temperature is elevated in the early postmortem period. *Human Pathol, 16:* 560, 1985.
9. Nelson, E.L.: Estimation of short-term postmortem interval utilizing core body temperature: A new algorithm. *Forensic Sci Internat, 109:* 31–38, 2000.
10. Knight, B.: The evolution of methods for estimating the time of death from body temperature. *Forensic Sci Internat, 36:* 47, 1988.
11. Weiner, P.D., and Pearson, A.M.: Inhibition of rigor mortis by Ethylenediamine Tetracetic Acid (EDTA). *Proc Sci Exp Bio Med, 123:* 185, 1966.
12. Lie, J.T., and Sun, S.C.: Ultrastructure of ischemic contracture of the left ventricle (stone heart). *Mayo Clinic Proc, 51:* 785, 1976.
13. Seelye, R.N., Nevalialainen, T.J., Gavin, J.B., and Wester, V.J.: Physical and biochemical changes in rigor mortis. *Biochem Med, 21:* 323, 1979.
14. Vanderwee, M.A., Humphrey, J.M., Gavin, J.B., and Arminger, L.C.: Changes in the contractile state, fine structure and metabolism of cardiac muscle cells during the development of rigor mortis. *Virchow Arch, 35:* 159, 1981.
15. Pappas, T.N., Taylor I.L., and Dabas, H.T.: Postprandial neurohormonal control of gastric emptying. *Am J Surg, 155:* 98, 1988.
16. Brophy, C.M., Moore, J.G., and Christian, P.E.: Variability of gastric emptying measurements in man, employing standardized radiolabeled meals. *Digestive Dis Sci, 31:* 799, 1986.
17. Kelly. K.A.: Motility of stomach and gastroduodenal juction. *Phys Gastrointestinal Tract, 1:* 393, 1981.
18. Adelson, L.: *The pathology of homicide.* Springfield, IL: Charles C Thomas, 1974.
19. Thommesen, P., Sgaard, P., Christensen, T., and Funch-Jensen, P.: Final gastric emptying of solid food in healthy subjects—Determined by x-ray examination and radionuclide imaging. *Rontgenblatter,* March 1990.
20. Bolondi, L., Bortolotti, M., Santi, V., Calletti, T., Gaiana, S., and Labo, G.: Measurement of gastric emptying time by real time ultrasonography. *Gastroenterology, 89:* 752, 1985.
21. Micozzi, M.S.: Experimental study of postmortem change under field conditions: Effects of freezing, thawing and mechanical injury. *J Forensic Sci, 31:* 953, 1986.
22. Brondum, N., and Simonsen, J.: Postmortem red discoloration of teeth. *Am J Forensic Med Pathol, 8:* 127, 1987.
23. Galloway, A., Birkby, W.H., Jones, A.M., Henry, T.E., and Parks, B.O.: Decay rates of human remains in an arid environment. *J Forensic Sci, 34:* 607, 1989.
24. Stewart, T.D.: *Essentials of forensic anthropology.* Springfield, IL: Charles C Thomas, 1979.
25. Gotouda, H., Takatori, T., Terazawa, K., Nagao, M., and Tarao, H.: The mechanism of experimental adipocere formational hydration and dehydrogenation in microbial synthesis of hydroxy and oxo fatty acids. *Forensic Sci Internat, 37:* 249, 1988.
26. Rayburn, W., Sander, C., Barr, M., and Rygiel, R.: The stillborn fetus: Placental histologic examination in determining a cause. *Ob Gyn, 65:* 637, 1985.
27. Moritz, A.R.: Classical mistakes in forensic pathology. *Am J Clin Pathol, 26:* 1382, 1956.
28. Pounder, D.J., and Jones, G.R.: Postmortem drug redistribution. *Forensic Sci Internat, 45:* 253, 1990.
29. Kenneth, G.V., and Smith, A.: *Manual of forensic entomology.* New York: Cornell Univ. Press, 1986.
30. Van de Voorde, H., and Van Dijck, P.J.: Determination of time of death by fungal growth. *Rechtsmedizin, 89:* 75, 1982.

Part 2

CHEMICAL CONSIDERATIONS

WILLIAM Q. STURNER

INTRODUCTION

THE GROWTH OF POSTMORTEM chemistry from early investigative studies to routine practice has advanced from the occasional complementary procedure to becoming an integral component at the time of the autopsy. These biochemical examinations often provide important data not only in determining the cause and mechanism of death and estimating the time since death, but also confirming many disease processes which represent a substantial portion of the medical examiner's caseload. It has been estimated that five to 10% of all cases can either be resolved or greatly aided in medical diagnoses as well as postmortem interval estimation by using chemical analyses of the body fluids.[1,2]

Postmortem chemistry had its beginning when blood was retained after death and examined for many substances. It was soon found that interpretations of some data from blood can be called into question due to autolysis producing interfering products and other postmortem alter-ations. Additional fluids have more recently been employed with the vitreous humor providing significant anatomic and chemical benefits, such as protection against early decomposition and thermal changes (Fig. III- 43).[3] This is often true for cerebral spinal fluid (CSF) which has also been extensively studied. Pericardial and synovial fluids have been tested less frequently with mixed results compared to other specimens, but have shown promise in other diagnostic areas.

Vitreous humor, along with serum and CSF, have received the most attention regarding scientific investigations over the past several decades and will be highlighted and discussed in detail. Landmark studies, especially those by Coe,[1,2,4] will often be referred to as well as the review of more recent work involving a variety of fluids and the documentation of some newer substances. Results from specific conditions such as SIDS will also be emphasized.

EVALUATION OF BIOCHEMICAL RESULTS

Evaluation of postmortem chemical studies from body fluids requires consideration of the following factors.

Time of Specimen Procurement

It is preferable that samples be obtained at the earliest possible time, with the optimal period ranging from shortly following death to the beginning of decomposition. Postmortem changes may significantly vary over time depending on environmental surroundings, with a refrigerated body preferred over one exposed to a warm temperature. Autolysis of blood, as indicated above, produces significant hemolysis, which modifies many results. CSF and vitreous humor, on the other hand, are usually clear and serous (watery), making them ideal for testing. These latter body fluids can, however, become opaque and discolored when putrefaction ensues.

Source of Fluid and Method of Removal

Early studies of enzymes, insulin, gases, and a variety of drugs displayed significant differences between samples from the right and left sides of the heart as well as between cardiac and femoral

128

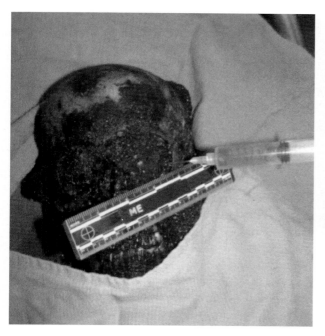

FIGURE III-43. Severely burned body with clear vitreous removed from eye.

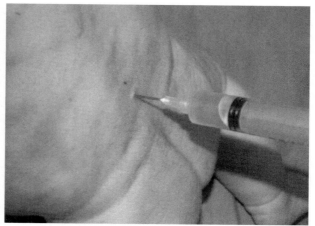

FIGURE III-44. Posterior view of infant with clear CSF from lumbar puncture.

blood.[1,2,4-6] Peripheral locations are now preferred as postmortem analysis has shown them to better reflect those levels found in the living state.[7,8]

Samples of vitreous humor should be obtained with a small (10–12 cc) syringe and a 20 gauge needle applying an easy but deliberate suction. Aggressive removal as well as the employment of vacuum tubes often results in retinal tissue fragments becoming dislodged, contaminating the usually clear specimen and potentially interfering with expected results. CSF amounts can vary from a few to more than 15 mL of fluid, whereas vitreous humor quantities are usually from 1 to 5 mL from each eye, although this can be somewhat less in the infant. CSF becomes the specimen of choice in child abuse cases when eyes are to be examined histologically, and a lumbar location represents the optimal site (Fig. III-44). It is necessary to remove all the vitreous from each eye as there are variations in solute concentrations near the retina as opposed to the center of the globe.[4] If the samples of vitreous obtained are viscous, centrifugation is recommended with use of the supernatant which passes more easily through the tubing of newer laboratory instruments.

Analytical Methodology and Normal Values

Values obtained from the various studies of serum, CSF, and vitreous humor can be affected by the analytical method employed.[9,10] This will not affect the interpretation of values for substances such as urea nitrogen but may do so for certain electrolytes, e.g. sodium. More recently, heat application has been utilized to improve the precision of electrolyte measurements.[11] With standard ranges of most substances documented in the literature, forensic scientists must be prepared to undertake similar methodology or understand the differences that may occur with procedures used in their own or other laboratories.

Variations of Vitreous Humor Levels in Different Eyes

Whereas many studies comparing chemical values of each eye show no significant difference when specimens are simultaneously withdrawn, others have reported that variations of some substances do occur. For example, the potassium level varied by more than 10% from mean values for each eye in 18.6% of a group when measured by an ion-specific electrode rather than flame photometry, which subsequent work has also demostrated.[12-14] The investigator must therefore take this into account, especially when obtaining fluids from separate eyes at varying intervals following death, since differences in the results may not necessarily represent the true picture of the postmortem change.

CARBOHYDRATES

Glucose

Early investigations have demonstrated that blood taken from the vena cava and the right side of the heart may have elevated glucose concentrations due to glycogenolysis in the liver with subsequent passage into nearby vascular channels.[1,2,4] It has been shown, for example, that blood obtained from an indiscriminate cardiac puncture can reveal an increased glucose suggesting a spurious antemortem diagnosis of diabetes mellitus. On the other hand, a low glucose concentration from right atrial blood with the additional finding of elevated ketones may indicate, along with autopsy findings and other supportive information, a condition of malnutrition and potential neglect.[4]

Increased levels of glucose occur in non-diabetics, even in samples of peripheral blood from various conditions such as cardiovascular disease and traumatic deaths including hanging, strangulation and electrocution.[1,2] An elevated catecholamine level from terminal stress has been postulated as the cause for this postmortem hyperglycemia, but similar findings have also been documented following resuscitation procedures. Coe has reported that in 1000 consecutive natural deaths, elevated glucose levels of 500 mg/dl (27.8 mmol/L) were found in 103 cases, none of whom had an antemortem diagnosis of diabetes, but wherein 87 of these patients were terminally resuscitated.[1] Other studies have revealed similar results, but suggested that uncontrolled diabetes could still be diagnosed from carefully examining the postmortem blood.[15] A serum glucose level alone, however, should not be used to diagnose diabetes mellitus.[4]

Newer studies on blood have proven useful when measuring glycosylated hemoglobin (HbA_{1c}), which is stable, and glycosated protein (fructosamine), which falls slowly after death.[16–20] The postmortem levels of these substances in normal patients decrease over time, whereas the concentrations in uncontrolled diabetic patients are sufficiently increased to be diagnostic. Investigations of these glycosates in vitreous humor have also been conducted.[21,22]

The difficulty in interpreting blood glucose values has led to examinations of CSF and vitreous. Glycolysis often results in a rather precipitous decrease of vitreous glucose in non-diabetics shortly following death but has little effect on high glucose concentrations in the uncontrolled diabetic patient.[23] Coe has shown in his aforementioned study that in non-diabetic patients measuring over 500 mg/dl of glucose in the peripheral blood, there was no case recorded in which the vitreous humor glucose level exceeded 100 mg/dl. Furthermore, in a complementary investigation testing several thousand vitreous specimens, glucose concentrations over 200 mg/dl were noted only in diabetic fatalities.[1] Thus, diabetic ketoacidosis can be readily confirmed by an elevated glucose and the presence of ketones in the vitreous humor.

Several reports have documented the sudden death of adults and children due to unsuspected diabetes mellitus, including an aketotic form showing a disproportionately elevated vitreous glucose with normal ketone levels.[24,25] A reliable diagnosis of diabetes can be made even after embalming as the vitreous will retain its antemortem glucose level.[26] In severely decomposed cases, blood and urine have been examined for acetone to diagnose ketoacidosis without the benefit of an accompanying vitreous glucose test.[27] Vehicular and other deaths potentially caused by hypoglycemia can be suggested from vitreous analysis but should be corroborated by analysis of an accompanying clinical blood sample.[28]

Other diseases have been studied with interpretation of glucose values used to support antemortem diagnoses. Elevated glucose levels have been observed when fatal hypothermia has been documented.[29-32] Slowing of glycolysis due to the low temperature and hyperglycemia resulting from stress are mechanisms that have been offered for this phenomenon. Research implicating hypoglycemia as a factor in SIDS and other infant deaths has not been successful, as glucose in the vitreous humor has generally been within normal limits.[4] Cases of neonatal diabetes and other metabolic conditions have been exceptions to this finding. Instances of accidental ingestion of foods with a high sugar content have resulted in a fatal hyperglycemic outcome.[33] Deliberate ingestion of a sugar solution in a depressed diabetic has also been reported.[34]

Lactic Acid

As indicated above, one is seldom able to identify hypoglycemia in the postmortem state because of significant glycolysis in all the body fluids following initial studies in the vitreous humor which suggested otherwise. To remedy this situation, it had been proposed that by combining the levels of glucose and lactic acid from spinal fluid specimens, the diagnosis of hypoglycemia could be made. Investigators further studied both diabetics and non-diabetics by measuring glucose and lactic acid in vitreous humor, and concluded that combined values over 375 mg/dl excluded hypoglycemia, whereas concentrations over 410 mg/dl were consistent with fatal decompensated diabetes mellitus.[35] They additionally suggested that values below 160 mg/dl might be diagnostic of hypoglycemia, but lacked individual data to confirm this concept. Other investigators performing similar studies were unable to improve upon these results.[36] The author's group described children without antemortem hypoglycemia whose combined values of lactic acid and glucose in vitreous humor were less than 100 mg/dl.[37] It appears from all these reports that an accurate postmortem diagnosis of antemortem hypoglycemia remains an elusive problem awaiting a more definitive solution.

Early studies of lactic acid have shown a dramatic and rapid increase in postmortem blood levels and a more regular early rise in CSF.[38] Jaffe also found concentrations in the vitreous humor to increase after death.[39] The study of lactic acid in infants referred to above included SIDS, respiratory infection and asphyxia, with the lowest combined levels (137 +/− 51 mg/dl) (15.4 +/− 5.7 mmol/L) found in the traumatic asphyxial cohort.[37] It was concluded that chemical analysis, coupled with case findings including the presence or absence of petechial hemorrhages, might be helpful in separating cases of SIDS from traumatic asphyxia.

Vitreous ascorbic acid levels decrease slowly over time, whereas vitreous pyruvic acid values decline rapidly following death,[39,40] but forensic applications for these substances have not been forthcoming. Inositol rises after death in CSF from a mean value of 2.7 ± 4.5 mg/dl to 72 mg/dl but shows substantial individual variations precluding its use in postmortem interval (PMI) determination.[41]

NITROGENOUS COMPOUNDS

Urea and Creatinine

The general stability of both urea and creatinine in the postmortem state, even with moderate decomposition, has been verified by old and recent studies of blood, CSF and vitreous humor.[1,42] As a result, the analyses of these substances have been useful when postmortem examination was limited or in supporting autopsy findings of renal disease, whether from natural causes including congenital defects or from chemical toxins.[4] Only minimal decrease of urea nitrogen occurs in vitreous humor following embalming so that uremic abnormalities can still be confidently determined.[26] Electrolyte measurements showing an imbalance accompanied by an elevated urea nitrogen are both required for a diagnosis of antemortem dehydration, a condition which cannot be supported solely by an increase in urea.[43]

Other Nitrogenous Compounds

In contrast to urea nitrogen and creatinine, non-protein nitrogen, ammonia and amino acids will increase in serum following death.[1] As a result, these compounds cannot be used to determine antemortem renal function or other diseases. Investigators including Schleyer, however, have employed these and additional markers to assess the PMI.[38] van den Oever noted a linear elevation in vitreous ammonia during the early PMI and proposed this as a possible indicator of the time since death.[44]

Free amino acids are present in the vitreous humor, and these substances have shown a rise in cases of sudden infant death.[45,46] However, they increased at varying rates for the different acids and appeared unreliable after 24 hours postmortem. Furthermore, an aminoacidopathy was not able to be established as an etiologic factor in SIDS cases.

Creatine was measured in CSF,[38] and more recently in vitreous,[47] both indicating a slow increase for up to 10 days. Glutamine was found to be elevated in CSF after liver failure,[1] but levels also rose with the PMI, rendering clinical interpretation equivocal.[4]

Oxypurines

Uric acid has been measured in postmortem serum, CSF, and vitreous humor.[48–50] A progressive elevation has been noted in most studies, but not in pooled frozen specimens, whereas varying levels found in synovial fluid appear to be more closely related to the cause of death.[51]

Xanthine has been shown to rise markedly in spinal fluid after death.[49,50,52] Vitreous xanthine levels have apparently not yet been reported. Hypoxanthine, on the other hand, has received significant attention, with studies noting elevated levels in extracellular fluids during hypoxia.[53] Further work has demonstrated much higher concentrations in SIDS cases than infants dying from other causes, suggesting a prolonged hypoxic state in the sudden infant death cohort,[54,55] but this has not been the experience of other investigators.[56,57] The former group has also used elevations of vitreous hypoxanthine as an estimate of the PMI during the first 24 hours, suggesting enhanced reliability as compared to potassium.[58] This phenomenon has also been examined and supported by James.[59] Madea, however, found better correlation with potassium than hypoxanthine.[60]

ELECTROLYTES

Sodium and Chloride

Serum concentrations of sodium and chloride fall shortly following death averaging as much as 1 mEq/L per hour. Because of the inability to rely on such changes, which are subject to variation in individual cases, it has become standard procedure to measure sodium and chloride in the vitreous humor where values remain nearly unchanged throughout the early postmortem period.[1,2] As a result, significant changes in sodium and chloride in antemortem serum are accurately reflected in levels obtained from vitreous humor which will, as a result, support a diagnosis of electrolyte imbalance.[61,62]

Coe has documented four distinct patterns (Table III-4) involving abnormal vitreous electrolytes:[4]

1. *Dehydration (hypertonic):* High sodium and chloride with a moderate increase in urea nitrogen.
2. *Uremia:* Normal sodium and chloride with markedly elevated urea nitrogen and creatinine.
3. *Low salt (hypotonic):* Decreased sodium and chloride with low potassium (15 mEq/L or less).
4. *Decomposition:* Low sodium and chloride with elevated potassium (20 mEq/L or more).

Potassium must be measured at the same time as sodium and chloride so that a true *low salt* pattern can be distinguished from decomposition, which also shows sodium and chloride decreases. Since potassium increases with time following death, a low potassium level will thus support the *low salt* diagnosis rather than postmortem autolysis.

TABLE III-4

PATTERNS OF ABNORMAL ELECTROLYTES

Category	Na+	Cl-	Urea	K+
Dehydration (hypertonic)	?	?	?	±
Uremic*	±	±		±
Low Salt (hypotonic)	?	?	±	?
Decomposition	?	?	±	

* Creatinine also markedly increased

It bears repeating that the analytical method employed for the measurement of sodium and chloride can affect the results and therefore the interpretation of the data. As discussed above, when comparing multiple instruments, the values indicative of an elevated sodium measured by flame photometry were found to be within the normal range when using an ion-specific electrode in the Ektacham system. Similar variations were noted for chloride but the changes were not significant for urea nitrogen.[12]

Electrolyte imbalance as a result of dehydration has been observed in infants with symptoms and/or documented findings of gastroenteritis.[63,64] Elevated sodium and urea nitrogen are the major chemical abnormalities found in these instances. In dehydration cases reportedly caused by ingestion of hyperosmolar formulas, hypernatremia has been the sole abnormality. Others have described hypochloremia in children and adults suffering from prolonged vomiting.[65] In adult patients, fatty liver and/or cirrhosis as a result of alcoholism can produce the *low salt* pattern.[66] In infants and adults who show evidence of malnutrition and dehydration but little else at autopsy, the use of vitreous humor to demonstrate electrolyte imbalance has helped to confirm these diagnoses. Such cases may display only external signs of dehydration such as sunken eye sockets and a decrease in skin turgor as well as *dryness* of the internal tissues.[67]

Salt intoxication has been described, as has water intoxication, resulting from forced ingestion as a form of punishment.[68] A case reported by Benz in which a three-year-old girl was made to eat food and drink liquid laden with table salt produced a vitreous sodium level of 210 mEq/L and a chloride of 167 mEq/L. Vitreous urea nitrogen was 30 mg/dl and the osmolarity was

442 mOsm/kg.[4] A diagnosis of salt poisoning should be suspected in any antemortem serum or postmortem vitreous sodium concentration over 200 mEq/L.

The author has examined a case of forced water intoxication in three siblings because "other types of punishment were ineffectual." The youngest, age 7, developed a seizure after ingesting *nearly a gallon* of water. Hospital admission blood data revealed a sodium of 118 mg% and chloride of 87 mg%. She died approximately one week following unconsciousness and coma.

Adult examples of water intoxication due to psychogenic polydypsia have been reported.[69] Others have been associated with cardiac medications:

A 58-year-old hypertensive woman was on a prescribed low-salt diet in addition to taking diuretics and digoxin, which she often renewed. Symptoms included weakness, nausea and some vomiting. She was found dead by neighbors at her residence where she lived alone. Moderate heart disease was noted at autopsy but there was no evidence of congestive heart failure. Vitreous chemistries revealed a sodium of 104 mEq/L, chloride 77 mEq/L, and potassium 6.2 mEq/L with a normal urea and glucose. Serum digoxin was 1.2 ng/ml in the peripheral blood with no other drugs detected. The final diagnosis was severe electrolyte imbalance caused by the low-salt diet and the diuretics.[70]

Potassium

Vitreous potassium concentrations have been shown to rise gradually and linearly with increasing time following death, allowing it to be employed as an estimation of the PMI. On the other hand, potassium breaks down in the cells of the body, including the blood, and rises precipitously following death thereby prohibiting serum levels from being used.[1] In CSF, potassium values rise more slowly but become unreliable after the twentieth hour postmortem.[46] A number of external factors influence the accuracy and validity of vitreous potassium including sampling (removal) procedures, analytical methodology, and the ambient temperature of the environment.[71]

Regarding sampling techniques, as previously mentioned, the entire globe must be emptied since fluid obtained near the retina may have different concentrations of solutes, including potassium, than liquid from the mid-portion of the

TABLE III-5

FORMULAS USING VITREOUS HUMOR K+ FOR PMI

PMI = 7.14 [K+] - 39.1		Sturner (1964)
PMI = 5.26 [K+] - 30.9		Medea (1980)
PMI = 4.32 [K+] - 18.35		James (1997)
PMI = 2.58 [K+] - 9.30 (all cases)		Muñoz (2001)
PMI = 3.92 [K+] - 19.04 (sudden deaths only)		Muñoz (2001)

eye.[4] Instrumentation comparisons have revealed that potassium values determined by flame photometry are less than those using an ion-specific electrode.[12] Thus, the rate of increase of potassium found in earlier studies tends to be lower than those performed in more recent investigations. In addition, and perhaps most importantly, environmental temperature has been shown to significantly affect the rate of change in the potassium increase, in contrast to earlier work indicating that this did not play a role.[71]

Internal factors also affect the elevation of vitreous potassium levels, including the age, duration of the terminal event and the level of urea nitrogen.[4,13] For example, vitreous potassium levels increase at a steeper rate in the infant as compared to the adult.[65,72] However, attempts to reduce pediatric data to a reliable graph or workable formula have as yet been unsuccessful. It has also been reported that individuals dying from sudden traumatic death have a more steady rise of potassium than those dying from a prolonged illness, the latter often reflecting recorded antemortem values.[13,73]

For these reasons, the possibility of error tends to be significant, especially as the time after death increases. Although some investigators have ceased to employ vitreous potassium for determining the PMI as a result of these findings, this test has been shown to be more reliable after the first 24 hours than any other chemical tests, especially when circumstances potentially affecting the results have been considered.[74]

Several formulas for the PMI have been developed (Table III-5), which differ when those factors described above have been taken into account. The slope of the rise in potassium determined by the author[73] was lower than that from more recent studies, including that of Medea et al., who found that their formula provided more reliable estimates.[75] The latter has been considered preferable unless the environmental temperature has been close to refrigeration levels during the PMI. In any event, the use of this formula under ideal circumstances provides confidence limits of plus or minus 20 hours for the first 100 hours after death. Recent work has provided additional data in support of this procedure, with new formulas developed, including further analysis on separation of hospital deaths from non-hospital fatalities.[76,77]

Case studies have indicated that vitreous potassium often provides a better estimate of the PMI than assessing the amount of decomposition, measuring body temperature, and even evaluating rigor mortis. Coe and Curran describe:

A teenage boy was discovered in the woods showing excellent preservation due to the environmental temperature remaining near freezing. The cause of death was multiple gunshot wounds. Rigor mortis was noted suggesting that the boy had been dead less than 48 hours. However, the vitreous potassium was over 25 mEq/L, consistent with the death interval being greater than 96 hours. Investigators subsequently discovered that the boy had been shot eight days prior to discovery. His stomach contents matched a meal provided by his mother two hours prior to his disappearance.[74]

Calcium, Magnesium, Phosphorus and Sulphur

Examination of postmortem serum initially showed that calcium remained constant in the early period following death, but additional investigations described a slow elevation during an increasing PMI.[78,79] Spinal fluid results revealed relatively stable values for up to 10 hours after death.[80] However, calcium in the vitreous humor, which averages between 6 and 8 mg/dl, rises slowly until decomposition.[81] Others felt that the increase found in patients dying from heart disease or asphyxia was helpful in establishing the PMI.[82] Vitreous levels tend to be independent from serum values so that even with an accurate diagnosis of antemortem hypocalcemia, there could be normal vitreous calcium concentrations.[61,83] Although studies of SIDS infants suggested that calcium was abnormal because of pathology or absence of the parathyroid glands, this finding has not been substantiated.[1]

An early and continuous rise in both serum and CSF magnesium levels has been noted.[1,2,80] Vitreous magnesium levels are dependent on age, with premature infants averaging 6 mg/dl (2.5 mmol/L).[81] Magnesium levels in infants are higher than those in adults, whose average is 2 mg/dl (0.82 mmol/L). This is probably the result of increased enzymatic activity in childhood associated with growth.[84,85] Thus, a gradual decrease in magnesium with advancing age has been determined to be physiologically normal. Reports have indicated a slow rise in postmortem magnesium with a lengthening PMI, but this was extremely variable and felt not to be reliable in estimating time of death.[81,82] Magnesium deficiency had also been suggested as a responsible factor for SIDS, but subsequent investigations have not supported this hypothesis.[84-86] Vitreous magnesium and CSF have been measured in two separate studies following immersion of human eyes in seawater, attempting to predict the length of time a decedent may have been submerged and whether a diagnosis of drowning could be supported.[87,88] An interpretation of this data seems to be dependent on water temperature,[89] and results from similar work by the author's group using bovine eyes appear neither to approximate a reliable time interval nor confirm the diagnosis of drowning.[90]

Inorganic and organic phosphorus values in serum and spinal fluid have shown an increase following death and vitreous inorganic phosphorus levels have also been measured.[91] Sulfate concentrations in serum and CSF remain constant in the early postmortem period, but in uremic fatalities, both serum and CSF values rise in direct relationship to the amount of urea or creatinine.[92]

Other Trace Metals

Selenium deficiency has been described in sudden and unexplained death in animals and was also considered as a potential factor for SIDS. However, selenium levels measured from infant fatalities due to recognized causes have been reported to be similar to those from sudden infant deaths.[93] Zinc levels were recorded in groups of older patients, with lower vitreous concentrations found in alcoholics compared with non-alcoholics.[94] This could not be substantiated by others who stressed the problem of contamination along with a postmortem rise in zinc; however, this latter study was performed using blood rather than vitreous.[95] Iron levels in vitreous humor were found to be less than those in serum, whereas a case report of iron poisoning revealed a six-fold increase in vitreous concentrations.[96] Strontium has been measured in serum from drowning fatalities and felt to be helpful in diagnosing saltwater, but not freshwater drownings.[97] However, these results have been questioned because of the statistical analysis.[98] Subsequent work has nonetheless confirmed the reliability of this test in freshwater fatalities.[99]

LIPIDS

Total serum cholesterol remains within a normal range following death, and postmortem levels have been shown by several authors to correlate closely in both high and low concentrations with antemortem values.[100-102] Considerable variation and unpredictability has been noted by others with cholesterol values increasing, decreasing, or remaining essentially unchanged during the first 24 hours after death.[103] Postmortem changes in cholesterol and other lipid levels have reportedly been affected by possible idiosyncrasy in the instrumentation systems.[104] Total cholesterol measurements have been employed to document familial hypercholesterolemia in spite of potential difficulties arising from these alterations.[105]

Changes after death have also been described in the study of postmortem triglycerides.[106] Additional lipids including total fatty acids, total lipoproteins, and beta lipoproteins were shown to be stable after death, supported by the determination of apolipoprotein-E phenotypes in postmortem serum.[107] Further investigations have reported irregular changes and proposed that any levels measured after the first day following death should be carefully interpreted.[104] Since most individuals are not in the fasting state at the time of death, elevated lipid concentrations should be evaluated with caution, and it becomes essential to correlate values with the contents of the stomach and upper intestinal tract. Thus, a meal ingested just prior to death might have been responsible for some of the earlier equivocal findings regarding the association of lipids and heart disease. However, a later study of lipids and lipoproteins showed little effect from either the PMI or recently ingested food on the results.[108]

PROTEINS

Measurements of total proteins as well as the albumin/globulin ratio after death are similar to that recorded in antemortem specimens except when significant hemolysis exists.[109,110] A slight fall in albumin with a modest increase in beta globulin has been described, with other fractions remaining generally unchanged. Immunoglobulins have shown a good correlation between values prior to and following death, although some qualitative differences have been observed.[111–113] Soluble proteins measured in vitreous humor were noted to be in the range of 40 to 80 mg/dl with the highest values occurring in the elderly.[114,115] Some proteins are unique to the eye whereas others have varying proportions in the blood and vitreous, but nearly all of the serum proteins can be detected in at least small concentrations in the vitreous humor.[116]

Electrophoretic studies have revealed that hypogammaglobulinemia is not related to SIDS, although some authors have documented higher levels of IgM in SIDS cases as compared to controls,[117–119] whereas others have found identical levels of IgM and IgE.[120] Postmortem electrophoresis has also confirmed clinical gammopathies including agammaglobulinemia and multiple myeloma, both of which had been diagnosed during life.[4]

IMMUNOLOGY

Postmortem fluids and tissues have undergone immunological techniques to document and characterize inflammatory and other diseases including myocarditis, syphilitic aortitis, Goodpasture's syndrome, meningococcemia, myasthenia gravis, and Reye's syndrome. Adenoviruses and respiratory syncytial (RS) viruses have been identified in the serum and vitreous, and hepatitis C virus and human immunodeficiency virus (HIV) have also been recovered by this technique.[4] Commercially available enzyme-linked immunosorbent assays (ELISAs) using Western blot analysis have shown exceptional specificity and sensitivity. Positive results were obtained when blood was drawn more than 24 hours following death, and even when serum analysis was not performed for several months.[4] The use of vitreous as well as aqueous humor as a fluid medium to demonstrate a variety of antibodies has been successful.[121–127]

The radioallergosorbent test (RAST) has been employed to identify the venom of bees which have allegedly caused death from anaphylactic shock.[128] This same technique has also substantiated fatal penicillin reactions as well as anaphylaxis resulting from certain foods.[129] Measurements of human mast cell tryptase will support anaphylactic reactions in the postmortem state.[130] A more recent study, however, urges caution when attempting to use an elevated tryptase alone to diagnose anaphylaxis.[131] Mast cell tryptase has also been reported to be significantly higher in a group of SIDS cases as compared to controls.[132]

Radioimmunoassay studies of spinal fluid from SIDS and control infants have documented differences in β-endorphin fractions.[133] Immunoassay analysis for human myoglobin has shown acceptable reproducibility in spite of hemolysis. This technique has been used in the assessment of antemortem injuries just prior to demise. The ratio of blood to spinal fluid levels of myoglobin was negatively correlated with increasing time following death.[134] An immunoabsorbent method has also been used for assaying postmortem thyroglobulin (Tg) in an attempt to support the diagnosis of mechanical asphyxia. However, no relationship between the PMI and serum Tg levels was observed. These values were also said to be reliable in specimens which were markedly hemolyzed.[135] Postmortem levels of neopterin, a derivative of pteridine, have been determined in serum. This substance increases with time following death but not with the uniformity required to use for the PMI estimation. Concentrations in urine are stable, reflect the antemortem findings in the serum, and have been judged to be helpful in the postmortem diagnosis of inflammation.[136]

BILE PIGMENTS

Although earlier studies found that antemortem and postmortem concentrations of serum bilirubin were similar, recent investigations revealed that some increase takes place following death. This change is relatively minor so that postmortem values generally agree with the amount of jaundice determined in the living patient.[4,78] Small amounts of bilirubin have also been detected in vitreous humor, CSF, and synovial fluids with considerable variations as compared to serum.[137] Urobilinogen has been found to pass from the blood into the spinal fluid whenever the blood level is elevated and the CSF-blood barrier is altered. CSF and urinary urobilinogen remain approximately equal. Urobilinogen in the urine remains unchanged after death so that postmortem values will reflect antemortem concentrations.[4]

Regarding the postmortem evaluation of liver function, low serum proteins with an inverted albumin/globulin ratio, elevated bilirubin, and abnormal levels of bile and urobilinogen in the urine are among the significant indicators of severe liver disease. Hepatic coma has been diagnosed by the determination of glutamine in the spinal fluid, with levels recorded three times as high in coma patients with liver failure compared to those without coma, even though the latter group contained patients with significant liver disease. Postmortem chemical examination for mild liver disease, however, is fraught with difficulty because of erratic hepatic enzyme elevations and the difficulty in interpreting small increases in bilirubin.[4]

ENZYMES

Enzymes provide little diagnostic value in postmortem cases, as serum elevations rapidly develop in amylase, transaminase, lactic dehydrogenase, creatinine phosphokinase, as well as alkaline and acid phosphatase.[138] Animal studies have demonstrated similar findings and revealed that this increase of enzymes is often temperature dependent. Notably, one enzyme which does not significantly change following a prolonged PMI, even at room temperature storage, is blood cholinesterase.[139] This permits a reliable analysis of this enzyme to detect poisoning by organic phosphate compounds, which cause a decrease in cholinesterase.[140] Total cholinesterase is stable for 10 days when refrigerated although there will be individual differences related to the length of the terminal episode.[141] More recent studies have examined specimens from simulated chemical weapons exposure.[142] Another enzyme with potential value is y-glutamyl transferase, which has been used in documenting chronic alcoholism after death as well as during life.[143] Carbohydrate-deficient transferrin (CDT) measured in vitreous has also shown promise in diagnosing alcoholism.[144,145]

Enzymes in the CSF, including transaminase, have likewise shown an increase following death, precluding interpretation of levels during life.[146] Initial studies in vitreous humor revealed variable or minimal amounts of detectable enzymes which were independent from serum values.[61,62] Later work has confirmed that y-glutamyl transferase shows little passage through the blood-vitreous barrier.[143,147] However, amylase does enter the vitreous and an increase in pancreatic amylase from acute hypothermia, including a preferential elevation of isoamylase in prolonged cases, has been reported.[148]

Postmortem vitreous increases of aminopeptidase and cathepsin-A in brain damaged patients have been reported, possibly assisting in case evaluation when autolysis precludes an adequate morphologic examination.[149] Enzymatic measurements in cases of SIDS have included transferase, creatine kinase, lactic dehydrogenase, and phosphoenolpyruvate carboxykinase (PEPCK), all of which show substantial variations.[150,151] High lactic acid dehydrogenase levels discovered during an unrelated study have been reported in cases of SIDS.[152]

Pericardial fluid analyses for enzymes, including lactic dehydrogenase and creatine kinase as well as their isoenzymes, have been performed to help establish the diagnosis of myocardial injury as a result of cardiac trauma and early myocardial infarction.[153,154] Additional reports have shown similarities in biochemical results among natural and violent deaths.[155] Troponin I has been evaluated in serum and more recently studied in pericardial fluid as a possible discriminator of sudden cardiac death, but with equivocal results.[156] An attempt to relate alkaline phosphatase, lactic dehydrogenase, and transaminase levels in synovial fluid to causes of death has met with limited success.[157] Amniotic fluid measurements of creatinine phosphokinase have been used to diagnose intrauterine fetal death.[158]

HORMONES

Pituitary growth hormone has shown a pronounced rise in the serum of infants shortly before succumbing to respiratory distress syndrome. This elevation was not dependent on glucose metabolism, acid-base balance or temperature.[159] Thyroid stimulating hormone (TSH) in the serum of both adults and infants is constant up to 24 hours following death making it a reliable test in assessing thyroid gland function.[160,161] The blood-vitreous barrier will be penetrated in some cases, but no relation was observed between postmortem serum and vitreous TSH.[162] Luteinizing hormone (LH) maintains its stability in the serum over 48 hours, with non-traumatic deaths showing lower concentrations than those dying violently. LH rarely passes through the blood-vitreous barrier.[163]

Serum cortisol in both adults and infants remains unchanged during the early postmortem period, averaging 18 mg/dl, and was noted to be similar in cardiac and peripheral blood.[164] This test can therefore help to exclude Addison's disease when hypoplastic adrenal glands or adrenal hemorrhage are found at autopsy. CSF levels of cortisol have been measured with values ranging from 1–17 ng/mL, with the average near 4 ng/mL.[165] Steroids have not been reported to penetrate the vitreous. 17-Hydroxycorticosteroids in postmortem serum are often elevated, with higher values noted after acute illnesses as compared to encephalopathies.[166] Serum concentrations of adrenaline and noradrenaline were found to be increased in normal subjects but were lower in cases of fatal trauma compared to sudden natural death.[167] Urinary catecholamines measured in fatal hypothermia cases revealed increased levels of both adrenaline and noradrenaline.[168,169] On the other hand, hyperthermia victims demonstrated elevated noradrenaline but low adrenaline concentrations.[170] Further experiments have not supported the usefulness of these biogenic amines as indicators of antemortem stress.[171]

Postmortem serum insulin levels in healthy patients are higher than antemortem values but large variations have been noted, with specimens from the right ventricle averaging some ten times greater than those obtained from the peripheral vascular system.[172] However, Coe has found that postmortem peripheral blood samples of insulin were lower than terminal antemortem specimens in most cases and that their level decreased as the PMI lengthened.[4] A number of reports involving suicides and homicides by insulin poisoning have been documented.[173-175] Others have discussed the techniques of insulin analysis along with the general subject of insulin toxicity.[176,177] Postmortem serum levels of C-peptide have been reported to be higher from the left side of the heart than the right side. These values decrease with an increasing PMI but there is considerable individual variation, with the rate of fall being 0.15 to 0.2 ng/mL/hour during the first 24 hours. Insulin and C-peptide penetrate the blood vitreous barrier to a minimal extent.[4] Measurements of C-peptide and insulin in overdose cases and in controls have recently been described.[178,179]

Thyroxin (T_4) has shown a postmortem decrease whereas patients exhibiting a slow death have also revealed low T_4 levels within three days prior to death. As a result, caution must be exercised when interpreting a low postmortem T_4 level as potential evidence of hypothyroidism.[160,180] Alternatively, a high postmortem level of T_4 and protein-bound iodine have helped to confirm a diagnosis of thyrotoxicosis.[181] Normal T_4 concentrations have been found in infants categorized as SIDS.[182] T_4 has not been shown to cross the blood-vitreous barrier.[162] Triiodothyronine (T_3) has been noted to both increase and decrease following death, thus hampering interpretation.[183] One SIDS study reported that a group of babies showed elevated levels of T_3.[184] Further investigations revealed that this change was unrelated to SIDS and could represent a postmortem artifact.[161,185-187] An unusual case of thyrotoxicosis has been diagnosed by a T_3 level following postmortem examination.[188] T_3 had not originally been found to penetrate the blood-vitreous barrier.[162] A newer postmortem study of thyroid hormones in blood and vitreous, along with thyroid gland histology, demonstrated T_3 and T_4 in femoral blood comparable to clinical values, and that those in the vitreous were lower than the blood results.[189] Serum parathyroid hormone (PTH) levels range from a stable postmortem level to a moderate elevation up to 17 hours after death.[183] Evidence of penetration of the blood-vitreous barrier by PTH has been reported.[4]

Postmortem serum testosterone from males who died suddenly averaged somewhat lower levels than suicidal deaths.[190] Melatonin values of infants who expired at night were decreased in SIDS cases compared to those dying from other causes suggesting a possible defect or an impairment of circadian rhythm.[191] Chorionic gonadotropin in both postmortem blood and urine showed concentrations corresponding to antemortem values in patients having tumors of the choriocarcinoma variety.[192] Serum prolactin has been found to differ according to the cause of death, with an elevation seen in postoperative cases, in the chronically ill, and in drug-induced suicides.[193] Prolactin in vitreous and spinal fluid has apparently not been studied.

MISCELLANEOUS

Blood gas analysis has been performed in canines in which fatal cardiac or respiratory arrest was induced under controlled conditions.[194] The PO_2 of systemic arterial blood in cardiac deaths was found to be more than 25 mmHg as compared with lower levels obtained in the respiratory group. A similar study has also been undertaken in humans at the hospital intensive care setting with similar findings.[1,2] PO_2 has been measured in a group of SIDS cases with lower levels found in this cohort as opposed to higher values for sudden *explained* infant deaths and in a random series of infant autopsy cases.[195] Postmortem oximetric profiles in various cases, excluding fire deaths, have been examined with only limited diagnostic value achieved.[196] In many adults, the appropriate blood specimen cannot be obtained, rendering blood gas analysis an inadequate test for routine use, although some fatalities due to cardiac arrythmia have been differentiated from instances of drowning.[4] Postmortem vitreous carbon dioxide content is quite stable, averaging a concentration of 15 mEq/L.[1]

The increasing acidity of blood during the PMI has been investigated, with the location of the sample influencing the amount of decrease in pH. Severely acidotic individuals differ from normal people to such an extent that determination of the acid-base status was felt to be useful during the first five hours following death.[1,2] The pH of cardiac blood has been evaluated in a small group of patients showing that during the PMI the concentrations fell from 7.0 to 5.5 over a period of 20 hours.[197]

Measurements of corticotropin-releasing factor in CSF during the first 12 hours after death revealed higher concentrations in suicidal fatalities than in a controlled population.[198] Other research relating to suicide has examined serotonin and its metabolite, 5-hydroxy indole acetic acid (5-HIAA). Some data showed 5-HIAA to be the same or higher in CSF from suicides as in normal individuals.[165,199] Other investigators, however, determined that both serotonin and its metabolite, 5-HIAA, are lower in suicidal patients than in controls.[200,201] Examination of tryptophan (TRP), serotonin metabolites such as 5-HIAA and other biogenic amine metabolites found that concentrations of 5-HIAA are higher in postmortem samples than in cisternal fluid from living patients. This study also showed that 5-HIAA and another amine, 3,4-dihydrox-

yphenylacetic acid (DOPAC) remained steady after death but TRP revealed a linear increase during the PMI.[202]

Other biochemical tests examining the time of death have been addressed. In the above study of monoamine metabolites in the CSF, the concentration of DOPAC increased during the PMI, but there was a scattering of individual data.[202] Investigations have further measured the third component of complement (C3), the rate being dependent on temperature with accuracy claimed under controlled conditions.[203] Changes in synovial fluid proteoglycans have also been suggested as useful in estimating the PMI.[204] None of these newer studies or calculations of other substances compare with vitreous potassium analysis which remains as the optimal biochemical test, especially in selected cases over longer postmortem intervals.[4] New techniques to measure vitreous potassium, such as capillary electrophoresis, have been utilized in forensic cases.[205,206] Studies documenting injectable potassium chloride have not been reported, although a fatal inadvertent spinal anesthetic administration has been described.[207]

Physical characteristics of serum and CSF have shown a shifting of the ultraviolet absorption curve in patients dying of hypoxia.[208] Fractions of serum esterase as determined by electrophoresis have revealed an increase in the concentration of some, with a diminution of others, while one new additional fraction has been determined.[138] Spinal fluid pleocytosis has been commonly observed after death, particularly in SIDS infants. The individual cells, predominantly lymphocytes and macrophages, are unable to be typed or compared after 12 hours. This phenomenon appears to be unrelated to any neurological condition or infectious agent.[209] Postmortem methemoglobin has been studied and expressed as a percentage of total hemoglobin. No relationship was found between recorded levels and the time of death or autopsy findings. Postmortem concentrations were deemed not to be reliable indicators of methemoglobinemia in the antemortem state.[210]

SUMMARY*

Routine chemical analysis of vitreous humor as well as serum, CSF, and newer fluid sources has become a commonplace procedure required in the general forensic autopsy. Vitreous studies of glucose, urea, sodium, chloride, and other chemical parameters provide medical information and often the diagnosis of conditions such as diabetes mellitus, uremia, and various types of electrolyte imbalance. Potassium measurement in the vitreous remains the most reliable chemical test for estimating the PMI in the majority of cases, with refinements of the procedure continuing to be described. Hormone analyses, enzyme studies and protein measurements may assist and even confirm additional diseases and other causes of death. A deficiency of some elements and abnormalities in others thought to be related to SIDS have not proven to be factors in this still enigmatic condition. The forensic pathologist must be cognizant of postmortem changes involving each of these substances and knowledgeable as to which procedures can provide accurate results in a given situation.

REFERENCES

1. Coe, J.I.: Postmortem chemistry of blood, cerebrospinal fluid and vitreous humor. In Wecht, C.H. (Ed.): *Legal Medicine Annual 1976*. New York: ACC, pp. 55–92, 1976.
2. Coe, J.I.: Postmortem chemistry of blood, cerebrospinal fluid and vitreous humor. In C.G. Tedeschi, W.G. Eckert and L.G. Tedeschi (Ed.): *Forensic Medicine*, vol. 2. Philadelphia: Saunders Co., pp. 1033–1060, 1977.
3. Harper, D.R.: A comparative study of the microbiological contamination of postmortem blood and vitreous humor samples taken for ethanol determination. *Forensic Sci. Int., 43* (1): 37–44, 1989.
4. Coe, J.I.: Postmortem chemistry update. *Am. J. Forensic Med. Pathol., 14* (2): 91–117, 1993.
5. Aderjan, R., Buhr, H., and Schmidt, Gg.: Investigation of cardiac glycoside levels in human postmortem blood and tissues determined by a special radioimmunoassay procedure. *Arch. Toxicol., 42* (2): 107–114, 1979.
6. Vorpahl, T.E., and Coe, J.I.: Correlation of antemortem and postmortem dioxin levels. *J. Forensic. Sci., 23* (2): 329–334, 1978.
7. Pounder, D.J., and Jones, G.R.: Postmortem drug redistribution–a toxicological nightmare. *Forensic Sci. Int., 45* (3): 253–263, 1990.
8. Prouty, R.W., and Anderson, W.H.: The forensic science implications of site and temporal influences on postmortem blood-drug concentrations. *J. Forensic Sci., 35* (2): 243–270, 1990.
9. Coe, J.I., and Apple, F.S.: Variations in vitreous humor chemical values as a result of instrumentation. *J. Forensic Sci., 30* (3): 828–835, 1985.
10. Daae, L.N.W., Teige, B., and Svaar, H.: Determination of glucose in human vitreous humor. *Z. Rechtsmed, 80* (4): 287–291, 1978.
11. McNeil, A.R., Gardner, A., and Stables, S.: Simple method of improving the precision of electrolyte measurements in vitreous humor. *Clin. Chem., 45* (1): 135–136, 1999.
12. Balasooriya, B.A.W., St. Hill, C.A., and Williams, A.R.: The biochemistry of vitreous humor. A comparative study of the potassium, sodium and urate concentrations in the eyes at identical time intervals after death. *Forensic Sci. Int., 26* (2): 85–91, 1984.
13. Madea, B., Henssge, C., Hönig, W., and Gerbracht, A.: References for determining the time of death by potassium in vitreous humor. *Forensic Sci. Int., 40* (3): 231–243, 1989.
14. Pounder, D.J., Carson, D.O., Johnston, K., and Orihara, Y.: Electrolyte concentration differences between left and right vitreous humor samples. *J. Forensic Sci., 43* (3): 604–607, 1998.
15. Gormsen, H., and Lund, A.: The diagnostic value of postmortem blood glucose determinations in cases of diabetes mellitus. *Forensic Sci. Int., 28* (2): 103–107, 1985.
16. Chen, C., Glagov, S., Mako, M., Rochman, H., and Rubenstein, A.H.: Postmortem glycosylated hemoglobin (HbA1c): Evidence for a history of diabetes mellitus. *Annals Clin Lab Sci, 13* (5): 407–410, 1983.
17. John, W.G., Scott, K.W.M., and Hawcroft, D.M.: Glycated haemoglobin and glycated protein and glucose

Acknowledgement: The assistance of Adam F. Craig, M.D., is sincerely appreciated.

concentrations in necropsy blood samples. *J Clin Pathol, 41* (4): 415–418, 1988.

18. Valenzuela, A.: Postmortem diagnosis of diabetes mellitus. Quantitation of fructosamine and glycated hemoglobin. *Forensic Sci. Int., 38* (3,4): 203–208, 1988.

19. Maruna, P., Skrha, J., and Strejc, P.: Serum fructosamine after death. *Diab. Med., 6* (5): 460, 1989.

20. Ritz, S., Mehlan, G., and Martz, W.: Postmortem diagnosis of diabetic metabolic derangement: Elevated alpha 1-antitrypsin and haptoglobin glycosylation levels as an index of antemortem hyperglycemia. *J. Forensic Sci., 41* (1): 94–100, 1996.

21. Peclet, C., Picotte, P., and Jobin, F.: The use of vitreous humor levels of glucose, lactic acid and blood levels of acetone to establish antemortem hyperglycemia in diabetics. *Forensic Sci. Int., 65* (1): 1–6, 1994.

22. Osuna, E., García-Víllora, A., Pérez-Cárceles, M.D., Conejero, J., Abenza, J.M., Martínez, P., and Luna, A.: Vitreous humor fructosamine concentrations in the autopsy diagnosis of diabetes mellitus. *Int. J. Legal Med., 112* (5): 275–279, 1999.

23. Sturner, W.Q., and Gantner, G.E.: Postmortem vitreous glucose determinations. *J. Forensic Sci., 9* (4): 485–491, 1964.

24. DiMaio, V.J.M., Sturner, W.Q., and Coe, J.I.: Sudden and unexpected deaths after the acute onset of diabetes mellitus. *J. Forensic Sci., 22* (1): 147–151, 1977.

25. Irwin, J., and Cohle, S.D.: Sudden death due to diabetic ketoacidosis. *Am. J. Forensic Med. Pathol., 9* (2): 119–121, 1988.

26. Coe, J.I.: Comparative postmortem chemistries of vitreous humor before and after embalming. *J. Forensic Sci., 21* (3): 583–586, 1976.

27. Smialek, J.E., and Levine, B.: Diabetes and decomposition: A case of diabetic ketoacidosis with advanced postmortem change. *Am. J. Forensic Med. Pathol., 19* (1): 98–101, 1998.

28. Sturner, W.Q., and Sullivan, A.: Hypoglycemia as the responsible factor in a truck driver accident fatality. *J. Forensic Sci., 28* (4): 1016–1020, 1983.

29. Bray, M., Luke, J.L., and Blackbourne, B.D.: Vitreous humor chemistry in deaths associated with rapid chilling and prolonged freshwater immersion. *J. Forensic Sci., 28* (3): 588–593, 1983.

30. Bray, M.: Chemical estimation of fresh water immersion intervals. *Am. J. Forensic Med. Pathol., 6* (2): 133–139, 1985.

31. Bray, M.: The eye as a chemical indicator of environmental temperature at the time of death. *J. Forensic Sci., 29* (2): 396–403, 1984.

32. Coe, J.I.: Hypothermia: Autopsy findings and vitreous glucose. *J. Forensic Sci., 29* (2): 389–395, 1984.

33. Sturner, W.Q., and DiMaio, V.J.M.: Fatal hyperglycemia and acidosis due to pancake syrup ingestion in a child with colonic interposition for esophageal structure from lye ingestion. *AACTION, 1* (1): 3–5, 1973.

34. Banaschak, S., Bajanowski, T., and Brinkmann, B.: Suicide of a diabetic by inducing hyperglycemic coma. *Int. J. Legal Med., 113* (3): 162–163, 2000.

35. Sippel, H., and Möttönen, M.: Combined glucose and lactate values in vitreous humor for postmortem diagnosis of diabetes mellitus. *Forensic Sci Int, 19* (3): 217–222, 1982.

36. De Letter, E.A., and Piette, M.H.: Can routinely combined analysis of glucose and lactate in vitreous humour be useful in current forensic practice? *Am. J. Forensic Med. Pathol., 19* (4) 335–342, 1998.

37. Sturner, W.Q., Sullivan, A., and Suzuki, K.: Lactic acid in concentrations in vitreous humor: Their use in asphyxial deaths in children. *J. Forensic Sci., 28* (1): 222–230, 1983.

38. Schleyer, F.: Determination of time of death in the early postmortem interval. In: *Methods of Forensic Science*, vol. 2. New York Interscience, John Wiley and Sons, pp. 253–293, 1963.

39. Jaffe, F.A.: Chemical post-mortem changes in the intra-ocular fluid. *J. Forensic Sci., 7* (2): 231–237, 1962.

40. Gantner, G.E., Caffrey, P.R., Sturner, W.Q., and Brenneman, C.: Ascorbic acid levels in the Postmortem Vitreous Humor. *J. Forensic Med., 9* (4): 156–159, 1962.

41. Nixon, D.A.: Cerebrospinal fluid inositol and its rise in post-mortem specimens. *J. Physiol., 129:* 272–280, 1955.

42. Fekete, J.F., and Brunsdon, F.V.: The use of routine laboratory tests in postmortem examinations. *Can. Soc. Forensic Sci. J., 70:* 238–254, 1974.

43. Andrews, P.S.: Cot deaths and malnutrition: The role of dehydration. *Med. Sci. Law, 15* (1): 47–50, 1975.

44. van den Oever, R.: Postmortem vitreous ammonium concentrations in estimating the time of death. *Z. Rechtsmed, 80* (4): 259–263, 1978.

45. Durham, D.G., Dickinson, J.C., and Hamilton, P.B.: Ion-exchange chromatography of free amino acids in human intraocular fluids. *Clin Chem, 17* (4): 285–289, 1971.

46. Patrick, W.J.A., and Logan R.W.: Free amino acid content of the vitreous humour in cot deaths. *Arch. Dis. Child, 63* (6): 660–662, 1988.

47. Piette, M.: The effect of the postmortem interval on the level of creatine in vitreous humour. *Med. Sci. Law, 29* (1): 47–54, 1989.

48. Sturner, W.Q., Dowdey, A.B.C., Putnam, R.S., and Dempsey, J.S.: Osmolality and other chemical determinations in postmortem human vitreous humor. *J Forensic Sci, 17* (3): 387–393, 1972.

49. Harkness, R.A., and Lund, R.J.: Cerebrospinal fluid concentrations of hypoxanthine, xanthine, uridine and inosine: High concentrations of the ATP metabolite, hypoxanthine, after hypoxia. *J. Clin. Pathol., 36* (1): 1–8, 1983.

50. Manzke, H., Krämer, M., and Dörner, K.: Postmortem oxypurine concentrations in the CSF. *Adv. Exp. Med. Biol., 195* (A): 587–591, 1986.

51. More, D.S., and Arroyo, M.C.: Biochemical changes of the synovial liquid in corpses with regard to the cause of death. 1: Calcium, inorganic phosphorus, glucose, cholesterol, urea nitrogen, uric acid, proteins, and albumin. *J. Forensic Sci., 30* (2): 541–546, 1985.

52. Praetorius, E., Poulsen, H., and Dupont, H.: Uric acid, xanthine and hypoxanthine in the cerebrospinal fluid. *Scand. J. Clin. Lab. Invest., 9:* 133–137, 1957.

53. Saugstad, O.D., Schrader, H., and Aasen, A.O.: Alteration of the hypoxanthine level in cerebrospinal fluid as an indicator of tissue hypoxia. *Brain Res., 112* (1): 188–189, 1976.

54. Poulsen, J.P., Rognum, T.O., Hauge, S., Øyasæter, S., and Saugstad, O.D.: Postmortem concentrations of hypoxanthine in the vitreous humor–A comparison between babies with severe respiratory failure, congenital abnormalities of the heart, and victims of sudden infant death syndrome. *J. Perinat. Med., 21* (2): 153–163, 1993.

55. Opdal, S.H., Rognum, T.O., Vege, A., and Saugstad, O.D.: Hypoxanthine levels in vitreous humor: A study of influencing factors in sudden infant death syndrome. *Pediatr. Res., 44* (2): 192–196, 1998.

56. Carpenter, K.H., Bonham, J.R., Worthy, E., and Variend, S.: Vitreous humour and cerebrospinal fluid hypoxanthine concentration as a marker of premortem hypoxia in SIDS. *J. Clin. Pathol., 46* (7): 650–653, 1993.

57. Belonje, P.C., Wilson, G.R., and Siroka, S.A.: High postmortem concentrations of hypoxanthine and urate in the vitreous humor of infants are not confined to cases of sudden infant death syndrome. *SAMJ, 86* (7): 827–828, 1996.

58. Rognum, T.O., Hauge, S., Øyasaeter, S., and Saugstad, O.D.: A new biochemical method for estimation of postmortem time. *Forensic Sci. Int., 51* (1): 139–146, 1991.

59. James, R.A., Hoadley, P.A., and Sampson, B.G.: Determination of postmortem interval by sampling vitreous humor. *Am. J. Forensic Med. Pathol., 18* (2): 158–162, 1997.

60. Madea, B., Käferstein, H., Hermann, N., and Sticht, G.: Hypoxanthine in vitreous humor and cerebrospinal fluid–A marker of postmortem interval and prolonged (vital) hypoxia? Remarks also on hypoxanthine in SIDS. *Forensic Sci. Int., 65* (1): 19–31, 1994.

61. Coe, J.I.: Postmortem chemistries on human vitreous humor. *Am. J. Clin. Pathol., 51* (6): 741–750, 1969.

62. Leahy, M.S., and Farber, E.R.: Postmortem chemistry of human vitreous humor. *J. Forensic Sci., 12* (2): 214–222, 1967.

63. Emery, J.L., Swift, P.G.F., and Worthy, E.: Hypernatraemia and uraemia in unexpected death in infancy. *Arch. Dis. Child, 49* (9): 686–692, 1974.

64. Huser, C.J., and Smialek J.E.: Diagnosis of sudden death in infants due to acute dehydration. *Am. J. Forensic Med. Pathol., 7* (4): 278–282, 1986.

65. Blumenfeld, T.A., Mantell C.H., Catherman, R.L., and Blanc, W.A.: Postmortem vitreous humor chemistry in sudden infant death syndrome and in other causes of death in childhood. *Am. J. Clin. Pathol., 71* (2): 219–223, 1979.

66. Sturner, W.Q., and Coe, J.I.: Electrolyte imbalance in alcoholic liver disease. *J. Forensic Sci., 18* (4): 344–350, 1973.

67. Coe, J.I.: Use of chemical determinations on vitreous humor in forensic pathology. *J. Forensic Sci., 17* (4): 541–546, 1972.

68. Zumwalt, R.E., and Hirsch, C.S.: Subtle fatal child abuse. *Hum. Pathol., 11* (2): 167–174, 1980.

69. DiMaio, V.J.M., and DiMaio, S.J.: Fatal water intoxication in a case of psychogenic polydipsia. *J. Forensic Sci., 25* (2): 332–335, 1980.

70. Coe, J.I.: Forensic aspects of cardiac medications. *Am. J. Forensic Med. Pathol., 2* (4): 329–332, 1981.

71. Coe, J.I.: Vitreous potassium as a measure of the postmortem interval: An historical review and critical evaluation. *Forensic Sci. Int., 42* (3): 201–213, 1989.

72. Mason, J.K., Harkness, R.A., Elton, R.A., and Bartholomew, S.: Cot deaths in Edinburgh: Infant feeding and socioeconomic factors. *J. Epidemiol. Commun. Health, 34* (1): 35–41, 1980.

73. Sturner, W.Q., and Gantner, G.E.: The postmortem interval: A study of potassium in the vitreous humor. *Am J Clin Pathol, 42* (2): 137–144, 1964.

74. Coe, J.I., and Curran, W.J.: Definition and time of death. In: Curran W.J.C, McGarry, A.L.M., and Petty, C.T.S. (Ed.): *Modern Legal Medicine, Psychiatry, and Forensic Science.* Philadelphia: FA Davis, pp. 140–169, 1980.

75. Madea, B., Hermann, N., and Henbge, C.: Precision of estimating the time since death by vitreous potassium–Comparison of two different equations. *Forensic Sci. Int., 46* (3): 277–284, 1990.

76. Gamero Lucas, J.J., Romero, J.L., Ramos, H.M, Arufe, M.I., and Vizcaya, M.A.: Precision of estimating time of death by vitreous potassium–Comparison of various equations. *Forensic Sci. Int., 56* (2): 137–145, 1992.

77. Muñoz, J.I., Suárez-Peñaranda, J.M., Otero, X.L., Rodríguez-Calvo, M.S., Costas, E., Miguéns, X., and Concheiro, L.: A new perspective in the estimation of postmortem interval (PMI) based on vitreous [K+]. *J. Forensic Sci., 46* (2): 209–214, 2001.

78. Coe, J.I.: Postmortem chemistries on blood with particular reference to urea nitrogen, electrolytes, and bilirubin. *J. Forensic Sci., 19* (1): 33–42, 1974.

79. Hodgkinson, A., and Hambleton, J.: Elevation of serum calcium concentration and changes in other blood parameters after death. *J. Surg. Res., 9* (10): 567–574, 1969.

80. Naumann, H.N.: Cerebrospinal fluid electrolytes after death. *Proc. Soc. Exp. Biol. Med., 98:* 16–18, 1958.

81. Farmer, J.G., Benomran, F., Watson, A.A., and Harland, W.A.: Magnesium, potassium, sodium and calci-

um in post-mortem vitreous humor from humans. *Forensic Sci. Int., 27* (1): 1–13, 1985.

82. Nowak, R., and Balabanova, S.: Determination of calcium and magnesium in postmortem human vitreous humor as a test to ascertain the cause and time of death. *Z. Rechtsmed, 102* (2–3): 179–183, 1989.

83. Dufour, D.R.: Lack of correlation of postmortem vitreous humor calcium concentration with antemortem serum calcium concentration. *J. Forensic Sci., 27* (4): 889–893, 1982.

84. Swift, P.G.F., and Emery, J.L.: Magnesium and sudden unexpected infant death. *Lancet, 2:* 871, 1972.

85. Blumenfeld, T.A., and Catherman, R.L.: Postmortem vitreous concentration (PVC) of Na, K, Cl, Ca and Mg in sudden infant death syndrome (SIDS). *Pediatr. Res., 9:* 347, 1975.

86. Sturner, W.Q.: Magnesium deprivation and sudden unexpected infant death. *Lancet, 2:* 1150–1151, 1972.

87. Adjutantis, G., and Coutselinis, A.: Changes in magnesium concentration of the vitreous humor of exenterated human eyeballs immersed in sea water. *Forensic Sci, 4*(1): 63–65, 1974.

88. Coutselinis, A., and Boukis, D.: The estimation of Mg2+ ion concentration in cerebrospinal fluid (C.S.F.) as a method of drowning diagnosis in sea water. *Forensic Sci., 7* (2): 109–111, 1976.

89. Bray, M.: The effect of chilling, freezing, and rewarming on the postmortem chemistry of vitreous humor. *J. Forensic Sci., 29* (2): 404–411, 1984.

90. Sturner, W.Q., Balko, A., and Sullivan, J.: Magnesium and other electrolytes in bovine eyeballs immersed in sea water and other fluids. *Forensic Sci, 8* (2): 139–150, 1976.

91. Devgun, M.S., and Dunbar, J.A.: Biochemical investigation of vitreous: Applications in forensic medicine, especially in relation to alcohol. *Forensic Sci. Int., 31* (1): 27–34, 1986.

92. Jensen, O.M.: Diagnosis of uraemia postmortem. *Dan. Med. Bull., 8* (suppl): 1–97, 1969.

93. Rhead, W.J., Saltzstein, S.L., and Cary, E.E.: Vitamin E, selenium, and the sudden infant death syndrome. *J. Pediatr., 81* (2): 415–416, 1972.

94. McDonald, L., Sullivan, A., and Sturner, W.Q.: Zinc concentrations in vitreous humor: A postmortem study comparing alcoholic and other patients. *J. Forensic Sci., 26* (3): 476–479, 1981.

95. Piette, M., Timperman, J., and Vanheule, A.: Is zinc a reliable biochemical marker of chronic alcoholism in the overall context of a medico-legal autopsy? *Forensic Sci. Int., 31* (4): 213–223, 1986.

96. Mittleman, R.E., Steele, B., and Moskowitz, L.: Postmortem vitreous humor in fatal acute iron poisoning. *J. Forensic Sci., 27* (4): 955–957, 1982.

97. Piette, M., and Timperman, J.: Serum strontium estimation as a medico-legal diagnostic indicator of drowning. *Med Sci Law, 29* (2): 162–171, 1989.

98. Hooft, P.J.: Serum strontium estimation as a drowning indicator: Statistical evidence revised. *Med. Sci. Law, 29* (4): 347, 1989.

99. Azparren, J.E., Vallejo, G., Reyes, E., Herranz, A., and Sancho, M.: Study of the diagnostic value of strontium, chloride, haemoglobin and diatoms in immersion cases. *Forensic Sci. Int., 91* (2): 123–132, 1998.

100. Naumann, H.N.: Postmortem liver function tests. *Am. J. Clin. Pathol., 26* (1): 495–505, 1956.

101. Enticknap, J.B.: Lipids in cadaver sera after fatal heart attack. *J. Clin. Pathol., 14:* 496–499, 1962.

102. Enticknap, J.B.: Fatty acid content of cadaver sera in fatal ischaemic heart disease. *Clin. Sci., 23:* 425–431, 1962.

103. Särikioja, T., Ylä-Herttuala, S., Solakivi, T., Nikkari, T., and Hirvonen, J.: Stability of plasma total cholesterol, triglycerides, and apolipoproteins B and A-1 during the early postmortem period. *J. Forensic Sci., 33* (6): 1432–1438, 1988.

104. Hart, A.P., Zumwalt, R.E., and Dasgupta, A.: Postmortem lipid levels for the analysis of risk factors of sudden death: Usefulness of the Ektachem and Monarch analyzers. *Am. J. Forensic Med. Pathol., 18* (4): 354–359, 1997.

105. Leadbeatter, S., and Stansbie, D.: Postmortem diagnosis of familial hypercholesterolaemia. *BMJ, 289* (2): 1656, 1984.

106. Sturner, W.Q.: Postmortem lipid studies: Attempts to correlate with death from arteriosclerotic heart disease in the young age group. *Forensic Sci. Gaz., 2* (1): 5–7, 1971.

107. Lehtimäki, T.: Determination of apolipoprotein E phenotypes from stored or postmortem serum samples. *Clin. Chim. Acta, 203* (2–3): 177–182, 1991.

108. Hiserodt, J.C., Perper, J.A., Koehler, S.A., and Orchard, T.J.: A comparison of blood lipid and lipoprotein values in young adults who die suddenly and unexpectedly from atherosclerotic coronary artery disease with other noncardiac deaths. *Am. J. Forensic Med. Pathol., 16* (2): 101–106, 1995.

109. Coe, J.I.: Comparison of antemortem and postmortem serum proteins. *Bull. Bell Mus. Pathobiol., 2:* 40–42, 1973.

110. Robinson, D.M., and Kellenberger, R.E.: Comparison of electrophoretic analyses of antemortem and postmortem serum. *Am. J. Clin. Pathol., 38* (4): 371–377, 1962.

111. Brazinsky, J.H., and Kellenberger, R.E.: Comparison of immunoglobulin analyses of antemortem and postmortem sera. *Am. J. Clin. Pathol., 54* (4): 622–624, 1970.

112. McCormick, G.M.: Nonanatomic postmortem techniques: Postmortem serology. *J. Forensic Sci., 17* (1): 57–62, 1972.

113. McCormick, G.M.: Serological aspects of environmental disease: The lung. Presented to the Society of Pharmacological and Environmental Pathologists, Chicago, IL, 1975.

114. Vilstrup, G., and Kornerup, V.: Protein fractions in corpus vitreum examined by paper electrophoresis. *Acta Ophthamol, 33* (1): 17–21, 1955.

115. Balazs, E.A., and Denlinger, J.L.: The vitreous. In: Davson, H. (Ed.): *The Eye,* 3rd ed. Orlando, FL: Academic Press, pp. 542–543, 1984.

116. Cooper, W.C., Halbert, S.P., and Manski, W.J.: Immunochemical analysis of vitreous and subretinal fluid. *Invest. Opthamol., 2* (4): 369–377, 1963.

117. Khan, W.N., Ali, R.V., Werthmann, M., and Ross, S.: Immunoglobulin M determinations in neonates and infants as an adjunct to the diagnosis of infection. *J. Pediatr., 75* (6 pt 2): 1282–1286, 1969.

118. Urquhart, G.E.D., Logan, R.W., and Izatt, M.M.: Sudden unexplained death in infancy and hyperimmunization. *J. Clin. Pathol., 24* (2): 736–739, 1971.

119. Urquhart, G.E.D., Izatt M.M., and Logan, R.W.: Cot death: An immune-complex disease? *Lancet, 1:* 210, 1972.

120. Clausen, C.R., Ray, C.G., Hebestreit, N., and Eggleston, P.: Studies of the sudden infant death syndrome in King County, Washington: IV. Immunologic studies. *Pediatrics, 52* (1): 45–51, 1973.

121. Gergora, Z., and Bruckova, M.: Attempts to demonstrate specific antibody responses in the vitreous body of the eye. *J. Hyg. Epidemiol. Microbiol. Immunol., 29* (1): 195–198, 1985.

122. Pepose, J.S., Pardo, F.S., and Quinn, T.C.: HTLV-III ELISA testing of cadaveric sera to screen potential organ transplant donors. *JAMA, 256* (7): 864, 1986.

123. Pepose, J.S., Pardo, F., Kessler, J.A., Kline, R., Donegan, E., and Quinn, T.C.: Screening cornea donors for antibodies against human immunodeficiency virus. *Ophthalmology, 94* (2): 95–100, 1987.

124. Klatt, E.C., Shibata, D., and Strigle, S.M.: Postmortem enzyme immunoassay for human immunodeficiency virus. *Arch. Pathol. Lab. Med., 113* (5): 485–487, 1989.

125. Tappero, P., Merlino, C., Cavallo, R., Vai, S., and Negro Ponzi, A.: Anti-HIV antibodies in postmortem vitreous humor. *Panminerva Med., 31* (4): 187–188, 1989.

126. Little, D., and Ferris, J.A.J.: Determination of human immunodeficiency virus antibody status in forensic autopsy cases in Vancouver using a recombinant immunoblot assay. *J. Forensic Sci., 35* (5): 1029–1034, 1990.

127. Grupenmacher, F., Silva, F.M., Abib, F.C., Grupenmacher, L., Silva, A.C., and Rodriques de Almeida, P.A.: Determination of cadaveric antibody against HIV in vitreous humor of HIV-positive patients: Potential use in corneal transplantation. *Ophthalmologica, 203* (1): 12–16, 1991.

128. Schwartz, H.J., Squillace, D.L., Sher, T.H., Tiegland, J.D., and Yunginger, J.W.: Studies in stinging insect hypersensivity: Postmortem demonstration of antivenom IgE antibody in possible sting-related sudden death. *Am. J. Clin. Pathol., 85* (5): 607–610, 1986.

129. Yunginger, J.W., Sweeney, K.G., Sturner, W.Q., et al.: Fatal food-induced anaphylaxis. *JAMA, 260* (10): 1450–1452, 1988.

130. Yunginger, J.W., Nelson, D.R., Squillace, D.L., et al.: Laboratory investigation of deaths due to anaphylaxis. *J. Forensic Sci., 36* (3): 857–865, 1991.

131. Randall, B., Butts, J., and Halsey, J.F.: Elevated postmortem tryptase in the absence of anaphylaxis. *J Forensic Sci, 40* (2): 208–211, 1995.

132. Platt, M.S., Yunginger, J.W., Sekula-Perlman, A., Irani, A.M., Smialek, J., Mirchandani, H.G., and Schwartz, L.B.: Involvement of mast cells in sudden infant death syndrome. *J. Allergy Clin. Immunol.,* (2 pt 1): 250–256, 1994.

133. Storm, H., Reichelt, C.L., and Rognum, T.O.: Beta-endorphin, human caseomorphin and bovine caseomorphin immunoreactivity in CSF in sudden infant death syndrome and controls. In: *The International Narcotics Research Conference (INRC) 1989.* New York: Alan R. Liss, pp. 327–330, 1990.

134. Miyaishi, S.: An enzyme immunoassay for human myoglobin and its application to forensic medicine. *Jpn. J. Legal Med., 45* (1): 6–25, 1991.

135. Tamaki, K., Sato, K., and Katsumato, Y.: Enzyme-linked immunosorbent assay for determination of plasma thyroglobulin and its application to postmortem diagnosis of mechanical asphyxia. *Forensic Sci. Int., 33* (4): 259–265, 1987.

136. Ambach, E., Tributsch, W., Rabl, W., Fuchs, D., Reibnegger, G., Henn, R., and Wachter, H.: Postmortem neopterin concentrations: Comparison of diagnoses with and without cellular immunological background. *Int. J. Legal Med., 104* (5): 259–262, 1991.

137. Naumann, H.N., and Young, J.M.: Comparative bilirubin levels in vitreous body, synovial fluid, cerebrospinal fluid and serum after death. *Proc. Soc. Exp. Biol. Med., 105:* 70–72, 1960.

138. Árnason, A., and Bjarnason, Ó.: Postmortem changes of human serum esterases. *Acta Pathol. Microbiol. Scand. [A], 80:* 841–846, 1972.

139. Petty, C.S., Lovell, M.P., and Moore, E.J.: Organic phosphorus insecticides and postmortem blood cholinesterase levels. *J. Forensic Sci., 3* (2): 226–237, 1958.

140. Ferslew, K.E., Hagardorn, A.N., and McCormick, W.F.: Poisoning from oral ingestion of carbofuran (furadan 4F), a cholinesterase-inhibiting carbamate insecticide, and its effects on cholinesterase activity in various biological fluids. *J. Forensic Sci., 37* (1): 337–344, 1992.

141. Moraru, I., Belis, V., Streja, D., Droc, I., and Ivanovici, V.: The study of blood cholinesterase in the cadaver in various kinds of death. In: *Proceedings of the Third International Meeting in Forensic Immunology, Medicine, Pathology and Toxicology.* London, England, 1963.

142. Klette, K.L., Levine, B., Dreka, C., Smith, M.L., and Goldberger, B.A.: Cholinesterase activity in post-

mortem blood as a screening test for organophosphate/chemical weapon exposure. *J. Forensic Sci., 38* (4): 950–955, 1993.

143. Piette, M., and De Schrijver, G.: Gamma-glytamyl transferase: Applications in forensic pathology: I: Study of blood serum recovered from human bodies. *Med. Sci. Law, 27* (3): 152–160, 1987.

144. Sadler, D.W., Girela, E., and Pounder, D.J.: Post mortem markers of chronic alcoholism. *Forensic Sci. Int., 82* (2): 153–163, 1996.

145. Osuna, E., Pérez-Cárceles, M.D., Moreno, M., Bedate, A., Conejero, J., Abenza, J.M., Martínez, P., and Luna, A.: Vitreous humor carbohydrate-deficient transferrin concentrations in the postmortem diagnosis of alcoholism. *Forensic Sci. Int., 108* (3): 205–213, 2000.

146. Fan, K.: 2′, 3′–cyclic nucleotide 3′–phosphohydrolase activity in postmortem human spinal fluids. *Neurosci. Lett., 19* (2): 229–233, 1980.

147. Devgun, M.S., and Dunbar, J.A.: Postmortem estimation of gamma-glytamyl transferase in vitreous humor and its association with chronic abuse of alcohol and road-traffic deaths. *Forensic Sci. Int., 28* (3–4): 179–80, 1985.

148. Devos, C., and Piette, M.: Hypothermia and combined postmortem determination of amylase and isoamylase in the serum and the vitreous humor. *Med. Sci. Law, 29* (3): 218–228, 1989.

149. Luna, A., Jimenez-Rios, G., and Villanueva, E.: Aminopeptidase and cathepsin A activity in vitreous humor in relation to causes of death. *Forensic Sci. Int., 29* (3, 4): 171–178, 1985.

150. Richards, R.G., Fukumoto, R.I., and Clardy, D.O.: Sudden infant death syndrome: A biochemical profile of postmortem vitreous humor. *J. Forensic Sci., 28* (2): 404–414, 1983.

151. Sturner, W.Q., and Susa, J.B.: Sudden infant death and liver phosphoenolpyruvate carboxykinase analysis. *Forensic Sci. Int., 16* (1): 19–28, 1980.

152. Badcock, N.R., and O'Reilly, D.A.: False-positive EMIT-st ethanol screen with postmortem infant plasma. *Clin. Chem., 38* (3): 434, 1992.

153. Luna, A., Carmona, A., and Villanueva, E.: The postmortem determination of CK isoenzymes in the pericardial fluid in various causes of death. *Forensic Sci. Int., 22* (1): 23–30, 1983.

154. Steward, R.V., Zumwalt, R.E., Hirsch, C.S., and Kaplan, L.: Postmortem diagnosis of myocardial disease by enzyme analysis of pericardial fluid. *Am. J. Clin. Pathol., 82* (4): 411–417, 1984.

155. Arroyo, A., Valero, J., Marron, T., Vidal, C., Hontecillas, B., and Bernal, J.: Pericardial fluid postmortem: Comparative study of natural and violent deaths. *Am. J. Forensic Med. Pathol., 19* (3): 266–268, 1998.

156. Cina, S.J., Thompson, W.C., Fischer, J.R. Jr., Brown, D.K., Titus, J.M., and Smialek, J.E.: A study of various morphologic variables and troponin I in pericardial fluid as possible discriminators of sudden cardiac death. *Am J Forensic Med Pathol, 20* (4): 333–337, 1999.

157. More, D.S., and Arroyo, M.C.: Biochemical changes of the synovial liquid of corpses with regard to the cause of death. 2: alkaline phosphatase, lactic acid dehydrogenase (LDH), and glutamic oxalacetic transaminase (GOT). *J. Forensic Sci., 30* (2): 547–551, 1985.

158. Kerenyi, T., and Sarkozi, L.: Diagnosis of fetal death in utero by elevated amniotic fluid CPK levels. *Ob. Gyn., 44* (2): 215–218, 1974.

159. Stubbe, P., Mentzel, H., and Wolf, H.: Growth hormone fluctuations in the paramortal period. *Horm. Metab. Res., 5* (3): 163–167, 1973.

160. Coe, J.I.: Postmortem values of thyroxine and thyroid stimulating hormone. *J. Forensic Sci., 18* (1): 20–24, 1973.

161. Ross, I.S., Moffat, M.A., and Reid, I.W.: Thyroid hormones in the sudden infant death syndrome (SIDS). *Clin. Chim. Acta, 129* (2): 151–155, 1983.

162. Chong, A.P.Y, and Aw, S.E.: Postmortem endocrine levels in vitreous humor. *Ann. Acad. Med. Singapore, 15* (4): 606–609, 1986.

163. Mendelson, J.H., Dietz, P.E., and Ellingboe, J.: Postmortem plasma luteinizing hormone levels and antemortem violence. *Pharmacol. Biochem. Behav., 17* (1): 171–173, 1982.

164. Finlayson, N.B.: Blood cortisol in infants and adults: A postmortem study. *J. Pediatr., 67* (2): 248–252, 1965.

165. Arato, M., Falus, A., Tothfalusi, L., Magyar, K., Sotonyi, P., and Somogyi, E.: Post mortem cerebrospinal fluid measurements in suicide. *Acta Med. Leg. Soc. (Liege), 36* (2): 120–125, 1986.

166. Done, A.K., Ely, R.S., and Kelly, V.C.: Studies of 17-hydroxycorticosteroids: XIV. plasma 17-hydroxycorticosteroid concentrations at death in human subjects. *Am. J. Dis. Child., 96:* 655–665, 1958.

167. Lund, A.: Adrenaline and noradrenaline in blood from cases of sudden, natural or violent death. In: *Proceedings of the Third International Meeting in Forensic Immunology, Medicine, Pathology and Toxicology.* London, England, 1963.

168. Hirvonen, J., and Huttunen, P.: Increased urinary concentration of catecholamines in hypothermia deaths. *J. Forensic Sci., 27* (2): 264–271, 1982.

169. Lapinlampi, T.O., and Hirvovnen, J.I.: Catecholamines in the vitreous fluid and urine of guinea pigs dying of cold and the effect of postmortem freezing and autolysis. *J. Forensic Sci., 31* (4): 1357–1365, 1986.

170. Kortelainen, M., Huttunen, P., and Lapinlampi, T.: Urinary catecholamines in hyperthermia-related deaths. *Forensic Sci. Int., 48* (1): 103–110, 1990.

171. Hirvonen, J., and Huttunen, P.: Postmortem changes in serum noradrenaline and adrenaline concentrations in rabbit and human cadavers. *Int. J. Legal Med., 109* (3): 143–146, 1996.

172. Lindquist, O., and Rammer, L.: Insulin in postmortem blood. *Z. Rechtsmed, 75* (4): 275–277, 1975.

173. Sturner, W.Q., and Putnam, R.S.: Suicidal insulin poisoning with nine day survival: Recovery in bile at

autopsy by radioimmunoassay. *J. Forensic Sci., 17* (4): 514–521, 1972.

174. Dickson, S.J., and Cairns, E.R.: The isolation and quantitation of insulin in postmortem specimens–A case report. *Forensic Sci., 9* (1): 37–42, 1977.

175. Hood, I., Mirchandani, H., Monforte, J., and Stacer, W.: Immunohistochemical demonstration of homicidal insulin injection site. *Arch. Pathol. Lab. Med., 110* (10): 973–974, 1986.

176. Kernbach-Wighton, G., and Püschel, K.: On the phenomenology of lethal applications of insulin. *Forensic Sci. Int., 93* (1): 61–73, 1998.

177. Fletcher, S.M.: Insulin. A forensic primer. *J. Forensic Sci. Soc., 23* (1): 5–17, 1983.

178. Iwase, H., Kobayashi, M., Nakajima, M., and Takatori, T.: The ratio of insulin to C-peptide can be used to make a forensic diagnosis of exogenous insulin overdosage. *Forensic Sci. Int., 115* (1, 2): 123–127, 2001.

179. Winston, D.C.: Suicide via insulin overdose in nondiabetics: The New Mexico experience. *Am. J. Forensic Med. Pathol., 21* (3): 237–240, 2000.

180. Bonnell, H.J.: Antemortem chemical hypothyroxinemia. *J. Forensic Sci., 28* (1): 242–248, 1983.

181. Simson, L.R.: Thyrotoxicosis: Postmortem diagnosis in an unexpected death. *J. Forensic Sci., 21* (4): 831–832, 1976.

182. Bader, M.: Normal thyroxine levels in sudden infant death syndrome. *JAMA, 248* (23): 3095, 1982.

183. Rachut, E., Rynbrandt, D.J., and Doutt, T.W.: Postmortem behavior of serum thyroxine, triiodothyronine, and parathormone. *J. Forensic Sci., 25* (1): 67–71, 1980.

184. Chacon, M.A., and Tildon, J.T.: Elevated values of triiodothyronine in victims of sudden infant death syndrome. *J. Pediatr., 99* (5): 758–760, 1981.

185. Peterson, D.R., Green, W.L., and van Belle, G.: Sudden infant death syndrome and hypertriiodothyroninemia: Comparison of neonatal and postmortem measurements. *J. Pediatr., 102* (2): 206–209, 1983.

186. Lee, W.K., Strzelecki, J., and Root, A.W.: Serum T_3 values and SIDS. *J. Pediatr., 101* (1): 161, 1982.

187. Schwarz, E.H., Chasalow, F.I., Erickson, M.M., Hillman, R.E., Yaun, M., and Hillman, L.S.: Elevation of postmortem triiodothyronine in sudden infant death syndrome and in infants who died of other causes: A marker of previous health. *J. Pediatr., 102* (2): 200–205, 1983.

188. Herman, G.E., Kanluen, S., Monforte, J., Husain, M., and Spitz, W.U.: Fatal thyrotoxic crisis. *Am. J. Forensic Med. Pathol., 7* (2): 174–176, 1986.

189. Edston, E., Druid, H., Holmgren, P., and Öström, M.: Postmortem measurements of thyroid hormones in blood and vitreous humor combined with histology. *Am. J. Forensic Med. Pathol., 22* (1): 78–83, 2001.

190. Roland, B.C., Morris, J.L., Sr., and Zelhart, P.F.: Proposed relation of testosterone levels to male suicides and sudden deaths. *Psychol. Rep., 59* (1): 100–102, 1986.

191. Sturner, W.Q., Lynch, H.J., Deng, M.H., Gleason, R.E., and Wurtman, R.J.: Melatonin concentrations in the sudden infant death syndrome. *Forensic Sci. Int., 45* (1, 2): 171–180, 1990.

192. Ludwig, J.: *Current Methods of Autopsy Practise.* Philadelphia: W.B. Saunders, pp. 220, 1972.

193. Jones, T.J., and Hallworth, M.J.: Postmortem prolactin as a marker of antemortem stress. *J. Clin. Pathol., 52* (10): 749–751, 1999.

194. Mithoefer, J.C., Mead, G., Hughes, J.M.B., Iliff, L.D., and Campbell, E.J.M.: A method of distinguishing death due to cardiac arrest from asphyxia. *Lancet, 2:* 654–656, 1967.

195. Patrick, J.R.: Cardiac or respiratory death. In: Bergman, A.B., Bechwith, J.B., and Ray, C. (Ed.): *Sudden Infant Death Syndrome: Proceedings of the Second International Conference on Causes of Sudden Death in Infants.* Seattle: University of Washington Press, pp. 131, 1970.

196. Maeda, H., Fukita, K., Oritani, S., Ishida, K., and Zhu, B.L.: Evaluation of post-mortem oxymetry with reference to the causes of death. *Forensic Sci. Int., 87* (3): 201–210, 1997.

197. Sawyer, W.R., Steup, D.R., Martin, B.S., and Forney, R.B.: Cardiac blood pH as a possible indicator of postmortem interval. *J Forensic Sci, 33* (6): 1439–1444, 1988.

198. Arató, M., Bánki, C.M., Bissette, G, and Nemeroff, C.B: Elevated CSF CRF in suicide victims. *Biol. Psychiatry, 25* (3): 355–359, 1989.

199. Endo, T., Hara S., Kuriiwa, F., and Kano, S.: Postmortem changes in the levels of monoamine metabolites in human cerebrospinal fluid. *Forensic Sci. Int., 44* (1): 61–68, 1990.

200. Stanley, M., and Stanley, B.: Postmortem evidence for serotonin's role in suicide. *J. Clin. Psychiatry, 51* (4) (suppl): 22–28, 1990.

201. Molcho, A., Stanley, B., and Stanley, M.: Biological studies and markers in suicide and attempted suicide. *Int. Clin. Psychopharm., 6* (2): 77–92, 1991.

202. Kärkelä, J., and Scheinin, M.: Tryptophan and biogenic amine metabolites in postmortem human cisternal fluid: Effects of postmortem interval and agonal time. *J. Neurol. Sci., 107* (2): 239–245, 1992.

203. Kominato, Y., Kumada, K., Yamazaki, K., and Misawa, S.: Estimation of postmortem interval using kinetic analysis of the third component of compliment (C3) cleavage. *J Forensic Sci, 34:* 207–217, 1989.

204. Hansen, L.M., Donnell, M., Robinson, S., Heimer, R., Molinaro, L., and Laposata, E.A.: Changes in synovial fluid proteoglycans as a possible marker of time of death [Abstract G25]. In: 42nd annual meeting, 1990, American Academy of Forensic Science, AAFS publication no. 90–92.

205. Tagliaro, F., Manetto, G., Cittadina, F., Marchetti, D., Bortolotti, F., and Marigo, M.: Capillary zone electrophoresis of potassium in human vitreous humor: Validation of a new method. *J. Chromatogr. B., 733* (1–2): 273–279, 1999.

206. Ferslew, K.E., Hagardorn, A.N., Harrison, M.T., and McCormick, W.F.: Capillary ion analysis of potassium concentrations in human vitreous humor. *Electrophoresis, 19* (1): 6–10, 1998.

207. Meel, B.: Inadvertent intrathecal administration of potassium chloride during routine spinal anesthesia: Case report. *Am. J. Forensic Med. Pathol., 19* (3): 255–257, 1998.

208. Laves, W.: Agonal changes in blood serum. *J. Forensic Med., 7:* 70–73, 1960.

209. Platt, M.S., McClure, S., Clarke, R., Spitz, W.U., and Cox, W.: Postmortem cerebrospinal fluid pleocytosis. *Am J Forensic Med Pathol, 10* (3): 209–212, 1989.

210. Reay, D.T., Insalaco, S.J., and Eisele, J.W.: Postmortem methemoglobin concentrations and their significance. *J. Forensic Sci., 29* (4): 1160–1163, 1984.

Part 3

FORENSIC ENTOMOLOGY

Neal H. Haskell

WITH THE DAWNING of the new millennium, the criminal justice system has increased its awareness of the usefulness of entomological evidence. This is due, in part, to the need for a more accurate estimation of the victim's time of death. In addition, the forensic entomologist, by using insect evidence, may be able to determine the origination of a body from a specific geographic area, sites of trauma on insect infested remains, toxicological analysis using the feeding insect larvae when human tissues are no longer available for such testing, and analysis of human blood meals from blood feeding insects for specific identification of a suspect or a victim.

Historical Background

Forensic entomology can be defined as the application of the study of insects and their arthropod relatives in legal proceedings. It has both civil and criminal components; but by strict definition is an applied science with recognized and accepted scientific principles within the field of entomology.

Despite the increased attention given to this field in recent years, forensic entomology is not new. The first documented case involving forensic entomology was a murder in thirteenth century China recorded in a forensic manual entitled *The Washing Away of Wrongs*.[1]

In 1235 A.D., the Chinese criminalist Sung Tz'u investigated the murder of a peasant worker whose body was discovered in a rice field. Noting the lack of physical evidence at the scene, and after fruitless questioning of the villagers, Tz'u requested that each farmer from the village bring his hand sickle for inspection. He arranged their sickles in front of each owner and after the passage of only a few minutes, flies appeared and congregated on only one sickle. The farmer who owned the sickle took this as a religious omen and immediately confessed.

Today, it would be obvious as it was to Tz'u that the flies were attracted to trace amounts of blood and tissue that remained on the blade. The unusually astute Tz'u is also credited with recognizing the utility of insect colonization patterns as possible indicators of antemortem wounds and the link between flies and maggots. He commented on the timing of insect colonization, now termed *insect succession*.

A review of the history of entomology points to the fact that Tz'u was over four hundred years ahead of his Western counterparts. The link between flies and maggots was not discovered in the Western world until 1668, with the now famous experiments of Francesco Redi disproving the theory of spontaneous generation. It is also interesting that the first use of insects in a death investigation from the West was not until March 22, 1850 when Dr. Bergeret d'Arbois investigated the case of an infant who had been plastered within a wall of a home near Paris, France. Dr. Bergeret utilized the insect evidence to determine that the remains had been placed within the wall in 1848, and that mites had deposited eggs on the remains in 1849, thus exonerating the current owners of any wrongdoing. The blame was shifted to the people who occupied the home in 1848. This case represents the first application of insect succession data in a death investigation.

Despite the earlier work of Dr. Bergeret, the researcher and author J. P. Megnin is generally credited with introducing the western world to the science of entomology. In 1894, Megnin published *La Faune des Cadavers: Application de l'entomologie a la médicine légale,* or as it is generally termed *The fauna of cadavers*. The purpose of this landmark work was to prove that the postmortem interval could be estimated by analysis of arthropods that inhabit the remains. Megnin described eight stages of human decomposition that he was able to identify from his empirical observations.[2] The eight stages set the groundwork for the many field experiments that followed involving the successional colonization of insects on human remains.

Although a great number of field studies have been undertaken to establish growth rates of insect larvae and succession patterns, entomology could not advance without the assistance of insect taxonomists. Insect taxonomists concern themselves with the identification and classification of insects based on identifiable characteristics unique to a specific species. Before entomologists can apply their knowledge to a legal investigation, they must first know the species of insect involved in the case. Most fly identification characteristics employed today for species determination were formulated in the late 1800s and early 1900s. There are two primary insect families from the fly group (Diptera) of medicolegal importance, the *Blowflies* (Family Calliphoridae), and the *Flesh Flies* (Family Sarcophagidae).

In 1916, J. M. Aldrich undertook the task of classifying and categorizing an entire group of flies for the purpose of their potential use in biological control. As a result of this work, he published a manuscript that detailed the identification of species within the family Sarcophagidae.[3] This manuscript focuses on one of the only distinguishing characteristics of the family, the genitalia of the male fly. Unfortunately, the sarcophagid larvae are not distinct enough or fully described to make identification based on their physical appearance. Identification of the many species in this family has always been problematic. This is why it is so critically important to not only preserve samples at the scene, but also to collect additional live samples for rearing to adult. It is not always possible to make a species level determination even with live reared adults. The advancement of DNA and protein techniques[4] and molecular technology will undoubtedly facilitate better identification of all life stages, but development of a genetic database of the numerous insect species, including the sarcophagids, is a very time-consuming and costly project. Due to limited resources, it may be some time before the full potential of molecular techniques are realized in insect identification.[4–9]

Entomology was advanced into the forefront of forensic science in 1935 with the infamous case of Dr. Buck Ruxton.[10]

Entomological evidence was crucial in determining the time of death when the remains of two dismembered bodies were discovered in a ravine known as *Devil's Beef Tub* in Dumfriesshire, Scotland. The remains were identified as Isabella Ruxton, the wife of Dr. Ruxton, and her personal nurse Mary Rogerson. Fly larvae on the remains were determined to be no older than 12 days. It was concluded that flies would have laid eggs on the bodies within 48 hours and therefore the remains had been thrown into the ravine at least 12 and no more than 14 days prior to their discovery. Based on the determination of the postmortem interval and other limited physical evidence, Dr. Ruxton, who never admitted his guilt, was found guilty and was executed by hanging.[11]

It was not until 1948 when D.G. Hall published *The Blowflies of North America* that entomology gained a solid foundation. Nothing so exhaustive as the detailed descriptions of flies of this family had been published before, or since. Interestingly, Hall published this work, in part, due to requests of the FBI and the Washington Metropolitan Police regarding the use of insects as evidence. D. G. Hall's monograph remains the standard reference work on blowflies.[12] Hall and Townsend published an additional in-depth investigation into blowflies, that was published as part of the *Insects of Virginia Series*. This publication has become an unofficial identification guide to the blowflies of the eastern United States.[13]

The publication of *Entomological Parasitology: The Relations Between Entomology and the Medical Sciences*[11] generated a great deal of attention to the subject of entomology and still remains one of the defining publications of this science. Throughout the mid-1960s, Jerry Payne undertook the task of gathering basic data to support the postmortem interval estimation technique of successional analysis. Payne detailed the changes that occurred during the decomposition of pig carcasses exposed to insects, and compared them with the changes observed in carcasses in which insect activity was excluded. Payne cataloged over 500 species of insects that inhabit carcasses in both terrestrial and submerged environments. Although many studies have been conducted and data compiled regarding arthropods in association with carrion, little has been obtained with a potential forensic application in mind. In the United States, one of the first studies that focused on the role of insects in the decomposition process of human remains, with a direct reference to its future forensic application, was by Rodriguez and Bass.[14]

Another landmark event in entomology was the publication by Smith, *A Manual of Forensic Entomology.*[15] It is a compilation of insect developmental data, case histories, and an excellent overview of the scope and application of entomology. For the first time, entomologists had a reference that detailed applications. At that time, one of the problems that still existed in the field was the fact that no book, manual, or guide existed that was written for the death investigator or crime scene technician. It was obvious that unless crime scene personnel were made aware of the scope of entomology, and how to properly recognize, collect and preserve evidence, the science could not hope to advance. In an attempt to increase the applicability, *Entomology and Death: A Procedural Guide* was published in 1990.[16] This text was directed towards those involved in the death investigation process and like Smith's book, it provided an overview of the scope and applications, with its main focus being proper collection and preservation techniques.

There are a number of methods entomologists can employ to determine the PMI.[9] The two most commonly used are distinctly different in their approach. In practice, they are complementary and not exclusive of one another.

One method utilizes knowledge of insect succession. A postmortem interval estimation can be made from the presence or absence of insects in combination on the remains. This method may not provide the precision necessary when short PMIs, such as 15 to 30 days, are involved. It is generally employed in cases with time intervals greater than 20 to 30 days and generally weeks to months, instead of days. Insect succession may also be used to demonstrate a season of the year and can estimate a postmortem interval back over several seasons. The drawback of this method is that it requires considerable empirical research, with the application limited to cases from geographic areas similar in climate and habitat to those in which the original succession research was conducted.

For instance, an entomologist could not readily apply succession data obtained from the west coast of the United States to a case from the east coast and expect a high level of confidence in the results. While it is possible that the insect succession could indeed be the same, a great deal of caution is recommended before conclusions are drawn due to the likelihood that major insect fauna and climatological conditions may be different. Therefore, depending on geographic area, specific terrain, climatological impact, and microenvironmental factors, the entomologist may need multiple data sets from within a particular region of the country. Thus, overall applicability of using succession data as an estimation of the postmortem interval during the initial few weeks after death can be limited due to the daunting task of data collection for specific environments.

The second primary approach of PMI determination is to utilize the rate of development of the insects on the body. One of the main advancements in the field is application of temperature-dependent development of insects to the estimation of the decedent's PMI.[17] The French scientist Reaumur was the first to recognize the temperature dependent development of insects in the early 1700s,[18] but it was not until the1950s that this principle was used to predict insect development.[19-21] Typically, this is one of the more accurate and precise methods an entomologist can utilize, but it also has important considerations and limitations.[9]

The basic premise of temperature dependent rates of insect development is that insects develop faster as temperature increases. These rates are bounded by what is described as their *thermal minimum, developmental minimum,* or *lower limit threshold temperature,* and an *upper lethal maximum temperature.*[9,21,22,25-29] This temperature response is described as the *S-shaped* growth curve.[30] Countless marine and terrestrial organisms exhibit this type of development, and it is commonly employed as a predicative indicator by natural scientists throughout the world.

One application of the temperature dependent development method to PMI estimation is to utilize the accumulated degree-day, or accumulated degree-hour, methodology. To apply this method properly, the species of insect in question must first be correctly identified, and climatological data must be collected from a nearby weather reporting station. The entomologist must understand how to correctly apply the developmental temperature thresholds and accumulated degree theory. This method may be misapplied because some entomologists may speak in terms of *degree hours,* when in actuality, they should limit themselves to *degree days* and weather stations may only report daily maximum and minimum temperatures instead of hourly temperature data. If hourly temperatures are not reported, then degree-hour calculation cannot be made.[17,26]

Although much literature on the topic has been published in scientific journals, there are only a few books available that are directed at the non-entomologist. Recently, Dr. Zakaria Erzinclioglu, one of Britain's most recognized entomologists, published his memoirs *Maggots, Murder, and Men.*[31] The work was not intended to expand scientific boundaries, but for the first time, a book was offered to those interested in the life and casework of a forensic entomologist. Quickly following the publication of Dr. Zakaria's book, M. L. Goff published *A Fly for the Prosecution,* which is directed towards the layperson with an interest in entomology. A work which did advance the scientific boundaries into the twenty-first century, *Forensic Entomology: The Utility of Arthropods in Legal Investigations,*[32] which featured chapters by entomologists in the United States and Canada.

Currently, much research is being devoted to improving the application of molecular techniques for both the identification of insect species as well as the recovery and genetic profiling of human tissue from insect contents.[8] Advancements are currently being made towards establishing basic statistics on the reliability of PMI estimations based on entomological evidence.[33-35] In addition, computer modeling techniques are being employed to reduce statistical error and to provide an alternative means of PMI estimation techniques. With a variety of analytical techniques at their disposal, entomologists are well prepared to assist those involved in the death investigation process when entomological evidence is recovered.

Applications of Forensic Entomology

Within the criminal justice system, the use of entomology is mainly associated with death investigations. When a dead body is found, there are multitudes of questions to be answered. Among the most important are: who is the victim; what was the cause and manner of death; where did the death occur; when did the death occur; and who are the suspects?

Currently, entomology is utilized to answer the question of how long the victim has been dead. This application has been the primary emphasis of most cases to date. Entomological evidence can also indicate where the death actually occurred. This application is based on geographic distributions of insect species. Additionally, entomology has been used to identify areas or sites of trauma on the remains when decomposition and maggot infestations are so advanced that the superficial tissues have been changed or totally destroyed. Insect larvae and puparia may be used to identify chemicals or drugs that have been introduced into the decedent's body before or at the time of death. These four applications of insect evidence are most commonly used in death investigations today.

Time of Death

Most death case investigations, specifically murder cases, are greatly enhanced if the time of death can be established. Suspects can be eliminated or implicated based on time of death information.

The use of a specific species' known growth and development for stages of its life cycle is the most precise method of estimating the time of death. The most common group of insects used for this specific application of the postmortem interval (PMI) estimation are blowflies (Family: Calliphoridae).

The calliphorids comprise 90 known species in North America with approximately 40 species available for use in PMI estimation. Blowflies usually are the first insects to colonize dead animals, with some species finding the dead animal

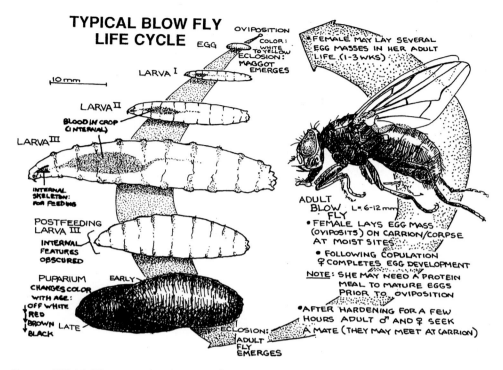

FIGURE III-45. The generalized blowfly (Calliphoridae) life cycle with an egg stage, three larval stages, a postfeeding larval stage and an adult stage. (after E.P. Catts, Catts and Haskell eds. *Entomology and Death*)

within seconds to minutes after death when temperatures are adequate to support flight activity.

The blowflies have a life cycle known as complete metamorphosis (Fig. III-45). The life stages of the blowflies include: (1) an egg stage; (2) a 1st instar larval stage; (3) a 2nd instar larval stage; (4) a 3rd instar larval stage; (5) a migrating larval stage; (6) a puparial stage; and (7) an adult stage. If the species of blowfly, the life stage, and the temperatures are known, a time estimation of initial colonization can be determined. This has been made possible by previous research on the duration of the life stages of many insect species at known temperatures in both laboratory and field studies.

Most research studies[36] with the exception of Greenberg,[37] indicate that blowflies are not active at night. Also, the species *Phormia regina* and *Cochliomyia macellaria* both delay their colonization from 12 to 24 hours at temperature in the 70s and 80s.[38,39]

The maggot infested, decomposing remains of a man were found under a pile of household items, in front of a garage within 15 feet of the street on Monday the 8th of August at approximately 12:00 noon. At autopsy, the cause of death was attributed to three stab wounds to the upper thorax. The victim was subsequently identified as the resident of the house. His wife, also a resident of the same address, became the primary suspect and was arrested for his murder. She claimed that she had last seen her husband around 10:00 PM on the evening of Saturday the 6th of August. This story would make the corpse about 36 hours old at the maximum time interval. Other information suggested that no one else had seen the husband since Thursday night at around 10:00 PM when the couple was leaving a local bar. At this time the couple was having a heated argument, with her screaming at him, "You SOB, I'm going to kill you!" If he had died sometime on the night or early morning hours of the 4th or 5th this would place the PMI at around 96 hours.

Insect specimens were recovered from the remains and shipped to a entomologist for examination and analysis. Two species of blowflies were identified from maggots retrieved from the body; the Black Blowfly *(Phormia regina)* and the Secondary Screw Worm *(Cochliomyia macellaria)*. The oldest life stage present was mature feeding 3rd instar larvae of *C. macellaria*. A representative sample had been recovered from the remains and included younger stages (early 3rd stage larvae, 2nd stage larvae and 1st stage larvae) of the same species. This assemblage of larvae suggested that a time interval much longer than 36 hours had passed. The remaining portion of the analysis and temperature data assessment was then conducted.

One method used for assessing temperatures is the quantification of hourly or daily temperatures to the units of either degree hours (DH) or degree days (DD). A degree hour is the hourly temperature less a base temperature giving the unit, degree hour. The base temperature is a temperature determined to be the lower developmental threshold, below which no growth and development take place. Once the units are determined, simply add each hour for the duration of time in question. This summation provides the units, accumulated degree hours (ADH). A degree day is the daily mean temperature less the base. As with ADH, add each day in question and this will yield the unit, accumulated degree days (ADD).[26] For this case there was a short period of time to study, and the hourly data were available, so the unit DH was chosen and used.

From experimental data, it was found that between 950 and 1150 accumulated degree hours are needed for *C. macellaria* to reach the mature feeding 3rd stage larvae. Therefore, when assessing the temperatures for the period, the entomologist would be looking for the range of time when this number of degree hours are accumulated. For this case, both above scenarios (wife's story v. other witness at bar) were evaluated. If the wife's story is true and her husband was killed during the early morning hours of August 6th, blowflies would not have colonized until after sunrise on the morning of the 6th. Energy unit accumulation would have ended when the larvae were collected at about noon on the 8th. The total ADHs present for this scenario would sum to only 450 (Table III-6). This total is hundreds less than what is needed to reach the 3rd stage maggot of *C. macellaria*.

Upon study of the second scenario, where the couple left the bar on Thursday August 4th at around 10:00 PM, colonization could have begun after sunrise on August 5th, so energy unit accumulation would begin at this point. By working backwards from the time the maggots were collected on August 8th and accumulating the degree hours, we reach 925 ADHs by midnight August 5th–6th with 1250 ADHs totaling by midnight August 4th 5th. Our needed ADHs is between 950 and 1150 (Table III-7). This value is reached prior to sunset on August 5th and would extend to sunrise of that same day. There is also a delay of some 12 hours or more for these two species of blowflies so death could have occurred even before midnight on August 4th with colonization during midday to late afternoon prior to sunset.

TABLE III-6

TOTAL ADH FOR PERIOD OF TIME FOR WIFE'S STORY OF LAST TIME SHE HAD SEEN HER HUSBAND

Date	ADH	Total ADH
8/8/94	196	196
8/7/94	250	446
8/6/94	0	0

TABLE III-7

TOTAL ADH FOR PERIOD FROM LAST KNOWN SIGHTING OF VICTIM LEAVING BAR ON THE EVENING OF AUGUST 4

Date	ADH	Total ADH
8/8	196	196
8/7	323	519
8/6	407	926
8/5	328	1254
8/4	0	1254

This evidence was presented to the court during a pretrial suppression hearing. The defendant watched as the entomological evidence was presented to the court. The next day, she accepted a plea agreement of 25 years in prison offered by the prosecutor to avoid the possibility of a longer sentence if she were to go to trial.

Another means of using an insect's specific life cycle to estimate time of death is to utilize its' specific seasonal distribution. Most insects are not found year-round, but only during portions of the four seasons. This is made even more specific by the geographic area in which a species is present.[40,41] Table III-8 lists several species of blowflies with their seasonal distributions for Indiana. Often when remains are recovered, many years have passed. Even after hundreds of years have elapsed between death and recovery, there still may be the puparial life stage of the blowfly remaining in or around the skeletal human remains. Though less precise than the above method mentioned, a confident estimate can be given to a season of year or possibly even the month when death occurred by careful examination of the empty puparial cases of the blowflies or other Diptera. This is seen in work conducted by Gilbert and Bass[42] in recovered Indian remains from the mid-1800s. In an earlier recovery of buried remains of Anasazi Indians dating to the mid-700s, analysis of the

TABLE III-8
SEASONAL OCCURRENCE OF BLOWFLIES
(CALLIPHORIDAE) IN NORTHERN INDIANA (1986)

Calliphorid Species	*Spring*	*Summer*	*Autumn*
Black Blowflies			
Phormia regina	X	X	X
Green Bottle Flies			
Lucilia illustris	X	X	X
Phaenicia coeruleiviridis	0	X	X
Phaenicia sericata	0	0	X
Blue Bottle Flies			
Calliphora colordensis	X	0	0
Calliphora livida	X	0	0
Calliphora vicina	X	0	X
Calliphora vomitoria	0	0	X
Calliphora terrae-novae	X	0	0
Cynomyopsis cadaverina	X	0	X

X - present   0 - absent

puparial cases indicated that death had occurred during summer and that the remains would have been exposed to open air for a period of several days before burial.[44]

In Indianapolis, three retired schoolteachers (a brother, sister and aunt) lived together however, only the male was seen about the small town. He told friends and neighbors that the two women were bedridden and he was caring for them. When the man was not seen for a number of days, neighbors became concerned, entered the house and found him dead on the living room floor. The bodies of two elderly women, were found in their beds, their bodies mummified.[45]

Recovery of pupae from one of two remains suggested October as the month of death for that particular individual while, absence of any blowfly activity on the second remains suggested a winter death. These times of the year were confirmed by documents (a diary, Christmas and birthday cards) recovered from the rooms where the women were found. While the month or season of death can be estimated with accuracy by this method, the specific year when death occurred is usually not possible to determine. Both women had died of natural causes and had been dead for approximately 10 years.

A second method for estimation of the PMI utilizes the concept of secession of different groups and species on decomposing remains as the carrion ages over time. As decomposition progresses, great changes take place in the soft tissues from a biochemical basis.[46] With these decompositional changes in the soft tissues of animals, comes a variety of odors being emitted due to the changes in the biochemistry. This brings about the attractability of the carrion to

different insect groups/species at different times postmortem.[2,47]

Through carrion studies in specific geographic areas and within specific habitats, the progression of decomposition, along with the changes in the insect fauna, can be established. This is known as successional patterns or seral waves of insects on carrion.

It should be noted that while both methods can be used for estimation of the postmortem interval, the specific species life cycle method is more precise when compared to the seral wave method. This is due to the variability of habitat, temperature and geographic area where the remains are discovered as opposed to where the empirical data study was conducted. Caution should be given to fixing specific short time intervals, a day or two, when applying this method. There is certainly nothing wrong with a several day or greater range when dealing with time of death greater than 30 days.

Geographic Location of Death

It is possible to determine a location of death of an individual by using insect evidence. This application of entomology is a more general determination than a specific one. However, there are exceptions where a specific geographic area may be identified from a particular species of insect.

The insects have what are called *ranges of geographic distributions* in which they reside. These ranges usually include like habitats or environments where temperatures and seasons are consistent with specific geographic areas of the world. On a global basis, there are those species found in the old world tropical areas (Tropical), the old world temperate areas (Palearctic), the new world temperate (Nearctic), and new world tropical (Neotropical).

For North America, calliphorid (blowfly) species number approximately 90. Of these 90 species about 40 may be used for forensic investigations. However, not all species are found from coast to coast. There are few species that are ubiquitous to the entire United States. *Phormia regina* (the Black Blowfly), *Phaenicia sericata,* and

Calliphora vicina are three species which can be found across the country, but their individual appearance is regulated by season of the year.

An example of a blowfly species with very limited distribution, *Phaenicia thatuna,* one of the green bottle flies, is found within about 50 miles of Coeur d'Alene, Idaho, at elevations of 3500 feet or more and only from July 1 to July 20.[12] If, for instance, a body was recovered in Illinois with *P. thatuna* on it, a reasonable conclusion would be that the body originated from that part of Idaho during July.

Other insect groups or other Arthropods (including spiders, ticks, mites, centipedes, millipedes, crabs, crawfish, and lobsters) may also have specific areas of geographic distribution.

A case from California where chiggers were recovered from crime scene responders investigating a murder. The species of chigger has a very limited geographic range of no more than a half mile in diameter of where the body was dumped. All crime scene personnel came from the scene with heavy infestations of the arthropod. When interviewed by detectives in the general course of the ensuing investigation, one of the suspects was scratching at chigger bites. After careful survey of the suspect's neighborhood, it was concluded that due to the absence of chiggers, where the suspect said he had been, the only location where the suspect could have contracted the chigger infestation was at the site where he had deposited the remains. After being presented with this evidence, the suspect confessed to the murder.[48]

Aquatic insects (Stoneflies, Mayflies, Caddisflies, and certain Diptera) are yet another group of insects that may provide connections between a suspect and a victim's remains. Many species of aquatic insects spend a great portion of their life cycle in water habitat as immature insects, feeding and growing. When they mature to the adult stage, they usually have a mass emergence (hatching) as adults, but are only present as an adult for a brief period of time. Certain adult aquatic insects have no mouthparts from which to feed and they will die shortly after they have mated and deposited their eggs. With this biology and behavior, a specific time frame can be identified relative to the adult of the species as well as a specific geographic region.

Areas of Trauma on the Remains

Blowflies are usually the first insects to find a body and begin colonization. The usual and preferred sites for initial colonization are the nose, mouth and eyes.[35] This is due in part to the attractant gases produced by the intestinal flora.[46] Also, the eyes, nose and mouth offer protection from predators, shading and moisture from which the newly hatched larvae can feed. Based on research in Tennessee,[50] it has been observed that blowfly larvae cannot penetrate adult human skin during the initial days of decomposition. Blowfly larval access to the muscles and organs must be through the natural body orifices. Human infants, however, do not have the heavy keratinization of the epidermal layer as is found in human adults, thus maggots are able to penetrate into the deeper soft tissues with little difficulty. As in adults, the nose, mouth, and eyes remain the preferred sites of entry, as are the pelvic openings, with an additional site being the umbilical area in the newborn.

The literature indicates that if large colonies of larvae are found in the vaginal area, and if the larvae are older than those in the face, or if there is exclusive colonization of the vaginal site, then some type of trauma is likely to have occurred in that opening.[36] Even during times when temperatures are high, there is a delay of colonization in the pelvic area. After several hours, however, the vaginal and anal areas will be colonized with sizable numbers of maggots.

When decomposition is advanced and all evidence of external trauma is destroyed, maggot colonization sites can provide clues as to where the trauma existed. The normal progression of tissue clearing of animal or human remains is sequential and consistent if there are no injuries present. This progression is dependent on the positioning of the remains, specifically what body parts may be in contact with the ground or with each other. For instance, if the body is laying on its side and an arm is resting under the torso, soft tissue clearing may take place on the arm in direct contact with the ground. This is due to the presence of moisture in the soil and the shading and protection of the arm from solar radiation by the torso.

The following describes the sequence of colonization for a subject in a supine position with the extremities spread slightly away from the torso:

Once the blowfly larvae have established in the face, and later in the pelvic area, the soft tissues of the head will be the first tissues to be cleared with the clearing extending to the neck region. Tissues in the pelvic area are reduced during this early stage of decomposition. As time progresses, the superior infestation will continue to feed down through the neck tissues and into the external and internal portions of the upper thorax. The maggots continue to feed as they move down into the lower thorax and upper abdominal areas. The inferior larval colony will remain primarily localized within the pelvic region and continues to clear the muscle and organ tissues there. There is little or no disturbance of the tissues of the upper and lower extremities due to inability of the larvae to penetrate adult human skin. Depending on temperature, the larvae that have reached feeding maturity by this stage of colonization have already migrated off the remains to pupate in the soil. Tissues in the lower abdominopelvic region are still moist, while remaining tissues in the extremities are dry and tough. Once the blowfly larvae leave, the body maintains this appearance for days or weeks. Other insect species continue to feed on the remaining dried tissues, with little physical changes in appearance over the next several weeks.

If antemortem or postmortem trauma has occurred to the remains, the above sequence may be altered. Environmental conditions, regional location, and variable temperatures can alter the drying of the remains, thus the amount of tissues the maggots are capable of successfully clearing. When a site of maggots are seen on the mid-torso, for instance, and blowfly colonization has begun only in the facial area, trauma in the area should be suspected. Examination of the underlying soft tissues may reveal a bullet track or knife wound.

If there is early colonization in the face and pelvic area and a heavy concentration of larvae is found on the soft tissues of the fingers, where the hand is away from the body trunk, examination of the fingers may reveal cuts or bullet wounds suggesting that the hand was thrown up in a defensive posture just prior to the attack.

Exposing the abdominal viscera, upper thoracic cavity, or the cranial vault through extensive blunt force, cutting or gunshot wound trauma provides enhanced attractability of the remains to searching female blowflies. When environmental conditions are favorable, hundreds of blowflies may be attracted in a matter of minutes to these wound sites and to the body organs thus exposed. This increased activity in conjunction with flies laying eggs within these exposed areas increases the speed in which clearing of organs, muscles, and other soft tissues from the skeletal structure of the body takes place. This rapid disappearance of tissue can give the impression of a longer PMI than is truly present. Therefore, it is essential to consider the age of the developing insects and the intervening temperatures, and not the physical appearance of the remains.

Toxicological Determinations from Insect Stages

Studies have shown that insect adults and larvae can be used to determine when chemical compounds are present in tissues.[51-58] These chemical substances range from heavy metals to drugs. The drugs or chemicals are ingested by the adult or larval specimen, then deposited into fat bodies within the insect or the protein of the exoskeleton (chitin). A quantity of larvae is collected, homogenized, then screened for the presence of these substances by a number of techniques, such as: gas chromatography, thin-layer chromatography, gas chromatography-mass spectrometry and high-performance liquid chromatography/mass spectrometry.[59]

Studies are ongoing regarding quantification of drug concentrations in insects versus concentrations of the chemicals in human tissues. Current application is limited to qualitative analysis of chemicals or drugs in the insect. The relationship between drug levels in insects compared to that in human tissues is unknown at the present time.

Postmortem Artifacts From Insects

A number of insects in both indoor and outdoor environments can leave superficial lesions or deeper impressions in living or dead humans. These artifacts, which resemble antemortem wounds, are created by a number of insect species from at least three major insect Orders. These artifacts may be confused with other trauma on the remains when these marks have had the opportunity to age, dry and darken. Insect lesions can resemble burns, human bites, scratches, or other types of superficial wounds. Information regarding the habitat where the remains were recovered is important. Size and orientation of the lesions may offer additional information as to what type of insect caused the damage.

For remains found in outdoor environments, the insect group most commonly encountered is ants. Under certain circumstances, cockroach and some type of beetle feeding may also be found. Ant artifacts will show superficial, small, often linear excavated areas of skin, usually on regions of the body where the skin is exposed (Fig. III-46). If there are substrates in contact with the skin, feeding may take place around them leaving a pattern.

In southern California, a body was found face down, partially covered by palm fronds, in a lot adjacent to an apartment building (Fig. III-47a–b). What was thought to be an extensive patterned injury from a shoe was noticed when the body was examined at the scene. However, it was subsequently shown that the patterned artifact was from large numbers of ants feeding from around and under the palm fronds.

There is considerable documentation of cockroaches feeding on both dead and living humans.[60-64] The feeding lesions of cockroaches appear slightly deeper than ant lesions and encompass a larger area. With heavy populations and enough time, extensive areas of skin can be eaten away by feeding cockroach larvae and adults (Fig. III-48).

In a documented case from Central Illinois, extensive areas of skin on the arms, hands and torso were eaten in less than four hours after death. The cockroaches ate only the exposed skin on either side of the forearm, and not the skin in direct contact with the floor on which the forearm was resting.

As with ants, cockroaches may also leave patterned injuries on skin.

The pattern on the lateral portion of the infant's torso was a result of fiber netting and structural support bar on the playpen restricting access to the skin in the area where the cockroaches were feeding (Fig. III-49). The initial impression at the autopsy was that of child abuse with antemortem wounds caused by beating. The close-up (see Fig III-49) and other photographs taken at the scene showed numerous feeding adult cockroaches on the playpen.

Most cockroach feeding cases occur indoors, but in one case, cockroach feeding created a puzzling series of wounds which initially could not be explained. The murder victim had been placed upon a pile of large sticks. Other sticks were placed over the body, partially concealing the

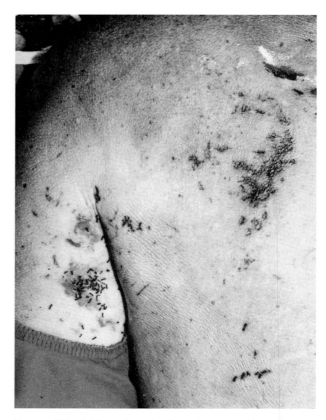

FIGURE III-46. Typical ant feeding on exposed human skin. A cluster of ants is seen on the back of the arm.

remains. When the body was found there was a large number of excavated areas with intermittent linear areas of undisturbed skin.

Further studies on cockroach and ant feeding are needed to devise not only the morphological characteristics of the artifacts, but a concrete test for positive determination of the wounds. There has been controversy between entomologists and pathologists over whether or not artifacts on remains are those of insects or from some other means. A definitive test may be possible by using group specific salivary proteins produced by cockroaches at the individual feeding sites. By swabbing across the site, presence or absence of cockroach salivary proteins could be established.

Other insect artifacts have been confused with trauma, conditions at the scene, or non-related substances found on bodies.

The body of a woman found in the Pacific Northwest had areas of petechial hemorrhage in the skin, but limited to areas not covered by clothing. Close examination revealed

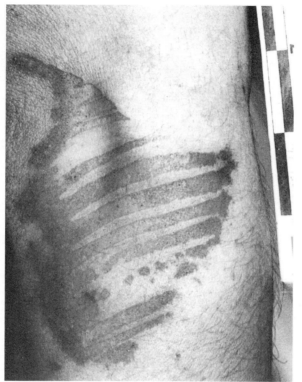

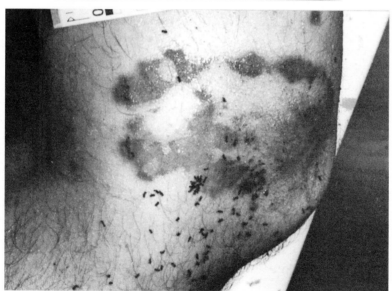

FIGURE III-47a–b. Patterned injury actually the result of ants feeding through palm fronds. (Courtesy of D. Greenlea, San Bernadino Police Department).

that these *pinpoint* hemorrhages were actually mosquito probing sites. Since the dead woman was still warm, a heavy infestation of mosquitoes probed the body, however, in the absence of capillary pressure no blood was drawn. The mosquitoes continued for a time in search of a site that would yield their needed food.[64]

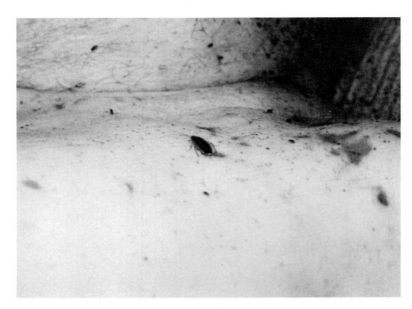

FIGURE III-48. Cockroach on decedent in mobile home with cockroach feeding artifacts. (Courtesy of Jasper County Indiana Sheriff's Department.)

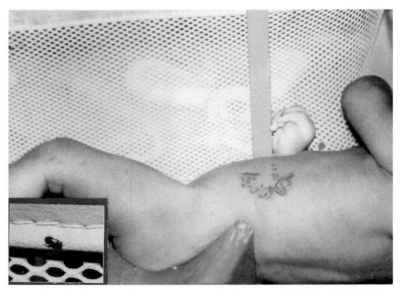

FIGURE III-49. Cockroach feeding artifacts on infant. Initially suspected of being the result of physical trauma. The insert shows a cockroach on the playpen. (Courtesy of Dr. D. Hawley, Indiana University School of Medicine.)

Seattle provided another interesting case involving insects. Direction of blood spatter and blood found under the cover page of a calendar that hung on the wall seemed inconsistent with a gunshot to the head which had killed the woman. After removal of the body from the scene, what had first appeared to be blood splatter artefact were actually found to be footprints of cockroaches which had been tracking through pools of blood.[64]

In yet another case, high velocity blood spatter observed at a scene seemed inconsistent with the circumstances surrounding the case. Upon analysis, the small dots of blood where finally identified as fly specks, the fecal and regurgitated materials of high concentrations of blowflies at the scene.

A stringy substance has been observed in cases of extended PMI from a number of states over the past three decades. In all cases, decedents had been dead for at least three months and more often over two years. The material resembles pencil sharpener shavings, but is tough to separate. In 1987 this substance, found on a Indianapolis case,[45] was identified (Fig. III-50a) by referring to an old case study from Denmark in 1962.[64] The material is the peritrophic membrane found to encase feces as it passes through the gut of certain beetle larva (Fig. III-50b). This membrane protects the inside of the intestine from damage caused by rough fecal materials. The importance of recognizing this membrane is that its presence suggests a prolonged PMI of months to years and that the remains must have been sheltered from the elements where degradation of the membrane would be significantly reduced.

Collection Procedures

Proper collection and preservation of insect specimens from human remains is imperative if meaningful answers are to be obtained. Accurate determination of specimens to species level can be accomplished only if morphological characteristics are intact and preserved for study. Can an entomologist draw an accurate conclusion from a single larva collected at the death scene? Possibly, but greater detail and precision can be achieved if adequate numbers of the insects are recovered for examination.

When conducting a death investigation, there are only two primary opportunities when the entomological evidence can be collected. The first is at the scene and the second is during the autopsy. It would be desirable to collect at both, to assure the greatest chance for recovery of all insect kinds present around, on, or inside the body. If both times of collection are not possible, then the scene where the body was recovered would present the most favorable opportunity to obtain the necessary specimens.

The death scene investigator will encounter a variety of habitats when investigating death scenes across the continent. These environments may comprise: high mountain areas; grassy plains; tropical forests; swamps; alpine meadows; river banks; car trunks; high plain deserts; drainage and irrigation ditches; lake shores; abandoned buildings; ponds; or shallow graves.

Collection of Data at the Death Scene

Primary to the collection of evidence at the death scene, whether entomological or otherwise, is the protection of the scene to preserve any and all evidence involved with the case.

The order of insect evidence recovery at the death scene can be divided into a number of stages:
1. Visual observations and notations of the scene.
2. Initiation of climatological data collection from the scene.
3. Collection of specimens from, and over the body before removal.
4. Collection of specimens from the surrounding area [up to twenty feet from the body] before removal of the remains.
5. Collection of specimens from directly under and in close proximity to the remains [three feet or less] after the body has been removed.

Recording the observations of insect activity on the remains prior to collection may prove useful to the investigation because once the collection is initiated, fast flying insects, highly mobile ground-crawling insects and sites of infestations may be altered or disappear.

Visual Observations of Insect Activity at the Scene

Visual observation and notation of insect activity in and around the remains can be of value even before the remains are examined. The scene investigator may accomplish this by:
1. Entering records on the *Death Scene Case Study Form* (Fig. III-51).
2. Recording the locations of major insect infestations associated with the body or surrounding areas. These infestations may be eggs,

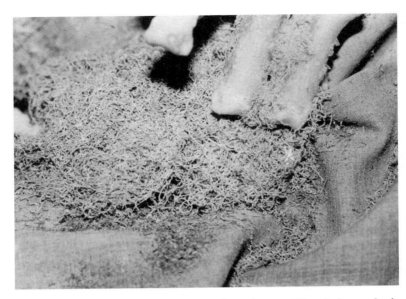

FIGURE III-50a. Peritrophic membrane from dermestid beetle larvae feeding on desiccated remains from long-term postmortem interval. (Courtesy of Dr. M. Clark, Indiana University School of Medicine.)

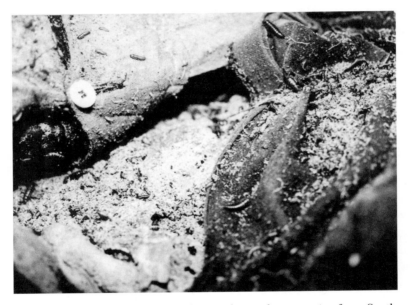

FIGURE III-50b. Peritrophic membrane observed on remains from South Carolina after extended postmortem interval. (Courtesy of E. Gardner, Charleston Police Department.)

larvae, pupae, or adult stages in any combination or by themselves.

3. Approximating the number and kinds of flying and crawling insects.
4. Recording immature stages of particular adult insects observed (flies or beetles). These stages may include eggs, larvae, pupae, empty pupal cases, cast larval skins, insect fecal material, and exit holes or feeding marks on the remains.
5. Recording any insect predation such as beetles, ants and wasps, or insect parasites.

DEATH SCENE CASE STUDY FORM

CASE STUDY # _____   DATE _____

NAME _____   AGE _____   SEX _____

DATE FOUND _____   DATE REPORTED MISSING _____

LAST SEEN ALIVE _____   LOCATION FOUND _____
                                                          City/County   State

INVESTIGATOR _____

SITE DESCRIPTION _____
_____

DEATH SCENE AREA
RURAL _____
    forest _____   tillable field _____   pasture _____   brush _____   roadside _____
    barren area _____   closed building _____   open building _____
    other _____
URBAN/SUBURBAN _____
    closed building _____   open building _____   vacant lot _____   pavement _____
    trash container _____   other _____
AQUATIC HABITAT _____
    pond _____   lake _____   creek _____   small river _____   large river _____
    irrigation canal _____   marine environment _____   other _____

EXPOSURE   open air _____   burial _____ (depth)   other_____

    Comments _____

ENCLOSED _____   shelter _____   plastic bag _____   auto _____   other _____

    Comments _____

REMAINS
CLOTHED _____   entire _____   partial _____   nude _____

    portion of body clothed _____
_____

    STAGE OF DECOMPOSITION fresh _____   bloat _____   active decay _____

    advanced decay _____   remains _____   saponification _____   other _____

    Comments _____

    EVIDENCE OF SCAVENGERS _____

    TRAUMA CONTRIBUTING TO INSECT ACTIVITY _____
_____

TEMPERATURES AT SCENE   ambient _____   body surface _____   ground surface _____
    under-body interface _____   soil _____ (10 cm, 20 cm depth)   maggot mass _____
    water temperature (if aquatic) _____   enclosed structure _____   [record temperatures
    (ambient, ground, soil) periodically each day at site for 2-5 days after body recovery]

NUMBER OF SAMPLES OBTAINED   preserved _____   live _____

WEATHER DATA _____
_____
_____

FIGURE III-51. Entomological Death Scene Case Study Form (from Catts and Haskell, eds. Entomology and Death).

6. Recording the position and orientation of the body: including the compass direction of the main axis, position of the body extremities, and position of the head and face in relation to other body areas; recording which body parts are in contact with the ground or other surfaces; recording where there would be sunlight and shade in the immediate area during a normal daylight cycle.

7. Recording insect activity within 10–20 feet of the body. Note flying, resting, or crawling insect adults, larvae and pupae within this area.

8. Recording any unusual naturally occurring, manmade, or scavenger- caused phenomena which could alter environmental effects on the body such as, trauma or mutilation of the body, burning, covering or enclosing of the body, burial, movement, dismemberment.

Written notations of the scene can be augmented with photographs and drawn sketches. Timed close-up photographs of the different stages or infestation sites of the insects found may provide important clues in analyzing the entomological information from the scene at a later date.

While video documentation is excellent for overall recording of the scene and observing entomological information from a gross perspective, fine details required in entomological investigations usually cannot be viewed by this procedure. A 35mm camera with a macro lens is the best tool for recording details of entomological evidence.

Collecting Climatological Data

Climatological or weather data are critical when analyzing entomological evidence from the death scene. The time required for insects to undergo their life cycle development is determined almost entirely by the temperature associated with those species present in a particular environment. Other climatological conditions, such as rainfall, full sun, snow cover, fog, also may influence the developmental rates or carrion feeding habits of the insects found at death scenes. Proper collection of data by the crime scene technician is essential to the investigation.

Since temperatures at the scene during the time when the remains were in place are of utmost importance, the following are suggestions for taking temperature readings *(the thermometer should be shaded from direct sunlight when taking all temperatures):*

1. Ambient air temperature can be evaluated by taking readings at one and four foot heights above the body.

2. Ground surface temperatures can be obtained by placing the thermometer on the ground immediately above any surface ground cover.

3. Body surface temperatures should be obtained by placing the thermometer on the skin. This will show heat loading of the remains through solar radiation.

4. Under-body temperatures, recommended for scenes during fall or winter, can be obtained by sliding the thermometer between the body and the ground. Ground heat may keep temperatures at or above freezing well into subfreezing ambient temperatures.

5. Maggot mass temperatures can be obtained by inserting the thermometer into the center of the maggot mass.

6. Soil temperatures should be obtained immediately following body removal at a ground point that was under the corpse mass. Also, soil temperatures should be taken at a point three to six feet from where the body lay. These should be recorded from three levels: directly under any ground cover (grass, leaves, etc.); at a soil depth of four inches; and at a soil depth of eight inches (primarily at scenes where there has been partial or full burial of the body).

Estimate the duration of exposure of the corpse to direct sunlight, broken sunlight and shade for the total daylight hours. This can be accomplished by observing overhead and surrounding vegetation, and buildings, etc. or the location of windows and noting their compass direction relative to the position of the remains. If there is any question as to this relationship, observation of the site periodically throughout a sunny day will provide additional information. When direct sunlight is shining on the body, the external temperature and some internal temperatures of the body, close to the surface, will be higher than when the corpse is shaded. These higher temperatures will be recorded even if the thermometer bulb is shaded and will reflect accurate temperature readings for the exposed remains.

Relative humidity has been found to be of little importance east of the Rocky Mountains due to adequate air moisture usually present on a continual basis.[39] In the more arid areas of the country, however, obtaining readings of relative humidity may answer questions as to why certain maggot stage development was not reached or maturation of the insects present was not accomplished.

After completing the insect collections and data recovery from the scene, weather data for the time period in question should be obtained. This time period extends from a few days prior to the estimate of the suspected time when death occurred (last seen alive) through a period of 3–5 days beyond the time when the body was discovered. Weather data retrieval can be accomplished by contacting the nearest National Weather Service (NWS) Station or other climatological data gathering agency. All data are eventually sent to NOAA, National Climatic Data Center, Asheville, NC, 28801-2696 and can be obtained in the form of published recorded material.

It may be important to conduct periodic temperature observations (3 to 4 readings over a 24-hour period for 3 or 4 days, particularly during times of temperature maximums and minimums) at the death scene after the body has been removed. This procedure will assess the correlation of the site temperatures with those of the closest NWS station.[26,66] Great differences can exist even in short spatial distances and the possibility for this type of error must be considered. By making periodic daily visits, including after dark, to the site over several days, accurate calibration can be made between the data of the NWS and death sites.

Collection of Specimens before Body Removal

Proper collection and preservation techniques, specimen labeling, and data recording are necessary.

An aerial insect net is essential during this stage of the entomological investigation for collecting fast flying adult insects over the remains. If flying insects are present over the body, aerial sweeping or trapping techniques for collecting can be employed. Flying insects associated with carrion are strong, fast fliers, thus, netting of these specimens requires some experience and practice. Following immobilization with a killing jar, the insects captured in the net can be transferred into vials (4 dram screw cap) of 75% ETOH (ethyl alcohol) by placing a small funnel into the vial and carefully dumping the contents of the net into the funnel. Some of the specimens may be placed into a dry vial for direct pinning. If stored in this dry condition, however, the insects must be processed in a few hours because excessive moisture on the insects as a result of condensation arising from within the closed vial can promote mold growth that will quickly damage or destroy the specimens. The sweep netting procedure should be repeated three to four times to ensure a representative sample of all flying insects present.

Many ground-crawling adult insects or larvae can be collected with forceps or fingers. Preservation should be conducted in the same manner as with adult flying insects. These include beetles, ants, bees and wasps, true bugs, springtails, and newly emerged flies.

A label should be placed into each collection vial immediately which gives the sample number, hour, date, case number, and county/city. Labels made with a graphite pencil will not be affected by solutions used to preserve the specimens. A duplicate label should be affixed to the outside of the vial. This double labeling procedure should be standard practice.

The sweep netting technique can also be used to capture insects resting on vegetation in the area surrounding the body. By sweeping the vegetation within 10–20 feet of the corpse, some of the adult insects may be collected.

Once the surrounding area has been processed, collection of specimens from the body can begin. Eggs and a mixed size sample of larvae (tens to hundreds) should be collected and preserved in one of the specified preservatives

TABLE III-9
SOLUTIONS FOR KILLING AND PRESERVING INSECTS

1. Ethyl Alcohol (Ethanol) 70–80% Solution

For killing and preserving adult specimens; for preserving larval specimens.

Ethanol (ETOH) usually is purchased in bulk at 95% concentration. To make a 70% solution from this, simply measure 70 units of the 95% ETOH and add enough water (distilled is preferred) to give a total of 95 units of mixed solution. An 80% solution is similarly prepared by adding enough water (15 units) to 80 units of 95% ETOH to give a total of 95 units of mix.

2. Hood's Solution:

For killing and preserving adult specimens; for preserving larval specimens.

75% Ethanol	95 ml
Glycerine	5 ml

3. Kahle's Solution:

For killing and preserving adult specimens; for preserving larval specimens.

95% Ethanol	30 ml
Formaldehyde	12 ml
Glacial Acetic Acid	4 ml
Water	60 ml

4. KAA:

For killing larval specimens only (not for preserving as it causes specimens to become overly brittle after approximately 12 hours).

95% Ethanol	80–100 ml
Glacial Acetic Acid	20 ml
Kerosene	10 ml
Dioxane	10 ml

After killing, specimens should be transferred from KAAD to 70–80% alcohol (ethanol).

5. X.A.:

For killing larval specimens.

Xylene	50 ml
95% Ethanol	50 ml

6. X.A.A.:

For killing larval specimens only (not for preserving). See comments for K.A.A.D.

Xylene	40 ml
Isopropyl Alcohol	60 ml
Glacial Acetic Acid	50 ml
Dioxane	40 ml

The solutions intended only for killing larval specimens are best used at the point of initial collection. The larvae should then be transferred into 75% ethanol within 10–12 hours after they have been placed in these killing agents. The longer they are left in the killing solutions (i.e., KAA and XAA), the more brittle they will become. If these are shipped to the entomology laboratory in the killing agents in less than a day after collection, then the entomologist can make the transfer to ethanol.

listed in Table III-9. The largest larvae observed should be collected and, if numbers permit, several dozen of these should be placed into the preservative solution (Fig. III-52). A second portion (2–3 dozen) of large larvae should be placed alive into plastic specimen cups containing damp paper toweling, or placed directly into previously prepared maggot rearing cups (Fig. III-53). It is important to rear the eggs, and the very small larvae, as well as the larger larvae, to adulthood to facilitate and confirm species identification of the eggs or larvae collected. By making compan-ion sample collections, confirmation of the species is insured. In addition, the date and time when the sample was preserved is recorded for calculating backwards to the time of initial colonization.

Specific areas of the body where concentrated insect activity most likely will be encountered during the earlier stages of colonization are the nasal openings, ears, mouth, eyes and trauma-tized areas of the body, where the skin is broken. Skin creases of the neck also may contain egg masses. Egg masses will also be found along the

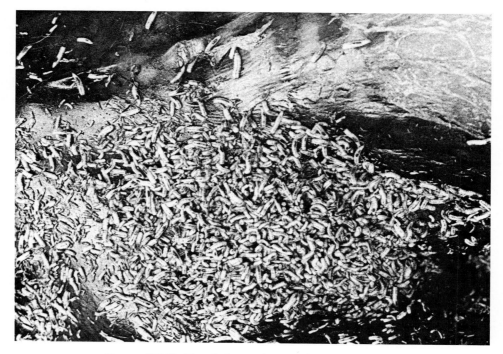

FIGURE III-52. Blowfly larvae (maggots) of different ages.

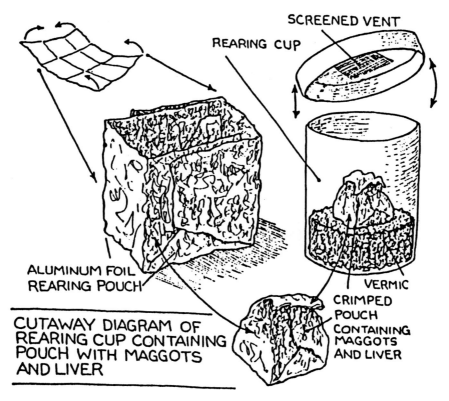

FIGURE III-53. Diagram of the maggot rearing cup (maggot motel) with beef liver pouch inserted for rearing fly eggs and larvae to adult specimens for identification confirmation. (From Catts and Haskell, eds. *Entomology and Death.*)

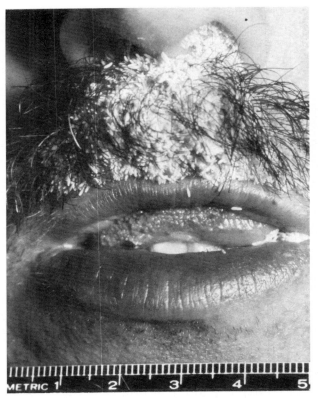

FIGURE III-54. Clusters of young maggots in left nostril and moustache.

hair line close to the natural body openings, open wounds and exposed genital and anal areas may contain egg masses and larvae (Fig. III-54).

Collection of Specimens after Body Removal

In cases where bodies are outdoors and are heavily infested, many adult insects, larvae, pupae, and other arthropods, will remain on the ground after the body is removed. The procedures described earlier should be followed for each of the different insect stages seen following removal of the body.

Migrating maggots should be collected as are feeding maggots, but additional information is necessary to prove the maggots are in the migration phase of their life cycle. The companion samples are made, but an estimate of the distance and compass direction from the body should be documented with these preserved and live samples. The distance from the corpse will determine that the larvae are in the migration phase of their life cycle.

Soil sampling is also recommended due to mature larvae moving away from the remains and burrowing into the soil to form the puparial stage of their life cycle. Soil samples should be approximately a four-inch deep cube or core of material from areas associated with different body regions such as head, torso and extremities. Soil samples of this size fit well into two pint or slightly larger cardboard (cylindrical ice cream type) or plastic containers or gallon size metal cans, such as those used in arson investigations. Additional soil samples (at least three in addition to those above) should be taken from adjacent to, and up to three feet or more from the body, noting the origin of each sample in reference to the body. The samples should be labeled in the same manner as the insect vials.

Collecting Materials and Equipment

1. Aerial insect nets (e.g. 15" or 18" diameter bags with 3' handles; 15" or 18" collapsible nets with variable handle lengths).
2. Screw cap collecting vials (4 dram size).
3. Wide-mouth (8 oz) pharmacy bottles with screw tops.
4. Forceps; medium-point dissecting curved forceps.
5. Styrofoam or cardboard containers with lids, 16 oz size. (maggot motel)
6. Plastic specimen cups, screw cap lid type, 4 oz size.
7. Paper labels, heavy quality paper, for placement inside of collection container.
8. Paper labels, adhesive backed, for placement on the exterior of collection containers.
9. Dark graphite pencil (#2), for marking paper labels.
10. Hand trowel or 4"–6" core sampling tool, for soil sampling.
11. Thermometer, electronic and/or mercury.
12. Solutions for preserving specimens (see Table III-9).
13. Data sheet–Death Scene Case Study Form.
14. Log Book - for recording location, scene data, date, etc.

Collection of Entomological Specimens During Autopsy and in Other Specific Environments

Specific collecting techniques and procedures in different environments will enhance the recovery of insect specimens. Although these are similar to general collecting procedures, there are instances when an added step is necessary or an additional observation must be made. The following suggestions for collecting at the autopsy or other types of environments will add reliability to the entomological evidence.

Collection of insect evidence at the autopsy is done in conjunction with the pathologist performing the autopsy. Most likely the corpse will be enclosed in a *body bag* when it arrives from the scene, particularly if the remains are in a state of advanced decomposition. In cases where the corpse is heavily infested with insects, the outer surface of the body bag may have larvae or adult insects on it. These insects should be collected and labeled using procedures described previously. Once the body bag is opened, the inner surfaces of the bag should be examined for insects. The insects may have crawled from the body due to changes in temperatures. They should be collected and labeled with notations as to which area of the body (head, torso, and extremities) they were near.

Many times remains are stored for some time in coolers or refrigeration units prior to autopsy. Notation should be made of both the total time the body was being refrigerated and at what temperature along with other information, such as temperature during transport of the body to the morgue, etc. Also, the temperature of the maggot mass should be recorded when the body is removed from the cooler. There may be little or no effect of the lower temperatures on insect development if the maggot mass was well established prior to the body being placed in the cooler. Maggot mass temperatures may be in the 85–95° F range even if the temperature in the cooler is around 30° F.

Once on the examination table, a detailed search for insect evidence can begin. If the body is clothed, a thorough examination of the clothing is essential and may yield a variety of stages and kinds of insects. Folds in the clothing where eggs, larvae, pupae, or adults may be sheltered should be gently opened. Moist patches on clothing are excellent areas to search; fly eggs are often laid in moist areas. The collection of seeds and other plant materials should be conducted for analysis by a botanist. In addition to plant parts, certain live stages of insects may be found in stems or seeds of plants that may give clues as to habitat, time, or geographic aspects in the case.

After the clothing has been examined and removed, areas of the body where concentrations of insect activity are found should be noted and photographed to show the extent of infestation and insect composition. Representative samples from each major infestation site should be collected.

Once the internal portion of the autopsy has begun, major sites of insect activity may include the skull with natural body openings, hair and scalp, respiratory tract, including inner nasal passages, esophagus, genital and rectal areas, and antemortem wound sites, as well as the chest cavity, pelvic area under mummified skin, or areas under desiccated skin of the limbs. Insects collected from any of these areas should be labeled and preserved, and their locations noted.

Collection of Specimens from Buried Remains

When remains are buried, insect fauna is limited greatly by the amount of soil covering the body.[47,67] Megnin,[2] Motter[68] and Leclercq[69] found that buried remains had their own insect fauna peculiar to a given type of environment. Burial slows the decompositional process due to lower, more constant temperatures at varying soil depths and by exclusion of some bacteria and the majority of insects which colonize surface carrion. Blowflies can be excluded access to buried remains by as little as one inch of covering.[67] Sarcophagid (flesh flies) and muscid larvae have been recovered from remains that have been buried deeper. Several of the smaller fly species, rove beetles and ants[70] have been collected from bodies covered with four inches of soil.[15]

Remains which are left exposed for a period of time, but buried later, may be colonized by species which are only capable of direct body access. The presence of such species may help establish a chain of events prior to burial, regarding the deposition of the corpse. For example, blowfly puparia recovered from 100-year-old Indian skeletal remains from South Dakota suggested the season of the year in which the remains were buried.[42] Similar conclusions were drawn from Anasazi remains which were 1100 years old and recovered from a grave in Farmington, New Mexico.[43]

Collection of Specimens from Enclosed Structures

Enclosed structures present several problems in the evaluation of insect colonization, development, and evidence collection. First, if the structure is tightly closed such as, newer automobiles with the windows and doors closed; tightly sealed rooms; metal containers with air seals; or newer, well-insulated, air conditioned houses, the chemical attractant cues needed for attraction of the initial colonizing insects does not dissipate as rapidly or in the same manner as do bodies in the open. The question arises as to how much time has elapsed before the odors emanate from the restrictive confines. In some circumstances, the odors never permeate from the container. However, even in such cases, extensive visual searches should be conducted at the scene to make certain no insect life stages are present.

Second, assuming the attractant odor has emanated from the structure or container, insects may still be excluded from direct access to the corpse. Thus, there may be considerable numbers of flies or other carrion insects outside the enclosed structure attempting to gain access to the corpse. The concentration of blowflies outside a structure or container (e.g. car trunk), should indicate that something inside the enclosure is dead and beginning to decompose. Flying insects should be collected by aerial netting, and ground-crawling insects should be hand collected. The duration of time that the remains have been in place may be indicated by certain assemblages of insects from a successional wave group.[2] This is due to the production of different odor attractants or other chemical cues associated with advancing decomposition. For example,

if only blowflies were found attempting to gain access, this may indicate a shorter PMI, whereas, the presence of phorid and muscid flies would suggest a more extended period of time.

Third, the enclosed structure probably does not have temperatures comparable to those reported from the local National Weather Service station. As explained in *Collecting Climatological Data,* temperatures in a particular outdoor habitat may be considerably different from those recorded at the NWS station, and independent temperature data must be collected from the scene to determine accurate environmental conditions. It is critical to know the microclimatic environmental conditions at the location where the insects' development is taking place to estimate accurately the duration of their developmental time. When dealing with enclosed structures this becomes even more critical. A car parked on a black asphalt surface with the windows closed, on a mild sunny day (75° F or 24° C), may exhibit temperatures 30–40° F (20° C+) degrees higher inside the passenger compartment or trunk than the ambient air temperature. This condition could accelerate larval development by several days, creating a considerable error in PMI estimation. By recreating the circumstances of the enclosed structure and recording temperature data, an accurate correlation may be obtained between the NWS data and the enclosed environment in question.

Collection of specimens from enclosed structures may require knowledge of some of the likely places where the fly larvae may migrate. In houses where the corpse is in advanced stages of skeletanization and mummification, it is possible that more than one generation of larvae have migrated off the remains, changed to pupae, and emerged as adults. Inspection of the edges of the room, as well as under the carpeting or carpet pad may reveal reddish to dark brown to black elongated fly puparia along the base board or in cracks or gaps in the wood. Often, postfeeding maggots may be found under carpeting, rugs, or other coverings that provide protection and seclusion for their transformation to the pupal stage.

The larvae may migrate to pupate into other rooms as well. A basement or crawl space under the structure will be an additional source of insects if the corpse is in advanced decomposition and fluids have seeped through flooring and into the space below. Larvae, pupae, or adults may be found in such areas. The same occurs in automobiles, where insect development will continue under floor mats and carpeting, between seats, and even under the upholstery which is in close proximity of the corpse. Larvae may also migrate into the car trunk to pupate, so this area must be inspected as well.

Because newly emerged adult flies and beetles seek light and the outdoors, the backside of window blinds, shades and curtains should be searched for these adult flying insects. Window sills and ledges on the inside of the structure may hold high numbers of adult flies or other species which have completed development on the remains, or have emerged from puparia, and are seeking natural outdoor habitat. If the enclosed area is too hot, the insects may die from exposure. Thus, empty puparia, puparia, or dead larvae or adults may be found inside closed structures.

When collecting specimens, dead dried samples should be handled carefully because of their fragility. They should be stored in fluid preservative to allow for rehydration. Following these procedures will provide additional important data to the investigation. The sum total of the evidence provides the pieces of the puzzle from which the overall picture of the event will be constructed.*

REFERENCES

1. McKnight, B.E. *The washing away of wrongs: Forensic medicine in thirteenth century China.* University of Michigan Press. Ann Arbor, 1981.
2. Megnin, J.P. La faune des cadavers: Application e l'entomologie a la médecine légale. *Encyclopédie Scientifique des Aide-Mémorie.* Maison Gauthiers-Villas et Fils, Paris, 1894.
3. Aldrich, J.M. *Sarcophaga and Allies.* Thomas Say Foundation. Lafayette, IN, 1916.
4. Wallman, J.F., and M. Adams. The forensic application of allozyme electrophoresis to the identification of blowfly larvae (Diptera: Calliphoridae) in southern Australia. *J. Forensic Sci., 46*(3): 681–684, 2001.
5. Sperling, F.A.H., Anderson, G.S., and Hickey, D.A. A DNA-based approach to the identification of insect species used for postmortem interval estimation. *J. Forensic Sci., 39:* 418–427, 1994.
6. Malgorn, Y., and Coquoz, R. DNA typing for identification of some species of Calliphoridae. An interest in forensic entomology. *Forensic Sci. Int. 28;102* (2–3): 111–119, 1999.
7. Vincent, S., Vian, J.M., and Carlotti, M.P. Partial sequencing of the cytochrome oxydase b subunit gene I: A tool for the identification of European species of blow flies for postmortem interval estimation [published erratum appears in letter from Wells and Sperling. *J. Forensic Sci.* (Nov): 45(6)]. *J. Forensic Sci.,* Jul, *45*(4): 820–823, 2000.
8. Wells, J.D., and Benecke, M. DNA Techniques for Forensic Entomology. *Forensic entomology: The utility of arthropods in legal investigation.* CRC Press, LLC. Boca Raton, FL, 2001.
9. Wells, J.D., and LaMotte, L. Estimating the Postmortem Interval. *Forensic entomology: The utility of arthropods in legal investigation.* CRC Press, LLC. Boca Raton, FL, 2001.
10. Glaister, J., and Brash, J.C. *Medico-legal aspects of the Ruxton case.* Edinburgh: Livingstone, 1937.
11. Leclercq, M. *Entomological parasitology: The relations between entomology and the medical sciences.* Pergamon Press. London, 1969.
12. Hall, D.G. *The blowflies of North America.* Thomas Say Foundation. Baltimore, MD, 1948.
13. Hall, R.D., and Townsend, L.H., Jr. *The blow flies of Virginia.* (Diptera: Calliphoridae). The Insects of Virginia, No. 11. Virginia Polytechnical Institute and State University Research Bulletin, No. 123, 1977.
14. Rodriguez, W.C., and Bass, W.M. Insect activities and its relationship to decay rates of human cadavers in East Tennessee. *J. Foren. Sci., 28:* 423–432, 1983.
15. Smith, K.G.V. *A manual of forensic entomology.* British Museum (Natural History), London and Cornell University Press. Ithaca, NY, 1986
16. Catts, E.P., and Haskell, N.H., Eds. *Entomology and death: A procedural guide.* Joyce's Printshop, Clemson, SC, 1990.
17. Hall, R.D. Perceptions and Status of Forensic Entomology. *Forensic entomology: The utility of arthropods in legal investigation.* CRC Press, LLC. Boca Raton, FL, 2001.
18. Reaumur, R.A.F. de. Observation du thermometre, faites a Paris pendant l'annee 1735, comparees avec cells qui ont ete faites sous la ligne a Isle de France, a Alger et en quelque-unes de nos isles de l'Amerique,

* Acknowledgments: I wish to thank Dr. Adam Craig, Susan Gruner, Jane Haskell and Buthene Haskell for their assistance and suggestions.

Mémoires de l'Academie Royale des Sciences de l'Institut de France, Paris, 1735.

19. Arnold, C.Y. The Determination and significance of the base temperature in a linear heat unit system. *Proc. Am. Soc. Horticult. Sci.* 74: 430–445, 1959.

20. Arnold, C.Y. Maximum-minimum temperatures as a basis for computing heat units. *Proc. Am. Soc. Horticult. Sci.* 76: 682–692, 1960.

21. Sharpe, J.H., and DeMichele, D.W. Reaction kinetics of pokilotherm development. *J. Theor. Biol.* 64: 649–670, 1977.

22. Byrd, J.H., and Butler, J.F. Effects of temperature on *Cochliomyia macellaria* (Diptera: Calliphoridae) development. *J. Med. Entomol.* 33: 901–905, 1996.

23. Byrd, J.H., and Butler, J.F. Effects of temperature on *Sarcophaga haemorrhoidalis* (Diptera: Sarcophagidae) development. *J. Med. Entomol.* 35: 694–698, 1997.

24. Byrd, J.H., and Butler, J.F. Effects of temperature on *Chrysomia rufifacies* (Diptera: Calliphoridae) development. *J. Med. Entomol.* 33: 901–905, 1998.

25. Catts, E.P., and Goff, M.L. Forensic entomology in criminal investigations. *Ann. Rev. Entomol.* 37: 253–272, 1992.

26. Higley, L.G., and Haskell, N.H. Insect development and Forensic Entomology. *Forensic entomology: The utility of arthropods in legal investigation.* Ed. J.Byrd and J. Castner, CRC Press, LLC. Boca Raton, FL, 2001.

27. Higley, L.G. and Peterson, R.K.D. Initiating sampling programs, in L.P. Pedigo and G.D. Buntin (Eds.), *Handbook of sampling methods for arthropods in agriculture.* CRC Press, LLC, Boca Raton, FL, 1994.

28. Higley, L.G., Pedigo, L.P., and Ostlie, K.R. DEGDAY: A program for calculating degree days and assumptions behind the degree day approach. *Environ. Entomol.* 15: 999–1016, 1986.

29. Wagner, T.L., Wu, H., Sharpe, P.J., Schoolfield, R.M., and Coulson, R.N. Modeling insect developmental rates: A literature review and application of a biophysical model. *Ann. Entomol. Soc. Am.* 77: 208–225, 1984.

30. Davidson, J. On the relationship between temperature and rate of development of insects at constant temperatures. *J. Anin. Ecol.* 13: 26–28, 1944.

31. Erzinçlioglu, Z. *Maggots, murder, and men: Memories and reflections of a forensic entomologist.* Harley, Colchester, UK, 2000.

32. Byrd, J.H., and J.L. Castner. *Forensic entomology: The utility of arthropods in legal investigations.* CRC Press, LLC. Boca Raton, FL, 2001.

33. LaMotte, L.R., and J.D. Wells. P-values for postmortem intervals from arthropod succession data. *Journal of Agricultural, Biological and Environmental Statistics,* 5: 58–68, 2000.

34. Schoenly, K. A statistical analysis of successional patterns in carrion-arthropod assemblages: Implications for forensic entomology and determination of the postmortem interval. *J. Forensic Sci.* 37 (6):1489–1513, 1992.

35. Schoenly, K., Goff, M.L., and Early, M. A BASIC algorithm for calculating the postmortem interval from arthopod successional data. *J. Forensic Sci.,* 37 (3): 808–823, 1992.

36. Hall, R.D., and Haskell, N.H. Forensic entomology–Applications in medicolegal investigations. In *Forensic sciences,* Ed. C. Wecht. Matthew Bender, New York, 1995.

37. Greenberg, B. Nocturnal oviposition behavior of blow flies (Diptera: Calliphoridae). *Jour. Med Ent.,* 27 (5): 807–810, 1990.

38. Hall, R.D., and Doisy, K.E. Length of time after death: Effect on attraction and oviposition or larviposition of midsummer blowflies (Diptera: Calliphoridae) and flesh flies (Diptera: Sarcophagidae) of medicolegal importance in Missouri. *Annals of the Ent. Soc. Am.,* 86: 589–593, 1993.

39. Haskell, N.H. Factors affecting diurnal flight and oviposition periods of blowflies (Diptera: Calliphoridae) in Indiana. Ph.D. dissertation, Purdue University, West Lafayette, IN, 1993.

40. Baumgartner, D.L. Spring season survey of the urban blowflies (Diptera: Calliphoridae) of Chicago, Illinois. *Great Lakes Entomologist,* 21: 130–132, 1988.

41. Haskell, N.H. Calliphoridae of pig carrion in Northwest Indiana: A seasonal comparative study. Master's thesis, Purdue University, West Lafayette, IN, 1989.

42. Gilbert, B.M., and Bass, W.M. Seasonal dating of burials from the presence of fly pupae. *American Antiquity,* 32: 534–535, 1967.

43. Kearns, T.M. Salvage Recovery of Prehistoric Human Remains from a Private Residence in Farmington, New Mexico. Western Cultural Resource Management, Inc., San Juan County, (F) 156, Farmington, NM, 1999.

44. Haskell, N.H. Report of diagnostic laboratory examination. Case Report requested by Western Cultural Resource Management. Farmington, NM, 1999.

45. Lord, W.D. Case studies in forensic entomology. In *Entomology and death: A procedural guide.* Catts, E.P. and Haskell, N.H., Eds. Joyce's Printshop, Clemson, SC, 1990.

46. Gill-King, H. Chemical and ultrstructural aspects of decomposition. In *Forensic taphonomy,* Haglund, W. and Sorg, M., Eds. 93–108, CRC Press, Boca Raton, FL, 1997.

47. Payne, J.A. A summer carrion study of the baby pig *Sus scrofa* Linnaeus. *Ecology, 46:* 592–602, 1965.

48. Webb, J.P., Jr., Loomis, R.B., Madon, M.B., Bennett, S.G., and Greene, G.E. The Chigger species *Eutrombicula belkini* Gould (Acari: Trombiculidae) as a forensic toll in a homicide investigation in Ventura county, California. *Bull. Soc. Vector Ecol., 8* (2): 141–146, 1983.

49. Merritt, R.W., and Wallace, J.R. The role of aquatic insects in forensic investigations. *Forensic entomology: The utility of arthropods in legal investigation.* J. Byrd and J. Castner, Eds., CRC Press, LLC, Boca Raton, FL, 2001.

50. Schoenly, K., and Haskell, N.H. Aquatic insects in forensic investigations. *Bulletin of National Institute of Justice,* Washington, D.C., 2000.

51. Sohal, R.S., and Lamb, R.E. Intracellular deposition of metals in the midgut of the adult housefly, Musca domestica. *J. Insect Physiol., 23:* 1349–1354, 1977.

52. Sohal, R.S., and Lamb, R.E. Storage excretion of metallic cations in the adult housefly, Musca Domestica. *J. Insect Physiol., 25:* 119–124, 1979.

53. Nuorteva, P., and Nuorteva, S.L. The fate of mercury in sarcosaprophagous flies and in insects eating them. *Ambio, 11:* 34–37, 1982.

54. Beyer, J.C., Enos, W.F., and Stajic, M. Drug identification through analysis of maggots. *J. Forensic Sci., 25:* 411–412, 1980.

55. Leclercq, M., and Brahy, G. Entomologie et medecine legale: Datation de la mort. *Journal de Medecine Legal, 28:* 271–278, 1985.

56. Gunatilake, K., and Goff, M.L. Detection of organophosphate poisoning in a putrefying body by analyzing arthropod larvae. *J. Forensic Sci., 34:* 714–716, 1988.

57. Introna, F., Jr., LoDico, C., Caplan, Y.H. and Smalek, J.E. Opiate analysis of cadaveric blowfly larvae as an indicator of narcotic intoxication. *J. Forensic Sci., 35:* 118–122, 1990.

58. Kintz, P., Godelar, A., Tracqui, A., Mangin, P., Lugnier, A.A., and Chaumont, A.J. Fly larvae: A new toxicological method of investigation in forensic medicine. *J. Forensic Sci., 35:* 204–207, 1990.

59. Goff, M.L., and Lord, W.D. Entomotoxicology: Insects as toxicological indicators and the impact of drugs and toxins on insect development. In *Forensic entomology: The utility of arthropods in legal investigations.* Byrd, J.H., and Castner, J.L., Eds. Boca Raton, FL: CRC Press, LLC, 2001.

60. Roth, L.M., and Willis, E.R. The medical and veterinary importance of cockroaches. *Smithsonian Misc. Coll., 134:* 10, 147 pp, 1957.

61. Keh, B. Scope and application of forensic entomology. *Ann. Rev. of Entomol. 30:* 137–154, 1985.

62. Froede, R.C. *Handbook of forensic pathology.* Northfield, IL: College of American Pathologists, 1990.

63. Denic N., Huyer, D.W., Sinal, S.H., Lantz, P.E., Smith, C.R., and Silver, M.M. Cockroach: The omnivorous scavenger. Potential misinterpretation of postmortem injuries. *Am. J. of For. Med. and Path., 18:* 2, 177–180, 1997.

64. Haskell, N.H., Hall, R.D., Cervenka, V.J., and Clark, M.A. On the body: Insects' life stage presence and their postmortem artifacts. In *Forensic taphonomy,* Haglund, W., and Sorg, M., Eds., Boca Raton, FL: CRC Press, 1997, pp. 415–456.

65. Voigt, J. Specific postmortem changes produced by larder beetles. *J. Forensic Med. 12:* 76–80, 1965.

66. Haskell, N.H., Grant, R.H., Hawley, D.A., and Mischler, J.E. "The estimation of heat unit requirements of developing larvae using statistical regression of temperature measurements from a death scene." American Academy of Forensic Science, 48th Annual Meeting, Nashville, Tennessee, 1996.

67. Rodriguez, W.C., and Bass, W.M. 1985. Decomposition of buried bodies and methods that may aid in their location. *J. Forensic Sci., 30:* 836–852, 1985.

68. Motter, M.G. A contribution to the study of the fauna of the grave. A study of one hundred and fifty disinterments with some additional experimental observations. *Jour. N.Y. Entomol. Soc. 6:* 201–231, 1898.

69. Leclercq, M. Entomologie et médecine légale. Etude des insectes et acariens nécrophages pour déterminer la date de la mort. *Spectrum 17:* 1–7, 1975.

70. Payne, J.A., King, E.W., and Beinhart, G. Arthopod succession and decompostiton of buried pigs. *Nature,* London *219* (5159): 1180–1181, 1968.

Part 4

EXHUMATION

MICHAEL M. BADEN

THE WORD EXHUMATION, from the Latin *ex,* out of, and *humus,* ground, is now used to include the disinterment of remains buried lawfully or unlawfully, and the disentombment of those buried above ground in mausoleums.

Traditionally, exhumations have been performed to permit autopsy or re-autopsy to determine cause of death for criminal justice or civil litigation purposes when information has become available that was not known at the time of burial. In recent years, there has been increased international and human rights interest in the exhumation of mass graves to identify the dead and to assist in determining whether war crimes have been committed. Advances in DNA technologies have also stimulated interest in exhumations to resolve questions of paternity and genealogy. Non-forensic exhumations are sometimes performed when bodies or cemeteries must be moved and to examine long-buried remains for academic purposes.

The Exhumation Request

The first issue the pathologist must address when an exhumation is suggested is whether this procedure will provide answers to the questions that led to the consideration of the exhumation. If the questions include the identity of the decedent, the cause of death or the presence of poisons, such as arsenic or thallium, the answer is *Yes*. If the body has been embalmed and the issue is the presence of alcohol, which was also present in the embalming fluid, the answer is *No*.

The most common question asked by family, police or attorneys when requesting exhumation is *What condition will the body be in?* The answer to that question is *I don't know until I see the remains.* The condition of the body cannot be specifically predicted because of the many unknown variables that affect the rate of deterioration of soft tissues and bone: How much rainwater or groundwater entered the casket? How well was the body embalmed? How advanced were decomposition changes and internal bacterial growth when the body was buried? Some bodies remain almost perfectly preserved after years of burial while others are severely deteriorated after a few days or weeks.

Medgar Evers, a Black civil rights leader, was shot in the back and killed in 1963 in Jackson, Mississippi. The autopsy report and bullet were lost. When his body was exhumed in 1991 to reconstruct the bullet track for trial purposes, it was in near perfect condition (Fig. III-55).

Further inquiry revealed that the body had been buried on the side of a hilly elevation in Arlington Cemetery, Virginia, that permitted rapid runoff of rain water, and that the embalmer had used "three times as much embalming fluid as usual" because the weather was very hot and the funeral parlor did not have air conditioning or refrigeration.

Byron De La Beckwith, a leader of the local White Citizen's Council and Ku Klux Klan, was convicted of Evers' murder 30 years after the shooting.

The editor has recently examined two exhumed bodies, one after 17 years of burial, the other after 24. Both bodies had previously been autopsied and were in an excellent state of preservation (Fig. III-56a–b). Figure III-56a had died of head injuries with extensive skull fractures and although the brain was not amenable for detailed findings, the skull was in such perfect condition that mechanism and manner of death were determinable. Also, identification could readily be made. Figure III-56b had died of multiple stab wounds and the body was exhumed to obtain specimens for DNA analyses. Facial features were impeccable and identification was made by the family at grave site. The remarkable feature for both these bodies was that the burial environment was dry and despite the many years that had passed, the casket seals were intact, preventing water from entering.

The author's experience, with more than 300 exhumations of lawfully and unlawfully buried bodies, shows that the three structures most resistant to decay are the skeleton, which preserves

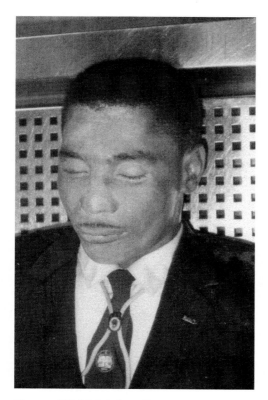

FIGURE III-55. Medgar Evers exhumed after 28 years of burial, in a remarkably good state of preservation.

traumatic injuries to bone from gunshot wounds, stab wounds or blunt force impacts; arteries, which preserve evidence of coronary and cerebral arteriosclerosis; and the teeth, which may be helpful in identification of the remains.

After the medical examiner testified at trial that the cause of death was a single gunshot wound to the back of the head, defense attorneys asked to have the one prosecution eyewitness disqualified because he had testified that he saw and heard two gunshots. The judge ordered a one-day recess in the trial so that the body could be exhumed and a determination made as to the number of gunshot wounds. The body had been buried for three years.

At exhumation, the body was identified by dental x-ray comparison; the remains were in excellent condition and re-autopsy confirmed that there were two entrance wounds to the back of the head as the eyewitness had stated (Fig. III-57).

Injuries that perforate the skin cause bleeding and are usually readily identifiable as suspicious deaths to be fully investigated. Such cases usually do not require exhumation. Deaths from asphyxia or poisoning that may present no obvious external manifestations to raise suspicion by the family, by the police or by the physician who issues the death certificate, and autopsies performed without proper examination of the neck organs or retention of tissues or fluids for toxicologic examination, more commonly lead to exhumation requests.

A series of sudden, unexplained New Jersey hospital deaths led to the exhumation of five bodies and the toxicologic identification of d-tubocurarine (curare), a muscle paralyzing drug that prevents breathing and causes fatal respiratory arrest, in three of the decedents. They had not received this drug therapeutically. A surgeon, called *Dr. X* by the media, was indicted for killing a rival surgeon's patients to embarrass him. A jury did not convict (Fig. III-58).

As the soft tissues are lost, the earliest skeletal structure to deteriorate is the thyroid cartilage which may be at issue if the possibility of strangulation has been raised. The hyoid bone can more often be recovered, particularly as it becomes calcified with age; the entire neck area must be carefully examined as the hyoid bone may have moved from its anatomic position due to deterioration of the surrounding soft tissues and during the disinterment process.

The disadvantages of examining exhumed bodies is that the passage of time, prior autopsy and the embalming process produce artifacts which must be distinguished from premortem injury. The advantage is that more information is available at the exhumation than when the body was buried or previously autopsied. The exhumation autopsy is a focused examination to determine whether the cause of death as certified is correct and whether there is evidence of another more competent cause, needle punctures, poisoning, strangulation, suffocation, based on new information: confessions, witness statements, a series of other deaths of spouses or of children or of patients in hospitals.

Exhumations have been critical in identifying health professionals who murdered hundreds of patients before suspicions were aroused. Dr. Harold Shipman in England may have killed as many as 300 of his elderly female patients at their homes by injecting them with morphine; Nurse Kristin Gilbert used epinephrine injections in hospital patients in Massachusetts; Dr. Michael Swango may have killed over 30

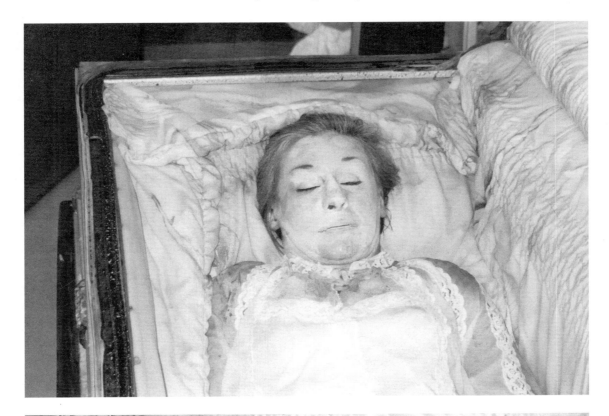

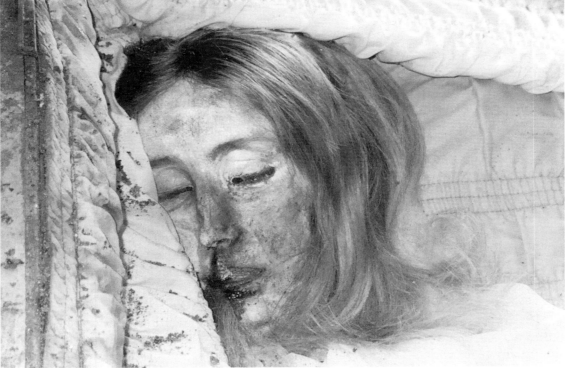

FIGURE III-56a–b. (a) Forty-two-year-old woman after 17 years of burial. (b) Twenty-nine-year-old woman after 24 years of burial.

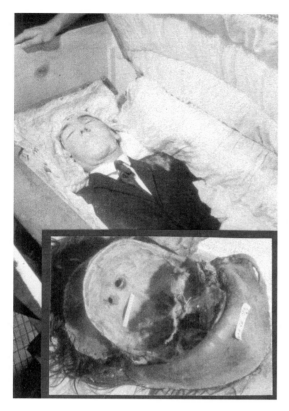

FIGURE III-57. Body exhumed after three years to settle conflicting testimony at trial regarding number of shots. Two beveled entrance gunshot wounds are clearly seen in the skull (insert).

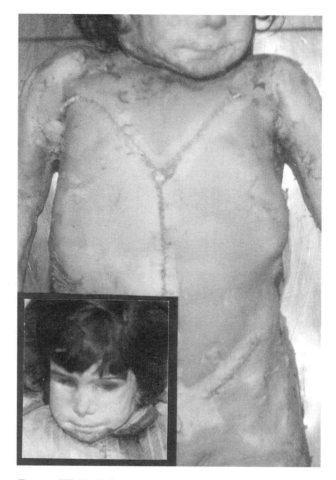

FIGURE III-58. Exhumation autopsy after 10 years revealed death was due to a muscle paralyzing drug.

patients in hospitals across the United States and in Zimbabwe using a variety of poisons including arsenic and nicotine.

Recent toxicologic advances now permit the extraction of poisons from small pieces of tissue saved for histologic purposes.

Florida Bay County Medical Examiner and forensic pathologist, William Sybers, M.D. was convicted in 2001 for the murder of his wife in 1991 after succinylcholine was identified in formalin fixed tissues that had been retained ten years earlier and processed into paraffin blocks for microscopy. The family refused to allow the police to exhume the body for a second autopsy.

An appeals court later reversed the conviction on the basis that the evidence about the poison was based on testing too novel to be accepted science.

Exhumation Process

The legal requirements to exhume a lawfully buried body vary widely in different jurisdictions and may be governed by federal, state, or local laws applicable to where the body is buried. The wishes of the next of kin, cemetery regulations and even the wishes of the owner of the burial site, may also apply. If there is disagreement, a judge is usually the decision-maker. In general, the law has traditionally permitted the next of kin to have greater authority to prevent an official autopsy after burial than before because concerns as to the sanctity of the sepulcher or grave prohibited disturbing the final resting place, except in the most extreme circumstances.

Exhumations are customarily performed in the early morning before cemetery visitors and media arrive and so that the body can be re-interred before nightfall, if the family wishes. The cemetery workers use the same earthmoving equipment for exhumation that they have available for inhumation. Many cemeteries now require that the casket be placed in a cement liner so that the grounds stay level as caskets collapse over time. These cement boxes present a barrier to water reaching the casket but should water get in, it cannot get out.

Arsenic and other chemicals may be a normal component in some soils with great concentration variations. Soil samples should be taken from around the casket for toxicologic analyses during the disinterment process. Should the remains show a poison to be present the soil can be tested to exclude the possibility that the poison was washed into the body after burial by rainwater or ground water.

The top of the cement liner is best removed at the grave site by chains and a backhoe to reveal the casket and whether water is present. The casket is then removed to the autopsy site, usually a medical examiner's office or funeral home.

Identification of the remains must be made carefully. The headstone and cemetery records and casket markings identify where the body should be, but the prosector must further confirm identification of the remains after the casket is opened by direct visualization, fingerprints, dental records, other X-ray comparisons, tattoos, scars, or if necessary, by DNA. Occasionally caskets move in soft soil after burial; or the wrong body may have been inadvertently removed from a hospital or mortuary and then buried with the wrong name. Rarely more than one body may be improperly and intentionally buried in a single burial plot.

The entire exhumation and autopsy process should be well documented by words and photographs, so that others may review the findings at a later time. The clothing may be useful for identification purposes and should be described in detail. Other contents of the casket may also assist in the identification of the body such as, photographs, jewelry, writings, dolls, or other keepsakes that may have been placed in the casket.

Samples of soil or water inside the casket should be collected for possible analysis if poisoning is suspected. The soft tissues of exposed areas of the body, usually from the face and hands, deteriorate the fastest. The portions of the body covered by plastic, such as the trunk or the internal organs saved in a viscera bag, if an autopsy had been performed, stay preserved for long periods of time, even decades. Waterproof embalming makeup may settle prominently on the bones of the face as soft tissues disappear. Mold growth, commonly Aspergillus species, may be striking and may show many colors: white, black, brown, and green on clothing and on skin. The mold tends to preserve, rather than destroy, underlying skin by keeping it dry and reducing bacterial growth.

The 32-year-old physician wife of an anesthesiologist was found dead in her bed in Miami, Florida. A private physician certified the death as due to arteriosclerotic heart disease. The body was exhumed seven months later. White mold growth had helped preserve the skin.

The heart was entirely normal and an injection site was identified in the left buttock which contained succinylmonocholine, a breakdown product of succinylcholine, a rapid acting muscle paralyzing drug that kills by preventing breathing. The husband was convicted of second-degree murder (Fig. III-59).

A 40-year-old construction worker complained of abdominal pains about six months before he died and shortly after he began working on the demolition of the old chemistry building at a local college. His health deteriorated without a diagnosis being made until a few days before death when toxicologic studies showed that he had been poisoned with thallium, which was available in the chemistry building and persuaded police that a co-worker had been poisoning him.

But after two years of a fruitless investigation, his body was exhumed to determine when the thallium was administered. Segmental hair analyses showed that he had received doses of thallium for 12 months, long before beginning work at the chemistry building. A large amount of thallium was also identified in the proximal duodenum which could only have been ingested when his wife gave him a McDonald's milk shake while he was in the hospital and just before he lapsed into terminal coma. She admitted that she had been poisoning him for a year for financial reasons by putting small amounts of rat poison in his iced tea (Fig. III-60).

Embalming Artifacts

Most bodies in this country are embalmed before burial, but not in other countries. The embalming process slows bacterial decomposition but introduces many artifacts that can be misinterpreted: skin incisions to permit arterial

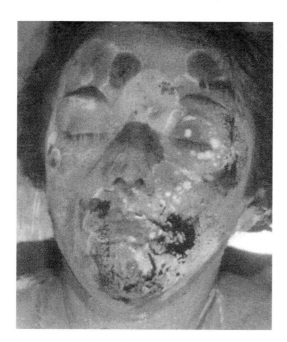

FIGURE III-59. Thirty-two-year-old woman exhumed after seven months showing postmortem growth of Aspergillus mold on left side of face.

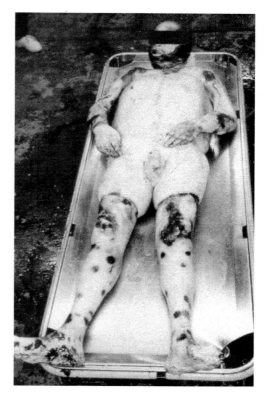

FIGURE III-60. Construction worker exhumed after two years of burial. The black areas are Aspergillus nigrans.

embalming for replacement of blood by embalming fluids should not be mistaken for stab wounds; an abdominal perforation, usually closed by a plastic embalmer's button, which permits cavity embalming through a long metal trocar, about one-half inch in diameter, should not be confused with a bullet hole; the multiple perforations of the abdominal and thoracic organs caused by the trocar should not be mistaken for premortem injury; tissue moved from one organ to another by the penetrating trocar should not be misinterpreted as tissue emboli; blood clotted during the embalming process should not be mistaken for premortem thrombus or embolus. On the other hand, a large pulmonary embolus in the pulmonary artery may well be fragmented by repeated jabs with the embalmer's trocar and the fragments of the clot washed away by the injected formaldehyde leaving no evidence of the cause of death. Air introduced during arterial embalming should not be misinterpreted to be a premortem air embolism.

An exhumation is a team effort in which the contributions of the toxicologist, serologist,

forensic dentist, forensic anthropologist, radiologist, photographer and crime laboratory often prove to be more important than the contribution of the pathologist alone.

Civil Litigation

Exhumation for civil litigation purposes may require evaluations as to whether a medical diagnosis or treatment was faulty; whether there were pre-existing illnesses that affected life expectancy; whether there was conscious pain and suffering and for how long; whether drugs of abuse were present when the automobile or workplace accident occurred; whether the injury was caused by a faulty appliance; and whether the proximate cause of death was a remote injury that some time later precipitated pulmonary embolism, aortic dissection or aneurysm, or myocardial infarction.

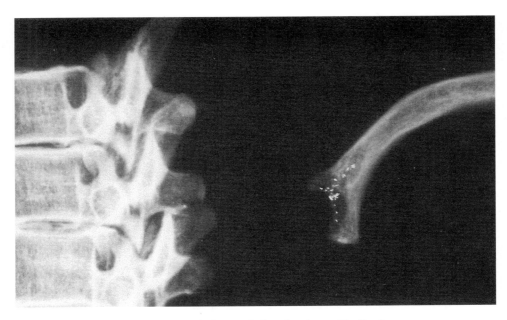

FIGURE III-61. X-ray of rib revealed pinhead metal bullet fragments.

Exhumations are increasingly being performed to determine paternity as in 1997 when the remains of French actor Yves Montand, who had died in 1991, were disinterred by court order at the request of his claimed illegitimate daughter. DNA proved he was not her father.

Unlawful Burials

The burial of a body to illegally dispose of it or to hide it is usually associated with rapid deterioration of the soft tissues; there may be evidence of animal activity if the body was near the surface, often with removal of some skeletal remains distributed over a wide area. Evaluation of insect activity and plant and root growth may assist in determining how long the remains had been at the site. Search for foreign materials that may have inadvertently been included with the remains at the burial site have sometimes revealed beer cans with fingerprints, traceable eye glasses, usable shoe prints beneath the body, clothing, and buttons left by the perpetrator. DNA analyses have proven to be of great value in identifying the unlawfully buried. Full body x-rays are of value for identification purposes and to search for radiopaque foreign materials such as bullets or shrapnel.

A 12-year-old girl had been missing for seven years when information was given to police by an informant that she had been shot in the back and buried in an apple orchard.

The completely skeletonized remains were recovered but no bullet was present. However, an internally beveled semi-circular gunshot wound of entrance was found in a posterior rib which on x-ray, showed small pinhead sized metal bullet fragments that confirmed the cause of death (Fig. III-61).

Recent exhumation of mass graves have assisted families in recovering the remains of loved ones as well as in the investigation of war crimes in Serbia, South Africa, El Salvador, Argentina, Guatemala, and other countries (Fig. III-62).

When bones are found in attics or wooded areas, or by scavenging dogs or during construction of homes, shopping malls or the like, it is necessary first to determine if the remains are human, remembering that decomposed bear paws can appear grossly and radiologically similar to decomposed human hands. If human, the next issue is to determine how old the bones are, whether of current investigative interest or from an old, forgotten burial site. Determination of race is also important and of great significance

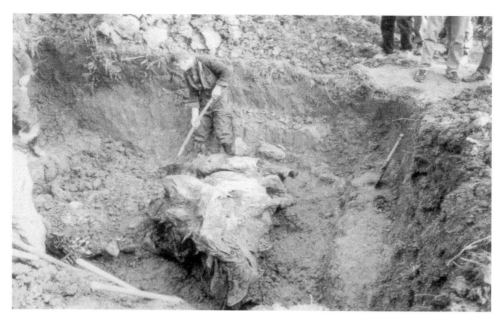

FIGURE III-62. Excavation of mass grave.

because in many jurisdictions, Native American Indian burial sites of any age cannot be disturbed and the excavation must stop.

Historic Interest

Exhumations may be performed to resolve old historic questions. The body of the twelfth President of the United States, Zachary Taylor, who died in office in 1850 of presumed natural causes, was disentombed from his mausoleum and examined in 1991 at the request of his descendants to determine whether he had been poisoned over a period of time with arsenic. Hair analyses proved that he had not been poisoned.

In 1918, a worldwide pandemic killed more than 20 million people. It was thought that the epidemic was due to an influenza virus but the causative agent was never confirmed. Recently, some of the victims have been exhumed from Norway's Arctic permafrost, where they had been buried, in an effort to identify the cause using new technologies.

James Starrs, Professor of Law and Forensic Science at George Washington University, has led multidisciplinary forensic teams that searched for the buried remains of Jessie James,

Billy the Kid, and other notable Americans and to determine the identity of the Boston Strangler, who was said to have killed eleven women in Massachusetts in the early 1960s.

The finding, exhumation and identification of the Romanov family members, who had ruled Russia for 300 years and who were murdered in 1918, solved one of the great mysteries of the twentieth century.

On July 17, 1918, Czar Nicholas and his wife Alexandra and their five children were killed by their Bolshevik captors at Lenin's orders. The captors were instructed to burn the bodies so that no remnants would be found. They realized after three days of trying to destroy the two smallest children, with little success, that the gasoline-fueled fires were hot enough to burn the bodies but not to destroy them, so they buried them secretly in the nearby Ural Mountains in Siberia.

The disputed remains were found and then exhumed in 1991. In 1993, at the request of the Russian government and American State Department, a team of American forensic scientists led by anthropologist William Maples and including forensic dentist Lowell Levine, microscopist Catherine Oakes and the author, confirmed the identification of Nicholas, Alexandra, and three children.

The skeletons were in good condition with some soft tissues that had turned to waxy adipocere still present. The American team on the basis of anthropologic and dental evaluations determined that Alexi, the only son and youngest child and 17-year-old, Anastasia were missing. The Russian team that relied upon photographic overlay tech-

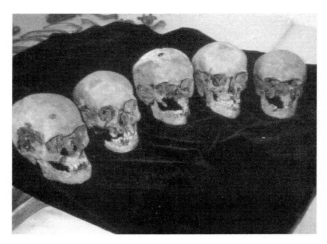

FIGURE III-63. Skulls of members of the missing Romanov family murdered in 1918.

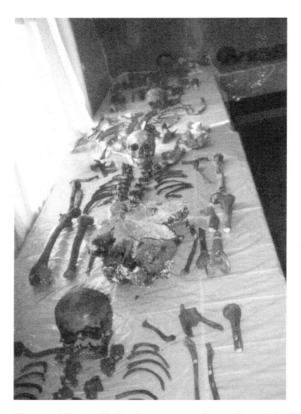

FIGURE III-64. Skeletal remains exhumed in 1991 confirmed to be Czar Nicholas, his wife and three of their five children.

niques concluded that the missing daughter was 19-year-old, Marie.

Subsequent mitochondrial and nuclear DNA analyses confirmed that the decedents were the Romanovs. The bodies could then be buried with their ancestors in the Saints Peter and Paul Cathedral in St. Petersburg, Russia (Figs. III-63 and III-64).

DNA obtained from a surgical pathology histologic slide of Anna Anderson, who had claimed to be the missing Anastasia, showed that she was not a Romanov.

The unautopsied body of a young woman entombed in an above ground mausoleum for 145 years was discovered to be in excellent condition when the cemetery had to be moved. The good state of preservation permitted DNA analyses for genealogic purposes and toxicologic, trace evidence, dental and anthropologic studies and study of the clothing and fabrics on the body. Histologic examination showed excellent preservation of cellular structures in the viscera (Fig. III-65).

Cremation

Cremation, or destruction of the body by fire, is becoming increasingly popular in the United States with more than 25% of all decedents now being cremated. The cremation process, requiring direct flame and temperatures of between 1600° F to 3000° F for 30 minutes to three hours, destroys all soft tissues and organic components of bone and reduces the adult body to about five pounds of calcified, inorganic, flame-resistant bone fragments. These irregular fragments are then crushed by a processor to produce a rather uniform fine ash, referred to as *cremains,* that may be saved in urns or dispersed. Cremation destroys DNA and almost all poisons, but not bullets. False teeth, dental implants, root canal pins and natural teeth often remain and may be of use in identifying the cremains and in determining whether there was commingling of ashes due to faulty cremation procedures.

For additional reading on the subject of embalming and preservation of the body, including mummification and what one may expect to find in an exhumation, the reader is referred to *Modern Mummies—The Preservation of the Human Body in the Twentieth Century* by Christine Quigley, 1998, McFarland and Co., Inc.,

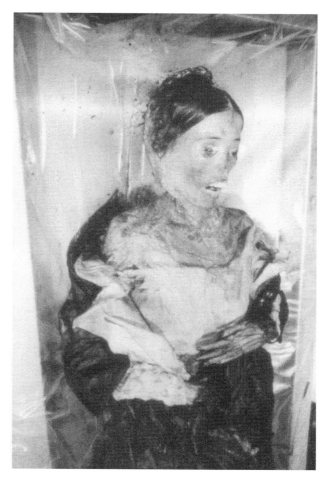

FIGURE III-65. Unautopsied young woman after 145 years entombment in an aboveground mausoleum. The excellent state of preservation was the result of drying due to lack of air in an airtight narrow metal coffin.

Publishers, Jefferson, N.C. 28640 and *Forensic Pathology* by Bernard Knight, Oxford University Press, NY, 1991.

Chapter IV

IDENTIFICATION OF HUMAN REMAINS

Part 1

DANIEL J. SPITZ

DIVERSE TECHNIQUES

POSTMORTEM IDENTIFICATION of human remains can be challenging depending on the nature of the remains. In most jurisdictions, it is the medical examiner's duty to determine the identity of the dead. For this reason a death involving an unidentified body should always be investigated by the coroner or medical examiner. In most medical examiner departments, approximately ten percent of the decedents are brought to the office unidentified due primarily to skeletization, decomposition, severe burning/charring or mechanical trauma involving the head and face.[1]

Although the role of body identification is typically that of the medical examiner, this task is best accomplished by using the combined efforts and resources of local law enforcement agencies together with the expertise of forensic pathologists and other forensic scientists or consultants. A team approach shortens the time required for identification and allows each forensic scientist an opportunity to provide information that may be vital to the investigation. The fingerprint examiner, forensic odontologist, serologist, trace evidence examiner, anthropologist, entomologist, forensic photographer, artist, and sculptor all bring skills that can help with identification. Other consultants, including the botanist, jeweler, clothier, and shoe merchant can, in certain cases, provide clues.

In general, identification of an unknown body consists of linking a decedent to an individual whose identity has been previously established. As will be discussed, identification may be accomplished in a variety of ways and with different degrees of certainty. For the majority of bodies examined by medical examiners, the decedent's identity is known by the time the body arrives at the medical examiner's office. In most cases, the body is tagged at the scene and appropriately labeled with the decedent's name, age, sex, and race. Acceptance of the identity of a body brought directly from the scene using only an identification tag attached to the body is generally appropriate, however, it should be understood that misidentification is more likely to occur with this approach.

The identification as determined by scene investigators should in certain circumstances be confirmed using visual identification by someone familiar with the decedent. A decedent's identity should be confirmed whenever there is the possibility of misidentification by scene investigators. It is recommended that identity confirmation be performed whenever more than one body is removed from a single scene. This situation most commonly occurs when there are multiple fatalities in a motor vehicle collision. Misidentification may not only result in injustice to the next of kin, but also liability on the part of the pathologist.

Some bodies received at medical examiner departments are brought in as *unknowns*. These unknown decedents are typically homeless individuals, bodies recovered from water, charred bodies or skeletonized remains. Bodies which are not viewable, such as, skeletonized remains, charred remains and fragmented or decomposed bodies, can be challenging to identify since visual identification of the decedent is generally not possible. Bodies that are not viewable for whatever reason should be identified using an accepted scientific method of identification. Decomposed bodies usually come to the medical examiner's office with a presumptive identification based on the scene investigation, however, definitive identification should be confirmed using one or more of the methods that will be discussed.

Accurate identification of human remains is crucial for a variety of reasons. Identification permits notification of next of kin which allows family members to begin the grieving process, make the necessary funeral and service arrangements and determine the final disposition of the remains. Only then may the next of kin proceed with the probate of wills and apply for disbursement of benefits and insurance. In addition, official documents certifying death cannot be completed until identification has been established. With regard to law enforcement, positive identification may be necessary for investigators to collect evidence, develop leads in the case, question possible witnesses, establish the corpus delicti of homicide and reconstruct the sequence of events of a crime. Rapid identification is important to homicide detectives because the lack of identification hampers the development of leads and decreases the likelihood of locating witnesses. In deaths where criminal conduct is not suspected, identity of a decedent often yields important information that helps investigators gain an understanding of the circumstances surrounding the decedent's demise which is often helpful for determining cause and manner of death.

In the event that a body is unable to be identified, the body may be buried but only after full body radiographs, dental x-rays and charting, fingerprints (if possible) and specimens for DNA analysis are collected. These items should be kept indefinitely or until the body is identified. Under no circumstances should an unidentified body be cremated, buried at sea, or donated for anatomical study.

Establishing the Remains as Human

When presented with unidentified remains, the medical examiner's first priority is to determine whether the remains are human. The correct determination as to the nature of the remains allows police investigators to not waste time and resources investigating decomposed or skeletonized animal remains. Accurate identification may be difficult when specimens are small, fragmented, or burned.

Residents of an apartment complex called police after noticing a foul odor emitting from a trash dumpster near their unit. The police who arrived on scene observed what appeared to be decomposing internal organs, but were unable to determine if the remains were human. The medical examiner summoned to the scene determined that the remains were non-human and most likely from a goat. Further investigation was deemed unnecessary based on the medical examiner's determination, however, an interview with an apartment resident led police to a man who was known to sacrifice chickens and goats for spiritual reasons. The remains of several other animals and numerous religious artifacts were found in his apartment.

When gross examination fails to distinguish human from animal remains, a simple study of red blood cell morphology on a smear or in tissue often allows for proper characterization. The red blood cells of birds, reptiles, and amphibians are oval and nucleated whereas the mature red blood cells of humans are round and non-nucleated. To determine species origin with certainty, serologic testing can be performed by using an extract of tissue set up against animal and human antisera. The technology of human leukocyte antigens (HLA) tissue typing, routinely performed in matching donated human organs to transplant recipients, has been transferred into forensic identity for the purpose of paternity testing, pedigrees and paleopathology. The major drawback of this powerful system is the requirement for viable lymphocytes, within 12 hours of death, which are usually not available in forensic cases.

As far as law enforcement is concerned the determination that remains are non-human is sufficient evidence to dissolve their interest in the case (Fig. IV-1). Human remains may or may not be of forensic significance, a determination that can usually be made depending on the scene investigation and circumstances surrounding how the remains were discovered. Broadly interpreted, bones of forensic significance generally means that the interval since death is less than fifty years with discovery being in an unauthorized area for burial. The condition of the bones largely depends on where they were found and

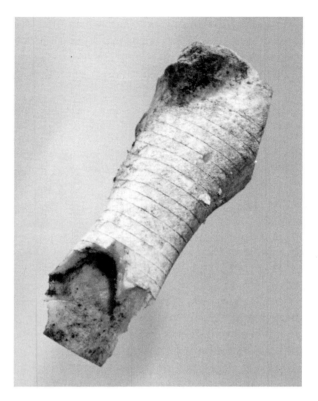

FIGURE IV-1. Bone found at an excavation brought to the medical examiner's office. The bone was of animal origin. The cuts suggest spiral slicing as done with ham.

the environmental conditions such as degree of wetness, dryness, and exposure to the elements and animals. Unburied bones typically show weathering, replacement of the marrow by soil, and stress fragmentation. Casketed bones are typically well preserved and are usually admixed with wood and coffin nail fragments, casket hardware and personal effects buried with the decedent. Local historical societies and land ownership records may identify old graveyards and family burial plots. Carbon (^{14}C) dating can distinguish bones originating from non-modern (prior to AD 1650), pre-modern (between 1650–1950), and modern (1950-present) periods.[2] Remains exhibiting signs of proper burial in a coffin generally do not require identification unless the circumstances demand identification for reinternment in a vandalized cemetery or for historical purposes.

Whenever bones are discovered, oftentimes while excavating a building site or a road, they are taken to the medical examiner for evaluation and determination of whether they are of human origin. Bones determined to be of animal origin are discarded. If the bones are of human origin, the area is searched and sifted for additional remains. Cadaver dogs have occasionally been used to locate human remains, including skeletonized remains, often buried such as following an earthquake or in graves.

To the untrained eye, small animal bones may be mistaken for infant bones, and larger animal bones may be confused with the bones of young children, especially when the head and pelvis are absent. The classic conundrum of the seemingly similar bear paw to the human hand or foot is easily solved by comparison of radiographs which should demonstrate the bear's typical sesamoid bones (Fig. IV-2a–b). Fleshed remains can be compared by a serologist using a panel of antisera to differentiate domestic and wild animals, while hair-bearing remains can be compared using exemplars of human and animal hair to establish the animal of origin.

Recently reported were two examples of non-human remains that were brought to the attention of law enforcement because they were thought to be human. In both cases, police investigators suspected a concealed stillbirth or neonaticide. One investigation was terminated after a pathologist determined that the remains were that of a soiled, partially dismembered plastic skeleton. In the other case, an apparent fetus was found in a landfill. Police took the specimen to a local woman's hospital where physicians felt the remains were that of a 16-week fetus. A fibroblast culture was initiated for comparison should a possible mother be found, however, the remains were subsequently examined by a pathologist who identified the specimen as a rubber fetus. The police investigation was terminated.[3]

A head-sized decomposed mass was discovered by hunters near a river bank. It bore long brown hair of fairly uniform length. Reporters heard of the find and the evening newspapers and television news reported that a decapitated head had been found. Local residents were upset and the police were deluged with phone calls and tips. Radiography of the find disclosed no underlying bony structures. A cross section revealed a woody core. The long stringy hair was actually fine roots.

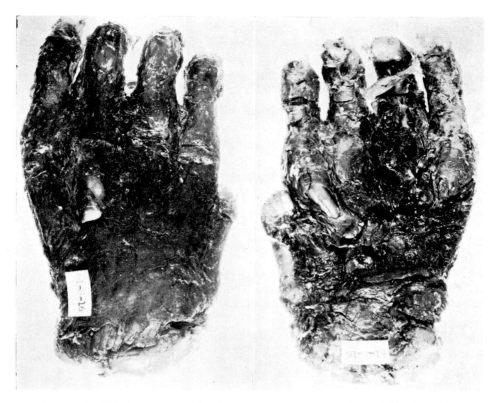

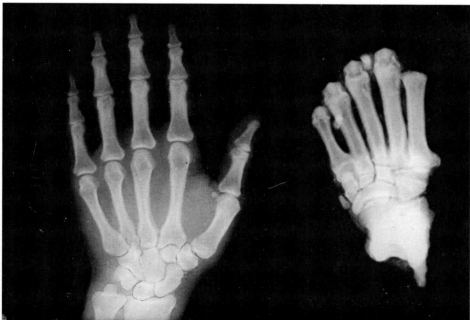

FIGURE IV-2a–b. (a) Bear paw resembling a human hand. (b) Radiographs identify differences in bony structure of the human hand (left) and the bear paw (right) which shows numerous sesamoid bones.

Children found a small skeleton in an abandoned house in a high crime area of town. Homicide detectives were dispatched and the medical examiner summoned. The bones appeared to be an infant lying on its side. After close examination and photographs, it was discussed how to best recover the bones causing the least disturbance. As the bones were moved, it was noted that there were an excessive number of vertebrae. An astute detective discovered a *tail* indicative of a small animal and not a human baby.

Identification of commingled human remains is a challenge for forensic investigators and usually requires a multidisciplinary approach to solve. The most common origin of commingled bones originate from uncovered old burial grounds, simultaneous deaths from mass disasters, deaths from wartime atrocities (mass graves), deaths from exposure while in a remote location (i.e., remains of world explorers/ trekkers) and from the disposal site of serial murderers. Clues to commingling are an excessive number of bones, discrepancies in the size of paired bones and vertebrae, and sex, age and race differences. Consultation with a forensic anthropologist will typically allow for separation of the skull and pelvic bones based on age, sex and race characteristics. In the event that the remains are consistent with a known missing person, postmortem radiographs and comparison with antemortem films may allow for positive identification. Forensic odontology techniques may be helpful separating commingled remains, especially if teeth with dental work are present and antemortem records are available for comparison. In virtually all instances, DNA can be isolated from skeletal remains. Nuclear DNA may be able to be isolated from recently skeletonized remains whereas mitochondrial DNA techniques may be necessary to obtain a DNA sequence from older, skeletonized remains.

Scene Investigation and Recovery of Remains

The identification of an unknown decedent begins at the scene where the body is found and proceeds forward and backward based on evidence collected from the scene (Fig. IV-3). It is during the scene investigation that valuable evidence may be collected. A meticulous search of the scene for personal effects may provide the

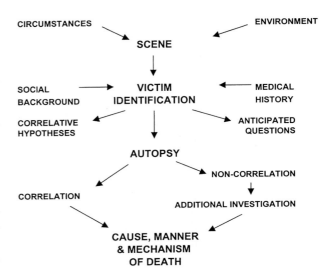

FIGURE IV-3. Algorithm showing multifaceted approach to human identification and how this interacts with scene investigation, autopsy, and cause and manner of death.

means to make a presumptive identity which can then help investigators gain the necessary information to make definitive identification. At the scene, clues as to what someone was doing at the time of their death or evidence of possible witnesses are the beginnings of the trail that may lead to identity and help solve cases that involve criminal activity.

A thorough scene investigation is imperative in any suspicious death and the importance of visiting the death scene of an unidentified body cannot be overstated. In most jurisdictions, the crime scene is controlled by the homicide detective with the medical examiner being in charge of the body. Both agencies working together render the greatest chance for proper death scene investigation, including the collection of evidence that will be helpful in identifying the victim. Viewing the scene with the body present and in some cases even after the body has been removed helps pathologists correlate what is observed at the scene with the autopsy findings. Unusual or atypical findings on the body are often easily explained if the pathologist is familiar with the environment from which the body is recovered.

A pathologist's preliminary findings and opinions help guide the police with their investiga-

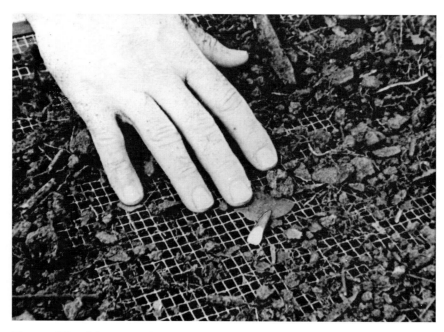

FIGURE IV-4. Sifting of soil in and around decomposed and skeletonized remains assists in recovery of teeth lost during decomposition. (Courtesy of Thomas W. Goyne, Division of Forensic Science, Richmond, VA.)

tion. An opinion regarding time of death is best made when the body is examined at the scene. For each crime scene, investigators have only one chance to properly collect evidence before the body is moved. For this reason, every death scene must be investigated with an open mind in the event that evidence of foul play is uncovered at some time in the future. It is only with a proper death scene investigation that evidence will not be lost, overlooked, or contaminated.

When at the scene of an unidentified body, recovery of the remains should proceed in an orderly manner beginning with photographic documentation. With regard to unidentified skeletal or decomposed remains, the pathologist can help guide investigators so that all bones, teeth and personal effects are recovered. Each death scene is different and the investigative approach should be modified based on the nature of the remains, the location of the body and the resources available to the investigators. Useful investigative techniques may include aerial photography, grid search of the immediate area, supplementary lighting, stripping of vegetation, ground search with metal detectors and a

return search for additional evidence once vegetation is dormant. Multiple searches offer the best chance to recover small bones, teeth, jewelry, clothing, buttons, contact lenses, or other personal effects any of which may be the key to determining the decedent's identity. Sifting of the ground near the decedent using a 3/16 inch mesh screen is the best way to recover such evidence (Fig. IV-4).

Should the case result in a court proceeding, security of the scene and the chain of custody will be important issues, necessitating established standard procedures for documenting the chain of custody. Grid diagrams and photographs document where items are found and may provide supporting evidence regarding cause and manner of death. To illustrate this point, the bullet from the chest of an individual who dies and decomposes will likely be found on the ground under the body. However, it is important to remember that the scene where a body is discovered may not be the scene where the death occurred. Determination that the crime took place elsewhere may be crucial in solving the case and in determining the identity of the victim.

Although decomposed and skeletonized remains present problems in personal identification, even viewable, well-preserved decedents may be difficult to identify when they are not local residents. An unidentified person's lack of close personal relationships may result in no missing person's report being on file, the usual starting place for possible identification. In such situations, cooperative-working relations with newspapers and other media will help in publicizing the need for persons with information to come forward.

SOURCES OF INFORMATION

The following records may contain information suitable for comparison with identification features developed by physical examination and forensic science analyses: Missing persons reports (local, state and National Crime Information Center (NCIC)), fingerprints (ten print cards or latents), medical records (civilian and military), dental records, radiographs, photographs, employment records, police records, passports, and school records.

National Crime Information Center (NCIC) Unidentified and Missing Persons Files

The Federal Bureau of Investigation (FBI) National Crime Information Center (NCIC), *Unidentified Persons* (UP) and *Missing Persons* (MP) files were established in 1983, in response to the Missing Children Act of 1982 (28 USC 534). The *Unidentified Persons* file receives and stores descriptive data on unidentified living persons, bodies, skeletons and body parts. The *Missing Persons* file receives entries from law enforcement agencies. Categories of persons eligible for entry into the UP/MP files are listed in Table IV-1. The files permit entry of numerous descriptors via law-enforcement agencies' NCIC terminal operator as listed in Table IV-2.

Information entered on unidentified dead persons is compared with data entered into the missing persons file after the estimated date of death of the unidentified body. Entries on missing persons are compared with unidentified dead persons whose date of death occurred after the missing person was last reliably seen alive. The computer generates a list of possible matches for investigators who then arrange for direct comparison of dental x-rays, skeletal radiographs and other identifying data. Entries of missing persons, unfortunately, have fewer dental, radiographic and blood group identifiers entered than submissions of unidentified persons where problems are more likely to be the lack of data or delayed entry necessitated by the several days to weeks needed to complete an identification work-up. When report forms or entry via local law enforcement agencies is not possible, families, coroners and medical examiners may enter cases through regional offices of the FBI. Federal legislation enacted in 1990 now requires entry of dental and other data on missing children after a 60-day screening interval (42 USC 5779).

Report guides containing forms and instructions are available through NCIC or a local FBI office. Publications detailing information about missing persons and unidentified dead persons are available to law enforcement agencies (Fig. IV-5). The initial entry form requests basic information including sex, race, height, weight and clothing description. As additional information, such as dental features and anthropologic data is obtained, the entry can be amended. Unfortunately, fewer than 4 percent of the missing person entries include dental characteristics, since reporting agencies often fail to record and preserve the dental records. Currently, approximately 65 percent of unidentified persons in the NCIC database include dental characteristics and radiographs. For missing persons, consent forms for medical and dental information, optometric information and lists of physical descriptors are provided for the next of kin to more closely describe the missing person.

The issue of personal identification has gained significant momentum following the assault on America on September 11, 2001 when two hijacked airplanes were deliberately crashed into

TABLE IV-1

UNIDENTIFIED AND MISSING PERSONS ELIGIBLE
FOR ENTRY INTO THE NCIC UNIDENTIFIED
PERSONS/MISSING PERSONS FILES

Unidentified Persons	Missing Persons
Unidentified deceased and body parts, skeletons	Disabled
	Endangered
Catastrophe victims	Involuntary (abduction or kidnapping)
Unidentified living persons, children, adults, amnesia victims	Juvenile
	Catastrophe (disaster victim)

TABLE IV-2

DESCRIPTORS THAT CAN BE ENTERED INTO
UNIDENTIFIED PERSONS/MISSING PERSONS FILES
FOR COMPUTER COMPARISON

Unidentified Persons	Missing Persons
** Body parts	Sex, race, birth year
Sex, race, estimated birth year	* Date of last contact
Date of death/found	Height/weight/build
Height/weight, eye/hair color	Hair color/style
Scars/marks/tattoos/moles	Scars/marks/tattoos/moles
Fingerprint classification	Fingerprint classification
Blood type	Blood type
Optometric prescriptions	Eye color/disorders/ optometric prescriptions
Fractures/deformities/ needle tracks	Artificial body parts, aids, medical devices/missing organs
Medical devices/missing organs	Deafness
Jewelry/clothing	Fractures/deformities/ needle tracks
Dental records	Jewelry/clothing
Other, miscellaneous (e.g. toxicology and diseases)	Dental records
Other physical characteristics	Other miscellaneous (diseases, medicines, etc.)
** Cause and manner of death	Other physical characteristics
Medical history	* Social security number
Toxicology	* License plate/vehicle
	* Occupation
	* Places frequented
	* Possible destination
	Medical history
	Toxicology

* MP only
** UP only

the Twin Towers in New York City killing over 3,500 people. As a result of this terrorist attack, interest has risen in establishing a National ID card system. Such a card would contain basic information about the holder, including social security number and would be linked to a Federal database containing detailed personal information such as, thumbprints and/or fingerprints, facial features, imprint of voice, eye patterns, handwriting samples and hand geometry. For fingerprinting the individual places his or her thumb on a small scanner, the computer then translates the print's unique curves into a series of mathematical patterns. Video scanners identify and process facial features, such as the eyes, mouth and size of face, into a virtual algorithmic map or constructed model. An imprint of the voice is recorded and broken into a variety of audio characteristics. A video scanner captures the patterns of one or more parts of the inside of the eye. A signature is applied onto a digital tablet and the structure of the letters, words and tendencies are analyzed. Hand geometry involves placing the hand on a surface with small protrusions to dictate where to place fingers then a video system records finger length, thickness and curvature. The information gathered by the scanner is automatically processed by a computer system and identity is immediately confirmed.

METHODS OF IDENTIFICATION

Identification of human remains should be done using one or more methods and the degree of certainty associated with the identification depends on how the identification is performed. The degree of certainty associated with identification is best classified as *definitive, presumptive,* or *speculative.*

Definitive identification is a legally sufficient identification based on objective comparison of antemortem and postmortem information. *Presumptive identification* describes a situation in which positive identification has more likely than not been established, however, all other possibilities could not be excluded. *Speculative identifica-*

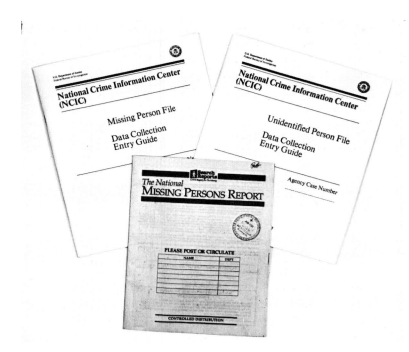

FIGURE IV-5. FBI-NCIC missing person and unidentified person data collection guides and the National Missing Persons Report.

tion carries the lowest degree of certainty and for all intents and purposes, renders the decedent unidentified.

The most common method of *definitive* identification is visual recognition of the decedent's face or body by someone with personal knowledge of the decedent's appearance. In addition to visual identification of a decedent, accepted scientific methods of definitive identification include comparison of fingerprints, dental records, radiographs, deoxyribonucleic acid (DNA) analysis, unique anthropomorphic features, and various types of physical evidence where an exemplar item such as a fingernail or hair can be authenticated as having originated from the unidentified decedent.

Methods of *presumptive* identification include recognition of clothing, unique tattoos, scars, or birthmarks. Evidence obtained from a scene that may be used to make a presumptive identification include various papers, medication bottles, or identification bearing the decedent's name. In certain circumstances, the fact that a decedent is found in his or her secure residence may be suf-

ficient information to make a presumptive identification. The use of serologic tests for determination of blood groups and proteins or human leukocyte antigens (HLA) may be used for forensic identity, but these methods have largely been replaced by DNA techniques.

In some situations, there is no single method available to definitively identify a decedent, but there is abundant evidence pointing to the decedent's identity based on the circumstances surrounding the death, investigation of the scene and examination of the body. Any one piece of circumstantial evidence would be insufficient to make a definitive identification, but the totality of the evidence when considered collectively is sufficient to determine the decedents identity beyond any reasonable doubt.

In cases where the decedent's identity may be challenged or where foul play is suspected, identification of a body should be made using an accepted method of definitive identification. This approach will hold up to any cross-examination in which the decedent's identity is questioned. It is now becoming increasing more common to resort to DNA sequencing to confirm the identity of a not viewable body whose family is available to provide a DNA sample for comparison.

The mummified and partially skeletonized remains of a young woman were found in a remote, wooded area. Adjacent to the body were several articles of clothing including a metallic green bikini top, two black platform shoes and a multicolored beach wrap with a distinctive design and inscription. Clothing removed from the body included a metallic green bikini bottom, which matched the bikini top and a black lycra halter top. Personal items recovered from around the body included an earring with a single white pearl, multiple clear stones and metal hoop clasp and several fingernails painted with blue-green polish. The cause of death was blunt head trauma and the manner of death was homicide.

The missing persons file was accessed and a likely match was made with a 19-year-old female who had been reported missing 17 days previously. The victim's family arrived from out of state and upon recognition of the decedent's personal effects specifically, the earring and the beachwrap, demanded the body be handed over to them. Being of Orthodox Jewish faith they wanted an immediate burial. Because of the nature of the case, definitive identity was essential and the body could not be released based on circumstantial evidence, no matter how convincing. Bone, teeth and soft tissue were submitted to the local crime lab together with samples from the victim's next of kin. Because the body was recently deceased, a swab of the bone surface yielded nuclear DNA that confirmed her identity.

Unidentified decedents require complete external and internal examination to document external scars, birthmarks, congenital abnormalities, evidence of prior injury, tattoos and occupational marks or injuries. Internal examination will reveal the surgical absence of organs and presence of disease that may be compared with antemortem medical records. Surgically implanted medical devices such as pacemakers, prosthetic cardiac valves and orthopedic hardware may be traced back to a specific individual. Pacemakers are inscribed with a model and serial number and the manufacture's name. This information can be traced by the company and the name of the person who received the pacemaker can be obtained. Other surgically placed devices including inferior vena cava filters and vascular grafts may provide important clues to the decedent's identity. In addition to providing points of identification, autopsy information is essential for determination of cause and manner of death. The body will not ever be in better condition

than at the time of initial examination so photographs of facial features, tattoos, scars and other distinctive physical features are indicated. The shape of ears many times assists in identifying unknown remains. Each person's ears are unique. Also, comparison of the hairline to a recent photograph may aid in identification (Fig. IV-6a–c). Full body radiographs of the remains as they are received will not only show bony injuries and anomalies, but the location of personal effects, metal fragments and other radiopaque evidence.

Visual Identification of the Deceased

Visual recognition is the most widely used method of identification. Depending on the identifier, visual recognition may be either *presumptive* or *definitive*. If the individual making the identification has not seen the decedent recently or has reservations regarding the identity, this method may only yield a *presumptive* identification. Personal recognition of a decedent can under certain circumstances be less reliable than fingerprints, dental comparison, or radiology. It relies on memory and the ability to make a rapid mental comparison of physical features under stressful conditions. Brothers, sisters, and mates have been known to misidentify accident victims even when collateral evidence such as an accident report, tentative identification by a witness, or driver's license comparison suggests a loved one is dead.

Another hazard associated with visual identification is denial. The situation may be so stressful or the remains altered by age, injury, disease, or change in lifestyle that identification is denied even if it is later confirmed by fingerprints or dental examination. It is most prudent to confirm a decedent's identity using a method other than visual recognition in all cases in which there is alteration of the body, a long interval since the person was last seen by the identifier, or a dramatic change in appearance of the individual. Furthermore, positive visual identification may be made fraudulently for purposes of disguising a homicide or for the purposes of collecting death benefits and insurance of a living co-conspirator.

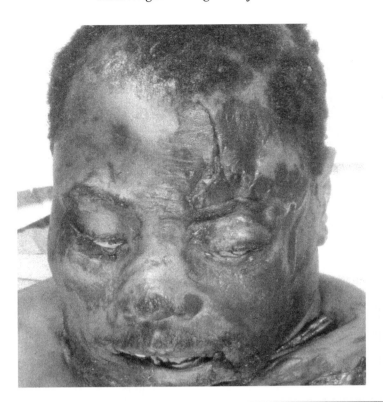

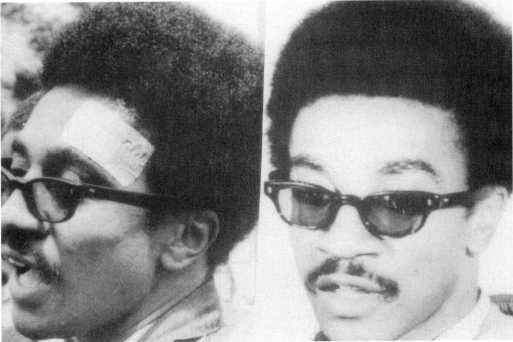

FIGURE IV-6a–b. (a) A markedly disfigured man was killed in an explosion. The question arose whether a particular individual might have been the victim. A news photograph (b) was obtained of the individual in question and showed a different shaped ear and a differently shaped hairline (c) excluding him as the victim.

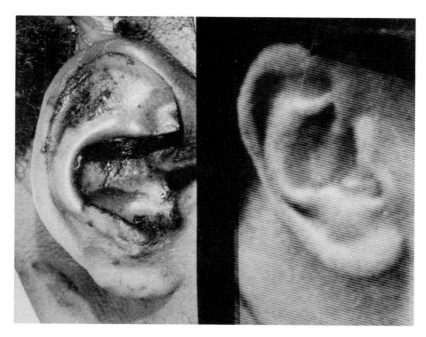

FIGURE IV-6c

A gasoline tanker was involved in a crash and became engulfed in flames. Charred fragmented remains, without teeth, sinuses or vertebrae were recovered from the cab of the incinerated vehicle. Investigators began collecting medical and military records to determine blood group and locate radiographs of the driver.

During the autopsy, the pathologist noted some bone ends were flat across as if sawed. Radiographs were inconclusive for confirmation of human bone configuration. Residual tissue was submitted for serologic identification of tissue of origin and for blood group. When set up against a panel of species specific antisera the tissue was identified as pig. The truck driver and a co-conspirator were charged and convicted of attempted fraud.

Visual identification of a decedent may be accomplished by direct or indirect visualization. Most medical examiner departments use an indirect viewing method either by Polaroid or digital photography or by a closed circuit video camera and monitor. Identification by closed circuit TV is best done in black and white as it is less traumatic. Direct visual identification is most commonly accomplished using a viewing room in which the body is viewed through a window. Direct visual identification with the decedent and the next of kin in the same room has become infrequent and is not permitted in most medical examiner departments. The possibility of spread-

ing communicable diseases and liability issues should an injury occur are the most common reasons for not permitting direct contact between the decedent and the individual doing the identification.

Polaroid and digital photographs have dual purposes. The photos may be shown to family members in a controlled, comfortable environment for purposes of identification and the photos may also be used by detectives performing neighborhood canvasses to find witnesses to a crime. The use of 35-mm photography is cumbersome for identification of viewable bodies since the time necessary for film development may delay the process. One of the advantages of digital photography is that a skilled photographer can manipulate the computer image and make a mutilated face presentable for the purposes of identification. Funeral directors, using restorative techniques with wax and make-up may accomplish the same. Loss of facial bone structure secondary to skull and facial fractures will distort a person's appearance and make visual identification difficult. In situations where the face is intact, but distorted secondary to fractures, adding support behind the fractures to reshape the head and

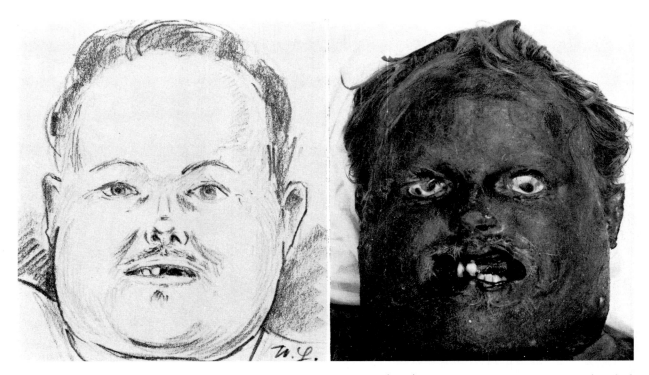

FIGURE IV-7. Mummified body of a thirty-four-year-old Caucasian male (right) kept refrigerated for over a year identified through an artist's sketch after publication in a widely distributed newspaper.

face may allow for visual identification. This technique has been successful in cases of suicidal shotgun wounds of the mouth.

Artist's sketches and Identi-Kit® reconstructions are two rapid methods of portraying an unidentified person in newspapers or on television in a public appeal for identification (Fig. IV-7). Photographic superimposition of postmortem skulls positioned in the same orientation as an antemortem photograph, or optical devices coupled with a television camera using computer software-aided evaluation of the skull to an antemortem photograph, permit comparison of photographs at varying angles to verify visage.[4,5]

Forensic sculptors working with skeletal remains and modeling clay can reconstruct facial features to permit identification (Fig. IV-8a–b). Skeptics of this procedure question the artists' objectivity. Computer programs are available to simulate aging so that if the interval between disappearance and death or discovery is long, a more accurate depiction of facial features is possible. The latter procedure is particularly helpful in the case of abducted living children who do

not know their real identity or unidentified dead children where the circumstances suggest survival for months to years after their disappearance.

Clothing and Personal Effects

Clothing and personal effects are easily accessible and often provide important clues to identity. In mass disasters, such as plane crashes, fires, or mass drownings, all clothing and personal effects should be left with the body until they can be documented, inventoried and photographed. Comparison of clothing and personal effects found on the decedent can be compared with descriptions obtained from the next of kin, thus providing investigators with a presumptive identity. In mass disasters, miscellaneous personal belongings and clothing that cannot be linked to a particular decedent should be displayed before the next of kin. Although this provides little help with direct identification, it helps determine who are the likely victims in the disaster. Having a

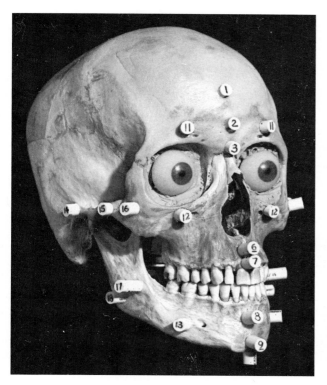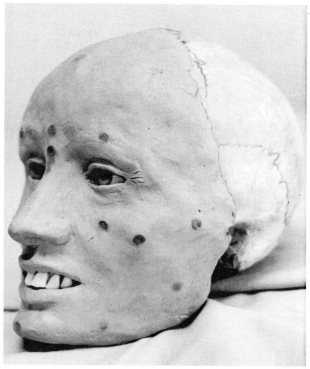

FIGURE IV-8a–b. (a) Facial reconstruction: Use of tissue depth marker guides in preparation for clay facial reconstruction. (b) A skull with clay molded to tissue marker depths to exhibit facial features. (Courtesy of Thomas W. Goyne, Division of Forensic Science, Richmond, VA.)

presumptive identity allows investigators to obtain fingerprint cards, dental records, and x-rays all of which can be used to afford a definitive identification.

The bloated body of a woman was recovered from the James River. The jeans and shirt showed a name in marking pen. A search of missing persons records disclosed a woman of that name missing from a mental hospital some 30 miles upstream. Hospital records included dental charts which confirmed identification and psychiatric history documenting her repeated wish to die by jumping off the Benjamin Harrison bridge.

Clothing may provide important clues as to the identity of a decedent. Laundry marks, uniforms and uniform logos will help investigators narrow down the list of missing persons. Careful examination of clothing may yield a name or other identifying information (Fig. IV-9). The type of clothing may provide clues as to what the decedent was doing at the time of death. Clothing may also help determine the social class or background of the decedent. Clothing measurements and size can be compared to standard size and weight tables providing good estimates of weight and height of skeletons or partial remains.[6] A complete description of clothing should include type of garment, size, color, condition, manufacturers label information, laundry marks, names and numbers. In accordance with the Federal Textile Fiber Products Identification Act, apparel and textiles of domestic manufacture without a corporate name label, have a label bearing a registration number (RN) or in the case of wool, a wool product label (WPL). The RN and WPL Encyclopedia list the name, address and phone number of thousands of manufacturers, wholesalers and importers of apparel and textiles by RN and WPL numbers.[7] The Federal Trade Commission (FTC) can also assist with tracking the importer or manufacturer of clothing. The clothing manufacturer's production information may give a time frame and site of sale to assist in tracking the origin of an unidentified person. In addition to providing clues as to the decedent's identity, clothing may be useful

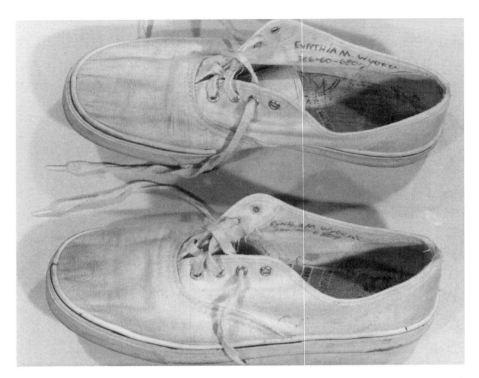

FIGURE IV-9. Use of clothing to render a presumptive identification. The name and social security number of the decedent had been written on the inside of the shoes. Marking of clothes with owner's name is commonly practiced in some schools and certain types of institutions.

with regard to manner of death determination. Clothing with bullet holes, stab cuts or tread marks are such examples.

Personal effects are often very helpful with respect to identification. The items that are most useful for this purpose include driver's licenses, credit cards, prescription medication, papers bearing the decedent's name, eyeglasses, watches and jewelry. Without a photographic identification, such as a driver's license, identification of a decedent using personal effects should be considered presumptive. It is possible that the personal effects may not actually belong to the decedent or that they were stolen or borrowed. Furthermore, the items may be planted on the decedent to mislead investigators and attempt to criminally interchange identity.

Jewelry and watches should be examined by a jeweler for the alphanumeric code, for example 47 AE, of the American Watchmakers Institute (Fig. IV-10). The Institute, at P.O. Box 11011, Cincinnati, Ohio can identify the watchmaker leading to repair records and the identification of the person submitting the watch for repair. Rings, lockets, belt buckles and bracelets may bear monograms or engravings of names, initials and dates. Keys may have distinctive features characterizing them as vehicle, house, or security keys. Successful unlocking of a house, car, or storage locker may render clues as to the decedent's identity, as well as provide information that may be helpful if the case is of criminal interest. Many personal effects will be made unrecognizable by extreme heat, however, military identification tags (dog tags) resist temperatures of 2000° F. Eyeglasses may be examined for comparison of prescriptions and the frames checked for manufacturing information and model number.[8]

A routine sweep of a Miami canal led to the discovery of an old model Chevrolet sedan found submerged and partially covered by mud and silt. Upon removal from the water, the car was identified as a Dade County Water and Sewer Authority vehicle. Police divers at the scene conducted a cursory search of the muck-filled vehicle and found human bones and clothing. Upon further excavation of the

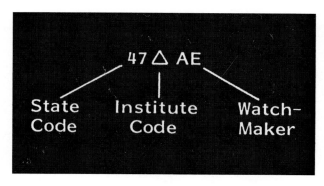

FIGURE IV-10. Code of the American Watchmakers Institute. (Courtesy of Ewell Hartman.)

vehicle the complete skeletal remains of a middle-aged, Caucasian male were discovered. In addition to the clothing and bones, numerous personal items including a silver watch, two rings and a wallet containing several credit cards inscribed with a name believed to be the decedent were recovered from the vehicle.

Review of county records led investigators to the name of the person who had been issued the vehicle and it was discovered that he was declared a missing person in 1979. Upon review of the original police report, it was discovered that the decedent was reported missing when he failed to return home after a night out with several friends. Reconstruction of the events associated with the case led to the determination that the decedent was likely on his way home when he lost control of his vehicle and entered the canal which paralleled the road. His body had remained undiscovered for 22 years.

A complete upper and a partial lower denture in addition to multiple natural teeth were recovered, however, no dental records were available for comparison. Based on the families identification of the numerous personal effects recovered from the vehicle (Fig. IV-11), the characteristics of the skeleton and the circumstances surrounding his disappearance, the name of the decedent was verified. Although DNA testing was not felt to be necessary to confirm his identity, at the request of the decedent's family, DNA testing was performed using the recovered teeth. Due to the age of the skeletal remains, nuclear DNA was unable to be sequenced, however, mitochondrial DNA sequencing confirmed the decedents presumed identity.

The decomposed body of a man was recovered in the Chesapeake Bay. A key with the Norwegian word for cook was found in the pocket of the seaman who had drowned six months earlier and helped establish identification (see Fig. III-31a).

Personal papers often bear writing that compares favorably with known antemortem exemplars. The first three digits of a social security number indicates the state of issuance and

should result in an inquiry regarding missing persons in that state.

Fingerprints and Footprints

Fingerprints remain the easiest and most reliable method of identification. Historically, identification by fingerprints has proven to be more reliable, less labor intensive and easier than bertillonage, which was Alphonse Bertillon's system of detailed and precise anthropomorphic measurements of prisoners, used to identify criminals in France.[9] During the eighth and ninth centuries in China, fingerprints were used to identify persons executing sales contracts and for the identification of immigrants and visitors. Church documents from the 1600s show signatures and thumb and fingerprints for identification. The identification of criminals by fingerprints began in the late 1800s and became the preferred method of identification of criminals in England and Wales in 1901, and in the United States after 1903. The history of fingerprints and fingerprinting is recounted by Polson.[10]

Based on the ideas of Dr. Henry Faulds in Japan and Sir William James Herschel in India, Sir Francis Galton, a cousin of Charles Darwin, published the results of his own research, *Fingerprints,* in 1892. During the same decade Juan Vucetich, a police official in Argentina and Inspector General of Police Edward Richard Henry in Bengal, India studied Galton's work and developed classification systems. Modifications of these systems are used for conventional fingerprint identification to this day. The national file for fingerprints at the Federal Bureau of Investigation (FBI) was developed in 1924. In addition, there are local, state and regional fingerprint files to which unidentified prints can be compared. Entry of fingerprints into the Unidentified and Missing Persons Files within the National Crime Information Center (NCIC) first occurred in the mid 1980s. The first automated fingerprint identification systems (AFIS) came on line in the late 1970s.

Fingerprints are present after the twelfth week of gestation. Whether burned, decomposed, mutilated or mummified, bodies often exhibit

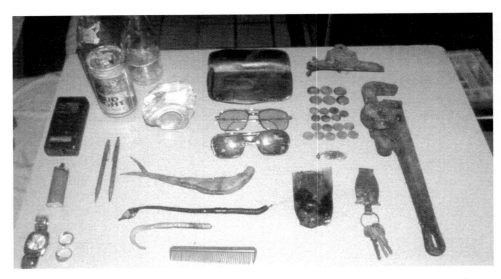

FIGURE IV-11. Miscellaneous personal items consisting of an engraved ring, wrist watch, car keys, and other items. The personal effects were identified by relatives and allowed for positive identification.

sufficient fingerprints or partial prints for identification. Even when damaged, recovery of usable finger and palmprints may be possible. Mummified fingers can be soaked in warm water until pliable and then injected subcutaneously with water or glycerol to raise the ridges and remove wrinkles. Fragile charred fingers should be amputated at the second joint taking care not to touch the fingerpad. Attempts to straighten contracted burned hands by pressing on fingertips may destroy fragile residual prints. In these situations, fingers can be effectively straightened by cutting the flexor tendons in the palm of the hand.

The epidermal layer may separate as a *glove of skin* in decomposed bodies, bodies immersed in water for extended periods, and in bodies with second-degree burns. Certain corrosive chemicals will have the same effect, as does immersion in gasoline, especially if a high octane. This *glove of skin* may provide fingerprints, as does the internal surface of the glove, in the reverse (Fig. IV-12a–b). Fingerprints from degloved skin are best obtained by placing the sloughed skin over a gloved hand and rolling the fingers in the usual fashion. If the skin is sloughed and unavailable, less distinct but adequate impressions may be obtained by printing the dermis. Attempts by fugitives to obliterate fingerprints by injury or grafting and thus frustrate

fingerprint identification have been mostly unsuccessful. Occasionally, in mason and cement workers, fingerprints may be sufficiently abraded to yield unreadable prints. In difficult cases, trained fingerprint examiners should be consulted. In the absence of local expertise, formalin fixed hands amputated at the wrist may be submitted to the Identification Division of the FBI for examination and possible identification. The hands or fingers should be fixed in 1% alcohol in an unbreakable container and sent to:

Federal Bureau of Investigation
Attention: Latent Fingerprints Section
Identification Division
935 Pennsylvania Ave., N.W.
Washington D.C. 20535
(202) 324-2163

Fingerprints, footprints, and palmprints of a decedent, when compared with antemortem tenprint fingerprint cards or single latent prints of a known missing person have been used to identify large numbers of disaster victims. They permit identification and reunion of multiple body parts and have the added advantage of being rapidly available from civilian and criminal fingerprint files, from the military, places of employment and as latents from personal effects.

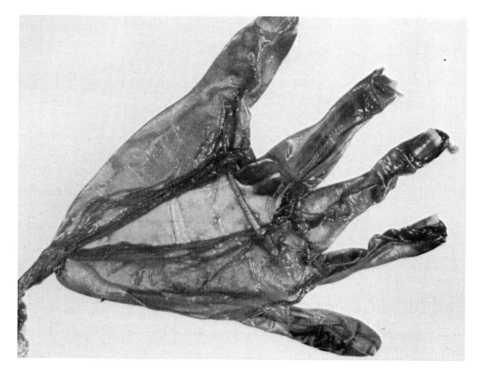

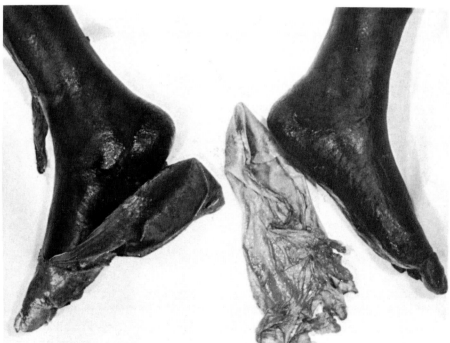

FIGURE IV-12a–b. De-gloving of the hand and foot skin of a decomposed body suitable for finger and footprinting. The same type of skin separation occurs in bodies recovered from water and in second-degree burns.

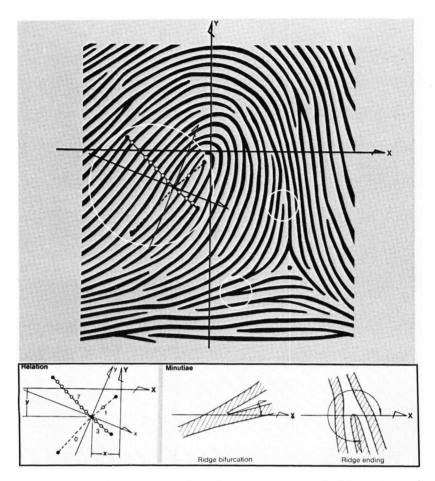

FIGURE IV-13. Minutiae oriented in relation to axes provide the position and direction of fingerprint features for comparison by AFIS. (Courtesy, NEC Technologies, Boxborough, MA 01719.)

Automated Fingerprint Identification Systems (AFIS)

Prior to the use of computers a single fingerprint from a decedent could not be searched as an unknown against fingerprint files, a procedure that required ten, or at a minimum, nine searchable prints. However, the development of computerized automated fingerprint identification systems (AFIS) permits rapid entry, comparison and identification. Automated systems depend on computer comparison of minutiae (Fig. IV-13). Minutiae are the location and orientation of fingerprint ridges at points of termination (ridge endings) or branching (bifurcations). Patterns of minutiae uniquely characterize individual prints and are the basis of comparison for identification.

Monozygotic twins share a higher number of similar minutiae, but are nevertheless not identical and able to be distinguished.

Automated systems customarily have three subsystems.[11,12] An input subsystem reads ten print cards, accepts input on latent prints, and receives descriptive data on offenders. The reader/scanner orients each print by assigning axes which are two perpendicular intersecting lines superimposed on the fingerprint image according to classification conventions programmed into the computer. The coordinates of each minutiae are expressed in relation to these axes. The matching subsystem handles fingerprint matching by aligning the coordinates and comparing the minutiae. It also stores minutiae data and descriptive information. The digital image retrieval subsystem stores and retrieves image data generating a list of candidates having a high degree of similarity. The system also displays prints for visual comparison and prints out hard copies. Although the computer selects possible matches, visual comparison by a fingerprint examiner is necessary to confirm the identity. Thus, a single complete or partial unknown print from a body or a latent print lifted at the crime scene can be used to identify the owner. The system can also compare latent print to latent print; so if the decedent or living person has a latent on file, a trail leading to a serial offender can be initiated.

Automated systems achieve identifications in minutes to hours as opposed to weeks to months using conventional manual search methods. A directory of individual cities, agencies and regional AFIS databases is available for investigators needing searches.[13] In exceptional cases, when fingerprint detail is fine enough even the ridges, pores, and edges of ridges may be compared.[14]

In many cases, shoes or socks cover a decedent's feet. This provides some protection from burning, postmortem animal activity and water damage, all of which may render the hands and fingers unsuitable for printing. In unidentified decedents unable to be fingerprinted, footprints may be taken for comparison with antemortem samples. Possible sources of antemortem footprints include the military, commercial airlines and birth records although the latter are usually of poor quality and difficult to compare. Occasionally, comparison of a photographic enlargement of a birth footprint, showing toeprints, ridge details and flexion creases, to that of an adult will affect identification or document a baby mix-up.

Lip prints are unique and may be compared if an antemortem exemplar can be found. The best source for a lip print exemplar is from glassware or cigarettes. Cigarette butts may yield other information such as DNA and in secretors, blood type. The ability to make a positive identification based on visual comparison of human ears or latent ear prints remains a controversial subject. Iannarelli describes a system utilizing the human ear for identification purposes,[15] however, these results have not been substantiated or repro-

duced in subsequent studies. The use of latent ear prints has been challenged in legal proceedings, and cases based on this evidence have been overturned. Ear shape biometrics have been used in several European countries, however, forensic experts still disagree on whether such evidence represents a true science. In short, further studies are needed before ear prints and ear shape evidence can be held to the same standard as fingerprints or DNA analysis.

A commercial airliner crashed and largely burned. Two elderly ladies on the passenger list remained unidentified. A search of body parts disclosed a segment of scalp, henna dyed hair and an ear. Photographs of the missing women were enlarged and the ears compared. One compared favorably as did hair recovered from her residence permitting identification.

The ridge detail of fingernails and toenails is sufficiently unique to permit identification by tool marks examiners if reliable exemplars can be found (Fig. IV-14).

Dental Examination and Comparison

Because teeth are the most durable structures of the human body, they are remarkably resistant to destruction and the effects of decomposition. Teeth are also so unique that no two sets are the same. These characteristics make comparison of dental features one of most reliable methods of identification and the most frequently used method of identification in cases of mass disaster associated with body charring and fragmentation. Since intraoral dental radiographs are an essential diagnostic tool in dental practice, they are commonly part of a patient's dental records. An in-depth discussion of dental charting and comparison is beyond the scope of this chapter and is detailed in *Chapter VI.*

When faced with a charred, decomposed or skeletonized body, it is imperative that care is taken to protect the teeth to allow for complete x-rays and dental charting. Because charred, blackened teeth are extremely fragile, it is important for scene investigators, body transport personnel, and the medical examiner to use caution to avoid further damage to the teeth. Studies indicate that when exposed to high heat, teeth may become

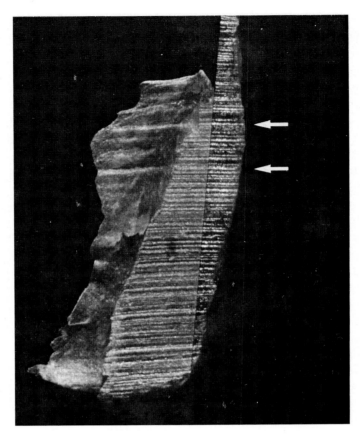

FIGURE IV-14. Torn fingernail recovered from a scene (left) and a known exemplar fingernail (right). Alignment of ridges (arrows) allowed successful match and victim identification. (Courtesy of Ann D. Jones, Division of Forensic Sciences, Richmond, VA.)

brittle at 400° F and disintegrate into ash at about 900° F (Fig. IV-15).[16] Facial soft tissue of a charred body may be lost leaving only a charred skull, however, depending on how much of the lips and perioral tissue remains, the teeth may be insulated from the high heat and remain intact. Insulated teeth and dental restorations are likely to withstand considerably higher temperatures and upon reflection of the charred perioral tissue the anterior teeth may be found in perfect condition (Fig. IV-16). In the majority of charred bodies, the posterior teeth are well preserved and can be used for dental comparisons.

At the scene of a decomposed or skeletonized body, a thorough, organized search should be undertaken in order to retrieve all teeth from under and around the body. Before the body is moved and the ground disturbed, the area around the decedent's head should be searched looking for any teeth which may have fallen out.

In most situations, forensic odontologists should be consulted when a body is to be identified using comparisons of antemortem and postmortem dental charts. Consultation with experienced odontologists will not only allow identification based on subtle bone structure and tooth characteristics, but will help forensic pathologists gain a working knowledge of the subject. With a basic understanding of dental x-rays, forensic pathologists should be able to make definitive identifications using antemortem and postmortem x-rays by comparing amalgam fillings (silver), bridgework, restorations and dental implants (Figs. IV-17 and IV-18). In cases where the comparison is equivocal and in all cases of suspected criminal activity, a forensic

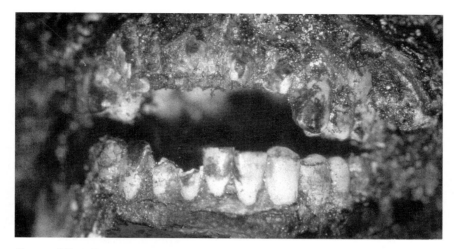

FIGURE IV-15. Disintegration of anterior teeth from prolonged exposure to extreme heat.

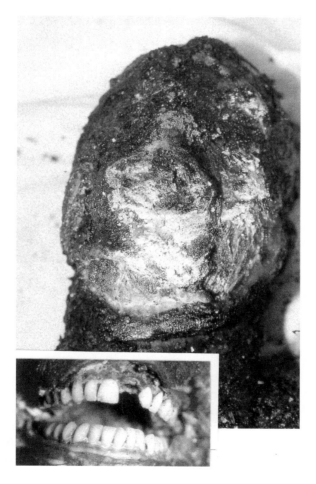

FIGURE IV-16. Unrecognizable charred head and face of a homicide victim recovered from the trunk of a burning vehicle. (Insert) Reflection of the perioral tissues allows visualization of the intact anterior teeth. The upper central incisor is most likely absent as a result of antemortem trauma rather than heat-related disintegration, since the adjacent teeth are in perfect condition and show no heat-related artifact.

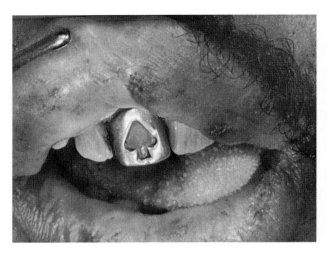

FIGURE IV-17. Identification based on dental records which described the unusual gold cap on the upper right central incisor.

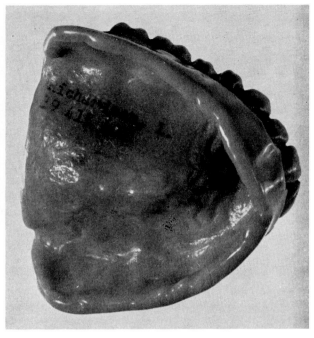

FIGURE IV-18. Dentures are quite resistant to the effects of trauma and heat. The dentures may be compared with antemortem dental charts or like in this case the name and identification number of the decedent may be inscribed on the dental plate.

odontologist should be consulted to confirm the identity. When faced with a complicated dental comparison and no dentist is available, both jaws should be removed and preserved.

Forensic odontologists can make a definitive identity by comparison of a multitude of dental features. Restorations, tooth configuration, residual tooth fragments, tooth impressions, fit of dentures (Fig. IV-19a–b) and photographic comparison of smile (Fig. IV-20) are a few methods which have been successfully employed. Dental charts, radiographs, skull radiographs, impressions, bite marks and dental appliance and laboratory records can also be used for comparison purposes.

Deciduous (primary) and permanent teeth erupt at different ages. Determination of an unknown decedent's age can be estimated based on examination of the teeth with respect to eruption of the primary or permanent teeth. Up to the age of 14 years, tooth development is one of the best parameters for age determination. From 14 to 23 years, dental development may be used, but skeletal indicators are more consistent. After the age of 24 age estimation using teeth characteristics progressively becomes less accurate.[17] The average age of tooth eruption is shown in Table IV-3.[18]

Dental records are often combined with medical records in federal and state hospitals and prisons. When a person disappears and foul play is suspected, dental records should be collected promptly either by permission from the next of kin or by local law, as permitted. Inactive records tend to be purged and destroyed, or lost when a dentist moves or dies. As seen with medical records, dental records are variable in quality and quantity. Some dentists chart only their own work, others chart the complete mouth and others only note work done on the billing sheet. Collecting the complete record, including charts, x-rays and billing information from every dentist who has treated the missing person improves the chances of inclusion or exclusion. Radiographs include the configuration of teeth adjacent to treated teeth perhaps permitting identification by concurrence of unusual root morphology of a normal tooth. Comparison of dental records is the most common and reliable method of identification of skeletons followed by radiologic identification.

Entry of dental characteristics of unidentified bodies into the NCIC unidentified and missing

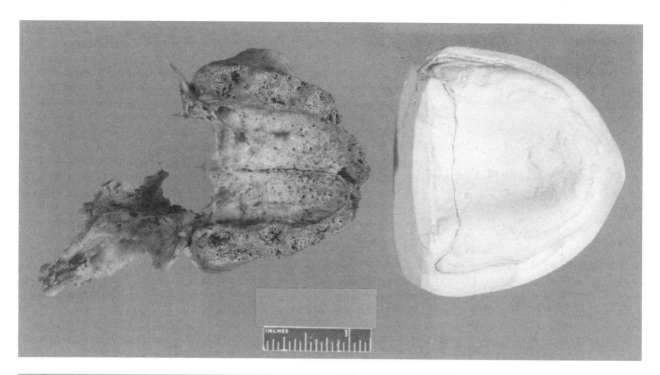

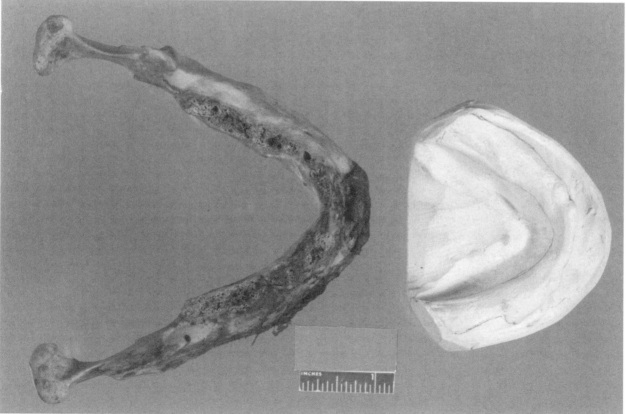

FIGURE IV-19a–b. Denture casts fit the upper and lower jaws and are suitable for comparison and identification. These molds are usually retained by dentists for many years.

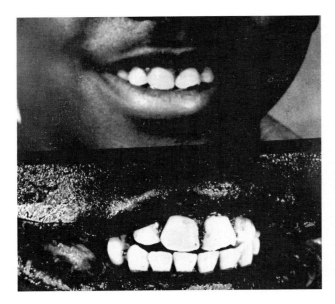

FIGURE IV-20. Dental identification by *smile*. Comparison of a denture of an unidentified decomposed body to a photograph of a *smiling* missing person shows match with frontal teeth.

TABLE IV-3
AVERAGE AGE OF TOOTH ERUPTION*

Deciduous Teeth	
Upper Central Incisors:	7–10 months
Lower Central Incisors:	5–9 months
Upper Lateral Incisors:	8–10 months
Lower Lateral Incisors:	15–21 months
Upper Canines (cuspid):	16–20 months
Lower Canines (cuspid):	15–21 months
First Molars:	15–21 months
Second Molars:	20–24 months
Permanent Teeth	
Upper Central Incisors:	7th year
Lower Central Incisors:	7th year
Upper Lateral Incisors:	8th year
Lower Lateral Incisors:	8th year
Canines (upper & lower):	11th–12th year
First Premolars:	9th year
First Molars:	6th year
Second Molars:	12th–13th year
Third Molars:	17th - 25th year

* Netter, F. Atlas of Human Anatomy. Ciba-Geigy, 1989.

persons files significantly reduces the number of futile exchanges of records between police agencies and medical examiners and promotes swift identification of distant missing persons. Computer software programs such as The Computer-Assisted Postmortem Identification (CAPMI) System receive and compare dental records of victims of mass disasters, enabling more rapid identification of air crash, flood and explosion victims.[19]

Radiographic Examination and Comparison

Radiographs present unique skeletal anatomic features analogous to a fingerprint and provide for a reliable means of identification when antemortem radiographs are available for comparison.[20] Evaluation of radiographs assumes a predominant role in cases of fire, decomposition, or mutilation. Radiographs are common in the practice of clinical medicine and are often on file at local hospitals. It is good practice to take full body x-rays of all unviewable bodies regardless of whether antemortem films are known to be available. In order to make a definitive identifi-

cation of an unidentified individual, careful comparison using antemortem and postmortem radiographs must be performed, however, there is currently no standard as to how the comparison should be done. Unlike fingerprints, there is no minimum number of comparison points that must match before identification can be made. It has been found that when comparing antemortem and postmortem radiographs, a positive match of one to four unique features without having any discrepancies is considered sufficient to make a definitive identification.[21] Although a single distinctive skeletal feature may allow for positive identification, the use of multiple points of comparison increases the degree of certainty.

Previous studies have reported 100% accuracy in human identification using comparison of antemortem and postmortem radiographs, however, a study by Kuehn et al. found that comparison of chest radiographs as a method of positive identification is accurate in only 80% of cases with variation depending on who is doing the identification. The investigators site the quality of the films as being the most significant limiting factor. The study also concluded that forensic anthropologists may be uniquely qualified to accurately compare antemortem and postmortem films, most likely because anthropologists commonly use shapes and contours of skeletal structures rather than bone pathology.[22]

The ability of a forensic investigator to make an identification by comparison of antemortem and postmortem radiographs partly depends on the quality of the films and the degree to which the postmortem radiograph matches the position of the antemortem x-ray.[22] It is best to try and duplicate the position shown in the antemortem film so that subtle changes will not be missed or obscured by angulation or bone rotation. Depending on the quality of the films and the bone(s) being compared, specialized expertise in radiographic interpretation increases the likelihood of an accurate comparison.[23]

Radiographs may be taken and successfully interpreted regardless of the bodies' state of preservation. Postmortem radiographs of a decomposed body may be readily recognized as such by the presence of gas formation throughout the soft tissue. This artifact should be ignored when comparing antemortem and postmortem x-rays. Radiographs not only allow visualization of the skeleton, but also identify surgically implanted orthopedic hardware (Fig. IV-21a–b), sternal wires (Fig. IV-22), pacemakers, intravascular devices (inferior vena cava filters and coronary artery stents), surgical clips, bullets and other metal fragments (i.e. knife tip). All of these features are suitable for comparison with antemortem films. Furthermore, x-rays will help locate personal effects not seen upon external examination of the body. Radiographs will also aid in identification by providing clues as to one's past injury and medical diseases. Although antemortem radiographs may not be available, a complete set of postmortem x-rays should be taken and kept on file in the event that antemortem x-rays surface after the body has been buried. This may prevent unnecessary exhumation of the body. In some situations, an identifying feature may not be known by the next of kin, but nevertheless, x-ray examination will often demonstrate unique skeletal characteristics that can be compared using old radiographs or medical records. Normal bone variation, congenital malformations, healed trauma and slow growing tumors are good examples of such conditions.

Postmortem radiographs showing sesamoid bones, fused ribs, or vertebrae, osteomas, and old clinically insignificant fractures may be of great value with regard to identification. Written radiology reports may not mention such abnormalities, and therefore the actual films should be obtained for direct comparison.

The vertebral column offers many unique features for comparison and is probably the most useful part of the skeleton for the purpose of comparing radiographs (Fig. IV-23). Each vertebra develops from three primary and five secondary ossification centers which allows for great individual variability in the size, shape and configuration of the bone.[24] Anatomic landmarks on the spine that are useful for comparison include the shape and configuration of the spinous processes and vertebral bodies, and the morphology of the arches and articular surfaces.[1] Definitive identification can be made by positive comparison of only one spinous process as long as no inconsistencies are noted, however, with good quality radiographs, multiple points of comparison are likely (Fig. IV-24a–b). The vertebral column commonly has age-related changes that allow for easy comparison. Degenerative changes in the form of vertebral osteophytes, ossification of intervertebral ligaments and herniated discs are typically unique to each individual and are thus invaluable with regard to identification.[25,26] Scoliosis and kyphosis of the vertebral column may be hard to assess in postmortem radiographs making these conditions difficult to compare with antemortem films. Consideration must be given to the length of time between the antemortem radiograph being used for the comparison and the postmortem radiograph.

The skull provides several anatomic structures that can be useful with regard to human identification. The four major sinuses of the human skull include the frontal, sphenoid, ethmoid, and maxillary. Of these structures, the frontal sinus has been found to be the most unique among individuals allowing definitive identification or exclusion.[27] Similar to fingerprints, the frontal

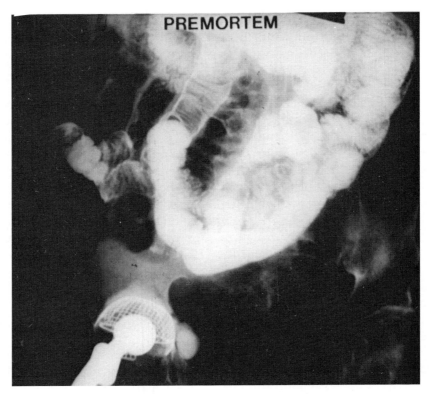

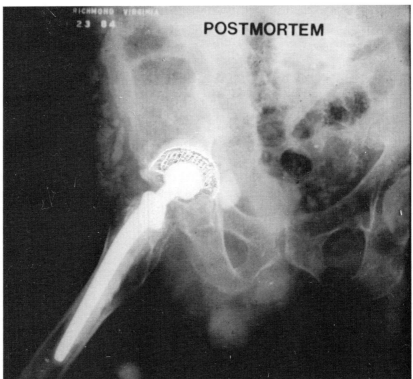

FIGURE IV-21a–b. Comparison using antemortem films taken during a gastrointestinal series (a) and postmortem films taken at the time of autopsy (b). The configuration of the femoral prosthesis and adjacent bone structures match.

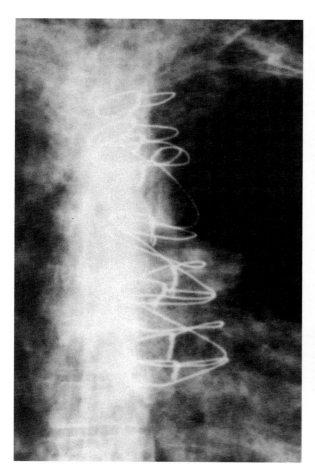

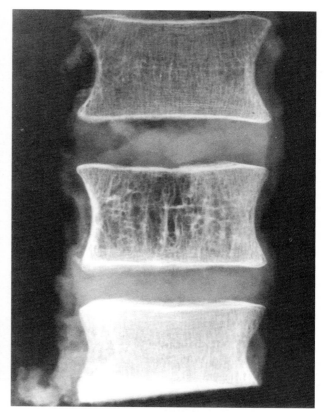

FIGURE IV-23. Lumbar vertebrae showing trabecular structure and osteoporosis.

FIGURE IV-22. Identification of a decomposed man by comparison of antemortem and postmortem chest radiographs which demonstrated identical configuration of sternal wires placed during coronary artery bypass surgery.

sinus is so distinct that the chances of two individuals having a frontal sinus with the same morphology is virtually non-existent.[28,29] The frontal sinuses are rudimentary at birth and although they may be partially developed by the end of the first year of life, they are not usually identified radiographically until six or seven years of age. The sinus is fully developed by early adulthood[30] at which time radiographic features are best visualized. For this reason, comparison of frontal sinus morphology is best done in individuals at least 20 years of age.[30,31]

In addition to frontal sinus anatomy, there are several other morphologic features of the skull that may be suitable for comparison. These include the mastoid air cells,[27,32] sphenoid bones, arterial and venous markings[27,32] and suture patterns.

The axial skeleton has been used for identification purposes and there are reports describing various features that have been used for comparison. These include specific bony anomalies, arthritic changes of vertebrae, appearance of the scapulae, sacroiliac and pubic joint configuration, and bone trabecular patterns.[1,26,30] The trabecular architecture of bone is subject to change over time as a result of bone demineralization associated with osteoporosis.[33] For this reason, the identity of an unknown individual should not be ruled out based solely on comparison of trabecular bone architecture.[30]

The largely decomposed remains of an elderly man were recovered from a remote wooded area. He was edentulous and no fingerprints were recoverable. Radiographs revealed

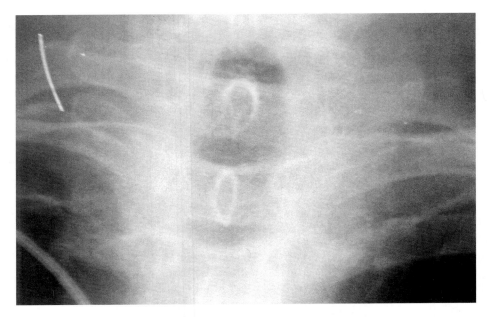

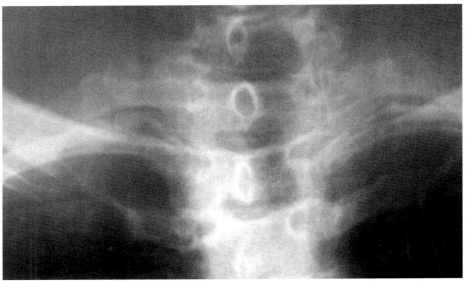

FIGURE IV-24a–b. Identification using comparison of antemortem (a) and postmortem (b) chest radiographs in which the shape and configuration of several spinous processes were matched.

a cluster of small metal surgical clips in the right lumbosacral region consistent with a lumbar sympathectomy during life. An elderly man was missing from a nearby county. Medical records, including radiographs of the pelvis of the missing man were obtained from a distant University Hospital. The records documented a sympathectomy several years earlier and the clips on the radiographs, when superimposed upon those of the dead man matched perfectly. Osteoarthritic spurs of the spine, arthritic changes in the hips and bone trabecular patterns also compared favorably.

A 13-year-old girl disappeared from a downtown city neighborhood. Several months later the partial skeleton of a young girl was discovered in a shallow grave in woods in a distant county. Dentition on the missing girl had changed since her last recorded dental check due to deciduous tooth loss and eruption of permanent teeth rendering attempts at dental identification unsuccessful. A skull film taken at age 6 was found and compared. Sinus development was insufficient on the antemortem film for comparison, but the meningeal vascular groove and diploic venous pattern on

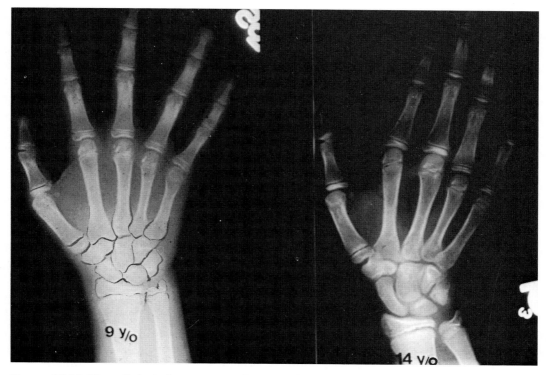

FIGURE IV-25. The radiological appearance of centers of ossification and epiphyseal closure distinguish a 9 year-old from a 14 year-old. Although radiological age and chronological age do not always coincide due to genetic and nutritional factors, radiological evaluation is invaluable in sorting out siblings and children recovered from mass disasters.

lateral skull films of the skeleton matched the patterns on the antemortem radiographs of the missing girl affording positive identification.[32]

When taking postmortem radiographs of children, it is important to take additional films and special views of the joints, especially the wrist and hand. This may enable comparison with standard ages of appearance of ossification centers and epiphyseal closure[34] (Fig. IV-25). Teeth follow a predictable sequence of eruption permitting aging by the odontologist within several months (see Table IV-3). A pediatric radiologist can often identify subtle findings suggestive of abuse or natural disease.

SKELETAL REMAINS

The complete examination of skeletal remains warrants consultation with a physical anthropologist. Should an anthropologist be in close proximity to the medical examiner's office, partially skeletonized remains are best examined prior to the bones being manipulated.

To facilitate transport to a distant consultant, decomposed remains may be reduced to bone. Soaking in a solution of household bleach, (sodium hypochlorite 4.5–6%) and sodium hydroxide, 5–10 g/liter, separates soft tissues from bone and placing in acetone overnight degreases them. An alternative method utilizes a combination of maceration of tissue over several days in water followed by soaking in enzyme detergent.[35] Bones should be defleshed gently to avoid causing scalpel cuts or other injury that may be misinterpreted on anthropologic examination. The chemical means of removing soft tissue from bone are very effective, but at the same time corrosive to bone. If time permits, the least damaging method of flesh removal is burial for several weeks. Placement in a beetle pit, if such is available, is by far the most advantageous, accomplishing tissue removal in less than 24 hours with no observable bone damage even to most delicate bony structures.

Separating postmortem artifact from premortem injury is essential to the interpretation of cause and manner of death. When presented with skeletal remains, the suspicion of foul play should always be considered. Subtle skeletal injury may not be apparent to the untrained eye although this type of evidence may be crucial to solving the case. For this reason, anthropological consultation should be sought even if no injuries are initially seen. The fewer findings the skeletal remains present, the more important it is to submit them for anthropological consultation. For detailed information regarding forensic anthropology refer to *Chapter V.*

Because human bones are remarkably resistant to the ravages of time and environment they permit personal identification and recognition of injury, disease, and markers of occupational stress many years after death. Even cremated remains may include fragments of femoral head, pelvis, skull and teeth sufficient to allow for determination of sex and race. Antemortem injury may sometimes be identified in these remains. If remains are fleshed, but decomposed, a practical quick consult for sex and age may be obtained by excising and defleshing the medial aspect of the clavicle, anterior iliac crest, pubic bone and sternal ends of ribs 1–7 for evaluation by an anthropologist.[36]

Determination of Sex

Sexing decomposed or mutilated bodies may be difficult depending on the degree of decomposition. Confirming the presence of residual breast, uterine, ovarian, prostatic or testicular tissue allows definitive determination of sex. Collateral evidence, such as radiographic demonstration of a contraceptive device in decomposed tissue is presumptive evidence of female while the finding of breast implants is not always conclusive.

Single measurement indices for sex include the diameters of the humeral, radial, and femoral heads. A diameter of the humeral head of 47 mm or greater is male; a diameter of 43 mm or less is female. Measurement of the maximum and minimum diameter of the adult radial heads and femoral heads discriminates between male and female more than 90% of the time. The maximal female radial head diameter measures 21 mm or less while males measure 24 mm or greater.[37] A femoral head vertical diameter of greater than 45 mm is characteristically male whereas this measurement in females is typically 43 mm or less. The development of sophisticated statistical tests and measurements has produced finer definitions of race, sex and height making discriminant function analysis by the anthropologist the best method to determine the sex, age and race of partial skeletons. In general, characteristics of the skull and pelvis can reliably allow determination of sex (Table IV-4) (Fig. IV-26).

Determination of Age

Well-preserved bodies present few problems in aging although there is a tendency to underestimate age of persons with youthful skin, especially Blacks. Estimates of age of decomposed or skeletonized remains require correlation of dental age as evidenced by the stage of tooth eruption (see Table IV-3), tooth wear, and alveolar ridge resorption. Radiological studies demonstrating the extent of cranial and epiphyseal unions, degenerative bone and joint changes add clues as to a decedents age.

Radiographs of the chest plate also exhibit characteristic age changes. Progressive ossification of the ribs at the costal cartilages correlates best with increasing age within 5–8 years of real age.[38] The ridge detail of the pubic symphysis permits estimates within five-year spans, most accurately for males. Plastic models representing the changes at various ages are available for study.[36] A study by Hutchinson and Russell found that epiphyseal fusion of various bones serve as landmarks for age estimation.[39] The

TABLE IV-4

DIFFERENTIAL CHARACTERISTICS OF THE SKULL AND PELVIS FOR MALES AND FEMALES

	Male	*Female*
Pelvis		
Subpubic arch	Less than 70°	Greater than 70°
Greater sciatic notch	Acute angle	Approximately 90°
Pre-auricular sulcus	Ill defined	Distinct
Obdurator foramen	Oval	Almost triangular
Body of pubis	Triangular	Square
Acetabulum	Large, AV 52mm	Forward Lateral, AV 46mm
Ilia	High, upright	Lower flaring
Superior inlet	Heart shaped	More elliptical
Skull		
Size	Relatively large	Relatively small
Frontonasal angle	Sharp, angular	Smooth curve
Supraorbital ridges	Prominent	Poorly developed
Forehead	Slopes backward	Nearly vertical
Surface cheek bone	Rough, concave	Smooth, flat
Mandible tip (chin)	Squarer	Pointed
Foramen magnum	Large, long	Smaller, rounder
Mastoid processes	Large	Small
Other Bones		
Sternum length (x-ray)	173mm+	121mm or less
Diameter femoral head	45mm+	43mm or less
Circumference radial head	69mm+	55mm or less

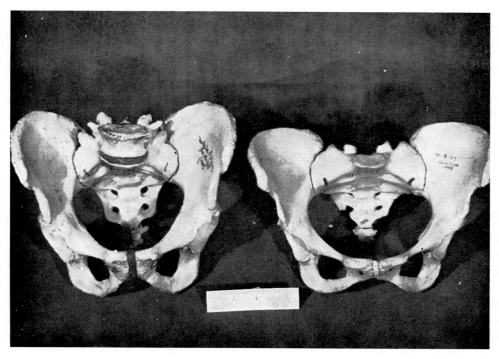

FIGURE IV-26. The wide pelvic inlet, subpubic angle and sciatic notch are characteristic features which distinguish the female pelvis (right) from the male pelvis (left).

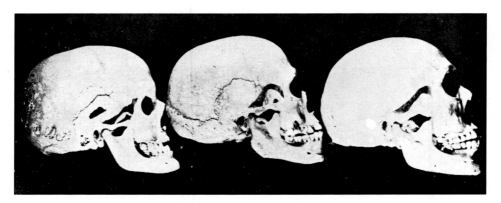

FIGURE IV-27. The racial differences of the skull, particularly the degree of prognathism are seen in these lateral views of Caucasian (left), Black (center), and Asian (right) skulls.

proximal epiphysis of the femur fuses before the distal epiphysis. Both fuse in the late teens or early twenties.

A less reliable method of age estimation, approximating decades, is based on closure of cranial sutures. Suture closure begins at the inner table of the skull progressing to the outer table. Therefore, the skull should be opened before assessing age. Studies of closure of cranial sutures are described by Krogman.[40]

Aging children and infants depends on the radiographic appearance of centers of ossification and the degree of closure of epiphyses correlated with dental characteristics. Krogman's and Fazekas' textbooks detail the aging of fetuses.[40]

Race

Although race determination may usually be determined by observation of the decedent's skin color and hair characteristics, this is becoming increasingly difficult as our society becomes more integrated. Race determination on skeletal remains is based on examination of the skull, pelvis and long bones. In most cases a forensic anthropologist is needed to develop an opinion as to the race of a skeleton because of the variability within races and the blending of many national and racial stocks in the United States. For example, Native Americans, Eskimos and Asians share several skeletal features. In general, the typical White skull shows a flat frontal profile, whereas Blacks show prognathism (Fig. IV-27). Orbital configuration in Blacks is squarish,

while Whites exhibit triangular and Asians show more rounded shapes. The White pelvis is broader and the symphysis lower than that of Blacks which tends to be more cylindrical. The long bones of the extremities in Blacks tend to be longer and straighter.

Estimates of Living Stature

When direct measurement is not possible, the standard regression formulae developed by Trotter and Gleser[40] using the length in centimeters of long bones will provide an estimate of height to plus or minus one inch. Of all the long bones, femur length correlates best with height (Table IV-5). If race is known, specific tables based on race and ethnicity have been compiled by Krogman.[40]

Eye and Hair Color

Eye color in the well-preserved body ranges from dark brown to maroon through green, blue and gray. The NCIC unidentified person file permits entry of fine distinction in eye color. After the corneas are clouded, eye color may be difficult to determine. If the postmortem interval is not too long, rewetting the corneas may clear them sufficiently to determine if the irides are dark or light. Hair is resistant to putrefaction and remains intact for years. A hair mat should be diligently sought in the vicinity of any skeleton. Hair examination can identify race as well as the effects of heat, bleaching, dying, cutting and the residues of gunpowder.

TABLE IV-5
ESTIMATION OF LIVING STATURE USING FEMUR LENGTH*

White Male:	2.32 (femur length in cm) + 65.53 = femur length in cm (+/- 3.94 cm)
Black Male:	2.10 (femur length in cm) + 72.22 = femur length in cm (+/- 3.91 cm)
White Female:	2.47 (femur length in cm) + 54.10 = femur length in cm (+/- 3.72 cm)
Black Female:	2.28 (femur length in cm) + 59.76 = femur length in cm (+/- 3.41 cm)

1 inch = 2.54 centimeters

Example:
Given a femur length (white male) of 50 cm.

$$= 2.32 \ (50 \ cm) + 65.53 = femur \ length \ (+/- \ 3.94 \ cm)$$
$$= 116 + 65.53 = 181.53 \ cm \ (+/- \ 3.93 \ cm)$$

Estimated Stature = 181.53 cm / 2.54 = 71.47 inches or ~ 5 feet 10 inches

Stature Range: 181.53 cm + 3.93 cm = 185.46 cm
181.53 cm − 3.93 cm = 177.60 cm
= 185.46 cm / 2.54 = 73.01 inches or ~ 6 feet 0 inches (maximum)
= 177.60 cm / 2.54 = 69.92 inches or ~ 5 feet 8 inches (minimum)

* From Bass, W.M. *Human Osteology: A Laboratory and Field Guide,* Third Edition, Missouri Archaeological Society, Columbia Missouri, 1987.

AUTOPSY EXAMINATION

Birthmarks, Congenital Defects, Tattoos and Scars

Any skin markings on an unidentified decedent's body should be measured, diagramed and photographed. Areas suggestive of old scars are candidates for histologic confirmation of increased collagen and perhaps old suture material in deeper layers. Tattoos may be anywhere and should be carefully documented. Tattoos are an expression of the personality of the decedent (Fig. IV-28), some sending clear messages about past experiences, lifestyle (jailhouse and hand-made tattoos), sexual and religious motifs (Figs. IV-29 and IV-30) and personal interests (Harley-Davidson motorcycle motifs). The decedent's name or initials, the name or initials of others, social security, military service and prisoner of war or concentration camp numbers (Fig. IV-31) are but a few of the tattoos that may lead to identification. Tattoos are recorded in police and FBI records and can thus be easily compared with those on a decedent. In the past, attempts to obliterate tattoos have resulted in unsightly, irregular scarring with some pigment usually still visible. Current laser technology allows for tattoo removal without significant scarring, however,

this procedure is quite expensive costing several hundred dollars to remove a small tattoo. If the body is darkly discolored or bloated, wiping away the darkened slipping epidermis often allows the tattoo to be seen more clearly (*see* Fig. XXV-24). Even in a non-decomposed body a tattoo can be enhanced by causing a second-degree burn, then wiping off the epidermis. High contrast photography, computer image enhancement and infrared photography may enhance some tattoo ink pigments, making faint, undecipherable tattoos more distinct. Recently applied tattoos may be recognized by their scaling (Fig. VI-32).

Scars come in all shapes and sizes. Some are associated with surgical procedures, some are the result of a traumatic injury and some are induced voluntarily. Certain scars are so unique that they can be used for identification purposes (Fig. IV-33). Hypertrophic scars (keloids) are more commonly seen in Blacks (Fig. IV-34a–b).

Internal Examination

Every unidentified decedent requires a complete autopsy and microscopic examination to document preexisting disease, such as hyperten-

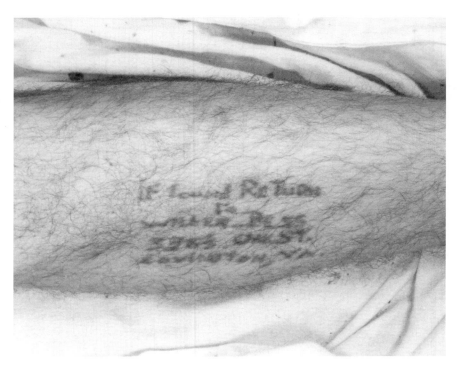

FIGURE IV-28. This individual was concerned that he may get lost.

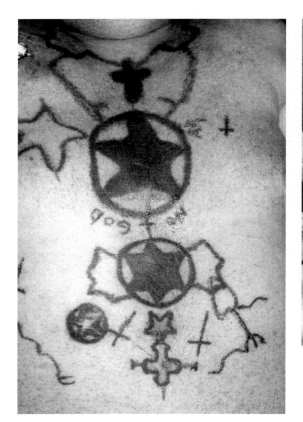

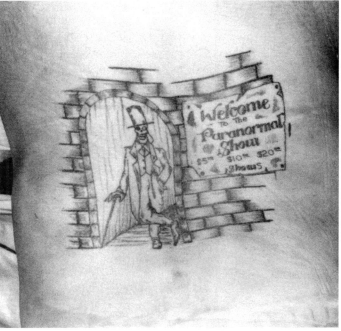

FIGURE IV-30. Tattoo suggestive of life style.

FIGURE IV-29. Multiple homemade Satanic tattoos (pentagram symbols, upside down crosses and "No God") give clues as to a decedent's personality.

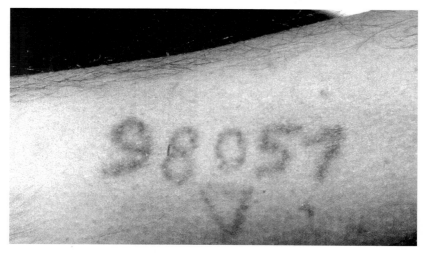

FIGURE IV-31. Tattoo from a concentration camp survivor.

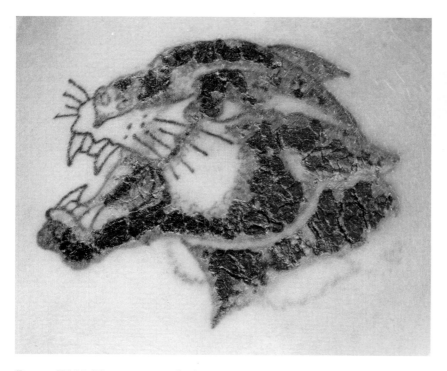

FIGURE IV-32. This is a tattoo which covers an old one. Extensive scaling is noted in the new dark areas.

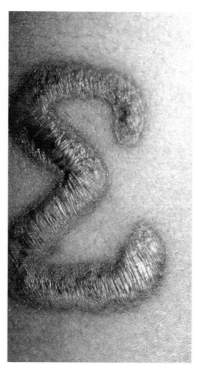

FIGURE IV-33. Scar formation from branding. This individual was in a college fraternity, branded with the Greek letter epsilon.

sion, diabetes, old strokes, Alzheimer's disease, surgical removal of organs, or perhaps drug therapy or abuse. Findings, such as old strokes or other neurologic diseases hint at mental disability.

Yellow fluorescence of the calvarium suggests tetracycline or major tranquilizer therapy, however, diabetes mellitus may also cause yellowish discoloration of the skull. Pathologic findings may be

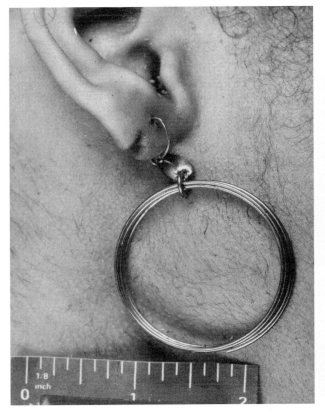

Figure IV-34a. Remote tear of an earlobe by an earring adjacent to earring in place.

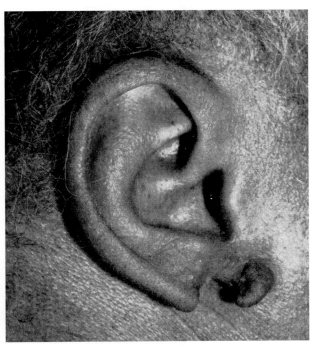

Figure IV-34b. Hypertrophic scar of ear lobe due to a tear caused by an earring.

comparable with medical records documenting blood group, medications and surgical procedures. Even burned or decomposed bodies may reveal valuable information for possible later comparisons. Desiccated tissues may be rehydrated using the method described by Zimmerman.[42] The technique of rehydration utilizes immersion of the tissue into Ruffer's solution of 50 parts water, 30 parts absolute alcohol, and 20 parts 5% sodium carbonate with adequate rehydration achieved in one to two days. Rehydrated specimens are then fixed in absolute alcohol for one to three days, embedded in paraffin, sectioned and stained according to standard techniques. Tissue should also be retained for toxicological analysis as well as for possible DNA testing.

Forensic Toxicology

Postmortem toxicological analyses can disclose information about the lifestyle and mental and physical health of an unidentified person. The presence of anticonvulsant medication in a decedent's body is evidence of a seizure disorder in life. Similarly, antidepressant use points to clinical depression and perhaps suicidal tendencies. The use of illicit drugs such as cocaine or heroin or designer drugs currently common in young adults may provide investigators with leads by indicating a decedent's habits and lifestyle. Bone, bone marrow, hair, bloodstains and maggots are unconventional, but suitable specimens for detecting drugs in decomposed or skeletonized remains.[43,44]

HAIR EXAMINATION

Human hair is useful for identification as well as for evaluation as physical evidence at crime scenes. Hair is durable and resists decomposition for long periods of time. It may be admixed with body fluids and stuck to the clothes of dead bodies or tangled in a mat at the scene of a decomposed or skeletonized body. Even incinerated bodies may have hair stubs or roots that may be recovered. On occasion, the finding of passively transferred pet hairs may complicate the identification process. The fewer hairs that are available, the more diligent should be the search to improve the probability that the recovered hair belongs to the decedent. Any foreign hairs recovered have a greater significance as physical evidence to link an assailant or a scene to a victim. Hair comparisons, when favorable, are usually described as consistent with a known sample or exemplar, unless an extremely unusual feature, genetic or acquired, is identified. The usual sources of exemplar hairs for comparison with an unidentified decedent's hair or for a source of mitochondrial DNA are hairbrushes and other grooming implements, bedding, clothing and plumbing fixture traps associated with the unknown or missing person.

A hair consists of the root or bulb, shaft and tip. The outer layer of the shaft consists of a cuticle composed of microscopic non-pigmented scale-like plates. The cortex forms most of the substance of hair and contains keratin and pigment granules. The pigment may be diffuse, granular or both and the degree of pigmentation varies from slight, when hair may appear colorless, to so dense that it obscures internal structures. Color is variable and is a summation of different tints. The cortex surrounds the medulla, a central or occasionally eccentric, hollow core (Fig. IV-35). The scale pattern of hair along with other features differentiates human from animal hair. The shape of a hair shaft may be round, oval or flattened and the density, shape and distribution of pigment granules characterize race.

When available, scalp hair is more useful than axillary, pubic or body hair for purposes of identification. On occasion, body hair, particularly axillary, pubic or perianal hair may provide additional clues to identification. Whereas, head hair provides phenotypic information as to race, body hair appears to provide more genotypic data which may be important when dealing with individuals of mixed racial families. In general, Caucasoid head hair tends to have an oval shape (cross section) with uniform distribution of fine or coarse pigment, depending on color. Hair of Black persons has the shape of a flattened ellipse, and has dense, but less regular pigment. Hair of Mongoloid persons, including American Indians, Eskimos and Asians is round and larger on cut section, and has dense, more uniformly distributed pigment (Fig. IV-36).

Although preliminary information can be obtained by gross and microscopic examination, hair analysis by a forensic scientist may reveal evidence of dying, bleaching and sex (if the hair root is well preserved). Determination of sex based on bleaching and permanent waving is risky given the high incidence of bleaching and waving by both men and women. Hair examination cannot be used to determine age. Comparison of unidentified hairs with exemplar hairs for consistency should be conducted by an experienced forensic scientist hair examiner. Neutron activation testing, which converts elements in hair into radioactive isotopes, permits comparison of the radiation emitted from an unknown hair with known standards. It provides a quantitative comparison of native and acquired cosmetic and environmental elements to further characterize the source of hairs. A recent study by Linch concluded that microscopic examination of head hair can be used to reliably opine that the hair originated from a decomposing body, however, the microscopic changes cannot be used to determine postmortem interval.[45] Many drugs can be detected by analysis of the hair shaft and allow for an approximate time-line of when the drugs were used.[44] Most laboratories will require at least 50 hairs for testing.

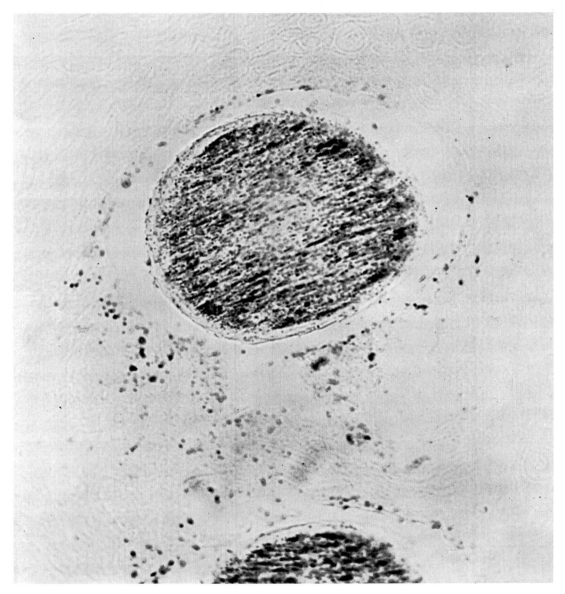

FIGURE IV-35. Microscopy of cross sections of hair not only shows the distribution of pigment in the cortex and thickness of the cuticle, but also the configuration of the hair shaft. This hair in cross section exhibits a relatively thick cuticle, dense pigmentation and a round shape, consistent with Asian origin.

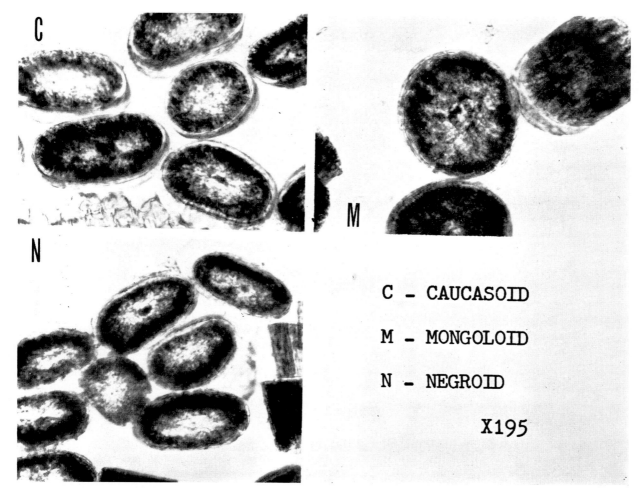

FIGURE IV-36. Comparison of cross sections of hair from Caucasoid (C), Mongoloid (M) and Negroid (N) persons.

DNA Analysis and Comparison

Deoxyribonucleic acid (DNA) has widespread application in forensic medicine and is now frequently used to aid in the identification of human remains. With the exception of monozygotic (identical) twins, each person's DNA is unique. The term *DNA fingerprint* is a description by analogy, comparing the uniqueness of the whorls and loops of an inked fingerprint to the uniqueness of an individual's DNA. For a detailed discussion of DNA analysis and application see *Part 2*.

REFERENCES

1. Kahana, T., Goldin, L., and Hiss, J. Personal identification based on radiographic vertebral features. *The American Journal of Forensic Medicine and Pathology, 23* (1): 36–41, 2002.
2. Taylor, R.E., Suchey, J.M., Payen, L.A., and Slota, Jr. P.J. The use of radiocarbon ^{14}C to identify human skeletal remains of forensic science interest. *Journal of Forensic Sciences, 34:* 1196–1205, 1989.
3. Byard, R.W., Ross, R.A., and Zuccollo, J. Potential confusion arising from materials presenting as possible human remains. *The American Journal of Forensic Medicine and Pathology, 22* (4): 391–394, 2001.

4. Fitzpatrick, J.J., and Macaluso, J. Shadow positioning technique: A method for postmortem identification. *Journal of Forensic Sciences, 36:* 480–500, 1991.

5. Nickerson, B., Fitzhorn, P., Koch, S.K., and Charney, M.A. Methodology for near-optimal computational superimposition of two-dimensional digital facial photographs and three dimensional cranial surface meshes. *Journal of Forensic Sciences, 36:* 480–500, 1991.

6. Fierro, M.F., and Loring G. *Handbook for Postmortem Examination of Unidentified Remains.* Appendix D. Tables of Proportionate Measurements, pp. 243–258. Skokie, Illinois, College of American Pathologists, 1986.

7. RN and WPL Encyclopedia. *The Salesman's Guide.* New York: National Register Publishing Co./Division of Macmillan, 1991.

8. Stahl III, C.J. Identification of human remains. In Spitz and Fisher (eds). *Medicolegal Investigation of Death,* 2nd ed. Springfield, IL: Charles C Thomas, 1980.

9. Thorwald, J. *The century of the detective.* New York: Harcourt Brace and World Inc., 1965, pp. 20–26.

10. Polson, C.J. Fingerprints and fingerprinting: A historical study. *American Journal of Police Science, 41:* 495–517, 1950.

11. Printak Inc., 1250 North Tustin Avenue, Anaheim, CA 92807.

12. *Automated Fingerprint Identification System (AFIS) Users Training Manual.* Boxborough, MA: NEC Information Systems, 1987.

13. Illinois Criminal Justice Information Authority, Automated Fingerprint Identification System (AFIS) Reference Guide. Illinois Criminal Justice Information Authority, 120 South Riverside Plaza, Suite 1016, Chicago, Illinois 60606-3997 (312-793-8550).

14. Ashbaugh, D.R. Ridgeology. *Identification News,* pp. 6–12, December 1985.

15. Iannarelli, A.V. *Ear identification.* Fremont, CA, Paramont Publishing Co., 1989.

16. Vale, G.L., and Noguchi T.T. The role of the forensic dentist in mass disasters. *Dental Clinics of North America, 21* (1): 123–135, 1977.

17. Titunik, I.R. Forensic dental identification of human remains. American Society of Clinical Pathologists, Check Sample. *Forensic Pathology, 41* (3): 29–48, 1999.

18. Netter, F. *Atlas of human anatomy.* Ciba-Geigy, 1989.

19. Lortaon, L., Rethman, M., and Friedman, R. The computer-assisted postmortem identification (CAPMI) system: A computer-based identification program. *Journal of Forensic Sciences, 33:* 977–984, 1988.

20. Atkins, L., and Potsaid, M.S. Roentgenographic identification of human remains. *JAMA, 240:* 2307–2308, 1978.

21. Fischman, S.L. The use of medical and dental radiographs in identification. *International Dental Journal, 35:* 301–306, 1985.

22. Kuehn, C.M., Taylor, K.M., Mann, F.A., Wilson, A.J., and Harruff, R.C.: Validation of chest x-ray comparisons for unknown decedent identification. *J. Forensic Sci., 39* (2):373–377, 1994.

23. Hogge, J.P., Messmer, J.M., and Doan, Q.N. Radiographic identification of unknown human remains and interpreter experience level. *Journal of Forensic Sciences, 39* (2):373–377, 1994.

24. Brogdon, B.G. Radiological identification of individual remains. In Brogdon, B.G., *Forensic Radiology.* Boca Raton, FL: CRC Press, 1998, 149–188.

25. Sauer, N., Brantley, R.E., and Barondess, D.A. The effect of aging and the comparability of antemortem and postmortem radiographs. *Journal of Forensic Sciences, 33:* 1223–1230, 1988.

26. Kahana, T., Ravioli, J.A., Urroz, C.L., and Hiss, J. Radiographic identification of fragmentary human remains from mass disaster. *The American Journal of Forensic Medicine and Pathology, 18:* 40–44, 1997.

27. Ribeiro, F de A. Standardized measurements of radiographic films of the frontal sinuses: An aid to identifying unknown persons. *Ear Nose and Throat Journal, 26:* 32–33, 2000.

28. Nambiar, P. Naidu, M.D.K., and Subramaniam, K. Anatomical variability of the frontal sinuses and their application in forensic identification. *Clinical Anatomy, 12:* 16–19, 1999.

29. Marlin, J.M., Clark, M.A., and Standish, S.M. Identification of human remains by comparison of frontal sinus radiographs: A series of four cases. *Journal of Forensic Sciences, 36:* 1765–1772, 1991.

30. Harris, A.M.P., Wood, R.E., Nortje, C.L., and Thomas, C.J. The frontal sinus: Forensic fingerprint? A pilot study. *Journal of Forensic Odontostomatol, 5* (1): 9–15, 1987.

31. Yoshina, M. Miyasaka, S., Sato, H., and Seta, S. Classification system of frontal sinus patterns by radiography: Its application to identification of unknown skeletal remains. *Forensic Science International, 34:* 289–299, 1987.

32. Messmer, J., and Fierro, M. Personal identification by radiographic comparison of vascular groove patterns of the calvarium. *American Journal of Forensic Medicine and Pathology, 7:* 159–162, 1986.

33. Rhine, S., and Sperry, K. Radiographic identification by mastoid sinus and arterial pattern. *Journal of Forensic Sciences, 36:* 272–279, 1991.

34. Greulich, W.W., and Pyle, S.I. *Radiographic atlas of the skeletal development of the hand and wrist,* 2nd ed. Stanford University Press, California, 1959.

35. Stephens, B.G. A simple method for preparing human skeletal material for forensic examination. *Journal of Forensic Sciences, 24:* 660–662, 1979.

36. Suchey, J.M. Race differences in pubic symphyseal aging patterns in the male. *Am J Phys Anthropol, 80:* 167–172, 1989.

37. Berrizbeitia, E. Sex determination with the head of the radius. *Journal of Forensic Sciences, 34:* 1206–1213, 1989.

38. McCormick, W.F., and Stewart, J.H. Age-related changes in the human plastron: A roentgenographic

and morphologic study. *Journal of Forensic Sciences, 33:* 100–120, 1988.

39. Hutchinson, D.L., and Russell, K.F. Pelvic age determination using actual specimens and remote images. *Journal of Forensic Sciences, 45* (5): 1224–1227, 2001.

40. Ubelaker, D. Dental Analysis. In Krogman, S.M., and Iscan, M.Y. *The human skeleton in forensic medicine,* 2nd ed. Springfield, IL: Charles C Thomas, 1986.

41. Bass, W.M. *Human osteology: A laboratory and field guide,* 3rd ed., Columbia: Missouri Archaeological Society, 1987, pp. 221–222.

42. Zimmerman, M.R. Paleopathology in Alaskan mummies. *American Scientist, 73:* 20–25, 1985.

43. Beyer, J.C., Enos, W.F., and Stajic, M. Drug identification through analysis of maggots. *Journal of Forensic Sciences, 25:* 411–412, 1980.

44. Suzuki, O., Hattori, H., and Asano, M. Detection of methamphetamine and amphetamine in a single human hair by gas chromatography/chemical ionization mass spectrometry. *Journal of Forensic Sciences, 29:* 611–617, 1984.

45. Linch, C.A., and Prahlow, J.A. Postmortem microscopic changes observed at the human head hair promixal end. *Journal of Forensic Sciences, 46* (1):15–20, 2001.

DNA

Lynne M. Helton

Numerous advances have been made in the last 15 years in terms of the technologies used for DNA analysis. The first use of DNA testing for forensic purposes came in 1985 after work by Dr. Alec Jeffreys, who discovered the first multilocus DNA probes.[1] His method examined more than one location of the DNA genome at one time. The term *genome* is used to describe the full complement of a person's DNA. The result of Jeffreys' work was a complicated multibanded pattern for each individual tested. The first forensic case to use this exciting technique was *Regina v. Pitchfork* in England. This sexual assault case, brought to conclusion by the voluntary testing of more than 5000 males, was made famous worldwide in the novel, *THE BLOODING* by author Joseph Wambaugh.[2] The semen donor was eventually identified using Jeffreys' method. Since that time, continuous advances have been made in DNA testing for forensic purposes.

DNA Structure

DNA molecules are found in the nucleus of cells, also referred to as nuclear DNA. If we could visualize DNA it would resemble a spiral staircase, and is considered a *double helix* structure. The basic unit of the DNA molecule is the nucleotide. A nucleotide is made up of three components: a sugar, a chemical base containing nitrogen, and phosphoric acid. In DNA, the sugar is 2'-deoxyribose; a pentose containing five carbon atoms.[3] The chemical bases are single or double ring structures that are attached to one carbon of the sugar molecule. A phosphoric acid group is attached to another carbon of the sugar which completes the nucleotide. Nucleotides are joined together end-to-end to form a linear DNA strand.

The chemical bases provide the variation in each nucleotide unit, while the sugar and phosphate portions form the backbone of the DNA molecule and do not change. Any one of four chemical bases can present in a DNA molecule. They are adenine (A) and guanine (G), which are double ring structures called purines. The other bases are thymine (T) and cytosine (C), which are single ring structures called pyrimidines.

The DNA molecule is a double stranded structure, with two strands of DNA linked together by bonds between two chemical bases, much like the rungs holding together the two sides of a ladder. When the two stands are linked together, the bases attached to each other are known as a base pair. Chemical bases must be complimentary to each other in order to form a base pair (Fig. IV-37). Adenine can only pair with thymine, and guanine can only pair with cytosine. Genetic information is stored in the varying combinations of A, T, G, and C along the length of a DNA molecule, much like computers store code by the varying combination of zeros and ones. In its entirety, the DNA molecule consists of approximately three billion base pairs.

Greater than 99% of DNA is the same between individuals. Human DNA is comprised of 50,000 to 100,000 genes that code for important proteins. Less than one percent of DNA varies between individuals. For forensic purposes, scientists use only areas that demonstrate great variability between individuals. These regions are non-coding regions, regions between genes or sometimes within a gene, and are scattered throughout the DNA molecule.

The variation (or polymorphism) between individuals can be seen as either length polymorphisms or as sequence polymorphisms. Length polymorphisms are fragments or sections of DNA that differ from each other by being longer or shorter depending on the number of base pairs. Sequence of polymorphisms are fragments of DNA that differ in the arrangement of bases along the length of the fragment.

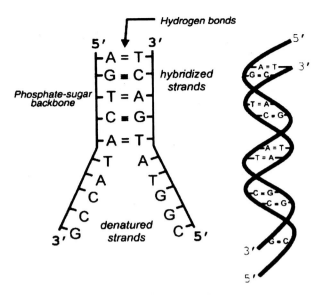

FIGURE IV-37. Base pairing of DNA strands to form a double-helix structure.

Early DNA Methods

By the late 1980s, the complex multibanded pattern obtained by the Jeffreys' method gave way to the examination of one genetic location *(locus)* at a time. This method, using probes to detect a variable number of tandem repeat (VNTR) markers, is known as *Restriction Fragment Length Polymorphism (RFLP)* testing. Large DNA fragments between 500 base pairs and 10,000 or more base pairs could be isolated and identified. The RFLP fragments represented *length polymorphisms* that occur in all individuals, with a tandemly repeated *core base repeat unit.* The base pair unit that was repeated again and again could be up to 80 base pairs long, resulting in DNA fragments of 500 to 10,000+ base pairs in length.[4]

An individual is either homozygous or heterozygous at each genetic location, that is, possessing either one or two DNA fragments or *alleles.* Recall that half our DNA is inherited from our mother and half from our father. An *allele* is defined as any one of the possibilities for a genetic location. A *homozygote* individual would have one DNA fragment at a genetic location. Using a computer-based measuring system, this RFLP DNA fragment could be *measured* as a certain

number of base pairs in length, i.e., 6350 base pairs. A *heterozygote* individual would have two DNA fragments at a genetic location, each with a differing number of tandem repeats. For example, one DNA fragment might be measured as 2,000 base pairs in length, and the other at 4,700 base pairs long. Although the RFLP typing system is not currently widely used, the concept of tandemly repeated core base pair units creating DNA fragments of *differing lengths* is the basis for the state-of-the-art DNA technology used today. This new technology is called STR (short tandem repeat) DNA analysis, and will be discussed later.

RFLP testing is considered a *continuous* allelic system because there is no set number of tandem repeats possible at any given genetic location. Typically, six genetic locations were used for RFLP testing purposes, providing excellent discrimination between individuals. However, the limitations of RFLP technology quickly became evident. RFLP testing required relatively large sample sizes of 200 to 400 nanograms (ng) of DNA for successful typing results at all genetic locations. That would require a semen stain about half the size of a dime, or a bloodstain about the size of a nickel. Samples like vaginal swabs with a trace amount of semen, or cigarette butts, another common example of small quantities of DNA, did not yield sufficient DNA for successful results with RFLP testing. Degraded DNA was also unsuitable for RFLP testing. Degradation of DNA samples over time, or due to environmental conditions, would often result in the DNA fragments of interest being randomly broken within the tandemly repeated sequence. Additionally, the technique was time-consuming and resulted in analysis times of weeks to months per case. On a practical note, the time requirements necessary for RFLP testing meant that it was not routinely possible to get DNA information quickly to the law enforcement community, either for investigative information, or for purposes of preliminary court proceedings prior to the actual criminal trial.

Forensic scientists looked to another form of DNA testing using the PCR (polymerase chain reaction) process to overcome the limitations seen with RFLP testing. The PCR process mimics the process carried out in the human body every day in order to sustain life, namely, the process where we create identical copies of our DNA molecule for each new cell that is created. This process is often thought of as molecular copying or *xeroxing.*

The PCR process is carried out in an instrument called a *thermal cycler* and allows for the exact copying of portions of a DNA molecule under very strict laboratory conditions. This process is also referred to as amplification, and allows for a specific region of DNA to be copied over and over again. The result is millions to billions of copies of a particular DNA sequence. The PCR process uses short pieces of DNA called *primers* that are created in the laboratory, most commonly a commercial laboratory, in order to target a specific region of DNA to be copied.

The first part of the PCR process requires that the double stranded DNA be separated into single strands, or *denatured.* Denaturation occurs when the hydrogen bonds keeping two DNA strands together are broken, like a zipper being unzipped. The DNA primer then attaches *(anneals)* to a region of the DNA just before the section of DNA to be copied. The last part of the PCR process involves the *extension* of the primer with the help of an enzyme called DNA polymerase (Fig. IV-38). DNA polymerase uses individual bases (A's, T's G's and C's) that are also ingredients in PCR process, and adds the complementary bases one at a time, in the correct order complementary to the original DNA sequence. A simple analogy is a child who is taking alphabet blocks from a pile, and placing them one at a time in a straight line. One complete cycle of the PCR process includes denaturation, annealing, and primer extension. Multiple cycles are performed (usually 25–30 cycles) to complete the PCR process. Without the ability to make copies of DNA samples, many forensic samples would be impossible to analyze.

Early PCR DNA Testing

One of the first most widely used PCR methods for forensic DNA typing was a *reverse dot blot* procedure. This method examined *sequence polymorphisms,* differences in actual DNA sequences, in persons using sequence-specific probes. This system is considered a *discrete* allele system because only a defined number of DNA types are possible at a given genetic location. Probes, synthetic pieces of DNA complementary to a specific DNA sequence, are permanently bound to *dots* on a paper-like typing strip.[5] More than one dot, small circular test area, was present on each typing strip. The probe would target, be complementary to, a specific amplified DNA region, causing the DNA to bind with the probe on the paper typing strip. A color reaction was used to visualize the bound probe/DNA sample, resulting in the formation of a blue color within the dot. This DNA typing system was the first commercial DNA kit available to forensic scientists. It combined the ability to obtain DNA types from small sample sizes with an increased speed of analysis.

The first reverse dot blot typing kit examined the HLA DQα (DQ alpha) genetic location. Then, an improved typing system was created for the DQα genetic location, which allowed better identification of all the possible genetic types. This improved typing kit was only available when purchased with a second new kit, AmpliType® PM, commonly known as Polymarker. The Polymarker kit allowed DNA types at five additional genetic locations to be examined at the same time using the same technique with the paper typing strip. These markers were not as discriminating as the DQα markers, with only two to three possible DNA types at each of the five locations. It was an attempt to increase the power of discrimination of this DNA typing method with all the advantages of PCR. However, the reverse dot blot systems had their disadvantages. They included difficulty in interpretation, especially with mixed DNA samples, and a much lower power of discrimination than with RFLP testing.

The AmpliType®PM (Polymarker) kit was important to forensic scientists because it was the first time that simultaneous amplification of more than one genetic location was performed. Today's advanced DNA testing capability combines the breakthrough of simultaneous amplifi-

Polymerase Chain Reaction

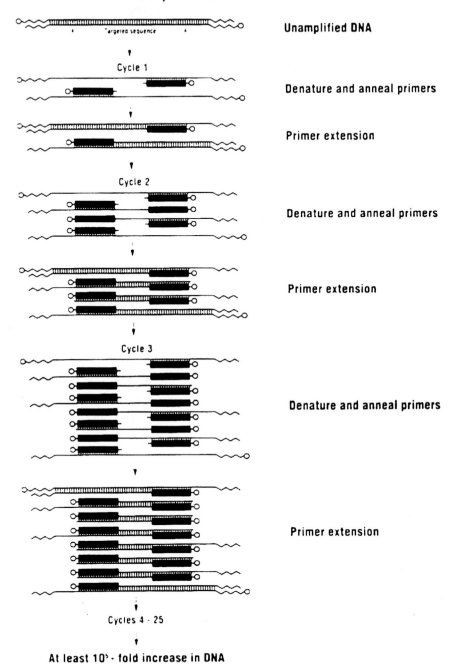

FIGURE IV-38. The polymerase chain reaction (PCR) is used to make exact copies of a DNA region of interest. The original DNA strand, called the template, is separated using high heat, and the effect is like unzipping a zipper. Very small pieces of DNA called primers attach near the site to be copied. The primer is extended, turned into a complete complementary DNA strand, with the help of a chemical. The chemical helper finds bases and plugs them in one at a time, like putting building blocks in a row, until the DNA strand is complete. The process is repeated over and over again until millions of copies of the DNA fragment are made.

cation with the discriminating power of short tandem repeat analysis using fluorescent primer technology. The concept of simultaneous amplification has now become known as *multiplexing*.

CURRENT FORENSIC DNA TECHNOLOGY

STR DNA Analysis

The state-of-the-art DNA typing method used today is known as STR DNA analysis. This technology is based on tandemly repeated DNA sequences with a *core base pair repeat unit* that is typically four base pairs in length. These repeats result in *short tandem repeat* (STR) DNA fragments (Fig. IV-39). The resulting small STR fragments range in size from approximately 100 base pairs to 400 base pairs in length, in comparison to the tandem repeat fragments up to 10,000 or more base pairs seen with RFLP analysis. The small sizes of the STR fragments (less than 400 bp) make STR markers an excellent choice for forensic applications where degraded DNA is common.[6] Better amplification of degraded DNA samples can be accomplished because only small pieces of DNA are required.

Beginning in 1996, the FBI coordinated an effort to establish a standardized core group of STR genetic locations for use with the national DNA database *CODIS* (**Co**mbined **D**NA **I**ndex **S**ystem). Standardizing the genetic locations used by forensic scientists means that data generated at every crime lab are compatible and can be compared. Specific features of the DNA database (CODIS) will be discussed later. At the conclusion of the FBI study, a core group of 13 genetic locations was chosen. The final choices were based on factors including the robustness of the location, the ability of certain locations to be accurately detected when amplified or copied at the same time, and the ability of the locations to provide good discrimination power between individuals.

STR locations can be amplified (copied) using the PCR process, and then analyzed by electrophoresis to separate the DNA fragments according to size. Electrophoresis is the migration of molecules when in an electric field. Amplification of several genetic locations at the same time occurs when several different primers are labeled with different fluorescent dyes. Each fluorescent primer specifically recognizes a desired STR site. Most commonly, capillary electrophoresis is carried out with an Applied Biosystems ABI Prism® 310 Genetic Analyzer for fragment separation. The 310 analyzer separates DNA fragments as they travel through a special polymer solution in a capillary column. This is compared to traditional techniques where DNA fragments migrate through a gelatin-type material. The 310 genetic analyzer simultaneously detects multiple fluorescent dyes after they are excited by a laser, and pass in front of a detection window in the capillary column. Detection of DNA types at multiple locations, even when the DNA fragments have similar lengths, i.e., similar numbers of tandem repeats, is possible when they are labeled with different dyes. This is known as multicolor analysis. STRs are considered a *discrete* allele system because there are only a defined number of DNA types possible at each genetic location.

The size, or length, of the STR fragments is determined by the number of repeat units. For

Short Tandem Repeats (STRs)

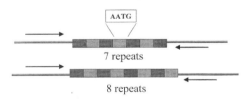

the repeat region is variable between samples while the flanking regions where PCR primers bind are constant

Homozygote = both alleles are the same length

Heterozygote = alleles differ and can be resolved from one another

FIGURE IV-39. The number of tandem repeat units in the repeat regions varies among individuals, making them useful markers for human identification.

example, one of the 13 CODIS genetic locations is D5S818. This location has simple repeats of the sequence AGAT.[7] There are 10 common DNA types, which are designated as 7, 8, 9, 10, 11, 12, 13, 14, 15, and 16. The genetic type 7 is considered to have 7 repeats of its *core* four base pair repeat (AGAT), and is a shorter DNA fragment than the type 15, which has 15 repeats of AGAT. The D5S818 genetic location has fragments ranging in size from 135bp to 171bp. Another STR marker, the D8S1179 location, has similar size DNA fragments (128bp to 168bp). Simultaneous analysis of these two locations can occur because amplification of the D5S818 locus is carried out with a primer labeled with one color fluorescent dye, while the D8S1179 primer is labeled with a different fluorescent dye. In this way multiple genetic loci can be co-amplified and individually detected. A combination of three different fluorescent dyes is typically used to accomplish this.

In forensic laboratories, STR analysis is carried out using commercially purchased DNA typing kits for the 13 core CODIS locations. DNA typing kits are available from two primary manufacturers. Currently, DNA typing for the 13 core loci is accomplished by using two typing kits in combination. Using two kits together, part of the 13 locations are amplified using the first kit, and the remainder of the locations are amplified using the second kit. One typing system utilizes PE Applied Biosystems AmpFlSTR® Profiler Plus™ and COfiler™ kits. The other typing system uses Promega Corporation GenePrint® STR Powerplex™ 1.1 and PowerPlex™ 2.1 kits.

The DNA fragments detected at each genetic location are represented on a chart called an electropherogram (Fig. IV-40). Using the PE Profiler Plus™ kit, three genetic locations are detected with a blue fluorescent dye, four locations are detected using a green fluorescent dye, and three locations are detected using a yellow fluorescent dye. One of the genetic locations detected with the green dye is Amelogenin, and allows for gender (sex) typing of the DNA sample. At this genetic location it is possible to detect the presence of the X and/or the Y chromosome. Females have only the X chromosome, while males have both the X and Y chromosomes.

Determining the sex of the DNA donor can provide probative information about the biological stain, especially in the case of bloodstain evidence.

Sources of DNA

Of specific interest to investigators are the kinds of crime samples from which DNA can be obtained. Blood, semen and vaginal secretions have been traditionally thought of as sources of DNA. With the advances in forensic DNA technology, it is possible to obtain DNA types from items not previously considered as *biological evidence*. This has meant that forensic DNA scientists and investigators alike must now *think outside the box* when considering what may be a source of DNA at a crime scene.

For instance, used condoms have routinely been recovered for semen evidence, so the semen donor can be associated with the condom. Now, it is possible to treat the inside and the outside of the condom as separate samples. The outside of the condom can be swabbed separately to recover female vaginal epithelial cells. Now both the victim and the suspect can be associated with the condom, which can be critical if the condom is in a location remote to the victim, i.e., the suspect's house.

Other exciting sources of DNA include crime samples containing skin cell DNA, which include skin cells from casual transfer situations. Studies have demonstrated that by holding an object for a matter of seconds, enough skin cell DNA may be deposited on an item to obtain a DNA result. Importantly, this could include weapon handles, which have most commonly been protected for fingerprints. Other potential sources of skin cell DNA include eyeglasses, watch bands, ligatures, fingernail clippings, and some clothing items, such as the inside surfaces of baseball hats or work gloves.

Items such as cigarette butts, drinking glasses, eating utensils, toothbrushes, pop cans, chewing gum and ski masks can provide a source of DNA from mouth (buccal) cells.

STR DNA types can only be obtained from hair in the event there is sufficient root material

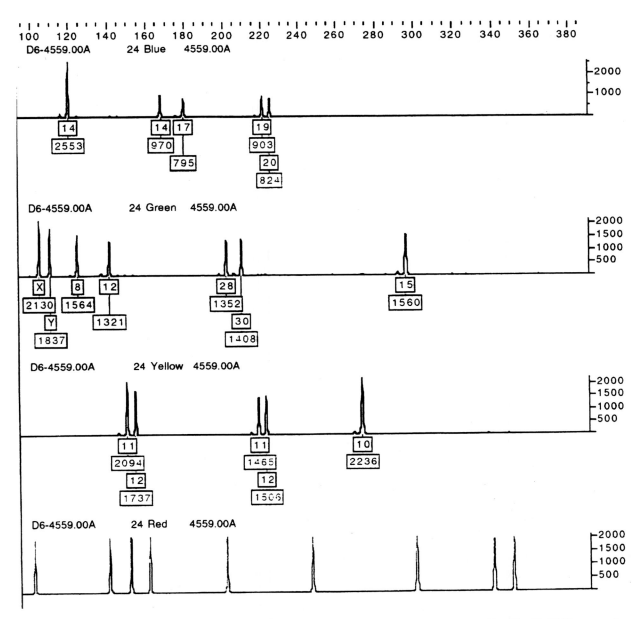

FIGURE IV-40. Electropherogram with DNA data generated by PE Applied Biosystems Profiler Plus™ DNA typing kit. Each peak represents a DNA genetic type at a given genetic location. Nine total genetic locations plus the gender location Amelogenin are represented. The detection of both the X and Y chromosomes, as indicated in the boxes directly underneath the first two peaks in the green region, indicates the DNA is from a male donor. DNA primers labeled with blue, green and yellow fluorescent dyes were used to amplify the fragments. The genetic types appear in the boxes directly underneath each peak. The first peak in the blue region is labeled 14, hence that DNA fragment has 14 repeats. In the next blue region, the DNA donor has two genetic types, labeled 14 and 17, fragments with 14 and 17 repeats. At each genetic location, the DNA types detected are indicated in the boxes below the peaks. All of the genetic types combined represent the complete DNA profile for the male DNA donor.

that is relatively fresh. This is commonly seen in forcibly pulled hair samples. Hair samples that do not contain root material (hence, no nucleat-

ed cells with DNA) may be candidates for mitochondrial DNA testing. Mitochondrial DNA testing will be discussed later in this section.

Finally, human tissue and bone specimens are also excellent sources of DNA. Commonly, abortus tissue is analyzed for criminal paternity testing purposes. It is important that the abortus or other tissue samples are not placed in a chemical fixative, such as formalin. The fixative will denature and destroy the DNA.

Tissue samples should be collected in clean sterile specimen containers, and frozen until submission to the DNA lab for testing. Bone and tissue samples are commonly collected for DNA analysis to aid in the identification of human remains. Deep muscle remains the best type of tissue sample for DNA testing. The best bone samples are typically flat bones, ribs, or a long bone like the femur. When the decomposition process has sufficiently degraded the DNA in blood, tissue and/or bone, mitochondrial testing may yield DNA results.

Interpretation of DNA Results

When two DNA specimens give the same DNA types at every genetic location, the DNA profiles are said to *match*. A complete DNA profile is defined as the total complement of DNA types detected at all the genetic locations tested. A partial DNA profile is defined as DNA types detected at some, but not all, of the genetic locations tested. Partial profiles are most commonly seen in very degraded DNA samples or in casual contact samples where insufficient skin cells are present to obtain DNA types at every genetic location.

When providing testimony as to a DNA match, the role of DNA scientist is to also provide some statistical estimate of the strength of the match. This estimate aids the jury in determining how much weight to assign to the DNA match. The more DNA comparison points (genetic locations) used, the tighter the match. Currently, a statement of identity is not made regarding a matching DNA profile. In other words, a DNA scientist will not say that "John Doe" *is the source of the DNA* on the item of evidence. Instead, the DNA scientist will provide an estimate of how frequently a DNA profile is expected to be seen in a given population. The estimate refers specifically to the DNA profile detected on the *evidence sample*.

Much in the same way that it is known how frequently the human blood groups (A, B, AB, and O) occur in different populations, it is also known how frequently DNA types occur in differing populations. For example, Type A blood occurs in approximately 42% of the Caucasian population, but is only seen in approximately 26% of the African American population. Therefore, Type A blood is seen in both populations but in differing frequencies of occurrence.

With regard to DNA, extensive population studies have been conducted to determine the frequency of occurrence of DNA types at each of the genetic locations used for DNA testing. The frequence of each DNA type is mathematically determined by counting the number of times that a given DNA type is seen, divided by the number of individuals examined. This is known as the *allele frequency*.[8]

Frequencies of DNA types have been determined for numerous different population groups around the world. Once the frequency of the DNA type is known, mathematical equations exist for determining the frequency of seeing two DNA types in that *exact combination* at a given location. This is known as the *genotype frequency*. For example, if DNA types 12,14 are identified at genetic location D5S1358 (recall 12 repeats and 14 repeats), then the frequency for the 12 and the frequency for the 14 are used to determine the frequency of *seeing them together* at that location.

Last, the final frequency for the *complete DNA profile* is determined by multiplying together all of the genotype frequencies for each genetic location. This is known as the combined frequency.[9] Using all 13 core CODIS locations, the frequency for a DNA estimate typically provides numbers in the quadrillions and quintillions. That means that when the frequency of occurrence of a DNA *evidence profile* in a population is one in 20 quadrillion, the expectation of seeing that profile in the population is exceedingly rare. When testimony is given that a DNA profile matches a given person, the jury can then decide how much weight to assign to the match.

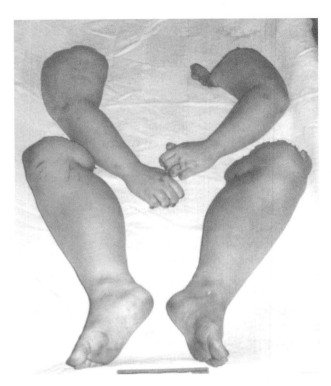

FIGURE IV-41a. Limbs recovered from a trash dumpster.

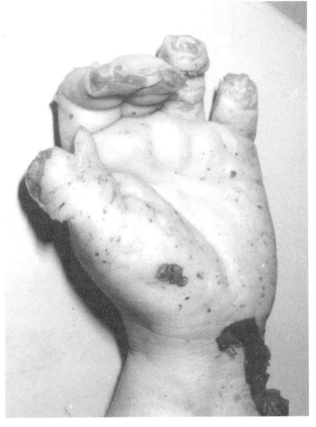

FIGURE IV-41b. Close up view of obliterated fingertips. The fingertips from both hands were removed.

A Forensic Case Study

A 35-year-old white female had been living in England with her sister after becoming estranged from her husband. She returned to the United States to be with her two teenage children and to finalize her divorce. Approximately 3 days after her return, and after an argument with her husband, she went to bed about midnight and was never seen again. Six days later, her sister called the local police department in the United States when she was not on her scheduled return flight to England. The missing person report quickly turned into a murder investigation.

Two days after she disappeared, a set of arms and legs were found in a plastic trash bag (Fig. IV-41 a). The limbs were recovered from a trash dumpster behind a restaurant in a neighboring community. The fingertips from both hands had been removed and/or obliterated (Fig. IV-41 b). Nine days after the limbs were recovered, a torso without a head was found, in a black plastic trash bag, in a field about 70 miles away, across the state line (Fig. IV-42). The limbs were provided to the medical examiner at the time of the autopsy of the torso. The medical examiner was able to physically match the limbs to the torso.

Seven days after the discovery of the torso, a consent search was performed of the missing woman's family home. A portion of the basement floor appeared freshly painted with a different color than the rest of the basement. Paint cans, and a paint pan containing a paint roller, were found

in the basement. The paint and roller were still tacky. Luminol spray was used by crime lab personnel to examine the basement floor. Chemical fluorescence was detected on more than one area of the floor, indicating the presence of blood. Areas of the freshly painted surface were chipped away to reveal fresh bloodstains in the concrete floor (Fig. IV-43). The bloodstains were collected for DNA comparison with the limbs and torso.

In addition to the bloodstains from the basement floor, the victim's toothbrush was recovered from the family home. The toothbrush was collected as an alternate known source of DNA from the victim. Additionally, known blood samples were collected from the husband and children of the victim for the purpose of conducting reverse paternity testing of the torso and limbs. STR DNA analysis was conducted on tissue samples from the limbs and torso, as well as biological material from the toothbrush. STR DNA testing was also performed on the bloodstains from the basement floor, and the known blood samples from the victim's family. The DNA profiles from the limbs, torso and basement floor matched the DNA profile from the victim's toothbrush (Fig. IV-44). Also, using the known DNA profiles from the husband and children, maternal types

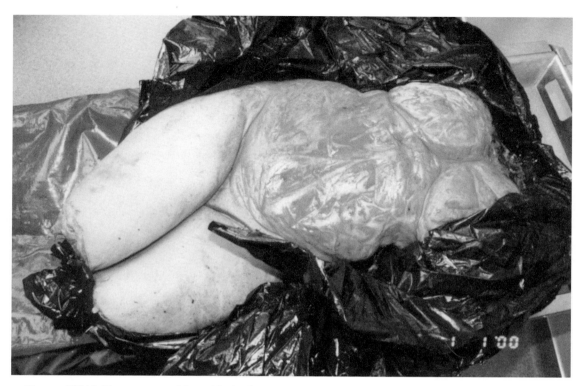

FIGURE IV-42. Torso removed from black plastic trash bag. Discoloration on upper torso is dried blood.

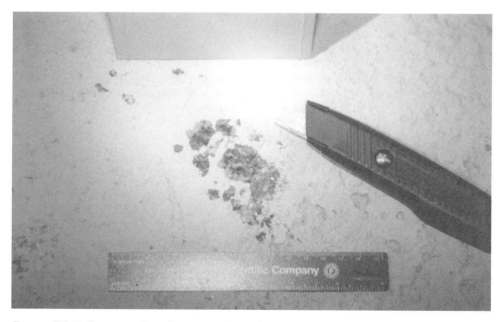

FIGURE IV-43. Basement floor from victim's residence. Light grey paint chipped away to reveal fresh bloodstains in pitting on concrete floor.

observed in the DNA from the children matched types in the DNA profiles from the limbs and torso.

The investigation generated additional compelling circumstantial evidence, including the fact that the husband

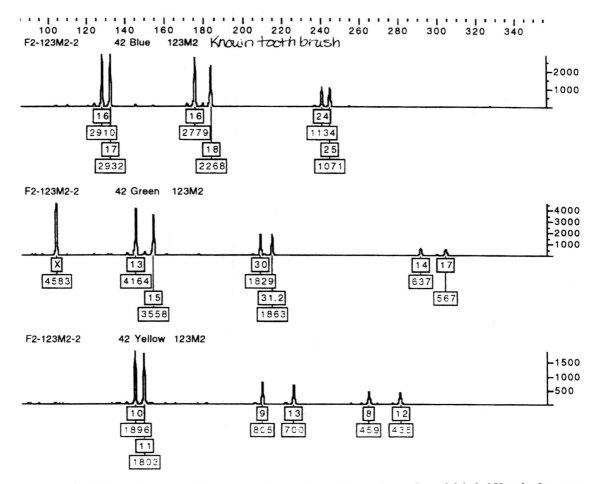

FIGURE IV-44. DNA profile detected from the victim's toothbrush. Note the single peak labeled X in the first green region (Amelogenin-gender typing). The presence of only the X chromosome is consistent with a female DNA donor.

had rented a van after his wife's disappearance. An eyewitness described a man matching the husband's description driving a similar van in the area the torso was discovered. Trace evidence examiners matched paint chips found in the plastic trash bags to paint from the basement floor. The husband was convicted of premeditated first-degree murder and sentenced to life in prison without parole.

Combined DNA Index System (CODIS)

The national DNA database (CODIS) exists as a way to match forensic evidence to convicted offenders, and potentially match evidence samples to each other, thereby establishing related cases. The database requires that testing be performed on the 13 core STR genetic locations agreed upon as the result of the extensive study coordinated by the FBI.

All 50 states within the United States have legislation allowing for the collection of DNA samples from persons *convicted* of certain classes of crimes. Samples cannot be collected from persons who are merely suspects in crimes. Most states are now going to legislation that calls for DNA samples to be collected from all convicted felons, including violent and non-violent felonies.

Crime statistics show that significant numbers of people convicted of burglary go on to commit more serious crimes, especially sexual assaults. There is currently much emphasis to make sure samples from these non-violent offenders are profiled and entered into the database. A person convicted of burglary, or another non-violent offense, may spend little, if any, time in jail. They are therefore able to commit another crime more quickly than someone convicted of a violent felony who is incarcerated for an extended period of time.

When a convicted offender profile is entered into the database, it is automatically compared to all the evidence profiles in the database. Conversely, when an evidence profile is entered into the database, it is compared against all convicted offender samples. Evidence samples are also compared against each other, in order to related cases. When one semen evidence profile is found to match another semen profile, two unrelated cases can be linked to the same perpetrator. If neither agency has a suspect, the match can still open investigative possibilities. If one of the agencies has already identified a suspect, the other agency has literally generated a suspect out of nowhere. Of course, that is also the goal of comparing evidence profiles to convicted offender profiles.

There are three *layers* of information sharing within the national database. Evidence profiles are first entered into the *Local database* at the crime lab doing the actual DNA testing. This is the first time, a comparison of evidence-to-evidence profiles is performed. At regularly scheduled intervals, local DNA profiles are then uploaded to the *State database,* where comparisons are again performed between all samples in the State database. Finally, profiles from the state database are uploaded to the *National database.* At this point, evidence and convicted offender samples are compared with samples from every other state. Each time new samples are entered into the Local, State, or National database, the comparisons take place all over again. DNA profiles are continuously being compared against all other new samples coming into the system.

Mitochondrial DNA Analysis

Mitochondria are small biological bodies, or organelles, found in all cells. The primary function of mitochondria is to provide energy for the cell to function.[10] Within each mitochondria there is a small spherical DNA molecule that is used only by that mitochondria. This DNA molecule does not contain a mixture of genetic information from both mother and father like nuclear DNA does. Instead, the mitochondrial DNA is inherited maternally, and the DNA sequence does not change from mother to child. For instance, all siblings in the same maternal line will have an identical mitochondrial sequence to their mother. The mother and all *her* siblings will have the same mitochondrial sequence as their mother, and so on. Therefore, the mitochondrial sequence is not unique to an individual, but common to a family maternal lineage. In that way, it is possible for a woman to have a brother, a son and an uncle, *her* mother's brother, with the same mitochondrial DNA sequence as herself.

As stated previously, mitochondrial DNA (mtDNA) is a spherical molecule, compared to the familiar double helix structure found in the nucleus of cells. It is approximately 16,569 base pairs in length, while nuclear DNA is about three billion base pairs long. The region of the mitochondrial DNA that is known to vary between individuals is found in an area of the DNA known as the *control region,* a segment of DNA that is approximately 1100 base pairs (Fig. IV-45). It is estimated that 1–2%, or one to two bases out of 100, are highly variable between unrelated individuals in this region of the mtDNA. On average, two unrelated individuals will have six to 12 differences in their mtDNA sequence. Therefore, mitochondrial DNA testing identifies sequence polymorphisms, as opposed to the length polymorphisms seen with STR testing.

Mitochondrial DNA is important to forensic DNA testing because it can be efficiently amplified even in severely degraded biological samples. This is due to the high copy number of mitochondrial DNA molecules found in each cell, as opposed to the single copy of DNA found in the nucleus of a cell. Hundreds of mitochondria can be found in a single cell, and each one has a DNA molecule. While it is possible to obtain mtDNA information from samples without nuclear DNA (such as a hair sample with no root material) or skeletal remains (where no nuclear DNA remains in tissue or bones), it is not the first choice for forensic DNA testing. This is because is does not allow for individualization of a sample. It is best used for human identification purposes, as in the case of a missing person.

Mitochondrial testing can establish that a deceased missing person is a biological relative

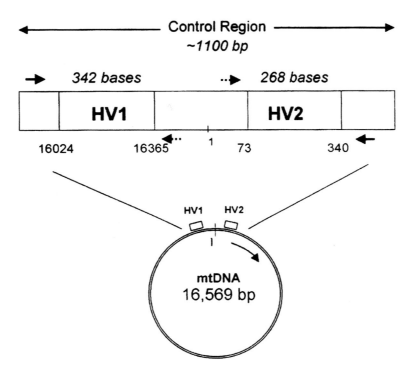

FIGURE IV-45. Circular mitochondrial DNA molecule illustrating the control region. Variation between individuals is seen within this region.

of living family members. A recent prominent case using mtDNA testing for human identification involved the analysis of human remains in the Tomb of the Unknown Soldier for the Vietnam War. Military intelligence pointed to the possibility that the remains in the tomb could either be those of U.S. Serviceman 1st Lt. Michael Blassie, or one other individual.

The remains were exhumed, and mtDNA testing was performed using known blood samples from the mother and siblings in both families. The results of the mtDNA testing showed that the mitochondrial sequence from the remains was identical to the mitochondrial sequence from the Blassie family, and did not match the other family.[11] The remains were re-buried in Arlington National Cemetery as those of Michael Blassie (Fig. IV-46). It would appear with today's technology, there will probably never be another unknown soldier. The U.S. Armed Forces DNA Identification Laboratory is the leader in mitochondrial DNA technology, and each and every serviceman and woman has a DNA sample on file for identification purposes.

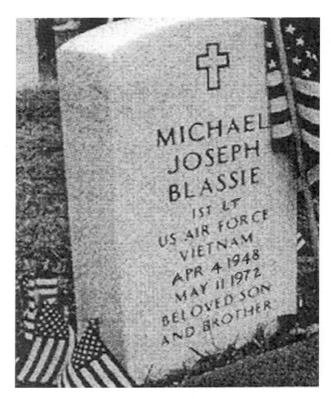

FIGURE IV-46. Remains of 1st Lt. Michael Joseph Blassie.

For forensic purposes, mtDNA testing can be a tool for obtaining DNA information from highly degraded samples such as decomposed remains. This testing can also provide genetic information for some hair samples. Although the DNA information will not result in an individual identification in some circumstances, it is better than no information at all.

REFERENCES

1. Jeffreys, A.J., Wilson, V., and Thein, S.L. Hypervariable 'Minisatellite' regions in human DNA. *Nature, 314:* 67–73, 1985.
2. Wambaugh, J. *The Blooding.* New York: William Morrow & Co., Inc., 1989.
3. Brown, T.A. *Genetics: A molecular approach,* 2nd ed. London: Chapman & Hall, 1992.
4. Inman, K., and Rudin, N. *An introduction to forensic DNA analysis.* New York: CRC Press, 1997.
5. Saferstein, R. Editor. *Forensic science handbook,* vol. III. Englewood Cliffs, NJ: Prentice Hall, 1993.
6. Butler, J.M. *Forensic DNA typing.* San Diego, CA: Academic Press, 2001.
7. *AmpFlSTR Profiler Plus™ User's Manual.* Foster City, CA: PE Applied Biosystems, 1997.
8. Holt, C.L., Stauffer, C., Wallin, J.M., Lazaruk, K.D., Nguyen, T., Budwole, B., and Walsh, P.S. Practical applications of genotypic surveys for forensic DNA testing. *Forensic Science International, 112:* 91–109, 2000.
9. National Research Council. *The evaluation of forensic evidence.* Washington, D.C.: National Academy Press, 1996.
10. Fourney, R.M. Mitochondrial DNA primer and forensic analysis: A primer for law enforcement. *Canadian Society of Forensic Science Journal, 31* (1): 45–53, 1998.
11. Holland, Dr. M.: Personal communication. Mitochondrial DNA sequence analysis in forensic casework methods and issues, 1999.

Chapter V

FORENSIC ANTHROPOLOGY

William M. Bass

PHYSICAL OR BIOLOGICAL anthropology is that field of science that studies man from his earliest beginnings, about five million years ago, to the present. Thus, the scientific study of the skeleton, both human and animal, is found in anthropology. The application of these skills to modern forensic cases is forensic anthropology.

Forensic anthropology is the field of science which focuses on the identification of more or less skeletonized remains, either human or animal, in a legal context. Forensic anthropology is a rapidly growing subspecialty. Beyond the elimination of non-human elements, the identification process undertakes to provide opinions regarding sex, age, race, stature, and such other characteristics of each individual involved, as may lead to his or her positive identification.

This definition takes into account certain practices in the forensic field stemming from the fact that identity depends primarily on the soft parts and only secondarily on skeletal parts. Coroners and/or medical examiners, whose duty it is to investigate unexplained deaths, are trained primarily to deal with fleshed remains.

When confronted with skeletonized remains, investigators turn to forensic anthropologists because of their greater osteological expertise.[1] Professional forensic anthropologists are certified by the American Board of Forensic Anthropology.

The forensic anthropologist is usually the last person in the human identification chain. Most often bodies can be identified by morphological features or fingerprints, but occasionally bodies burned or decomposed beyond recognition require the expertise of a trained osteologist. One of the first and basic texts in forensic anthropology is that by Krogman,[2] with a more modern revision by Krogman and Iscan.[3]

This chapter will cover seven areas of forensic anthropology:

- is the bone human or animal?
- length of time since death
- age at death of the skeleton
- determination of sex of the skeleton
- determination of race of the skeleton
- estimation of stature from the skeleton
- other means of identification

IS THE BONE HUMAN OR ANIMAL?

The initial question facing the forensic investigator is *"are the remains human?"* This is not always as easy as it may seem and many have misdiagnosed the species of a bone(s), especially confusing bear (Ursus) paws with human (Homo) hands. An expert osteologist can give much more information than identifying bones as human. The identification of non-human bones should also include the genus and, if possible, the species. Bones found in a forensic context are often small or fragmentary. There are additional problems with burned and almost always frag-

mentary remains. J. L. Angel, a renowned anthropologist at the Smithsonian Institute in Washington, D.C., reported that about 10% of the bones brought to him for evaluation were determined to be of animal origin.[4]

Since 1954, we have identified skeletal remains in the areas of forensic and physical anthropology. Since coming to the University of Tennessee in 1971, we have conducted two studies[5,6] of the types of skeletons that have been presented by law enforcement agencies for identification. A summary of the cases submitted for identification

240

from 1972–1994 indicates that 25–30 percent are non-human. This higher percentage than that reported by Angel is thought to be the result of many training classes for law enforcement agents, popularized literary accounts of forensic investigations involving skeletal remains, media attention and television coverage of forensic cases. Of the 23 species of non-human bones submitted for identification, the most common in Tennessee have been the remains of deer, dog, pig and cow followed by, chicken, horse, bear, calf and rabbit.[7]

Unfortunately, most guides to animal bone identification have been prepared for or by archaeologists[8-10] and are of limited use in a forensic setting because they deal primarily with wild animals. Skeletons of small animals are often mistaken for the remains of human fetuses or newborns. Fortunately, most animals are not the size of adult humans. Anthropoid ape bones closely resemble those of man but the chances of a non-human primate skeleton turning up in a forensic context is remote. In human fetuses, newborns, and children, the epiphyses have not united thus, the ends of the shafts (diaphyses) will be rough, unattached. The difference then is one of size and maturity (Fig. V-1). If a skeleton is found that includes tail bones, it is not human.

Misidentification of bear paws has been reported in the forensic literature.[11,12] Either gross examination or superior x-ray views of a bear paw should reveal deep v-shaped grooves on the distal end of each metatarsal. If tissue remains, the presence of two sesamoid bones at the distal end of each metatarsal will be seen in a bear paw. Humans have sesamoids at the distal end of the first metatarsals and metacarpals only.

LENGTH OF TIME SINCE DEATH

One of the first questions asked by an investigator is *"how long has this decaying body or skeleton been here?"* This is a complicated and difficult question since little comparative data exist and there are many yet unresolved issues. The few articles which exist in anthropological literature on the time interval since death have been summarized by Bass[13] and Rodriguez and Bass.[14] Payne[15] conducted a summer carrion study of the baby pig *(Sus scrofa)* where he found *"a definite ecological succession occurred among the fauna of carrion. Each stage of decay was characterized by a particular group of arthropods, each of which occupied a particular niche. Their activities were influenced by physical properties of carrion, rapidity of putrefaction, time of day, and weather."* He found six stages of decomposition which were delimited for carrion exposed to arthropods: flesh, bloated, active decay, advanced decay, dry, and remains. Rodriguez and Bass recently observed the decay rate of human cadavers in all seasons of the year in east Tennessee. The succession of insects and the time of their appearance for spring and summer is presented in their article.[14]

THE DETERMINATION OF AGE AT DEATH
OF A SKELETON

A basic knowledge of human biology, growth and development, and the aging process is needed to identify the gradual changes that occur in the skeleton from birth to old age. The following is a short summary to be used as a guide; experience is one of the best teachers.

Aging can be divided into two major categories, maturation and degeneration.

Maturation

A good comparative dental chart of dentition has been prepared by Schour and Massler[16] with ages from a larger sample size by Ubelaker.[17] Man has two sets of teeth, deciduous and adult (Fig. V-2).

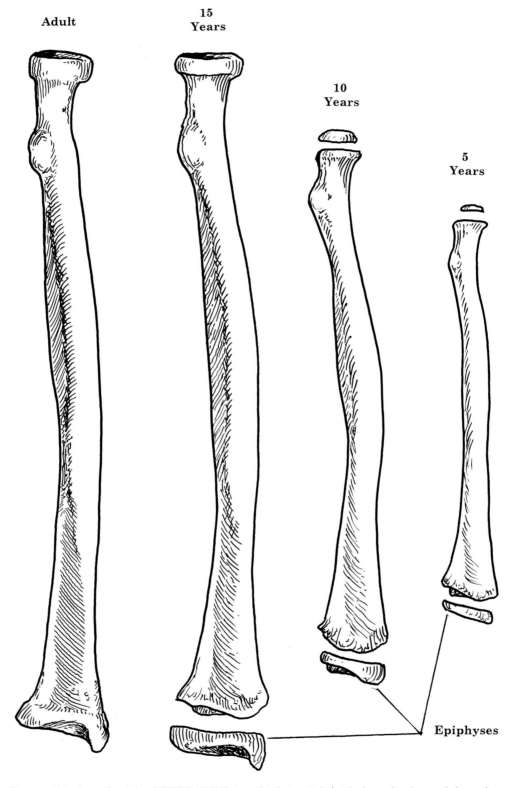

FIGURE V-1. Growth of the *LEFT RADIUS* from birth to adult (with the palm forward the radius is on the thumb side between the wrist and elbow).

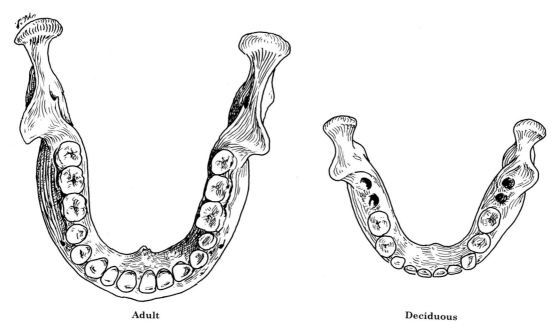

Adult   Deciduous

FIGURE V-2. Dentition.

Deciduous (Baby or Milk Teeth)

- Approximately six months of age: lower central incisors erupt.
- Approximately 24 months of age: all 20 deciduous teeth are usually erupted. The second deciduous molars are the last to erupt.
- Approximately two to six years: retain deciduous teeth. As the skeleton grows, children develop spaces between the teeth (once erupted, teeth do not get larger but the bone does grow).

Adult Teeth

Adult teeth are larger and whiter than deciduous teeth. Deciduous teeth have a thinner enamel covering over the dentine, thus they appear more yellow.

- Approximately six years: first adult tooth, the six-year molars appear behind the 20 deciduous teeth.
- Approximately 6-1/2 to 11-1/2 years: period of mixed dentition where the deciduous teeth are replaced by adult teeth.

- Approximately 12 years: second molars erupt. Usually all deciduous teeth have been lost by age 12.
- Approximately 18 years: third molars, wisdom teeth, may or may not erupt. Genetically, we are losing our third molars and in many people they are impacted or never erupt. Any number (from one to four) of the third molars may be missing.

Epiphyses

During the growth process there are 806 centers of ossification which unite into 206 bones in the adult skeleton. By approximately age 13 in girls and age 15 in boys, the epiphyses begin to unite to the diaphyses, or shaft. The sequence of epiphyseal union occurs at the elbow, hip, ankle, knee, wrist, and shoulder with union occurring first at the elbow and last at the shoulder. Epiphyseal union of the medial clavicle and anterior iliac crest from a large sample of modern forensic cases has been reported by Suchey et al.[18]

Age 13 to 17 years is the most active period of epiphyseal union. This is the period of the cir-

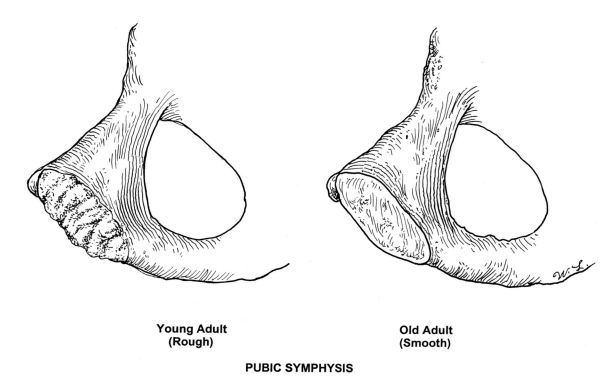

Young Adult
(Rough)

Old Adult
(Smooth)

PUBIC SYMPHYSIS

FIGURE V-3. Changes in the pubic symphysis from young adult with a *rough* surface to an old adult with a *smooth* surface.

cumpubertal spurt in growth with the major growth of the body terminating with the closure of the epiphyses.

At circa age 25, the last epiphysis to unite is the sternal end of the clavicle.[17]

During the growth process, age can be determined by measuring the length of the long bones and comparing with published standards.[17] Aging standards of fetal skeletal material has been published by Fazekas and Kosa.[19]

Degenerative Changes or Degeneration

Following the end of the growth period, signaled by closure of most of the epiphyses, the skeleton begins a slow process of wearing out (Fig. V-3). These degenerative changes appear in the early twenties and are present in increasing degrees until death. Additional studies by Iscan, Loth, and Wright,[20] and Stewart and McCormick[21] have focused attention on the age and sex ossification patterns of the sternal end of the ribs. For human identification purposes, the three best

areas to estimate age at death of an adult are the pubic symphysis, osteon counting, and osteoarthritic lipping.[22–24]

Changes in the Pubic Symphysis

Standards for males were first published in the 1920s by T. Wingate Todd, an anatomist at Western Reserve University.[25] Because cadaver populations contain mainly older individuals, little data existed on young males until 1957 when Tom McKern and T. Dale Stewart published data obtained on young American males killed during the Korean War.[26] It was not until the early 1970s that data on changes in female pubic symphyses were published by B. Miles Gilbert.[27]

Standards for comparison of pubic symphyseal changes are available in the forensic anthropological literature. Essentially as one grows older, the face of the pubic symphysis changes from one that is *rough* with an appearance of *mountains* and *valleys* to one that becomes smoother with the mountains wearing off and the valleys filling up (see Fig. V-3). To determine age at death, a comparison of the unknown specimen is made with published standards which exist for both males and females. One caution, however, is that with older age, changes of the pubic symphysis become more obscure and determination of age at death in the sixties and seventies with a plus or minus five-year range is difficult. More accurate methods of age estimation have recently been reported by Suchey and associates.[18,28]

Osteon Counting

A microscopic method developed by Ellis R. Kerley in the 1950s to determine age at death from the microscopic structure of bone[22] has proven to be quite accurate. This method requires sectioning a long bone, usually the femur, at its midshaft, cutting, grinding, and polishing a thin section (80 microns) and viewing this section through polarized light. Standards for the amount of lamellar bone, osteons, osteon fragments, and haversian and non-haversian canals have been published. Revisions of Kerley's method have been reported.[23,24]

Osteoarthritic Lipping

It is known that as people age, their skeletons reflect the various stresses encountered throughout life. A gross quantification of these changes, especially in the vertebral column, has been published by Stewart and allows estimation of age of older individuals.[1]

Using all of the aforementioned methods, other indicators, and experience in observation, the age at death can be fairly accurately determined (Fig. V-4).

THE DETERMINATION OF SEX OF THE SKELETON

It is difficult, if not impossible, with the present state of knowledge to determine the sex from the skeletons of preteens. Skeletal sexual criteria manifest themselves at puberty and are not clear in skeletons below the age of 12 to 15 years.

The best area to determine the sex of an adult skeleton is from the pelvis, second best the skull, and lastly from the rest of the skeleton.

The Pelvis

Women have broader hips than men and this width of the pelvis can be found in three different areas.

Length of Pubic Bone

When the innominate bone is held so that the pubic portion can be viewed from either the anterior or posterior aspect, the examiner can notice that the female has a long pubic portion and much wider subpubic angle than the male (Fig. V- 5).

Width of the Sciatic Notch

Generally, the notch is narrow in males and broad in females. If the examiner's thumb is inserted into the sciatic notch, the notch should be relatively filled in a male allowing for little lateral movement, whereas, in a female with a wider or broader notch, lateral movement of the thumb is possible. Considerable variability in this trait has been observed; occasionally males have wide notches. Therefore, it is best not to base your judgment of sex on this one criterion. The more criteria that can be used, the more accurate will be the determination.

Bone Buildup on the Sacroiliac Joint

One method of obtaining width is to add bone along the sacroiliac joint. Starting in the unarticular area posterior to the sacroiliac articulation in a male, the examiner can normally draw a pencil across the sacroiliac articulation of the ilium. This portion of the ilium where it articulates with the sacrum is flat in males. There is a buildup of

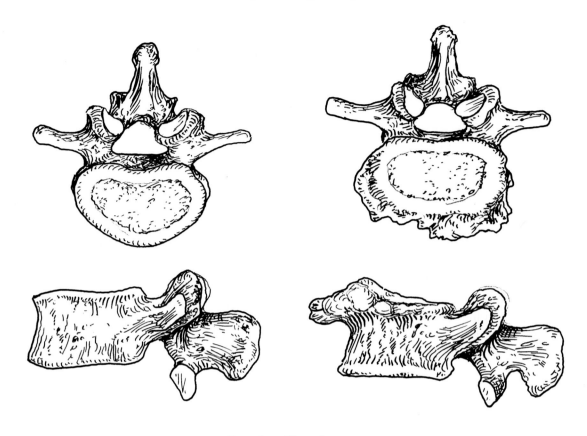

Lumbar Vertebrae

Young adult   **Old adult with osteoarthritic lipping**

FIGURE V-4. Changes around a joint surface from the build-up of osteoarthritic lipping with age.

bone in this same area in a female so that beginning at the same areas as above, the pencil encounters a ridge of bone in the sacroiliac articular area (Fig. V-6).[7,29]

Skull

Sex differences in the skull are mainly due to sexual dimorphism where the male is larger, more rugged, and muscle attachments are more marked; whereas, the female is smaller, more gracile, and smooth.

Males have larger mastoid processes, well-marked supra-orbital ridges, prominent muscle markings in the occipital region, and metrically a larger mouth.

Females usually have a smooth forehead with little or no supra-orbital ridges and because of less physical activity have shallow muscle markings on the occipital bone.

The chin in a male is usually square; the chin comes to a point in a female.[7]

It is difficult to determine sex from anthropometric measurements of the teeth. However, anthropometric measurement of the skull have been used successfully by Giles and Elliot to establish multivariate statistical procedures to determine the sex of unidentified bodies, using

**Public Portion of
Left Innominate**

Front View

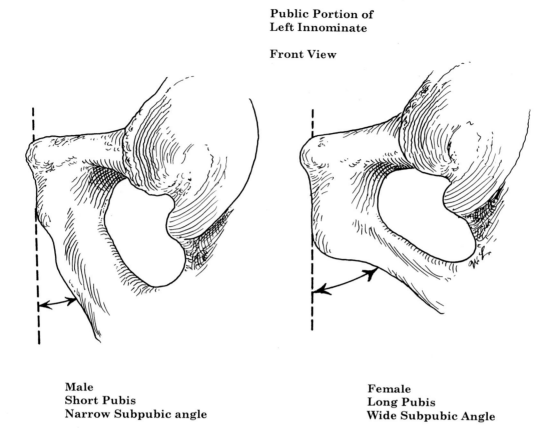

**Male
Short Pubis
Narrow Subpubic angle**

**Female
Long Pubis
Wide Subpubic Angle**

FIGURE V-5. Pubic portion (front view) showing the differences between a male, (with a short pubis) and a female (with a longer pubis).

the skull.[30] Giles also has a discriminate function test for sex discrimination of the mandible.[31]

The Rest of the Skeleton

Without the pelvis or the skull, sex determination of the skeleton is more difficult. Observable differences are due mainly to sexual dimorphism; males are usually larger in size because they normally reach puberty two years later than girls and thus grow two years longer. Overall size is the main criteria but specific areas should be looked at, as follows.

Maximum Diameter of the Head of the Femur

Measure the maximum diameter of the articular surface. A measurement below 43 mm sug-

gests a female, above 45 mm a male.[7,32] This is also true of the humerus with approximately the same measurements.

Width of the Ala of the Sacrum

In some cases, the width of the articular area of the sacrum for the fifth lumbar vertebra in a male will be greater than half the width of the entire sacrum. A male's larger skeletal structure requires bigger articular areas. The ala in females are less than half of the width of the sacrum.[33]

Length of the Sternum

The gender predictive value of sternal length has long been known: an article by Stewart and McCormick on measurements of sternal lengths

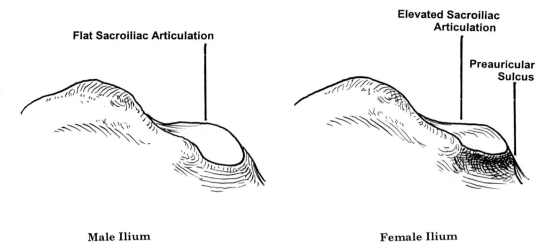

Flat Sacroiliac Articulation

Elevated Sacroiliac Articulation

Preauricular Sulcus

Male Ilium   **Female Ilium**

FIGURE V-6. Illustration of differences in the sacro-iliac articulation between males and females.

on chest plate x-rays for 617 autopsied adults from the United States gives valuable data for U.S. forensic cases.[34] A combined manubrium mesosternal length of 121 mm or less included only females, and sternal lengths of 173 mm and above included only males. They were able to predict sex, with approximately 80% accuracy, using the following ranges: female up to 142 mm and male greater than 158 mm. Sex determination was questionable for sternal lengths 143 mm to 157 mm.

Jit and associates report on sexing the human sternum.[35] Their data, based on Asian Indians, give smaller measurements than those from American and European populations.

Septal Apertures of the Humerus

The presence of a supra condyloid foramen in the distal end of the humerus, what Ales Hrdlička called septal apertures in 1932, is seen more frequently in females.[7] The sternal foramen has been found to occur about twice as often in men as in women.[36]

Caution is warranted when determining sex of a skeleton on the basis of associated clothing or personal items. The literature contains many examples where the true identity of a person was confused by substitution of clothing of the opposite sex.

THE DETERMINATION OF RACE OF THE SKELETON

Race is one of the most difficult determinations that the forensic anthropologist will encounter. Only two areas of the skeleton can, at present, be used to determine race, the skull, specifically the face, and the femur. Some research has been done on anterior-posterior femoral curvature but presently results are not definitive.[37]

In a skull, with little or no damage to the facial skeleton, the following criteria can be used to determine race.

Anthropometric Measurements

In 1962, Eugene Giles and Orville Elliot published information on the use of anthropometric measurements in a multivariate statistical analysis to determine race from skull examinations.[38] This procedure allows a discrimination between Caucasoids (Whites), Negroids (Blacks), and Mongoloids (American Indians). More recently Ousley and Jantz[39] have used anthropometric measurements of recent forensic cases to set up

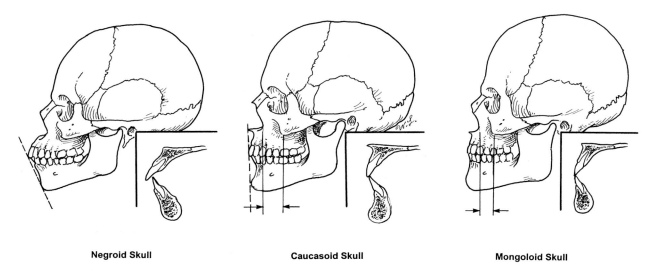

Negroid Skull   **Caucasoid Skull**   **Mongoloid Skull**

FIGURE V-7a–c. (a) Shape of Negroid (Black) skull with prognathism and no nasal sill. (b) Shape of a Caucasoid (White) skull with a nasal sill and receding maxillary bones. (c) Slope of a Mongoloid (also American Indian) skull with projecting maxillary bones and an edge-to-edge bite in the incisor region.

computer forensic discriminate functions for both sexes and major racial groups.

Prognathism in Negroid Skulls

Prognathism is the protrusion of the alveolar regions of the mandible and maxilla. It is common in Negroid individuals, is seen slightly in Mongoloids, and only occasionally in Caucasoids (Fig. V-7a–c). A quick test is to occlude the lower jaw in its proper dental occlusion, and with a pencil attempt to touch the base of the nasal aperture and chin at the same time. If this can be done, the skull is usually Caucasoid. Negroid individuals have a protrusion of the alveolar portion of mandible and maxilla, thus in Blacks the pencil will not touch the base of the nose and the chin at the same time (see Fig. V-7a).

Nasal Sill, in Caucasoid Skulls

Observe carefully the base of the nasal aperture. With a pencil resting against the maxilla just below the nasal opening, try to run the pencil gently into the nasal opening. In Caucasoids there is usually a dam or nasal sill which will stop the pencil (see Fig. V-7b). In Negroid skulls there is no dam or nasal sill and the pencil will glide easily into the nasal aperture.

Flat Face, in Mongoloids

Hold the skull with the occipital region in one hand with the face up. Balance a pencil across the nasal aperture. Now try to insert a finger between the pencil and the cheek bone under the lateral edge of the eye. If a finger can be inserted without knocking off the pencil, the skull is probably Caucasoid. This is difficult, if not impossible, to do with Mongoloid skulls (see Fig. V-7c). Mongoloid (including the American Indian) is the only race that is *cold adapted*. They have flat, usually round, faces whereas the nose and the face of Whites come to a point along the midline.

Those in biological anthropology believe that the geographic races seen around the world have derived their various anatomical and physical characteristics as a result of *climatic adaptation*. Humans are animals that have adapted to the climatic zone in which they were born and follow the zoological rule proposed by Allen which states *"the extremities of warm-blooded animals tend to be shorter in cold climates in order to conserve body heat"* and the ecological rule by Bergmann that states *"that within a species of warm-blooded animals, those living in colder climates tend to be larger than those in warmer climates."*

Before humans moved from one geographic area to another, the Black or Negroid races inhabited only the warmer areas such as Africa and Melanesia. The Caucasoids or Whites adapted to a more moderate climate with heavy cloud cover (Europe) and thus, did not need the dark skin to protect them from ultraviolet radiation. Mongoloid racial groups adapted to the colder parts of the earth, Northern Asia such as Mongolia and Siberia and the Eskimo of North America. They have flat broad faces, the nose does not stick out, short arms and legs and a short trunk which enabled survival in a cold environment.

Edge-to-Edge Bite in Incisor Region, in Mongoloids

When most people occlude their teeth, they will have an overbite: a situation where the upper or maxillary incisors are in front of the lower or mandibular incisors. Mongoloids, and especially American Indians, have an edge-to-edge bite in the incisor region. Look for wear on the occlusal (biting) surface of the incisor teeth on skulls with the incisor teeth present. If wear is present, i.e., the enamel is worn off exposing the dentine, then the skull is probably American Indian.

Distal Femur

Craig[40] in 1994 conducted a significant doctoral dissertation research project on the racial differences of the distal femora of 423 modern Blacks and Whites. She used lateral radiographs of the knee and drew a line parallel to the posterior shaft of the femur. She drew a second line on the x-ray directly through Blumensaat's line. Craig states that in a sagittal section of the femur, the intercondylar shelf can be seen as a line of dense cortical bone that actually forms a *roof* of the intercondylar notch. This area of dense bone can also be seen in a lateral radiograph of the knee, as a relatively radiopaque line. This line was first described by Blumensaat in 1938. She

then determined the intercondylar shelf angle by simply measuring the angle created by these two lines.

Craig found that the mean for the intercondylar shelf angle in Whites is 146.2 degrees and the mean for Blacks is 137.8 degrees. The sectioning point is 141 degrees. Eighteen percent of the sample overlapped across the sectioning point.

The following case exemplifies the value of age, sex, and race criteria. A recent telephone call from an insurance company requested aid in the identification of a policyholder, a 34-year-old white male who had gone to Monterrey, Mexico with a friend and rented a Chevrolet Suburban. Three days after their arrival the vehicle was found burned a few miles outside of the city with a charred body in the driver's seat.

The friend had gone to the Mexican authorities and said that his friend, the 34-year-old white male, had rented the Suburban and was the only one who drove it and he asked for some of the burned remains to take back to the U.S. for burial. The policy holder, however, had a seven million-dollar policy and the insurance company did not want to pay unless a positive identification could be made.

The burned Chevrolet Suburban had been impounded by the police. Investigation of fire scenes usually requires careful excavation using archaeological techniques. In a fire, the arms and legs are the first to burn because of their relatively small size. As the fire progresses steam pressure inside the skull causes it to break open unless there is a preexisting opening such as a gunshot, a stab wound, or fracture. In an intense fire or in the case of cremation, the skull will fragment (Fig. V-8). If the fire continues, the thoracic cavity is the next to disintegrate followed by the pelvis and pelvic organs.

A fire scene is no different than a crime scene. Therefore, the same rules of preservation and examination apply. Initial inspection of the Chevrolet Suburban showed that the fire had started in the area of the right rear quarter panel, and was probably intentionally set. This was not a regular car fire that started in the motor compartment.

Charred remains of an adult human were recovered from the driver's seat area and revealed extensive degenerative bone changes with osteoarthritic lipping, predominately in the lumbar area (Fig. V-9). Osteoarthritic lipping around vertebral joint surfaces begins in the early thirties and increases with age. In the case in question age was consistent with someone in their fifties or sixties, not 34.

Teeth are remarkably fire resistant. While the rest of the body was charred and disintegrated, teeth on the floorboard included shovel shaped incisors with edge to edge occlusal wear, both classic Mongoloid and/or American Indian genetic traits.

Excavation of the vehicle proved that the individual in the Suburban at the time of the fire was a 50-plus-year-old, probably a Mexican peasant, since Mexican peasants are

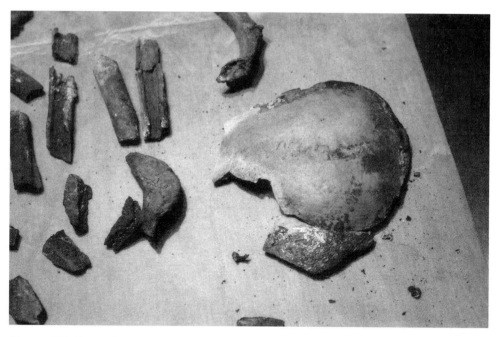

FIGURE V-8. Burned human remains from a car fire with a large unburned section of top of the cranial vault on the right, suggesting body was upside down with head on floor at time of fire.

basically American Indians with some European admixture. Examination and x-ray of the burned remains failed to determine the manner of death.

The 34-year-old was arrested in Boston working as a financial planner and was found guilty of insurance fraud and sentenced to Federal Prison. The charred body in the vehicle remains unidentified.

Estimation of Stature from the Long Bones

A number of formulas exist which enable calculation of stature from long bones. In general, most calculations are based on the maximum length of the long bones. Probably the best method to use on skeletal material from the United States are the formulas developed by Trotter and Gleser on Caucasoids, Negroids, Mongoloids, and Mexicans.[41,42] Calculation of stature from long bones is not difficult if an osteometric board, or improvised but exact device, is used.

Other Means of Identification

The skeleton is a record of the life of the individual. Insults to a body such as trauma causing either healed or unhealed fractures, dental caries and in many cases the filling of these cavities, some diseases, malnutrition, and some occupations will leave their marks on the teeth and bones.[43]

Many people break bones during their lifetime. These fractures will usually leave their marks. A skeleton exhibiting numerous old healed fractures of the nose and maxilla, possibly mandible, suggests a person whose lifestyle led them to participate in fights. In addition, the metacarpals, phalanges, and carpal bones should be carefully checked for old healed fractures also suggesting wounds from fighting. The pattern, of such healed fractures, often suggests the social status of the individual.

In today's population, most bone fractures are set by medical personnel. If x-rays are still available, these x-rays will offer a means of positive identification using before and after death views of the same bone.

One of the best means of making a positive identification is from the dentition. However, the name of a missing person must be supplied and one must have records to compare with the

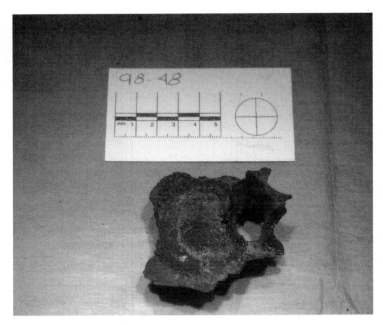

FIGURE V-9. A burned lumbar vertebra with extensive osteoarthritic lipping suggestive of an adult of 50+ years. The jagged edges of the lipping extend outward from the vertebral center which is the weight-bearing portion of the vertebra.

unknown skeleton. When recovering a skull, special care should be taken to recover the front teeth (incisors). These are single rooted teeth and often fall out when the tissues decay and are often left at the scene. Incisor teeth are important in the identification of children under three or four years who have not had dental care. Genetic anomalies of the shape and size can often be matched with a photograph of a smiling child.

Any disease that affects the skeleton can be determined after death. Knowledge of paleopathology, possessed by most forensic anthropologists, can aid in determining positive identification. Many occupations can affect the skeleton. A skeletal series of American Indians from southern Louisiana who moved about the swamp by boat had massive shoulders and arms from canoeing. The use of tobacco pipes can be seen in dental wear and often tobacco stains will indicate smoking or the use of smokeless tobacco. Copper jewelry will leave a greenish-blue stain on the bone. Care should always be taken to recover related jewelry items.

Handedness (the preference for the right or left side) can also be ascertained. The preferred side receives the major blood supply; thus, the muscles are better developed and their attachments to the bones are increased. Handedness can only be determined when bones of both upper limbs are present for comparison. Bones from the preferred side are larger and longer. This carries over to differences in shoe size and sleeve length.

Summary

The skeleton is the most durable system of the mammalian body and remains intact or in fragmentary condition long after all other systems have been destroyed through decay, fire, or other methods. Forensic anthropologists can use their knowledge of the skeleton and its variations to provide information that can lead to positive identification. The skeleton varies through life due to maturation, growth, and degenerative changes. Also, healed fractures, dental caries, and diseases that leave their mark on bone can all aid in a positive identification. Methods used in the differentiation between human and non-human skeletal remains, ascertaining length of time since death and age at death, and determining sex and stature of human skeletal remains are ways a forensic anthropologist can determine identification. The forensic anthropologist can also provide additional forensic information because the skeleton is a permanent record of much that has happened to a person during life.

REFERENCES

1. Stewart, T.D.: *Essentials of forensic anthropology.* Springfield, IL: Charles C Thomas Publisher, 1979.
2. Krogman, W.M.: *The human skeleton in forensic medicine.* Springfield, IL: Charles C Thomas Publisher, 1962.
3. Krogman, W.M., and Iscan, M.Y.: *The human skeleton in forensic medicine,* 2d edition. Springfield, IL: Charles C Thomas Publisher, 1986.
4. Angel, J.L.: Bones can fool people. *FBI Law Enforcement Bulletin, 43:* 17–20, 1974.
5. Bass W.M., and Driscoll, P.A.: Summary of skeletal identification in Tennessee, 1971–1981. *J Forensic Sci., 28:* 159–168, 1983.
6. Marks, M.K.: William M. Bass and the development of forensic anthropology in Tennessee. *J. Forensic Sci., 40:* 729–734, 1995.
7. Bass, W.M.: *Human osetology: A laboratory and field manual,* 4th edition. Missouri Archaeological Society. Columbia, 1995.
8. Olsen ,S.J.: *Mammal remains from archaeological sites. Part I. Southeastern and Southwestern United States.* Papers of the Peabody Museum of Archaeology and Ethnology, Cambridge, MA: Harvard University, vol. 26, pp xii–162, 1964.
9. Cornwall, I.W.: *Bones for the archaeologist.* New York: Macmillan, 1956.
10. Gilbert, B.M.: *Mammalian osteo-archaeology: North America.* Missouri Archaeological Society, Columbia, 1973.
11. Stewart, T.D.: Bear paw remains closely resemble human bones. *FBI Law Enforcement Bulletin 28:* 18–21, 1959.
12. Hoffman, J.M.: Identification of nonskeletonized bear paws and human feet. In Rathbun, T.A., and Buikstra, J.E. (eds): *Human identification: Case studies in forensic anthropology.* Springfield, IL: Charles C Thomas Publisher, pp. 96–106, 1984.
13. Bass, W.M.: Time interval since death, a difficult decision. In Rathbun, T.A., and Buikstra, J.E. (eds): *Human identification: Case studies in forensic anthropology.* Springfield, IL: Charles C Thomas Publisher, pp. 136–147, 1984.
14. Rodriguez, W.C., and Bass, W.M.: Insect activity and its relationship to decay rates of human cadavers in East Tennessee. *J Forensic Sci., 28:* 423–432, 1983.
15. Payne J.E.: A summer carrion study of the baby pig Sus Scrofa Linnaeus. *Ecology, 46:* 592–602, 1965.
16. Schour, I., and Massler, M.: *Development of the human dentition,* ed 2, chart. Chicago, American Dental Association, 1944.
17. Ubelaker, D.H.: *Human skeletal remains: Excavation, analysis and interpretation.* Chicago: Beresford Book Service, 1978.
18. Suchey, J.M., Owings, P.A., and Wiseley, D.V.: Skeletal aging in unidentified persons. In Rathbun, T.A., and Buikstra, J.E. (eds): *Human identification: Case studies in forensic anthropology.* Springfield, IL: Charles C Thomas Publisher, pp. 278–297, 1984.
19. Fazekas, I.G., and Kosa, F.: *Forensic fetal osteology.* Budapest: Akademiai Kiado, 1978.
20. Iscan, M.Y., Loth, S.R., and Wright, R.K.: Age estimation from the rib by phase analysis: White males. *J. Forensic Sci., 29:* 2094–1104, 1984.
21. Stewart, J.H., and McCormick, W.F.: A sex and age-limited ossification pattern in human costal cartilages. *Am J Clin Pathol, 81:* 765–769, 1984.
22. Kerley, E.R.: The microscopic determination of age in human bone. *Am J Phys Anthropol, 23:* 149–164, 1965.
23. Kerley, E.R., and Ubelaker, D.H.: Revisions in the microscopic method of estimating age at death in human cortical bone. *Am J Phys Anthropol, 49:* 455–546, 1978.
24. Kerley, E.R.: Microscopic aging of human bone. In Rathbun, T.A., and Buikstra, J.E. (eds): *Human identification: Case studies in forensic anthropology.* Springfield, IL: Charles C Thomas Publisher, pp. 298–306, 1984.
25. Todd, T.W.: Age changes in the pubic bones: The male white pubis. *Am J Phys Anthropol, 3:* 285–334, 1920.
26. McKern, T.W., and Stewart, T.D.: Skeletal age changes in young American males, analyzed from the standpoint of identification. Technical Report EP-45. Headquarters Quartermaster Research and Development Command. Natick, MA, 1957.
27. Gilbert, B.M., and McKern, T.W.: A method for aging the female os pubis. *Am J Phys Anthropol, 38:* 31–38, 1973.
28. Suchey, J.M., Wiseley, D.V., Green, R.F., and Noguchi, T.T.: Analysis of dorsal pitting in the os pubis in an extensive sample of modern American females. *Am J Phys Anthropol, 51:* 517–540, 1979.
29. Iscan, M.Y., and Derrick, K.: Determination of sex from the sacroiliac joint: A visual assessment technique. *Florida Scientist, 47:* 94–98, 1984.
30. Giles, E.O., and Elliot, O.: Sex determination by discriminant function analysis of crania. *Am J Phys Anthropol, 21:* 53–68, 1963.
31. Giles, E.O.: Sex determination by discriminant function analysis of the mandible. *Am J Phys Anthropol, 21:* 129–135, 1964.

32. Dittrick, J.: Sexual dimorphism of the femur and humerus in prehistoric Central California skeletal samples, thesis. California State University, Fullerton, 1979.

33. Anderson, J.E.: *The human skeleton: A manual for archaeologists.* Natural Museum of Canada, 1962.

34. Stewart, J.H., and McCormick, W.F.: The gender predictive value of sternal length. *Am J Phys Anthropol, 4:* 217–220, 1983.

35. Jit, I., Jhinger, V., and Kulkarui, M.: Sexing the human sternum. *Am J Phys Anthropol, 53:* 217–224, 1980.

36. McCormick, W.F.: Sternal foramena in man. *Am J Phys Anthropol, 2:* 249–252, 1981.

37. Stewart, T.D.: Anterior femoral curvative: Its utility for race identification. *Hum Biol, 34:* 49–62, 1962.

38. Giles, E.O., and Elliot, O.: Race identification from cranial measurements. *J Forensic Sci, 7:* 147–157, 1962.

39. Ousley, S.D., and Jantz, R.L.: FORDISC 2.0 Personal Computer Forensic Discriminant Function. Anthropology Department. University of Tennessee, Knoxville, 1996.

40. Craig, E.A.: Intercondylar shelf angle: A new method to determine race from the distal femur. *J Forensic Sci, 40:* 777–782, 1995.

41. Trotter, M., and Gleser, G.C.: Estimation of stature from long bones of American whites and Negroes. *Am J Phys Anthropol, 10:* 463–514, 1952.

42. Trotter, M., and Gleser, G.C.: A re-evaluation of estimation of stature based on measurements of stature taken during life and of long bones after death. *Am J Phys Anthropol, 16:* 79–123, 1958.

43. Capasso, L., Kennedy, K.A.R., and Wilczak, C.A.: *Atlas of occupational markers on human remains.* Edigrafital S.P.A. Teramo, Italy, 1999.

Chapter VI

FORENSIC ODONTOLOGY

Part 1

BITE MARK IDENTIFICATION

RICHARD R. SOUVIRON

Introduction and History of Forensic Odontology

THE USE OF TEETH and dental structures for the identification of unknown remains has a long documented history. The teeth and dental apparatus are virtually indestructible and will remain intact almost indefinitely.[1-6] Dental structures have been used by archeologists and anthropologists for centuries. The first known recording of dental identification was made by Junker, who used two molars linked together by gold wire for identification of body parts located in a tomb at Giza. In the eighteenth century Paul Revere, a practicing dentist, used a bridge he constructed to identify General Earl Warren who was killed at the battle of Bunker Hill and buried in a mass grave.[7-9] The Webster Parkman case of 1849 was the first documented case in which dental identification was used in the courts of the United States.[4]

Dr. Oscar Omodeo published the first textbook describing the science of Forensic Dentistry in 1898, *L'Art Dentaire En Medicine Legale*. It was not until 1966, that the next textbook devoted entirely to Forensic Dentistry was published by Gustafson.[10] This text was followed closely by the publication by Luntz and Luntz, *Hand Book for Dental Identification*.[9] Since the mid twentieth century there have been numerous chapters in text such as this on the use of forensic odontology. However, the most complete and detailed text available today is *The Manual of Forensic Odontology*, Third Edition, edited by Bowers and Bell, 1995, a publication of the American Society of Forensic Odontology.

The basis for dental identification is the statement that *"no two sets of teeth are identical."* When taken in toto a computer analysis of the dental structures reveals more than 2.5 billion different possibilities in charting the human dental structure.[11] Even in identical twins the dental structures are different.[12,13] The adult dentition has 32 teeth, including the third molars, with five surfaces on each tooth, a total of 160 possible combinations. Combined with root formations and alveolar boney structures, it is easy to understand the 2.5 billion possibilities. When considering dental restorations, root canals, root canal fillings, post and core, pins, anatomic anomalies, enamel pearl, dens in dente and anomalies such as fractured and chipped teeth, the combination of possibilities may exceed 2.5 billion.

Generally speaking, the greater the amount of body destruction, the greater the importance of dental identification. Enamel, which is 98% inorganic, is the hardest, most durable part of the human body. Until the recent advent of DNA identification, fingerprint and dental were the major scientific methods of identification where the body was subject to severe traumatic injury, incineration, decomposition or skeletanization. In cases where there has not been total tissue destruction dental identification may be helpful where no fingerprint records exist. Dental, fingerprint and DNA are the most reliable forms of body identification. Numerous identification errors exist based upon visual identification and/or personal effects.[12-16] The emotional trauma pro-

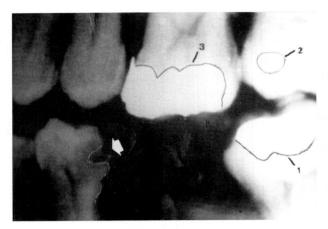
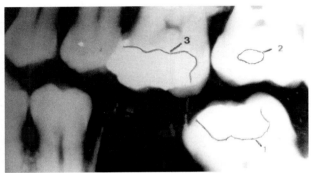

FIGURE VI-1a–b. (a) Postmortem x-ray (bitewing) of decomposed body. Note large decay (arrow) on lower second bicuspid. (b) Antemortem x-ray depicting the change in a lower right bicuspid with decay occurring subsequent to the fillings and prior to death. Antemortem, has no decay on bicuspid but positive identification is made.

duced to the next of kin during visual identification should be a consideration when other identification means, such as dental or fingerprint identification, exist. Civil aviation disasters emphasize the importance of positive identification by methods other than visual, i.e., dental and/or fingerprints.

Dental identification is performed by comparing antemortem dental records with postmortem records. Dental x-rays are the most reliable for comparison identification (Fig. VI-1a–b). In addition to x-rays, dental charts and family photographs are used routinely in performing identification. In the event of an unknown body, antemortem dental records may be available from the U.S. Department of Justice National Crime Information Center, if a missing person report had been filed.[17–19]

POSTMORTEM DENTAL EXAMINATION

Postmortem dental examinations are usually performed at a coroner or medical examiner office. Occasionally, the examination may be performed at a funeral home or at an exhumation site.

Three major components of a postmortem dental examination are photographs, x-rays and dental charting. The dental x-ray is the most reliable form of dental identification when antemortem x-rays are available.[20–22] When antemortem x-rays are not available, an antemortem photograph of the anterior teeth, a smiling photograph, if enough anomalies are present, may provide positive identification (Fig. VI-2). Dental chart comparisons, in most situations, are the least reliable of the three identification modalities.[23,24] Should an unknown decomposed or burned victim be released for burial (no cremation should be permitted), jaw resection and preservation may be performed at the discretion of the medical examiner or coroner. This prevents needless exhumations should identification leads occur.

CRIME SCENE, CRASH SCENE, DISCOVERY SITE

The recovery of body parts from the crime scene, crash scene, or discovery site is the responsibility of the medical examiner/coroner and his staff. Police and fire agencies are not trained in

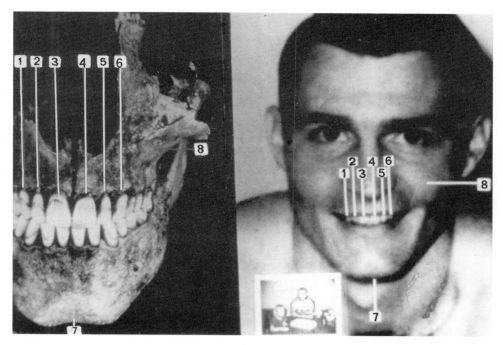

Figure VI-2. Dental identification was thought impossible when a skull with 32 perfect teeth was discovered. A family of a missing person supplied a smiling photograph sufficient to match with the teeth.

recognizing dental parts. Often a combination of high impact trauma and fire complicate aviation crash investigations. Teeth will be scattered along with the body parts. Proper dental evidence recovery at the scene means the difference between a rapid identification or a prolonged agonizing process. When skeletanization occurs, teeth, particularly the maxillary and mandibular anterior teeth, will separate from their sockets. These teeth have conical shaped roots. When the periodontal ligament, which holds the teeth in place, deteriorates, the teeth may fall out and often maggot and beetle activity will bury the teeth several centimeters below the surface. A large ground area beneath the skull should be dug to the level of unstained soil and retained for sifting at the medical examiner facility. Animal activity at the scene will scatter the skull and teeth. In homicide cases, dental evidence is sometimes removed by the perpetrator to prevent identification of the victim. More commonly, the heads and hands of individuals are removed to prevent identification.

Police officer, Gerald Schaffer who was convicted of kidnaping and murdering 28 young girls wrote about his murders detailing his efforts for removal of the head and teeth to prevent body identification. Officer Schaffer was trained in the importance of body identification for the investigation and prosecution of homicide cases.

In another homicide case, a body was found floating in a remote South Florida canal. A perforating gunshot wound of the abdomen was present. The hands and head were missing (Fig. VI-3a). Weeks later the body was identified by use of an antemortem photograph which demonstrated a peculiar pattern of birthmarks on the left arm. Ten years later a skull was found with no skeletal remains in the same vicinity (Fig. VI-3b–c). Original dental records safeguarded in the medical examiner case file readily established identity. The skull had also been perforated by a bullet. The hands were never found.

It cannot be emphasized enough that a crime scene search must be thorough and complete in order to recover all possible dental evidence. Positive identifications have been made as a result of a single tooth being found at the death scene.

In this case, the victim had been missing for eight years. After Hurricane Andrew in August of 1992, a large pond in

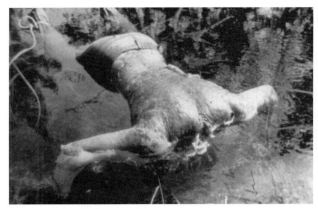

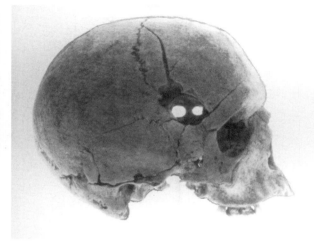

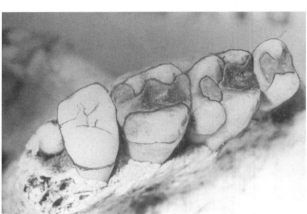

FIGURE VI-3a–c. (a) Headless and handless body found in a South Florida canal. (b) Ten years later a partial skull and half of a lower jaw were discovered in a remote South Florida area. (c) The dental records from the ten-year-old case match to the skull.

Homestead, Florida was drained and cleaned. Within the pond workers found an intact van with a license eight years old. The driver was totally decomposed and parts of the body had been removed by crabs and fish. The maxilla, but not the mandible was recovered. When first brought to the Medical Examiner's Office no front teeth were present. Crime scene investigators traced the van to the missing individual. He had no dental records, no dental treatment but did have a smiling photograph taken shortly before his disappearance. No identification was possible until front teeth could be found. While sifting through the slime and debris in the van, crime scene personnel located a single central incisor (Fig. VI-4a). The fit into the root socket was a perfect match and the unusual half moon-shaped incisal chip matched exactly to the same tooth and chip in an antemortem photograph (Fig. VI-4b). The identification was made.

DNA evidence may be obtained from teeth years or even centuries after death from mummified pulpal material. However, the process is costly and time consuming but maybe the only means left for positive body identification if dental and/or fingerprint comparison are not possible.

When teeth are removed antemortem, repair begins immediately. Within weeks of the dental extraction bone begins to form in the socket and within months the socket may be completely filled with bone. However, the outline of the previous root may remain radiographically evident for years after the extraction. In postmortem avulsion of teeth the sockets will have sharp edges and remain open and obvious.

ANTEMORTEM DENTAL RECORDS

In the case of mass disaster, such as an airline crash, a manifest of individuals on the flight is available.[25–26] In hotel fires, train and other such disasters there is usually a limited population

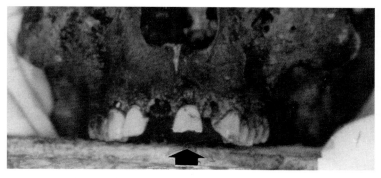

FIGURE VI-4a. A skeleton inside a van was found submerged in a lake after eight years. Anterior maxillary teeth had fallen out. The left upper cental incisor was found in mud inside the van. Identification was made by comparison with an antemortem photograph. The central incisor with visible fracture was replaced in its socket.

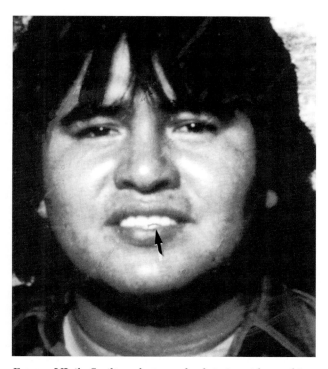

FIGURE VI-4b. Smiling photograph of victim with matching tooth deformity.

group based upon registration or manifest. In these cases, the forensic dentist and medical examiner do what they always do except, they have to do more of it and do it quicker.

Obtaining antemortem records is not the responsibility of the forensic dentist. However, many times it will be necessary for the dentist to consult with the victim's dentist to help interpret records, request a specific type of x-ray or to obtain clarification of the records that have been received. The dentist should be an integral part of the investigative staff in obtaining antemortem records in all civil or military-type disasters.

With the advent of computers the categorizing of antemortem and postmortem dental records and their eventual recovery for comparison has been made much easier and faster.[27-30] The use of CAPMI-4 (computer aided postmortem identification version 4) and WIN-ID are two programs available to provide for recording and rapid access of the antemortem and postmortem material. Our experience is that one or two highly skilled and experienced forensic dentists should input the data to minimize errors. Computerization of the antemortem records is most useful to hasten the identification process when victim numbers exceed 30.

Current dental identification procedures are complicated by a great reduction of tooth decay associated with public water fluoridation programs. Many young individuals experience only orthodontic dental care. A large population group has not had any orthodontic or restorative dentistry performed.

When antemortem dental records are nonexistent or contain no radiographs then the use of a smiling family photograph has proven to be extremely beneficial both from a standpoint of accuracy and speed of identification. Almost everyone has posed for a smiling photograph. Such photographs, when obtained by the investigators, should have the individual's name on the back of the photograph and a date when the photograph was taken. A photograph taken 20 years prior to death would not be as valuable as a photograph taken within the last year or two. The smiling photograph is most effective and most accurate when the population group is limited and other identifiable personal effects, drivers license, voters' registration cards and so forth are in association with the remains. Visual body identification has a greater propensity for error. With criminals, visual identification may be deliberately erroneous to conceal a crime for multiple reasons, including insurance fraud. Sometimes a bombing or arson victim is the perpetrator. His cohorts may deny that he was present to further complicate the identification. Dental and smiling photograph comparisons help to eliminate the possibility of such misidentification.

Lacking fingerprint, DNA, or unique physical anthropological evidence, dental x-ray comparisons are the most accurate means of body identification. Preparation of postmortem x-rays should be standard procedure on all dental structures even with edentulous jaws or single loose teeth.[31-33] Later, comparison opportunities may arise.

Postmortem, panoramic x-ray studies of skeletanized or decomposed individuals are extremely difficult to obtain. Far more practical and less expensive is the use of dental periapical x-rays. When preparing postmortem x-ray examinations it is recommended that Kodak double pack film be used to gain an extra set of original x-rays. When obtaining antemortem x-rays, it is important that the x-ray be documented as to the name of the individual, the date when it was taken and right versus left. Copied x-rays do not possess the Kodak orientation indentation. With such copies right or left determination may prove to be difficult, if not impossible.[34-36]

COMPARISON OF ANTEMORTEM AND POSTMORTEM DENTAL RECORDS

When comparing ante and postmortem dental records, proper orientation as to maxillary and mandibular right and left is important. As noted by the use of computer methodology, some 2.5 billion possibilities exist in comparison of dental structures.[37-39] However, if there are no dental restorations present the possibilities are greatly reduced. In these cases bone trebecular pattern, anomalies in the jaw bone (exostosis, Tori, abscesses, unusual radiolucent or radiopaque areas) are used for comparison.[40-43] Root formations, enamel pearl, dens in dent or auxiliary canals may be present and will serve as a basis for a positive identification. When dental restorations exist the comparison becomes much easier. The fact of a filling matching with the charted antemortem record by itself does create a positive identification. However, the structure of the preparation of the tooth, as revealed by the x-ray, often will be unique (see Fig. VI-1a–b). Therefore a single restoration may make a positive

identification. Many times superimposition of the antemortem and postmortem x-ray may be done.

Major discrepancies may appear between the antemortem and postmortem dental x-rays or charts. Examples such as teeth being present antemortem and not present postmortem are a function of dental procedures i.e., extractions. Restorations that change size from antemortem to postmortem may readily be explained by dental treatment prior to death but after the antemortem x-ray. It is therefore extremely important not to co-mix the antemortem and postmortem dental x-rays.

Comparison by dental chart or written record is recognized as a means of positive identification but does not produce the degree of accuracy of DNA or dental x-ray or an unusual smiling photograph. Dental charts are usually handwritten by a dentist or assistant and may be extremely difficult to interpret.[24,44] Where unusual procedures were performed that were detailed in the antemortem record and these same anomalies (root canals, restorations, pins and posts) are present postmortem, a positive identification may be made.

In the following case, the killers attempted to cover their crime by returning to the scene several times to destroy the dental evidence. They were partially successful but eventually resorted to placing dynamite on the remains and *blowing up the body.* However, a small piece of the lower jaw with three teeth was recovered some thirty feet from the explosion site (Fig. VI-5). These were the only teeth which were recovered. The suspected victims' military records were obtained. The dental records matched the postmortem x-ray of the three teeth and a positive identification was made.

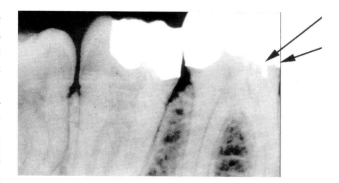

FIGURE VI-5. Postmortem x-ray showing amalgam and pins (arrows). Antemortem dental x-rays were not available but a military dental chart was. Dental charting of pin placement and amalgam restoration in the mandibular first molar coincide with the postmortem x-ray.

AGE, RACE, AND SEX DETERMINATION

The forensic dentist serves as part of the team with the coroner or medical examiner and anthropologist. An anthropologist can be helpful in determining age, race, and sex of a badly decomposed or skeletanized individual. In cases where only the skull and mandible remain the teeth, especially in young individuals up through the age of thirteen, can be accurate in age determination up to give or take six months. The basis of these identifications is primarily x-ray of the postmortem specimen and comparison with the dental aging charts in the text Massler and Schour or Furuhata, *Forensic Odontology* (1967), Thomas. As an individual approaches mid-teens to mid-twenties, dental age determination becomes more difficult and may be based upon closure of the root apices of the third molar and to a lesser degree of accuracy the eruption of the third molar. More studies and research need to be performed in this area. The latest and best information available is produced by Dr. Harry Mincer, and published in the *Journal of Forensic Sciences.*[45]

Age determination by dental means loses accuracy after the late twenties through middle age. Age determination at this point is done by *guesstimating* the individuals age, taking into consideration wear of the teeth, bone loss, and height of alveolar ridges in edentulous individuals.[46-48] If the victim is unknown, police may be misled by a poor dental age estimate and overlook a likely person. If the police receive missing person inquiries, let the forensic dentist be given the opportunity to exclude on the basis of dental opinion.

Teeth may also be used in aiding the anthropologist and medical examiner in race and sex determination. The classic is the shovel-shaped incisors which are a predominant feature in the Native American, Inuit, and Asian race.[49] The presence of a fourth molar, maxillary and mandibular diastemas are more prevalent in the black race than in either the white or Asian. Determination of the sex of skeletal or decomposed remains is more anthropological than dental. Consultation between and with the physical anthropologist, forensic odontologist and medical examiner produce the most accurate estimates of age, race, and sex.[50-51]

THE MASS DISASTER

The definition of mass disaster varies between death investigative jurisdictions. In some an incident producing five bodies or more from a single episode is a mass disaster. In other jurisdictions that have higher case loads for dental identifications, thirty or more from a single incident would be considered a mass disaster. Regardless of the individual's definition of a *mass disaster,* when numerous victims result from a single incident in which there is high impact trauma and fire with extensive body destruction, mass disaster techniques should be employed.

Forensic dentists in many areas of the United States and Canada have formed mass disaster teams or dental disaster squads, etc.[52] The teams consist of three groups, antemortem, postmortem and comparison sections. The antemortem team is responsible for consulting with the medical examiner and medical examiner investigators, categorizing the information received from the antemortem dentist, consultations with the family and antemortem dentist when obtaining the records (including the smiling family photograph).[53] A forensic dentist team member, knowledgeable with computers and the CAPMI-4 or WIN-ID programs should enter the antemortem records into the computer.[27] The forensic dental literature is replete with guidelines and procedures for forming mass disasters teams.[52,54]

The postmortem dental team should be experienced dentists, preferably forensic dentists with qualifications in body identification, to examine, chart, photograph and x-ray the postmortem material. The comparison team should consist of the chief forensic odontologist for the jurisdiction who should have the final responsibility for comparison of postmortem and antemortem dental records and be responsible for the establishment of the positive identification.[53] In cases where no antemortem dental records exist and the comparison has to be made from a family photograph matched to postmortem x-rays and photographs, such comparison technique should be performed by a board certified forensic dentist, reviewed and concurred with by at least two other qualified colleagues.

SMILING PHOTOGRAPH IDENTIFICATION

The appearance of one's smile can be altered dramatically by changing the position and the color of the upper anterior teeth. This can be done in several ways. Gold teeth can be purchased along with a complete set of upper removable anterior teeth from mail order sources. Dentists also have the ability to provide an individual with gold, steel or porcelain removable jacketed teeth (Fig. VI-6a–c). The knowledge of this technique has been used by criminals to disguise their appearance.

PROSTHETIC DEVICE IDENTIFICATION

Many people, particularly institutionalized and even the homeless, may possess complete upper and lower dental prostheses. When confronted with a totally edentulous individual for identification, accurate photographic records should be made with and without the prosthesis in place. The prostheses should also be photographed outside the mouth. The under surface of the prosthesis may contain vital information for the identification. Ideally the prosthesis will contain the name of the individual or a code number that may be traced (Fig. VI-7). Prosthetic devices may be switched during hospital or nursing home care. This problem should be taken into consideration when dealing with complete removable prostheses.

Full dentures are made from various materials and the teeth of the full dentures can be either plastic, composite or porcelain. The commercial teeth will have numbers and designations on the lingual surfaces or the under surface that may provide valuable information to the investigating odontologist.

The jaws of the deceased with or without teeth should be examined carefully for lesions and a full series of x-rays prepared. Retained root tips,

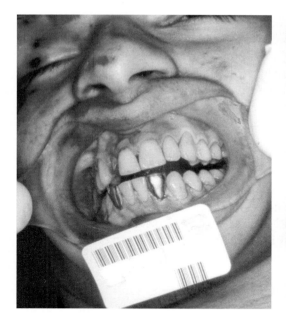

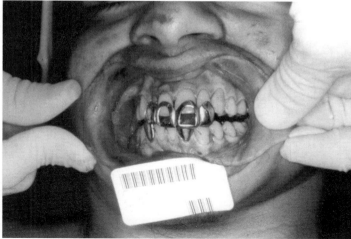

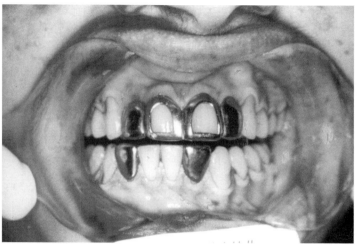

FIGURE VI-6a–c. Dental apparatus can be used specifically to mask an identity. (a) Suspect with natural maxillary incisors. (b) Gold shell crowns found at crime scene being placed over teeth. (c) Perfectly fitted, gold crowns in place and used as an effective disguise and can be placed and removed at will.

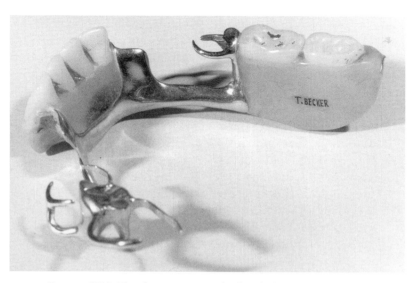

FIGURE VI-7. The denture is inscribed with the wearer's name.

impacted teeth, supernumerary teeth and other radiographic anomalies including bullet fragments found within the jaw bone can be used for comparison with antemortem films or medical records. The partial denture or removable bridge usually does not contain identification numbers or the name of the individual but may be very specific as to its attached teeth. Preparation or precision rests will be located on the support teeth and indeed the denture may be fitted directly into the mouth to determine that it belongs to a particular victim. If no antemortem records exist a dentist may recognize his work. As a last resort photographs or even the entire denture or bridge may be sent to the *dentist of record* for identification.

Fixed prostheses such as bridges and crowns and implants are a much more specific means of identification (Fig. VI-8). With general acceptance of implants for replacing missing teeth, antemortem records for dental comparison are usually available. In excess of 23 different implant systems are available in the United States. Radiographic examination of the implanted prosthesis and consultation with a manufacturer will narrow the field in cases of unknown individuals.

Because of the high cost of implant prostheses the social economic level of the unknown victim, more likely than not, would be high. The exceptions would be persons that receive implants in dental schools and other teaching facilities. Laboratory prescriptions to the dental laboratory are another means of cross-referencing identifications. In most cases individuals that have extensive fixed crown and bridge work along with dental implants have a dentist of record and antemortem records are usually complete. Identification can be made quite quickly. In comparison, the full denture wearer may not have visited a dentist in decades. Antemortem records may be non-existent. There may, however, be unusual characteristics in the denture that can be compared with an antemortem smiling photograph such as a broken front tooth, a space between the teeth, or a gold decorative crown.

In summation, the dental x-ray followed by the smiling photograph and/or dental chart are used to determine body identification, especially in deaths where there is decomposition, skeletanization, incineration, or high impact trauma. Dental identification is used most often where decomposition and skeletanization render fingerprints and DNA impractical or impossible.

BITE MARK EVIDENCE

Bite marks are patterns produced when teeth contact a softer material. Bite marks have been described as tool marks. Similarities exist in their examination. At crime scenes bite marks may be found on inanimate objects such as apples, chewing gum, cheese, moon pies, cookies, etc. Teeth may leave marks on steering wheels, dashboards and even hoods of automobiles. The biter may be the attacker, the victim, or both. Teeth marks on the hands and forearms of the attacker may indicate defensive wounds and on the knuckles of hand or fingers when the victim was struck in the mouth. In many cases, bites are left by animals, predominantly dog, on humans. Animal bites may be ante- or postmortem. The differentiation between animal bites and human bites will be discussed later in this chapter.

During the latter half of the twentieth century, analysis and utilization of bite mark evidence has truly made a major contribution to the criminal justice system. The first known bite mark that reached the appellate court level in the United States is *Doyle vs. Texas* in 1952. (Doyle vs State, 159 page 1, Texas Criminal 310,311,263S.W.2nd d, 779,1954). This concerned a bite mark in cheese, not human flesh. Approximately 20 years ensued before the next major bite mark case occurred. This case set a legal precedent in the United States in several respects. The bite was inflicted in skin. The bite was inflicted in an area (nose) of the body in which a three-dimensional replica of the suspect's teeth could be generated. Comparison evidence was obtained from the suspect with the use of a search warrant.

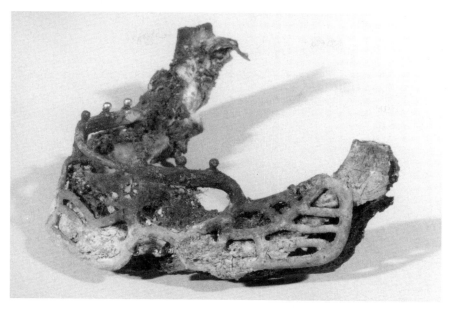

FIGURE VI-8. Lower jaw of charred body showing extensive implant device. Totally unburnt and easy to identify.

California vs. Marx[55,56] has been used as a standard for admissibility of bite mark. As of this writing there are several hundred bite mark cases that have reached the appellate court level or higher in most states. Although somewhat outdated, an excellent legal history resource article is *Forensic Dentistry and the Law: Is Bite Mark Evidence Here to Stay?* by De La Cruz.[57]

Subsequent to the Marx case, the most controversial case in forensic dentistry occurred with the introduction of bite mark evidence by the Prosecution in People vs. Malone, 43 Illinois. App. 3d 385,356 NE. 2nd 1350 1976. Seven forensic dental experts testified (four for the Prosecution and three for the Defense) and 1,300 pages of bite mark testimony were generated, a record not broken to this day.

Again, bite mark evidence became prominent when utilized in the conviction and death sentence of Theodore Robert Bundy in Miami, Florida in 1979.[58] Television and newspaper coverage throughout the United States catapulted bite mark evidence into national prominence as a new emerging forensic science (Fig. VI-9a–b).

As a result of many controversial bite mark issues within the forensic odontology communi-

ty, the American Board of Forensic Odontology established guidelines for bite mark evidence in 1984. These guidelines were further refined and updated in 1994. In addition to guidelines, a set of published standards for *bite mark terminology* was developed and approved by the American Board of Forensic Odontology (ABFO). The guidelines and standards for bite marks, as well as body identification, have been published in the *Manual of Forensic Odontology*[59] and in the *Journal of American Dental Association*.[60]

The forensic odontology community has continued to refine and improve its methodology and research in documentation of bite mark evidence. Comparison of known bite mark standards with unknowns and additional research in DNA, photography and computer digitalization has greatly increased the reliability of bite mark evidence. In 1999, the American Board of Forensic Odontology established a proficiency testing program for bite mark evidence. As of this publication the proficiency testing is voluntary. Within future years it is predicted that proficiency testing for bite mark experts will be required in order to obtain recertification by the American Board of Forensic Odontology.

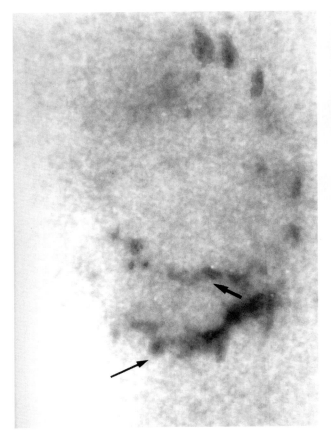

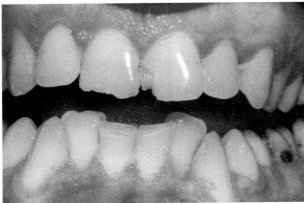

FIGURE VI-9a–b. (a) Bite mark corresponds with teeth of Theodore Bundy. Bite mark reveals a double lower tooth bite mark with crooked teeth. *Top of picture:* Three drag patterns consistent with sharp broken edges of upper teeth. (b) Teeth of Theodore Bundy taken from newspaper photograph of Bundy's smiling face.

BITE MARK VS. FINGERPRINT

As a result of high profile cases with bite mark evidence linking the attacker to the victim, such evidence has been compared in lay publications to fingerprints. Terms such as *"positive identification," "positive match"* and the bite mark was left by the suspect *"indeed and without a doubt,"* have been addressed in the ABFO bite mark guidelines and determined to be unacceptable.[61] Nevertheless, within the criminal justice system, police, prosecutors, defense and especially news media refer to bite marks with the same level of certainty for identification as fingerprints. However, nothing could be further from the truth. Indeed bite mark evidence is vastly different from fingerprint evidence.

Fingerprints and DNA will produce a *positive* identification. A fingerprint cannot be altered or changed into another classifiable pattern with time or with mechanics. The Federal Bureau of Investigation has maintained fingerprint files with literally millions of fingerprints classified with the name and identification of individuals. Specialists work full-time with fingerprint identification and matching. Fingerprints have a long history in the criminal justice system dating back to the early 1900s. With fingerprints there is a point scale and depending upon the agency there is a specific number of points of comparison that would render a positive match between the latent print and the suspect. With computerization rapid identifications may be made with fingerprints. DNA likewise does not change with time, indeed DNA evidence can be obtained from body parts such as the dentinal pulp that are centuries old.

Bite marks *do not* render positive identifications when related to the *world population.* Although it is a generally recognized scientific fact that no two sets of teeth are alike, i.e., they are unique,[62] the bite pattern left by these teeth cannot produce an accurate enough recording in skin or food stuffs to eliminate a world population group. Conversely, it is recognized that bite mark evidence can be 100% exclusionary in certain situations.

Unlike a fingerprint, the teeth of a suspect can be changed by means of dental restorations, self-inflicted mutilation, or even extraction. There is no national depository of bite marks that can be used as a standard to measure individuality. There are no recognized number of specific points of comparison in order to make a match. Indeed there is no *positive match* with bite marks. According to the terminology of the standards of the ABFO the highest degree of certainty is *"reasonable medical certainty, extremely probable, a high degree of certainty which means virtually certain no reasonable or practical probability that someone else could have done it."* As a result of no national depository for bite marks (highly impractical because of the ability to change the teeth) rapid computerization for comparisons is not possible. It takes a great deal of time for a forensic odontologist to analyze and compare bite mark evidence.

With the negative comparison between bite mark, DNA, and fingerprint evidence propounded in the previous paragraphs, there is much positive to be said about bite mark evidence when compared with fingerprints or DNA. Most important is that a *good* bite mark may yield clues as to the dental profile of a suspect. For instance, gaps between the teeth, a tooth out of line, a missing tooth, a chipped tooth, all can be recorded whether it is skin or an object such as chewing gum, cheese, or bologna.

Unlike a fingerprint, a bite mark is a sign of violence when left in human flesh, whether it was inflicted defensively or offensively. Bite marks can be an aid in determining the age of a biter. The differentiation between the deciduous dentition (baby or milk teeth) and that of the adult or mixed dentition can give some clue as to the chronologic age, i.e., child, young adult, or adult perpetrator.[63] This is of special significance in cases of suspected child abuse where the allegation is often made by an adult perpetrator that another child in the home has inflicted the bite mark.

A bite mark, if inflicted hard enough, will produce a permanent injury. There have been documented cases of bite mark injury pattern existing for months or years resulting in patterned scarring (Fig. VI-10a–b). This particular point can be extremely important in non-homicide cases where battery was involved. One of the requirements for aggravated battery, which carries a far more serious sentence than a simple battery, is the production of a permanent injury. Finally, in court, fingerprints or DNA evidence is explained totally by a forensic expert (a side-by-side comparison) to the jury. With bite mark evidence the jury can actually compare 1:1 photographs and the suspect's teeth models (direct comparison). This is done in several ways, by the use of acetate overlays (discussed later in this chapter), direct placement of the models to the bite mark, 1:1 photograph (Fig. VI-11a–b), and production of test bite marks in media such as wax, styrofoam, or *silly putty* to illustrate certain class and individual characteristics of the bite. Many times the jury will perform their own experiments with this evidence in order to confirm or reject the testimony of the prosecution or defense expert.

BITE MARK RECOGNITION AND ANALYSIS

The recognition of an injury as a bite mark is the first step. The medical examiner, criminologist, crime scene investigator, emergency department nurse, physician, or police have the first opportunity to *discover* a bite mark. Much like a fingerprint or DNA, if the evidence is not recognized, recorded, and preserved it is of little or no value. In addition to the recognition of a pattern injury being a bite mark, the forensic dentist should be called to the scene or the medical examiner's office as quickly as possible to record this evidence. Portions of bite mark evidence are

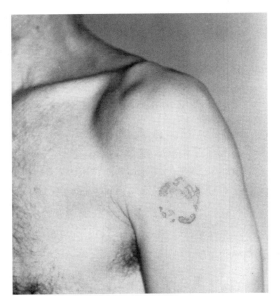

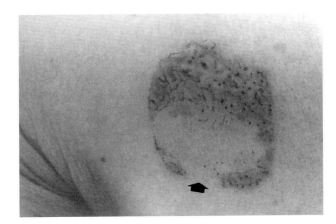

FIGURE VI-10a–b. (a) Persistent bite pattern over a year old in a living person. (b) Pattern indicates a space (arrow) in the lower anterior part of the mouth, a missing or partially missing tooth.

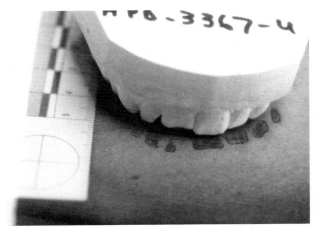

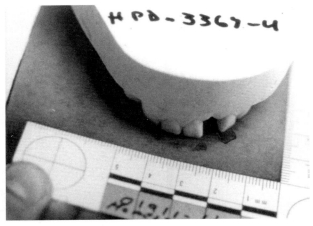

FIGURE VI-11a–b. Comparison of suspect's model with 1:1 photograph of bite mark. (a) Maxillary model over life sized photograph of the bite mark. (b) Mandibular model with missing lower tooth conforms with the skin pattern injury.

ephemeral. The changes occur rapidly if the bite is inflicted on a living individual. However, it may not change much in a decedent except for decomposition and livor. Autopsy incisions through or near the bite will distort the evidence. A team approach is needed in all cases involving bite mark evidence.

The analytical approach to bite mark evidence follows certain steps. First, is the pattern injury artifact or indeed a mammalian bite mark? If a mammalian bite, is it human or animal? If human, determine which pattern represents upper teeth and which lower teeth. Pathologists may find this difficult. Next is to determine the dental profile of the perpetrator. The forensic dentist, not necessarily the pathologist or police, may detect patterns of dental anomalies in the bite mark (Fig. VI-12a–c). Spaces between the upper front teeth, rotated or out of place teeth, a specific missing individual tooth or even the

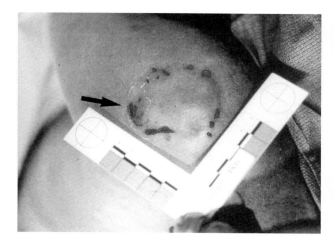

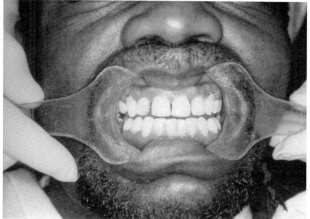

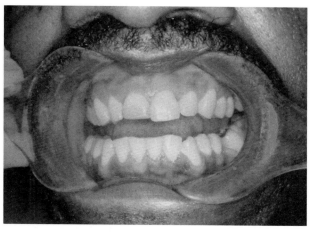

FIGURE VI-12a–c. (a) The left upper central incisor has produced a prominent mark (arrow) indicating a shortened or missing right upper central incisor. (b) A suspect is excluded because both upper central incisors are the same length. (c) Another suspect with a fractured right upper central incisor can be excluded.

presence of all the teeth are important in eliminating individuals as suspects.

The most important and difficult aspect of the evaluation of bite mark evidence is the initial analysis of the pattern injury. Postmortem insect activity, laying in gravel, EKG pads, or other medical devices can produce pattern injuries that will mimic a bite mark. Even dentists have confused serpiginous ant bite patterns with human bites. Dog bites are often an early consideration where pattern injuries are found on the deceased.

Once the pattern injury is determined to be a human bite, the next step is initial photographic documentation. Photographs should be taken before the body is cleaned or the bite pattern disturbed. Orientation photographs are essential.

The closer views should be both plain and with a proper scale. The use of the ABFO #2 scale is recommended in all bite mark cases. It will help determine size, color balance (grey scale) and parallax.[64]

The second step is the collection of salivary DNA. This is covered in great detail later in the chapter.

Following the collection of the DNA samples additional photographs are taken. Occasionally a bite occurs in an area where the change of position of an extremity will alter the bite pattern (Fig. VI-13a–c). Photographs should be taken of the bite with the extremity at both extremes of position and midway. One does not know the dynamics of the struggle at the time the bite was

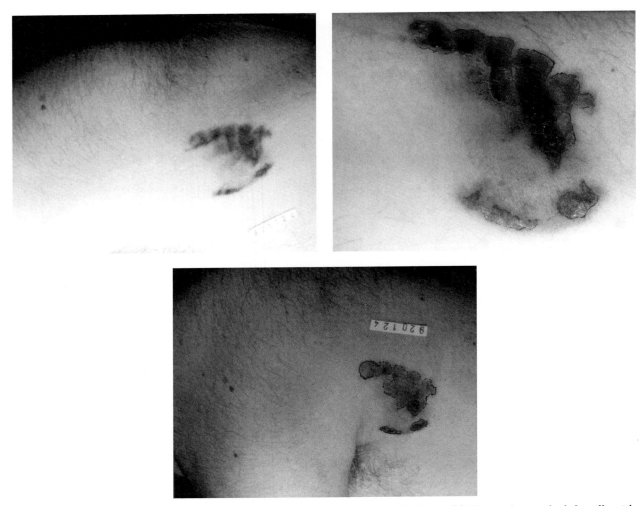

FIGURE VI-13a–c. Distortion of bite pattern by postmortem manipulation of the body. (a) Bite mark near the left axilla with arm raised. (b) Closer view. (c) Arm at side. There is a change in the width and appearance due to arm manipulation.

inflicted so consider all the possibilities. Body areas with flaccid, loose tissue are most susceptible to distortion from any pattern injury, especially a bite mark. The amount of tissue taken into the mouth before the bite is inflicted will dramatically alter the static pattern on the tissue (Fig. VI-14). The action of the victim will also influence the final tissue pattern of the bite. The examiner must be aware of these dynamics and factor them into his analysis. The use of reflective ultraviolet light, color photography, digital photography, infrared photography will be discussed later in this chapter. Follow-up photographs taken on a daily basis, on both living and deceased victims, may provide additional evidence for a more accurate evaluation. A hard

bite inflicted on a living victim results in profound changes over time, beginning with swelling and extravasation of blood into the area followed by fading and color changes that occur during the healing process with eventual crusting followed by pigment loss. The different stages of healing may reveal better clarity for individual tooth characteristics.

The forensic dentist should perform a detailed accurate analysis of both individual and class characteristics. The forensic dentist should be able to differentiate between the maxillary and the mandibular arches, make direct measurements from the skin using dividers or calipers and record individual characteristics such as spaces between teeth, crooked, protruding, bro-

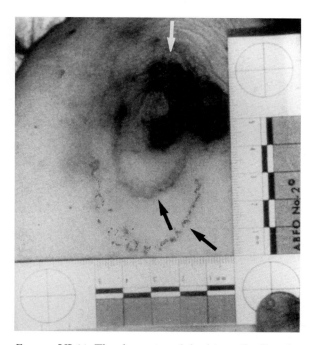

FIGURE VI-14. The dynamics of the bite will affect the static tissue pattern. Bite on breast shows lower teeth with double bite. Upper teeth (white arrow) caused severe contusion, laceration and distortion. Individual teeth identification not possible. Lower double teeth bite mark (black arrows) leaves identifiable pattern. One bite appears half again as large as the other.

ears. There was an alternate theory that perhaps an alligator was also involved and responsible for the death. This theory was subsequently disapproved by close analysis of the bite mark and claw patterns. Lion, grizzly bear, shark, and alligator have been responsible for human death but these are relatively rare. Distinguishing between the bite being the cause of death or postmortem activity is the ultimate responsibility of the coroner or medical examiner.

The human bite mark has characteristics that may be described as two oval or semilunar arches or half rings approximating each other. In many bite mark cases, one or the other arch does not mark. There are several explanations for this. The dynamics of the bite may produce more prominence on the right or the left side. A single arch bite may result, particularly if such things as clothing, or hard objects, as a finger, are interposed over one of the arches. Movement or twisting of a victim during the time that he is being bitten alters the configuration of the bite.

Individual tooth characteristics, when identifiable are used to establish the dental profile of the biter. In a *good* bite mark both the maxillary and mandibular teeth will mark. However, exact measurements may rarely be made of the incisal width of the teeth which created the pattern. Even in the clearest bite patterns, bleeding (bruising) tends to obliterate exact outlines. Nevertheless, spaces between the teeth may readily be demonstrated. Sharp, pointed or broken teeth will register. A missing tooth will not register, but crowding, protruding, flattened, rotated and angled teeth will. All of these individual characteristics are extremely important for documentation during the examination and will be used by the examiner in creating a dental profile (Fig. VI-16a–b).

A difficult, yet important, aspect is the aging of the pattern injury. Reference literature indicates great discrepancy in bite marks inflicted on living individuals as to the effect of healing and age determination of the bite.[65–68] Skin color, site of the bite, biting pressure and health of the victim create variables in the patterns which affect age estimation. When the wound is inflicted at or near the time of death the pattern injury will remain unchanged for a much longer period of

ken, or missing teeth. In his final analysis the forensic odontologist maybe able to establish a dental profile, which will be valuable for the police investigator and add to the credibility of the examiner.

Class characteristics denote the arch form. Human bite marks leave a pattern injury that is distinguished from that of most animals. The human canine or cuspid teeth located at the corners of the mouth do not as a rule protrude much past the plane of occlusion of the centrals and lateral incisors. In animal bites (canine, feline, bear, etc.) the canine basically is the fourth tooth, not the third from the mid-line and is used for gripping, holding, and indeed killing the victim. Dog bites are by far the most common animal bites left on humans (Fig. VI-15a–b). Although dog bites are the most common animal bite the forensic dentist will encounter they usually do not result in death. In Figure VI-15c, the victim was attacked and killed by three pit bull dogs resulting in severe facial damage especially to the

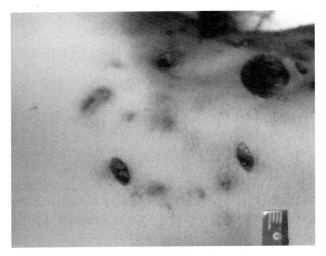
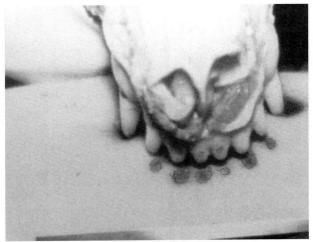
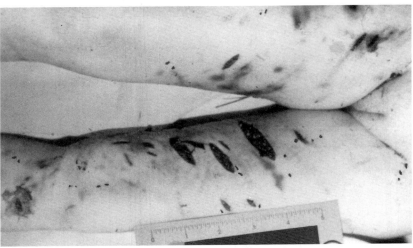

FIGURE VI-15a–c. Dogs leave both teeth and claw marks. (a) Bite pattern. (b) Upper jaw of dog fits the bite pattern. (c) Multiple dog bites and claw marks on victim.

time. Microscopic slide analysis should be part of the analysis in the deceased victim because the time of the bite reference death may become an issue. The pathologist should be aware that older literature references are most valuable when age estimates are expected to be based upon microscopic changes. Blood extravasation, without tissue crush, provokes no neutrophilic reaction. Robertson and Mansfield[69] demonstrate a five-day bruise which is indistinguishable from a fresh bruise.

When death occurs, all vital reactions stop. If the bite was inflicted immediately prior to death or immediately after death, indentations, the third dimension, will remain in the skin. This may be extremely helpful in determining the time of infliction of the bite in reference to the time of death.

PRESERVATION OF BITE MARK EVIDENCE

Preservation of bite mark evidence is critical. In a living victim photographic evidence is the most important means of preservation. Normally impressions and lifting of the bite pattern on a

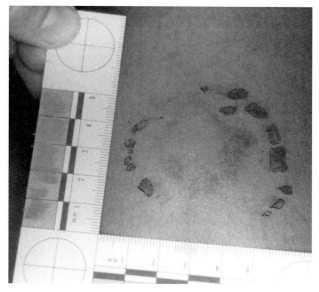

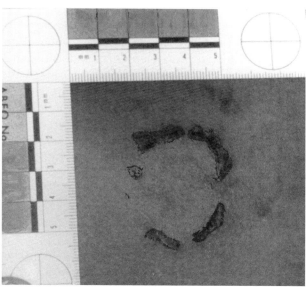

FIGURE VI-16a–b. Amount of flesh taken into mouth and variable sites affect the appearance and especially the width of the bite pattern. (a) Left arm (b) Right shoulder. Victim survived and described the attack. The key dental profile is on the shoulder. A lower right central incisor is missing or broken off and upper left central and lateral incisors are chipped.

living subject are futile because of the delay of the examination following the infliction of the bite.

When the bite is inflicted at or about the time of death the preservation process is five fold:

First and most important is photographic preservation of the bite mark with the ABFO scale in place.

Second is the swabbing of the bite wound for salivary DNA. No salivary DNA evidence can be expected if the bite was inflicted through clothing or other such media. The investigator should be aware of this and be very careful in preserving any garment that might have been placed in the area of the bite.

Third, following photography and saliva DNA sample collection, is the lifting of the bite mark with fingerprint powder. The dusting of the bite with carbon powder or other standard fingerprint technique, the lifting of the bite mark with tape or even better with the footprint lifter will preserve the *bite print* (Fig. VI-17a–b). The bite print having been lifted can be analyzed visually and well preserved for later analysis.[70] Additionally, fingerprint powder has been shown to pick up indentations in the skin which were not readily visible to the naked eye.[71] This is important in determining the length of time between the infliction of the bite and the time of death.

The fourth step is the three-dimensional impression of the bite wound. This is performed today very readily and quickly with the use of 3M-Express® polyvinylsolixate (PVS) impression material.[72] Once the material has been applied utilizing the mixing tube and dispensing gun, a backing media is applied to the tacky material. It can be a perforated acrylic tray, Hexclite orthopedic mesh, or dental stone, all of which will prevent distortion of the impression. Once the material has set and been removed from the body, the indentations and actual outline, if present in the skin, will be duplicated and preserved. It should be noted that the impression is a negative of the actual bite and a dental stone pour into the PVS material will produce a positive of the skin and bite. If there are no indentations in the skin obviously there will be no recording of indentation with the footprint lifter or with the impression material.

The fifth step is the actual removal of the tissue. This is usually done under the direction and approval of the chief medical examiner. Extreme

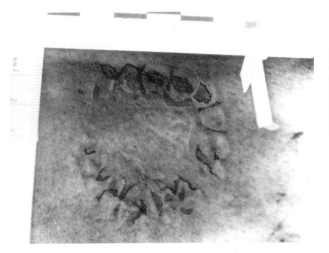
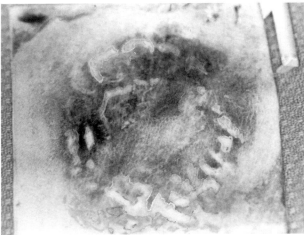

FIGURE VI-17a–b. Pattern enhancement with fingerprint powder. (a) Retention of pattern with the footprint lifter. (b) The lifted pattern reveals indentations of the flesh indicating a perimortem or postmortem bite without vital reaction.

caution should be taken if a body is viewable and the marks are in a sensitive area such as the cheek, forehead, chin, or lips. Consultation with the medical examiner, family members, the detectives and the prosecutor may be indicated before excision of the bite wound is performed. The funeral director should also be aware of this procedure and its importance to the overall investigation.

The analysis and transillumination of the bite tissue sample may aid in a more accurate opinion.[73] The procedure for removing the tissue after the impressions have been made is as follows. The tissue is cleaned and a *support ring* is formed around the bite mark. If the tissue is removed from the body without a support ring there is a 20–40% distortion factor, depending upon the area of the body. The most effective method of stabilizing the tissue is to perform a customized dental acrylic support ring (Fig. VI-18a–c). This can be molded and shaped to the body and once it sets it is extremely hard. The superior and inferior medial and lateral areas are marked with an indelible pen both on the acrylic ring and on the tissue itself. The ring is then removed, cyanoacurate (crazy glue) is applied to the ring, it is placed back onto the tissue in exactly the same location in which it was made. To further secure the tissue to the support ring it is sutured in place with either interrupted or mattress-type sutures. At no point should the tissue ring be closer than one centimeter to the bite. Once the ring is secured to the tissue an incision is made on the outer edge of the ring and the entire epidermis, dermis, and subcutaneous fat and muscle layers are removed. Photographs should be taken of the underside of the tissue as well as the bite mark. This demonstrates the depth of bleeding and the relative amount of pressure necessary to have caused this injury. The tissue will be used for additional photography analysis with transillumination. Once the forensic odontologist has completed the bite mark tissue analysis it may be preserved with 10% formalin, refrigerated, placed in Keiserlings solution, or it can be frozen. A section may be removed for histopathology study and correlation with tissue reaction of other injuries on the victim.

In homicide cases, where the victim is to be cremated, prepare a dental impression and dental photographs of the victim's teeth. The victim may have bitten the attacker during the altercation. There may also be bite marks on the victim that could have been self-inflicted. The forensic odontologist must be able to explain all the possible contingencies. Saliva samples and blood for DNA study should be taken from the victim.

Vale and Noguchi reported 67 bite mark cases and recorded the percentages of bites on different areas of the body. The highest percentage, 37.3%, involved the arms. If fingers and hands were included, the percentage rose to 43.3%.

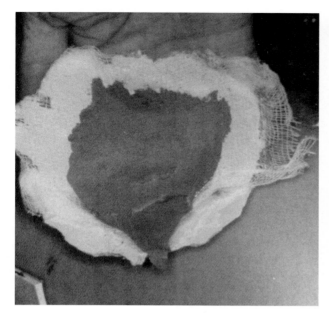
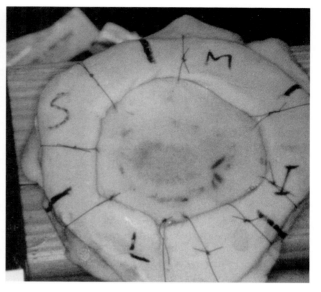
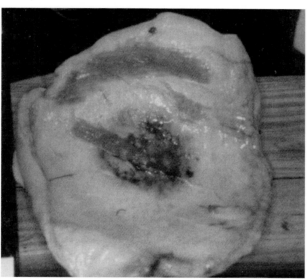

Figure VI-18a–c. Various techniques. (a) Three-dimensional impression with rubber base material and dental stone backing. (b) Removal of tissue using acrylic ring and sutures. (c) Removal of tissue into the muscle layer reveals deep hemorrhage indicating a painful crushing type trauma.

The breast is next in frequency, 22%. Multiple bites existed in 40%. With males as the bite victims, 50% were located on upper extremities or back.[74]

BITE MARKS ON INANIMATE OBJECTS

Investigators should consider the possibility of partially eaten food discarded at the crime scene. Numerous literature citations and especially the initial Doyle versus Texas appellate case relate to bite patterns of evidentiary value other than in skin. Most common food substances with the perpetrator's teeth marks are apple, chewing gum, cheese, sausage and other firm foods.[75] Styrofoam® cups, pencils and other non-food objects have been found with teeth marks. With perishable items extreme care should be taken to rapidly record and preserve this evidence. Criminalists and crime scene investigators have developed methods for doing this. Some, but not all, include the use of cyananoacrilate, freezing, photographic preservation and dental impression materials.

A Moon Pie® was found at the scene of a triple homicide (Fig. VI-19). It was important to know if the attacker or one of the victims had left the half-eaten moon pie. Rapid differentiation between the potential biters was based on the dental profile of the individual who bit the Moon Pie®. He had a left central incisor out of line *buck*

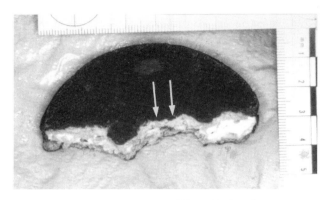

FIGURE VI-19. Bite pattern in Moon Pie® indicating protruding upper anterior teeth, *buck toothed* appearance (white arrows).

tooth. None of the three victims had such a dental anomaly and were excluded.

RECOVERING BITE MARK EVIDENCE FROM THE SUSPECT

If a suspect realizes or is told that he has inflicted a bite wound on his victim he will have the advantage of altering his teeth. Hence, confidentiality in bite mark cases is essential. In order to obtain dental impressions and bite mark evidence from a suspect the rights of the suspect must be taken into consideration. Bite mark evidence has been challenged constitutionally under the Fourth, Fifth and Sixth Amendments.

The Fifth Amendment protects citizens against *self-incriminating testimony*. However, the argument of self-incrimination as a result of a dental impression being taken, would not constitute *testimony* under guidelines established by the U.S. Supreme Court which states that physical evidence *does not* constitute *testimony*. Specifically, this was argued and a decision rendered by the Supreme Court in *Holt vs. United States*.[76] Additionally, in *Schmerber vs. California,* the Supreme Court of California concurs that taking of dental impressions, as physical evidence, is not a violation of the Fifth Amendment of self incrimination.[77]

The Fourth Amendment dealing with search and seizure provisions likewise does not consider the taking of physical evidence from an individual a violation of his constitutional rights, if the taking of the impressions is based on probable cause with a lawful arrest.

Likewise, the Sixth Amendment dealing with the defendants right to counsel occurs only during *critical stages* of criminal proceedings.[78] When the bite mark is deemed to be of evidentiary value and an analysis of that bite is able to produce a dental profile, the investigative authorities will have probable cause, enabling the prosecutor to obtain dental records, i.e., photographs, teeth impressions and bite records, thus satisfying the defendants constitutional rights under the Fourth, Fifth and Sixth Amendments.

In order to obtain dental impressions and bite mark evidence from a suspect, one of three procedures may be followed:

CONSENT FROM THE SUSPECT—The suspect must be notified in advance to sign a consent. If he refuses, valuable time may be lost and he may alter his teeth.

A COURT ORDER—Probable cause is a prerequisite for a court order. A court order has the disadvantage of being heard in open court with the defense attorney arguing to prevent the taking of impressions based upon the Fourth and Fifth Amendments to the Constitution.[79–82]

SEARCH WARRANT—Again probable cause is needed. The forensic odontologist's evaluation of the bite mark is needed to demonstrate unusual patterns that may have been produced by similar anomalies in the suspect's teeth. A smiling photograph or direct observation of the suspects teeth will present the comparison standard. The dental opinion may present the prosecuting attorney with evidence of probable cause to obtain a search warrant. The search warrant directs the suspect to voluntarily or involuntarily submit himself to taking of the dental records. All search warrants or court orders should contain the phrase *"reasonable force where necessary."* Most of the time the suspect is already in jail. The use of reasonable force has proven necessary on occasion where this author has found it necessary to restrain a suspect.

The examination of the suspect covers multiple facets, photography, recovery of saliva for DNA, careful examination with charting and impressions. The exact detailed procedure for obtaining salivary DNA from a suspect is discussed later in this chapter. The forensic odontologist should prepare complete oral photographs using proper macrophotographic lenses, with and without cheek retractors and the ABFO #2 scale in some of the photographs. An identification label should appear in one or more photographs so that all may be identified as to source. When completed the photographic survey should clearly record the labial, facial, occlusal, incisal and lingual aspects of the teeth, the arch configurations and any anatomic variants such as tori. Sufficient scales and identification labels are needed to permit one-to-one photographic reproductions, measurements and assured identification.

The dental examination should note abnormalities such as periodontal disease, pharmacologically induced gingival hyperplasia, mobility of the teeth, recent extractions particularly in the upper or lower anterior portions of the mouth. Fractures of the anterior teeth, if they exist, must be evaluated to determine, if possible, their age.

A wax bite or polyvinylsoloxilate bite record is taken from the suspect. The bite should be taken in protrusive as well as centric. Dental impressions of both arches are prepared with polyvinylsoloxilate (PVS). The advantages of polyvinylsoloxilate are accuracy, durability and ability to produce numerous models. If PVS is not available, Jeltrate® may be used. Models from Jeltrate® impressions must be prepared soon thereafter and only one set of models should be made from each impression. The forensic dentist should have at least three working sets of models for each jaw. One set should be the first pour *pristine* models and should be kept secure and unused. Another initial or first pour set is the actual working model. The incisal edges are marked to use for the computer acetate overlays. A third initial set should be kept in reserve in case the working model is broken, lost, or destroyed. The diagnostic models that are taken from the suspect must be poured with dental stone and not plaster of Paris. No bubbles or other defects should exist on the biting edges of the models. Great care should be taken in this regard to compare the models to intraoral photographs of the actual teeth to assure complete accuracy.

EVALUATION AND COMPARISON

Bite mark analysis, evaluation and comparison to the suspect is accomplished primarily by a series of techniques that vary among forensic odontologists. Some use clear acetate tracings (discussed subsequently), both hollow and solid volume. Life-size (1:1), as well as two or three times life-size tracings or computer generated acetates of the incisal edges, are compared with a corresponding size photograph of the bite mark. ABFO #2 scale should appear in all acetate exemplars as well as the bite mark photograph to document clearly that the size of the photograph and acetate examples are the same.

Test bites of the suspect's teeth in dental wax (Aluwax®, baseplate wax, etc.) are measured accurately with calipers and transferred to the bite mark 1:1 photograph. Conversely measurements from the bite mark can be transferred back to the test bites. Styrofoam® has been used and has advantages over wax as it is less affected by temperatures and more durable during transport. Styrofoam® does not render detail as sharp as wax. It is more useful to demonstrate class as opposed to individual characteristics. *Silly putty* has been used to produce test bites. If feasible, test bites using the suspect's models, may be reproduced on cadavers and actual skin bites compared to the victim's bite.

Subjectivity as well as objectivity occur during bite mark comparison with the suspects dental models. Some characteristics may not be readily apparent or interpreted. Numerous techniques may be needed to arrive at an interpretation. Much time is needed for the examiner to arrive at his/her final conclusion as to a suspect's teeth, vis-a-vis the bite mark. This is not a rapid process but requires time and patience from all parties, dentists, medical examiner, police, prosecutors and the courts.

ANCILLARY INFORMATION

At one time, the thinking was that ancillary case investigative information might be detrimental to the objectivity of the forensic dentist's opinion. It was thought that the bite mark photographs and suspect's models should be studied without any supplemental information. However, the history of the incident, the crime scene photographs, autopsy report and photographs are all useful to assist the forensic dentist in evaluation of the bite mark. Scene photographs depicting the victim, body position, clothing type and relationship to the bite are all very important in the interpretation of bite mark patterns.

Prejudicial criminal information about the suspect or the victim are not needed. When a forensic dentist is asked to give a second opinion, highly recommended in major crime cases, the second opinion dentist must be given the opportunity to review *all original* materials studied by the initial forensic odontologist. Duplicates may be distorted during copying and/or transportation. All crime scene photographs, the autopsy report and photographs should be furnished to the second opinion odontologist in order to assure a fair and proper interpretation.

OPINION

The final conclusion is the greatest challenge for the forensic odontologist. It has been stated numerous times that no two sets of teeth are alike, therefore no two sets of teeth can leave the same bite mark. This has never been proven with in vitro studies. The only research of bite prints involves wax impressions. No two sets of natural teeth pressed into wax leave exactly the same imprint. Wax is not the same as human flesh.[83]

In many criminal investigations the population group is limited to a small community group, parents, friends, spouse or ex-spouse, etc. In this situation the bite mark evidence may be more specific. When a bite mark is from the *general population* it is impossible to state with cer-

tainty that the suspect, to the exclusion of everyone in the world, left this bite pattern. Bite marks, unlike fingerprints and DNA, do not have a large classified population group to assess the degree of probability or even reasonable dental certainty in a formal opinion. The circumstances surrounding the event along with the physical evidence of the bite mark must be put into perspective by authorities. An advantage of bite mark evidence, unlike DNA or fingerprints, is that the jury will have the physical evidence to examine. The fact remains that for exclusionary purposes bite mark evidence may be positive. For specific inclusion, bite mark evidence may only be to a level reasonably certainty, high degree of probability but not 100% to the exclusion of the entire world population. Nevertheless, bite mark/suspect comparison can be very specific if the population group is limited.

SUMMARY

The major contributions of bite mark evidence to the criminal justice system is twofold: The determination of dental characteristics of the unknown perpetrator plus, the subsequent linking of the suspect to the victim as to approximate time of infliction of the bite mark relative to time of death, unique tooth pattern links and DNA relationships. Often overlooked in the literature is that bite marks are extremely specific for the exclusion of a suspect. This has great value for police investigators, the ability to eliminate a suspect early in the investigation.

When the limitations and advantages of bite mark evidence are considered in the totality of the case, bite prints/marks will continue to be valuable evidence for both the defense as well as the prosecution.

Editorial Comment

Two recent cases in Michigan involving bite mark evidence brought into question the reliability of standard bite mark comparison. Two defendants, Moldowan and Cristini, both convicted of sexual assault based on bite mark evidence had their convictions overturned. The Michigan Supreme Court determined that "bite mark analysis does not have the mathematical precision attached to DNA."

Courts are now re-examining previous convictions based on dental evidence. It would appear that identification based on bite mark analysis is too subjective to afford reliability beyond a reasonable doubt.

Acknowledgments

I would not have been able to have written this chapter without the assistance of several individuals. First, Mr. Lenny Wolfe, Chairman of the Forensic Imaging Department, Miami Dade County Medical Examiners Office and his entire staff. My secretary, Nichole Hardin for many hours of typing and retyping this manuscript. Mrs. Sandy Mannis for her expertise in proofing the manuscript. Professor Carol Henderson for her assistance with the legal aspects of bite mark evidence. Most important of all Dr. Joseph Davis, Chief Medical Examiner, Miami Dade County, Florida. Dr. Davis has provided me with the opportunity, the education and training and the encouragement to pursue this most exciting and interesting aspect of dentistry. He provided his expertise in contributing information to this chapter. Dr. Davis has set an example for all of us to follow in the field of forensics and has provided motivation for me to continue this endeavor.

Richard Souviron, D.D.S.

P.S. I forgot my wife of 25 years who has put up with my trips to the morgue during family occasions, holidays such as Christmas and New Years. She has been encouraging and supportive throughout this entire effort.

REFERENCES

1. Rosenbluth, E.S.: A legal identification. *Dent Cosmos, 44:* 1029, 1902.
2. Gustafson, G.: *Forensic odontology.* London: Staples Press, pp. 30, 111, 118–131, 140–164, 1966.
3. Reid, R.: On the application of dental science in the detection of crime. *J. Br. Dent. Assoc., 5:* 556, 1884.
4. Campbell, J.M.: Professor J.W. Webster eliminates Dr. George Parkman. *Dent. Mag. Oral Topics, 75:* 73, 1958.
5. Cleland, J.B.: Teeth and bites in history, literature, forensic medicine and otherwise. *Aust. J. Dent., 48:* 107–123, 1944.
6. Fry, W.K.: The Baptist Church cellar case. *Br. Dent. J., 75:* 154, 1943.

7. Forbes, E.: *Paul Revere and the world he lived in.* Sentry edition. Boston: Houghton Mifflin, 1942.

8. Luntz, L.: Historic forensic odontology, Int. Microform. *J. Leg. Med.* Vol. 7, no. 3, 1972.

9. Luntz, L., and Luntz, P.: *Handbook for dental identification.* Philadelphia: J. B. Lippincott Co., 1973.

10. Gustafson, G.: *Forensic odontology.* New York: American Elsevier Publishing Co., 1966.

11. Spitz and Fisher: *Medicolegal investigation of death.* Springfield, IL: Charles C Thomas Co., IV: pp. 118–121, 1980.

12. Sognnaes, R.F.: Talking teeth: The developing field of forensic dentistry can increasingly aid the legal and medical professions in problems of identification. *Am. Sci., 64* (4): 369–373, 1976.

13. Keiser-Nielson, S.: Dental identification: Certainty v. probability. *Journal of Forensic Sciences, 9:* 87–97, 1977.

14. Grant, E.A., Pendergast, W.K., and White, E.A.: Dental identification in the Norronic disaster. *J. Can Dent Assoc, 18:* 3, 1952.

15. Knott, N.J.: Identification by the teeth of casualties in the Aberfan disaster. *Br Dent J, 122:* 144, 1967.

16. Keiser-Nielson, S.: Proposed minimum requirements for establishing identity by teeth. *Int. Microform J. Leg. Med., 4* (4), card 7, F3-11, 1969.

17. Haglund, W.D.: The National Crime Information Center (NCIC) Missing and Unidentified Persons System Revisited. *Journal of Forensic Sciences, 38* (2), March 1993, pp. 365–378.

18. Bell, G.L.: Testing of the National Crime Information Center Missing/Unidentified Persons Computer Comparison Routine. *Journal of Forensic Sciences, 38* (1), January 1993, pp. 13–22.

19. NCIC Offline Search statistics as of 1/19/95.

20. Luntz, L.L.: Dental radiography and photography in identification. *Dent Radiogr Photogr, 40:* 83, 1967.

21. Gustafson, G., and Johanson, G.: The values of certain characteristics in dental identification. *Acta Odontol Scand, 21:* 367, 1963.

22. Cottone, J.A., and Standish, M.S.: *Outline of forensic dentistry.* Year Book Medical Publishers, Inc., 1982.

23. Knudson, K.G., and Cottone, J.A.: Complete dental charting: A medicolegal obligation. *Dental Student,* Jan: 46–54, 1984.

24. Delattre, V.F., and Stimson, P.G.: Self-assessment of the forensic value of dental records. *Journal of Forensic Sciences, 44* (5): 906–909, 1999.

25. Eckert, B.: The forensic disaster at Tenerife, the worlds greatest fatal aircraft accident. *Journal of the Forensic Sciences, Vol. 9,* pp. 236–238, 1977.

26. Dailey, J.C., and Webb, J.E.: Forensic odontology task force organization. *Military Medicine, 153,* pp. 133–137, 1988.

27. Lorton, L., and Langley, W.H.: Postmortem identification: A computer-assisted system. *Research Report,* U.S. Army Institute of Dental Research, Walter Reed Army Medical Center, Washington, D.C., 1984.

28. Siegel, R., Sperber, N.D., and Trieglaff, A.: Identification through the computerization of dental records. *Journal of Forensic Sciences, 22:* 434–442, 1977.

29. Cohen, M., Schroeder, D.S., and Cecil, J.C.: Computer-assisted forensic identification of military personnel. *Military Medicine, 148:* 153–156, 1983.

30. Morlang, W.M.: Mass disaster management update. *California Dental Association Journal, 14:* 49–57, 1986.

31. Standish, M.S., and Stimson, P.G.: Symposium on forensic dentistry: Legal obligations and methods of identification for the practioner. *The Dental Clinics of North America, 21* (1), 1977 .

32. Law, C.A., and Bowers, C.M.: Radiographic reconstruction of root morphology in skeletonized remains: A case study. *Manual of Forensic Odontology.* Edited by Bowers and Bell, 1995.

33. Mincer, H.H.: Salvaging improperly exposed or incorrectly processed radiographs. *Manual of Forensic Odontology,* Bowers and Bell, 1995.

34. *Publication D3-8; Kodak X-Omat Duplicating Film Technique Guide.* Health Sciences Division, Eastman Kodak Company, Rochester, New York.

35. Langland, O.E., Sippy, F.H., and Langlais, R.P.: Copying or duplicating radiographs. *Textbook of Dental Radiology,* 2nd ed. Springfield, IL: Charles C Thomas, pp. 314–317, 1984.

36. *Publication M3-148: Kodak Rapid Process Copy Film.* Health Sciences Division, Eastman Kodak Company, Rochester, New York.

37. Gustafson, G., and Johanson, G.: The values of certain characteristics in dental identification. *Acta Odontol Scand, 21:* 367, 1963.

38. Frykholm, K.O.: On the possibility of estimating the degree of statistical probability in odontological identification of unknown persons. *Sven. Tandlak. Tidskr., 51:* 531–536, 1964.

39. Keiser-Nielson, S.: Possible combinations between a given number of remaining or missing teeth. *Tandlaegebl., 70:* 663–665, 1966.

40. Hrdlicka, A.: Mandibular and maxillary hyperostoses. *Am J Phys Anthropol, 27:* 1–67, 1940.

41. Levesque R.P.: Torus palatinus: A clinical survey. *Georetown Dent J., 31,* 12–15, 1965.

42. Johnson, C.C., Gorlin, R., and Anderson, V.E.: Torus mandibularis: A genetic study. *Am J Hum Genet, 17:* 432–442, 1965.

43. Matthews, G.P.: Mandibular and palatine tori and their etiology. *J Dent Res, 13:* 245 (abstr. 102) 1933.

44. Knudson, K.G.: Complete dental charting: A medicolegal obligation. *Dental Student, Jan 62* (4), 1984.

45. Mincer, H.H., Harris, E.F., and Beryyman, H.E.: The A.B.F.O. study of third molar development and its use as an estimator of chronological age. *Journal of Forensic Sciences, 38* (2), 379–390, 1993.

46. Massler and Schour. The appositional life span of the enamel and dentine forming cells. *J. Dent. Res., 25,* 1946.

47. Costa, R., Jr.: Age determination of human remains. In Angel and Zimmerman, *Dating and age determination of biological materials.* London: Croom Helm Ltd., 1968.

48. Ubelaker, D.: *Human skeletal remains,* 2d ed. Washington, D.C.: Taraxacum, 1989.

49. Hooten, E.A.: On certain Eskimoid characteristics on icelandic skulls. *Am J Phys Anthropol, 1:* 53–76, 1918.

50. Liversidge, H.M., and Molleson, T.I.: Developing permanent tooth length as an estimate of age. *Journal of Forensic Sciences, 44* (5) 917–920, 1999.

51. Maples, W.R.: An improved technique using dental histology for estimation of adult age. *Journal of Forensic Sciences, 23* (4), 764–670, 1978.

52. Warnick, A.J.: Forensic Dental Identification Manual endorsed and sponsored by the Michigan Dental Association, 1989.

53. Bowers, M.C.: The crash of Alaska air flight 261. *ASFO-News Bulletin,* Spring 2000.

54. Warnick, A.J.: Dentist aid in the identification of crash victims. *Journal of the Michigan Dental Association, 69,* October, 553, 1987.

55. *People vs. Marx,* 54 Cal. App. 3d 100, 126 Cal. Rptr. 350 (Dec. 29, 1975)

56. Vale, G.L., et al.: Universal three dimensional bitemark evidence in a homicide case. *Journal of Forensic Sciences,* July, 642, 1976.

57. De La Cruz, R.A.: Forensic dentistry and the law: Is bite mark evidence here to stay? *American Criminal Law Review, 24,* Spring 4, 1987.

58. *Bundy, Theodore R. vs. State of Florida,* Supreme Court of Florida, No. 57772, June 21, 1984.

59. Bowers, C.M., and Bell, G.L.: *Manual of forensic odontology.* Colorado Springs: American Society of Forensic Odontology, 1995.

60. American Board of Forensic Odontology: Guidelines for bitemark analysis. *Journal of American Dental Association, 112,* 383–386, 1986.

61. Bowers, C.M., and Bell, G.L.: Supra, pp. 345–353.

62. Rawson, R.D., et al.: Statistical evidence for the individuality of the human dentition. *Journal of Forensic Sciences, 29,* 245–253, 1984.

63. Moorees, C.F.A.: The dentition of the growing child. Massachusetts, Harvard Univ Press, pp. 79–110, 1959.

64. Hyzer, W., and Krauss, T.C.: The bitemark standard reference scale-ABFO No. 2. *Journal of Forensic Sciences, 33* (2), 498–506, 1988.

65. Robertson, I., and Mansfield , R.A. Antemortem and postmortem bruises of the skin. *Journal of Forensic Medicine, 4* (1):2–10, 1957.

66. Bowers, C.M.: The visual aging of bitemarks, beyond the pale of forensic odontology. *News of the American Board of Forensic Odontology, 3* (1):9–12, 1995.

67. Langlois, N.E.I., and Gresham, G.A.: The ageing of bruises: A review and study of the colour changes with time. *Forensic Science International, 50:* 227–38, 1991.

68. Robertson, I., and Hodge, P.R.: Histopathology of healing abrasions. *Forensic Science, 1:* 17–25, 1972.

69. Robertson, I., et al.: Supra, pp. 8–9.

70. Rao, V.J., and Souviron, R.R.: Dusting and lifting the bite print: A new technique. *Journal of Forensic Sciences, JFSCA, 19* (1), Jan. 326–330, 1984.

71. Souviron, R.R., and Silver, W.M.: Odontoglyphics–A different system for recording bitemarks. Oral Presentation, *American Academy of Forensic Sciences,* Reno Nevada. February 2000.

72. Benson, B.W. et al.: Bitemark impressions: A review of techniques and materials. *Journal of Forensic Sciences, 33* (3), 1238–1243, 1988.

73. Dorion, R.B.J.: Transillumination of bitemark evidence. *Journal of Forensic Sciences, 32* (3), 690–697, 1987.

74. Vale, G.L., and Noguchi, T.T.: American distribution of human bite marks in a series of 67 crimes. *Journal of Forensic Sciences, JFSCA, 28* (1) Jan. 61–69, 1982.

75. *Seivewright vs. State of Wyoming,* Supra.

76. *Holt vs. United States,* 218 U.S. 245 (1910)

77. *Schmerber vs. California,* 384, U.S. at 765.

78. *Robinson vs. Percy,* 738 F2.d 214, 219 (7th Cir. 1984)

79. *Schmerber vs. California* 384, U.S. at 768. Supra (1966).

80. *People vs. Milone,* 43 III App. 3d 385, 392–95, 356 N.E. 2d 1350, 1355–60 (1976).

81. *State vs. Sapsford,* 22 Ohio App. 3d 1, 1–2, 488 N.E. 2d 218, 220 (1983).

82. *State vs. Asherman,* 193 Conn. at 716, 478 A. 2d at 242 (1984).

83. Levine, L. Bite Mark Workshop, Odontology Section, AAFS. February 20, 1999, Orlando, Florida.

84. Rawson, R. et al., supra.

Part 2

ADVANCED TECHNIQUES IN DENTAL IDENTIFICATION AND BITE MARKS

DAVID SWEET

DNA FROM HARD TISSUES

TEETH AND BONES are the hardest substances in the human body and have been recognized as valuable sources of forensic DNA evidence. Methods to recover this evidence have included sectioning, fragmenting, or crushing the samples to allow the DNA present inside the embedded cells to be extracted and purified. Recently, a technique called *cryogenic grinding* has been adapted to samples of teeth and bone to enable this process to be completed in a sterile and controlled environment (Fig. VI 20a–d).

Cryogenic grinding involves pulverization of the tooth or bone sample in a freezer mill using liquid nitrogen to freeze the sample at extremely low temperatures rendering it brittle. A plunger moving back and forth inside a sterile tube under the influence of the freezer mill's alternating magnetic field impacts the sample against a metal anvil at each end of the tube. After six minutes, the tooth or bone sample is reduced to a fine powder. This increases the surface area sufficiently to allow lysis buffers to break open the cellular and nuclear membranes liberating genomic DNA into solution. Subsequently, the DNA can be recovered, purified and submitted to PCR-based DNA analysis.

Once the DNA profile is obtained from the questioned sample it is compared to either direct or indirect reference samples to identify its origin. A direct sample is obtained from the person who is believed to be the decedent, such as from a personal item used by the person during their life or from a biological sample that is known to originate from the person. Examples of direct reference samples include clothing, personal hygiene items, jewelry, biopsy specimens, blood samples, etc. Indirect samples are usually obtained from family members so that paternity testing of these samples can establish if the deceased person is biologically related to the people who supplied the indirect samples.

A 1998 case from British Columbia shows how DNA from teeth can be compared to a direct reference to establish a person's identity. The skeletal remains of a woman were discovered in a remote park by a couple walking their dog. A wallet containing credit cards and a driver's license were used to establish tentative identification of the decedent as one "HK." HK had been missing for approximately 39 months. She had recently moved to Canada from Japan, where extensive dental treatment had been completed. Unfortunately, dental records for HK were not available from her dentist and, since she was estranged from her family, indirect reference samples were also unavailable.

DNA was extracted using cryogenic grinding from two molar teeth that were present in the lower jaw. A DNA profile of the skeletal remains was obtained. Known reference samples for HK were obtained from 1993 and 1994 Pap smears stored at the British Columbia Cancer Agency. The Provincial Coroners Service found these samples through a search of the missing woman's medical records. DNA was extracted from the Pap smears. Therefore, a genetic profile that was known to come from HK was obtained. Comparison of the profiles from the teeth and Pap smears showed that there was a match. In this case, the wallet and documents found at the scene provided information about the possible identity of the victim and DNA evidence was sufficient to establish a positive identification.

It is important for investigators to recover and preserve biological samples using the best possible methods to maximize the results of DNA testing. As a general rule when dealing with teeth or bone samples, the exhibits should be kept cold and dry to minimize the effects of bacterial contamination and DNA degradation. Similarly, the exhibits should be submitted to the DNA laboratory expeditiously to enable testing procedures to begin as soon as possible. Teeth and bones can be refrigerated if submission to the laboratory will be within 1–2 days. Freezing the exhibits is

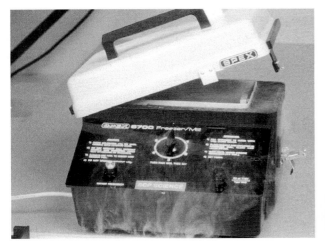

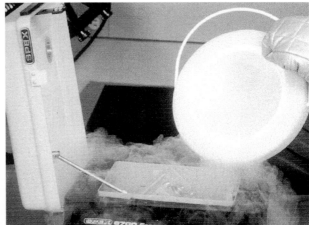

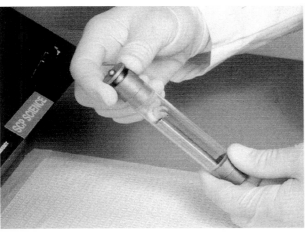

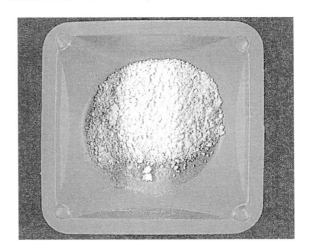

FIGURE VI-20a–d. Using a freezer mill and cryogenic grinding it is possible to reduce a sample of tooth or bone to powder. This exposes embedded cells, which enables DNA to be extracted and purified. (a) Freezer mill, (b) liquid nitrogen to freeze the sample and make it brittle, (c) sterile cylinder with ferromagnetic plunger, tooth sample and metal anvils, and (d) powder produced after grinding for six minutes.

suggested if the time before submission is prolonged.

DNA from Bite Marks

Consideration of human bite marks as physical evidence and comparison of the injury pattern to suspects' teeth is similar to forensic *toolmark* investigation. Exemplars can be obtained using informed consent or a judicial warrant to seize dental impressions from suspects to enable comparison of the shapes, sizes and configuration of the teeth to the injury. Recently, it has been shown that salivary DNA of sufficient quality and

quantity is deposited during biting and can be recovered from the injury, distinguished from the DNA of the victim's skin and compared to known reference samples that are made available from suspects. Now, in most jurisdictions, it is possible to obtain DNA reference samples from suspects using judicial warrants, which provides an opportunity to compare the DNA profile from saliva found at the bite site to the DNA profile of the suspect. In this way, it is possible to establish if there is a match and determine the likelihood that the suspect is the saliva contributor.

In 1995, as a result of a comprehensive research project dealing with saliva deposited on

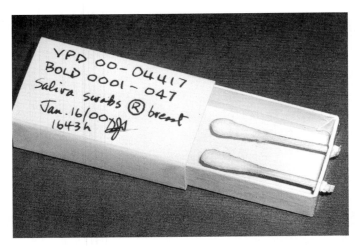

FIGURE VI-21. Storage of saliva swabs prior to submission to the laboratory for analysis is very important. After initial air-drying of the moist swabs, it is recommended that they be packaged in evidence containers that allow air to circulate keeping the exhibits dry. This figure shows a cardboard slider box that is effective for this purpose. Note that it is labeled according to established continuity of evidence guidelines.

human skin, we developed a new technique for the collection of biological evidence from dried stains. We called the *double swab technique*. This method was first presented for collection of saliva from bite marks on human skin. However, today, it has been used for other types of stains, and has enhanced the recovery of DNA from stains of saliva, blood, semen, etc. The method involves swabbing of the stain with a wet swab (sterile, distilled water) and medium pressure. The dried cells within the stain are rehydrated by the water, which loosens them from the surface of the substrate. This is followed by use of a dry swab with light pressure to act as a sponge to collect the water left on the skin. Both swabs must be thoroughly air-dried. This can be accomplished at room temperature for a minimum of 45 minutes before packaging the swabs for submission to the laboratory. Or, after initial drying the swabs can be placed in an evidence box or paper evidence envelope, which will allow air to continue to circulate and further dry the swab heads (Fig. VI-21). It is important not to seal the swabs in plastic evidence containers as the humid environment inside the container may promote bacterial growth and DNA degradation.

It has been shown that saliva stains on human skin can deteriorate over a period of time, depending upon environmental conditions. Humidity, temperature and decomposition of the skin at the site of the bite mark may affect the recovery of salivary DNA from bite marks. Research has shown that at room temperature sufficient saliva for DNA typing can be recovered up to 72 hours after deposition on the skin. However, in hot, humid conditions this time interval may be reduced; in cold, dry conditions the evidence may last significantly longer.

With the advent of alternate light sources to search for stains of bodily fluids, it is now possible for investigators to locate dried stains of blood, saliva and other fluids when they are not readily apparent. Stains of saliva that have been deposited during kissing and sucking can now be recognized. It is recommended in cases where sexual violation of the victim occurs that locations on the body that are usually the target of sucking or kissing, such as the breasts, groin, neck, lips, etc. be scanned for potential biological evidence. The double swab technique can be used to recover saliva deposited in these areas.

Surprisingly, it has been reported that salivary DNA evidence was successfully recovered from a bite mark on a body that was submerged in a slow-moving river for almost six hours. Apparently, the saliva was so sticky that it held the cells on the skin's surface until they were later recovered at autopsy and submitted for DNA typing. It appears that one cannot predict exactly where or when DNA evidence may be available in a given case. It is recommended that efforts be directed to collecting *every* potential source of evidence. Only after DNA typing is performed can one be certain of the final result.

Bite marks are sometimes perpetrated through clothing. This may render the pattern of the bruises and abrasions on the skin indistinct or of such quality that physical comparison may not be possible. Collection of salivary DNA from the clothing that was directly over the bite mark may provide a valuable source of biological evidence that can be compared to potential suspects, even when a comparison of the teeth to the injury is not possible. Cuttings from the article of clothing and extraction of DNA from the stain that is present on the fabric may prove fruitful. However, the same guidelines that were suggested for handling biological exhibits from teeth and saliva swabs must be used with clothing containing saliva stains. The clothing should be protected from UV light sources, heat, humidity and other environmental insults to maximize the potential yield of DNA evidence.

Objects found at the crime scene may also exhibit marks from human teeth. Hold-up notes from bank robberies, notebooks, pencils, pens and other inanimate objects may contain both physical and biological evidence from teeth and saliva. It has proven difficult to extract DNA from bitten foodstuffs, but this is currently the focus of continuing research. Recently, for the first time, salivary DNA was successfully recovered and analyzed from a bite on bacteria-rich cheese. This is significant because bacteria produce a group of enzymes called nuclease, which degrade DNA.

Two men broke into a house and stole various valuable items. Upon returning home, the residents discovered furniture overturned, food and condiments from the kitchen spread around the house and knives stabbed into a wall. A block of yellow cheese with a single bite mark was discovered in the living room. When the suspects were arrested, there was sufficient evidence to charge them with possession of stolen property. However, it was difficult to link them directly to the crime scene. Investigators focused their attention on the recovered block of cheese and sought the help of a forensic odontologist to compare the bite mark to the suspects' teeth.

As soon as the cheese was brought to the forensic laboratory the double swab technique was used to recover any biological evidence from the surfaces contacted by the upper and lower lips during biting. The swabs were frozen and stored at B20EC. Impressions were produced from the physical evidence recorded in the bite mark and a warrant was obtained to seize dental exemplars from one of the suspects whose teeth appeared to be similar to the pattern of the bite mark. The warrant could not be executed because the suspect was unable to contact his legal counsel for advice. The expert and the police were concerned that the suspect might attempt to change his teeth by filing them or damaging them in some other way. Since this could eliminate any potential matches to the bite mark, it was determined that attempts to obtain a DNA profile from the swabs should be made.

A complete DNA profile consisting of nine genetic loci plus the gender-specific locus was obtained from the swabs. A warrant was then obtained from a judge to seize a blood sample from the suspect, which was completed without incident. Comparison of the DNA profile from the cheese to that from the suspect determined that either the suspect was the saliva contributor or someone else with an identical DNA profile was the contributor. The likelihood of someone else selected at random having the same DNA profile as the suspect was calculated to be 1 in 159 trillion. The suspect was convicted of break-and-enter and robbery.

REFERENCES

1. Sweet, D., and Hildebrand, D.P.: Recovery of DNA from human teeth by cryogenic grinding. *J Forensic Sci, 43* (6):1199–1202, 1998.
2. Gill, P., Ivanov, P.L., Kimpton, C., Piercy, R., Benson, N., and Tully, G., et al.: Identification of the remains of the Romanov family by DNA analysis. *Nature Genetics, 6:* 130–135, 1994.
3. Sweet, D., Lorente, J.A., Lorente, M., Valenzuela, A., and Villanueva. E.: An improved method to recover saliva from human skin: The double swab technique. *J Forensic Sci, 42* (2): 320–322, 1997.
4. Sweet, D., Lorente, J.A., Lorente, M., Valenzuela, A., and Villanueva, E.: PCR-based typing of DNA from

saliva recovered from human skin. *J Forensic Sci, 42* (3): 447–451, 1997.

5. Sweet, D., Hildebrand, D., and Phillips, D.: Identification of a skeleton using DNA from teeth and a Pap smear. *J Forensic Sci, 44* (3): 630–633, 1999.

6. Sweet, D., and Shutler, G.G.: Analysis of salivary DNA evidence from a bite mark on a submerged body. *J Forensic Sci, 44* (5): 1069–1072, 1999.

7. Sweet, D., and Hildebrand, D.: Saliva from cheese bite yields DNA profile of burglar: A case report. *Int J Legal Medicine, 112* (3): 201–203, 1999.

Part 3

ADVANCED PHOTOGRAPHIC TECHNIQUES

GREGORY S. GOLDEN

WHAT HAPPENS AROUND US from day-to-day is seen through eyes that are limited to a visible portion of the spectrum. Research has shown that many animals see better at night than in daylight because their visual acuity allows them to see not only in low light conditions, but also the radiation emerging from their environment. By employing blocking filters, laser lights, panchromatic films, and certain digital chips, we, too, can capture images that are normally beyond the realm of detection with our human eyes.

Among the advanced techniques available for crime scene and forensic photographers in general are Reflective Ultra Violet (UVA), Infra-Red (IR), and fluorescence, also known as Alternate Light Imaging (ALI). These methods differ from each other in many aspects including protocol, armamentaria, and range of the spectrum utilized to produce the image. The visual results of each technique are also completely unlike the other. Since this chapter deals primarily with Bite Mark Evidence, which is predominantly a pattern injury inflicted to living tissue, an area of photography where Infra-Red is less successful, the contrasting areas of UVA and ALI will be discussed.

REFLECTIVE ULTRA VIOLET (UVA)

Ultraviolet or UV radiation is divided into three separate groups of waves.[1] Short wave UV consists of radiation from 200 to 280 nanometers in length. This range is typically used in sterilization procedures. Medium wave UV is that portion that extends from 280 to 320 nanometers. Without protection from short and medium wave UV, our skin burns in the sunlight. Long wave UV is comprised of radiation that is 320 to 400 nanometers in length. This is the range of ultraviolet radiation most useful to photography.

The technique of UVA photography is well understood in many fields of interest. Archaeological photographers use UVA to provide information about ancient objects, revealing coloration and writings obscured by the passage of time.[2] The field of dermatology has utilized UVA for years to help locate and identify skin disorders.[3] Apropos to forensic investigation, UVA photography can show surface details in bite marks and pattern injuries that are not readily observable under normal lighting conditions.

Virtually any size professional camera can be utilized to make ultraviolet photos. The most popular format is 35-millimeter. Lenses, on the other hand, are more specific. Most recently manufactured macro-lenses are coated with the chemical "fluorite" which is designed to block UV transmission. It is highly recommended that one use a non-coated quartz lens with this application. The UV-Nikkor 105mm f/4.5, meets this criteria however, is no longer manufactured. The special quartz crystal lenses made by Zeiss for Hasselblad and other companies. These lenses transmit 75% of the ultraviolet radiation reflected from the image and eliminate the need to correct the focal shifts that occur during the UVA and IR techniques.[4]

Filtration of all other light outside the long UVA range is necessary. This is accomplished with either a Wratten or Kodak # 18-A filter placed in front of the lens. In close-up photography, it will be necessary to have a strong light source such as a strobe-type flash. The Nikon SB 140 was designed with UVA photography in mind and supplies ample quantities of UV radiation during exposures. The entire system can be mounted on a tripod.

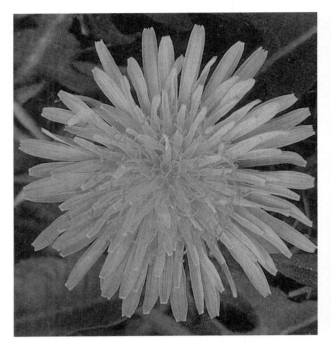 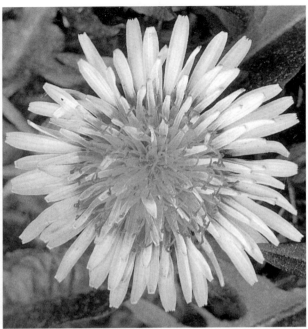

FIGURE VI-22a–b. (a) Dandelion taken with normal lighting conditions. (b) Same dandelion as in Figure VI-22 a taken with color film and UVA. (Photographs provided with permission of Bjφrn Rφrslett.)

Since long UVA has no visible color, the films predominantly used for this technique are of the Panchromatic black and white group. Kodak T-Max with an ISO of 400 is an ideal film for documentation of bite marks and pattern injuries. While color UVA photography has been described as "problematic" and "difficult at best," there are some successful results available for color UVA primarily limited to fields other than forensic investigation. Of the recent research that has been done with color emulsion, so far the most acceptable film found for capturing color UVA images is Fuji RTP® combined with a Nikon® FF filter.[5]

Figure VI-22a–b are of a dandelion, taken under normal lighting and UVA conditions in that order. Although these published images are in black and white, Figure VI-22a in color shows a yellow flower. The UVA photo in Figure VI-22b is of the same flower, only now the outer half of the petals are white and the inner portion of the flower is bright red.

What makes UVA photography in bite mark injuries so useful is the degree of enhancement it provides to the surface detail of the skin. Subdermal bruising in bite marks can be so extensive that details of the teeth left in the epidermis are obscured by extravasation of blood throughout the underlying tissues. UVA photography can show surface detail, revealing inter-dental and sometimes intra-dental features. When distinctive, these surface clues can be very useful in determination of suspects.

Figure VI-23a is a photograph of a bite mark on the breast of a homicide victim, taken with normal flash photography. Figure VI-23b is the same photo taken with UVA technique. Figure VI-23c compares the anterior incisors of the suspect to the injury. Note the consistencies between the angles of the incisors and the marks on the breast.

ALTERNATE LIGHT IMAGING, (FLUORESCENCE)

The spectral principle responsible for what happens in fluorescent photography is called the *Stokes Shift,* after its discoverer, Professor G.G. Stokes.[6] A brief explanation of what occurs when

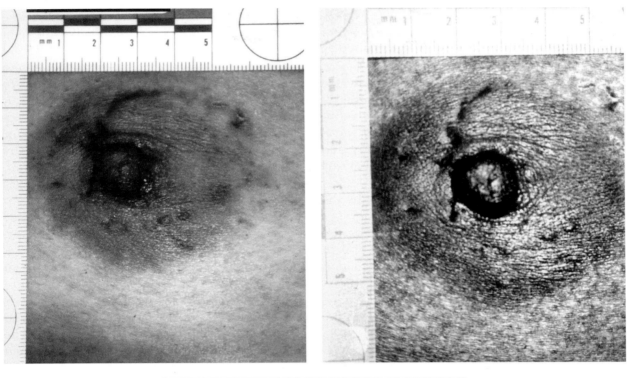

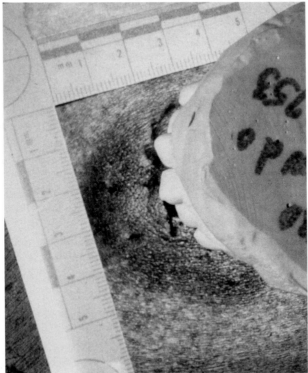

FIGURE VI-23a–c. (a) Bite on breast of a rape/homicide victim. Normal flash illumination. (b) Same bite mark utilizing UVA technique. (c) Comparison of suspect's dentition to Figure VI-23b.

a high intensity, narrow band of filtered visible light strikes an object must be understood for comprehension of this phenomenon at a physical level.

Most of the light striking an object is reflected from its surface. Some light energy is absorbed at the atomic level and remitted at a longer wavelength than the incident light. This longer wavelength light is the fluorescent light energy and can be observed by using filters that block the incident light. Once blocked, only the longer wave fluorescent light passes through to the observer's eye or the film emulsion.

Almost anything in nature can be made to fluoresce, depending on which wavelength of light stimulates the highest level of atomic excitation in the illuminated object.[7] Research on the bioluminescence of skin has detected a peak excitation at 430–450 nanometers which is near the UVA range but is actually visible blue light.[8,9]

There are instances when it is to the investigator's advantage to be able to observe bruises below the surface of the skin. An aged bite on a living victim that no longer has any distinguishing surface features or one that reveals no individual tooth characteristics can frequently be visibly enhanced with the ALI technique.

Field study of ALI has uncovered numerous uses for this fascinating approach to forensic photography, especially in locating many forms of trace evidence. Finding blood, fibers, illicit drugs, gunshot residue, latent prints, and alterations in questioned documents are some of the reasons an investigator will use this technique in verification and collection of trace evidence.

There are several companies that manufacture forensic light sources. Depending upon the needs of the criminologist, an appropriate unit can be located and purchased through many of the forensic supply vendors that retail the tools for investigative work. A fundamental principal regarding forensic light sources is that the higher the light output, the better the photographic results. Recent advances in bulbs, power units, and light cables have made it feasible under most conditions to capture a successful fluorescent image on slide or print emulsion film. It is recommended that a liquid light guide or direct output optics be used for best results.[10] Fiber-optic type cables originally developed for this equipment work fine for scanning but do not provide the light output necessary for good photographic results.

Film speeds and exposure factors will vary with each situation. In most cases, however, using ALI with a modern forensic light source, the photographer should be able to capture an adequate image with 100 ISO film. Exposure times should range between 1/4 sec. to 2 seconds at f/4 to f/5.6 aperture with the light source and camera at distances of 12 to 24 inches from the subject. Prior to all exposures, the camera should be mounted on a sturdy tripod, focused, and with the lens oriented at a perpendicular angle to the injury before through-the-lens light meter readings are taken with the appropriate filter in place.

Variables such as darker skin coloration and motion in live subjects; i.e., child abuse victims, require films of a higher speed such as 400–1600 ISO. Unlike UVA, ALI must be accomplished in total darkness except for the illumination of the light source. Any ambient light will interfere with the image, particularly in the higher speed films.

As a rule, photographers entering this field of science should become familiar with their camera equipment, its capabilities, and the appropriate exposure settings prior to actual casework. Pre-testing, under controlled conditions, is highly recommended. Many instructional courses are available throughout the country on a regular basis.

DIGITAL APPLICATIONS

This topic would be incomplete without including some mention of digital applications to UVA and ALI techniques of forensic photography. Digital cameras have always been able to capture images of any object using visible light for illumination, no matter what the color. The technology employs chips called "Charged Coupled Devices" (CCD's). These chips have always been adequate for ALI, however most early 35mm digital cameras were unable to detect UVA radiation. Fortunately, there are now CCD's that do have the capability to record UVA and IR images. In fact, digital photographic research in the fields of biophotonics, DNA sequencing, photomedicine, and photodynamic therapy (PDT), utilize the latest generation digital cameras and colored lasers to unveil the dynamics and the direction of modern medicine through UVA and ALI techniques.[11]

Each new technological innovation in digital cameras that is unveiled to the consumer marketplace brings with it associated useful features, advantages, and benefits. There are also some unfortunate downsides. Most of the well-known camera manufacturers saw the handwriting on the wall long ago and have since marketed some type of digital camera for public distribution. There are hand-sized single frame and videocams available and endoscopic/microscopic versions of each, depending upon the field of research and application.

Sales prices vary with the sophistication of the digital unit. A rule of thumb is that the higher the resolution capability, more storage capacity, and more superior optics that are available, the more pricey the equipment will be. Digital cameras currently range in price from a few hundred dollars to six figures for the highly sophisticated equipment. As the technology evolves, it is anticipated the price will spiral downward as new models replace current ones. Hopefully, just like computers, everyone will ultimately be able to afford one.

Speaking of computers, keep in mind that digital cameras generally are required to interface with one. Whether it is a network, PC, laptop, or palm pilot, an appropriate data transfer port will be necessary, as well as the software to download and manipulate the images. Imaging software applications are also available at a wide range of prices, depending upon the level of complexity.

In summation, these advanced photographic methods, although entirely different in their protocols and results, are immensely important adjuncts to the field of forensic investigation. It is crucial that they be employed whenever possible. By ignoring their existence, it is unlikely that the totality of available evidence will ever be accumulated.

REFERENCES

1. Huda, A.: UVA, UVB, and UVC and their possible effects. *Health Phy 2000, 78,* May (5 Suppl): S75.
2. Eliadis, E. Archaeological Photography, UV Photography web page article, 1996, http://users.hol.gr/~eliad/uvtheo.htm.
3. Kochevar, I.E., Pathok, M.A., and Parrish, J.A.: *Photophysics, photochemistry, photobiology: Dermatology in general medicine,* 4th ed. New York: McGraw-Hill.
4. Nieuwenhuis, G., *J. Biol. Photography,* 1991, p. 17.
5. Rorslett, B.: web page http://www.foto.no/nikon/uvfilms.html.
6. Stokes, G.G.: On the change of refrangibility of light. *Philosophical Transactions* of the Royal Society of London, pp. 385–396, 1853.
7. Guilbault, G.: *Practical fluorescence.* New York: Marcel Dekker, 1973.
8. Devore, D.: Ultraviolet absorption and fluorescence phenomena associated with wound healing. *Thesis for Doctor of Philosophy,* University of London, Dept. of Oral Pathology, Oct. 1974.
9. Dawson, J.B.: A theoretical and experimental study of light absorption and scattering by in vivo skin. *Phys. Med. Biol., 25,* No. 4, 1980.
10. Melles Griot, Laser and Electro-Optics Group, 2051 Palomar Airport Rd., 200, Carlsbad, CA 92009, E-mail: sales@carlsbad.mellesgriot.com.
11. Digital Imaging vs. Film. *BioPhotonics International, Photonic solutions for biotechnology and medicine.* Pittsfield, MA: Laurin Publishing Co. Inc., April/May 2000.

Part 4

THE USE OF DIGITAL ANALYSIS IN BITE MARK IDENTIFICATION

C. MICHAEL BOWERS AND RAYMOND J. JOHANSEN

CONCEPTS OF DIGITAL COMPARISON ANALYSIS

Q and K Evidence

FORENSIC DENTISTS TESTIFY in court regarding certain types of medical evidence involving teeth. This includes bite mark analysis and the identification of human remains. The basis of many opinions is the direct superimposition of Questioned (Q) and Known (K) samples that have sufficient identification value to demonstrate features of common origin or establish an exclusionary result. In all but the most routine cases, these direct analysis methods demand rigorous attention to scale dimensions and the detection of photographic distortion in these images of forensic interest, for example radiographs, photographic slides, negatives, prints, and digital images.

The forensic dental techniques are generally analogous to the physical comparison of Q and K evidence found in fingerprint, ballistics and toolmark studies. These disciplines have the criminalist using a comparison microscope to place the Q and K evidence samples side by side. The loops, whorls, striations, indentations, accidental and class characteristics present in the evidence samples may then be visually compared. What is difficult to assess in the crime lab and dental lab are the dimensional parameters of the evidence samples. In dentistry, the traditional ruler and protractor measurements and shape comparison processes are manually derived from evidence photographs and dental stone casts of a suspect's teeth. These methods can vary between examiners and are therefore, somewhat subjective in nature. Alternatively, some crime lab analysts ignore size comparisons and focus on similarities in class and individual features. In both situations, the possibility of error arises from subjective examiner methods and partial selection of the available physical information. It is clear that additional tools and protocols are needed. The advent of digital technology has provided the opportunity to improve the quality of our comparative analyses.

Advantages of the Digital Image Format and Analysis

- Speedy transmission of digital information.
- Large amounts of digital information can be stored in a very small space.
- Digital images can be enhanced quickly and easily.
- Chain of custody issues are easily handled with digitization.
- Digital information can easily be duplicated and shared worldwide.
- Handling of digital information has proven to be very reliable.
- Standardization of procedures is simplified.

The recent development of easily available digital imaging software (i.e., Adobe® Photoshop®) and image capture devices such as scanners and digital cameras has created an opportunity to better control these variables. This also allows the forensic examiner to turn the computer monitor into a comparison microscope with the added benefit of the following functions:

1. Accurate means of measuring physical parameters of crime scene evidence.
2. Correction of common photographic distortion and size discrepancies.
3. Help eliminate examiner subjectivity
   - better control of image visualization
   - standardization of comparison procedures.

4. Better reproducibility of results between examiners.
5. Electronic transmission and archiving of image data.

6. Fabrication of exemplars of the evidence and comparison techniques.
7. Accurate and meaningful demonstrations in court.

FEATURES OF DIGITAL EVIDENCE

This section describes the steps necessary to create a digital comparison. The examples are from a typical forensic dentistry bite mark evaluation. The application of these methods may also be useful to other areas of forensic investigation that require image comparison information.

Image Formats

There are a number of formats in which forensic investigators receive two-dimensional bite mark evidence, i.e., images of the injury pattern. These include floppy disks, zipped (compressed) computer files, Zip Disks (100MB or 250 MB storage capacity), compact disks (CD) and email attachments. These formats are already digitized and thus are simple to manage. Most often, the evidence is in the form of photographic prints, slides or negatives and must first be scanned in order to carry out a digital analysis. The resolution of the resultant scanned images must be appreciated since it is a critical factor, impacting the accuracy of the subsequent steps.

Resolution

The detail of a digital image is represented by the number of dots per inch (dpi) for scanners and digital cameras. Higher resolution not only produces a sharper image but also allows the image to be enhanced in a variety of ways not available with a lower resolution image. The rule of thumb is to work with as high a resolution image as the computer and printer can accommodate.

Adobe® Photoshop® is a popular software program which allows for a multitude of imaging features, functions, enhancements and metric analysis procedures. The initial working image seen on the monitor may be too small to accurately analyze. The image can be enlarged using the Zoom tool to see details more clearly. The image may be viewed, in increments, up to 1600% on the computer monitor using this tool. The only limitation to the enlargement is the resolution of the image. Lower resolution images tend to become pixilated (fuzzy) at higher magnification and difficult to work. This emphasizes the need for a high-resolution image (at least 300 dpi), as previously mentioned. This is especially true when working with images of very small detailed objects or patterns. When measuring important elements of an image it is advisable to use the highest Zoom setting your monitor will accommodate.

Digital Control of Photographic Distortion

The tools within Photoshop® can be used to detect and correct for certain angular distortions of an image caused by poor photographic technique (Fig. VI-24). This is an extremely important step as it forms the foundation for the comparison procedures that follow.

A photograph is a graphical representation of the objects within the range of the camera's lens. The degree to which this graphic exactly reproduces those objects is influenced by many variables. When bite marks are photographed or dental x-rays are used as evidence, attempts are made to carefully control perspective variables in an effort to obtain an accurate representation of the bite mark or dental restoration for later comparative analysis. Unfortunately, these efforts are not always successful and distortion is often introduced into the image.

Photography of bite marks and similar types of two and three-dimensional physical evidence should have the following features:

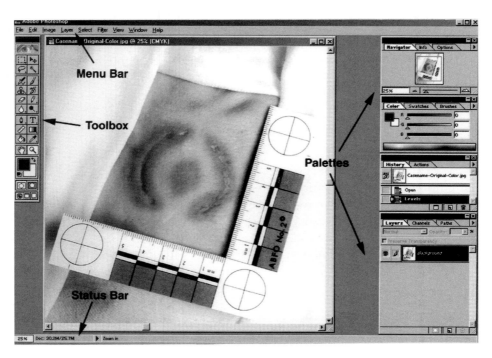

FIGURE VI-24. Photoshop® screen with bite mark image.

- Presence of a scale (or some appropriate measuring device) oriented on the same plane as the bite mark or evidence sample.
- The orientation of the camera back (film plane) to the scale is parallel.
- The scale is on the same plane as the bite mark thus eliminating parallax distortion. (The scale is used to reproduce a life-size image of the object. Its displacement below or above the object will make this later process inaccurate.)

Correcting for Photographic Distortion

If it has been determined that significant distortion exists, it must be corrected before the bite mark photograph is resized and/or enhanced. Only then can a meaningful comparison analysis be accomplished. Too often in the past, this step has been ignored, leading to inaccurate results. Due to the ease with which this can be digitally accomplished, correction of photographic distortion should be standard in all comparative analyses. There are four categories of photographic distortion.

TYPE I DISTORTION: Occurs when the scale and bite mark are on the same plane but the camera angle is not parallel to them (Fig. VI-25a). This is also called "off-angle" distortion. This type of distortion can be digitally corrected (Fig. VI-25b).

When the image of the scale is brought back to its original size and shape, the image of the bite mark will also be corrected (rectification). This assumes that the scale itself is on a single plane and there is no parallax distortion relative to the bite mark.

TYPE II DISTORTION: If the scale is not on the same plane as the bite mark (type II distortion), rectifying the scale will adversely affect the proportions of the injury pattern. In situations like this it is best not to try to rectify the scale but do the later resize (1:1) procedure based on the scale *as is*.

The amount of parallax distortion present will obviously affect the accuracy of the results. The weight given to the results will contribute to the ultimate decision in the case. The investigator must decide what amount of distortion is accept-

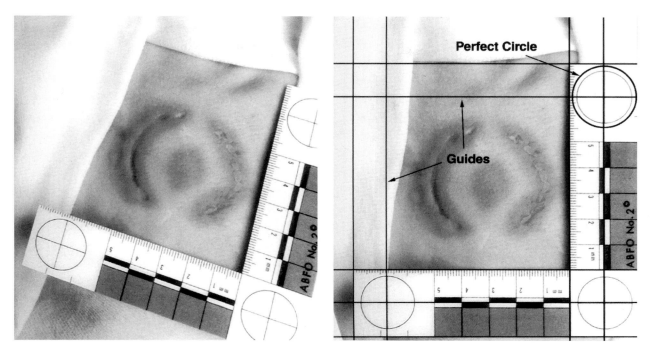

FIGURE VI-25a–b. (a) Type I distortion. (b) Type I correction.

able in order to produce a meaningful comparison.

TYPE III DISTORTION: In some cases, one leg of a two-dimensional scale will have perspective distortion but the other leg will not. This is Type III distortion. Notice the scale in Figure VI-26. In this illustration, the horizontal leg of the scale is distorted but the vertical leg is not. Here, we can use the non-distorted leg to do the resizing procedures with accurate results. This would be similar to performing a resize based on a one-dimensional scale in the image.

TYPE IV DISTORTION: In this instance, the scale itself may be bent or skewed (Fig. VI-27). There can be forensic value if the scale is relatively flat in the area directly adjacent to the bite mark. Peripheral scale inaccuracies can be discounted. Use only the area next to the mark for the resizing procedures. Do not use the entire scale.

The above scenarios encompass most of the physical distortion seen in bite mark and other evidentiary photographs. When detected and properly corrected, the resulting image modification will result in an accurate resize and a meaningful comparison.

Limitations to This Method

It is important to realize which type of distortion, if any, is present within the original bite mark photograph. This often can be a difficult task and requires some experience. Also of concern is the fact that we are using a two-dimensional object (the scale) to help analyze three-dimensional images. In some instances, this is not a problem if, for example, the bite mark is on a relatively flat surface.

The final analysis of each case depends upon the quality of the evidence presented. In cases where all the variables are carefully controlled and distortion correction is successful, a greater certainty of opinion is possible. In some cases, the quality of the bite mark photograph may be so poor that it precludes a meaningful analysis altogether.

Photographic Standards

The above discussion should emphasize the need to follow strict protocol, including the use a tripod, whenever possible, when photographing bite mark injuries and other types of physical evi-

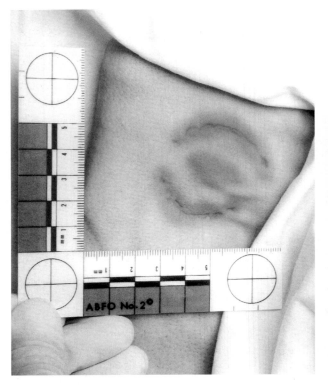
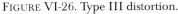

FIGURE VI-26. Type III distortion.

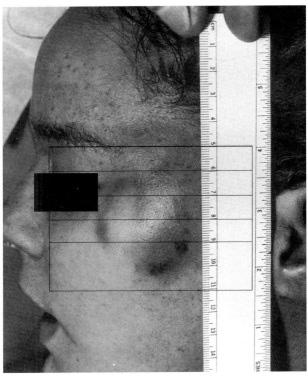

FIGURE VI-27. Type IV distortion.

dence. As mentioned, the transitory nature of some evidence samples can sometimes mean there is only one opportunity to photographically document the evidence.

DIGITAL ANALYSIS OF TWO AND THREE DIMENSIONAL EVIDENCE

Resizing the Image to Life-size

In order to resize the photograph of the bite mark to life-size or larger (2X, 3X, etc.) there must be an item of known size within the image. Ideally this is a ruler or scale. A ratio (resize ratio) is established between two values. The first is the relative size of the known object within the image, or in other words, what the computer *thinks* the image size is of this item. The second value is the real life-size dimension of that same object. This ratio is then used to adjust the image size. Digital resizing of an image is easily accomplished; thus eliminating the need to have a photographic laboratory involved in the evidence chain of custody. This not only simplifies procedures but also saves processing time and main-tains examiner continuity throughout the examination.

Image Enhancement

At this stage, the bite mark image can be digitally enhanced to show details, which may otherwise be obscured. It is important to realize that these enhancement procedures do not change the content of the image. They simply allow existing elements of an image to be better visualized. Digital technology allows the investigator to exercise better control over crime scene images.

Some argue that this increased control may allow unethical investigators the opportunity to alter image evidence to better support their opinions. Digital information is simply an exemplar of actual physical evidence. Exemplars are not evidence. They are exhibits presented to support the opinion of the individual giving testimony. Any misuse of digital imaging is the result of the human condition and not the fault of the technology. It is ethical to digitally enhance something that is present in order to better visualize certain features.

Computer-Generated Overlay Fabrication

In forensic dentistry, transparent overlays are fabricated from images generated by scanning the suspect's dental casts (Fig. VI-28). Other methods of image capture work equally well if the evidence sample does not lend itself to scanning. For example, if the evidence sample is too large to be scanned or too fragile to be moved, conventional or digital photography can be used to capture the image.

Non-metric Analysis of the Bite Mark and Suspect's Dentition

Once the bite mark image and the overlay are completed, a non-metric analysis can be carried out. This involves superimposing the overlay onto the bite mark injury and investigating points of concordance or discrepancy.

The relevant areas of the overlay image are selected and brought into the bite mark image using the familiar *drag and drop* (Windows and Macintosh commands) maneuver. This new *Comparison Image* is made up of a number of superimposed but separate image layers. A typical bite mark comparison image would include the bite mark image as the Background layer, the maxillary arch overlay layer and the mandibular overlay layer (Fig. VI-29). Each of these layers can be individually enhanced and/or moved.

Compound Overlay

More information than just the outlines of the biting teeth can be gathered from the suspect's scanned dental casts. If individual characterization is present, this should be included in the

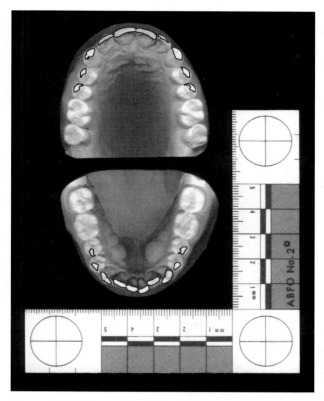

FIGURE VI-28. Scan of models with biting edges selected by the computer.

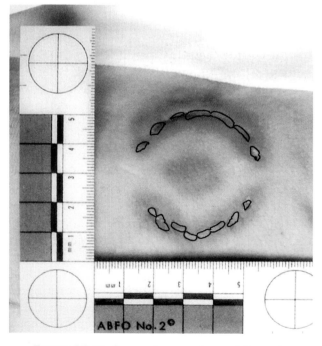

FIGURE VI-29. Comparison overlay on bite mark.

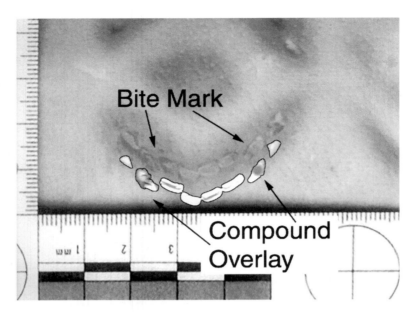

FIGURE VI-30. Compound overlay.

computer generated overlay along with the tooth outlines.

Chipping, wear facets, unusual anatomy, and dental erosion are some examples of the features that can be visualized and recorded using Photoshop® and the digital image. This type of overlay is referred to as a *compound overlay*. The compound overlay contains not only the perimeter outlines of the teeth but also images of the individual features within the outlines (Fig. VI-30).

These features can be described as the topography of the teeth surfaces. They are three-dimensional in nature and are considered individual variables useful in this analysis. In the scanned image of the dental casts, these features are displayed as variations in the value of each color or grayscale portion of the tooth. The closer a portion of tooth is to the scanner surface, the lighter it appears in the image. Darker features can be viewed as farther away or recessed from the primary biting edge.

When only a partial bite mark exists and identification is otherwise difficult, the compound overlay can be extremely valuable. In these cases, identification comparisons can often be made based on these individual features of a single tooth. With a high resolution image and a high zoom setting, these features can be visualized up close and then compared with the injury or Q sample.

Recording the Analysis

The comparison processes can be recorded on videotape, or compatible presentation software. Many of the newer computers sold today come with multimedia hardware and software that allow the user to create digital video clips on the desktop which can be played back on a data projector during a presentation of the evidence. Various stages of the comparison can also be printed when hard copies are desired for verification and demonstrative purposes.

Metric Analysis of Bite Mark Injuries

The use of digital imaging allows the examiner to establish physical data parameters for bite mark cases. The application of certain Photoshop® tools and functions will provide the dental examiner with concise physical evidence data that will create linear and angular information useful to support the final conclusions regarding a case.

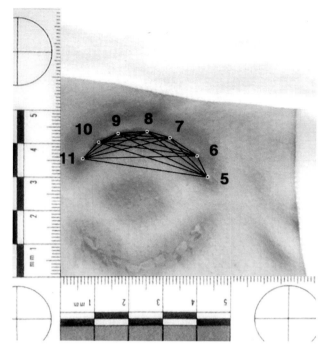

FIGURE VI-31. Spatial analysis of bite mark.

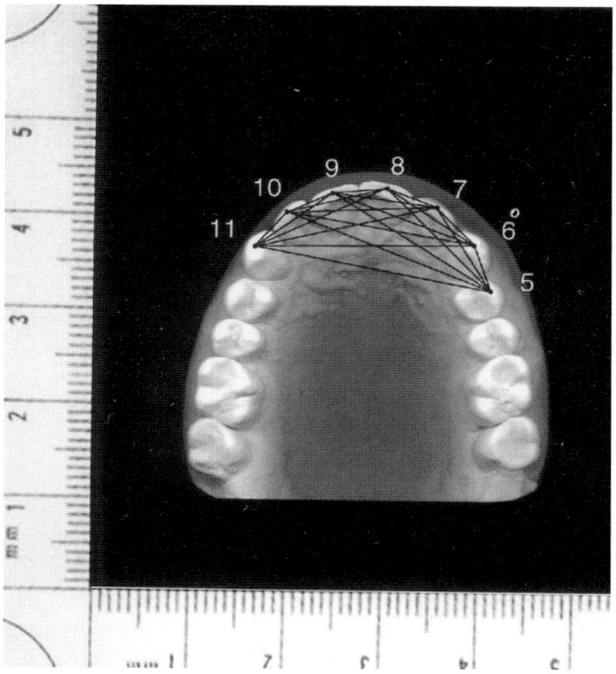

FIGURE VI-32. Spatial analysis of suspect.

Step One: Spatial Analysis of Bite Mark Injury

It is recommended that the injury pattern (Q) be completely analyzed before the dentition of a suspect (K) is evaluated. This parallels other protocols in forensic science and establishes hard data sets for this Q sample before commencing the analysis of the suspect's teeth. This insures a measure of blinded neutrality in the total analysis. The aforementioned photographic distortion may be controllable, but the other significant distortion factor in bite mark analysis is the acknowledged stretching and elasticity of skin injuries. The use of linear and angular measurements for all tooth marks provides the investigator the two-dimensional features present in the bite mark (Fig. VI-31). Examiners will also produce subjective documentation due to the visual vagaries of bruising and inflammatory (if present) response of skin injury patterns. This metric data is recorded and called the *Metric Profile* of the bite mark injury. The degree of identification value to these profiles is the subject of courtroom debate. The degree of variation between the bite mark profile and the subsequent suspect's metric pro-

file is the arena where differences will occur between odontologists. It is desirable, therefore, to measure as many physical parameters as possible. The individualization and discrimination value of the analysis should increase as more are measured.

Step Two: Analyzing the Suspect Dentition

Identical steps are then performed using the scanned images of the suspect's dental stone casts. The same linear and angular measurements are taken on the corresponding teeth and a metric profile for the Known sample is established (Fig. VI-32).

Step Three: Comparison Data

The K (suspect's dental casts) and Q (bite mark) metric profiles are mathematically compared. This allows quantification of data in a scientific manner. This data can then be entered into an existing dental database and used to establish frequencies of occurrence of similar profiles in a much larger sample population (Fig. VI-33).

Tooth Numbers	Questioned (Q) Data Points Distance (cm)	Questioned (Q) Data Points Angle (degrees)	Known (K) Data Points Distance (cm)	Known (K) Data Points Angle (degrees)	△ (%)
5-11					
5-10					
5-9					
5-8					
5-7					
5-6					
6-11					
6-10					
6-9					
6-8					
6-7					
7-11					
7-10					
7-9					
7-8					
8-11					
8-10					
8-9					
9-11					
9-10					
10-11					

$$\triangle = \frac{\text{Data Points Distance (K)} - \text{Data Points Distance (Q)}}{\text{Data Points Distance (K)}}$$

Note: A negative value for delta indicates the "Q" sample is larger than the "K" sample.

FIGURE VI-33. Comparison data table.

CONCLUSIONS

Human identification from dental structures can benefit from digital techniques. Bite mark identification can benefit considerably more. Bite mark analysis has suffered much of the same criticism as other pattern analysis disciplines have throughout their existence. That is, the subjective nature of its evidence interpretation and the associated perception of its lack of scientific theory. Although most courts in the world have upheld the principles and conclusions of traditional bite mark analysis, oftentimes the opinions of the forensic experts involved are in direct disagreement. What is lacking is a modern protocol that produces reliable, objective and reproducible results. The authors suggest that dental investigators consider using digital analysis to assist in reaching these goals.

Chapter VII

SUDDEN AND UNEXPECTED DEATH FROM NATURAL CAUSES IN ADULTS

BARBARA A. SAMPSON, VERNARD I. ADAMS, AND CHARLES S. HIRSCH

EVERY UNEXPECTED DEATH has an actual or potential medicolegal aspect, and in most countries such deaths come under the scrutiny of a medicolegal investigative official, who may be called a coroner, medical examiner, medical investigator or by some other title. He has the responsibility for establishing the cause and the manner of death in these unanticipated fatalities and also in those in which violence of some type is known or alleged to have played a part.

That sudden, unexpected and violent deaths are uniquely important to society is indicated immediately by the fact that they fall under the jurisdiction of a special medicolegal government official. Medical interest lies in accurate establishment of the nature of the fatal disease or injury and correlation of this information with the circumstances surrounding death. Legal importance derives from the availability and utilization of precise and objective medical data for the administration of justice, whether it be a civil action for wrongful death, workmen's compensation, insurance benefits under an accidental death policy and the like, or a criminal prosecution for some degree of homicide.

This chapter deals with several medicolegal problems that arise when death occurs suddenly or unexpectedly solely from natural causes in an adult. Reference will be made to traumatic situations and incidents for purposes of illustration, but the emphasis here is on those deaths that result entirely from disease.

UNEXPLAINED DEATHS

Clinically unexplained deaths fall into two categories: (1) those that occur in patients who have been studied extensively during prolonged, complex illnesses without a satisfactory diagnosis having been established; (2) those that follow an illness of such brief duration that there has been little or no opportunity for medical observation or studies to provide a reasonable explanation for what has occurred.

The more unexpected the death, the more likely it is to be unexplained. Experience has taught that it is more difficult to make a correct diagnosis in persons taken acutely ill who die shortly after admission to the hospital than in persons dying under almost any other circumstances. A meager or absent history combined with a hasty, incomplete physical examination and insufficient time to carry out informative tests in a dying and/or uncooperative patient often lead to deductions that are, at best, haphazard speculations.

CIRCUMSTANCES SURROUNDING SUDDEN AND UNEXPECTED NATURAL DEATHS

Sudden and unexpected deaths occur in persons with varying medical backgrounds, including those in whom a diagnosis of potentially lethal disease has never been made. Generally, with the exceptions noted in the following section, these victims have harbored some preexisting chronic disease of which they were unaware. Such lack of awareness can result from absence of preceding symptomatology or because clear-cut manifestations of illness have been ignored, minimized, misinterpreted, or rationalized.

At the opposite extreme are unexpected deaths occurring in the course of well-documented chronic diseases that have either progressed rapidly to a stage incompatible with life or have triggered the development of quickly fatal sequelae or complications.

SUDDEN DEATH AND UNEXPECTED DEATH

The terms *sudden* and *unexpected* have different meanings for different people. Death from peritonitis complicating a perforated peptic ulcer 48 hours after the onset of acute abdominal pain in a previously healthy adult might well be considered sudden and unexpected by his family and friends. The physicians in attendance would probably not consider such a death as either sudden or unexpected.

The death of a forty-eight-year-old man with a reliable history of hypertension and arteriosclerotic heart disease who collapses and dies instantaneously while playing golf is only relatively unexpected. His cardiovascular disease renders him vulnerable to sudden death at any moment. Such relatively expected or predicable deaths, to phrase it differently, resulting from chronic disease that seems to offer no immediate threat to the patient's life, comprise the most common category of unexpected death.

From the medicolegal point of view, the unexpected aspect of death is more important than its rapidity. It is the dramatic intrusion of the unexpected that is so often responsible for arousing the suspicion of violence. Many deaths that occur while the patient is under medical observation and care, indeed, while he is confined to the hospital, are sudden but hardly unexpected. The slowly deteriorating victim of a previously diagnosed carcinoma of the lung who dies immediately following bleeding from the air passages is a case in point. This spectacular termination of the patient's life is an anticipated manifestation of the natural course of the disease, and its occurrence occasions little surprise among those familiar with the behavior of this frequently encountered cancer. The medicolegal officer has little or no official interest in this type of death, despite its suddenness, if the decedent has been under the care of a physician who can (and will) sign the death certificate.

Absence of medical attention or failure of the physician to establish the correct diagnosis and prognosis of a potentially fatal illness help create situations where the abrupt appearance of death may be considered as totally unexpected. The forensic pathologist occasionally encounters sudden and unexpected deaths resulting from large intracranial tumors in persons who have been under observation and treatment for psychoneurosis, hysteria, or psychosis. Here, the attending physician has ascribed the presence of such symptoms as headache, vomiting and emotional lability to some unresolved conflict when they were actually produced by the tumor of the brain or its surrounding membranes.

In this context, the either/or fallacy of diagnosis deserves brief comment. In making his diagnosis on the basis of history, clinical observation and laboratory studies, the physician is strongly inclined to ascribe subjective and objective abnormalities either to this disease or to that disease. However, there are very few diseases whose presences are mutually exclusive, and in many instances two separate and distinct clinical entities are present in the same patient and perhaps in the same organ. Neurotic and psychotic patients are not immune to serious organic disease, and many sudden and unexpected deaths in these unfortunate individuals are the result of the families and physicians being misled by the psychiatric background and emotionally disturbed aspects of the overall presenting clinical picture.

disease and injury. However, the autopsy cannot provide a record, in real time, of the electrophysiological disturbances culminating in electrical silence of the brain and heart. Unless that record is provided by physiologic monitoring of a dying person, the pathologist must deduce the dying process by using clues from numerous sources, only one of which is the autopsy. Equally important are the evaluations of the history, circumstances surrounding death, and the fatal environment. Additional insights can be derived from toxicological and other chemical laboratory studies and from microbiological cultures.

At this point, a brief discussion of electrical communication in and between the heart and central nervous system is in order. The heart, when considered as an electrically activated organ, consists of tissues which function as insulators and tissues which conduct electrical impulses. Impulses can be generated and transmitted not only by specialized conduction tissue in the sinus node, atrioventricular node, His bundle, and bundle branches but by working myocardium as well. Insulating tissue, including adipose and fibrous tissue, is found in the cardiac skeleton separating the atria from the ventricles. The bulk of the heart is formed by contractile working myocardium.

Working myocardium is capable of generating a repetitive electrical impulse at any level of the heart, but that capacity is more highly developed in the specialized conduction tissue. Normally, the coordinated contraction of all the working myocardial cells depends on the organization imposed by the specialized cells. The automaticity of the sinus node is dominant and overrides the automaticity of the atrioventricular node and of the working myocardium.

The orderly propagation of the contractile wave front depends on the continuous overriding of potential ectopic pacemakers and on the absence of re-entry or circus pathways, either within the ventricles or between the atria and ventricles. When an ectopic ventricular focus takes over and drives the rest of the ventricular myocardium in an orderly fashion, premature ventricular contractions or sustained ventricular tachycardia are produced. In the presence of circus pathways, the ectopic signal can generate an uncoordinated wave front and ventricular fibrillation ensues. Because ventricular fibrillation and some forms of ventricular tachycardia produce no net forward pumping of blood, they are lethal if not corrected.

Ventricular ectopy can be viewed as the result of an irritable ventricle. Ventricular irritability is increased by hypertrophy, ischemia, sympathetic discharge, ethanol intoxication, hyperthyroidism and numerous drugs, including monoamine oxidase inhibitors, tricyclic antidepressants, caffeine, theophylline and other sympathomimetic agents such as epinephrine, norepinephrine, and agents found in diet pills and nasal decongestants.

The obverse of myocardial irritability is myocardial depression. Depressed myocardial cells have lessened contractile strength, diminished oxygen demand, slowing of the cell-to-cell propagation of electrical impulses, diminished amplitude of the electrical impulses, and a diminished rate of pulse generation. A beneficial effect of myocardial depression is reduced oxygen demand, which lessens the risk of ischemia and ectopy. A major danger of myocardial depression is failure of electrical impulse propagation, especially across the atrioventricular node, which functions not so much to facilitate conduction as to delay conduction and restrict it to one channel. Failure of impulse propagation across the atrioventricular node results in atrioventricular block. The ventricular response to atrioventricular block varies from the tolerable emergence of a dominant pacemaker in the His bundle to no response at all, resulting in cardiac standstill and death. The loss of a supraventricular impulse generator may permit the expression of a circus pathway and lethal ventricular tachyarrhythmia.

Myocardial depression can be caused by parasympathetic discharge, myxedema, hypothermia, and hyperkalemia. In the laboratory, an isolated heart supplied with oxygen and nutrients will continue to beat because of the automaticity of the sinus node. In the body, however, the heart is not an isolated organ. It has both sympathetic and parasympathetic innervation, which strongly influence the activity of both working and specialized conducting myocardium. The electrochemical discharge from the central nervous system to the heart and blood vessels can be strong enough or imbalanced enough to produce cardiac standstill, ventricular fibrillation, or emptying of the heart and central vessels by virtue of vascular redistribution.

The exact locations in the central nervous system of all the vasomotor centers which control autonomic discharge to the heart are not known, but the critical areas seem to reside in the region of the third ventricle, the midbrain, and the medulla oblongata. Sympathetic discharge flows down the intermediolateral columns of the spinal cord, and leaves the cord in the thoracic and lumbar regions by way of the chains of sympathetic ganglia running adjacent to the vertebral column. From the upper thoracic ganglia and from the stellate ganglion in particular, efferent branches pass into the mediastinum and along the base of the heart to innervate the myocardium and cardiac blood vessels. Parasympathetic discharges originating in the vasomotor centers exit the brain by way of the vagus nerves, which descend into the mediastinum and innervate the heart.

Theoretically, mechanical trauma anywhere in the pathways described above can induce profound electrical disturbances of the heart. Indeed instantaneous death, so sudden as to simulate sudden death by heart disease, can result from trauma or natural disease involving the central nervous system. Some examples include transverse fractures of the floor of the skull which run near the base of the third ventricle, fractures of the posterior fossa of the skull, dislocations of the neck, extremely forceful facial impacts that cause hyperextension of the head with resulting pontomedullary lacerations, and gunshot wounds of the brain or spinal cord. Each of the foregoing can be associated with instantaneous lethal disruptions of cardiac function and can be conceptualized as the equivalent of central cardiac concussion. Likewise, spontaneous subarachnoid arterial hemorrhages quickly form bloody tamponades in the cisterns at the base of the third ventricle and along the medulla, which can cause instantaneous death. Congenital malformations

of the craniocervical articulation can allow compression of the upper spinal cord or lower medulla with the same result.

Cessation of cardiac function causes unconsciousness in less than 15 seconds, paralysis of central respiratory centers within a few minutes, and irreversible cessation of cerebral function within approximately five minutes. On the other hand, respiratory arrest produces a somewhat slower death. The cerebral response is similar to that produced by cardiac arrest. The cardiac response is different and has been characterized as slow cardiac cessation.[7]

Respiratory arrest produces systemic hypoxia and acidosis. A heart free of disease can beat for several minutes. The first cardiac response to hypoxia is tachycardia. Then, bradycardia ensues and slow ventricular pacemakers take over. Finally, cellular metabolism is so disturbed that electromechanical dissociation ensues. In electromechanical dissociation, electrical discharge from the heart is still detectable, but there is no pulse and no blood flow. When the heart is diseased, the foregoing sequence, which is not invariable by any means, is often abbreviated by the early occurrence of ventricular tachycardia, ventricular fibrillation, or cardiac standstill.

The location of the respiratory centers is known in greater detail than is the location of the vasomotor centers. Nuclei in the medulla generate the basic respiratory rhythm. Centers in the dorsal pons fine-tune the basic rhythm.[8] Signals from the respiratory centers travel caudally through the upper spinal cord and exit mainly via the phrenic nerves. The phrenic nerves take origin mainly from the C-4 roots, with some contribution from C-3 and C-5. The phrenic nerves travel through the neck and along the sides of the pericardial sac to reach the two leaves of the diaphragm. Respiratory arrest can be caused by physical or chemical lesions involving the medulla oblongata, cervical spinal cord, phrenic nerves, neuromuscular junctions, and the muscles of respiration including the diaphragm.

Up to this point, our discussion has centered on intercellular communication by electrochemical impulses and derangements of this communication system. Sudden cessation of vital functions can also be effected by derangements of intracellular physiology. For example, the cyanide anion poisons the cytochrome oxidase system in mitochondria and thus prevents the utilization of oxygen. This derangement is so profound that effective cellular function and intercellular communication fail immediately. Alterations induced by abnormal metabolism of sugar, electrolytes, other endogenous substances, and countless drugs and poisons can cause similar lethal intracellular dysfunction.

Approach to the Heart in the Evaluation of Sudden Cardiac Death

Systematic examination of the heart should always include the thorough evaluation of the coronary arteries, myocardium, and heart valves. Our approach is to serially section the coronary arteries at an interval small enough to assess the entire luminal segment. In routine cases, slices of myocardium approximately 1.0 cm thick are made from the apex toward the base of the heart to approximately 2 cm from the atrioventricular valves. This allows examination of much of the myocardium. Then the valves are exposed by opening the heart *along the lines of blood flow.* In addition, histologic examination of the conduction system may be performed.

Sudden Cardiac Death: Function vs. Structure

All sudden cardiac deaths are mediated by acute derangements of physiologic function. Occasionally, the functional derangement is obvious, as in the case of ruptured myocardial infarcts with hemopericardium and tamponade. Usually, however, since the functional derangement is electrical, it leaves no footprints at autopsy and must be inferred from the presence of morphologically manifested chronic cardiac disease, involving either the conduction system, the coronary arteries, the myocardium, or the heart valves. The functional derangement, usually a ventricular tachyarrhythmia, occurs in the setting of transient electrical destabilization of the heart. Such a destabilization is usually the product of a predisposing chronic anatomic substrate and acute transient risk factors.[3] The anatomic substrates are familiar as *anatomic* or etiologic causes of death. Virtually any chronic disease of the heart can be an anatomic substrate for sudden cardiac death.

The transient risk factors are time-dependent, often reversible functional changes, such as altered autonomic tone, coronary artery spasm, and increased platelet adhesiveness. In exceptional instances, transient risk factors alone may produce lethal functional derangements with no detectable anatomic substrate whatsoever. Such deaths usually occur in a highly charged emotional situation. In other words, when functional changes are severe enough, fibrillation can occur in the absence of structural disease.

Lown has clearly demonstrated that psychological stress can directly lower the fibrillation threshold of the heart by means of increased sympathetic tone. In his discussion of transient risk factors, he suggests *the focus (of study) should be shifted from the heart as target to the brain as trigger,* and reports that stimulation of the hypothalamus can induce cardiac arrhythmias.[4]

Functional Disturbances of the Conduction System

Sudden cardiac deaths result when an electrically unstable heart is subjected to a transient change in its autonomic stimulation or electrolyte environment. Usually a predisposing chronic cardiac disease is demonstrable as the morphologic substrate for sudden death. In this section, however, we discuss functional sudden deaths, in which there is no anatomic substrate demonstrable by customary techniques or autopsy examination.

For some of these diseases, a handful of pathologists interested in the study of the conduction system have described a variety of abnormalities of the conducting bundles and surrounding tissue.[9-11] Interpretation of these abnormalities is difficult because the same abnormalities can be incidental findings in the hearts of persons dying of violent causes. For example, persistence of the dispersed fetal patterns of the atrioventricular node and His bundle and sclerosis of the atrio-ventricular nodal artery area are easily found in routine sections of hearts of persons dying from obviously non-cardiac causes.[12] It is possible that these findings are at one end of the spectrum of normal developmental variations and that they have the potential to make the heart electrically unstable. With this in mind we discuss functional deaths without anatomically defined disease.

Vagal Inhibition

Deaths from vagal inhibition of the heart are defined as sudden deaths that occur within seconds or a minute or two after minor trauma or peripheral or internal stimulation of a relatively simple and ordinarily innocuous nature. Investigation of the circumstances surrounding death discloses that such stimulation probably initiated a fatal cardiovascular inhibitory reflex.

A variety of incidents have been incriminated as precipitating factors for deaths from inhibition, i.e., a blow to the larynx or upper abdomen, a kick in the scrotum, pressure on the carotid sinus, cannulation of the cervix, etc. Therefore, death from vagal inhibition is usually considered accidental, inasmuch as it is initiated by microtrauma defined as an injury so slight that it does not produce a wound.

Spontaneous Ventricular Fibrillation

In rare instances, ostensibly healthy, robust persons have the functional equivalent of fatal syncope without demonstrable cause. The investigation of such deaths fails to uncover relevant medical history. Reliable eyewitnesses often provide statements that are compellingly indicative of innocent circumstances surrounding death. Complete, competent autopsies, including appropriate microscopic and toxicologic studies, disclose no abnormalities. Deaths of this sort usually occur during or after exercise or during intense emotional experiences.

That an episode of emotional stress, whether it be anger, fear, joy, or apprehension, can precipitate ectopy and even lethal ventricular arrhythmias in persons with organic heart disease is common knowledge. Less well known is the fact that such emotionally mediated adrenergic surges can have identical effects in hearts with no demonstrable anatomic lesion. Some authors have pointed out that such common lay terms as *scared to death* and *frightened to death* can be literally true when the immediate response to unusual and extraordinary fright is overwhelming.

The logical conclusion, after exclusion of reasonable alternatives, is that these victims had electrically unstable hearts. Since the rhythm responsible for the majority of instantaneous cardiac deaths is ventricular fibrillation, the designation *spontaneous ventricular fibrillation of undetermined etiology* is reasonable. One report described five patients with ventricular fibrillation and one with ventricular flutter, who were successfully resuscitated and studied by cardiologists. None had overt heart disease detectable by standard clinical means, but four had inducible ventricular fibrillation when subjected to programmed electrical stimulation.[13]

It is becoming increasingly possible to better define some instances of spontaneous ventricular fibrillation. For example, the Brugada syndrome is a rare, autosomal dominant disorder with characteristic electrocardiographic abnormalities of right bundle branch block and ST segment elevation in leads V1 to V3. It can cause ventricular fibrillation and sudden cardiac death. Some of these mutations have mapped to a cardiac sodium channel.[14]

Sudden and Unexplained Death in Sleep in Asian Men

These are called Pokkuri (sudden unexpected occurrence) Disease in Japan, Bangungut (nightmare) in the Philippines, and Nonlaitai (sleep-death) in Laos, Cambodia, and Vietnam.[15] This entity is well known in the Orient, but has only recently been recognized in North America. Polymorphic ventricular tachycardia and ventricular fibrillation have been unequivocally documented in some of the victims.[16] The deaths occur almost exclusively in young men during sleep. It is most common in December and January. Several theories are postulated. Responsible arrhythmias seem to occur during night terrors, which, unlike nightmares, occur during non-REM sleep and from which the victim cannot be aroused. Heart rate can precipitously rise to extraordinarily high levels during night terrors, indicating that the heart is subjected to a sudden surge of adrenergic current.[15] Pathological studies have revealed minimally increased heart weights and a variety of non-specific variations in the conduction system.[17,18] The incidence of this form of sudden death seems to decrease in immigrants to the United States, raising the possibility of a role for environmental factors.[19] Recent studies have shown EKG abnormalities in some of the survivors of these events.[17]

Long QT Syndromes

These disorders are characterized by a prolonged period of recovery from depolarization of the heart and a pronounced tendency to syncope and sudden death, mediated by ventricular tachyarrythmias. Diagnosis is hampered by the inconsistency of the electrocardiographic findings and the wide range of *normal* QT intervals. The most common form of this syndrome (also termed Romano-Ward Syndrome) is inherited in an autosomal dominant fashion, and 5 genes have been associated with it.[20–22] The defect is in cardiac ion channels, including subunits of 4 potassium channels and a sodium channel. A sixth locus on chromosome 4 is still being defined. Many of the mutations are missense mutations and effect various parts of the gene, complicating potential genetic screening. The potassium channel mutations result in loss of function, causing a total reduction in the current carried. In contrast, the sodium channel mutations result in a gain of function due to defective inactivation of the channel. The molecular definition of these diseases may allow better treatment with agents capable of modulating specific channel properties.

A second, much rarer but more lethal form of Long QT Syndrome is Jervell and Lange-Nielsen Syndrome. This usually has an autosomal recessive pattern of inheritance and is associated with congenital deafness. Homozygous mutations in a cardiac potassium channel have been identified.[23]

Pre-Excitation Syndromes (Wolf-Parkinson-White Syndrome)

Normally, the atria are electrically connected to the ventricles only through the His bundle. This syndrome is characterized by the presence of an extra-atrioventricular conduction path which allows re-entry of the conduction impulse and promotes the induction of ventricular tachycardia and ventricular fibrillation. The accessory pathways can cross the atrioventricular sulcus of either the right or left chambers or septum. Septal pathways can be found between atrial and ventricular myocardium, between the proximal atrioventricular node and the ventricular septum, or from the proximal atrioventricular node in the His bundle. Histopathologic documentation requires thousands of tedious step sections unless the accessory pathway has been localized by electrocardiogram. The diagnosis is made clinically. If an accessory pathway is demonstrated at autopsy in a victim of a sudden cardiac death with no clinical diagnosis of pre-excitation, the proper diagnosis is spontaneous ventricular fibrillation, since the pathway may or may not have been active. Wolf-Parkinson-White syndrome associated with hypertrophic cardiomyopathy occurs with an autosomal dominant mode of inheritance and has been genetically linked to chromosome 7q3.[24]

Sick Sinus Syndrome

Most instances of sick sinus syndrome are secondary to surgery in the region of the sinoatrial node. Occasional cases of spontaneous sick sinus syndrome occur. They are characterized by sinus bradycardia, syncope, and rarely, sudden death. Histopathologic investigation has been limited.[25,26]

Structural Disturbances of the Conduction System

Lev's Disease

Replacement fibrosis of the bundle branches bears the eponymous designation Lev's Disease. Bundle branch fibrosis is commonly present in aged hearts and hypertrophied hearts with premature sclerosis of the basal septum.[27] However, it is uncommonly diagnosed because of the infrequent autopsy examination of the bundle branches. This situation is easily rectified as left bundle branches are easily found in any casual transverse section of the anterior basal aspect of the ventricular septum.

Microscopic Abnormalities

Even casual sections of the region of the atrioventricular node will disclose minor anomalies in many victims of sudden cardiac death. It is possible that these anomalies provide a congenital substrate for electrical instability. Since the same anatomical variants can be found in hearts of persons dying suddenly from violent causes, we do not believe that death can be ascribed to many of these variants, with a reasonable degree of certainty, unless there are supportive clinical data.

The foregoing variants included persistent fetal dispersion of the atrioventricular node, ectopic nodo-fascicular (His Bundle) tracts, and ectopic atrioventricular tracts.[28] A frequent finding is the presence of striking sclerosis of the atrioventricular nodal artery, especially in the ventricular septum, distal to the arterial perforation of the central fibrous body. Such sclerosis is common in the presence of left ventricular

hypertrophy, but is found frequently in otherwise healthy persons who die from violence. Many other such minor variants have been reported. The potential of these variants to cause electrical instability has been debated.

Microscopic hemorrhages are found frequently in the atrioventricular node and the His bundle. Such hemorrhages are so frequent that we interpret them as autopsy artifacts unless there is vital reaction or gross evidence of mechanical trauma.

Collagen Vascular Disease

Ankylosing spondylitis, scleroderma, and rheumatoid arthritis can involve the cardiac valves with extension of the inflammatory process into the atrioventricular node or His bundle. Inflammatory involvement of the ventricular endocardium can affect the left bundle branches.

Infiltrative Diseases

In cases of hemochromatosis, amyloidosis, sarcoidosis, or any type of myocarditis, it is prudent to focus histologic examination on the conduction system. For example, a granuloma interrupting the His bundle is more significant than a similar granuloma in working myocardium.

CORONARY ARTERIES

The second component of the heart to consider is the coronary arteries They are subject to several diseases which may result in sudden cardiac death. These include arteritis, coronary dissection, and congenital abnormalities. However, by far the most common cause of sudden and unexpected death in the Western world is arteriosclerotic heart disease.

Arteriosclerotic Heart Disease

Arteriosclerotic heart disease usually kills by either of two principal mechanisms: pump failure or sudden arrhythmia. An uncommon mech-

anism of death is cardiac tamponade from rupture of a recent infarct.

Pump failure occurs with hearts that appear to be relatively stable electrically. After multiple ischemic insults, the left ventricle can have one or more infarcts, diffuse global subendocardial fibrosis, and dilation with congestive failure. When congestive failure is severe, all organs, including the heart, are underperfused. This may lead to pulmonary congestion and edema, chronic passive hepatic congestion, splenic congestion, peripheral edema and, ultimately, ischemic acute renal tubular necrosis and hypoxic encephalopathy. The left ventricle experiences global hypoxia which, when severe enough, finally generates ventricular ectopy or a bradyrhythm. In an electrical sense, these persons can be thought of as surviving their arteriosclerotic heart disease. The vast majority of them die in the hospital and come to autopsy in the practice of the hospital-based pathologist.

When arteriosclerotic heart disease kills before the onset of congestive heart failure, the mechanism is a sudden arrhythmia induced by myocardial ischemia, with or without the additional trigger effect of transient risk factors. This mode of death may be thought of as electrical failure, and it manifests as sudden death in those persons with electrically unstable hearts. Electrical instability, as manifested by sudden death rates, is increased by arterial hypertension, and electrical instability has been experimentally and epidemiologically linked with left ventricular hypertrophy.[29,30] Most persons dying from arteriosclerotic heart disease outside the hospital die of sudden electrical failure. Many of them have hypertension-induced left ventricular hypertrophy, and they are more properly said to have died of hypertensive *and* arteriosclerotic cardiovascular disease. Sudden arrhythmias tend to occur in persons who were not previously in distress. Such persons collapse in the bathtub, on the toilet, during intercourse, while operating motor vehicles, while speaking, while eating, during sleep, and during or after exertion; that is, at any time and in any place. Most of the arrhythmias are ventricular tachyarrythmias, most commonly ventricular fibrillation.[29] The sudden onset of ventricular fibrillation has been likened to turning off a light switch.

Ischemia is a common basis for the arrhythmias in persons experiencing sudden death. The ischemia is produced by the fixed atheromatous obstructions seen at autopsy and by compounding functional disturbances known as transient risk factors. It is the functional factors that explain why a 75% obstruction caused by a plaque in a coronary artery is compatible with life one minute and is deadly the next. These functional factors include transient elevations of blood pressure, which increase afterload and increase oxygen demand; increased neural sym-

pathetic discharge associated with increased oxygen demand; sympathomimetic irritation of the heart by caffeine, cocaine and epinephrine with increased oxygen demand; coronary artery spasm at the site of a fixed obstruction; platelet embolization from an ulcerated plaque leading to localized myocardial ischemia and irritability; and transient thrombosis at the site of a fixed obstruction. Finally, as our understanding of cerebral control over the heart increases, emotions are receiving increased attention as transient risk factors that precipitate sudden death in susceptible persons. These transient risk factors, which are the difference between live persons with arteriosclerotic heart disease and dead persons with arteriosclerotic heart disease, are hardly ever demonstrable at the autopsy table. Their presence must be inferred from the terminal circumstances.

It used to be thought that all sudden deaths from arteriosclerotic heart disease were due to coronary thrombosis with acute myocardial infarction. It was assumed that the infarcts occurred but were undetectable at autopsy in the early hours of evolution. It is true that although biochemical and functional myocyte abnormality may begin immediately after cessation of blood flow, death does not begin until 30–40 minutes later (as determined by electron microscopy), and cannot be detected by routine histology for 4–6 hours.[31] However, since the advent of cardiopulmonary resuscitation and cardioversion, numerous survivors of cardiac arrest have been studied by serial electrocardiograms and cardiac enzymes. Only a small minority develop signs of an infarct. The majority simply evince profound electrical instability.[29]

Arrhythmias also may develop during reperfusion of ischemic myocardium, from circus rhythms permitted by loops of viable myocardium coursing between islands of dead myocardium, or by ischemic zones with slowed impulse propagation. Such complex interfaces have been demonstrated for human and experimental infarcts.[32]

What are the key elements for the basis of the opinion that a person has died from arteriosclerotic heart disease? Arteriosclerotic disease is a very common finding at autopsy. Coronary sclerosis develops over a period of decades, and its presence is compatible with a vigorous life. Therefore, the mere demonstration of obstructive coronary atheromata is insufficient to render the opinion that coronary artery disease was responsible for the death. Likewise, even a recent myocardial infarct, important for its indication of recent disease activity and probable increased electrical instability, does not render a person immune from other causes of death.

The answer to our rhetorical question lies in the consideration of the terminal circumstances and in the reasonable exclusion of other diseases or injuries that can cause sudden death. What is reasonable depends on the circumstances. Consider the following hypothetical cases.

A 57-year-old postal worker with a history of recent chest pain is found dead on the floor of the kitchen by his wife ten minutes after she last saw him alive. The autopsy revealed a 450 gm heart with a 90% occlusion of the proximal left anterior descending coronary artery by atheromatous plaque. He has no other important disease or injury. His death is certified at the time of autopsy as hypertensive and atherosclerotic cardiovascular disease.

Consider the same 57-year-old man, this time found dead in a hotel room in the city in which he resides. The autopsy findings are identical. However, in this scenario, the circumstances are unusual, and the degree of certainty supporting the working hypothesis of death due to hypertensive and atherosclerotic heart disease is much lower than in the first scenario. A negative toxicological work-up may be necessary to achieve a reasonable degree of medical certainty that his death was due to heart disease.

Very few out-of-hospital sudden deaths from arteriosclerotic heart disease are preceded by classic symptoms of angina pectoris. Sometimes there is a history of palpitations, syncope, or vague chest pains.[6] In our experience, when such persons experience pain, it is often perceived as shoulder, neck, or abdominal pain or *heartburn*. Just as nitroglycerin pills are an investigative clue to the existence of a documented history of heart disease, antacid tablets often provide a clue to the presence of undiagnosed atypical angina.

A 48-year-old man was prescribed a non-steroidal, anti-inflammatory drug for a clinical diagnosis of shoulder bursitis. After his sudden demise, the autopsy revealed normal shoulder joints and coronary atherosclerosis.

A 63-year-old was found dead in his bathroom. In his pocket was a roll of antacid tablets. He never consulted a doctor. The autopsy revealed arteriosclerotic heart disease and a normal stomach.

The most common anatomic manifestation of arteriosclerotic heart disease at the time of death in out-of-hospital fatalities is uncomplicated coronary atherosclerosis, with no recent or healed myocardial infarcts. Recent occlusive thrombi are present in only a minority of instances.[2] The frequency of detection of plaque fissures with mural thrombi, microscopic cholesterol emboli, and evidence of acute myocardial ischemia will depend on the intensity of microscopic studies. Fiber waviness is a sign of irreversible ischemic injury that may be seen early. Coagulation necrosis, edema, and hemorrhages then appear. Contraction band necrosis may or may not be present. It is a manifestation of ischemia and has been found in the advancing wave front of acute infarction and in reperfused myocardium following ischemia.[33] Inflammatory cells follow in a predictable sequence to result finally in granulation tissue and fibrosis.

The roles that hypertension and diabetes play in accelerating coronary atherosclerosis have been well documented.[5] Atheromas in distal epicardial ramifications occur commonly with these diseases.

A common non-specific finding in deaths from arteriosclerotic heart disease is congestion. Victims of heart attacks typically have engorgement of the cardiac chambers and central capacitance vessels, and they evince pronounced postmortem lividity, often with a strikingly purple head. These changes probably are a consequence of agonal unbalanced autonomic discharge rather than hypervolemia.

The one form of sudden death from coronary disease whose mechanism is self evident is that resulting from a ruptured myocardial infarct, a catastrophic complication seen more often in women than in men and increasing in frequency with age.[34] This most commonly occurs four to seven days after the onset of the infarct. When the rupture involves the interventricular septum or a papillary muscle, death usually follows within a few hours as a result of acute myocardial failure. When the rupture traverses the left ventricular wall and communicates with the pericardial space, death from cardiac tamponade takes place within minutes from rapid accumulation of blood within the sac. Rupture is favored by elevated intraventricular pressure resulting from physical activity, hypertension or a valvular lesion. The entire thickness of the ventricular wall is usually involved by the infarct, and the infarct generally has evoked a marked acute inflammatory infiltrate.

A surprising feature of some ruptured myocardial infarcts is that they occasionally are observed in persons who have been carrying on normal or only slightly restricted activity for several days prior to their sudden fatal collapse. Thus, a major transmural infarct may elicit neither sufficient symptoms nor physical signs to indicate the presence of severe myocardial injury. Ruptured myocardial infarcts have been found relatively frequently in ambulatory institutionalized psychotic patients.[35] This prevalence is reasonably explained by postulating that mental illness may either make the patient oblivious to his bodily symptoms or interfere with his ability to communicate. Moreover, objective signs of serious illness may be overlooked in a large mental hospital with limited medical personnel. Nonetheless, the same apparently paradoxical situation occurs in non-psychotic persons. While absence of pain and other symptoms may result from a high pain threshold (silent infarct), it is difficult to understand the failure of severe acute disease to evoke shock and other clinical phenomena characteristically associated with severe myocardial damage. This is an example of the great discrepancy that may exist between the gravity of an organic lesion and the comparatively trivial clinical manifestations associated with it.

The most frequent errors committed by inexperienced or careless pathologists in the evaluation of arteriosclerotic heart disease involve emphasizing the study of the myocardium at the expense of the coronary arteries. The following errors are common:

- Failure to examine the sinuses of Valsalva to detect obstruction or hypoplasia of the coronary ostia.
- Sampling the coronary arteries at arbitrary intervals, i.e., 10 mm, 5 mm, or 3 mm. Sampling will often miss solitary stenoses. The optimal interval between cross-cuts depends on the caliber of the vessel and the presence of luminal obstruction. The cross-cuts must be close enough so that the entire luminal segment can be inspected by looking through it.
- Failure to examine the full length of epicardial arteries. The distal portion of the right coronary artery is a common site of atheromata.
- Failure to examine all the coronary arteries. Almost all pathologists will examine the proximal part of the left anterior descending artery. It is astonishing how many ostensibly well-trained pathologists omit examination of the right, left main or left circumflex arteries. If the aorta and pulmonary artery are cut long, the transverse sinus will be retained with the removed heart. In this situation the left main artery is inaccessible until the aorta is separated from the pulmonary artery. The left circumflex artery, in contrast to the right coronary artery, runs quite deep in the coronary sulcus, can be partly obscured by the overhanging left atrial appendage, and can be missed by shallow cross-cuts. The obtuse marginal branches of the circumflex artery and the diagonal branches of the ramus intermedius branches on the free wall of the left ventricle are commonly involved with atheromata, and their examination should not be neglected.

Non-Atherosclerotic Coronary Artery Disease

Morphologically normal coronary arteries can undergo lethal spasm; more often the spastic arterial segment is the seat of atherosclerotic narrowing.[36] Atherosclerotic obstruction or congenital narrowing of the coronary ostia can be accompanied by perfectly normal coronary arteries. Congenital hypoplasia of the coronary arteries is accepted by most forensic pathologists as a legitimate diagnosis, although no diagnostic criteria have been established for the entity. Congenital anomalies of the distribution pattern of the epicardial arteries have been associated with sudden death, particularly when the takeoff of the artery is at an acute angle to the sinus of Valsalva.[37] Arteritis, which in other organs would lead to chronic symptoms, can first manifest itself as sudden death when it involves the arterial supply of the heart.[36] Atherosclerotic aneurysms of the coronary arteries are uncommon. Dissecting aneurysms of the coronary arteries are uncommon also, but merit special attention here because of their predilection for women and because of their association with the peripartum period.[36] For all of the foregoing entities, the mechanism of death includes regional hypoperfusion of the heart and ventricular arrhythmias.

MYOCARDIUM

We will now focus on diseases that mainly effect the myocardium. Cardiomyopathies can be classified as hypertrophic, dilated and restrictive. In addition, many systemic diseases may involve the heart. The most common disease of the left ventricle, however, is simply hypertrophy.

Left Ventricular Hypertrophy

A heavy heart is, with few exceptions, an electrically unstable heart. With the possible exception of the physiologic cardiac hypertrophy of athletes,[38] left ventricular hypertrophy, regardless of etiology, is associated with ventricular ectopy, ventricular tachyarrythmias and sudden death.[29,39-41] This association is independent of coronary atherosclerosis. The etiology of this electrical instability is unknown.[42]

Concentric left ventricular hypertrophy is caused in part by increased afterload; that is, by pumping against high pressure downstream in the systemic circuit. Concentric hypertrophy of the left ventricle involves symmetric thickening of the ventricular septum and free wall with no enlargement of the chamber.[40] The most common etiology of concentric left ventricular hypertrophy is systemic arterial hypertension. Less frequent etiologies are aortic valvular stenosis, thyrotoxicosis, and isometric exercise. Left ventricular hypertrophy with ventricular dilation, known clinically as eccentric hypertrophy because of the left-shifted cardiac shadow on the roentgenogram, is found when the heart is subjected to both increased afterload and increased preload.[40] Preload refers to the volume of blood drained from the central veins and pumped into the ventricle from the atrium. When central blood volume is increased, the end-diastolic pressure of the left ventricle rises, which causes chamber dilation. The ventricular wall then hypertrophies in response to increased wall tension, so that the ratio of wall thickness to chamber diameter is preserved. Eccentric hypertrophy as defined above is seen with obesity.

A pseudohypertrophy pattern is produced in compensation for myocardial infiltration or regional necrosis. Total mass is increased, but functioning mass is unchanged due to the presence of non-contractile tissue.[40]

Asymmetric septal hypertrophy involves inordinate thickening of the ventricular septum relative to the left ventricular free wall. It is seen in classic cases of hypertrophic cardiomyopathy and occasionally in hypertensive hearts. Left ventricular hypertrophy accompanied by pronounced dilation can be seen with decompensation of any of the disorders mentioned above and with arteriosclerotic heart disease, valvular insufficiency, myocarditis and other cardiomyopathies.

Arterial Hypertension

Before the era of echocardiography, hypertension was viewed as a risk factor for the development of arteriosclerotic heart disease and indirectly for sudden death. It now is recognized that left ventricular hypertrophy itself is a powerful risk factor for sudden death, independent of arterial pressure or coronary sclerosis. Furthermore, hypertrophy is not a late complication of hypertension. Hypertrophy in response to an increased load can occur in weeks. Hypertrophy of the left ventricle is thought to be a function of increased afterload and of undefined neuro-humoral factors, which may include increased sympathetic tone, activation of the renin-angio-tensin-aldosterone system and renal kallikrein-kinin system, and endothelial factors.[43] Studies indicate that cardiac hypertrophy in hypertensive persons is not restricted to the left ventricle. The right ventricle is also thickened, and the pressures in the pulmonary circuit are increased, possibly because of the same neurohumoral factors.[44]

Ethanol has received attention as an agent capable of producing chronic arterial hypertension.[45,46] Curiously, when alcohol is withdrawn, the blood pressure drops almost immediately. It is possible that a substantial proportion of cases of hypertension are due to alcoholism.

The practical importance of this discussion is to emphasize that hypertensive heart disease, as manifested by ventricular hypertrophy, even in the absence of coronary atherosclerosis, is a competent cause of death.[42,47,48] The list of common cardiovascular manifestations of hypertension in medicolegal practice includes not only sudden death, but also congestive heart failure, enhanced coronary atherogenesis, intracerebral hemorrhages, dissecting aneurysms, and renal vascular disease. Angina in hypertensive patients without hypertrophy has been related to elevated resistance of the coronary microvasculature.[49] In those with hypertrophy, increased mass and wall tension are accompanied by increased oxygen demand. We commonly observe fibromuscular sclerosis of mural cardiac arteries in hypertensive subjects, especially in the basal septum and the papillary muscles.

Obesity

Obesity causes cardiomegaly by two mechanisms. First, as a consequence of increased body mass, the blood volume is increased. The heart responds by dilating and hypertrophying in concert with the dilatation. Second, obese persons are prone to hypertension and, therefore, can have ventricular hypertrophy out of proportion to chamber dilatation.[40] Their hearts tend to be electrically unstable. Obesity is discussed in greater detail elsewhere in this chapter.

Age

The heart weight increases gradually with increasing age, independent of documented hypertension. The cause is unknown.[40]

Idiopathic Concentric Left Ventricular Hypertrophy

In any medicolegal autopsy practice, there will be a large number of subjects with concentric left ventricular hypertrophy who have no valvular disease and no history of hypertension. A substantial minority will have no significant narrowing of the coronary arteries by atherosclerosis. In many cases, there is no medical history of hypertension because the deceased never visited a physician. In many more cases, occasional casual blood pressure readings obtained in physicians' offices were normal. Some pathologists classify these cases as hypertrophic cardiomyopathy or concentric left ventricular hypertrophy. It is our opinion that the vast majority represent cases of hypertension which were not diagnosed antemortem. Our opinion is based on the following:

- Hypertension is a disease of vast prevalence. Hypertrophic cardiomyopathy is an unusual, specific genetic disorder.
- Casual office readings of blood pressure cannot be relied upon to detect all hypertensive subjects. A normal blood pressure determination at one time means only that the subject was normotensive at that time. In other words, in terms of numbers of pulses measured, the casual cuff reading samples a very small number of pulses in comparison to the total number of pulses. For example, the cuff readings are taken over a period of perhaps a dozen heartbeats. In 6 weeks, the heart will beat approximately 4 million times.
- Continuous ambulatory monitoring of blood pressure reveals that blood pressure is highest while the subject is at work, not while at the doctor's office.[50] Hypertension is not a static characteristic, and many persons with hypertension are normotensive during much of the day.

- Blood pressure changes from second to second. Heart mass changes over a period of weeks or months.
- The heart may be hypertrophied before the blood pressure rises above the 2-standard deviation definition of normal. This has been demonstrated in teenage children of hypertensive parents.[51]

Cardiomyopathies

Cardiomyopathies are either primary diseases of heart muscle or myocardial manifestations of systemic diseases. These may be divided into hypertrophic, dilated and restrictive. Each type can cause sudden death.

Dilated Cardiomyopathy

Dilated cardiomyopathy is the most common form of cardiomyopathy (Fig. VII-1). The hearts are boggy and globular with biventricular dilation, patchy myocardial fibrosis, myocyte hypertrophy and degeneration and replacement fibrosis of myofibers. It can be caused by end-stage congestive failure due to myocardial disease. Examples of the latter include alcoholic (or other toxic) cardiomyopathy, myocarditis and the muscular dystrophies. *Ischemic cardiomyopathy,* a term popular with cardiologists, is ventricular dilatation due to arteriosclerotic heart disease. We advocate strongly that pathologists eschew the use of ischemic cardiomyopathy as a substitute for a pathologic diagnosis, because the term is etiologically non-specific. Any congenital, inflammatory, neoplastic, traumatic, or degenerative disorder that causes myocardial ischemia can cause an ischemic cardiomyopathy. It seems to us greatly preferable to make an etiologic diagnosis whenever possible. As a means of communicating more effectively with clinical colleagues, the pathologist may wish to preface a specific pathologic diagnosis with a functionally descriptive modifier: i.e., ischemic cardiomyopathy due to arteriosclerotic heart disease.

Alcoholic cardiomyopathy of acute onset usually is caused by the cardiotoxic effect of ethanol. There are no specific pathologic findings in the

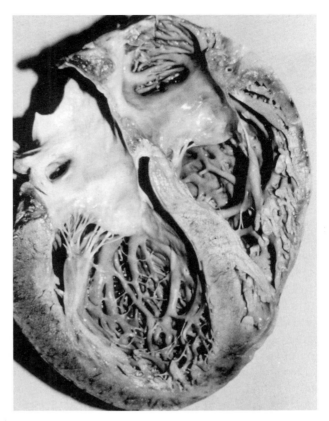

FIGURE VII-1. Idiopathic dilated cardiomyopathy. This four-chamber view shows marked dilation of all chambers.

heart to distinguish this entity from idiopathic dilated cardiomyopathy. Clinically, the distinction between idiopathic dilated cardiomyopathy and alcoholic heart disease is made by observing the patient in an alcohol-abstinent state. Alcoholic cardiomyopathy responds to removal of the noxious solvent from the body with hemodynamic improvement; idiopathic dilated cardiomyopathy does not. Clearly, this diagnostic test is impossible to apply in an autopsy practice. In the absence of antemortem studies, it is our practice to label a dilated cardiomyopathy as alcoholic if there are other anatomic stigmata of chronic alcoholism, such as cirrhosis, fatty change of the liver or pancreatitis, or if there is a reliable history of heavy drinking.

Peripartum cardiomyopathy is a poorly described disorder occurring in relation to pregnancy. It is morphologically indistinguishable from other variants of dilated cardiomyopathy.[52]

Most cases of cardiomyopathy due to muscular dystrophy will have been diagnosed clinically.[53] Duchenne's muscular dystrophy, for example, begins in childhood and only rarely presents as sudden unexpected death in an adult with no medical history. The heart usually has myocardial fibrosis.[54] Myotonic dystrophy, in contrast, is an adult-onset disease, which can present as sudden death with no prior medical diagnosis.[55] The anatomic findings in the heart consist of non-specific fatty and fibrous replacement. It is an autosomal dominant disease caused by an expansion of a trinucleotide repeat in the 3′ untranslated region of the myotonin protein kinase gene.[56] The diagnosis is suspected by the detection of the typical hatchet facies, non-muscular body habitus, and striking fatty replacement of the tongue, strap muscles and temporalis muscles. This diagnosis can be confirmed by telephone when the decedent's spouse or friends relate that he had difficulty opening jars, holding pencils, or performing similar manipulations.

However, for the majority of cases, dilated cardiomyopathy has no specific etiology and the term *idiopathic dilated cardiomyopathy* is applied. It is becoming clear that at least 20% of cases of dilated cardiomyopathy are heritable.[57] Many genetic loci have been identified, and the mutations are heterogeneous. The genes involved effect myocyte force generation, force transmission and energy production. Modes of inheritance include autosomal dominant and recessive, X-linked, and mitochondrial. One form that is autosomal dominant is caused by mutations in lamin A/C, components of the nuclear envelope.[58] Mutations in cardiac actin, a cytoskeletal protein, and desmin,[59] a muscle-specific intermediate filament also have been identified. Another X-linked form has mutations in the promoter region of dystrophin, the gene responsible for Duchenne and Becker muscular dystrophy.

Arrhythmogenic Right Ventricular Cardiomyopathy

This is a rare, autosomal dominant disease with variable penetrance which can result in heart failure, rhythm disturbances, and sudden death.[60,61] The hallmark is marked thinning of the wall of the right ventricle with fatty and fibrofatty replacement (Fig. VII-2a–b). A small number of cases with involvement of the left ventricle have also been reported. Six genetic loci have been linked to this disease, and the gene ARVD2 has recently been identified as the ryanodine receptor, the major calcium-release channel in the myocardial sarcoplasmic reticulum.[62]

Hypertrophic Cardiomyopathy

Hypertrophic cardiomyopathy is a very specific term that refers to an autosomal dominant disease caused by a mutation in one of the genes that encodes a protein that is part of the contractile apparatus of the cardiac sarcomere. The identified genes include beta-myosin heavy chain, alpha-tropomyosin, cardiac troponin T, troponin I, myosin binding protein-C, regulatory myosin light chain, essential myosin light chain, cardiac actin, and titin.[63,64] The classic form of hypertrophic cardiomyopathy is manifested by asymmetric hypertrophy of the left ventricle, in which the width of the ventricular septum exceeds that of the left ventricular free wall (Fig. VII-3a). Microscopically, the ventricles have a strikingly disorganized pattern of myofibers, most pronounced in the ventricular septum, and best demonstrated by transverse sections of the high interventricular septum (Fig. VII-3b). These individuals can have irritable ventricles and are prone to ventricular ectopy, tachyarrythmias, congestive heart failure, and sudden death.

There is marked clinical heterogeneity in this disease, which is related to the particular mutation. For example, 35% of these patients have a mutation in beta-cardiac myosin. They have a high degree of penetrance and are easily demonstrated early by echocardiogram. Mutations in troponin T cause a disease with less hypertrophy and sometimes near normal left ventricular wall thickness; however, there is a high rate of sudden cardiac death.

The importance of making the diagnosis of a familial cardiomyopathy is obvious as family members should be alerted and offered clinical

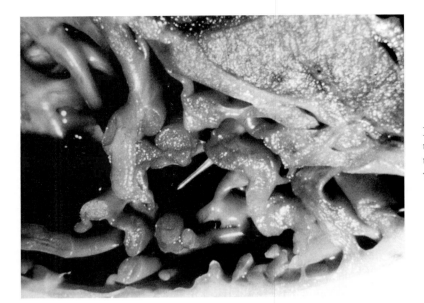

FIGURE VII-2a. Arrhythmogenic right ventricular cardiomyopathy. Note the marked thinning and fatty replacement of the right ventricular wall.

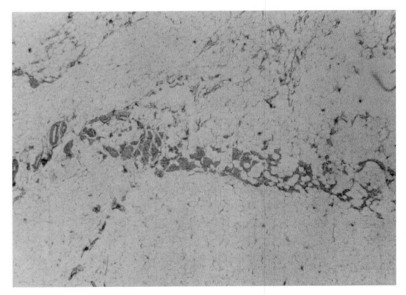

FIGURE VII-2b. Arrhythmogenic right ventricular cardiomyopathy (x10, Hematoxylin and Eosin). There is an almost complete absence of myocytes and an abundance of adipose tissue in this section of the right ventricle. This condition use to be referred to as adipositas cordis.

screening. Routine genetic screening is not yet feasible as there are already many causative genes identified, each with many different mutations. Also the mutations have variable penetrance, and there is evidence supporting a role for modifier genes and the environment in determining phenotype. However, the recent, rapid developments in high throughput DNA technology make such screening a realistic goal.

Restrictive Cardiomyopathy

Restrictive cardiomyopathies hemodynamically simulate pericardial constriction. Examples of systemic diseases whose myocardial involvement can produce a restrictive cardiomyopathy include amyloidosis, hemochromatosis and glycogen storage disorders. In the evaluation of deaths due to the foregoing diseases, microscop-

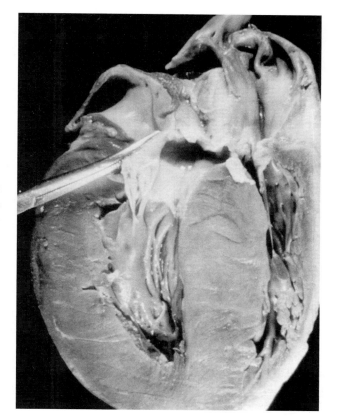

FIGURE VII-3a. Hypertrophic cardiomyopathy. There is marked asymmetric left ventricular hypertrophy and a characteristic fibrous endocardial plaque along the aortic outflow tract.

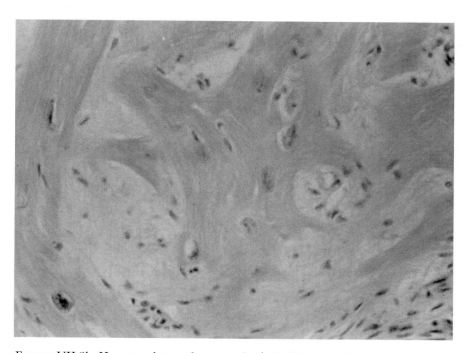

FIGURE VII-3b. Hypertrophic cardiomyopathy (×40, Hematoxylin and Eosin). There is marked myofiber disarray and interstitial fibrosis.

ic study of the specialized conduction tissue may be illuminating. Loeffler's endomyocarditis and endocardial fibroelastosis (which affects young children) are two other causes of restrictive cardiomyopathy of unknown etiology. Familial restrictive cardiomyopathies have also rarely been reported.[65,66] Histopathology shows only non-specific, patchy fibrosis.

Myocarditis

Myocarditis may be active, resolving (healing) or resolved (healed). It can occur as a complication of many infectious processes brought on by a wide variety of etiologic agents: bacteria, viruses, fungi, protozoa and even helminths. It may also occur as a result of local autoimmune reactions or hypersensitivity reactions. The histologic response may be specific as, for example, with the Aschoff nodule of acute rheumatic myocarditis or non-specific, as with viral and autoimmune myocarditis. The inflammatory process may be clinically apparent during the height of the primary disease, or it may first make itself manifest during the convalescent phase. It may be a complication of an obvious, grave systemic disease, follow what appears to be a mild respiratory infection, or be of unascertainable origin.

Clinically, the diagnosis of myocarditis is usually made in the presence of such symptoms as chest pain, dyspnea, and signs of cardiac failure, with confirmatory changes in the electrocardiogram. In the presence of a fulminating, complex primary infection, evidence of myocardial damage is often obscured. If the myocardial lesions are focal or primarily interstitial and do not involve the conduction apparatus, clinical recognition may be difficult.

Sudden and unexpected pump failure and shock can occur. In other instances, the lethal mechanism is initiated by damage to the conduction system or the establishment of ectopic foci of myocardial irritability, which in turn give rise to a fatal ventricular arrhythmia. When the result is sudden cardiac death, grossly, the heart may appear normal. Occasionally, a hint of disease is suggested by flabbiness to palpation or the presence of myocardial petechiae. The diagnosis of myocarditis is made on the basis of microscopic study of the myocardium, which reveals cellular infiltration of various types and of varying degrees of severity, accompanied by myocardial fiber degeneration and necrosis and by interstitial edema in a pattern not typical of ischemic necrosis.[67]

In few other causes of sudden death is the necessity of microscopic study so important in establishing the presence of a fatal lesion in the absence of gross abnormalities as it is in myocarditis. Because myocarditis is frequently non-uniform and focal rather than uniform and confluent, histological examination of only a few samples of myocardium is inadequate to exclude myocarditis. In unusual instances, we have observed unequivocal myocarditis in only two or three of several samples of myocardium, with the remainder being normal. Microscopic study of the specialized conducting tissues is often rewarding,[68] as is sampling of working myocardium from all four chambers.

Viral myocarditis can occur at any age, and it can occur in association with infection by the human immune deficiency virus prior to the onset of the fully developed acquired immune deficiency syndrome. Myocarditis is common in persons dying of the acquired immune deficiency syndrome, and in some instances may reflect direct infection of cardiac lymphocytes and macrophages by the human immune deficiency virus.[69]

However, a postmortem diagnosis of death from myocarditis should be approached with caution in the absence of antecedent clinical documentation of illness. Just as the presence of severe coronary atherosclerosis does not categorically establish that it was responsible for death, so a finding of focal or diffuse myocarditis does not exclude the participation of other diseases, injuries, or toxins. Myocardial foci of lymphocytic infiltration are observed occasionally in random histologic sections of hearts obtained from individuals whose death is clearly unrelated to myocarditis, i.e., immediately fatal gunshot wound of the head. Accordingly, myocarditis should be regarded as the cause of death only in the context of complete anatomic, circumstantial, and chemical studies.

Sarcoid Heart Disease

Myocardial sarcoidosis can cause sudden and unexpected death.[70] Porter[71] reported that 22 of 33 cases of sarcoid myocarditis terminated in this fashion, and that one-fourth of the victims had had no premonitory symptoms. Almost all victims of myocardial sarcoidosis have similar granulomata in other organs.

Variation in myocardial localization of the granulomata accounts for differences in the clinical picture. Several types of arrhythmias and electrocardiographic findings have been described, including different degrees of heart block and conduction delay, paroxysmal atrial and ventricular tachycardias, and S-T segment and T wave changes.

Clinically, symptomatic patients may present with angina pectoris, palpitations, or syncope. As with other forms of myocardial disease, sudden death has been ascribed to interference with conduction or the initiation of intolerable arrhythmias.

Rheumatic and Rheumatoid Heart Disease

Acute rheumatic fever is now rare. It produces a myocarditis which can involve the conducting system. Collagen vascular diseases such as ankylosing spondylitis or rheumatoid arthritis can include severe acute granulomatous and plasmacytic inflammation of the ascending aorta, aortic valve and coronary ostia, leading to coronary insufficiency or thrombosis. Rheumatic and rheumatoid carditis heal, leaving deformed valves which then give rise to valvular stenosis and insufficiency and compensatory ventricular hypertrophy with its attendant electrical instability.

Heart Valves

The final components of the heart we will discuss are the heart valves, which are subject to a number of congenital, acquired, and degenerative diseases.

Calcific Aortic Stenosis

Aortic stenosis is the most common valvular disease. When the first edition of this book appeared, aortic valve stenosis was a frequent cause of sudden death in medicolegal practice. Since then, cardiac surgery has blossomed to the extent that most of these stenotic valves are removed and replaced with prosthetic valves, theoretically permitting regression of left ventricular hypertrophy and reduction of the risk of sudden death. Complications which ensue from the placement of artificial valves generally are treated in the hospitals. Stenotic calcified aortic valves that require surgical removal may be congenitally bicuspid; some are post-inflammatory or have senile-type calcification without commissural fusion.[72] With all types of stenosis, the left ventricle develops concentric hypertrophy and, simultaneously, electrical instability. Most sudden deaths are due to ventricular irritability. Rarely, calcific deposits may involve the tissue between the right and non-coronary cusps, with impingement of the His bundle leading to heart block. With deformity of the aortic valve, blood flow to the coronary ostia may be impaired, with consequent increased ventricular irritability.

Mitral Valve Prolapse

Prolapse of the mitral valve occurs in five to 10% of the general population. It is found in teenagers, young adults and the elderly. Patients have an increased incidence of atypical chest pain, hyperventilation, and other non-specific disorders. Marfan syndrome and other connective tissue disorders are overrepresented in series of patients with the floppy mitral valve.

The terms mitral valve prolapse, floppy mitral valve, and mid-systolic click are not synonymous. While most such clicks are due to a floppy mitral valve, dysfunctional papillary muscle and cardiomyopathy can cause clicks with murmurs. Likewise, mitral valve prolapse is usually due to the floppy mitral valve syndrome, but it can be

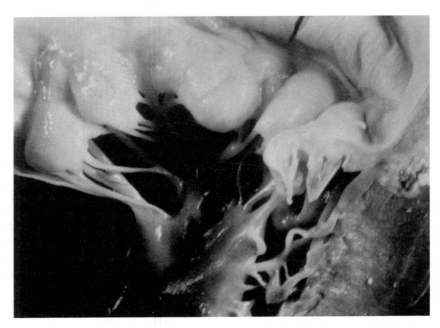

Figure VII-4. Myxomatous mitral valve. The marked redundancy and thickening of the mitral valve leaflets are characteristic. There is also calcification of the mitral annulus.

due to myocardial disease.[73] The anatomic basis for most instances of mitral valve prolapse is mucinous or myxoid degeneration of the cardiac skeleton.[74]

Grossly, affected hearts have baggy redundancy of the mitral valve leaflets, with parachute-like hooding between chordal attachments. The leaflets are often thickened (Fig. VII-4). Microscopically, the thickening corresponds to thickening of the zona spongiosa, which normally has a loose myxoid structure, and by mucinous infiltration of the zona fibrosa of the valve. Friction between coapting leaflets is responsible for the frequent occurrence of fibrosis of the valve edges. Similarly, the chordae tendineae can rub along the ventricular endocardium and produce fibrinous and fibrous friction ridges which can eventually entrap isolated chordae tendineae. Mucinous degeneration of cardiac nerves and intramural myocardial arteries has been demonstrated. In a minority of cases, the tricuspid and aortic valves are affected. Rarely, the pulmonary valve is affected.[73]

The major complications of mitral valve prolapse are bacterial endocarditis, mitral insuffi-

ciency with or without rupture of chordae tendineae, cerebral vascular thromboembolism, and sudden death. In a few patients with floppy mitral valve who died suddenly, monitoring revealed ventricular tachycardia degenerating to ventricular fibrillation.[75]

The survival curves of populations with floppy mitral valves are indistinguishable from the survival curves of the general population. Thus, the incidence of sudden death in this disorder is extremely low. A study from the Mayo Clinic reported a statistical 5-year freedom from sudden death of 98%.[76] However, the population with the condition is extremely large. Therefore, deaths due to mitral valve prolapse are not rare in a busy medicolegal practice. Although it is an accepted cause of sudden cardiac death, the mechanism is unknown.

Calcification of the Mitral Annulus

Senile calcification of the mitral annulus is common, particularly in elderly women. In such cases, the calcific deposits can impinge on the atrioventricular node or His bundle. Rarely, they may also affect valve function and may provide a nidus for thrombus formation or infective endocarditis.

Syphilis

Syphilitic aortic valvular damage that leads to insufficiency and regurgitation can also cause sudden death. The strain on the left ventricle with this type of valvular damage is even greater than that produced by stenosis, and the myocardial hypertrophy can reach truly enormous proportions, with the heart attaining a weight in excess of 1 kg. Here, too, coronary filling is compromised as a result of diastolic reflux, and the coronary ostia are frequently narrowed as a consequence of scarring from luetic mesaortitis.

Carcinoid Valvular Disease

Carcinoid syndrome can effect the heart valves, causing thickening of mainly the right-sided valves.[77] This is due to a plaque-like deposition on the valve and can result in stenosis and sudden death. Similar pathology is related to ergotamine therapy.[78]

Hemorrhage

Escape of blood through a defect or rent in the wall of a diseased blood vessel is a frequent mechanism of sudden, rapid death. The interval from onset of symptoms to exitus usually ranges from a few minutes to several hours. The underlying disease processes vary widely in etiology, and the primary sites of damage are located in the head, chest and abdomen. Arteries are more commonly involved, but fatal venous bleeding is not rare.

Lethal Mechanisms in Hemorrhage

Hemorrhage can produce several different physiologic disturbances, any one of which can be fatal:

Rapid loss of about one-third of the circulating blood volume in the average, healthy adult results in hypovolemic shock. During the course of the bleeding, progressively increasing disproportion between the capacity of the circulatory apparatus and the volume of circulating blood initiates such compensatory mechanisms as hemodilution, vasoconstriction and tachycardia in an effort to maintain equilibrium. If blood loss continues, compensation ultimately breaks down, and blood pressure falls to shock levels, with resultant cerebral and myocardial ischemia and death from global hypoxia.

Hemorrhage can kill quickly by creating increased pressure in or on a vital organ to the extent that its functional capacity is fatally compromised. This is the lethal process in hemopericardium (pericardial tamponade) and in spontaneous subarachnoid or intracerebral hemorrhage. Sufficient bleeding into the trachea or bronchi can result in rapid death from asphyxia, with the blood acting as a mechanical barrier to respiratory exchange. This type of hemorrhage is a common terminating mechanism in bronchogenic carcinoma and pulmonary tuberculosis.

When fatal hemorrhage involves the respiratory or gastrointestinal tracts, there is usually obvious clinical evidence of the terminal event in the form of hemoptysis, hematemesis or melena. If fatal bleeding takes place in some other site, no external manifestations may be present, and correct antemortem diagnosis must be based on proper evaluation of clinical and laboratory findings.

Deaths from hemorrhage are among the most readily diagnosed conditions encountered at autopsy. The presence of large quantities of blood in a body cavity, in the retroperitoneal space or within the substance of an organ usually permits the pathologist to make a prompt identification of the underlying disease, the site of the fatal vascular defect, and the mechanism of death.

Cerebrovascular Diseases

Although fatal hemorrhages occur in many different, widely scattered sites, several areas are especially vulnerable to this common lethal mechanism. Chief among these is the central nervous system.

Spontaneous intracranial hemorrhages fall into several fairly well-defined categories.

Intracerebral hemorrhage (apoplexy), usually attributable to a combination of arterial hypertension and arteriosclerosis, is the cerebrovascular catastrophe encountered most frequently in the middle-aged and older persons. The usual source of hemorrhage is rupture of a lenticulostriate branch of the middle cerebral artery with subsequent bleeding into the basal ganglia and adjacent structures. Occasionally the pons or cerebellum is the primary site of bleeding.

Progressive extravasation of blood into the cerebral parenchyma leads to mounting intracranial pressure, brain swelling and herniations with resultant cardiac or respiratory arrest. Rupture of the intracerebral hematoma into a cerebral ventricle or through the cortex permits escape of blood into the subarachnoid space. If the arachnoid is torn by the force of the hemorrhage, blood enters the subdural space, thus simulating a traumatic lesion from which the spontaneous hemorrhage must be differentiated.

Spontaneous subarachnoid hemorrhages account for approximately 4 to 5% of all rapid and unexpected natural deaths. The source of bleeding is generally perforation or rupture of a saccular berry aneurysm, located almost always at the bifurcation of one of the constituent vessels of the circle of Willis or of one of its major branches, which permits blood to accumulate rapidly on the undersurface of the brain. As bleeding continues, blood advances along the fissures, into the major cisterns and thence into the fourth ventricle, forming a bloody cerebral tamponade. Aneurysms frequently rupture into the cerebral parenchyma or into the subdural space. In fact, subdural and/or intracerebral hemorrhage without concomitant subarachnoid bleeding may be produced by a ruptured aneurysm.[79]

Estimates of the rapidity with which death ensues following rupture of berry aneurysms depend upon the source of the study population. Study of patients dying in hospitals tends to exclude sudden death, and persons surviving longer than one day are less likely to be autopsied at a medicolegal facility. Germane to the present context is Freytag's[79] analysis of 250 consecutive deaths due to ruptured intracranial aneurysms. These individuals were autopsied at the Office of the Chief Medical Examiner of Mary-

land; 60% had no survival and an additional 29% lived less than one day. The longest survival in her study was seven weeks. Some individuals survive their initial bleeding episode only to die with a recurrence. Former bleeding, which in most instances was asymptomatic or mildly symptomatic leakage from a fatally ruptured aneurysm, is common. When they occur such sentinel hemorrhages usually precede the fatal rupture and hemorrhage by several days.

Spontaneous subarachnoid hemorrhages, unlike the intracerebral variety, do not require the presence of associated hypertension for their occurrence. The preexisting vascular defect responsible for their genesis ruptures readily under normotensive conditions. Nevertheless, 25% of patients with ruptured cerebral aneurysms are hypertensive.[80]

Postmortem search for the offending aneurysm should be made while the brain is fresh, i.e., prior to fixation in formalin. Otherwise the extravasated blood that surrounds the vessels congeals and makes the task of demonstrating the vascular defect extremely difficult. Multiple aneurysms are present in approximately 12% of persons dying from spontaneous subarachnoid hemorrhage.[79]

Grossly the aneurysms are eccentric or rounded evaginations measuring from 1 to 2 mm to several centimeters in maximum dimension. Histologically the wall reveals absence of normal layering with degenerative changes in media and intima. Stehbens[81] states that the architectural differences between the uninvolved portion of the arterial wall and the aneurysm can probably be explained by the expansion that takes place in forming the saccular outpouching. Phagocytosed blood pigment is frequently visible in the adventitial portion of the aneurysm wall, indicating previous leakage. The presence of arteriosclerotic changes in the aneurysmal wall does not imply an arteriosclerotic origin of the lesion but rather degeneration superimposed on the congenital lesion or organization of mural thrombi.

Other Causes of Fatal Spontaneous Intracranial Bleeding

In addition to the common type of berry aneurysm responsible for the great majority of spontaneous subarachnoid hemorrhages, other varieties of cerebrovascular malformation can also lead to fatal bleeding into the subarachnoid space. Angiomas and arteriovenous malformations are said to account for about 9% of all spontaneous subarachnoid bleeding.[80]

Arteriovenous malformations are clearly the result of maldevelopment secondary to faulty differentiation of intercommunicating embryonal arterial and venous channels. These lesions are, in reality, enlarged arterial and venous pathways with one or more arteriovenous anastomoses, located usually on the surface of the cerebral hemispheres. Occasionally they extend into the subjacent cerebral parenchyma in wedge-shaped fashion. The neighboring or intervening brain tissue frequently presents anomalous neural development, necrosis or gliosis secondary to compression by the malformation or to circulatory deprivation as a result of the blood being drawn away by the arteriovenous shunt.[80]

Mycotic aneurysms, which develop following lodgement of septic emboli at points of bifurcation in the circle of Willis or distally in its major branches, can be responsible for fatal cerebrovascular rupture. Infected vegetations from heart valves damaged by congenital or acquired disease (subacute bacterial endocarditis) are the usual source of the bacteria-containing thrombotic masses that produce a localized destructive, suppurative arteritis, which ultimately goes on to complete mural destruction.

Fusiform arteriosclerotic cerebral aneurysms are almost always associated with gross, generalized cerebral atherosclerosis and are readily differentiated from other types of aneurysms. Luetic cerebral aneurysms are rare.

CVA and CVE

At this juncture a caveat is in order against use of the term *cerebrovascular accident (CVA)* when referring to cerebral hemorrhage, thrombosis or embolism. This is a particularly unfortunate appellation because the word accident carries with it the implication of mishap, misadventure or negligence and can lead to serious misunderstanding on the part of lay relatives and friends of

the decedent. If a catchall phrase is used for this group of cerebrovascular catastrophes, the term *cerebrovascular event (CVE)* is preferable. Best of all is use of the specific diagnostic term that accurately describes the lesion: cerebral hemorrhage, thrombosis or embolism. Cerebral thrombosis or embolism frequently causes sudden incapacitation but seldom results in sudden death.

Diseases of the Aorta

Inasmuch as the aorta carries more blood at higher pressure than any other vessel, exsanguinating hemorrhage occurs more often from mural disease in this major conduit than in any other vascular channel. Occasionally, spontaneous perforation of a major branch of the aorta (splenic artery, iliac artery, etc.) damaged by disease is the source of fatal blood loss.

Atherosclerotic Aneurysm of the Aorta

Progressive arteriosclerotic degeneration of the aorta with weakness and thinning of the wall leads to formation of fusiform or saccular aneurysms, largely filled with necrotic thrombotic debris. These can rupture resulting in hemorrhage, which usually proves fatal within a few hours following onset of symptoms. Because most arteriosclerotic aneurysms of the aorta are located in its abdominal portion, bleeding is initially retroperitoneal with subsequent rupture into the peritoneal cavity. Occasionally the defect in the aneurysm is located on its anterior surface and communicates directly with the peritoneal cavity. In these instances the fatal course is usually more rapid because bleeding proceeds more quickly into the peritoneal cavity than into the retroperitoneal space.

In addition to the two foregoing sites, arteriosclerotic abdominal aortic aneurysms may rupture into other structures. Communication of the rent in the aortic wall with the inferior vena caval lumen can cause death from acute high output heart failure as a consequence of sudden creation of a major arteriovenous fistula. Aortoduodenal fistulas also have been reported, with the clinical picture simulating bleeding peptic ulcer.

Aortic Dissection

Aortic dissection is one of four possible complications of spontaneous aortic laceration.[82] Spontaneous aortic lacerations are caused by an imbalance between the tensile strength of the aortic wall and the pressure head of the aortic blood column. Accordingly, the major risk factors for spontaneous aortic laceration are systemic hypertension and congenital weakness of the aortic wall, best exemplified by Marfan's syndrome. Marfan's syndrome results from mutations in the fibrillin gene which encodes for a component of the extracellular matrix.[83] Fully 90% of persons with aortic dissections have left ventricular hypertrophy with no etiology demonstrable except hypertension. Roberts has stated that if hypertension were to be controlled, aortic dissections, except those related to Marfan's syndrome, would be prevented.[84]

As used here, the term spontaneous aortic laceration denotes a tear involving the intima and the inner media. The four complications of aortic laceration comprise perforation directly through the adventitia; incomplete dissection, otherwise known as a medial tear; complete dissection, with formation of a cleavage plane in the media occupied by a turbulent hematoma; and degeneration of an aortic dissection to a saccular aneurysm.[82] The cleavage plane of aortic dissections creates a false, sleeve-like lumen with outer and inner walls. The plane is usually located so that the outer wall derives from the outer fourth of the aortic wall, and the inner wall from the inner three-fourths of the aortic wall. Consequently, when the head of pressure in the false lumen creates another rupture, the easiest path is through the adventitia rather than back to the true lumen.[84] The former type of rupture leads to rapid hemorrhage, usually into the pericardial sac or, less often, into the left pleural cavity, and rarely the right pleural cavity. The latter type of rupture produces a double-barreled lumen, which can eventuate in chronic complications related to ischemia in the perfusion beds of the aortic branch arteries. Exsanguination into a major body cavity and cardiac tamponade, with sudden death, are common sequelae of aortic

dissection, although aggressive and early surgical treatment saves some patients.

The concept that aortic dissection is a complication of cystic medial necrosis now has few adherents. Larson and Edwards examined specimens from 158 aortic dissections and found medial necrosis in only a minority.[85] The findings of medial necrosis are, in all likelihood, simply age-related and represent the histologic sequelae of years of injury and repair consequent to hemodynamic forces.[86,87]

The majority of dissections originate from a tear in the ascending aorta, usually in the tubular portion, but occasionally in the sinus portion.[82] Some of these remain localized to the ascending aorta, whereas many extend past the arch to end near the ligamentum arteriosum. Only a minority extend to involve the abdominal aorta. A few dissections are confined to the abdominal aorta.

Iatrogenic aortic dissections can occur as a consequence of cross-clamping, cannulation or incision of the aorta.[88]

In addition to rapid and life-threatening hemorrhage into a body cavity, re-rupture into the true lumen, and formation of a saccular aneurysm, aortic dissections can produce aortic insufficiency due to loss of commissural support for the aortic valve and to obstructions of coronary, arch, or abdominal arteries. The outside of the arch tends to be more involved, so that right coronary involvement exceeds left. In the abdomen, left intercostal arteries and the left renal artery tend to experience narrowing more than their counterparts on the right.[82]

In sudden death due to aortic dissection, the lethal mechanism can arise from pump collapse due to tamponade, hemorrhagic shock with circulatory collapse and global cardiac ischemia, regional cardiac ischemia due to coronary impingement by adventitial hemorrhage, and coronary insufficiency, caused by stripping of the sinuses of Valsalva from their supports.

Syphilitic Aneurysm of the Aorta

Spirochetal invasion of the aortic media during the secondary stage of syphilis, with subsequent damage to elastic and muscular tissue in this area, is the foundation for the development of a fusiform or a saccular aneurysm years later. The weakening of the vessel wall as a consequence of the inflammatory destruction of those elements that confer strength and elasticity leads to mural thinning and outpouching in the thoracic area. Subjected to the constant recurring physiologic stress of systolic pressure, the weakened area becomes thinner and thinner until it can no longer withstand the demand imposed on it and it ruptures, with resultant rapidly fatal hemorrhage. Bleeding is usually internal, with the blood accumulating in one of the pleural cavities (usually the left) or in the pericardial sac. If the aneurysm ruptures into the lung or a major bronchus, death is accompanied by hemoptysis, and when the aortic defect communicates with the thoracic esophagus, hematemesis is a prominent feature of the terminal episode. Rapidly lethal extracardiac shunts can be produced by rupture of syphilitic aortic aneurysms into the superior vena cava or pulmonary artery.[89]

Diagnosis of the luetic origin of the aneurysm is based on its location in the thoracic aorta (arteriosclerotic aneurysms of the aorta are rare above the level of the diaphragm) and the gross and microscopic stigmata of syphilis. Longitudinal intimal striations and wrinkling *(tree barking)* seen with the naked eye point to the syphilitic etiology of the lesion, and this impression is confirmed by the histopathologic criteria of the disease, which include destruction of the medial elastic fibers, with scarring and vascularization, and endarteritis obliterans of the adventitial vasa vasorum accompanied by perivascular infiltration with lymphocytes and plasma cells.

Gastrointestinal Bleeding

Peptic ulcers of the stomach and duodenum and esophageal varices are the two most frequent sources of fatal acute gastrointestinal hemorrhage. In the former two, the hemorrhage is arterial and originates from a vessel that has been encroached upon and eroded by the progressively enlarging ulcer. The eroded artery may be visible to the naked eye in the base of the ulcer.

Fatal venous bleeding in the gastrointestinal tract is most often the result of long-standing cirrhosis with portal hypertension and formation of esophageal varices. Postmortem demonstration of the source of esophageal bleeding is usually difficult because the formerly distended venous channels are now empty and collapsed. The presence of large quantities of blood in the stomach and intestine together with a granular or hobnailed liver point to this diagnosis in the absence of other lesions capable of producing lethal bleeding into the upper digestive tract. In addition to portal cirrhosis, other diseases that create portal hypertension give rise to esophageal varices and can terminate in similar fashion.

All other causes of unexpected, fatal acute gastrointestinal hemorrhage constitute but a small fraction of deaths from this mechanism. They include such diseases as ulcerating benign and malignant gastric and intestinal tumors and the Mallory-Weiss syndrome, the latter referring to hemorrhage from gastroesophageal lacerations induced by violent vomiting.

Respiratory Tract Bleeding

Bleeding originating in the respiratory tract, including the pharynx, can lead to death in one of two ways. The hemorrhage may be sufficiently voluminous to result in exsanguination and fatal hypovolemic shock, a sequence of events that occurs when the source of the bleeding is a comparatively large artery whose wall has been destroyed by some extravascular disease. The latter may be primarily infectious (i.e., tuberculosis, lung abscess, bronchiectasis) or neoplastic (i.e., bronchogenic or other type of respiratory tract carcinoma). Respiratory tract bleeding can be fatal even though the quantity of blood lost is far too small to cause hemorrhagic shock. Even moderate degrees of bleeding into the tracheobronchial tree can lead to speedy asphyxia as a result of the intraluminal blood being churned into a thick froth by the respiratory efforts of the victim. Bloody froth of this type is an effective barrier to the passage of air into and out of the trachea and its branches.

Miscellaneous Intraperitoneal Hemorrhages

Implantation of the fertilized ovum in some site other than the endometrial cavity, usually the uterine tube, results in the development of an ectopic (i.e., extrauterine) pregnancy, thus providing the basis for potentially exsanguinating intraperitoneal hemorrhage. Progressive growth of the fetus and other products of conception eventually leads to tubal stretching and rupture, with resultant brisk intra-abdominal bleeding, which is usually fatal if surgical intervention is not instituted promptly. At autopsy the characteristic findings include hemoperitoneum and a uterine tube showing intraluminal and intramural hemorrhage, chorionic villi and a fetus of six to 12 weeks gestational age.

Other infrequent causes of fatal intra-abdominal bleeding include such entities as spontaneous rupture of a large cavernous hemangioma of the liver, a hepatoma or a liver with peliosis, and mesenteric or diaphragmatic varices from portal hypertension. Spontaneous rupture of a spleen enlarged as a result of infectious mononucleosis, typhoid fever or malaria can also precipitate lethal intraperitoneal hemorrhage.

Chronic Alcoholism

Chronic alcoholism is a common addictive disorder associated with a multitude of psychological, physiologic and pathologic derangements. These derangements have lethal potential by a variety of mechanisms, some well defined and others poorly understood. Our concern here is with the physiologic and pathologic consequences of excessive alcohol ingestion, particularly those capable of causing sudden death, regardless of the presence or absence of a substance abuse disorder.

Deaths from alcoholism can be divided into those in which intoxication or an alcoholic lifestyle function as risk factors for violent incidents, those in which alcoholism is the proximate cause of death, and those in which alcoholism is both a risk factor for violence and a factor medically contributory to death. This discussion is limited to deaths in which alcoholism is a proximate or contributory medical cause. Specifically, we will not attempt to cover the larger range of fatalities caused by injuries of all sorts in persons whose judgment, coordination, and reflexes are impaired by ethanol intoxication.

As a solvent of somewhat lesser polarity than water, ethyl alcohol (ethanol) distributes throughout the aqueous compartments and cellular membranes in ways that are just beginning to be understood. The membranes most pertinent to a discussion of sudden death are those in the central nervous system and the heart.

For example, in binge drinkers, whose usual operating level of blood ethanol is zero, ethanol can function as a cardiac irritant that commonly produces atrial arrhythmias and occasionally produces ventricular arrhythmias.[90] Alcoholics accustomed to continuous intoxication can drink until intercellular communication fails in the respiratory centers, or they can experience seizures or sudden cardiac death when their blood alcohol falls to negligible concentrations.

Ethanol is capable of causing disturbances of cellular metabolism. The most common manifestation of such disturbances occurs in the liver where shifts of equilibrium in the fatty acid and carbohydrate cycles result in the accumulation of fat in hepatocytes. The fatty change is reversible, but can be followed by alcoholic steatohepatitis and ultimately by irreversible cirrhosis. The development of cirrhosis is governed by the amount and duration of ethanol consumption and by individual susceptibility to the toxic effects of ethanol. Acute pancreatitis evolves by unknown mechanisms. Wernicke's encephalopathy, due to concomitant thiamine deficiency, can cause sudden death due to alterations of autonomic function. When the target organ is the heart, alcoholic cardiomyopathy ensues.[91]

Some alcoholic deaths are easily understood on the basis of laboratory findings, whereas others are easily misunderstood and miscertified. In the past, the roles of cardiac irritability, alcoholic cardiomyopathy and postural asphyxia have been underappreciated. On the other hand, hepatic fatty change and cirrhosis have been accepted for years as competent causes of death, often with no real foundation in fact.

Fatty change, also known as fatty metamorphosis, has long attracted the attention of pathologists because it is a striking pathologic lesion. It is certainly associated with sudden death, but no convincing arguments have been advanced to explain how it could cause sudden death, although speculations are numerous. Cirrhosis of the liver, by itself, does not explain the sudden deaths of alcoholics. The scar tissue is metabolically unimportant, and nodules of regenerative liver tissue can perform all of the metabolic tasks of normal liver tissue. Certainly cirrhosis can initiate a lethal train of events; in such instances there is clear evidence of hepatic failure or of exsanguinating hemorrhage from ruptured varices. However, in the absence of liver failure or some other lethal complication of cirrhosis, we regard the hepatic alterations as no more than pathologic markers or the underlying fatal disease, chronic alcoholism.

In addition to its role as a cardiac irritant[92] and as a poison capable of inducing a cardiomyopathy with poor contractile function, ethanol can induce a sustained elevation of systemic arterial blood pressure.[46] This form of hypertension responds rapidly to cessation of drinking. As with any form of hypertension, chronic hypertension due to alcoholism leads to cardiac hypertrophy.

Ethanol is metabolized by alcohol dehydrogenase to acetaldehyde. Alcoholics, like diabetic persons and starved persons, can produce large amounts of acetone. Recent work indicates that the acetone can be converted to isopropyl alcohol by alcohol dehydrogenase.[46] This occurs when the concentration of acetone is sufficient to drive the reaction toward isopropanol. The same enzyme would normally catalyze the oxidation of isopropanol to acetone. Thus, the concomitant finding of isopropyl alcohol and acetone need not always indicate the ingestion of rubbing alcohol. The relative concentrations of the two compounds in each analyzed specimen and the concentration in gastric fluid are important in differentiating between an exogenous and an endogenous origin of isopropanol. Thus, if the acetone concentration is higher than the isopropyl alcohol concentration in most of the analyzed body fluids and the gastric fluid has concentrations suggesting mucosal secretion rather than ingestion, endogenous production is favored.

Central pontine myelinolysis is a cause of sudden death in alcoholics which is usually certified by hospital physicians. This disorder is probably a consequence of intravenous treatment of hyponatremia.

At this point we present several case histories that exemplify common medicolegal problems and their appropriate solutions.

Case 1. A single unemployed man who customarily drank all day every day was found dead in a comfortably heated bus station. He had been observed sleeping on the floor not long before. The autopsy revealed a 120-lb. anicteric man with fatty cirrhosis and a 420-gram heart without dilation or coronary atherosclerosis. The blood ethanol concentration was 0.03% and toxicological testing was otherwise negative. The cause of death was certified simply as chronic alcoholism. The omission of cirrhosis and fatty change as immediate causes of death was deliberate, since their possible role was speculative. The most likely mechanism of death was a ventricular arrhythmia, due either to hypertensive ventricular hypertrophy or non-dilated cardiomyopathy.

Case 2. A 110-lb. woman known to be a heavy drinker was found dead at home. The autopsy revealed bronchopneumonia and a soft dilated 390-gram heart without coronary atherosclerosis. Microscopy revealed non-specific changes of cardiac hypertrophy and no evidence of myocarditis. The blood ethanol concentration was 0.05% and no drugs were detected. Death was certified as bronchopneumonia due to chronic alcoholism with alcoholic cardiomyopathy.

Case 3. An alcoholic man was rushed to the hospital in shock. His blood pressure declined despite therapy and he died. The autopsy revealed a 2,000 mL hemoperitoneum, cirrhosis of the liver and varices of the diaphragm. DiMaio has reported several instances of spontaneous hemoperitoneum in cirrhotics, with no apparent source. In the case described here, we believe that the hemorrhage probably originated from the diaphragmatic varices, and certified the death as due to ruptured diaphragmatic varices with hemoperitoneum due to cirrhosis of liver due to chronic alcoholism. This case provides an instructive contrast to the far more common instances of exsanguinating gastrointestinal hemorrhage due to ruptured esophageal varices.

Case 4. A heavy drinker was found dead in his house under apparently natural circumstances. The autopsy revealed an edematous hemorrhagic pancreas, peripancreatic fat necrosis, and acute inflammation of the peritoneum. The blood ethanol concentration was 0.02%. The death was certified as acute pancreatitis due to chronic alcoholism.

Case 5. A 37-year-old alcoholic woman was found dead in her house. She had complained to her children of feeling unwell for three days prior to death. The autopsy revealed cirrhosis, steatohepatitis and chronic pancreatitis. The blood ethanol concentration was 0.04%. Acetone and isopropyl alcohol were found in blood, brain and gastric content. In all specimens, the acetone concentration equaled or exceeded the isopropanol concentration. Follow-up investigation by the police revealed no evidence to suggest ingestion of rubbing alcohol. The isopropanol was considered to be a metabolite of acetone. Death was certified as due to chronic alcoholism.

One of the idiosyncrasies of death certification is manifested by the conventions of certifying deaths due to acute ethanol intoxication. If a chronic alcoholic person dies with a high blood ethanol concentration, we interpret the intoxication as an acute exacerbation of a chronic disease and certify the manner of death as natural. On the other hand, if an impulsive person rapidly drinks a bottle of whisky to win a bet or a dare and dies from the ensuing ethanol intoxication, we believe that the death is an accident.

If the chronic alcoholic dies from drinking methanol or isopropanol, the manner of death is accident.

Chronic Intravenous Narcotism

Intravenous drug abusers are subject to death not only from accidental acute intoxications but also from a variety of infections. Fatalities for which the immediate cause is a disease, as a consequence of chronic drug abuse, are classified as natural deaths. Bronchopneumonia, human immunodeficiency virus infection, type B or C viral hepatitis, tuberculosis and bacterial endocarditis are common sequelae of the addict lifestyle. Human immunodeficiency virus (HIV) infection, hepatitis B or C infection, and endocarditis are directly attributable to the use of shared unsterile needles and syringes. Tuberculosis is more a product of the addict lifestyle and acquired immune deficiency. Bronchopneumonia can result from septic seeding from skin-popping ulcers or can ensue as a result of diminished tidal volume during opiate intoxication.

The term chronic intravenous narcotism and chronic drug abuse can stand alone as competent causes of death if the immediate mechanism is not ascertainable. Such situations can arise if the body is decomposed or if an intoxicating agent has physicochemical characteristics which make it undetectable by ordinary laboratory techniques.

Human Immunodeficiency Virus (HIV) Infection and the Acquired Immune Deficiency Syndrome (AIDS)

Three major routes for the transmission of the human immunodeficiency virus have been defined. Intravenous transmission occurs among intravenous drug abusers, hemophiliacs and blood transfusion recipients. Sexual transmission occurs not only among homosexual men but between heterosexual partners as well. Maternal infection is transmitted to the fetus during vaginal delivery.

Intravenous drug addicts comprise the majority of HIV-related deaths in medicolegal practice, largely because their lifestyle brings them within medicolegal jurisdiction. Many addicts have undiagnosed HIV-related disease. Some have been diagnosed at one hospital, but enter another hospital with their final illness and give no history.

A diligent search for opportunistic infection in these deaths is of paramount importance from a public health perspective. This may require cultures at the time of autopsy (especially when tuberculosis is suspected) and histologic sections should be routine. For example, Pneumocystis pneumonia is readily diagnosed by characteristic gross and hematoxylin-eosin microscopic appearances. Special stains for organisms can be valuable. Multifocal leukoencephalopathy and HIV encephalitis are often first diagnosed at autopsy.

Diagnosis of HIV-related disease by the medical examiner requires a prepared mind. We find it useful to test for seroconversion in all autopsies.

Morbid Obesity

Obesity increases the risk of sudden death in several ways. Hypertension is a risk of obesity; its presence increases the risk of hypertensive cerebral hemorrhage, dissecting aortic aneurysm and cardiac hypertrophy. Obese persons are at increased risk for diabetes mellitus and all of the complications of that disease. Venous stasis of the lower extremities is common and results in an increased risk of pulmonary embolism. The finding of a fatty liver in an obese person need not indicate an alcoholic etiology; fatty metamorphosis can be produced by the obesity itself. When the adipose deposits involve the chest walls and neck, ventilation can be impaired. The risk of postural asphyxia is increased in obese persons.

Obstructive Sleep Apnea

Obstructive sleep apnea is common in those with short fat necks. In this condition, diminished nocturnal pharyngeal muscle tone and thickening of the cervical soft tissues combine to produce obstructive airway collapse during inspiratory efforts. The *apnea* refers to the lack of airflow past the nose and mouth, not to central respiratory depression. During the *apnea* episodes, which can occur hundreds of times each night, the arterial blood becomes hypoxic until the hypoxemia leads to *sleep arousal.* Ventricular irritability is increased during the hypoxic episodes, but there is no detectable difference between the death rates of those with obstructive sleep apnea and controls.[93]

Pulmonary Embolism

Acute thromboembolic occlusion of one or more major pulmonary arteries has long been recognized and feared as a cause of sudden death in patients confined to bed. The preceding thrombogenesis responsible for the fatal embolus is usually initiated by a combination of bed rest or immobilization of a limb in a cast, with consequent slowing or stagnation of the circulation and changes in the blood composition, which favor the development of a phlebothrombotic process in the major veins of the legs or pelvis.

The finding of pulmonary thromboembolism as an immediate cause of death demands a search for the proximate cause. A history of recent lower extremity trauma or surgery or cast removal should be sought. The most common natural proximate causes are cardiovascular disease with impaired circulation, malignant tu-

mors, pregnancy and morbid obesity. Genetic susceptibility to venous thrombosis is increasingly being recognized, and should be suspected when the decedent is young or has a recurrent or family history of thrombosis or multiple stillbirths or abortions.[94] In general the mutations impair the control of the clotting cascade. The most common inherited thrombophilia is resistance to activated protein C (factor V Leiden).[95] Another nucleotide substitution in this gene causes another common thrombophilia.[96] Homocystinuria causes both venous and arterial thromboses.[97]

The mechanism by which pulmonary emboli produce sudden death depends, in part, on the size of the occluding clot, the diameter of the occluded vessel, and whether the vessel is a central conduit or a branch artery in the pulmonary circuit. When the right ventricle or the pulmonary artery are obstructed, the venous blood is dammed, the venous capacitance vessels become distended, forward flow through the pulmonary circuit to the left side of the heart and the aorta slows to a trickle, and mechanical cardiovascular collapse ensues. Typically, the heart generates electrical waveforms, but no peripheral arterial pulses can be felt.

When sudden death closely follows the obstruction of smaller radicles of the pulmonary arteries, a more complex group of physiologic disturbances has been described. Generalized pulmonary vasospasm, triggered by impaction of the embolus and mediated reflexly by the autonomic nervous system, leads to a sudden sharp increase in blood pressure in the lesser circuit with simultaneous marked dilatation and overdistension of the right ventricle. Associated with the cardiopulmonary dysfunction is systemic shock with peripheral hypotension and interference with coronary filling and coronary flow. The entire complex of cardiopulmonary vascular disturbance results in immediate cessation of vital function.

Most pathologists are careful to search for emboli in the pulmonary arteries. However, some thromboemboli can lodge in the right atrium and ventricle and never migrate to the pulmonary trunk. These cardiac emboli easily fall out of the inferior vena cava as the heart is removed during autopsy and can be totally missed. Careful observation during removal, or ligature of the vena cava before removal of the heart, or in situ dissection are necessary if cardiac thromboemboli are not to be overlooked.

Other Types of Embolism

Non-pulmonary thrombotic emboli are rarely, if ever, suddenly fatal. Occlusion of a major cerebral artery by an embolus arising from a mural thrombus in the left atrium or left ventricle or from a vegetation on the mitral or aortic valves usually leads to a relatively prolonged clinical course before death supervenes, the interval from embolism to exitus ranging from hours to days. Saddle emboli lodged at the bifurcation of the aorta or occlusive emboli in the major branches of the aorta (superior mesenteric, carotid, femoral) usually create recognizable syndromes that do not fall into the category of sudden and unexpected death.

Central Nervous System Causes of Sudden and Unexpected Death

Cerebral parenchymal and meningeal diseases of widely varying etiologies (infectious, neoplastic or idiopathic) can cause sudden and unexpected death. (Unexpected, rapid deaths from cerebrovascular catastrophes have been discussed earlier in this chapter.) The mechanism of death (central cardiorespiratory failure or paralysis) may be evoked by direct damage to the cerebral vital centers by the disease process itself, or it may arise secondary to increased intracranial pressure produced by space-occupying lesions, by cerebral edema and swelling or by a combination of both.

Invasion of and damage to vital areas within the brain by a virus occasionally produces quickly fatal encephalomyelitis. Rupture of a brain abscess is frequently followed by speedily lethal diffuse, purulent meningitis or ependymitis. Syphilis in the form of acute luetic meningitis, acute luetic cerebral arteritis, or general paresis is

yet an additional possible cause of sudden and unexpected death.

Intracranial Tumors

The majority of primary intracranial tumors, whether cerebral or meningeal in origin, usually give rise to progressively increasing signs and symptoms, which frequently extend over periods of months or years. The disabling character of the clinical response in such instances is ordinarily severe enough to induce the patient to seek medical aid, and when death supervenes under these circumstances, it is usually not of the sudden, unexpected or unattended type that falls within the jurisdiction of the medicolegal functionary. Nonetheless, sudden and unexpected deaths from intracranial tumors are not rare in forensic pathologic practice.[98] Such deaths can be precipitated by any one of several different mechanisms.

Gliomas that infiltrate and replace cerebral tissue in silent areas of the brain can attain comparatively large dimensions without producing symptoms of sufficient magnitude, significance or clarity to justify or stimulate clinical study and are thus ignored by the patient. Their early manifestations may appear in the emotional or psychic spheres and be regarded erroneously as indicating mental or emotional instability or functional psychosis. Meningeal tumors pressing on silent areas can enlarge slowly for many years without producing noteworthy subjective or objective changes because of compensatory cerebral mechanisms.

Distinctive clinical phenomena often appear first when the tumor has created a critical level of increased intracranial pressure. This point may be reached either as a result of a sudden increase in the volume of the intracranial contents that does not allow time for compensatory mechanisms to go into operation or because gradual enlargement of the tumor has taxed the compensatory mechanisms beyond their limits. In either event, death may ensue very quickly.

Abrupt, sudden increase in volume of the intracranial contents can come about either as a result of edema in and around the tumor or from sudden hemorrhage into the tumor, the latter event occurring most often with glioblastoma multiform. This malignant glioma characteristically contains many atypical blood vessels, which may rupture spontaneously or following minor trauma. Moreover, this tumor has a tendency to replace cerebral parenchyma as it grows, thus delaying the appearance of significantly increased intracranial pressure until the neoplasm is quite large.

Sudden swelling of a cystic tumor or pressure from a neoplasm in the region of the hypothalamus, aqueduct of Sylvius or fourth ventricle can cause sudden death from central disruption of autonomic control of cardiorespiratory function.

In addition to killing suddenly as a direct result of their internal expansion and encroachment, intracranial tumors may be responsible for sudden (violent) death indirectly by precipitating fatal traumatic incidents as a consequence of ataxia, dizziness, mental confusion or seizures, which often precede diagnostic clinical symptoms from intracerebral new growths.

Metastatic brain tumors are, on rare occasion, responsible for the types of situations just described. The most frequent primary sites for these tumors are lung and breast.

Epilepsy

Epilepsy, regardless of etiology, can cause sudden and unexplained death in several different ways, including initiation of fatal mishaps during a seizure in which loss of consciousness or of muscular control permits the occurrence of traumatic incidents (i.e., drowning, motor vehicle accidents) or results in obstruction of the respiratory tract due either to aspiration of gastric contents or to the position of the individual following the attack. Epileptics with significant stenosing coronary atherosclerosis can die suddenly of acute coronary insufficiency as a result of severe muscular exertion, hypoxia and hypertension precipitated by a violent seizure.

Epilepsy in and of itself can be responsible for sudden and unexpected death, sometimes with a single tonic convulsion.[99–101] Seizures limited to the autonomic nervous system without motor involvement (paroxysmal autonomic dysfunction) have been invoked as the mechanism of death in some epileptics found dead in bed without evidence of a major convulsion having taken place. Absence of tongue biting or fecal and urinary incontinence does not exclude the occurrence of epileptic convulsions, a fact well and amply documented by witnessed fatal seizures. Cardiac and respiratory exhaustion can follow in the wake of prolonged and repeated epileptic convulsions *(status epilepticus)*.

Although death may occur during the first major epileptic convulsion, a sound diagnosis of epilepsy as a cause of death cannot be based solely on the presence of some type of convulsive phenomena during the agonal period. Such indications of cerebral irritability are non-specific and occur with many different lethal processes.

Gross and microscopic examination of the brain in known epileptics frequently shows no characteristic changes or lesions that permit the pathologist to make an objective diagnosis of epilepsy. Many victims of epilepsy have anatomically normal brains. If death is to be ascribed to this disease, there should be a history of convulsions (fits, fainting spells), ideally supported by abnormal electroencephalographic tracings. In many instances it is quite difficult to obtain the details of previous convulsive episodes because the family desires to avoid the social stigma that is often associated with the diagnosis of epilepsy. In the absence of witnesses to the terminal episode, the verdict of death from epilepsy should be based on a reliable history and the performance of a complete autopsy that discloses no other anatomic or chemical cause of death.

The victims of fatal seizures in medical examiners' autopsy populations are often abusers of ethanol and drugs. Toxicological analysis for phenobarbital, phenytoin and other anti-convulsants often shows that in known epileptics deaths are associated with non-detectable or low concentrations of anti-seizure medications.[101] Seizure deaths can, however, occur in persons with therapeutic drug levels.[102]

A non-specific autopsy finding, common in autopsies of persons dead from seizure disorders, is pulmonary edema. Neurogenic pulmonary edema has been proposed as a possible mechanism of death in seizure disorders.[103]

Respiratory Tract Disease

Sudden and unexpected deaths occur with a variety of acute and chronic pulmonary disorders and as a result of several different lethal mechanisms. Reference has already been made to exsanguinating and asphyxiating pulmonary hemorrhages and to pulmonary embolism.

Lobar and Bronchopneumonia

Lobar pneumonia and extensive confluent bronchopneumonia account for the single largest group of victims dying unexpectedly from acute pulmonary disease. Lobar pneumonia may be primary, or it may be associated with and follow a severe viral disease such as Asian influenza.[104] In contrast, for bronchopneumonia, there is almost always an identifiable underlying condition. Chronic alcoholism, chronic drug abuse, cardiovascular disease, old age, and viral respiratory infections are the common predisposing factors. The mechanism of death is a combination of hypoxia and endotoxic depression of cardiac function. The observer is impressed with the striking discrepancy between the classical textbook description of the clinical manifestations demonstrated by the patient with grave pneumonia, i.e., shock, prostration, marked dyspnea and the like, and the fact that many persons with extensive pneumonia are able to be up and about and to carry on in some fashion up to the moment of collapse and death.

Pulmonary Tuberculosis

Pulmonary tuberculosis is an example of a chronic infectious pulmonary disease that is encountered occasionally as a cause of sudden and unexpected death. The lethal mechanism may be hemorrhage or toxicity. Once more we are confronted with the paradoxical situation where the victim has somehow managed to remain ambulatory despite the presence of far-advanced, active caseating and cavitating disease, thus creating a serious public health menace. When the cause of such a death is established by the medical examiner, he or she must immediately notify the public health authorities so that a search can be instituted promptly for contacts who may have been infected by the decedent. Lung culture is imperative to determine the drug sensitivities of the infectious organisms.

Chronic Bronchitis and Pulmonary Emphysema (Tobacco Lung Disease)

The finding at autopsy of hyperinflated lungs which remain persistently inflated after opening of the pleural cavities usually indicates the presence of small airway disease, in the form of asthmatic bronchitis or the chronic bronchitis and respiratory bronchiolitis of tobacco abuse.

Tobacco abusers who die with severe bronchitis and emphysema usually have arteriosclerotic heart disease as well, owing to the common risk factor of tobacco abuse. When both diseases are present, the decision as to which is primary and which is contributory rests on the medical and scene histories. Oxygen tanks, inhalers and a story of wheezing point to lung disease as being primary in the causation of death; chest pain and antacids point to heart disease.

Bronchial Asthma

A modest proportion of all deaths from chronic asthma is provided by fatalities that occur rapidly and acutely. The majority of patients who die quickly and unexpectedly from bronchial asthma usually do so during an acute asthmatic paroxysm. Such deaths are the result of widespread airway occlusion and do not necessarily correlate with the apparent severity of the preceding asthma attack.[105]

The bronchi and bronchioles become obstructed by a combination of factors, including the presence of tenacious, viscid mucoid exudate, edematous swelling of the mucosa and submucosa, and spasm of the airway musculature. These mechanically obstructive changes may be superimposed upon and complicated by chronic emphysema and right ventricular failure from chronic cor pulmonale. As the acute process progresses, ventilatory capacity is reduced and arterial hypoxemia develops. Hypercapnia is a grave sign but is uncommon. More typically, the arterial carbon dioxide tension is slightly below normal.[106]

At autopsy the lungs of persons dying of an acute asthmatic paroxysm are voluminous, pale and distended and often present shallow indentations resulting from pressure of the overinflated organs against the ribs. The trachea and bronchi may contain large quantities of thick, inspissated mucoid exudate, which effectively plug their lumens, or the obstruction may be largely due to inflammatory constriction of edematous distal airways.

Microscopic study establishes the presence of similar material in bronchioles as well, and in all sites the mucus frequently contains a liberal admixture of goblet cells and eosinophilic leukocytes. Other stigmata of chronic asthma usually include hyaline thickening of the basement membranes of the bronchial mucosa, bronchial and bronchiolar smooth muscle hyperplasia, hyperactivity of the mucous glands and abundant peribronchial infiltration by a pleomorphic cellular exudate in which eosinophils and neutrophils are prominent elements.

The majority of sudden deaths in asthmatics involve sudden and simultaneous loss of vital signs and consciousness, indicating a cardiac mechanism such as ventricular fibrillation. One obvious candidate for an intermediate mechanism leading to ventricular fibrillation would be generalized hypoxia from impaired ventilation, coupled with cardiac electrical instability due to cor pulmonale or other chronic cardiac disease. Respiratory failure as defined by carbon dioxide retention is a late complication and is more typical of hospital deaths than of out-of-hospital deaths.

In the absence of cardiac disease, we postulate that arterial air embolism to the vertebral or coronary arteries may ensue as a result of pulmonary overdistension, rupture of alveoli and bronchi, and the generation of extra-alveolar pulmonary air which finds its way to the pulmonary veins. Supporting this postulate are the microscopic observations noted above, the documented occurrence of air-trapping and arterial air embolism in SCUBA divers who inadvertently overdistend their lungs, and the acknowledged risk of arterial air embolism in the absence of breath-holding in divers with asthma or chronic bronchitis and emphysema.[107]

Primary Pulmonary Hypertension

This diagnosis is made by microscopic study of the lungs, which reveals thickening of small arterial walls, and plexiform angiopathy. The only autopsy clue to the necessity of a careful microscopic study of the lungs may be the presence of right ventricular hypertrophy. The diagnosis must be considered in cases of sudden unexpected death, especially those involving women, for whom the disease has predilection. The nature of the terminal cardiac electrical disturbances has not been well-described.[108]

Alimentary Tract Disease

Sequelae, complications and exacerbations of several chronic diseases in different portions of the gastrointestinal tract are occasionally responsible for unexpected and rapid rather than sudden deaths. Fatal hemorrhages originating from active chronic gastric or duodenal peptic ulcers or from ruptured esophageal varices secondary to hepatic cirrhosis have already been described. Perforation of a peptic ulcer with subsequent generalized fibrinopurulent peritonitis and shock can be a speedily fatal complication of this common disease. So, too, strangulated inguinal, femoral, umbilical or internal hernias whose signs and symptoms have been ignored can quickly progress to gangrene of the compromised intestine with resultant shock, peritonitis, and death. Lethal endotoxin shock can ensue so rapidly that peritonitis is not evident. Peritonitis can ensue from fecal retention; in the elderly a stercoral ulcer may not be demonstrable.

Acute Pancreatitis

Although acute pancreatitis is a disease with commonly recognized lethal potentialities, it is not ordinarily considered as a cause of sudden death. However, in some instances the clinical course is truly hyperacute and fulminating, with death supervening extremely rapidly if not instantaneously. Such abbreviated terminal episodes have been ascribed to preceding alcoholic debauches,[109] but they occur also in teetotalers. The etiology and pathogenesis of the diffuse, destructive inflammatory process is not yet completely established, but the lethal mechanism is one of overwhelming shock with violently disturbed electrolyte and protein levels.

MISCELLANEOUS CAUSES OF SUDDEN, UNEXPECTED AND RAPID NATURAL DEATH

There still remains a heterogeneous group of unexpected natural deaths not readily classifiable in any of the preceding categories. Chief among these are fatalities from bacterial infections in which there exists marked virulence of the microorganism, low host resistance or various combinations of both factors. Included in this consideration are untreated or neglected infection such as suppurative pyelonephritis.

Other examples of rapid deaths from infectious causes have been given earlier in this chapter, i.e., lobar pneumonia.

Waterhouse-Friderichsen Syndrome

The classic model of fulminating, fatal bacterial disease is the so-called Waterhouse-Friderichsen syndrome, of which Herrick said, *"No other infection so quickly slays."* The syndrome is characterized by bloodstream invasion by a virulent organism, most frequently the meningococcus, and bilateral adrenal hemorrhages. Intense cyanosis and cutaneous hemorrhages ranging in severity from a few scattered petechiae to large confluent, reddish purple macules are common. Hemorrhagic lesions also may be present in the oral cavity and conjunctivae.

Microscopically the dermal lesions reveal interstitial extravasation of erythrocytes or hemorrhagic foci of acute exudative inflammation. The adrenal changes vary broadly in degree from capillary engorgement through focal cortical hemorrhages to diffuse destructive hemorrhagic necrosis of cortex and medulla, converting the organs into bags of blood.

Clinically the patient presents a toxic, febrile illness of acute onset, soon followed by severe circulatory collapse and death. The entire course of the disease from apparent health to death may transpire in a few hours, much too short an interval for the development of a full-blown meningeal inflammatory response. The lethal mechanism is probably a combination of overwhelming bacterial toxemia and acute adrenal insufficiency, which produces profound shock.

In persons with hemorrhagic adrenal glands and no gross evidence of meningeal suppuration, blood cultures or antigen-detection tests are definitely in order, since meningococcemia can kill before the overt appearance of suppurative meningitis. Whenever meningococcal infection is suspected, emergency room and ambulance personnel, co-workers and the family of the deceased depend on the pathologist for an etiologic diagnosis in order to plan antimicrobial prophylaxis.

We highly recommend antibody-based latex agglutination tests for the detection of antigens to the meningococcus and other common agents of meningitis. Theses slide tests use urine or cerebrospinal fluid and take approximately 30 minutes to complete, as compared to 1 to 3 days for recovery and identification of an organism by culture. Our experience has been that microbiology laboratories are usually eager to provide such dramatic public service.

In infants, the appearances of adrenal hemorrhages can be mimicked by involution of the fetal adrenal cortex. Involutional hyperemia is not accompanied by edema, in contrast to the adrenal hemorrhage accompanying bacterial meningitis.

Hemophilus Influenza Type B Epiglottitis

Infection produced by other toxic, virulent organisms such as *Hemophilus influenza, type B,* can be fatal even though the bacteria remain localized and do not find their way into the bloodstream. Examination of cervical viscera is essential to disclose the acute suppurative epiglottitis and laryngitis, the most prominent anatomic manifestation of colonization by this death-dealing organism. The patient may have complained only briefly of a sore throat prior to unexpected collapse and death.

Epiglottitis is a well recognized infection in children, in whom the etiologic agent is almost always *H. influenza.* With widespread vaccination against this organism, the rate of infection in children has decreased dramatically. However, adults too are susceptible to this infection.[110] In adults other responsible organisms include *S. pneumoniae, H. parainfluenzae* and *S. pyogenes.*[111]

Metabolic and Endocrine Causes

In the absence of anatomic abnormalities or exogenous chemical agents that can be implicated as having caused death, consideration must be given to the possibility or probability of the presence of some metabolic disturbance in body chemistry or endocrine function that can lead to sudden death. Into this group fall such entities as the two extremes of faulty blood glucose regulation, hypoglycemia from hyperinsulinism arising from a functional adenoma of the islets of Langerhans and acutely developing diabetic ketoacidosis. The former diagnosis is made in the presence of a pancreatic tumor that has the characteristic histologic appearance of an islet cell adenoma and that contains large quantities of insulin.

Death can be ascribed to diabetic acidosis when large quantities of glucose and acetone are found in the urine, vitreous humor and cerebrospinal fluid at autopsy. The analytic specimen of choice is vitreous fluid.[112] On the other hand,

hypoglycemia cannot be diagnosed on the basis of a vitreous glucose determination, because vitreous glucose concentrations can drop to zero within one hour after death.[113]

Most complications of diabetes are treated in the hospital. Necrotizing fasciitis and mediastinitis can result from trivial infections that smoulder in the diabetic. In medical examiner practice, diabetes mellitus is most often diagnosed anamnestically when it is listed as a contributory cause in deaths due to arteriosclerotic heart disease.

Pituitary insufficiency has been implicated as a cause of sudden and unexpected death in young women who have previously suffered an infarct of their adenohypophysis following postpartum hemorrhage.[114] Such sudden deaths are usually preceded by indications of anterior pituitary hypofunction in the form of failure of lactation, amenorrhea and depressed thyroid activity, and they occur under conditions of stress. The responsible mechanism is probably adrenal insufficiency secondary to decrease in ACTH secretion by the damaged hypophysis.

Toxic thyroid nodules, myxedema and adrenal insufficiency of diverse etiologic origins have also been described as causes of sudden and unexpected death. Adrenal insufficiency should be considered in persons who are steroid dependent and who are subjected to the stress of an acute disease or injury.

Anaphylaxis

Anaphylactic reactions result from immunologic memory of previously encountered antigens.[115] Anaphylactoid reactions are identical in findings and outcome, but are produced by pharmacologic rather than immunologic degranulation of mast cells. When lethal, both types of reactions usually produce obstructive airway edema, wheezing, cutaneous hives, and vascular collapse and edema owing to increased vascular permeability.

Malignant Tumors

Only occasionally do lethal malignancies escape the notice of clinical physicians. In medicolegal practice, undiagnosed malignancies resulting in death are almost always seen in the homeless or the poor. Neoplasms of the lung, bowel, and breast are most frequently encountered.

Chronic Inanition and Cachexia

Wasting and dehydration may be caused by diseases easily diagnosed at autopsy, such as cancer, tuberculosis or the acquired immunodeficiency syndrome. However, inanition is often due to the inability of the decedent to care for him or herself. In these instances, the proximate cause of death must be sought by inquiry. Possibilities include endogenous depression, schizophrenia, Alzheimer's disease, and mental retardation.

Chronic Renal Failure

The best postmortem test for chronic renal failure, other than a medical history, is the measurement of urea nitrogen and creatinine in vitreous fluid. Anatomical examination of the kidneys permits the labeling of the type of disease, but is a poor way to judge renal function.

Most deaths from chronic renal failure are certified by treating physicians. Occasionally, the medical examiner will investigate deaths which occur during outpatient dialysis; most of these are due to cardiovascular disease. Rarely, a subcutaneous arteriovenous dialysis shunt can be picked until it bleeds, leading to arterial exsanguination.

Sickle Cell Disease

Sickle cell disease is characterized clinically by chronic hemolytic anemia, episodes of abdominal and joint pain, recurrent infections and thrombotic events. Infection, hypoxia, acidosis and dehydration can precipitate extensive intravascular sickling in these patients, with resultant sudden death. The occurrence of rapidly fatal intravascular sickling following physical exertion at relatively high altitude has been reported in military personnel with sickle trait.[116]

In the postmortem diagnosis of sickle cell disease, the history and circumstances are of more importance than the autopsy findings, since erythrocytes will routinely sickle in formalin. Hemoglobin electrophoresis can be helpful if there is no reliable medical history.

Old Age

Old age is listed in the *International Classification of Diseases* and is a competent cause of death for certification purposes. We generally reserve this diagnosis for persons over the age of 90 with minimal autopsy findings or no significant medical history. In old persons, the physiologic mechanisms for maintenance of homeostasis have a reduced capacity to respond to exogenous changes in temperature, diet, hydration and microbial flora. Upper respiratory and urinary infections, which would not be life-threatening in young persons, can lead to sepsis and death in the elderly.

The elderly heart develops tortuosity of epicardial vessels and ventricular hypertrophy. The ventricles appear short in contrast with the left atrium, which is dilated as a consequence of decreased left ventricular compliance and with the aorta, which is also dilated. The mural arteries become sclerotic and calcified, even when epicardial vessels are patent. The mitral annulus often calcifies, especially in women. Amyloid deposits are common.[116] The bundle branches undergo fibrosis, dropout or both. In view of all these anatomic changes, we believe that the elderly heart, in all likelihood, has less electrical stability than the young heart, exclusive of considerations of chronic disease, making it more susceptible to arrhythmogenic stimuli such as sepsis.

Complications of Labor and Delivery

Occasional instances of sudden death from amniotic fluid embolism or uterine rupture were noted in Luke and Helpern's study of medicolegal autopsies on young persons.[117]

REFERENCES

1. Goldstein, S.: The necessity of a uniform definition of sudden coronary death: Witnessed death within one hour of the onset of acute symptoms. *Am Heart J, 103:* 156–159, 1982.

2. Virmani, R., and Roberts, W.C.: Sudden cardiac death. *Hum Pathol, 18:* 485–492, 1987.

3. Myerburg, R.J.: Sudden cardiac death: Epidemiology, causes, and mechanisms. *Cardiology, 74:* 2–9, 1987.

4. Lown, B.: Sudden cardiac death: The major challenge confronting contemporary cardiology. *Am J Cardiol, 43:* 313–328, 1979.

5. Kannel, W.B., and McGee, D.L.: Epidemiology of sudden death: Insights from the Framingham Study. *Cardiovasc Clin, 15:* 93–105, 1985.

6. Panidis, I.P., and Morganroth, J.: Initiating events of sudden cardiac death. *Cardiovasc Clin, 15:* 81–92, 1985.

7. Davis, J.H., and Wright, R.K.: The very sudden cardiac death syndrome–A conceptual model for pathologists. *Hum Pathol, 11:* 117–121, 1980.

8. Berger, A.J., Mitchell, R.A., and Severinghaus, J.W.: Regulation of respiration (first of three parts). *N Engl J Med, 297:* 92–97, 1977.

9. Bharati, S., and Lev, M.: Arrhythmogenic ventricles. *Pacing Clin Electrophysiol, 6:* 1035–1049, 1983.

10. Bharati, S., and Lev, M.: Congenital abnormalities of the conduction system in sudden death in young adults. *J Am Coll Cardiol, 8:* 1096–1104, 1986.

11. Okada, R., and Kawai, S.: Histopathology of the conduction system in sudden cardiac death. *Jpn Circ J, 47:* 573–580, 1983.

12. James, T.N.: Normal variations and pathologic changes in structure of the cardiac conduction system and their functional significance. *J Am Coll Cardiol, 5:* 71B–78B, 1985.

13. Lemery, R., Brugada, P., Della Bella, P., Dugernier, T., and Wellens, H.J.: Ventricular fibrillation in six adults without overt heart disease. *J Am Coll Cardiol, 13:* 911–916, 1989.

14. Chen, Q., Kirsch, G.E., Zhang, D., Brugada, R., Brugada, J., Brugada, P., Potenza, D., Moya, A., Borggrefe, M., Breithardt, G., Ortiz-Lopez, R., Wang, Z., Antzelevitch, C., O'Brien, R.E., Schulze-Bahr, E., Keating, M.T., Towbin, J.A., and Wang, Q.: Genetic basis and molecular mechanism for idiopathic ventricular fibrillation. *Nature, 392:* 293–296, 1998.

15. Melles, R.B., and Katz, B.: Night terrors and sudden unexplained nocturnal death. *Med Hypotheses, 26:* 149–154, 1988.

16. Hayashi, M., Murata, M., Satoh, M., Aizawa, Y., Oda, E., Oda, Y., Watanabe, T., and Shibata, A.: Sudden nocturnal death in young males from ventricular flutter. *Jpn Heart J, 26:* 585–591, 1985.

17. Gotoh, K.: A histopathological study on the conduction system of the so-called "Pokkuri disease" (sudden unexpected cardiac death of unknown origin in Japan). *Jpn Circ J, 40:* 753–768, 1976.

18. Kirschner, R.H., Eckner, F.A., and Baron, R.C.: The cardiac pathology of sudden, unexplained nocturnal death in Southeast Asian refugees. *JAMA, 256:* 2700–2705, 1986.

19. Munger, R.G., and Booton, E.A.: Bangungut in Manila: Sudden and unexplained death in sleep of adult Filipinos. *Int J Epidemiol, 27:* 677–684, 1998.

20. Priori, S.G., Barhanin, J., Hauer, R.N., Haverkamp, W., Jongsma, H.J., Kleber, A.G., McKenna, W.J., Roden, D.M., Rudy, Y., Schwartz, K., Schwartz, P.J., Towbin, J.A., and Wilde, A.M.: Genetic and molecular basis of cardiac arrhythmias: Impact on clinical management parts I and II. *Circulation, 99:* 518–528, 1999.

21. Splawski, I., Tristani-Firouzi, M., Lehmann, M.H., Sanguinetti, M.C., and Keating, M.T.: Mutations in the hminK gene cause long QT syndrome and suppress IKs function. *Nat Genet, 17:* 338–340, 1997.

22. Abbott, G.W., Sesti, F., Splawski, I., Buck, M.E., Lehmann, M.H., Timothy, K.W., Keating, M.T., and Goldstein, S.A.: MiRP1 forms IKr potassium channels with HERG and is associated with cardiac arrhythmia. *Cell, 97:* 175–187, 1999.

23. Neyroud, N., Tesson, F., Denjoy, I., Leibovici, M., Donger, C., Barhanin, J., Faure, S., Gary, F., Coumel, P., Petit, C., Schwartz, K., and Guicheney, P.: A novel mutation in the potassium channel gene KVLQT1 causes the Jervell and Lange-Nielsen cardioauditory syndrome [see comments]. *Nat Genet, 15:* 186–189, 1997.

24. MacRae, C.A., Ghaisas, N., Kass, S., Donnelly, S., Basson, C.T., Watkins, H.C., Anan, R., Thierfelder, L.H., McGarry, K., and Rowland, E., et al.: Familial Hypertrophic cardiomyopathy with Wolff-Parkinson-White syndrome maps to a locus on chromosome 7q3. *J Clin Invest, 96:* 1216–1220, 1995.

25. Ector, H., and Van der Hauwaert, L.G.: Sick sinus syndrome in childhood. *Br Heart J, 44:* 684–691, 1980.

26. Sugiura, M., and Ohkawa, S.: A clinicopathologic study on sick sinus syndrome with histological approach to the sinoatrial node. *Jpn Circ J, 44:* 497–504, 1980.

27. Davies, M.J., Anderson, R.H., and Becker, A.E.: *The conduction system of the heart.* London: Butterworths, 1983, 230–242.

28. Cohle, S.D., and Lie, J.T.: Histopathologic spectrum of the cardiac conducting tissue in traumatic and noncardiac sudden death patients under 30 years of age: An analysis of 100 cases. *Anat Pathol, 3:* 53–76, 1998.

29. Anderson, K.P.: Sudden death, hypertension, and hypertrophy. *J Cardiovasc Pharmacol, 6:* S498–503, 1984.

30. McLenachan, J.M., Henderson, E., Morris, K.I., and Dargie, H.J.: Ventricular arrhythmias in patients with

hypertensive left ventricular hypertrophy. *N Engl J Med, 317:* 787–792, 1987.

31. Vargas, S.O., Sampson, B.A., and Schoen, F.J.: Pathologic detection of early myocardial infarction: A critical review of the evolution and usefulness of modern techniques. *Mod Pathol, 12:* 635–645, 1999.

32. Reimer, K.A., and Ideker, R.E.: Myocardial ischemia and infarction: Anatomic and biochemical substrates for ischemic cell death and ventricular arrhythmias. *Hum Pathol, 18:* 462–475, 1987.

33. Armiger, L.C., and Smeeton, W.M.: Contraction-band necrosis: Patterns of distribution in the myocardium and their diagnostic usefulness in sudden cardiac death. *Pathology, 18:* 289–295, 1986.

34. Wikland, B.: Death from ASHD outside hospitals: A study of 2,678 cases in Stockholm with particular reference to sudden deaths. *Acta Med Scand, 184:* 129, 1968.

35. Jetter, W.W., and White, P.D.: Rupture of heart in patients in mental institutions. *Ann Int Med, 21:* 783, 1944.

36. Cohle, S.D., Graham, M.A., and Pounder, D.J.: Nonatherosclerotic sudden coronary death. *Pathol Annu, 21:* 217–249, 1986.

37. Virmani, R., Chun, P.K., Goldstein, R.E., Robinowitz, M., and McAllister, H.A.: Acute takeoffs of the coronary arteries along the aortic wall and congenital coronary ostial valve-like ridges: Association with sudden death. *J Am Coll Cardiol, 3:* 766–771, 1984.

38. Maron, B.J.: Structural features of the athlete heart as defined by echocardiography. *J Am Coll Cardiol, 7:* 190–203, 1986.

39. Myerburg, R.J., Kessler, K.M., Bassett, A.L., and Castellanos, A.: A biological approach to sudden cardiac death: Structure, function and cause. *Am J Cardiol, 63:* 1512–1516, 1989.

40. Messerli, F.H.: Clinical determinants and consequences of left ventricular hypertrophy. *Am J Med, 75:* 51–56, 1983.

41. Haider, A.W., Larson, M.G., Benjamin, E.J., and Levy, D.: Increased left ventricular mass and hypertrophy are associated with increased risk for sudden death [see comments]. *J Am Coll Cardiol, 32:* 1454–1459, 1998.

42. Huser, C.J., and Hirsch, C.S.: Sudden cardiac death caused by hypertension independent of coronary atherosclerosis. American Society of Clinical Pathologists Check Sample, FP 88-6, *Forensic Pathology,* vol. 30, 1988.

43. Carretero, O.A., and Oparil, S.: Essential hypertension. Part I: Definition and etiology. *Circulation, 101:* 329–335, 2000.

44. Nunez, B.D., Messerli, F.H., Amodeo, C., Garavaglia, G.E., Schmieder, R.E., and Frohlich, E.D.: Biventricular cardiac hypertrophy in essential hypertension. *Am Heart J, 114:* 813–818, 1987.

45. Beilin, L.J., and Puddey, I.B.: Alcohol and hypertension. *Clin Exp Hypertens [A], 14:* 119–138, 1992.

46. Saunders, J.B.: Alcohol: An important cause of hypertension [editorial]. *Br Med J (Clin Res Ed), 294:* 1045–1046, 1987.

47. Kragel, A.H., and Roberts, W.C.: Sudden death and cardiomegaly unassociated with coronary, valvular, congenital or specific myocardial disease. *Am J Cardiol, 61:* 659–660, 1988.

48. Messerli, F.H.: Hypertension and sudden cardiac death. *Am J Hypertens, 12:* 181S–188S, 1999.

49. Brush, J.E., Jr., Cannon, R., Schenke, W.H., Bonow, R.O., Leon, M.B., Maron, B.J., and Epstein, S.E.: Angina due to coronary microvascular disease in hypertensive patients without left ventricular hypertrophy. *N Engl J Med, 319:* 1302–1307, 1988.

50. Devereux, R.B., Pickering, T.G., Alderman, M.H., Chien, S., Borer, J.S., and Laragh, J.H.: Left ventricular hypertrophy in hypertension. Prevalence and relationship to pathophysiologic variables. *Hypertension, 9:* 1153–1160, 1987.

51. Culpepper, WSd., Sodt, P.C., Messerli, F.H., Ruschhaupt, D.G., and Arcilla, R.A.: Cardiac status in juvenile borderline hypertension. *Ann Intern Med, 98:* 1–7, 1983.

52. Roberts, W.C., Siegel, R.J., and McManus, B.M.: Idiopathic dilated cardiomyopathy: Analysis of 152 necropsy patients. *Am J Cardiol, 60:* 1340–1355, 1987.

53. Hoogerwaard, E.M., van der Wouw, P.A., Wilde, A.A., Bakker, E., Ippel, P.F., Oosterwijk, J.C., Majoor-Krakauer, D.F., van Essen, A.J., Leschot, N.J., and de Visser, M.: Cardiac involvement in carriers of Duchenne and Becker muscular dystrophy. *Neuromuscul Disord, 9:* 347–351, 1999.

54. Frankel, K.A., and Rosser, R.J.: The pathology of the heart in progressive muscular dystrophy: Epimyocardial fibrosis. *Hum Pathol, 7:* 375–386, 1976.

55. Phillips, M.F., and Harper, P.S.: Cardiac disease in myotonic dystrophy. *Cardiovasc Res, 33:* 13–22, 1997.

56. Shelbourne, P., Davies, J., Buxton, J., Anvret, M., Blennow, E., Bonduelle, M., Schmedding, E., Glass, I., Lindenbaum, R., and Lane, R., et al.: Direct diagnosis of myotonic dystrophy with a disease-specific DNA marker. *N Engl J Med, 328:* 471–475, 1993.

57. Schonberger, J., and Seidman, C.E.: Many roads lead to a broken heart: The genetics of dilated cardiomyopathy. *Am J Hum Genet, 69:* 249–260, 2001.

58. Fatkin, D., MacRae, C., Sasaki, T., Wolff, M.R., Porcu, M., Frenneaux, M., Atherton, J., Vidaillet, H.J., Jr., Spudich, S., De Girolami, U., Seidman, J.G., Seidman, C., Muntoni, F., Muehle, G., Johnson, W., and McDonough, B.: Missense mutations in the rod domain of the lamin A/C gene as causes of dilated cardiomyopathy and conduction-system disease [see comments]. *N Engl J Med, 341:* 1715–1724, 1999.

59. Li, D., Tapscoft, T., Gonzalez, O., Burch, P.E., Quinones, M.A., Zoghbi, W.A., Hill, R., Bachinski, L.L., Mann, D.L., and Roberts, R.: Desmin mutation

responsible for idiopathic dilated cardiomyopathy. *Circulation, 100:* 461–464, 1999.

60. Corrado, D., Fontaine, G., Marcus, F.I., McKenna, W.J., Nava, A., Thiene, G., and Wichter, T.: Arrhythmogenic right ventricular dysplasia/cardiomyopathy: Need for an international registry. European Society of Cardiology and the Scientific Council on Cardiomyopathies of the World Heart Federation [In Process Citation]. *J Cardiovasc Electrophysiol, 11:* 827–832, 2000.

61. Thiene, G., Nava, A., Corrado, D., Rossi, L., and Pennelli, N.: Right ventricular cardiomyopathy and sudden death in young people. *N Engl J Med, 318:* 129–133, 1988.

62. Tiso, N., Stephan, D.A., Nava, A., Bagattin, A., Devaney, J.M., Stanchi, F., Larderet, G., Brahmbhatt, B., Brown, K., Bauce, B., Muriago, M., Basso, C., Thiene, G., Danieli, G.A., and Rampazzo, A.: Identification of mutations in the cardiac ryanodine receptor gene in families affected with arrhythmogenic right ventricular cardiomyopathy type 2 (ARVD2). *Hum Mol Genet, 10:* 189–194, 2001.

63. Seidman, C.E., and Seidman, J.G.: Molecular genetic studies of familial hypertrophic cardiomyopathy. *Basic Res Cardiol, 93:* 13–16, 1998.

64. Towbin, J.A.: Molecular genetics of hypertrophic cardiomyopathy. *Curr Cardiol Rep, 2:* 134–140, 2000.

65. Fitzpatrick, A.P., Shapiro, L.M., Rickards, A.F., and Poole-Wilson, P.A.: Familial restrictive cardiomyopathy with atrioventricular block and skeletal myopathy. *Br Heart J, 63:* 114–118, 1990.

66. Aroney, C., Bett, N., and Radford, D.: Familial restrictive cardiomyopathy. *Aust N Z J Med, 18:* 877–878, 1988.

67. Aretz, H.T., Billingham, M.E., Edwards, W.D., Factor, S.M., Fallon, J.T., Fenoglio, J.J., Jr., Olsen, E.G., and Schoen, F.J.: Myocarditis: A histopathologic definition and classification. *Am J Cardiovasc Pathol, 1:* 3–14, 1987.

68. Inoue, S., Shinohara, F., Sakai, T., Niitani, H., Saito, T., Hiromoto, J., and Otsuka, T.: Myocarditis and arrhythmia: A clinico-pathological study of conduction system based on serial section in 65 cases. *Jpn Circ J, 53:* 49–57, 1989.

69. Anderson, D.W., Virmani, R., Reilly, J.M., O'Leary, T., Cunnion, R.E., Robinowitz, M., Macher, A.M., Punja, U., Villaflor, S.T., and Parrillo, J.E., et al.: Prevalent myocarditis at necropsy in the acquired immunodeficiency syndrome. *J Am Coll Cardiol, 11:* 792–799, 1988.

70. James, T.N.: Sarcoid heart disease. *Circulation, 56:* 320–326, 1977.

71. Porter, G.H.: Sarcoid heart disease. *N Engl J Med, 262:* 1350, 1960.

72. Subramanian, R., Olson, L.J., and Edwards, W.D.: Surgical pathology of pure aortic stenosis: A study of 374 cases. *Mayo Clin Proc, 59:* 683–690, 1984.

73. Lucas, R.V., Jr., and Edwards, J.E.: The floppy mitral valve. *Curr Probl Cardiol, 7:* 1–48, 1982.

74. Scheuerman, E.H.: Myxoid heart disease: A review with special emphasis on sudden cardiac death. *Forensic Sci Int, 40* (3): 203–210, 1989.

75. Cheitlin, M.D., and Byrd, R.C.: Prolapsed mitral valve: The commonest valve disease? *Curr Probl Cardiol, 8:* 1–54, 1984.

76. Nishimura, R.A., McGoon, M.D., Shub, C., Miller, F.A., Jr., Ilstrup, D.M., and Tajik, A.J.: Echocardiographically documented mitral-valve prolapse. Long-term follow-up of 237 patients. *N Engl J Med, 313:* 1305–1309, 1985.

77. Ross, E.M., and Roberts, W.C.: The carcinoid syndrome: Comparison of 21 necropsy subjects with carcinoid heart disease to 15 necropsy subjects without carcinoid heart disease. *Am J Med, 79:* 339–354, 1985.

78. Hauck, A.J., Edwards, W.D., Danielson, G.K., Mullany, C.J., and Bresnahan, D.R.: Mitral and aortic valve disease associated with ergotamine therapy for migraine. Report of two cases and review of literature. *Arch Pathol Lab Med, 114:* 62–64, 1990.

79. Freytag, E.: Fatal rupture of intracranial aneurysms. *Archives of Pathology, 81:* 418, 1966.

80. Pool, J.L.: Diagnosis and recent advance in the treatment of subarachnoid hemorrhage. *JAMA, 187:* 404, 1964.

81. Stehbens, W.E.: Histopathology of cerebral aneurysms. *Arch Neurol, 8:* 272, 1963.

82. Murray, C.A., and Edwards, J.E.: Spontaneous laceration of ascending aorta. *Circulation, 47:* 848–858, 1973.

83. McKusick, V.A.: The defect in Marfan syndrome [news; comment]. *Nature, 352:* 279–281, 1991.

84. Roberts, W.C.: Aortic dissection: Anatomy, consequences, and causes. *Am Heart J, 101:* 195–214, 1981.

85. Larson, E.W., and Edwards, W.D.: Risk factors for aortic dissection: A necropsy study of 161 cases. *Am J Cardiol, 53:* 849–855, 1984.

86. Schlatmann, T.J., and Becker, A.E.: Pathogenesis of dissecting aneurysm of aorta. Comparative histopathologic study of significance of medial changes. *Am J Cardiol, 39:* 21–26, 1977.

87. Schlatmann, T.J., and Becker, A.E.: Histologic changes in the normal aging aorta: Implications for dissecting aortic aneurysm. *Am J Cardiol, 39:* 13–20, 1977.

88. DeSanctis, R.W., Doroghazi, R.M., Austen, W.G., and Buckley, M.J.: Aortic dissection. *N Engl J Med, 317:* 1060–1067, 1987.

89. Edwards, J.E.: Pathology of sudden death. *Minn. Med., 48:* 1519, 1965.

90. Panos, R.J., Sutton, F.J., Young-Hyman, P., and Peters, R.: Sudden death associated with alcohol consumption. *Pacing Clin Electrophysiol, 11:* 423–424, 1988.

91. Rubin, E.: Alcoholic myopathy in heart and skeletal muscle. *N Engl J Med, 301:* 28–33, 1979.

92. Gould, L., Reddy, C.V., Becker, W., Oh, K.C., and Kim, S.G.: Electrophysiologic properties of alcohol in man. *J Electrocardiol, 11:* 219–226, 1978.

93. Gonzalez-Rothi, R.J., Foresman, G.E., and Block, A.J.: Do patients with sleep apnea die in their sleep? *Chest, 94:* 531–538, 1988.

94. Seligsohn, U., and Lubetsky, A.: Genetic susceptibility to venous thrombosis. *N Engl J Med, 344:* 1222–1231, 2001.

95. Bertina, R.M., Koeleman, B.P., Koster, T., Rosendaal, F.R., Dirven, R.J., de Ronde, H., van der Velden, P.A., and Reitsma, P.H.: Mutation in blood coagulation factor V associated with resistance to activated protein C. *Nature, 369:* 64–67, 1994.

96. Poort, S.R., Rosendaal, F.R., Reitsma, P.H., and Bertina, R.M.: A common genetic variation in the 3'-untranslated region of the prothrombin gene is associated with elevated plasma prothrombin levels and an increase in venous thrombosis. *Blood, 88:* 3698–3703, 1996.

97. Mudd, S.H., Skovby, F., Levy, H.L., Pettigrew, K.D., Wilcken, B., Pyeritz, R.E., Andria, G., Boers, G.H., Bromberg, I.L., and Cerone, R., et al.: The natural history of homocystinuria due to cystathionine beta- synthase deficiency. *Am J Hum Genet, 37:* 1–31, 1985.

98. DiMaio, S.M., DiMaio, V.J., and Kirkpatrick, J.B.: Sudden, unexpected deaths due to primary intracranial neoplasms. *Am J Forensic Med Pathol, 1:* 29–45, 1980.

99. Freytag, E., and Lindenberg, R.: 294 medicolegal autopsies on epileptics–Cerebral findings. *Archives of Pathology, 78:* 274, 1964.

100. Hirsch, C.S., and Martin, D.L.: Unexpected death in young epileptics. *Neurology, 21:* 682–690, 1971.

101. Leestma, J.E., Walczak, T., Hughes, J.R., Kalelkar, M.B., and Teas, S.S.: A prospective study on sudden unexpected death in epilepsy. *Ann Neurol, 26:* 195–203, 1989.

102. Schwender, L.A., and Troncoso, J.C.: Evaluation of sudden death in epilepsy. *Am J Forensic Med Pathol, 7:* 283–287, 1986.

103. Terrence, C.F., Rao, G.R., and Perper, J.A.: Neurogenic pulmonary edema in unexpected, unexplained death of epileptic patients. *Ann Neurol, 9:* 458–464, 1981.

104. Oseasohn, R., Adelson, L., and Kaji, M.: Clinicopathologic study of thirty-three fatal cases of Asian influenza. *N Engl J Med, 260:* 509, 1959.

105. Hetzel, M.R., Clark, T.J., and Branthwaite, M.A.: Asthma: Analysis of sudden deaths and ventilatory arrests in hospital. *Br Med J, 1:* 808–811, 1977.

106. Boushey, H.A., and Nichols, J.: Asthma mortality. *West J Med, 147:* 314–320, 1987.

107. Kindwall, E.P., and Nemiroff, M.J. Pulmonary over-pressure accidents. In: Davis, J.C., ed., *Hyperbaric and undersea medicine weekly update.* San Antonio: Medical Seminars Inc., 1981.

108. Brown, D.L., Wetli, C.V., and Davis J.H.: Sudden unexpected death from primary pulmonary hypertension. *J Forensic Sci, 26:* 381–386, 1981.

109. Berman, L.G., Dunn, E., and Straehley, C.J.: Survey of pancreatitis. *Gastroenterology, 40:* 94, 1961.

110. Strausbaugh, L.J.: Haemophilus influenzae infections in adults: A pathogen in search of respect. *Postgrad Med, 101:* 191–192, 195–196, 199–200, 1997.

111. Khilanani, U., and Khatib, R.: Acute epiglottitis in adults. *Am J Med Sci, 287:* 65–70, 1984.

112. DiMaio, V.J., Sturner, W.Q., and Coe, J.I.: Sudden and unexpected deaths after the acute onset of diabetes mellitus. *J Forensic Sci, 22:* 147–151, 1977.

113. Coe, J.I.: Use of chemical determinations on vitreous humor in forensic pathology. *J Forensic Sci, 17:* 541–546, 1972.

114. Israel, S.L., and Conston, A.S.: Unrecognized pituitary hemorrhage (Sheehan's syndrome). *JAMA, 148:* 189, 1952.

115. Delage, C., and Irey, N.S.: Anaphylactic deaths: A clinicopathologic study of 43 cases. *J Forensic Sci, 17:* 525–540, 1972.

116. Jones, S.R., Binder, R.A., and Donoghue, E.M., Jr.: Sudden death in sickle-cell trait. *N Engl J Med, 282:* 323–325, 1970.

117. Luke, J.L., and Helpern, M.: Sudden unexpected death from natural causes in young adults. A review of 275 consecutive autopsied cases. *Arch Pathol, 85:* 10, 1968.

Chapter VIII

INVESTIGATION OF DEATHS IN CHILDHOOD

Part 1

FETICIDE AND NEONATICIDE

WERNER U. SPITZ
(REVISED BY DANIEL J. SPITZ)

THE DEATH OF A CHILD OFTEN CREATES a difficult diagnostic challenge for forensic pathologists. Such cases may be further complicated when the death involves a fetus or neonate. In these cases, special consideration must be taken to determine (1) viability of the fetus and (2) whether the child was a live birth or an *in utero* death (stillbirth). In deaths associated with trauma, it is essential to document all injuries, and to interpret how they were inflicted. With this in mind, a comparison of the injuries and circumstances surrounding the death can be made. Deaths involving children must take on a multidisciplinary approach that should include a detailed autopsy by a forensic pathologist and a thorough police investigation with statements taken from the parents or caregiver regarding how the injuries occurred. A visit to the scene by the forensic pathologist may be beneficial. When a child dies in the hospital, the treating physicians and radiologists may add vital clinical information to the case.

Homicide involving young children may be classified based on age and includes the death of a fetus (feticide), neonate (neonaticide) and infant (infanticide). In general, a fetus is classified as an unborn baby, neonates are less than 30 days of age post delivery and infants are between one month and 1 year of age. This section will deal primarily with feticide and neonaticide.

Studies have shown that most homicides involving neonates are committed by a parent (filicide) or stepparent and in the majority of neonatal deaths the mother is the guilty party.[1] The United States Justice Department reports that between 1990 and 1999, the number of children under the age of 5 killed by a parent fluctuated between 350 and 400 per year except for 1991 in which the total was slightly over 400. In 1999, the total number of homicides involving children under the age of 5 was 485 with 205 involving children less than 1 year of age.[2] With regard to young children, those under the age of one are most at risk for homicidal violence and neonates, especially those less than 24 hours old, are the most vulnerable. In general, the younger the child the more likely a parent is responsible for the death.

Several studies have cited the unfortunate likelihood of misdiagnosed neonatal homicides and there are a number of factors that may be responsible for such underreporting. In babies born outside of a hospital, the birth is not recorded and thus the death generally occurs without the benefit of a police investigation. A second explanation is that a neonatal homicide can occur without the use of force and thus there are no visible injuries on the body. This obviously makes determination of homicide more difficult. It is believed that between 2–5% of deaths classified as sudden infant death syndrome may actually be due to child abuse or neglect.[3,4] Some researchers believe that this number may actually be as high as 10–20%.[5]

Unexpected child deaths occurring around 2–3 months of age have been known to occur for centuries. Hippocrates was known to have said, "The state of childhood is most exposed to danger around the fortieth day."[5] Over the years, investigation of these deaths has generally yielded few findings leaving them classified as sudden infant death syndrome. Sudden infant death peaks in the third month of life and is much less common within the first 30 days and after the first year of life. Only with a meticulous police investigation coupled with a complete autopsy, including microscopic and toxicologic examination, will cases involving foul play be uncovered.

Fetal Deaths

Feticide is the death of a fetus whose birth is precipitated by an injury feloniously inflicted upon its mother.[6] The fetus may die as a result of premature birth following injury to its mother, as a direct result of the injury, to the fetus or placenta, or from a combination of injury and immaturity.

Within the last 10 years, some state laws have obviated the need for determining viability of a fetus before ruling homicide in these cases. An example is ORC 2903 et. seq. of the Ohio Criminal Code which now specifies that *"no person shall cause the death of another or the unlawful termination of another's pregnancy."* ORC 2903 includes the death of the fetus during any portion of its gestation, however, in some jurisdictions fetal viability is the deciding factor regarding prosecution. One must ascertain the statutory or common law in their jurisdiction regarding the legal definition of fetal viability. Skeletal bone age, crown-heel or crown-rump length, weight, head circumference, gyral development of the brain, and the level of glomerulogenesis or lung development may be used to approximate the gestational age of a fetus and determine the likelihood of viability.[7-10] If the fetus is macerated, tables relating limb measurements to gestational age are helpful.[7,9,10]

Viability of a fetus depends primarily on the gestational age, which is the best indicator of maturity. In many jurisdictions, all fetal deaths at more than 20 weeks gestation unattended by a physician must be reported to the medical examiner.

In Florida, statute 782.09 states that *"the willful killing of an unborn child by any injury to the mother of such child which would be murder if it resulted in the death of such mother, shall be deemed manslaughter, a felony of the second degree."* According to Florida law, criminal charges may be brought upon a mother who knowingly and intentionally injures or kills a fetus she is carrying. Florida also uses what is called the *born alive rule* which states that in certain situations (typically vehicular homicide) a fetus must be born alive for it to have all the rights of a *human being.* Under the born alive doctrine, a fetus that suffers prenatal injury at the hands of a third party and is later born alive is capable of supporting certain civil or criminal charges against the third party.[11]

A 28-year-old primipara (estimated gestation of 29 weeks) was stabbed in the abdomen. Injury to the mother's liver resulted in maternal and fetal shock. The mother's injuries were surgically repaired, but the massive blood loss caused premature labor. A 1,275 gram male neonate was delivered. The neonate developed multisystem organ failure and expired 18 hours post delivery. The autopsy showed anoxic changes in the brain and heart, and changes associated with shock in the liver, kidney, and intestine. The lungs were hemorrhagic and had early hyaline membrane formation. Since the death of the fetus occurred as a result of maternal injuries and immaturity brought on by premature labor, the manner of death was classified as homicide.

Once a fetus is born alive, it is considered a person in all jurisdictions. Irrespective of the length of gestation, if a child shows any signs of life, even if momentary, including respiration, heartbeat, or pulsation of the umbilical cord, the birth is considered a live birth and a birth certificate is filed. Birth is considered complete when the child is altogether (head, trunk, and limbs) outside the body of its mother, even if the cord is uncut and the placenta is still attached. A stillbirth or fetal death is a death prior to complete expulsion or extraction from its mother or a product of conception which has advanced through the twentieth week of gestation.[12] Intrauterine death is indicated by the fact that after separation from its mother the fetus does not breathe or show any other evidence of life, i.e., heart beat, pulsation of umbilical cord or movement of the voluntary muscles.[12] Under those circumstances a fetal certificate must be filed. Fetal certificates do not cite the manner of death, however, in cases where a stillbirth was the direct result of a criminal action by a third party, the autopsy findings must be conveyed to the prosecutor for possible legal action.

An 18-year-old primipara with an estimated gestation of 20 weeks had a domestic altercation with her male companion who struck his fist and knee into her lower abdomen. The woman noted a loss of fetal movements and had an onset of painful uterine cramps. Heavy vaginal bleeding ensued, and she was admitted to the hospital for treatment. Fetal heart tones were absent, and ultrasonography showed a dead fetus with 100% placental abruption. A stillborn female fetus was delivered followed by the placenta which showed evidence of severe abruption. A drug screen using maternal urine was negative. Intrauterine fetal demise was due to placental abruption following blunt impact to the mother's abdomen.[13] In this case, a fetal death certificate should be completed, however, the case should be referred to the prosecutor.

Neonaticide

Although Black's Law Dictionary defines infanticide as the murder or killing of a child soon after its birth, we distinguish such deaths in the first 30 days of life as neonaticide, and infanticide as death occurring between one month and one year of life. Some authorities define neonaticide as death within the first 24 hours.[14] In the majority of instances, neonaticide is committed by the mother in an attempt to hide a recent pregnancy,[15,16] or less commonly during a psychotic episode which sometimes occurs during the postpartum period (postpartum depression/psychosis). A study by Resnick concluded that most neonaticides that occur during the first 24 hours of life are committed because the child is unwanted due to rape, illegitimacy, or because the child is seen as a threat to the mother's way of life or ambitions. Unlike women who kill their older children, mothers who commit neonaticide are usually not mentally ill or psychotic.[17]

Resnick categorized mothers who kill their children into one of five categories.[17]

1. *Altruistic:* Women who kill their children to relieve real or imagined suffering.
2. *Accidental:* Women who beat their children to death, but who do not have a clear intent to murder.
3. *Revenge:* Women who kill their children to retaliate against their spouse.
4. *Unwanted Children:* Women who kill an unwanted child; usually to eliminate their responsibility.
5. *Psychotic Episode:* Women who kill without a clear motive.

The killing of a newborn baby during the first 24 hours of life is almost always committed by the mother, whereas in homicides involving neonates older than 24 hours the father is slightly more likely to be the guilty party. In almost all cases of neonaticide, a parent or caregiver is the prime suspect and in some cases both parents are suspected of being involved with the death.

In general, the mother who murders or abandons her newborn child is young, unmarried and received little or no prenatal care. Typically efforts are made to conceal the pregnancy and the delivery is often done alone. In most cases no plans or preparations are made for the birth. Many young mothers charged with neonaticide have no support network and commit the act because of religious pressures or family disapproval.[18]

Potter found several common characteristics of mothers who abandon a newborn child.[19]
- Childbearing at an early age
- Average intelligence
- Typically lives at home with her parents
- Conceals pregnancy from friends and relatives (pregnancy interpreted as weight gain)
- No preparations are made for the birth
- No help is obtained during labor or delivery
- When confronted with the death, almost all mothers initially claim that the baby was stillborn
- Usually conceals the infant's body and placenta
- Most obtain postpartum medical care

A 1998 study by Overpeck et al. found that 95% of neonates killed during the first day of life were not born in a hospital, compared to 8% of all infants killed during the first year of life.[1] In these cases, where the birth is not recorded, it is necessary for the pathologist to complete a birth certificate as well as a death certificate. Except in straightforward cases where homicidal violence is obvious, diagnosis requires experience as well as detailed information regarding prenatal care and the circumstances surrounding the birth and death (Fig. VIII-1).

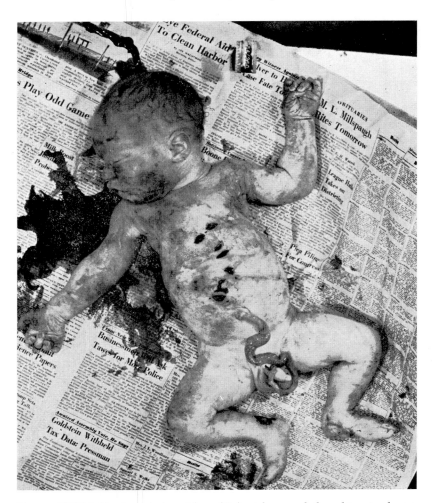

FIGURE VIII-1. Newborn baby with multiple stab wounds found in a trash can wrapped in newspaper.

Several issues need to be addressed by the forensic pathologist in cases of suspected neonaticide.

1. Can the fetus/neonate be identified as belonging to the mother?

   This is accomplished by examining the mother for evidence of recent delivery. Fetal blood may be alternatively placed in a plastic tube or on appropriate transport paper and sent to a certified DNA laboratory along with a tube of suspected mother's blood, both obtained under chain of custody, for comparison. A court order may be required to obtain a sample of the mother's blood.

2. Was the child born alive?

A mother confronted with the death of her newborn child will usually claim that the child was stillborn and that she disposed of the body because she was scared. The ability to prosecute such a case is generally based on whether the child was born alive.

Determination of whether the child was born alive is a critical factor when evaluating an abandoned neonate. Factors used to determine live birth include the presence of (a) food in the stomach, (b) air in the lungs, or (c) vital reaction of the umbilical cord stump.

(a) The presence of food in the stomach indicates antemortem swallowing and is absolute proof of a live birth.

(b) A lung that is expanded with air, i.e., a lung that has breathed, is doughy, pink and crepitant, and completely fills the pleural cavity. Impressions of the rib cage are sometimes seen on the lung surface. Many respirations are required before full expansion of the lung occurs. Before complete expansion of the lung it has a mottled pink to dark-red appearance due to the presence of lung tissue that is unexpanded and airless. A lung that has not breathed is shrunken, dark purple-red and firm. Whether there is air in the lung is best assessed using the hydrostatic (float) test. This test involves placing the lung tissue in a water bath and observing whether the tissue floats or sinks. The float test should be initially performed by placing the entire chest block (heart, lungs and trachea) in the water. Each lung should then be evaluated separately in addition to small sections from each lobe. When immersed in water, the airless lung tissue will sink. Lungs that sink are consistent with a child that did not breathe. Lung tissue containing air will float, indicating that the child took one or more breaths. This test must not, however, be regarded as absolute proof of a live birth since postmortem gas formation due to decomposition will keep a piece of lung afloat even if breathing did not occur. A small cube of liver may serve as a control. If the liver tissue floats, the test results are invalid. Artificial respirations either by intubation, bagging or mouth-to-mouth resuscitation may also give a false positive result. In general, decomposition and cardiopulmonary resuscitation (CPR) make this test unreliable. The float test should only be performed in water since using formaldehyde or alcohol may give false positive results.

In certain situations the live born, breathing neonate will have lungs that do not float. If a delivery occurs in a toilet bowl, bucket or bathtub filled with water, the neonate, if breathing may inhale water while submerged. Death in this case results from drowning and since air is not inhaled the lung flotation test is negative. As the postnatal interval shortens, evaluation of the float test becomes increasingly difficult. Although a neonate born in a toilet bowl and allowed to drown may have a negative float test, a live born

neonate may have bloody water in its stomach as a result of swallowing while submerged. Such a finding is convincing evidence that the child was alive upon submersion.[20]

Microscopic examination of a lung that has not breathed will have diffuse primary atelectasis (Fig. VIII-2). A lung that is expanded typically has open alveoli (Fig. VIII-3). Microscopic examination may be used in conjunction with other tests to support one's opinion, but should not be used as the sole criterion to distinguish intrauterine fetal demise from a live birth.

In cases of water submersion, microscopic examination of the lungs may demonstrate foreign particles which are inhaled as a result of immersion while trying to breathe. Such foreign particles may consist of cellulose and other indigestible substances which make up fecal matter. It must be emphasized that inhalation of amniotic fluid, which may occur in the course of normal delivery, will also result in the presence of particulate material in the lungs, including meconium. It is imperative that aspirated amniotic fluid or meconium be recognized and distinguished from elements of extraneous origin.

Maceration is conclusive evidence that a fetus died *in utero*. Normally, the intact amniotic sac does not contain bacteria and thus *in utero* decomposition is not putrefactive. When a fetus dies *in utero,* decomposition begins almost immediately, however, such changes may be difficult to recognize if delivery occurs shortly after death. Early postmortem changes include softening of the body tissues and loss of muscle and skin tone. More definitive evidence of intrauterine fetal demise is the presence of maceration which usually is evident within 4–6 hours after intrauterine death. Features of early maceration include a brown-red discoloration of the skin, muscles and viscera due to postmortem hemolysis. Continued maceration results in skin slippage and bullae which develop as fluid accumulates between the dermal and epidermal layers. In general, desquamation occurs *in utero* within 6 hours after death,[21] and involves the majority of the body surface by 24–36 hours. The fetal body cavities will contain serosanguinous fluid which should not be confused with pleural or abdominal hem-

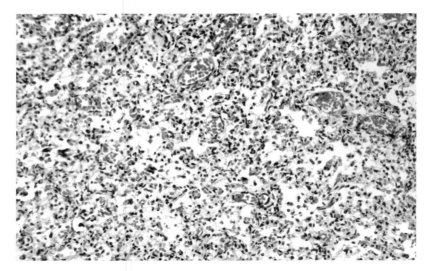

FIGURE VIII-2. Photomicrograph of a lung showing primary atelectasis in a stillborn fetus.

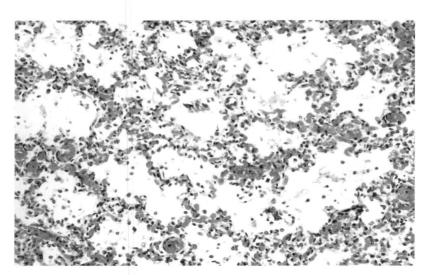

FIGURE VIII-3. Photomicrograph of a lung showing open alveoli in a live born neonate.

orrhage. With prolonged postmortem retention, the fetal soft tissues begin to be absorbed. The brain becomes liquified within a few days and allows for overlapping of the cranial sutures which may cause the head to have an abnormal shape, clearly discernible radiologically. The brain of an early macerated fetus is often soft, but can still be salvaged for examination provided special care is taken upon removal.[10,22] Floating the head in water as the brain is removed is one method that is useful to minimize postmortem artifact. Maceration may obscure microscopic and gross findings, however, evidence of pulmonary infection and congenital malformations can still be diagnosed in fixed and properly stained sections.

(c) Vital reaction of the umbilical cord stump or associated with an injury is proof of live birth. As with the umbilical cord, an inflammatory reaction that occurs with an injury can be used to

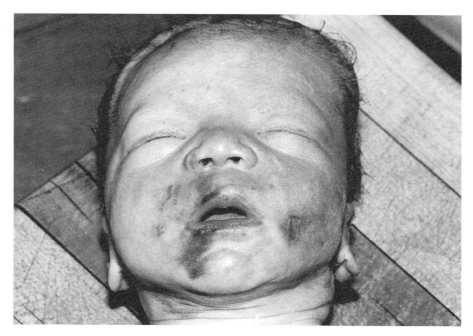

FIGURE VIII-4. Smothering of a newborn. The bruises and abrasions are caused by pressure of a hand against the baby's face.

reliably answer the live or stillbirth question. A microscopic tissue section showing inflammation, hemorrhage, or necrosis may be helpful in making this determination.

The presence of air in the stomach and intestine of a newborn may indicate that the child was born alive, but this finding is often unreliable and easily misinterpreted. Swallowing that occurs after delivery will result in air in the stomach and intestine, however, this is often artifactually created with cardiopulmonary resuscitation (CPR) and with postmortem gas formation associated with decomposition. In the case of intrauterine infection, the gastrointestinal tract may contain gas from bacterial growth, thus giving a false positive result. In general, the determination of a live or stillborn infant should not be solely based on the presence of air in the gastrointestinal tract.

Petechiae on the pleural surface of the lungs or epicardial surface of the heart is a non-specific finding that should not be used to determine whether a neonate was born alive. Petechiae seen in a stillborn fetus are believed to be secondary to intrauterine stress.

Asphyxia is the most common cause of death associated with neonaticide. Asphyxia is typically caused by smothering, strangulation, or suffocation using a hand or pillow to cover the neonate's mouth or by placing the baby in a plastic bag. In these situations, death is caused by anoxia due to interference with oxygen delivery to the brain. Bruises or abrasions may be found on the baby's cheeks, nose or lips, and although the injuries may be faint and superficial they are important to recognize (Figs. VIII-4 and VIII-5). Less frequently, there are injuries to the oral mucosa or frenula as a result of pressure applied over the mouth. The presence of such injuries is of considerable significance and may be the only autopsy finding suggestive of neonaticide. Neonates and young infants have an increased proportion of subcutaneous fat which congeals as the body cools. This often creates artifactual indentations or furrows in the soft tissues of the anterior neck (see Figure VIII-33). This postmortem artifact must be recognized to avoid an erroneous diagnosis of ligature strangulation.

Blunt impact injuries associated with homicidal violence may include abdominal injuries and/or head trauma. Craniocerebral trauma may or may not include skull fractures. Blunt abdominal injuries typically include lacerations of the

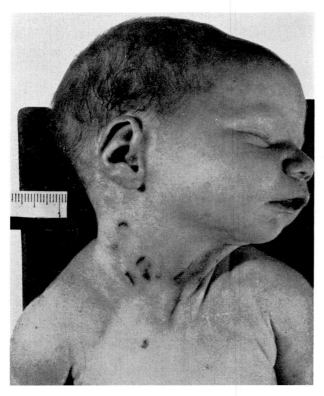

FIGURE VIII-5. Fingernail marks on the neck of a newborn suggestive of manual strangulation. The teenage mother claimed that the injuries were inflicted during her attempts to deliver the baby by herself.

liver, spleen, stomach and small intestine, mesentery and occasionally the adrenal glands and kidney. Often suspects of child abuse claim that a child's chest or abdominal injuries are the result of CPR. A study by Price et al. determined that intra-abdominal injuries are virtually never caused by chest compressions associated with CPR.[23] Skull fractures are often difficult to interpret in a neonate. A newborn's skull is soft and pliable and therefore fractures appear quite different from those in an adult. A linear fracture in the thin membranous bone of a newborn's skull may be better characterized as a ragged tear. Fetal skull development and anatomy should be understood to avoid mistaking a cranial suture for a skull fracture.

Another common method of neonaticide is drowning which usually is done by forcefully immersing a child into a toilet bowl or bathtub. The majority of drownings in neonates and infants are accidental and occur when the child is carelessly left unattended in the bathtub or near a swimming pool. Homicidal drowning in neonates is difficult to diagnose since in most situations no injuries are evident. Statements taken from the parents or caregiver should always be compared with the autopsy findings in order to uncover any inconsistencies. The autopsy should also include a careful search for acute, healing or remote fractures or other injuries. A homicidal drowning involving a neonate or infant is usually only classified as such if the act is witnessed or if a confession is obtained.

In 1984, Mitchell and Davis reported a series of 18 spontaneous births into toilets that occurred from 1956 to 1981 in Dade County, Florida. In one case, the infant was delivered into a toilet and left for one hour. Autopsy demonstrated an apparently previously viable neonate with a stomach full of bloody water which was inhaled from the toilet. The evidence of swallowing was considered proof of a live birth. The mother later told detectives that she was "glad to be rid of the child." Determining manner of death in these cases is difficult since ignorance and willful neglect are not easily separated entities. In this case, the history and autopsy findings combined with the mother's statement presented enough evidence to classify the death a homicide.[20]

Recently, attention has been given to neonates who die because of abandonment. In these circumstances, the child is placed into a dumpster, trash can or occasionally in an open field or wooded area. The child dies because of adverse environmental conditions (hyperthermia or hypothermia) or dehydration. Neglect of a newborn that results in death due to exposure should also be classified as a homicide. Healthy neonates are hardy and in moderate temperatures may survive several days without food or water[24] unless their constraint within a bag, dumpster, or trash bin results in respiratory compromise. Attempted disposal of the remains of a newborn child may strengthen evidence of neonaticide (Fig. VIII-6).

Death as a result of blood loss does not usually occur if the umbilical cord is not tied after

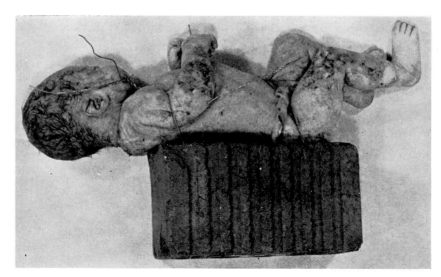

FIGURE VIII-6. This body of a neonate attached to cement block with wire was recovered from the Baltimore Harbor.

delivery. The initiation of breathing which occurs at birth causes circulatory changes which include cessation of placental blood flow. Tearing of the umbilical cord before or during delivery is associated with massive hemorrhage which can result in fetal death.

The umbilical cord may tear as a result of loading with as little as 11 or 12 pounds of weight. Therefore, the finding of a torn umbilical cord is not necessarily an indication of severe, deliberate ripping or tearing. Inspection of the severed edges of the umbilical cord may provide information regarding whether the cord was cut or torn. Cuts of the umbilical cord with dull scissors may be incomplete, i.e., not through and through, the edges may be abraded and crushed, sometimes irregular. If drying has set in, soaking the umbilical stump in tepid water may still permit a meaningful examination. Microscopic study of the severed edge may be helpful in identifying reactive vital changes such as hemorrhage, inflammation, or necrosis. The appearance of the stump may be used to estimate the time elapsed since the cord was severed. The umbilical stump begins to dry almost immediately after it is clamped and becomes yellow-brown and leathery over the next several days. In general, the stump falls off between 5 days and two weeks post-delivery. An umbilical cord tied with string

or something other than the usual umbilical clamp is evidence that a baby was delivered outside the hospital (Fig. VIII-7a). An umbilical stump with an inflammatory (vital) reaction or evidence of healing is proof of a live birth (Fig. VIII-7b).

Precipitous deliveries, in which the child is forcibly ejected from the uterus may result in injuries from impact with the ground or drowning if the birth occurs into a toilet or bathtub. In theory, this should be more common in multiparous women who have a large birth canal and deliver small or premature neonates. This is a rare event and a certain amount of skepticism is warranted. Features associated with prolonged or difficult labor such as swollen, hemorrhagic scalp tissues (cephalohematoma) may be used to refute this claim.

Although rare, several bizarre neonatal and infant homicides have been reported. These include injecting air into the fontanel of a newborn, forcing a child to eat pepper, biting a child to death, and causing an opiate overdose by rubbing morphine on the nipples and allowing the baby to breast-feed.[25]

Currently 26 states have enacted laws stating that mothers may take a neonate to a specific location, typically a hospital or church, and give the child up for adoption without being questioned. It

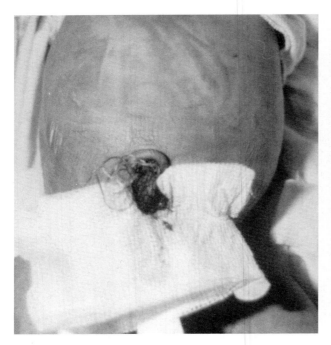 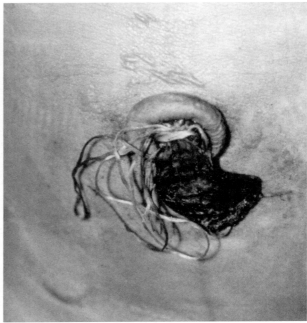

Figure VIII-7a–b. Abandoned newborn baby found in a duffel bag adjacent to a heavily traveled road. The umbilical cord was tied with green dental floss indicating that the child was most likely not born in a hospital. The umbilical stump showed evidence of healing which is proof of a live birth.

is believed that if a mother can rid herself of an unwanted child without having to identify herself, cases of neonaticide/infanticide will decrease.

A description of all the injuries that may occur in the course of delivery is beyond the scope of this chapter. In general, a normal spontaneous vaginal delivery may be associated with minor scalp hemorrhage or small cephalohematoma, but is not associated with skull fractures or significant intracranial injuries. A 1999 study by Towner et al. found that intracranial hemorrhage was rare in all neonates regardless of how they were delivered. Infants delivered by vacuum extraction, forceps or via cesarean section had higher rates of subdural hemorrhage as compared to babies born by spontaneous vaginal delivery.[26] Instrumentation, i.e., forceps, used in difficult deliveries has been associated with head and neck injuries and skull fractures, but for all practical purposes, injuries related to a difficult delivery that result in significant morbidity or mortality are symptomatic immediately or shortly after delivery.[27] The bones of the newborn skull are soft and poorly mineralized allowing for

considerable distortion without resulting in a fracture. Although rare, skull fractures are most commonly associated with forceps and usually consist of a small linear fracture of the parietal bone. Epidural hemorrhage may be associated with the fracture, but the hemorrhage is usually small and of little or no clinical significance. The defense of a suspect accused of neonatal homicide is often that the injuries were caused as a result of birth trauma. This should be scrutinized if the child initially appears normal and becomes symptomatic days or weeks following the birth. In cases of neonatal trauma, it may be valuable to consult with the obstetrician and/or pediatrician to get detailed information regarding the delivery and initial physical examination of the child. In cases of home delivery, physical examination of the mother by a gynecologist is often helpful, since it may establish conditions capable of explaining an abnormal delivery.

Although the possibility of neglect or abuse must always be considered, it should be recognized that the death of a neonate or infant may be secondary to natural causes or due to injuries

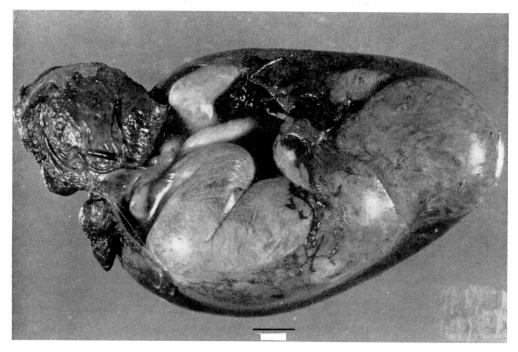

FIGURE VIII-8. A duffel bag containing the body of full-term, normally developed fetus enclosed in its amniotic sac was found abandoned in a communal bathroom in a woman's college. The baby died of asphyxia due to failure to rupture the amniotic membranes. This was considered to be a natural death, since it could not be expected that the mother would have the knowledge to rupture the membranes immediately following the birth. The sac was opened at autopsy.

sustained from a true, unforeseeable accident. Occasionally in these situations the mother may attempt to dispose of the body because of fear of being implicated in the death (Fig. VIII-8). It is imperative to correlate the autopsy findings with a statement obtained from the mother to determine the plausibility of her story.

In any neonate that dies, the possibility of death due to natural causes must be considered. The placenta should be obtained in order to document gross or microscopic abnormalities. Acute chorioamnionitis, acute or chronic villiositis, or deciduitis suggest an infectious process. If there is concurrent pulmonary or central nervous system inflammation, an intrauterine infection should be diagnosed. Several umbilical cord conditions may be associated with fetal demise either *in utero* or at the time of delivery. Microscopic sections of the umbilical cord should be evaluated to look for signs of infection (funicitis). The presence of a large retroplacental hematoma, organ hypoperfusion and shock support a diagnosis of placental abruption. The presence of a true knot in the umbilical cord and/or focal cord necrosis coupled with amniotic fluid aspiration favors a diagnosis of intrauterine asphyxia.

Congenital sepsis with pneumonia may be diagnosed by culture of the subamniotic space of the placenta, blood, or lung. Immunohistochemical techniques permit identification of some viruses including cytomegalovirus (CMV), although this and most other viruses can generally be diagnosed using routine H&E stain. Microscopic sections of lung showing numerous squames and/or meconium aspiration is seen in intrauterine hypoxia (see Fig. XX-33), however, this may be precipitated by both natural and unnatural conditions and is seen in both stillbirths and neonates born alive. Microscopic examination of the lung, placenta, liver, and spleen may demonstrate increased extra-medullary hematopoiesis. This finding raises the possibility of intrauterine hypoxia, hemolytic anemia of erythroblastosis or alpha thalassemia.

Several hematologic abnormalities, including sickle cell disease and thalassemia may be diagnosed using hemoglobin electrophoresis which is a routine test in most hospital laboratories.

Pulmonary malformations may be manifested by the presence of pulmonary agenesis or hypoplasia, cyst formation, sequestration, lymphangiectasia, or cystic adenomatoid malformation.[7] Microscopic sections of lung may reveal hyaline membrane formation, congenital malformations, or acute pneumonia. These findings support a diagnosis of natural death.

Various congenital malformations of the brain, heart, lung, and kidneys are natural causes of fetal and neonatal death that should be recognized. Classifying various syndromes and complex congenital anomalies is best accomplished by consulting a pediatric pathologist or one of several authoritative texts.[28]

Fetal Abuse by the Mother—Use of Illicit Drugs

In some jurisdictions, criminal prosecutions have proceeded relating to the use of illicit drugs by the mother. In general these have been unsuccessful. ORC 2903.09 (Ohio) precludes prosecution in those circumstances wherein an act or omission by a mother while she is or was pregnant results in the death of the unborn. In part, this legislation follows social and legal policy relating to *Rowe* v. *Wade*.[29] In Florida, a mother who uses illegal drugs and causes injury or death to her fetus is generally not charged criminally with child abuse. In these situations, civil action may be taken in an attempt to terminate the parental rights of the mother.

A newborn baby (Baby Boy Blackshear) (2000, 90 Ohio St. 3d 197), was noted to be jittery by the hospital's medical staff. A toxicology screen of the newborn's urine was positive for cocaine metabolites. The mother was also tested and found to have cocaine in her system. The trial court ruled that an unborn fetus is considered a person under the Ohio criminal code. Consequently, an unborn fetus is a *child* under ORC 2151.031. Therefore, harm which occurred prior to birth may constitute abuse. The Supreme Court ruled that the issue is not whether a fetus is a child, but whether a fetus has legal and constitutional rights. The Court opined that Juvenile Courts were created, in part, to protect those rights and empower the state to provide for the care and protection of children. Therefore, when a newborn screen yields a positive result of an illegal drug due to prenatal maternal drug abuse, the newborn is, for purposes of ORC 2151.031 (d), per se, an abused child, and parental rights may be terminated.

Pregnant women who abuse drugs may continue to abuse their children following delivery.[30–32] Injuries, neglect and failure to thrive have been described in over 50% of children who were exposed to illicit drugs *in utero*.[33]

In cases of intrauterine fetal demise in mothers who are known drug users, it is important for the forensic pathologist to take the necessary specimens for toxicological analysis. All body fluids available including vitreous, urine, blood and bile in addition to brain and liver tissue should be collected. For many years various neurologic deficits in young children were believed to be due to maternal cocaine use, however, recent studies have shown no direct link between so-called *crack babies* and maternal cocaine use.[34,35] Certain conditions, including placental abruption, and premature rupture of membranes have continued to be statistically associated with cocaine use while pregnant, however, establishing a definitive cause and effect relationship between these conditions and cocaine use is difficult. In general, fetal death or injury as a result of maternal drug use is a controversial topic which in most cases is difficult to prove. In addition, constitutional issues may preclude criminal prosecution in many of these cases.[36]

Consecutive Neonaticide or Infanticide

In 1988, Funayama and Sagisaka reported a series of consecutive infanticides in Japan. One case involved a mother who killed six neonates over an eight-year period and 11 others involved women who killed three or more neonates between 1979 to 1986. All suspects were the natural mothers of the murdered neonates and 11 of the 12 women were married. The babies were killed immediately after delivery by various methods of asphyxia including strangulation, smothering, or suffocation. One mother delivered three babies in the bathtub causing their death from drowning.[37] In 1994, a follow-up study by Funayama detailed five cases of repeated neonaticide over a 10-year period (1983–1992) in

Hakkaido, the northern most island of Japan. In all five cases, four or more neonates were killed by their natural mother shortly after delivery. None of the mothers were diagnosed with mental illness and the rational for their actions seemed to be economic. Once again, asphyxia was the most common cause of death.[38] In several countries including Japan, neonaticide is not severely punished and in most cases prison time is not part of the sentence. Consecutive neonaticide is much less common in Europe and the United States and carries a much harsher sentence.

Although the killing of a newborn is homicide and charged as a felony in the United States and in most other countries, neonaticide and infanticide is practiced in some cultures, including certain Indian families in the Andes mountains of southern Peru. In these cases, it is typically religious beliefs that drives a parent to kill.[39]

Consecutive neonaticide or infanticide is rare in the United States, however, over the years there have been several cases where multiple children have been killed over a period of time. In many of these multiple deaths, SIDS is determined to be the cause of death. Reinvestigation of several of these cases has uncovered evidence of homicide and in some situations a parent has confessed to the killings. Cases such as these have prompted changes in the criteria for the diagnosis of SIDS. Although causes of possible SIDS should be evaluated on a case-by-case basis, many experts now believe that two or more unexplained sudden infant deaths in the same family, in which a full workup fails to identify the cause of death, should not be classified as SIDS. In such situations, the second death should be classified as undetermined and the first case should be closely reevaluated. Any subsequent sudden unexplained childhood deaths in the same family should be viewed as highly suspicious. In this situation all three deaths are most likely unrecognized homicides.

REFERENCES

1. Overpeck, M.D., Brenner, R.A., Trumble, A.C., Trifiletti, L.B., and Berendes, H.W.: Risk factors for infant homicide in the United States. *N. Engl J Med., 339* (17): 1211–1216, 1998.
2. Federal Bureau of Investigation, Crime in the United States, Washington, DC, 1999.
3. American Academy of Pediatrics. Distinguishing sudden infant death syndrome from child abuse fatalities. *Pediatrics, 107:* 437–441, 2001.
4. Emery, J.L.: Infanticide, filicide and cot death. *Arch Dis Child., 60:* 505–507, 1985.
5. Emery, J.L.: Child abuse, sudden infant death syndrome and unexpected death. *Am J Dis Child., 147:* 1097–1100, 1993.
6. Adelson, L.: Pedicide revisited. *Am J For Med Path., 12:* 16–26, 1991.
7. Stocker, J.T., and Dehner, L.P.: *Pediatric pathology.* Philadelphia: J.B. Lippincott Co., 1992.
8. Keeling, J.W.: *Fetal and neonatal pathology.* New York: Springer-Verlag, pp. 34–37, 1987.
9. Fierro, M.F.: Infanticide, abandoned fetuses and newborns. In Foede, Richard C. (ed.), *Handbook of forensic pathology.* Northfield, IL: American Society of Clinical Pathologists, pp. 98–106, 1990.
10. Wigglesworth, J.S.: *Perinatal pathology, Vol. 15, Major problems in pathology.* Philadelphia, PA: W.B. Saunders Co., pp. 39, 86, 1984.
11. West Florida Statutes, Annotated, Chapter 782, Homicide; Statute 782.09, Killing of unborn child by injury to mother. West Group, 2001.
12. Ohio Revised Code Annotated. Title 37: Health, Safety and Morals. Section 3705.01(B). *Fetal death.* Cincinnati, OH: Anderson Publishing Co.
13. Ribe, J.K., Teggatz, J.R., and Harvey, C.M.: Blows to the maternal abdomen causing fetal demise: Report of three cases and review of the literature. *J For Sciences, 38:* 1092–1096, 1993.
14. Resnick, P.J.. Murder of the newborn: A psychiatric review of neonaticide. *Am J Psychiat., 126:* 1414–1420, 1970.
15. Sorenson, S.B., and Peterson, J.G.: Traumatic child death and documented maltreatment history. *Am J Public Health, 84:* 623–627, 1994.
16. Kunz, J., and Bahr, A.: A profile of parental and homicide against children. *J Fam Violence, 11:* 347–362, 1996.
17. Resnick, P.J.: Child murder by parents: A psychiatric review of filicide. *Am J Psychiat., 126:* 325–334, 1969.
18. Guileyardo, J.M., Prahlow, J.A., and Barnard, J.J. Familial filicide and filicide classification. *Am J For Med Path., 20* (3): 286–292, 1999.
19. Potter's Pathology of the Fetus and Infant. Gilbert-Barness E. (ed.) *Systemic pathology.* St. Louis, MO: Mosby, 1997.

20. Mitchell, E.K., and Davis, J.H.: Spontaneous births into toilets. *J For Sciences, 29* (2): 591–596, 1984.

21. Wigglesworth, J.S.: The macerated stillborn fetus, in *Perinatal pathology,* 2nd ed. Philadelphia, PA: W.B. Saunders Co., pp. 78-86, 1996.

22. Sparks, D.L., Coyne, C.M., et al.: Recommended technique for brain removal to retain anatomic integrity of the pineal gland. *J For Sciences, 42:* 100–102, 1997.

23. Price, E.A., Rush, L.R., Perper, J.A., and Bell, M.D.: Cardiopulmonary resuscitation-related injuries and homicidal blunt abdominal trauma in children. *Am J For Med Path., 21* (4): 307–310, 2000.

24. *Time, 126:* 14, 38, October 7, 1985.

25. Lewis, C.F., Baranoski, M.V., Buchanan, J.A., and Benedek, E.P.: Factors associated with weapon use in maternal filicide. *J For Sciences, 43* (3): 613–618, 1998.

26. Towner, D., Castro, M.A., Eby-Wilkens, E., and Gilbert, W.M.: Effect of mode of delivery in nulliparous women on neonatal intracranial injury. *N Engl J Med, 341:* 1709–1714, 1999.

27. Menticoglou, S.M., Perlman, M., and Manning, F.A.: High cervical spinal cord injury in neonates delivered with forceps: Report of 15 cases. *Obstet Gynecol, 86:* 589–594, 1995.

28. Jones, K.L.: *Smith's recognizable patterns of human malformation,* 4th edition. Philadelphia, PA: W.B. Saunders Co., 1988.

29. Rowe v. Wade, 410 U.S. 114, 1973.

30. Nolte, K.B.: Cocaine, fetal loss and the role of the forensic pathologist. *J For Sciences, 36:* 926–929, 1991.

31. Sturner, W.Q., Sweeney, K.G., et al.: Cocaine babies: The scourge of the '90s. *J For Sciences, 36:* 34–39, 1991.

32. Jaudes, P.K., and Edem, E.E.: Outcomes for infants exposed inutero to illicit drugs. *Child Welfare, 76:* 521–534, 1997.

33. Reece, R.M.: Fatal child abuse and sudden infant death syndrome. In Reece, *Child abuse: Medical diagnosis and management.* Baltimore, MD: Williams and Wilkins, 1996.

34. Hurt, H., et al.: Are there neurologic correlates of inutero cocaine exposure at age 6 years? *J Pediatrics, 138* (6): 1–6, 2001.

35. Addis, Am, et al.: Fetal effects of cocaine: An updated metaanalysis. *Reproductive Toxicology, 15* (4): 341–369, 2001.

36. Ferguson v. City of Charleston. No. 99-936, March 2001.

37. Funayama, M., and Sagisaka, K.: Consecutive infanticide in Japan. *Am J For Med Path., 9* (1): 9–11, 1988.

38. Funayama, M., Ikeda, T., Tabata, N., Azumi, J.I., and Morita, M.: Case report: Repeated neonaticides in Hokkaido. *Forensic Science International, 64:* 147–150, 1994.

39. De Meer, K.: Unexplained deaths in infancy. *Lancet, 353:* 749, 1999.

Part 2

THE ABUSED CHILD AND ADOLESCENT*

Marvin S. Platt, Daniel J. Spitz, and Werner U. Spitz

MAN'S INHUMANITY TO MAN in its most extreme form, mistreatment and murder of his off-spring, has been well documented throughout each era of recorded time. There has been virtually no conceivable form of inhumanity to children that has not been documented, including: Closeting in dark rooms, restraint to beds, suspension by their wrists from shower curtain rods, prolonged exposure to extremes of temperature, including forcing children to be seated unclad on blocks of ice, burning with cigarettes and forcing children with wet pants to be seated on stoves or radiators or immersed in hot water until extensive burns result. Deaths have also been caused by inhalation of pepper and by starvation.

Federal and state laws now define child abuse, neglect, and dependence and outline the care expected of parents and caregivers. Federal law PL 93-247 (1978), now amended and codified as 42 USCS Section 5106, defines child abuse and neglect in Section 5106g (4) as *"the physical and mental injury, sexual abuse, or exploitation, negligent treatment or maltreatment of a child under age 18 by a person who is responsible for the child's welfare under circumstances which indicate that the child's health or welfare is harmed or threatened."* [1]

Six patterns of child abuse are recognized: physical abuse, nutritional deprivation, sexual abuse, intentional drugging or poisoning, neglect of medical care or safety, and emotional abuse.[2] Of these, approximately 70% constitute physical abuse, 25% sexual abuse, and 5% underfeeding or neglect. Each year in the United States approximately 1 to 2% of children are reported to be abused and/or neglected. In 1997, approximately 3.2 million reports of child maltreatment were made to child protective service agencies.[3] About 10% of injuries to children under five years of age, who are seen in hospital emergency rooms, are due to abuse. The mortality is about 3% percent and has been reported to range from 2,000–4,000 deaths per year.[2] About one-third of the cases involve children who are under one year, one-third involve children between the ages of one to six years, and one-third are over six years of age. Premature infants have a greater risk of being abused. In some areas, firearms have become an increasing instrument of abuse and death.[4]

Although the recognition of abuse is usually straightforward, a young child with fresh bruises, healing fractures, and a history that inadequately explains the injuries, the diagnosis of child abuse may be difficult. The first problem is the false or misleading history that is often provided. A history of seizures, decreased movement of a limb, being hit by an older child, or self-inflicted injuries are frequently proposed by the caregiver(s). Another factor that influences recognition of abusive injuries includes a physician's experience with child abuse and family violence.[3] Jenny and Hymel[5] report on the failure of physicians to recognize abusive head injuries and errors in the interpretation of computed tomographic scans and skeletal radiographs. Often physicians fail to inquire about abuse to avoid offending or falsely accusing the family.

Herman-Giddens[6] recognized an underreporting of child abuse mortality in the United States. In a study of 259 child homicides evaluated in North Carolina, 84.9% resulted from child abuse. The State Vital Records system underrecorded deaths from battering or abuse by

---

* Part 2 is dedicated to the memory of James T. Weston who contributed this section to the first and second editions of this book (1973 & 1980). Dr. Weston was an early advocate of child death investigation who developed many of the original protocols still being used in child abuse investigation.

58.7%. Black children were killed at a rate three times higher than white children and males made up 65.5% of the known assailants. Biological parents accounted for 63% of the perpetrators of fatal child abuse.

Kairys[7] noted that there is no uniform national surveillance system for child abuse. Most states code child abuse only if there is a history of prior abuse and not all states have system-wide child fatality review boards.

Jenny and Hymel[5] noted that certain factors serve as clues for child abuse. Some such factors include: younger than six months of age, minority race, parents not living together, history of unexplained seizures, altered mental status, and abnormal respiratory status. Other evidence which should raise the possibility of child abuse includes recurring cases of unexplained injuries or death while with the same caregiver, simultaneous death in twins, dehydration in infants and young children, and child fatalities related to religious motivated medical neglect.[8]

Child mortality review committees have increased awareness of child maltreatment and in some cases have uncovered cases of child abuse. The Missouri statewide child fatality review panel[9] showed that 31.5% of childhood deaths resulting from trauma were due to caregiver maltreatment making it the leading cause of death in Missouri children younger than five years of age. Despite the implementation of an organized program in forensic medicine in Kentucky, some children continue to be abused, in part, because of a statutory emphasis on returning the child to their family.[10]

The Law

The death of any infant, child, or adolescent is under the purview of the medical examiner or coroner in most areas in the United States. Hanzlick[11] notes that 58% of the United States population is served by medical examiners, but one-fourth of the population is served by authorities who have no training or experience in infant death investigation.

Each state has enacted legislation that requires the reporting of known or suspected child abuse

to the proper authorities. In Michigan (MCL 722.622) the list of those required to report is lengthy and includes physicians, dentists, technicians, school staff, and social workers, to name a few. This responsibility also rests with the pathologist who conducts an autopsy on an abused child, whether or not such abuse was the cause of the child's death. Many states now have criminal statutes making child abuse a felony.

Failure to immediately report such suspicions of child maltreatment is a misdemeanor in most states. Furthermore, if the treating physician or the pathologist should fail to report such findings to proper authorities, and there is subsequent injury or death to another child in the same family, he/she can be held liable for civil damages arising out of the injury to the subsequent child.[12] Michigan law states *"A member of the staff of a hospital, agency, or school shall not be dismissed or otherwise penalized for making a report regarding this act or for cooperating in an investigation."* The instability of such families and the hostility of one parent that may develop against the other following abuse may also set the stage for civil litigation. Some states also have a provision within their child abuse statutes whereby if one parent is guilty of child maltreatment, the other parent, if living with the family, may also be considered culpably negligent in not reporting the abuse.[13]

The pathologist should be an advocate for children in addition to being an unbiased, objective observer for the society in which he/she practices. If a child or adolescent was intentionally harmed, it should be determined how the injury was inflicted and who was responsible. If injury or death was the result of an accident, was it preventable? If death was by natural means, could the disease process have been diagnosed earlier? If the disease was inherited, should the family be counseled so as to pursue adequate care of the other children?

When a child is injured or killed as a result of an accident or an intentional act, the medical examiner/coroner's expertise is often needed in court to help the jury understand the injuries and the circumstances surrounding the death. If the victim was not killed, the medical examiner/coroner usually has no jurisdiction in the case, but may advise as an expert witness whether the injuries are consistent with abuse or accident.

Medical science and the judicial system are entering into an era dominated by *evidence-based medicine.* To what extent this notion will be characterized is not yet clear. However, it will become an integral component of the judicial system, and judges and expert witnesses must address the implications of the Daubert and Kuhmo decisions of the United States Supreme Court.[14] Risinger notes how "observer effects" can undermine the expert witness in the search for evidence.[15]

Child Abuse Workup

A successful child abuse investigation requires a thorough and diligent examination. This threshold can be gained by attention given to the clinical history, physical examination of the victim, adequate processing of the scene, radiographic information, and complete analysis of the autopsy findings. In all circumstances, appropriate documentation of each of these elements is essential. An overview of this process is presented in Table VIII-1.

Clues which raise the possibility of child abuse and/or neglect include the following:

1. The history is inconsistent with the clinical or autopsy findings. For instance, the parent or guardian delayed in obtaining medical attention for the injured child. The degree and type of injury does not fit the history of a short distance fall. The alleged activities of the child do not match the child's age/development or scene findings.

2. The majority of abused children are under three years of age and most are less than one year.

3. Evidence of repetitive or cumulative injuries upon physical examination of the skin, soft tissues, and bones. The skin and soft tissues may show symmetrical injuries, patterns or impressions from instruments of abuse, burns by cigarettes or radiators, or immersion injury from scalding water. Old scars and healing bruises on the buttocks and back should raise suspicion, whereas, bruises on the shins, knees and

TABLE VIII-1
WORKUP OF CHILD ABUSE CASE

1. History from caregiver, family, neighbors, other witnesses, corroborate data with physician or clinical medical history.
2. Physical examination of victim for clues of abuse.
3. Scene investigation where child was injured.
4. Documentation of history and physical examinations.
5. Evidence gathering from physical examination and scene investigation:
   a. Skin: patterns of abuse and wounds; date lesions, diagram and photograph. Photos must contain scale, victim case number, and date.
   b. Diagram and photograph bite marks on skin and genitalia. Obtain forensic odontologist consultation if possible. Photograph to scale. Swab fluid or blood for secretor substance, DNA fingerprints.
   c. Examine vagina, rectum and mouth for possible sexually induced lesions. If sexual abuse is considered, obtain samples as outlined in (5d) and Table VIII-2. Diagram and photograph all sexually induced lesions.
   d. If sexual abuse is evident, obtain aspirates and swabs from vagina, rectum and mouth for sperm motility and morphology, acid phosphatase and P30 glycoprotein of semen. Examine for motility without delay. Store other samples in refrigerator and convey to police crime laboratory by accepted chain of custody procedures.
   e. Radiological findings: Obtain whole body films. Document and date all fractures, patient number and date. Consult with radiologist.
   f. Obtain blood for typing, toxicological studies and DNA fingerprints.
   g. Obtain urine for toxicological and metabolic studies. Freeze sample at $-20°$ C.
   h. Convey all items by chain of custody procedures.
6. If victim is deceased, do complete autopsy. Photograph significant lesions.
   a. Document items from 5 above.
   b. Obtain heart, spleen, blood and lung samples for bacteriological studies (and viral studies, if possible).
   c. Obtain frozen portions of liver, kidney, brain, gastric contents, lung and muscle for special studies if indicated.
   d. Take tissues from all organs, fix in formalin and process slides for microscopic examination.
   e. Date all lesions where possible (especially skin bruises, subdural hematomas, visceral contusions and injury sites).
7. Report case to police and required state agencies (including child protective services).
8. Review data and reinvestigate statements and scene if inconsistent findings are noted.
9. Execute a complete report.

bony prominences are often the result of accidental childhood injuries. Fingertip injuries appear as round to oval bruises on the chest, abdomen and back. They are caused by grabbing and squeezing of the child's body and are often associated with rib fractures, which may be acute or in various stages of healing.

4. A radiographic skeletal survey may show old and/or new fractures. Rib fractures should immediately raise questions, as should fractures of long bones, especially spiral fractures. Skull fractures, depending on the location and appearance, may also be suspicious. Imaging studies may show evidence of a duodenal hematoma, intestinal perforation, pancreatic pseudocyst, and/or lacerations of the liver or spleen.

5. Central nervous system injuries, such as acute or chronic subdural hematoma, retinal hemorrhages, subarachnoid hemorrhage, diffuse axonal injury, cerebral contusions and coma may all be associated with abuse, however, the injuries should be interpreted only after being made aware of the circumstances associated with the injuries. Inconsistencies between the type and distribution of trauma and the mechanism of injury as described by the caregiver should increase the level of suspicion.

6. Genital or anal injuries involving infants or children are suggestive of sexual abuse.

7. Evidence of starvation, dehydration, loss of weight, retarded growth and development and poor hygiene may be the result of negligent care and should be fully investigated.

Written workup procedures are available in California, Colorado, New Mexico, and Illinois. Copies of these can be obtained from the American Bar Association.[16,17]

A more recent workup resource is available in the "Guidelines for Death Scene Investigation of Sudden Unexplained Infant Deaths" as recommended by the Interagency Panel on Sudden Infant Death Syndrome. This document can be obtained from the U.S. Government Printing Office.[18]

The Sudden Unexplained Infant Death Investigation Report Form (SUIDIRF) contains a glossary of abbreviations and page-by-page instructions. Although the document is used for the workup of sudden infant death syndrome (SIDS) cases, much of the information is applicable to investigating any infant death, including child abuse. The document is not copyrighted and may be modified according to the needs of any forensic office.

The SUIDIRF is available in an electronic format on the CDC Worldwide Web server at Http:\\www.cdc.gov\ or from the CDC file transfer protocol server at Ftp.cdc.gov. These websites change over time thus, the reader is advised to pursue these with care and persistence.

Clinical History

Most child abuse cases surface when an injured child is brought to the emergency room or is found dead at home. Approximately 40% of abused children are not brought to the hospital for medical attention until the morning after injury; another 40% are brought in one to four days later.[19] Most injuries are caused by parents, live-in friends, guardians, or babysitters, and only rarely by a sibling or other child.[20]

It is important to recognize that battering occurs in all socioeconomic, intellectual and educational strata of society, although many indicted parents or caregivers have certain sociopsychological characteristics. Such individuals tend to be lonely, unhappy, angry people and under severe stress. They are often physically and emotionally exhausted *(apathy-futility syndrome)*[21] or may have been abused as children themselves. The abuse may be precipitated by a family crisis, such as loss of a job, loss of the family home, marital strife, or birth of another child.[21,22] Only 10% of battering and neglectful parents are considered mentally ill.

Drug and alcohol abuse within the household is a common factor associated with child abuse. Alcohol is involved in 54% of all reported cases of child abuse and 67% of those are associated with sexual abuse. The caregiver's use of marijuana, heroin, and cocaine induces child abandonment, deprivation of food and hygienic amenities, sadism and ritualism, and newborn addiction.

Children may have certain personality traits that incite the abuser, including being irritable, stubborn, or hyperactive. They may exhibit offensive behavior, intractable crying, poor sleeping habits and excessive wetting or soiling. Some children have perplexing diseases, such as chronic diarrhea or vomiting, cerebral palsy or eczema.

Often a clear delineation between children dying of neglect and deprivation and those who die as a result of repetitive injury is not apparent. It is not unusual for the repetitively mistreated child to be within the lower percentile of weight and stature and, when seen clinically, to present evidence of psychological withdrawal or organic brain dysfunction. The repetitive pattern of injury may be passively acknowledged by siblings and the opposite partner of the marriage. Child abuse may continue for months or years before resulting in the child's death.

Most abused children are male and their age ranges from several months to 10 or 11 years. The majority are at the age in which parents anticipate, but fail to achieve toilet training or cessation of repetitive crying.

Two other instances of repetitive abuse involve infants who have been repetitively shaken and the Münchausen syndrome by proxy. In the former entity, best classified as shaken (impact) syndrome, the infants have distinct anatomic findings which suggest this type of abuse. In the latter, the infants and children are frequently brought to the doctor or hospital with various medical complaints in order to receive unnecessary tests and treatment. These entities are described in greater detail below.

Scene Investigation

The Sudden Unexplained Infant Death Investigative Report Form (SUIDIRF) serves as a model for scene investigation and is now increasingly used by death investigators (see Table VIII-3, Part 3).

Wagner[19] described several elements necessary for an appropriate scene investigation. These include isolation, i.e., securing the scene, determining where the assault took place, collection of evidence with special emphasis on trace evidence, scene and body photographs and recognition of possible contaminants. All findings should be documented and the chain of custody preserved.

Additionally, the home should be evaluated for its state of repair, degree of cleanliness, furnishings, presence of food, heating, insect and rodent infestation, and neighborhood. Suspicious objects such as weapons (belts, rods, sticks, knives, firearms), as well as tools, furniture, utensils, cigarettes and drug paraphernalia should be documented and impounded after making note of their appearance. Photographs with a scale are advantageous when photographing possible weapons. All body fluids and tissue including blood, semen, hair, nails, tissue, saliva, urine, vomitus and the decedent's clothing should also be retained for analysis. All impressions such as fingerprints, footprints, tire tracks, palmprints, and bite marks should be preserved.

Witness statements should be obtained from family members, neighbors, friends, school contacts, hospitals, clinics, and physician's offices. It is advantageous to tape and transcribe all interviews. The witness should be identified by name, position, relationship to victim, address, telephone number, and occupation. In cases of sexual abuse a history and physical examination should be obtained from the live victim. Estimation of the time of injury or death is important. Whether this is a single episode of abuse, or one of multiple episodes, should be addressed. The mechanism of injury, and determination of whether the history is corroborated by scene findings, is one of the first questions to be answered.

Any injury without an adequate explanation, especially in an infant, should raise concerns about intentional injury or neglect. When an explanation for the injury is obtained this should be correlated with the autopsy findings to see if the mechanism of injury is consistent with the trauma. When autopsy findings are not in keeping with the preliminary investigative report, investigation of the circumstances must be pursued. A frequent explanation for the injury offered by the parents is that of a fall down stairs, a fall from a crib or bed, or blunt trauma from a toy. In some cases, examination of the body yields evidence of repeated abuse, however, the caregiver will commonly attribute all of the injuries to a single accidental event. Delay in seeking medical care, especially for significant injuries, needs to be carefully evaluated because this is a common factor in cases of abuse.

When child abuse is suspected, the findings must be shared with appropriate child protective agencies so that the welfare of the remaining siblings is protected. However, experience has shown that even in families with multiple children, often only one is singled out for abuse.

Radiographic Findings

Radiographic evidence of skeletal trauma occurs in approximately one-third of abused children.[23] The radiologist may be first to document pre-existing trauma in a child suffering from acute injuries. Intentionally inflicted fractures are common in children under four years of age, while school-age children more commonly sustain accidental fractures.

When a child is evaluated in the hospital or doctor's office, the acute signs of bone injury include swelling, redness and/or tenderness. Bone deformity, limitation of movement, guarding of a limb or decreased movement of the injured extremity may indicate a fracture. Remote skeletal injuries are frequently detected on routine radiographic evaluation for an unrelated problem.

When evaluating a living child who is suspected of being abused, full body radiographs should be taken at the time the child is initially seen and an additional set two weeks later. Acute rib fractures are often not seen unless the fracture is displaced, healing rib fractures are associated with callus formation which makes them easy to appreciate on x-ray.

An autopsy will detect fractures of the skull and ribs, however, it is possible to overlook acute and healing fractures of the extremities and rib fractures that are adjacent to the costovertebral junction. For this reason full body radiographs should be done preferably prior to autopsy. Although x-ray will typically identify acute and healing fractures, this should never replace direct examination of all fractures during autopsy. Consultation with a radiologist or anthropologist may help in these cases.

For living or deceased children suspected of being abused, it is unwise to obtain a *babygram* (i.e., a single full body x-ray on a 14 x 17 inch film) when attempting to identify skeletal injuries. It is good practice to obtain multiple x-rays from different angles covering the entire body. Computed tomography (CT) is useful in detecting rib fractures near the costovertebral and costochondral junctions as well as vertebral fractures. All postmortem films should be carefully reviewed prior to the autopsy, and if available, it is recommended that all antemortem films also be reviewed.

Twisting, pulling, and wringing are the common ways in which a child sustains an extremity fracture. Aggressive grabbing or squeezing of the chest often causes rib fractures and a blunt impact is the typical mechanism associated with a skull fracture. These types of injuries are most frequently seen in children under one year of age.

As Kleinman suggests,[24] it is wise to excise the fractured bone and in some cases its contralateral mate to demonstrate the injury and show the asymmetry between the fractured and intact bones. If there are multiple rib fractures, the ribs can be resected with the vertebral articulation intact such that the vertebral body and both rib arcs are removed *en bloc*. Fractured vertebrae should be resected together with the intact vertebrae above and below the fracture site. In some circumstances, after the bone is excised, and soft tissues removed, additional x-rays may be useful to demonstrate the fractures. Of course, this can be done on a formalin fixed specimen. This is especially helpful when evaluating a child with multiple acute and callused rib fractures. Whereas, color autopsy photographs may be considered inflammatory and not admitted in court, x-ray films are usually acceptable and can provide the jury with a visual image of the skeletal injuries.

All resected specimens should be placed in ten percent buffered formalin. When fully fixed, the bone can be decalcified and the section cut in a plane so that the tissue can be properly oriented in a cassette for tissue embedding. This insures optimal microscopic slide preparation and radiologic and histologic correlation.[24] The sections should be stained with hematoxylin and eosin and in some cases with special stains.

In non-fatal cases of child abuse exhibiting skeletal trauma, fractures of the extremities are

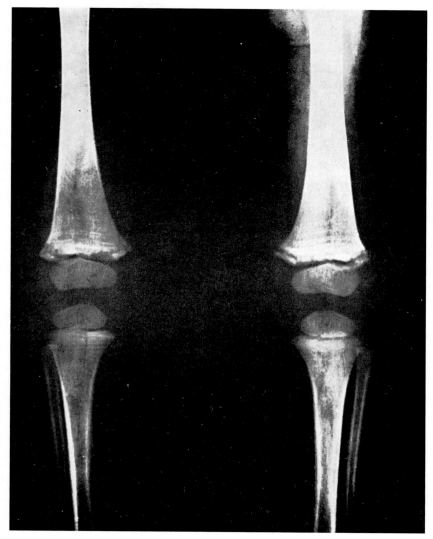

FIGURE VIII-9. AP radiographic view of the knees in a child, demonstrating metaphyseal fragmentation of the distal end of each femur, most prominent at the margins. Incomplete *bucket handle* appearance, a rather specific sign of trauma, is present at these metaphyses. There are transverse dense lines in the distal ends, indicating previous growth disturbance. New subperiosteal bone formation is present in the left proximal femur, indicating trauma of recent origin. Cortical thickening is present in the other long bones, especially the left tibia, evidence of more remote injury. Other metaphyseal fractures were present in this patient. (Courtesy, Dr. Frederick N. Silverman, University of Cincinnati College of Medicine.)

most common (77%), followed by fractures of the skull (34%) and ribs (19%).[23] The classic radiographic appearance of abuse-related long bone injury consists of a small chip fracture of the metaphysis, or a somewhat larger bucket handle fracture (Fig. VIII-9). In the extremities of infants or young children, epiphyseal-metaphyseal fractures are considered highly suspicious for abuse since the forces necessary to produce such fractures do not generally occur in accidental trauma at this age.[23-25] These fractures most commonly arise when a young child is grabbed by a limb and forcefully pulled or jerked.

Diaphyseal fractures are more frequent than epiphyseal-metaphyseal fractures and are statistically more frequent in non-accidental trauma.

Diaphyseal fractures are generally classified as spiral or transverse, each of which is associated with a specific mechanism of injury. Spiral fractures are usually caused by twisting or wringing of an extremity and in a non-walking child are suggestive of abuse. Spiral fractures have been seen following accidental falls indicating the importance of correlating the circumstances with the injury. Transverse fractures are produced by a direct blow or bending of the bone. These fractures are quite common and are usually accidental in nature.

Another occasionally encountered radiographic finding in abused children is separation of the periosteum from the underlying bone. In infants, the periosteum is loosely adherent to the bone and can be easily separated by twisting or wringing, as one does to wring water out of a towel, allowing blood shed from torn blood vessels to accumulate in the subperiosteal space. Subperiosteal hemorrhages should be differentiated from subperiosteal rarefaction which can be a physiologic phenomenon.[24,26] In circumstances where there is a true fracture, calcification of the subperiosteal hemorrhage becomes visible at the periphery after approximately ten to 14 days. By four to six weeks after injury, the subperiosteal calcification becomes solid and starts to smooth out and remodel. Periosteal separation and subperiosteal hemorrhage is usually a consequence of twisting or wringing of the soft tissues and is seen most commonly in the arms and thighs (Fig. VIII-10).

Rib fractures are a common finding in abused children. In the absence of major identifiable trauma or intrinsic bone disease, unexplained rib fractures indicate abuse. Oftentimes, both acute and healing (callused) rib fractures are seen in the same child. In cases of repetitive trauma, it is common to have acute and callused rib fractures as well as acute fractures through an area of callus. Posterior rib fractures are particularly suggestive of child abuse and are thought to result from aggressive grabbing and squeezing of the child[24,27] (Figs. VIII-11 and VIII-12). Rib fractures are rarely seen after resuscitative efforts and chest compressions associated with cardiopulmonary resuscitation should not be considered a legitimate explanation for rib fractures in an otherwise healthy child.[28,29]

The most common cause of death in child abuse is head injury. Falls from baby chairs, tables, sofas, or beds rarely cause skull fractures except perhaps, uncomplicated linear fractures. The skull fractures that may be seen with short distance falls are typically not associated with significant brain injury unless an epidural hemorrhage complicates the fracture. Fractures of the skull base or complex calvarium fractures associated with neurologic symptoms are more indicative of abuse, unless associated with significant accidental trauma such as, motor vehicle collisions.

A study by Belfer et al.[30] found occult fractures in twelve percent of children who presented with intracranial injuries. In an abused child, the presence of one fracture places the child at risk for having multiple fractures. Belfer found that 25% of children with a clinically evident fracture had at least one occult fracture identified by skeletal survey.

Skull fractures and intracranial injury can result from abusive or accidental trauma. In some cases, the presence of other injuries is helpful in determining the mechanism of injury. Craniocerebral injuries when coupled with rib or long bone fractures or visceral injuries involving the duodenum, pancreas, mesentery, liver, or spleen, should be considered abusive until proven otherwise.[31]

Vertebral body compression fractures, spinous process fractures and repeated fractures of the same bone are hallmarks of abuse.[24,27,32]

Computerized tomography (CT) and magnetic resonance imaging (MRI) are increasingly being used to detect abdominal trauma and intracranial injuries[24,27,33] (Fig. VIII-13). CT has been used for evaluation of bone and soft tissue lesions, and the MRI is most helpful to accurately depict vascular and soft tissue lesions of the brain and spinal cord. Acute subdural and subarachnoid hemorrhage is easily seen with CT, however, small quantities of subdural blood may not be detected. MRI will identify small collections of blood in the subdural space and is much more sensitive than CT for detecting parenchymal brain injury from shearing forces (Fig. VIII-14a–b). Retinal hemorrhages may be seen with CT or MRI, but only if very severe.

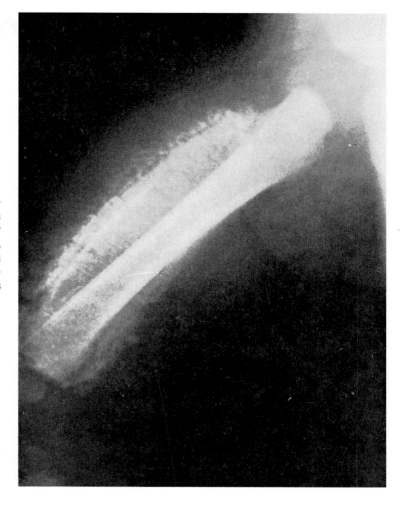

FIGURE VIII-10. X-ray of a large ossified sub-periosteal hematoma of the left femur in an eighteen-month-old child. This type of injury is usually due to *wringing* of the extremity, which causes separation of the periosteum from the bone and bleeding. It is noted especially in children, where the periosteum is somewhat more loose than in adults.

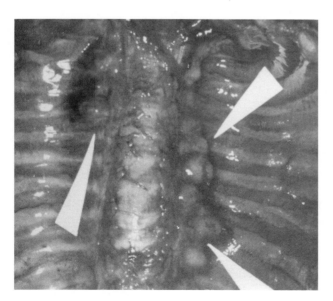

FIGURE VIII-11. Posterior rib fractures due to chest compression.

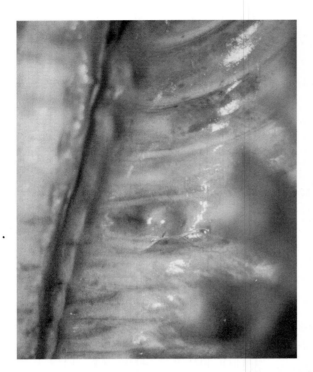

FIGURE VIII-12. Clustered areas of petechiae of the chest due to chest compression.

FIGURE VIII-13. Computerized tomography (CT) of skull showing space occupying lesion in left subdural space with slight compression of the brain (arrows), but no shift of the midline structures. (Courtesy, D. Steiner, M.D., Children's Hospital Medical Center of Akron.)

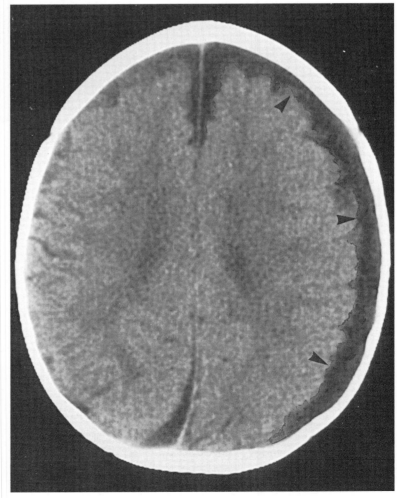

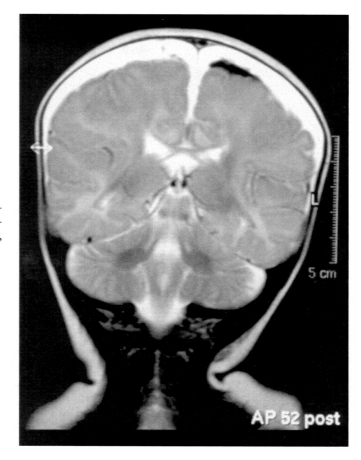

FIGURE VIII-14a. MRI of skull showing subdural hemorrhage at vertex and outer hemispheric fissure. (Courtesy, D. Steiner, M.D. and Kenneth Swanson, M.D., Children's Hospital Medical Center of Akron.)

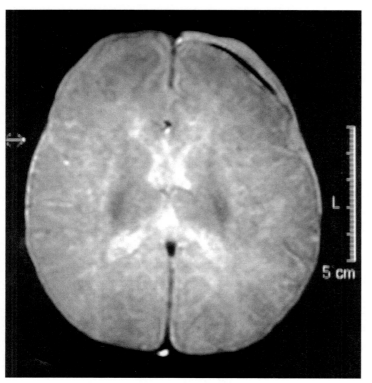

FIGURE VIII-14b. MRI of skull. T_2 gradient of ECHO sequence which shows hemosiderin deposition (black line) along the edge of the subdural hemorrhage. (Courtesy, D. Steiner, M.D. and Kenneth Swanson, M.D., Children's Hospital Medical Center of Akron.)

Radionuclear scans (scintigrams) can demonstrate unsuspected skeletal fractures, injuries to abdominal viscera, and evidence of osteomyelitis, which may follow injury to bone and soft tissue. Ultrasonography can be used to identify duodenal hematomas, pancreatic pseudocysts, or non-opaque foreign bodies in the vagina or bowel. This procedure is popular for it is neither invasive nor radiation producing.

Other radiographic findings may be helpful in the diagnosis of child abuse. Calcification is a well-known sequel of fat necrosis and may be found in the neck following neck compression or in an extremity in an area of soft tissue injury. Anorectal injuries following sexual abuse may result in rectal perforation which can be diagnosed by the presence of free air under the diaphragm or by air on radiopaque colon studies. Perforation of the pharynx or esophagus may lead to a cervical or intrathoracic abscess which can be radiographically diagnosed.

Skeletal trauma which receives no therapy or medical intervention may undergo a different healing progression when compared with fractures that are treated at the time the injury occurs (Fig. VIII-15). Aging of fractures that have not been medically treated is often difficult. Excellent radiographic photographs of these entities are described by Brill, Winchester, and Kleinman.[34] It is important that normal anatomic variations be distinguished from skeletal trauma when reviewing radiographs of suspected cases of abuse.[34,35]

Autopsy Findings

External Examination

A complete autopsy should be performed in all unexplained infant or childhood deaths. The absence of overt trauma on the body surface bears no relationship to the presence of internal trauma. Careful examination of the body surface for trace evidence may afford clues as to the assailant or the nature of the weapon used to inflict the injury. All trace evidence must be carefully documented, preserved and submitted for appropriate laboratory examination in accordance with chain of custody guidelines. Initial documentation should include diagrams and detailed photography of the child. All injuries should be photographed using a ruler or other scale.

Inspection of the body should note the nature of the clothing and the degree of cleanliness, as well as external characteristics of the child, including height, weight, development, head, chest and abdominal circumferences and state of nutrition. However, we have seen cases where severely neglected, undernourished children with pock-like diaper rash and/or injuries on the body surface were impeccably dressed, lying in their crib with brand new sheets and blankets. One such case had the store tags still attached to the bedding. Any postmortem changes such as body temperature, rigor and livor mortis, and the presence of postmortem insect activity should be noted. The extent of putrefaction should be correlated with the available history regarding the time and circumstances of the death. These may substantiate or negate initial statements of those who were with the child concerning their care at or before the time of death. Discrepancies between the distribution of livor mortis and the terminal position of the body requires follow-up investigation.

The state of nutrition as reflected by the amount of subcutaneous fat, the degree and extent of diaper rash and associated secondary complications such as, infection, scarring or loss of skin pigmentation should be documented. Insect infestation, including fresh bites or secondary infection in older bites, may indicate neglect.

The external examination should include a detailed description of all acute and remote injuries, noting size, shape, location, color, and the degree of healing. As a general rule, any pattern on a child's body is suspicious of representing a deliberately inflicted injury. Injuries that suggest a pattern are particularly important as the possible weapon can often be identified based on wound characteristics. If possible, the patterned injury should be photographed together with the suspected weapon to better illustrate how the pattern was caused.

The location of each wound on the body should be described with reference to known anatomic landmarks. A commonly asked ques-

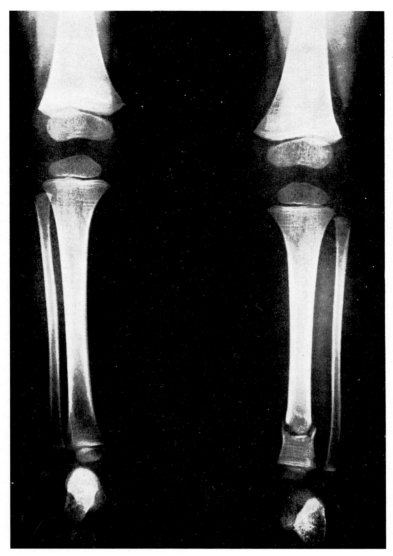

FIGURE VIII-15. AP radiographic view of the lower legs in a child, revealing an old fracture at the distal left tibia, with bone resorption and shortening. No medical attention was sought; hence, no immobilization or other therapy was afforded. (Courtesy, Dr. Frederick N. Silverman, University of Cincinnati College of Medicine.)

tion is: How many blows were dealt to the body? It is important to remember that one impact may cause two separate wounds depending on the type of weapon used and the location of the injury. Two, parallel, linear, train track-like bruises are often observed following a beating with a stick, rod, or belt as outlined in Chapter X. The two bruises are caused by a single blow and the distance between the parallel lines corresponds to the diameter of the rod or width of the belt.

Belt buckles are commonly used to beat a child and leave characteristic patterns on the skin. It is sometimes possible to measure or overlay the buckle with the injury to show how the pattern was made. Occasionally, the imprint of a chain, where the pattern reflects the size and shape of the links can be identified. A common patterned injury is the characteristic loop welt inflicted with a coiled rope or electrical cord (Fig. VIII-16a–b). Rings on the assailant's fingers may

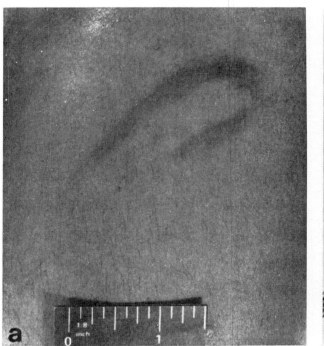
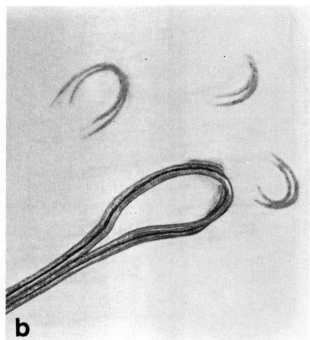

FIGURE VIII-16a–b. (a) Close-up of a bruise produced with a looped extension cord. (b) Diagram showing loop injuries.

also produce a patterned imprint. Occasionally, fragments of the instrument used for the beating are deposited on or beneath the skin, enabling matching with the weapon.

Defense injuries on the hands and arms result from attempts to ward off an assailant's blows. The defensive injuries should be compared with the principal injuries as they may be in the same stages of healing (Fig. VIII-17).

Bite marks (Fig. VIII-18) are often reported on abused children. Wounds that resemble human bite marks are best examined by a dentist, preferably a forensic odontologist. The wound should be photographed together with a scale. Although, in many instances, bite marks are inflicted by abusive adults, they may be caused by the child himself, especially if they are on the hands and arms.[36] Thus, bite marks on the upper extremities must be compared with impressions of the child's own dentition. A swab of the bite area may allow determination of the blood type from saliva and allow for collection of epithelial cells for DNA analysis. Blood samples of the victim and the accused must be obtained in order to serve as adequate controls in such analyses.

Traumatic alopecia occurs when the hair is forcefully pulled out, resulting in patchy areas of baldness. Subgaleal hemorrhage may be associated with hair pulling and does not always indicate a direct impact to the head.

Accidental bruises are commonly found on the forehead, knees, shins, and other bony prominences of toddlers and school aged children. Children in this age group frequently fall or play aggressively resulting in these types of injuries. Injuries caused by abuse may also involve these areas of the body, however, injuries to the chest, abdomen, buttock and lower back are more likely. Fresh fingertip bruises on the abdomen, chest, arms, or shoulders suggest that the baby was grabbed, squeezed and possibly shaken.

The buttocks and the soles of the feet may reveal acute or healing injuries not suspected by external examination (Fig. VIII-19a–b). Deep bruises of the buttocks are invariably due to severe beating. Each buttock should be incised and the skin undermined and examined for hemorrhage in the subcutaneous fat or deep muscles. Mongolian spots, which are birthmarks, may

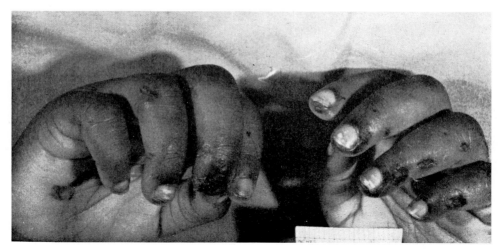

FIGURE VIII-17. Defense injuries of fingertips, showing necrosis, sustained in an effort to ward off blows to the head.

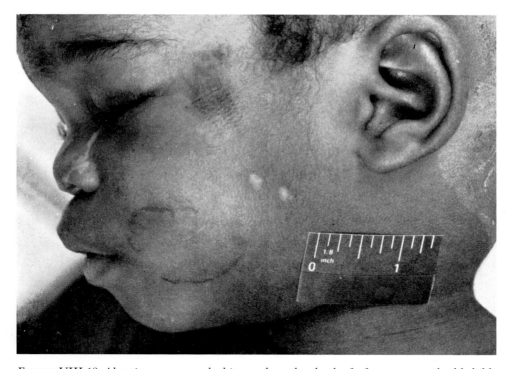

FIGURE VIII-18. Abrasions, scars, and a bite mark on the cheek of a fourteen-month-old child.

resemble a bruise especially when multifocal. They are seen commonly in Black and other pigmented infants, however, they lack anthropologic significance. They are usually seen on the lower back or buttocks (Fig. VIII-20). Incision of the pigmented area will show no hemorrhage in the subcutaneous tissue. Microscopic examination of a Mongolian spot will be negative for acute hemorrhage, hemosiderin-laden macrophages and iron deposition.

Incisions of the wrists and arms with undermining are advantageous for extending the area

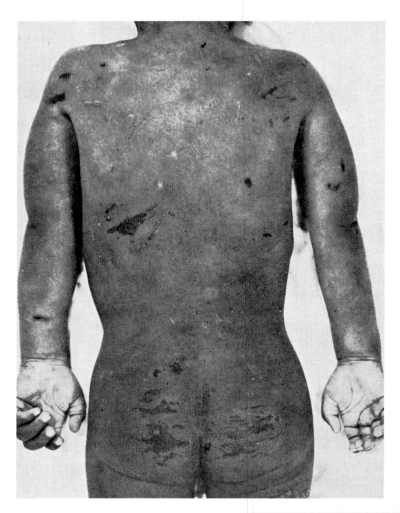

FIGURE VIII-19a. Back view of a battered two-year-old child. Note injuries due to beating in various stages of healing.

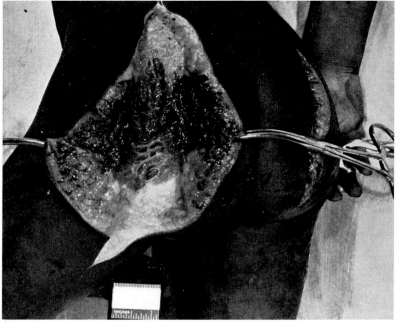

FIGURE VIII-19b. Incision of the wounds in Figure VIII-19 (a) showed deep fresh hemorrhage and deep scarring indicating prolonged mistreatment.

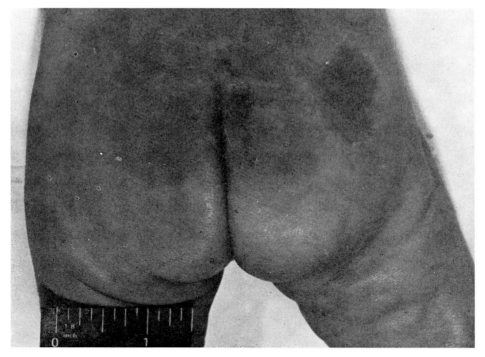

FIGURE VIII-20. Large *Mongolian spot* on the buttocks and sacral region of a two-month-old black child. In some areas the pigmentation is more pronounced, resembling a bruise.

examined without making multiple cuts in the skin. Undermining of a single midline incision of the back, shoulders and nape of the neck may reveal deep bruises not visible upon external examination. Examination of the posterior neck should be done on all children suspected of being abused. The posterior neck muscles, cervical vertebrae and associated ligaments are often injured in children who are shaken or who sustain a blunt head impact. The cervical spinal cord is also best examined from the posterior approach.

Examination of the body orifices may show mucosal tears in the mouth, laceration or bruising of the upper or lower frenulum (Fig. VIII-21), and chipped, loosened, or dislocated teeth. In association with these injuries, there may be patterned injuries of the face, chest, and abdomen in various stages of healing (Figs. VIII-22 and VIII-23). The female genitals may disclose evidence of penetration by a penis or finger or evidence of insertion of a foreign object. Man-

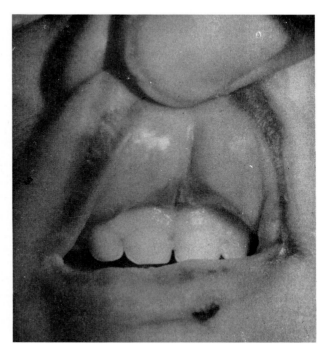

FIGURE VIII-21. Laceration of the frenulum, a common finding in physically abused children.

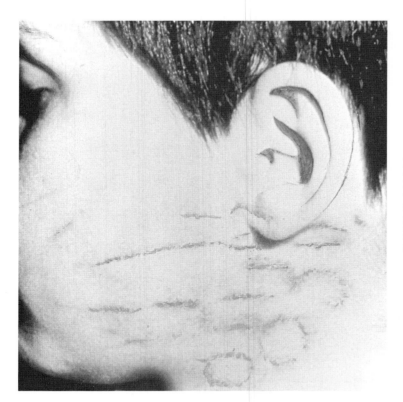

FIGURE VIII-22. Recent slap injury of face. Note the pattern of the fingermarks with capillary hemorrhages at the edges. Deeper hemorrhage and swelling would be seen the next day in the blanched areas. (Courtesy, D. Steiner, M.D. and Audio Visual Department, Children's Hospital Medical Center of Akron.)

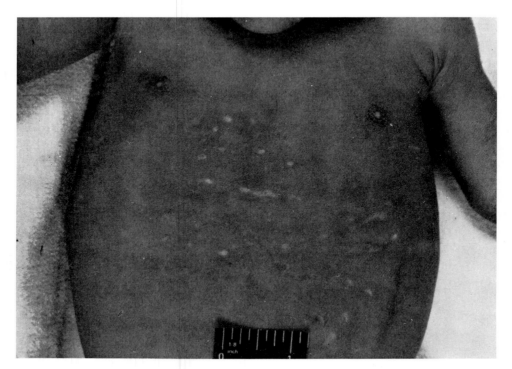

FIGURE VIII-23. Residual scars from previous beatings in a six-month-old child.

ifestations of earlier or repeated sexual penetration include healed mucosal tears, scarring, venereal warts and infection. Anal and vaginal dilatation without associated injury is usually a postmortem artifact caused by loss of muscle tone.[37,38] If there is suspicion of penetration of any of the body orifices, appropriate specimens for detection of sperm or seminal fluid should be collected.

The color of bruises in the skin undergoes a series of variable, but ongoing changes.[39,40] In general, a contusion is initially bluish-red to dark-purple and proceeds to green, then to yellow to brown. Unfortunately, these changes do not always occur in a predictable pattern in all people and cannot be reliably used to date an injury. The color of a bruise depends on several factors such as, time since inflicted, the natural skin pigmentation of the child, depth, size, tissue vascularity, and collagen thickness. Bruises should be documented by appropriate color photography using a scale. The pattern, shape, color, location and measured size of a bruise should be noted in the written record.

At best, the forensic pathologist can determine that the bruises are recent if they are red, blue or purple, and remote if they are green or yellow. Bruises which are maroon or brown are difficult to interpret and associate with an acute or healing injury. Although, it is alleged that postmortem hemorrhage may occasionally occur,[41] microscopic examination to demonstrate an inflammatory response in the tissue indicates that the bruise was inflicted during life. The inflammatory response is not immediate and is therefore not helpful when death occurs at or around the time of injury. Neutrophils are usually seen in the tissue within several hours after the injury. Hemosiderin-laden macrophages typically appear within one to two days, however, the timing when this occurs varies and cannot be used to determine the exact time of injury.[42] In general, it is appropriate to offer a time frame rather than an exact time an injury occurred.

It has been postulated that abrasions may be valuable for the purpose of injury dating.[41,43] Unfortunately, the data which support this theory are more than 30 years old and have not been reproduced by other investigators. Future corroboration of these concepts would be helpful.[44]

Upon completion of the postmortem examination, and ideally after a period of 12 to 24 hours of refrigeration, it is of value to re-examine a child's body. Bruises not seen at the time of the autopsy often become noticeable the next day, especially, if the body is turned face down to allow for gravity settling of the blood. For this reason, Jim Weston would turn over all bodies of children he examined. It was remarkable how often bruises appeared in various stages of coloration, when no evidence of injury existed initially. Drainage of the visceral blood during the autopsy and continued settling of the peripheral blood allows progressive blanching of the skin. This enables better delineation of superficial bruises and may reveal patterned injuries not noted earlier. The initial examination of a body may reveal only obscure minor swelling of the face or scalp associated with minimal or no discoloration. Upon subsequent examination following the autopsy, the contusions caused by knuckles and/or fingertips may become manifest.

Internal Examination

A complete internal examination is necessary to rule out any chronic disease that may have caused failure to thrive or contributed to a child's poor nutritional status and development.

Internal examination may demonstrate subcutaneous and/or intramuscular hemorrhages in the absence of conspicuous external trauma (see Fig. VIII-19a–b). Bruises of the scalp may not be apparent until it is reflected during the autopsy. Reflection must be far enough downward to permit exposure of the lower occipital scalp and soft tissues of the upper neck. In the front, the reflected scalp should be taken down to the level of the eyebrows.

Dissection of the subcutaneous tissue and muscles of the thorax, buttocks, and lower extremities may show hemorrhage not discernible on the skin surface. This examination can be expedited by reflecting the skin from a single midline incision.

Microscopic examination is important for dating injuries in the soft tissue, bone and is also helpful in distinguishing antemortem from postmortem trauma or artifact. For example, a child with fatal abusive head injuries also had a small liver laceration which was alleged to have been caused by resuscitative efforts. Microscopic examination of the liver laceration demonstrated acute hemorrhage in addition to numerous neutrophils and hemosiderin-laden macrophages. These microscopic findings indicated that the liver injury was inflicted while the child was alive and not the result of cardiopulmonary resuscitation. Of course, a detailed history of the events preceding the death must be obtained before

arriving at this conclusion. Theoretically, the child could have sustained fatal head trauma which required CPR, and life support for several hours. Autopsy would have then shown a torn liver with the vital reaction as above, yet the child sustained its liver injury as a result of CPR.

Microscopic examination of rib and long bone fractures can add important evidence to the timing of the injury. When evaluating injuries for the degree of healing, it is important that preexisting natural disease and/or repeated injury to the same area of the body be considered. Certain preexisting conditions and repetitive abuse may significantly retard the process of wound healing.

SPECIFIC TYPES OF INJURY

1. Overt homicide
2. Pediatric Head Trauma:
   • Shaken Baby (Impact) Syndrome
   • The Pediatric Skull and Brain
   • Short Distance Falls
   • Lucid Interval
   • Spinal Cord Injury
   • Biomechanical Mechanisms of Head Trauma
3. Abdominal and Chest Injuries
4. Other Forms of Abuse
   • Asphyxiation
   • Burns
   • Drowning
   • Poisoning
   • Subtle Abuse
5. Münchausen Syndrome by Proxy (MSBP)
6. Sexual Abuse
7. Child Neglect
8. Psychological and Emotional Abuse

Overt Homicide

Occasionally, children are the victims of overt homicide. Adelson[4] described the use of firearms particularly in homicide-suicide deaths, when a parent kills their children and themselves. Other modalities used in these circumstances include stabbing, drowning, and strangulation.

Pediatric Head Trauma

Shaken Baby (Impact) Syndrome

Seventy-five to 80% of all fatally abused children die of head injuries.[45] The mechanism associated with *shaken baby (impact) syndrome* is forceful shaking, causing the head to jerk back and forth followed by impact, against a surface such as a wall or floor, sometimes a piece of furniture, other times a firm cushion or other type of upholstery.

A recent position paper that discusses abusive head injuries in children is supported by the Board of Directors of the National Association of Medical Examiners.[45] The paper discusses some of the controversial issues associated with pediatric head trauma, particularly those which deal with *shaken baby (impact) syndrome.*

The American Academy of Pediatrics Committee on Child Abuse and Neglect has also issued a recent statement on this issue (Shaken Baby Syndrome: Rotational Cranial Injuries-Technical Report).[46] The Committee emphasizes that intracranial injury in a child younger than one year of age supports a presumption of child abuse. The statement is more clinically oriented and presents a good review of the history, epidemiology, clinical features, radiology, and management of surviving infants. However, since some abused children ultimately die from their injuries, the statement does not give due recognition to the role of the Medical Examiner or Coroner in taking jurisdiction in fatal cases, in ruling the cause and manner of death, or in the relationship of the Medical Examiner or Coroner with pediatricians in the community.

First described by Caffey in the early 1970s, *shaken baby syndrome* introduced the idea that serious or fatal head injury could be inflicted by aggressive shaking.[47,48] A constellation of findings associated with this mechanism was described and included subdural hematoma, subarachnoid hemorrhage, brain swelling and retinal hemorrhages. Examination of the child's body often demonstrated absence of injuries to indicate that the child sustained an impact to the head, i.e., no scalp contusions or lacerations and no skull fractures. Furthermore, these cases were complicated by the fact that the parents or caregiver denied abusing the child.

When evaluating traumatic head injuries in the pediatric population, whether during a clinical examination or at autopsy, it is important to not only recognize skull and brain injuries, but also to have the interpretative skills necessary to determine the likely causative mechanism of injury. When testifying as to the degree of impact, statements such as: *"forces equivalent to thirty miles per hour"* or *"a fall from a three-story building"* have been used to serve as an analogy for the jury. These statements are not supported by scientific facts.

The term *shaken baby syndrome* has become subject of much controversy and some investigators are now of the opinion that vigorous shaking of a child cannot cause the injuries once believed to be associated with this mechanism. Skeptics believe that a head impact is necessary to sustain the characteristic intracranial injuries previously associated with shaking. A more recent trend is to use the term, *shaken baby (impact) syndrome* when faced with a child who has abusive intracranial injuries with or without evidence of a blunt impact to the head.

As mentioned previously, whether the injury is the sole result of shaking or shaking plus head impact remains a vigorously debated topic. The lack of an impact site on the child's head indicates that either no impact occurred or the impact was against a soft surface such as a bed or couch. When the impact is against a hard, solid surface, the impact site typically consists of a scalp bruise, galeal or subgaleal, and swelling with or without skull fracture.

Those who believe a head impact is necessary to cause intracranial injury often refer to a study by Duhaime.[49] Using mechanical models, Duhaime demonstrated that it was difficult or impossible to achieve peak acceleration from shaking alone to account for the observed intracranial injuries. In this study, forces greater than 10 G could not be produced by shaking a one-month-old infant model, while forces over 300 G were generated when the head was impacted. This degree of force was shown to be in the range in which traumatic unconsciousness, subdural hematoma, and direct cerebral injury could occur. The model used by Duhaime to determine how much force could be transferred to an infant's head consisted of a doll with a rubber neck and the model used to determine the force necessary to produce shear injury in the brain was derived from studies on adult primates.[50] Although these studies have added to our understanding of brain injury mechanics, the data obtained from these models cannot be extrapolated to humans because neither model truly resembles an immature human infant skull and brain.[45]

On the other hand, many experts believe that aggressive shaking of an infant can itself cause death.[45,51–56] Evidence in support of this opinion includes witness accounts and detailed confessions in which shaking without impact is described. The absence of an impact site is also used to add credence to shaking without impact as the mechanism of injury, however, it is generally accepted that the presence of an impact site partially depends on the nature of the impacting surface. Also, infants typically do not show the characteristic contrecoup contusions that are seen in adults who sustain an occipital scalp impact.[57]

Determination of whether shaking or shaking with impact is the mechanism of injury will require continued research and cooperation between clinicians, pathologists and biomedical engineers. As the debate continues, it is most important to understand that subdural hematoma, subarachnoid hemorrhage, diffuse axonal injury, brain swelling and retinal hemorrhages can be seen in children who are both shaken and those who sustain a head impact. The mechanism of injury associated with both shaking and impact results in rotational forces that cause shearing injury to the brain and it is likely that both situations play a contributory role.[45] The presence of a scalp bruise or skull fracture indicates an impact, however, coexistent shaking cannot be excluded. The lack of an impact site indicates the possibility of shaking alone or shaking in addition to an impact against a soft surface.[45]

In abused children with head injuries, it is most appropriate to classify the cause of death based on autopsy findings, such as, craniocerebral injuries, rather than listing the cause of death by using what is suspected to be the injury mechanism, i.e., shaken baby or shaken impact syndrome.

Duhaime[58] recommends that abusive head injury be considered when any of the following are found:

• Acute or remote fractures
• Depressed, multiple or basilar skull fractures
• Craniofacial contusions or swelling
• Intracranial injury, including subdural, subarachnoid, intracerebral and retinal hemorrhages
• A history that changes frequently
• Conflicting statements from witnesses/caregivers
• A history that is incompatible or inconsistent with the injuries

Shaken baby (impact) syndrome accounts for an estimated 10–12% of all childhood deaths resulting from abuse.[59] The outcome of shaken baby (impact) syndrome is that between 7–30% of children die, 30–50% of children have severe neurologic deficits and 30% have a chance at full recovery.[45]

The classic shaken baby (impact) syndrome typically involves an infant that is less than six months of age, but it can be seen in children who are several years old. External injury is seen in 25–50% of cases,[45] with the most common injuries being fingertip bruises on the arms or thorax. Internal examination may show some or all of the following intracranial injuries: subdural hematoma, subarachnoid hemorrhage, diffuse axonal injury, cerebral edema and retinal and/or perioptic nerve hemorrhages.[51,59-62]

Skull fractures are definitive evidence of a head impact. Skull fractures must be evaluated together with other injuries, the circumstances associated with the incident and statements taken from witnesses and suspects. Linear fractures of the parietal bone may be seen in short distance falls, however, these fractures are rarely associated with significant intracranial injury or neurologic sequelae, unless complicated by subdural or epidural hemorrhage. Although linear fractures may be caused by abusive head trauma, multiple, complex, or depressed fractures that involve the parietal or occipital bones and the base of the skull are more common in abused children. Separation of cranial sutures so called, suture diastasis, is not due to skull fracture, but results from swelling of the brain. It may take several days until separation of the sutures occurs.

Stomping may result in comminuted fractures of the skull, including the base of the skull and calvarium, separation and overlapping of the cranial sutures, and extrusion of crushed, creamy brain matter between overlapping bones. The nature and magnitude of these injuries eliminates a fall or blow with a blunt object as the causative mechanism (Fig. VIII-24). Since death is rapid in such cases, scalp hemorrhage may not be extensive.

The mechanism of injury by stomping is identical to that which occurs in a child run over by an automobile. The findings at autopsy are the same. If the stomped area is in the hairy scalp, only a bruise or small laceration or no injury at all may be evident. If the facial area is involved, the pattern of the sole or heel of the shoe may be depicted on the skin. The other side of the face, the side facing the ground, is severely abraded and bruised, predominately over bony prominences. The type of surface making contact with the body will leave its mark on the skin. For example, cement will typically leave parallel lines of abrasion similar to *brush burns,* gravel will

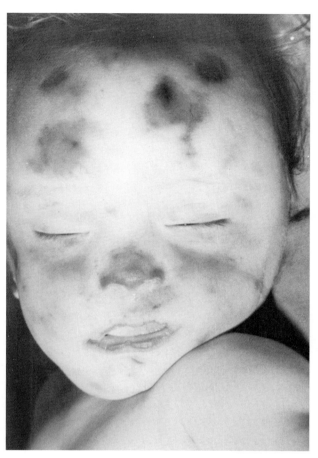

FIGURE VIII-24. Infant who sustained stomping of the back of the head into a shag rug. Note the symmetry of the injuries indicating full facial contact.

cause small defects and a woven fabric will be imprinted in the skin showing the weave pattern. After crushing has occurred, the contour of the head or chest for that matter, will usually be reestablished, due to the great resilience of a child's skeleton.

The mechanism and injury pattern of stomping are discussed further in Chapter X.

Subarachnoid hemorrhage in the setting of head trauma occurs when blood vessels within the arachnoid membrane are torn. It is commonly associated with abusive head trauma and usually consists of patchy areas of thin hemorrhage over the cerebral hemispheres, along the falx cerebri or tentorium. Although not well visualized by MRI initially, it may become evident after two to three days when additional small areas of bleed-

ing become apparent. Non-contrast CT scan remains the most accurate diagnostic tool initially, but after several days, MRI is the gold standard, since it is more sensitive to small areas of hemorrhage.[63]

Traumatic subarachnoid hemorrhage may or may not be limited to the area of impact, whereas, the hemorrhage related to a ruptured aneurysm or vascular malformation is concentrated at the rupture site.[64,65] Ruptured cerebral artery aneurysms typically cause extensive subarachnoid hemorrhage centered at the base of the brain.

Subdural hemorrhages are commonly seen in abusive head injury and are evident at autopsy in more than 90% of these cases.[45] The bleeding occurs when there is rupture of one or more bridging veins or the venous sinuses secondary to injuries associated with rapid acceleration/deceleration induced strains,[66,67] or translational forces. Occasionally a subdural hematoma may develop following a cerebral contusion or laceration. Laceration of a small artery at the surface of the brain may rarely cause subdural hemorrhage. When this occurs the subdural blood accumulates rapidly.[68]

The subdural hemorrhage seen in shaken baby (impact) syndrome may be unilateral or bilateral and is most frequently located over the cerebral convexities with a tendency to extend into the posterior interhemispheric fissure.[63] The presence of subdural hemorrhage in the posterior interhemispheric fissure is commonly seen with abusive head injury, but it is not diagnostic for abuse.[63,69] The subdural hemorrhage associated with abusive head trauma in children often consists of a widely distributed thin film of blood. It is not of significant volume to be considered space occupying, usually less than 10 mL and commonly only 2–3 mL, but rather serves as an indication that the brain had been subjected to shearing forces. Some subdural hematomas are large enough to cause increased intracranial pressure, mass effect and herniation of the brain. This type of bleeding typically occurs when there is laceration of the sagittal or transverse sinus. If blood within the subdural space organizes and forms layers, it becomes what is called a chronic subdural hematoma.

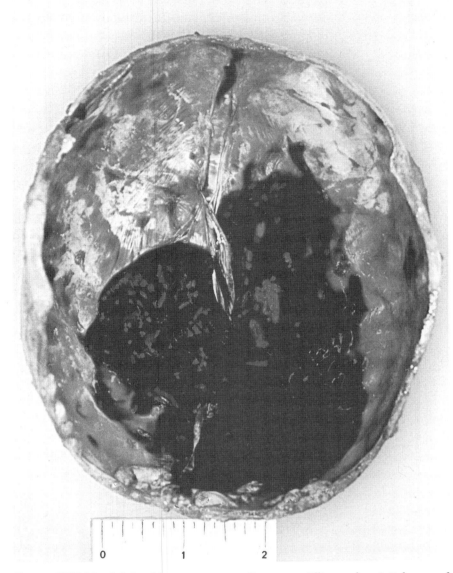

FIGURE VIII-25a. Subdural hematoma extending over midline and occipital areas of cerebral hemispheres. (Courtesy, Medical Examiner Office, Summit County, Ohio.)

The presence of a subdural hematoma in an infant or child, either acute or chronic, suggests abuse, however, other possible explanations must be considered. Although rare, natural diseases may cause or be associated with subdural bleeding, including cerebral artery aneurysms, vascular malformations, meningitis, and coagulation and hematological disorders such as, leukemia, sickle cell anemia, disseminated intravascular coagulation (DIC), hemophilia, von Willebrand's disease and idiopathic thrombocytopenic purpura (ITP). Subdural hemorrhage is rarely seen in a newborn infant after prolonged labor.

The age of a subdural hematoma may be assessed from the degree of neovascularization, fibroblastic proliferation and collagen deposition within the organizing hemorrhage as described in Chapter XIX (Fig. VIII-25a–c). Based on the gross and microscopic appearances of the sub-

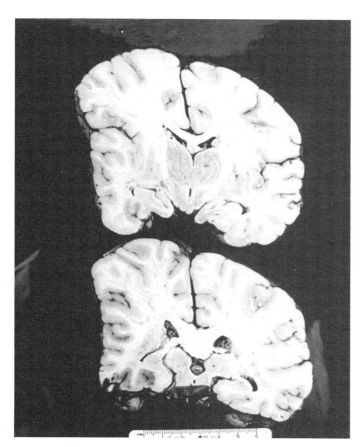

FIGURE VIII-25b. Another case in which a subdural hematoma caused compression of a cerebral hemisphere. (Courtesy, D.P. Agamanolis, M.D., Children's Hospital Medical Center of Akron.)

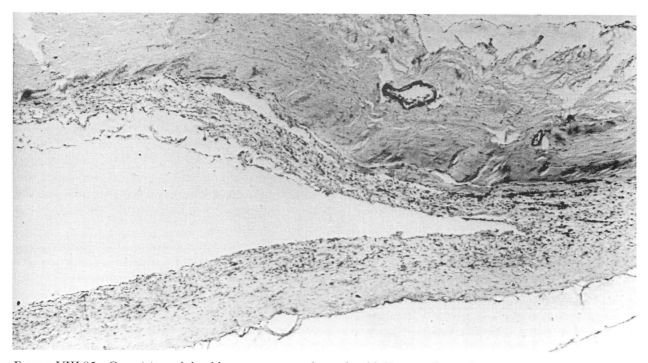

FIGURE VIII-25c. Organizing subdural hematoma, several months old. Notice collagen deposit at inner and outer membranes, with residual fibroblast and capillary responses. (Courtesy, D.P. Agamanolis, M.D., Children's Hospital Medical Center of Akron.)

dural hemorrhage, the forensic pathologist is often able to render an opinion as to the approximate age of the subdural and address the significance of the findings. With chronic subdural hematomas, it is not possible to determine the exact age of the hemorrhage, however, a reasonable time span can usually be estimated.

Occasionally, an acute subdural hematoma accompanied by abrupt onset of neurologic symptoms following minor trauma is postulated to have occurred from rebleeding of a chronic subdural membrane. Such rebleeding suggests abusive head trauma, since chronic subdural hematomas that are at risk for rebleeding are usually only seen in children with brain atrophy or surgically shunted hydrocephalus.[70] Furthermore, a rebleed believed to have come from a pre-existing chronic subdural membrane should immediately prompt the question: What caused the initial subdural hemorrhage? Several authors have recently debated the concept of rebleeding from a chronic subdural hematoma (CSDH).[71,72] In general, when a chronic subdural hematoma is diagnosed after work-up for non-specific neurologic symptoms, it is difficult or impossible to determine when the child would have become symptomatic. Furthermore, when an acute subdural hematoma is diagnosed in a child who was previously asymptomatic, it should not automatically be assumed that rebleeding from a chronic subdural membrane is responsible for the new hemorrhage.

A residual, well-organized subdural space with two fibrous lamina and a thin film of hemosiderin may be seen following the birth of an infant, and is not proof of a rebleeding CSDH.[46] The dura of infants and young children is abundantly cellular and contains proliferating fibrous tissue and hematopoetic cells, including macrophages, some of which contain hemosiderin. The presence of hemosiderin laden macrophages may be misinterpreted as a thin chronic subdural membrane by those unaware of the normal microscopic appearance of an infant's dura.

The diagnosis of acute bleeding in a chronic subdural hematoma should only be suspected if characteristic gross and microscopic findings are observed. A chronic subdural membrane should

be seen grossly and several sections examined microscopically. Microscopic examination will typically demonstrate recent hemorrhage in a background of vascular lakes, fibrovascular response, endothelial proliferation (neovascularity), acute and chronic inflammation, and hemosiderin deposition. The diagnosis of a rebleed in a chronic subdural hematoma should never be made solely based on microscopic examination in which a cellular dura with scattered hemosiderin-laden macrophages is seen.

Computerized tomograms (CT) of the brain may detect small amounts of interhemispheric subdural blood which may be missed at autopsy, however, autopsy examination is more sensitive than CT in detecting small convexity subdural hemorrhages. MRI can detect subdural hemorrhages of different ages, but it should not be used to estimate the age of the injury. Also, MRI should not be used to determine that a chronic subdural hematoma has rebled.[72] Errors in using MRI to estimate the time of injury can occur because a MRI may show a multilayered hemorrhage when in actuality the subdural blood is acute.[72] This occurs when an acute subdural hemorrhage bleeds profusely and forms a multilayered image on MRI. Errors also arise when there is a vascular lesion of the meninges or dural space which can mimic rebleeding of a CSDH.[73,74]

Occasionally, a subdural hematoma or intraparenchymal hemorrhage is said to be secondary to a coagulopathy. Hulka[75] and Hymel[76] have shown that pediatric abusive head trauma patients who die from parenchymal brain injury have prolonged prothrombin time and activated coagulation functions, however, it was also determined that these changes were secondary to the head trauma and not caused by an underlying bleeding disorder.

Since the presence of intracranial hemorrhage may raise the issue of a disease-related coagulopathy, we advise clinicians to obtain a CBC, platelet count, prothrombin time, and activated PTT on admission. We inquire if there is a family history of bleeding early in the course of the investigation. Normal findings remove this issue from consideration. We know that 10–20% of patients with head trauma and direct brain injury are known to develop coagulopathy[59,75,76] due to tissue thromboplastin activation of the coagulation pathway. This should be taken into account with the findings. Toxicological studies should be done on all cases.

In summary, when a chronic subdural hematoma is found, the questions that must be asked include: Is the initial subdural hematoma due to a previous accidental injury, previous abuse, or natural disease? Is there evidence of a fresh or healing skull fracture? In the event of a death where a rebleed is diagnosed, the forensic pathologist and neuropathologist must workup the case as in any other injured child. In a study by Feldman,[77] none of the accidental head injury cases had chronic or mixed acute and chronic subdural hematomas. In general, a rebleed in a chronic subdural hematoma should be investigated as abusive head injury.

Epidural hemorrhage is virtually always traumatic in origin, however, it is unusual in infants and children because the dura in this age group is tightly adherent to the inner surface of the skull. The tight adherence of the dura minimizes the potential epidural space and limits blood accumulation. Since the vascular grooves on the inner surface of the skull are not well-developed in young children, the middle meningeal artery is mobile and can be displaced rather than being torn. Epidural hemorrhage is associated with a skull fracture in approximately 40% of children as compared to 85% of adults.

Primary Diffuse Brain Injury

Cerebral concussion and *diffuse (traumatic) axonal injury* are classified as primary diffuse brain injuries with concussion generally being considered the beginning of the spectrum of progressively worsening brain injury. Both conditions are associated with altered consciousness and widespread brain dysfunction. The mechanism of injury consists of angular or rotational acceleration induced strains causing shearing injury to the brain.

Cerebral concussion was initially described as brief reversible neurologic dysfunction following closed head trauma,[78] however, it is now understood that the sequelae of cerebral concussion may or may not be reversible and that depending on the degree of neurologic dysfunction, death may occur. In all cases of cerebral concussion, little or no brain injury is detectable, either with neuroimaging techniques or at autopsy. Despite no detectable injury to the brain, most cases are associated with evidence of a head impact consisting of a scalp contusion or laceration and/or skull fracture. In some cases, focal subarachnoid hemorrhage is seen. Depending on the survival interval and the age of the child, axonal injury may be seen on microscopic examination.

Generally speaking, *diffuse axonal injury (DAI)* is considered a more severe form of cerebral concussion. A diagnosis of DAI is important in children because it may help establish the time that the injuries were inflicted.[79] Studies on children who sustained DAI from accidental head injuries found that all children demonstrated an immediate decrease in their level of consciousness.[80,81] More specifically, depending on the degree of axonal injury, these children demonstrate lethargy, unconsciousness, respiratory depression, apnea and/or seizures.[82,83] Survival time following DAI depends on the severity and distribution of axonal injury, however, in cases associated with respiratory depression or apnea, death probably occurs within minutes to hours outside of a hospital setting. Therefore, children diagnosed with DAI who die or have significant neurologic dysfunction are symptomatic at the time of the injury.[79] Correlating this with a case of suspected child abuse, there is a high likelihood of the perpetrator being with the child at the time the child becomes symptomatic.

Although axonal injury cannot be seen grossly, an indicator of DAI is the presence of vascular injury characterized by punctate or linear streak hemorrhages in the cerebral white matter. The hemorrhages typically become more prominent in children who survive for several days, however, because blood vessels in young children are very elastic and resistant to shear injury, the tissue hemorrhages are often not seen even though there is injury to the adjacent axons. The areas of the brain most susceptible to axonal injury include the corpus callosum, parasagittal white matter, dorsolateral quadrants of the rostral pons and surrounding the fourth ventricle and cerebral aqueduct. Microscopically, DAI appears as swelling of axons and axonal retraction balls (see Fig. XX-20) with axonal swelling being the more immediate manifestation of injury.[84]

In the majority of infants and young children who sustain shearing injuries to the brain, it is not possible to demonstrate the intraparenchymal hemorrhages associated with vascular injury or retraction balls or swollen axons that characterize DAI. It is virtually impossible to demonstrate the axonal pathology of DAI using light microscopy and hematoxylin and eosin staining techniques unless the survival period following the injury is at least 18–24 hours.[45] Should survival time be prolonged, the likelihood of seeing axonal swelling and axonal retraction balls is increased, but not guaranteed. In general, the younger the child, the smaller the axons making identification of axonal injury more difficult.[85] The use of beta amyloid precursor protein[86–88] or silver stains[89,90] may allow visualization of axonal retraction balls and axonal swelling in young children.[91] Although DAI may not be seen in all cases, the presence of subdural hematoma, subarachnoid hemorrhage and retinal hemorrhages should be considered markers of axonal injury and prompt a detailed investigation into the circumstances of the death.

Although DAI is typically associated with traumatic brain injury secondary to shearing forces, swollen axons and axonal retraction balls may be seen in non-traumatic hypoxic/ischemic encephalopathy.[84,88,92] The pattern of the axonal pathology may help determine whether the etiology is traumatic or secondary to hypoxia,[84,88] however, further research is necessary before this is fully understood.

In a study by Geddes et al.,[84] 37 infants (9 months or less) all of whom died from abusive head injury were evaluated together with 14 control infants who died from other causes. Evaluation of the abused children found that apnea was the most common symptom, being recorded in 75% of cases. Examination of the brains from these children demonstrated that hypoxic encephalopathy was the most common histologic finding. Only two children had evidence of diffuse traumatic axonal injury, whereas, 11 of the abused children and none of the controls were found to have axonal injury in the brain stem and spinal nerve roots indicating that the craniocervical junction sustains localized trauma from abusive head injury. The mechanism of injury was believed to be stretching of the tissue from cervical hyperextension/flexion. Based on these findings, it was postulated that the brain stem injury resulted in apnea which lead to hypoxic brain damage and brain swelling with death occurring from increased intracranial pressure. The authors concluded that the diffuse brain injury responsible for loss of consciousness in the majority of abused children is hypoxic rather than traumatic. In a separate but related study by Geddes et al.,[88] 53 cases of non-accidental head injuries were evaluated. Thirty-seven of the cases involved infants less than nine months of age and 16 of the cases involved children between the ages of 13 months and eight years. Traumatic axonal injury was found in only three cases, whereas axonal injury believed to be secondary to hypoxic brain damage was found in 21 cases. Eleven of the infants (less than nine months of age) had evidence of axonal injury localized to the craniocervical junction or cervical spinal cord. Conclusions drawn from this study included that diffuse traumatic axonal injury is uncommon in abusive head injury in children and that the apnea commonly seen in infant victims of non-accidental head trauma is most likely secondary to hypoxic brain damage.

Cerebral contusions, both coup and contrecoup are common in adults, but are rare in infants.[57] Lindenberg and Freytag[93] described tissue tears in the brain at the cortex-white matter junction in infants less than five months of age (Fig. VIII-26), which they termed contusion tears. When present, these injuries are usually in the orbital, temporal and first frontal convolutions and are caused by shearing forces acting on the poorly myelinated infant brain. Healing of such injuries occurs by gliosis, leaving small areas of yellow discoloration, occasionally small cystic

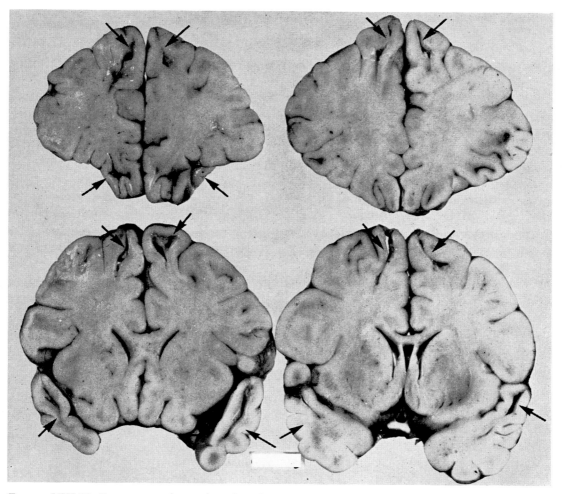

FIGURE VIII-26. Recent tears (arrows) in the white matter of the orbital lobes and two week old tears (arrows) in the white matter of the anterior temporal lobes and first frontal convolutions. Impact fracture through both parieto-occipital regions. (Photo courtesy of Dr. Richard Lindenberg, From *Arch Pathol, 87:* 298, 1969, reprinted with permission.)

spaces and hemosiderin deposits with surrounding reactive astrocytosis on microscopic examination. Overall, contusion tears are rare, but when present are virtually always seen together with subarachnoid and subdural hemorrhage.

Increased intracranial pressure following trauma can be caused by epidural or subdural hematomas, cerebral edema, or intraparenchymal hemorrhage. Cerebral edema may develop secondary to any significant head injury and is most prominent in a child whose head injuries lead to brain death. Cerebral edema develops within seconds following injury to the brain, however, should death ensue at or near the time

of impact, edema may be minimal or absent. Cerebral edema by itself is not sufficient to make a diagnosis of shaken baby (impact) syndrome.

Following severe head injury, the brain begins to swell. In children, the brain's initial response to trauma is to increase blood flow, whereas, the microvasculature in adults constricts resulting in decreased cerebral blood flow.[59,94] The initial intracranial swelling is thought to be produced by vasodilatation caused by the loss of cerebral auto-regulation and the response to elevated catecholamines.[83] Intracranial hypertension, systemic hypertension, apnea, and coma may rapidly ensue.[82,83,94-96] The work by Geddes demonstrated axonal injury to the brainstem and/or cervical spinal cord as a cause of apnea and subsequent hypoxic encephalopathy.[84,88]

If cerebral blood flow and tissue oxygenation is compromised, hypoxic-ischemic encephalopathy results. Brain swelling causes flattening of the cerebral gyri, narrowing of the sulci; notching of the parahippocampal gyri (unci), cingulate gyri or cerebellar tonsils; compression of the lateral ventricles and increased brain weight. The unfused cranial sutures may separate i.e., diastasis, however, this is not always seen. As brain swelling continues, herniation of the unci, cingulate gyri and/or cerebellar tonsils may occur. This is typically associated with brain death, but herniation is not seen in all brain dead infants. Microscopic examination will demonstrate eosinophilic neuronal degeneration, nuclear pyknosis and subsequent neuronal necrosis which is cell death. Ischemic changes are commonly seen in the periventricular white matter which is an area in the infant brain particularly susceptible to anoxia and ischemia. It is important to understand that global cerebral hypoxia may result in axonal pathology similar to that seen with severe shearing injury to the brain.

Retinal hemorrhages (Figs. VIII-27and see XX-20) are seen in 70–85% of infants and young children with severe rotational brain injuries,[45] however, they may also be observed in a variety of other situations and should therefore only be interpreted together with other autopsy findings and the circumstances surrounding the case.

The pathogenesis of retinal hemorrhages is not precisely understood, although several mechanisms have been proposed. These include elevated intraocular venous pressure with increased pressure in the central retinal vein, cycles of rapid acceleration and deceleration causing direct retinal trauma or traction caused by movement of the vitreous, chest compression causing elevated jugular venous pressure[97] and increased intracranial pressure. Retinal hemorrhages caused by increased intracranial pressure are rare. When present they are usually few and located at the posterior pole of the retina. Retinal hemorrhages are commonly associated with abusive head trauma,[59] although they may occasion-

ally be seen in motor vehicle accidents, vaginal delivery, and accidental falls.[98] Non-traumatic causes of retinal hemorrhages include spontaneous subarachnoid hemorrhage, bleeding disorders, thrombocytopenia, hyperviscosity, acute leukemia, meningitis, increased intracranial pressure and systemic infections.[99-102] Resuscitation as a cause of retinal hemorrhage is rare.[99,103,104] A study by Gilliland et al.,[99] on a series of 169 children found no cases of retinal hemorrhages caused by resuscitation attempts.

It has been postulated that the eyes of infants are particularly vulnerable to injury from shaking because the globes are able to move within the eye sockets due to the pliablity of the infant sclera.

Questions as to the incidence, severity, extent and time of persistence of retinal hemorrhages in newborns were addressed by Emerson et al.[105] who conducted ophthalmological examinations on 149 healthy newborn infants within 30 days of birth. The authors found that approximately 35% of newborns have retinal hemorrhages following an uncomplicated spontaneous vaginal delivery and that bilateral retinal hemorrhages were common. In all positive cases, the hemorrhages were intraretinal except one which was subretinal. By two weeks following delivery, 85% of the hemorrhages had resolved and virtually all hemorrhages had resolved by 30 days post delivery.

Retinal hemorrhages, subdural hematoma and occasionally skull fractures can result from a complicated delivery, however, the symptoms of such trauma would be seen at or around the time of delivery. Neurologic symptoms associated with intracranial injury presenting days to weeks following a normal spontaneous vaginal birth should not be attributed to birth trauma.

As mentioned previously, retinal hemorrhages may be seen in both abusive and accidental head trauma, however, the appearance and distribution of the hemorrhage may help distinguish between these two possibilities. Retinal hemorrhages associated with abuse are typically multifocal or diffuse and commonly extend to the periphery. The hemorrhages may be subhyaloid, submembranous, within the nerve fiber, subretinal, choroidal, or intrascleral.[59]

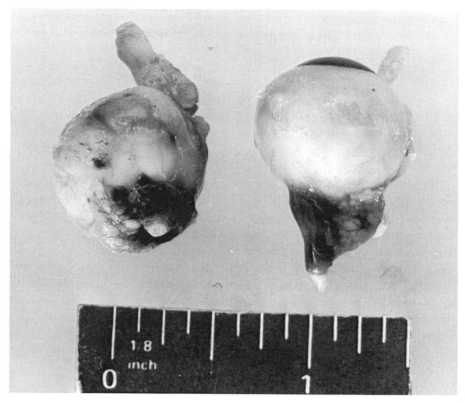

FIGURE VIII-27. Eyeballs of a *Shaken Baby*. Hemorrhages are noted at the back of the eyes, around the optic nerves.

Other forms of ocular injury that may be associated with abusive head trauma include vitreous hemorrhage, optic nerve hemorrhage (see Figs. VIII-27 and XX-20), retinal detachment, retinoschisis, which is traumatic splitting of the retina, infarction of the optic nerve, cataracts, dislocated lenses, and optic nerve atrophy.[60–62] Retinal detachment and retinoschisis should be diagnosed using indirect ophthalmoscopy rather than at autopsy. The artifact created by removing and bisecting the globes make postmortem diagnosis of these entities virtually impossible. The presence of a positive iron stain in retinal or optic nerve sections indicates that injury occurred previously,[62] perhaps within the previous 3–4 days.[106] The mechanism of traumatic retinal detachment associated with abusive head injury is most likely acceleration/deceleration of the head which causes movement of the vitreous which in turn puts traction on the retina.

Optic nerve sheath hemorrhages accompany retinal hemorrhages in 70% of abusive head injury.[61] Isolated optic nerve hemorrhage may be seen in association with traumatic or naturally occurring subarachnoid or subdural hemorrhage,[69] or occasionally when there is increased intracranial pressure from causes other than abuse.

Whenever a child is suspected of being abused, the ocular fluid should not be drawn from the eye. Although chemical analysis of the vitreous fluid may be important to diagnose dehydration, in cases of abuse, examination of the retina is usually more important. Aspirating the ocular fluid prior to examination of the retina may cause artifacts that are difficult to interpret. Prior to removing any tissues associated with the eyes, it is important to examine the external surface of the eyelids, periorbital skin, bulbar and palpebral conjunctivae, and corneas.

Once the brain and dura are removed, both eyes should be examined from the posterior approach after removal of the orbital roofs (see Chapter XXV). This allows direct, in-situ examination of the optic nerves and optic tracts. Removal of the eyes from the anterior approach should only be done in non-traumatic cases where intraorbital pathology is suspected. Once the orbital roofs are removed, dissection of the orbital fat exposes the optic nerves and globes. Cutting of the orbital muscles and conjunctivae allows removal of the eyes. Any pathologic changes involving the globes or optic nerves should be photographed prior to fixation. The globes should be left intact and fixed in 10% formalin for 24 hours. Formalin will usually discolor the tissue, however, the color can be restored if the tissue is placed in a 70% alcohol solution for several days. After fixation each eye should be cut in a horizontal plane making sure to cut through the optic nerve. Following gross examination of the retina, a section of each eye should be submitted for slide preparation.[107]

The Pediatric Skull and Brain

Comparison of craniocerebral injuries seen in adults and children is unreliable since the anatomy of the adult skull and brain is different from that of an infant. Recent mechanical testing demonstrated that the adult skull is eight times stronger than that of a newborn.[108] At the time of impact, the immature skull will bend inward at the impact site causing deformation and injury of the brain.[108,109]

There are many anatomic differences between infants and adults which allow for head and neck injuries commonly seen in abused children. Infants have a large head to body ratio and weak neck muscles making them more prone to acceleration/deceleration injuries. At birth, the brain is about 25% of the predicted adult weight and the weight of a child's head in approximately 10–15% of the body weight compared to approximately 2–3% in adults. The bones of the infant skull are thin and the skull is pliable because the cranial sutures are unfused and the fontanels are open. Also, the base of the infant skull is relatively flat due to immaturity of the orbital roofs and sphenoid bones. As the basilar skull develops, definition of the bones of the anterior, middle and posterior cranial fossae limits rotational movement of the brain within the cranial cavity. Infant brains are soft due to incomplete myelinization of the white matter and because the immature brain has a greater water content than the brains of older children and adults. The soft consistency of the brain renders axons more susceptible to injury following rotational movement.

With the infant skull and brain being significantly different from that of older children and adults, the diverse brain injury patterns seen in young children and adults must be viewed as more than coincidental. Several studies have concluded that the aforementioned anatomic differences render the immature skull and brain vulnerable to the shearing injury commonly associated with abusive head trauma.[50]

Short Distance Falls

When infants or young children fall out of beds or cribs or off changing tables from heights less than 36 inches, few suffer serious or life-threatening injuries.[58,77] Williams[110] reviewed a large number of infants and small children who were injured during witnessed falls and concluded that short distance falls are unlikely to produce serious or life-threatening trauma. Chadwick et al.[111] essentially corroborated Williams' findings, although their study included seven deaths among 100 children reported to have fallen four feet or less. In five of these cases, there were associated injuries implicating child abuse, and in the children who fell five to nine feet, there was no incidence of death.

Plunkett[69] searched the Consumer Product Safety Commission (CPSC) database to obtain a series of children who died as a result of head injuries sustained in falls of less than 10 feet associated with playground equipment. A total of 18 deaths were found over an 11.5 year period. Since the CPSC reports that approximately 120,000 children are evaluated in emergency departments each year for injuries associated with falls from playground toys, more than 1.3

million such emergency department visits would have occurred over the 11.5 year period used for the study. These numbers yield a rate of 1.3 deaths per 100,000 such falls. This study thus suggests that fatal craniocerebral injuries are rare following short distance falls.[112]

Although valuable information can be gained from this series, there are several limitations associated with the study. It has been shown that the biophysics of head injury in infants is fundamentally different from that in older children and adults.[77] Because none of the children who died were less than 12 months of age, meaningful conclusions regarding head injuries in the very young cannot be made. Furthermore, seven of the 18 children did not have an autopsy examination thus, the possibility of occult injuries or undiagnosed disease processes were not considered. Lastly, this study deals primarily with children whose bodies were in motion prior to sustaining a head impact. The angular acceleration/deceleration and/or centrifugal forces associated with swings and other similar playground toys may serve to increase the severity of the injury. Although, these are not cases of shaken (impact) baby syndrome, the mechanism of injury associated with the majority of these children reinforces the concept that rotational forces followed by impact increases injury severity as compared to falls associated with pure translational forces.

In general, falls that involve a height of less than five feet rarely cause significant or life-threatening head injury.[58,77,111] Essentially, all children sustain injuries from common, household accidents, which typically involve short distance falls. Although, such accidents usually cause minimal or no injuries, depending on the circumstances, uncomplicated, linear skull fractures may occur. These types of fractures are rarely associated with significant brain injury or a poor neurologic outcome, unless accompanied by extradural hemorrhage. Typical household falls primarily involve translational rather than rotational forces, and thus the type of force necessary to cause shearing injury to the brain are not generated.[45,57,58,113,114] Child abuse must be excluded in all pediatric deaths that are alleged to occur after a short distance fall.

In summary, when investigating deaths of children who have sustained head trauma, there is no substitute for a complete postmortem examination with correlation of the autopsy findings to the investigative circumstances, i.e., do the injuries fit the circumstances as alleged? With accidental and abusive head injuries, there are few absolutes making it important to judge each case individually using all available information.

Lucid Interval

When did the injury occur is a common question asked of forensic pathologists. This can often be answered by interpreting the injuries and the presenting symptoms. Knowing when neurologic symptoms will develop following head trauma can be difficult, however, understanding that certain brain injuries are associated with characteristic neurologic symptoms allows for an accurate assessment as to the time the injuries were inflicted. It is often important to determine when the injuries were sustained so as to include or exclude possible suspects based on who was with the child at the time of injury.

A lucid interval is the time between injury and the development of neurologic symptoms. Some pediatric head injuries are associated with immediate neurologic symptoms,[54] while other head trauma is associated with a lucid interval of variable duration.[69,115]

The likelihood of having a lucid interval depends primarily on the amount of shear injury to the brain and the region of the brain that sustains the injury, in addition to other factors such as, the presence of a subdural or epidural hematoma, traumatic axonal injury in the brainstem or spinal cord and brain swelling.

In 80% of children with head trauma, symptoms occur within one hour following injury.[59,69,115] Head injuries in young children that result from shear forces to the brain causing DAI are generally not associated with a lucid interval, especially if severe neurologic injury or death results.[45,79–81] This includes infants and young children who are victims of shaken baby (impact) syndrome.[51,52,54,116] Neurologic symptoms that are typically associated with traumatic axonal injury from shearing include an immediate decrease in the level of consciousness, seizure activity, respiratory irregularities and apnea.[82,83,94]

In the study by Plunkett,[69] one of the 18 children who sustained head injuries after falling from playground equipment had evidence of DAI. The child was immediately unconscious and later died.

Some craniocerebral injuries that ultimately result in neurologic impairment or death may be associated with a lucid interval. These injuries include subdural or epidural hemorrhage with or without skull fracture. The subdural hematoma in these situations is usually of large volume causing compression of the brain and brain swelling. This differs from the thin, often bilateral subdural hemorrhage that occurs with shearing injury and DAI.

A study by Kim et al.[117] investigated 729 children less than 15 years of age who sustained fall-related trauma. The cases were classified into two groups; those who fell from heights of less than 15 feet (low level) and those who fell from 15 feet or higher (high level). Four deaths occurred from falls less than 15 feet (1%). In all four of these cases, the admission Glascow Coma Scale score was 3 and abnormal findings were demonstrated on CT scan.

Spinal Cord Injury

In all cases of suspected child abuse, examination of the posterior neck should be performed. Grossly evident neck injuries are uncommon in abused children, however, injuries that may occur include cervical spine fractures, spinal cord contusions and cervical sprains.[59,63,70,115] The vertebral column in young children is largely cartilaginous allowing for spinal cord injury without an associated injury to the spinal column.

When examining the cervical spinal cord, a commonly encountered artifact is epidural blood staining which should not be mistaken for hemorrhage or injury.[118] The presence of subdural blood around the cervical spinal cord is a significant finding, however, it does not necessarily indicate that there was an injury to the neck. In many cases of pediatric head trauma in which there is a sub-

dural hematoma, posterior neck dissection will show subdural blood around the cervical spinal cord. This most likely occurs as intracranial subdural blood seeps downward into the spinal canal giving the mistaken impression of an independent subdural hemorrhage. Posterior neck dissection should focus on establishing whether the intracranial and spinal subdural are connected.

Spinal cord injuries associated with child abuse usually fall under the classification of spinal cord injury without radiographic abnormality (SCIWORA). SCIWORA is primarily seen in children since, the spinal ligaments and unossified bone in this age group may be deformed to the point where spinal cord injury occurs without causing a cervical fracture or ligamentous injury. In children suspected of being abused, axonal injury may be seen at the craniocervical junction if the tissue is stained with beta amyloid precursor protein. Survival time of at least 2–4 hours is needed before such injuries become visible.[88]

The mechanisms that may account for cervical injuries in children include (1) hyperextension-flexion which occurs as the head rapidly moves forward and backward, (2) distraction of the neck which occurs when the head is held stationary and the weight of the body causes strain on the cervical spine, and (3) rotation of the head which occurs as the head is rotated or bent laterally.

Biomechanical Mechanisms of Head Trauma

In order to accurately interpret craniocerebral injuries in children, it is necessary to become familiar with the biomechanics and pathophysiology associated with pediatric traumatic head injury.

The brain and spinal cord are enclosed in a semirigid bone vault, a flexible, but firm dural membrane, a thin, highly vascular arachnoid membrane, and bathed by cerebrospinal fluid. Within this neural mass, there permeates an arborizing, fragile, vascular tree. Each of these structures interrelates in a close, intense dynamic that forms a volume-pressure equilibrium.

When a force acts upon an area of the head, stress is induced and a mechanical load is created. A mechanical load may be static or dynamic. A *static load* occurs when a force is applied gradually as would occur with a slow crushing or squeezing injury, longer than 200 milliseconds (msec). A *dynamic load* occurs when a force occurs rapidly as would occur with rapid contact or motion injuries, less than 50 msec. Dynamic loading may be classified as contact or non-contact with contact forces being what is seen with an impact to the head *(impact loading)* and non-contact forces being generated from inertial forces associated with rapid cranial acceleration or deceleration *(impulse loading).*[89] Both contact and non-contact dynamic forces are what typically cause the craniocerebral injuries in adults and children.

Contact forces (impact loading) are caused by impact, however, there is often a combination of contact and inertial forces when there is a blow to the head.[89,119] Both of these forces are significant and result in the craniocerebral injuries seen in abused children. The impact may cause scalp injury and skull deformation with in-bending of the skull at the impact site. If the degree of skull deformation exceeds the tolerance of the skull, a fracture results.[119] The brain may sustain coup contusions, lacerations and extradural hemorrhages. Contact forces may also cause craniocerebral injuries away from the impact site including basilar skull fractures, contre-coup contusions and parenchymal hemorrhage, all of which are rare in infants and young children.

Noncontact forces (impulse loading) are caused by cranial acceleration/deceleration. The head is either set in motion or a moving head is stopped without being struck or impacted.[119] The brain may be injured in one of two ways. Movement of the brain within the skull may cause bridging veins to rupture resulting in subdural hemorrhage and shearing of the brain. With rapid acceleration or deceleration of the head, the skull moves slightly faster, or slower, than the brain which causes a deformation or strain wave at the brain surface that propagates into the deeper brain tissues.

Three types of impulse loads may occur: translational acceleration, rotational acceleration, or angular acceleration, which is a combination of translational and rotational acceleration. Translational loads occur when the head's center of gravity, the pineal gland, moves in a straight line, often in an anterior-posterior direction. In rotational strain, the head rotates about its center of gravity, and in angular or combined loads, the head moves both in translational and rotational formats. The strain that is generated may cause tension with elongation, compression, or shearing with tearing injury of the brain tissue.

The brain injury that occurs as a result of both contact and noncontact forces are what are classified as primary traumatic craniocerebral injuries.[89,119]

Although linear anterior-posterior head movement commonly occurs in translational mechanical loading, one should recognize that the head can also move at a 45-degree angle from its resting position in an X-Y plane or, alternately, a 45-degree angle in a three dimensional X-Y-Z space. In addition, a mechanical load can cause various injuries to the head since anterior, lateral, and obliquely placed mechanical loads affect the skull, brain, and blood vessels at different locations and positions.

The most significant strain, and ultimately the greatest injury to the brain, is caused by impact and non-impact induced angular or rotational head acceleration/deceleration loads. These phenomena lead to tearing of bridging veins causing subdural hemorrhage and DAI as the sheering force propagates deeper into the brain tissue. The culmination of these injuries is the development of secondary cerebral injuries including cerebral hypoxia and ischemia and cerebral edema. Ultimately the brain suffers from metabolic derangements, pressure/volume dynamic changes, dysfunction of cerebral blood flow autoregulation, fluid shifts in the brain tissue, and cell membrane channel dysfunction. In its worse scenario, the brain cells cannot undergo proper aerobic and anaerobic oxidative functions which result in depressed ATP energy sources, and disruption in ionic membrane functions. The cells become fluid-filled, swell, undergo hypoxic and ischemic changes, and ultimately irreversible necrosis and death. The cardiac and respiratory centers and autonomic functions are affected by the brain injury and cease to function. A vegetative state, coma, multiorgan system failure, and death are the ultimate outcomes.

When investigating head injuries in children, it is more important to be able to distinguish abusive from accidental head trauma than it is to know whether abusive head injuries in infants and young children are caused by shaking only or shaking with head impact. Mechanisms of injury associated with shaking and shaking with head impact are known to result in rotational forces that cause shearing injury to the brain and thus it is likely that both mechanisms play an important role in the pathogenesis of pediatric brain injury.

Abdominal and Chest Injuries

Abdominal organ injury is second in incidence to head injuries as the cause of death in abused children.[63,120,121] Four to 15% of all abdominal trauma is due to child abuse and abdominal injuries caused by abuse have a 40% fatality rate. The outcome associated with abusive abdominal injury is worse than that from accidents. This is most likely due to delays in treatment, false histories and the younger age of the child. All children with visceral injuries should receive a complete workup including a skeletal survey and a CT scan of the head, chest and abdomen.

When investigating the death of a child who has sustained fatal abdominal injuries, a complete autopsy examination is essential to document the nature and extent of the trauma. The autopsy findings should be correlated with the scene investigation and circumstances surrounding the traumatic event in order to determine whether the injuries are consistent with an accidental or abusive mechanism. Accidental abdominal trauma is commonly associated with motor vehicle collisions, pedestrian accidents, bicycle handlebar impacts,[122] certain types of falls and sporting accidents. Unintentional injury victims are usually of grade school age, whereas, infants and toddlers are more commonly victims of abuse.[52,63]

Common abusive abdominal injuries are lacerations of the liver or spleen followed by intestinal perforation, intramural hematoma of the duodenum, rupture of an intra-abdominal blood vessel, pancreatitis, and kidney and bladder injuries. Rarely seen is chylous ascites associated with an injury to the thoracic duct.

A blow to the abdomen may cause a laceration of the mesentery frequently associated with injury to the duodenum, small intestine, pancreas or retroperitoneum (Fig. VIII-28). Liver injuries commonly occur in the midline because this is the area that is compressed between the impacting force and the vertebral column. An impact to the left upper abdominal quadrant may result in injury to the spleen. Splenic trauma typically consists of a subcapsular hematoma or laceration with associated intra-abdominal hemorrhage. Subcapsular hematoma sometimes results in delayed rupture.

In cases of abusive abdominal trauma, the stomach and duodenum are the most commonly injured organs. Gastric ruptures commonly occur in the anterior wall along the greater curvature,[123,124] and the risk of rupture is increased when the stomach is distended. Any portion of the duodenum may be damaged. The typical injuries are traumatic rupture, intramural hemorrhage or bowel obstruction. The mechanism of duodenal injury consists of high-energy compressive forces, or acceleration/deceleration forces at the point of fixation. The compressive forces are usually the result of a punch or kick which crushes the duodenum between the impacting force and the spinal column. The head of the pancreas is in close proximity to the duodenum and may be injured by the same mechanism. Occult pancreatic injuries can lead to pancreatitis and pancreatic pseudocysts, conditions which in an infant should be attributed to abuse until proven otherwise.

The jejunum and ileum are rarely injured by abusive abdominal trauma. The jejunum and ileum are mobile and not easily compressed, however, depending on the force, injuries similar to those seen in the duodenum can occur. Delayed complications of intestinal injury include obstruction and intussusception which can occur following a bowel contusion. Rupture of a hollow organ such as the esophagus, stomach, duodenum or small and large intestine can

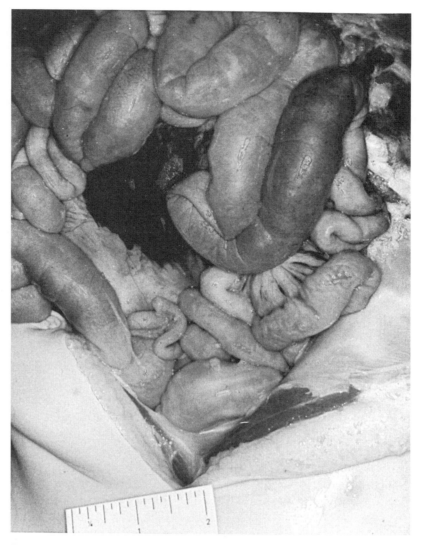

FIGURE VIII-28. Mesenteric laceration and hemorrhage. These lesions are frequently associated with injury to the duodenum, small bowel, pancreas, and retroperitoneum. (Courtesy, Medical Examiner Office, Summit County, Ohio.)

result from a blunt impact such as a punch or kick. Rupture of a hollow viscus, giving rise to chemical or bacterial peritonitis, frequently becomes evident within 24 hours following perforation, but depending on the injury, symptoms may be delayed for several days.[120] The symptoms of peritonitis include fever, abdominal pain, vomiting, and poor feeding. Although the colon is rarely injured in child abuse, sporadic cases have been reported.[120]

The kidneys and adrenal glands are infrequently associated with abusive trauma in chil-dren, although the incidence as reported in the literature varies widely.[125] The kidneys and adrenal glands are relatively protected by their location in the deep retroperitoneal space. Injuries to both organs consist of contusions or lacerations or hemorrhage in the surrounding retroperitoneal adipose tissue. The mechanism of injury is usually a direct impact with compressive forces.[125] Adrenal gland injuries resulting from both accidents and abuse are usually associated with other intra-abdominal trauma.[120] Adrenal hemorrhages may be seen in children diagnosed with sepsis, particularly in association with Waterhouse-Friderichsen syndrome. These hemorrhages are usually bilateral and are secondary to infection rather than trauma.

When an injured infant is evaluated, the presence of bruises on the chest or abdomen may suggest abuse, however, in most cases injuries on the external surface of the body are not present even when there is significant internal organ damage. The abdominal wall is mobile and yields to forceful blows, allowing the skin to escape bruising.[120] Furthermore, the abdominal organs of children are more susceptible to injury from blunt impact than those of adults because they have flexible ribs, large abdominal organs in relation to body size, absence of abdominal fat and lax abdominal muscle tone.[120] Round to oval bruises, usually approximately dime size, on the chest, abdomen or back are typically fingertip bruises caused by aggressive grabbing or squeezing. Symptoms that may be associated with abdominal trauma include vomiting, abdominal distention, pain and signs of shock (blood loss). Laboratory test results that may indicate abdominal injury include increased white blood count (leukocytosis), elevated pancreatic and hepatocellular enzymes, and hematuria. The onset of symptoms depends on which organs are injured and the extent of injury. In general, with significant abdominal injuries, symptoms worsen with time.

Some children are severely beaten through blankets or clothing and present with little or no external evidence of trauma. In such cases, internal examination will demonstrate the fatal injuries and help determine that the injuries are consistent with abuse. Autopsy findings in such cases commonly consist of lacerations of the liver and/or spleen, and occasionally rib fractures. The young age of the child often allows severe trauma without necessarily causing fractures. Such findings are usually the result of abuse, however, statements taken from the child's caregiver are important to correlate the injuries with the alleged mechanism.

Although, abusive chest injuries are less common than abdominal injuries,[126,127] a blow to the chest can cause a contusion or laceration of the heart, cardiac dysrrhythmia and cardiac arrest. Victims of chest trauma are typically struck with a fist, stomped, and/or kicked.

Cohle, Hawley, et al.[126] described six cases of homicidal cardiac lacerations. Five of the cases involved infants with the typical cardiac injury consisting of a right atrial laceration. Four of the victims had rib fractures. Cardiac rupture commonly results from compression of the heart between the sternum and the vertebral column, but may also occur from compression of the abdomen, puncture by a fractured rib, or rupture of a resolving, but necrotic previous contusion. Most victims with abusive chest trauma have other evidence of abuse, including abdominal and/or head trauma.

Cardiac injuries are most commonly seen in cases of accidental trauma rather than abuse. As with cardiac lacerations, contusions may be caused in motor vehicle accidents or by various crushing injuries. A localized blunt impact to the chest may cause sudden death due to cardiac arrthymia. This condition, also known as commotio cordis or cardiac concussion, is diagnosed when sudden death occurs following blunt chest trauma that leaves no visible injuries to the heart. A bruise in the chest wall may or may not be present. Most such cases are accidental and involve adolescent children engaged in sports. The impact may be from blunt objects such as, baseballs, bats, hockey sticks and hockey pucks. The victim dies suddenly because the blow interrupts the cardiac electrical cycle during the upstroke of the T-wave or at the peak of the QRS complex.[128] Denton and Kalelkar[127] described two male children who died of abusive commotio cordis. The scene investigation and comments made by the caregiver were critical in the workup. External findings in such children may include evidence of poor nutrition and dehydration, as well as recent and remote bruises in the skin indicating ongoing abuse and neglect. Radiographs may show remote or recent fractures. Internal examination should include a careful search for injuries with examination of the subcutaneous tissue of the chest, thymus, abdomen, back and extremities. Sections of the anterior chest and abdominal wall should be examined microscopically. The tissue may show acute hemorrhage associated with the impact. Sections of the heart, particularly the anterior wall of the right and left ventricles, may show similar findings.

A common defense provided by an individual charged with killing a child is that the chest and/or abdominal injuries were caused by resuscitative efforts, i.e., chest compressions. A study by Price et al.[121] concluded that primary blunt abdominal injuries in children due to cardiopulmonary resuscitation occur rarely, if at all.

Rib fractures are commonly seen in abused children. Rib fractures may or may not be associated with fingertip contusions on the chest or back. Although an infant's ribs are resilient, a localized force as would be exerted by grabbing or squeezing is the typical means by which a child sustains rib fractures. Rib fractures are often seen together with abusive head trauma.

Rib fractures associated with abuse may involve any portion of the rib with the posterior aspect, near the costovertebral junction being the most common location. In an abused child, rib fractures are often bilateral, multiple and of different ages indicative of repeated episodes of trauma.

As a rib fracture begins to heal, connective tissue proliferates forming what is known as a callus which serves to bridge the ends of the fracture. The callus is larger than the actual fracture site so that the ends of the fractured bone stay together in the early stages of healing. The callus size does not correlate with the age of the injury, and varies depending on the degree of bone displacement, viability of the overlying periosteum, degree of immobilization, the presence or absence of a foreign body at the fracture site and the nutritional status of the infant.

In general, acute rib fractures may be displaced or non-displaced. Displaced fractures are often associated with lacerations of the pleura and may cause injury to the lung or heart. Acute fractures show a variable amount of hemorrhage at the fracture site, however, microscopic examination may show hemorrhage up to several weeks following the injury. Microscopic examination of recent fractures will commonly show edema, fibrin clot, fibrinous exudate and acute inflammatory cell infiltrate. As the rib begins to heal, a callus can be seen as early as 5-7 days in immature human bone. The callus will have a variety of microscopic appearances depending on the degree of healing. Common findings include fibroblastic and chrondroblastic proliferation, neovascularization, new bone growth, loss of bone marrow elements and bone necrosis with increased osteoclastic activity. Eventually, the fracture gap is obliterated, bone marrow elements return and bony union occurs. This process generally occurs in weeks to months for an uncomplicated fracture. Finally, the rib will undergo some degree of remodeling in which the fracture callus is gradually transformed into normal bone. Remodeling can continue over a period of months to years.[129]

When evaluating rib fractures, it is important to examine each callus for the presence of a superimposed acute fracture. This indicates repeated episodes of trauma to the same region of the body. It is recommended to excise all rib fractures, decalcify the bone and submit the fracture site for slide preparation. This approach will often allow estimation of the age of the fracture. When rendering opinions as to the age of fractures, the possibility of repetitive injury disrupting the normal healing process should be considered.

As with abdominal injuries, studies have shown that rib fractures in infants and young children are extremely rare following attempted cardiopulmonary resuscitation, and that when present typically involve the anterior aspect of the rib near the sterno-chondral junction.[130]

Birth-related trauma is another explanation given by caregivers accused of child abuse. Birth trauma rarely causes intra-abdominal injury with the most common injury being a subcapsular hematoma of the liver. In most situations, the hematoma is not clinically significant, however, delayed hemorrhage from rupture of the hematoma has been reported to occur up to a week following delivery.[131] Rib fractures are rare following vaginal delivery, and although clavicular fractures occasionally occur, they are typically not clinically significant.

Other Forms of Abuse

Asphyxiation

Asphyxiation is a common cause of child abuse especially in infants. There may be no external or internal injuries associated with an asphyxial death, however, in all infant deaths, the forensic pathologist should examine the body for evidence of possible suffocation or smothering. Findings that may be significant include petechiae of the face and conjunctivae, scleral hemorrhages, abrasions on the face, particularly around the nose and mouth and bruises or lacerations of the lips, oral mucosa or frenula. Petechial hemorrhages in the thymus, epicardium, and pleura are non-specific, often stress related, and are commonly seen in children who die of natural causes.

Investigation of the circumstances surrounding a death is of critical importance when injuries are absent or non-specific. Multiple episodes of sublethal asphyxiation are suggestive of Münchausen syndrome by proxy. Any childhood death should prompt a search into the family's history with regard to previous infant deaths. A family who has had a child die of what was classified as sudden infant death syndrome, that now is faced with a second unexplained infant death should be investigated for the possibility that both deaths were due to homicide.

Burns

Approximately 10% of physical abuse in children involve burns and of all pediatric burn victims, an estimated 10–25% are deliberately inflicted. The mortality rate of inflicted burns is 30–50%, whereas the mortality rate of accidental burns is 2%. Risk factors associated with abusive burns include age less than four years, black race, male gender, and being the youngest of multiple siblings.

Burns caused by hot solid objects are generally second or third degree burns and typically involve one surface of the body. The shape and pattern of the burn is important, for it may indicate an instrument. Approximately, one-third of all burns in children are contact burns such as, from a lighted cigarette, stove, radiator or iron. Stove and radiator grate burns frequently are linear or checkerboard shaped, whereas burns from an iron are triangular (Fig. VIII-29a–b). Lighted cigarettes produce circular burns which are punched-out, crater-like lesions (Fig. VIII-30).

Scalding by hot water is the most common type of inflicted burn. Burns associated with immersion in hot water depend on the temperature of the water and the duration of exposure. The skin of children younger than age five and that of adults greater than age 65 is more susceptible to burn injury, primarily because the skin is thinner in these age groups. In addition, there is variation between different parts of the body due to skin thickness and vascularity. In general, infants and young children sustain second and third-degree burns in less than 1 second in water at or above 140° Fahrenheit (60° Celcius). With water temperature of 131° Fahrenheit (55° Celcius), second-degree burns are typically sustained within 2 seconds and third-degree burns within 5 seconds. Water temperature of 122° Fahrenheit (50° Celcius) will cause second-degree burns in approximately 11 seconds and third-degree burns in 20 seconds, 113° Fahrenheit (45° Celcius) will cause second-degree burns in approximately 2 minutes and third-degree burns in approximately 8 minutes.[132]

Immersion of a child into scalding water causes a straight, horizontal line of injury on the buttocks, thighs, or waist (Fig. VIII-31a-c). Usually the hands are spared and because the knees and feet are often flexed in response to pain, the back of the knees and front of the ankles may also be spared. If the buttock is immersed into the water, but pressed against the bottom of the tub, the central aspect may be spared or burned to a lesser degree than the surrounding skin. The same would hold true for a child held underwater by an individual using their shoe. The outline of the shoe or the pattern of the sole may be recognizable within the burn. Deliberate immersion into scalding water will cause a *straight burn line* by the water level. In contrast, burns sustained from accidental immersion are more irregular and of varying severity, often with burned and un-

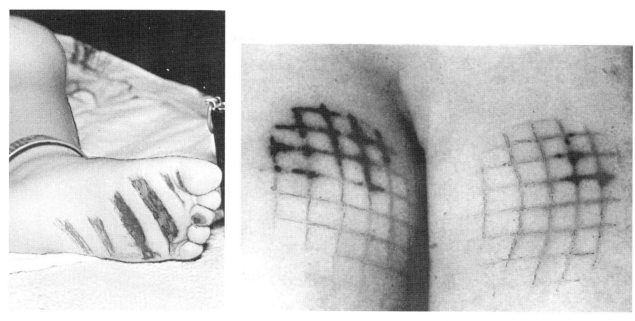

FIGURE VIII-29a–b. Examples of burn from an electrical stove and furnace grate. (Courtesy, D. Steiner, M.D. and Audio Visual Department, Children's Hospital Medical Center of Akron.)

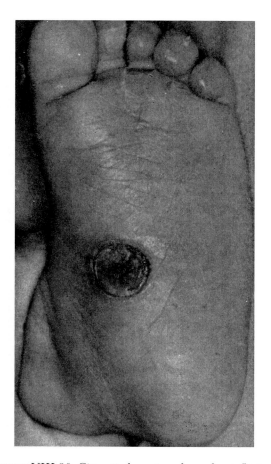

FIGURE VIII-30. Cigarette burn two days after infliction.

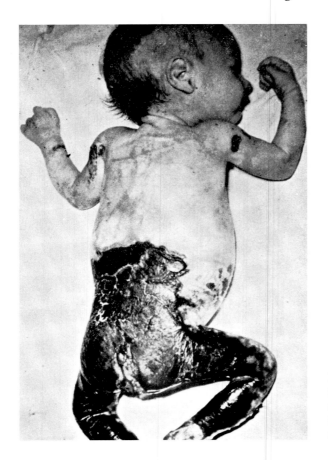

FIGURE VIII-31 (a) Extensive third degree thermal burns on a three-and-one-half-month-old child, suffered by immersion in a pan of hot tap water. (b) Extension of burns into the soles of the feet, the basis for initially doubting the presenting allegation of an overturned pan of water.

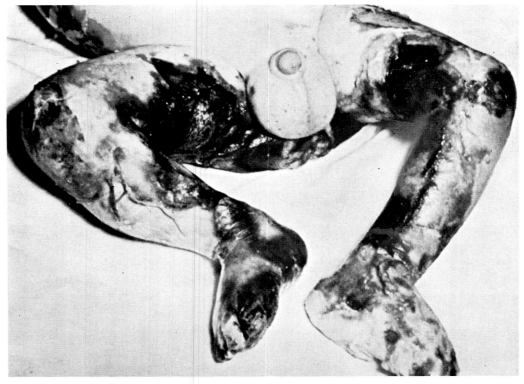

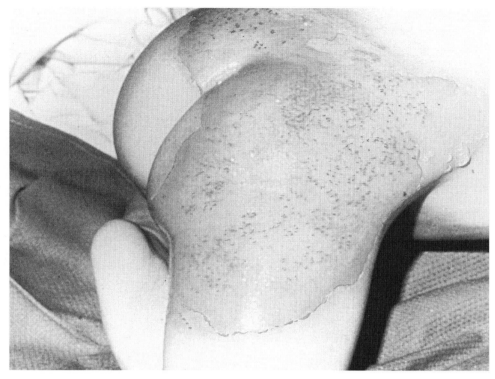

FIGURE VIII-31c. Second degree immersion burn inflicted as punishment.

burned skin in the same general area. A child who falls into a tub containing hot water or turns on a hot water faucet will have burns on the hands and knees. Scattered small splash burns are common. In a child standing in a tub containing hot water, the soles of the feet may be spared as a result of pressure against the tub.

The age and development of the child must be considered when evaluating the circumstances. Most children are able to turn a faucet by 24 months. Scald burns from tap water are preventable by lowering the water heater temperature to less than 120 degrees Fahrenheit.

Drowning

A less frequent form of abuse is deliberate drowning of an infant or child. Children are usually older (15–30 months) and the autopsy findings are typically the same as those of accidental drowning.

In 1994, a mother in South Carolina drowned her two young boys and claimed they were abducted. After many days, she confessed to letting her car roll into a lake with the two boys in the back seat. Both boys were unable to escape.

In June 2001, a Texas mother killed her 5 children by methodically drowning each of them one after the other. The ages of the children ranged from 6 months to 7 years. Postpartum depression and psychosis are believed to have played a role in the killings.

All cases of infant or child drowning require careful investigation and drowning in a bath tub is especially suspect whenever it occurs.

Poisoning

Poisoning is a relatively uncommon form of child abuse. Children have been fed large amounts of salt, salicylates,[133] diuretics, sedatives, narcotics,[134] cocaine, phenothiazides, psychotropic drugs and insulin. Scene investigation and history may point to poisoning. For instance, there may be drug paraphernalia, disarrayed medications, or evidence of parental drug use in the home. Evidence of neglect or non-organic failure to thrive is often present in children who have been abused in this manner. In all suspected cases, complete autopsy with collection of blood, urine, ocular fluid, gastric and small intestinal contents, and brain should be performed. Liver and kidney should be retained if blood and urine is unavailable. If the child was hospitalized prior to death, blood and urine samples from the time of admission should be obtained.

Comprehensive qualitative and quantitative toxicological analyses which include testing for lead are recommended. Any unnatural eating habits, known to occur in pica and contaminated water should be ruled out.[133,134]

Subtle Abuse

Zumwalt and Hirsch[135] draw attention to subtle forms of child abuse. They describe cases wherein children died as a result of excess salt feeding, dehydration, smothering, and hyperthermia in which the determination of abuse was attained only by suspicion and close attention to the scene and autopsy findings.

Occasionally a child will expire following trauma that is not ordinarily considered lethal. Cardiac arrthymia associated with stress cardiomyopathy has been proposed as the mechanism of death in these circumstances, however aspiration, seizure disorder, gram negative septic shock, drowning, and electrocution must be ruled out.[51,52] Non-fracture associated fat emboli should also be considered.[136]

Certain autopsy findings or artifacts may be mistaken for evidence of child abuse. Common among these are Mongolian spots. Bruises and swelling of the wrists or ankles from tight-fitting clothing may be mistaken for restraints (Fig. VIII-32). Other artifacts that may be mistaken for abuse include creases in the skin of the neck simulating a ligature mark (see Fig. XIII-33), facial mottling or lividity thought to be antemortem bruises, and bruises or abrasions on the face and chest which are secondary to attempted resuscitation.[137] Wounds due to medical intervention may also cause confusion with antemortem abusive injuries. Among these are cutdowns in the skin for vascular access, and lancet wounds which may be mistaken for stab wounds (Fig.

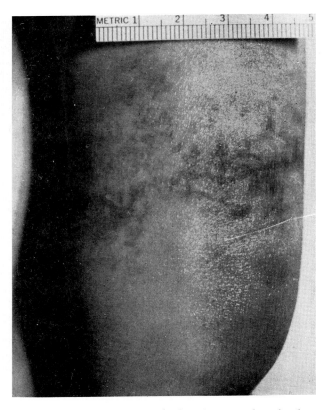

FIGURE VIII-32. Bruises on the legs from overly tight elastic bands on plastic pants may occur in children with capillary fragility. This may be mistaken as evidence of restraints.

VIII-34). Further, we have seen two parallel lines on the skin of the face after removal of strips of adhesive tape used to secure an airway. The parallel lines at the top and bottom of the tape simulated injury, because the skin in between was reddish discolored as a result of irritation. Some individuals are hypersensitive to tape adhesive resulting in sloughing of the epidermis when the tape is removed.

Münchausen's Syndrome by Proxy (MSBP)

Münchausen's syndrome by proxy (MSBP) was first described by Meadow in 1977 and is another form of covert child abuse. Reviews of this subject by Rosenberg may be found in Helfer[138] and Reese.[139] MSBP is defined as a cluster of symptoms and/or signs in which:

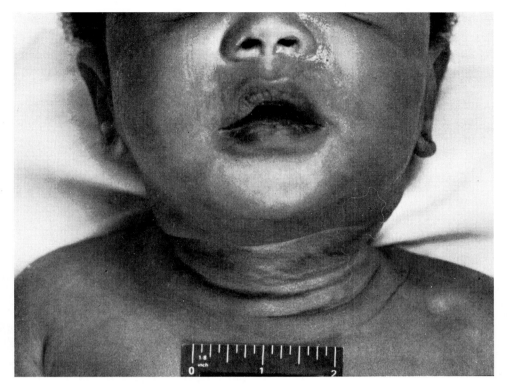

FIGURE VIII-33. Congealing of subcutaneous fat may cause indentation of the skin to resemble an imprint of a noose or ligature.

- The illness and symptoms of the child are fabricated and/or produced by a parent or caregiver.
- The child is repetitively taken to the doctor or hospital for medical assessment and treatment and is subjected to multiple unnecessary medical procedures.
- Knowledge about the cause of the child's illness is denied by the perpetrator.
- The child's acute symptoms abate when the child is separated from the perpetrator.

As of 1996, over 250 cases of MSBP have been reported worldwide with most occurring in Great Britain and the United States. This number probably represents only a small portion of the total number of cases since many go undiagnosed or unreported. Boys and girls are equally at risk with infants and toddlers being the typical age group affected.

Over 70 signs, symptoms, and laboratory findings have been associated with MSBP,[139] but the most commonly fabricated or induced symp-

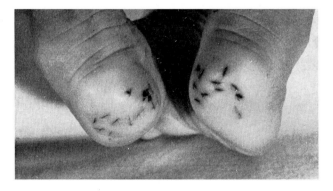

FIGURE VIII-34. Lancet stabs in a baby's heels inflicted to obtain blood samples for laboratory analyses during earlier hospitalization.

toms include seizures, bleeding, apnea, diarrhea, vomiting, fever, and rash. In addition to giving drugs to children, parents have been known to add blood to the child's secretions, give laxatives to induce diarrhea, overheat the body, falsify thermometer readings, and injure the skin to imitate dermatological lesions.

The short-term morbidity of these children is primarily related to the unnecessary workup-related diagnostic and therapeutic procedures. Long-term morbidity, defined as pain and/or illness that causes permanent disfigurement or impairment, involves at least 8% of the victims. Some victims have long-term psychologic morbidity which probably increases this number. Approximately 9% of the children die, usually from overt hostile acts such as suffocation or poisoning. When infants expire, it is important to distinguish the death from sudden infant death syndrome. A detailed investigation, including a history of the child's illness and a thorough autopsy will help in uncovering the true nature of the case.

Between 93 and 98% of the perpetrators are women, usually the child's mother, typically middle class, in all social, and economic strata, educated in some aspects of medicine or nursing. The perpetrators are often litigious and tend to sue doctors or medical institutions for wrongful death, malpractice, or malicious reporting of child abuse. A common motive is the desire to be the center of attention and to be connected with doctors and nurses. Other motives include dislike of the child, a desire to outwit doctors, and to extract financial reward in the course of their actions.

A diagnosis of MSBP is difficult and challenging. Although children may initially have an organic illness, the fact that the perpetrator overemphasizes the symptoms and engages in doctor shopping and repetitive clinic/emergency visits should prompt the physician to add MSBP to the differential diagnosis. MSBP must be considered in families with multiple cases of sudden infant death syndrome. A definite diagnosis of MSPB can be made when the perpetrator is either caught in the act or recorded by videotape. Evidence in support of the diagnosis includes laboratory documentation of drugs or poisons in the victim's body. In most cases, MSBP is a diagnosis made by exclusion and therefore a detailed review of the child's medical records should be included in the workup. If a dramatic improvement in the child's health emerges following separation from the caregiver with recurrence once returned, this diagnosis must be seriously entertained. Intervention to prevent serious harm or death is necessary when evidence in favor of MSBP is compelling. Even if the abused child is permanently removed from the home, attention must be given to other children in the household and to subsequent children born into the family.

Sexual Abuse

The tragedy of sexual abuse is played within different, sometimes interrelated, scenarios. On the one hand, it may be part of the physical abuse to which the child is subjected, whereas, in other circumstances it is ancillary to a specific homicidal action, i.e., murder-rape. The incident may occur within or outside the family constellation. Kempe[140] defines child sexual abuse as the involvement of children and adolescents in sexual activities they do not understand, to which they cannot give informed consent, or that violates social taboos. One should be wary of using age as a criterion since this threshold may be inconsistent with the statutory rape laws of many states.

Epidemiology and Clinical History

Childhood sexual abuse involves an estimated 1–2% of children in the United States. The median age of victims is 11 years, but episodes do occur in the first year of life. Girls are abused more often than boys. In 1986, the National Incidence and Prevalent Study of Child Abuse and Neglect concluded that 2.5 children per 1,000 were sexually abused each year, resulting in a total of 155,900 cases annually.[141] Since all cases of sexual abuse are not reported, the incidence is probably higher. Many of the perpetrators are known by the victim with family members accounting for 30–50%. Adult perpetrators have no typical personality profile. Heterosexual, bisexual, and homosexual adults can all be abusers.[141] Adolescents are perpetrators in at least 20% of the cases.

Many state rape laws criminalize some sexual activities between adolescent and adult partners.

Thus, physicians should be aware of state laws requiring reporting of sexual activity between adults and adolescents to child protective agencies, if the sexual activity is construed as abuse or neglect.[142]

There are three types of sexual abuse that should be recognized.[141-144] *Child molestation* refers to (a) touching or fondling of the genitals of a child, (b) asking the child to fondle the adult's genitals, (c) forced exposure to sexual acts or pornography. State law defines the age of the child when these acts are considered felonies or misdemeanors. *Sexual intercourse* includes vaginal, oral, or rectal penetration in non-assaultive circumstances. *Rape* is assaultive forced intercourse.

Incest is a legal term which identifies a sexual offense between an assailant and victim who are related and could not be legally married.[144] Most state laws include sexual acts with adopted or stepchildren in this category. Incest most commonly involves daughters and fathers and approximately 90% of incest victims are female. Approximately one-third of the victims are less than 6 years of age, one-third are ages 6–12, and one-third are 12–18 years.[144] Incest is frequently repeated with successive daughters. The incidence of stepfathers who victimize their stepdaughters is approximately five times greater than among natural fathers. Incest occurs in all socioeconomic and ethnic groups.[145]

Pedophilia involves non-violent sexual contact with a child by an adult. It usually consists of fondling, genital viewing, or oral-genital stimulation. The family or child usually knows the offender. As with incest, approximately 90% of the victims are female.

The crime of rape requires that the assailant use force to penetrate the victim. Penetration with or without ejaculation may take place in the vagina, mouth, or rectum. The act is assaultive, coercive, and non-consensual. Over 50% of all rapes involve victims less than 19 years of age and 30% of cases involve adolescents.[145]

In an infant or young child, injury to the genitalia or the presence of a sexually transmitted disease strongly indicates sexual abuse. Even when a young child is able to verbalize that sexual abuse has taken place, his or her ability to pro-

vide a true and accurate account of the incident(s) is often questioned. In preadolescence, the victims are frequently abused by relatives, but as they are exposed to more people, the risk of abuse by known individuals who are not related increases.[142] Adolescents make up 25–50% of all non-adult victims of sexual abuse.[141] Developmentally disabled or handicapped children are potential victims of sexual abuse.

The cornerstone of a proper evaluation is the medical history. Dejong and Rose[147] note that physical evidence is not essential for conviction and that successful prosecution depends on the quality of the verbal evidence and the effectiveness of the child victim's testimony. This notion has been corroborated by Lauritsen.[148] The elements of a proper historical evaluation are documented by Finkle and Dejong.[141]

Sometimes alert physicians become suspicious of sexual abuse during a history and physical examination. Alternatively, children may be brought for an assessment by child protective services or a law enforcement worker. Children who experience sexual abuse usually do not volunteer the events, but present with clinical or medical conditions which raise suspicion.[143] Symptoms that may be associated with ongoing sexual abuse include:
- Sleep and appetite disturbances
- Withdrawal, depression, guilt
- Hysteria or conversion neuroses
- Suicidal ideation
- Genital trauma or infection
- Sexually transmitted diseases (gonorrhea, syphilis, chlamydia, herpes, venereal warts, bacterial vaginitis [gardnerella], HIV)
- Recurrent urinary tract infections
- Pregnancy
- Promiscuity or prostitution
- Substance abuse

Physical Examination

A forensic pathologist may examine both deceased and living victims of sexual abuse. All children alleged to be sexually abused should have a complete physical examination, regardless of when the alleged act occurred.[141] The

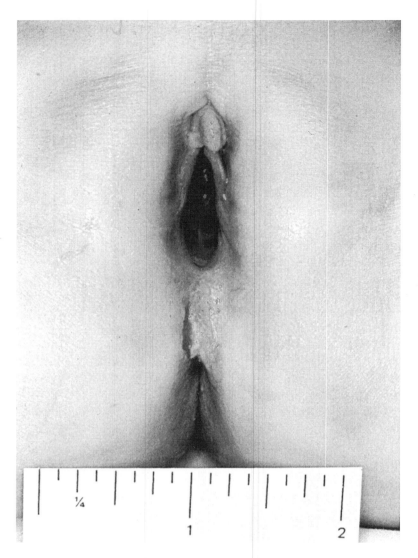

FIGURE VIII-35. Penetration trauma of child's vagina. Note the laceration of the perineum and laceration and contusions of hymen and vaginal introitus. (Courtesy, Medical Examiner Office, Summit County, Ohio.)

examination must be performed by personnel who are skilled in the recognition of injuries and collection and preservation of evidence. When there are no acute signs of injury, the body should be examined for evidence of healing injuries or chronic changes in the genital or anal anatomy. Chronic residual trauma may be evident weeks to months later.[141]

The child should be prepared for the examination and fears diminished. Preparation of the child and various positions used during the examination are well documented by Finkle and Dejong[141] and Reichert.[149] The vagina should be visualized to demonstrate mucosal hemorrhage or lacerations (Fig. VIII-35). Any vaginal dis-

charge should be documented and swabs collected. The hymen is visualized noting the shape and the presence of acute or remote injuries. The findings in chronic molestation include multiple healed hymenal lacerations, a spacious introitus, leukorrhea and cervicitis. In male children, the penis and scrotum should be examined for acute injuries and any urethral discharge should be swabbed for culture and microscopy.

A 1991 guideline of The American Academy of Pediatrics[141] recommends that certain findings are consistent, but not diagnostic, of sexual abuse. These include: (1) chafing, abrasions, or bruising of the inner thighs and genitalia; (2) scarring, tears, or distortion of the hymen; (3) a decreased amount or absent hymenal tissue; (4) scarring of the fossa navicularis; (5) injury to or scarring of the posterior fourchette; and (6) scarring or laceration of the labia minora.

The anatomy and terminology of all structures should be familiar to the examiner. Distinctions between normal, variations of normal and abnormal findings depend upon proper training and experience. Excellent color photographs are described by Finkle and Dejong,[141] Dejong and Rose,[147] and Gardner.[151] Photographs by Bays[152] describe normal variations and diseases that can be misinterpreted as abuse. Berenson describes the hymen of newborns and infants up to one year of age.[153]

The normal hymen is usually symmetric and has a fine smooth inner edge. It may have some bumps and irregularity, but disruptions in the posterior aspect are rarely found in children who have not been abused. Measurement of the vaginal introital diameter (hymenal orifice) was once popular for evaluating a child suspected of being sexually abused. A diameter in excess of 0.4 cm was highly suspect, however, this technique is no longer accepted due to the variability of the hymenal orifice depending upon the body position, tissue distensibility, and the state of relaxation.[141]

Within the last ten years, the colposcope has achieved widespread acceptance as the instrument of choice to improve visualization of the anal and genital regions of living victims.[141] The instrument can provide between four and thirty-fold magnification and can be adapted for video attachment. It may have built in red-free filters that cast a green light, enhancing visualization of mucosal injury. Photographic documentation of all abnormal findings should accompany every examination.

The anal anatomy should also receive close scrutiny. Acute anal injuries such as mucosal lacerations are easily recognized, but McCann[154] observed that a variety of perianal findings seen in abused children are non-specific (Fig. VIII-36). These include perianal erythema, perianal pigmentation, venous congestion, skin tags, and dilatation. McCann[37] and Stephens[38] also caution that the anal sphincter may relax after death

allowing the anus to dilate. Anal orifice size may vary with the age of the child, the amount of traction applied to the buttock, postmortem interval and a history of central nervous system injury prior to death.

Other findings in acute sexual abuse include perineal contusion, perihymenal erythema, bite marks and the presence of seminal fluid or blood group secretor products on the skin or genital area. Bite marks may occur on any area of the body, although in cases of sexual assault, they are common on the breasts, genitals, or buttocks. The bite marks should be photographed and the central area should be swabbed for serological and DNA evidence. Consultation with a forensic odontologist is recommended when a possible bite mark is present. Defense injuries such as bruises, abrasions, scratches, or lacerations on the forearms and hands of the victim are of particular significance.

If the rape occurred within 72 hours of the physical examination, sexual battery specimens should be obtained (rape kit). If the examination occurs after 72 hours, specimens are generally not taken, but the victim should receive prophylactic antibiotics and tests for gonorrhea, syphilis, HIV, human papilloma virus (HPV), and pregnancy. A speculum examination of the vagina is indicated when the victim is post-pubertal or when there is non-menstrual vaginal bleeding or major trauma to the external genitalia.

Although most victims are female, boys may be sodomized or forced to practice oral sex. Whenever such acts are suspected, the mouth, genitals, and ano-rectal areas of the victim should be examined and specimens collected.

The diagnosis of a sexually transmitted disease in a prepubertal child has long been considered an important clue to the possibility of abuse, however, some genital infections such as gonorrhea, HPV and chlamydia can be transmitted at or before birth. Venereal warts on the vulva and vaginal introitus caused by HPV, is sexually transmitted, although in very young infants it may occur from maternal transmission. It is uncertain whether bacterial vaginosis or genital mycoplasma are sexually transmitted diseases.[141]

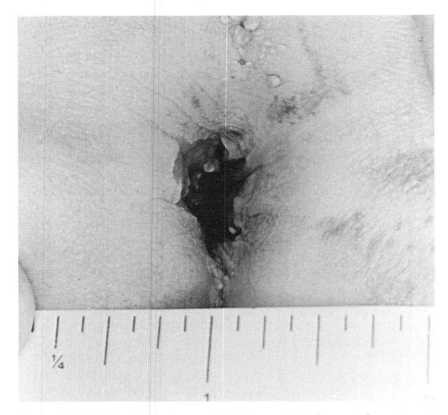

FIGURE VIII-36. Penetration trauma of child's anus. Note the recent lacerations at 2, 4, 6, 9 and 10 o'clock and venereal warts above. (Courtesy, Medical Examiner Office, Summit County, Ohio.)

Laboratory Derived Evidence

Multiple specimens from alleged rape victims, whether dead or alive, must be obtained for laboratory analysis. A prepackaged kit facilitates and organizes the sexual battery workup (Table VIII-2).

It has become a common occurrence for sexual assault victims to be drugged for the purpose of anamnestic rape. This is facilitated by using one of several recreational drugs to intoxicate the victim without the victim's knowledge. Benzodiazepines are frequently implicated and flunitrazepam (Rohypnol) has received much media attention. Benzodiazepines are readily available and mix well with ethanol. Anterograde amnesia ensues such that, the victim may be conscious but does not remember the ordeal. Gamma hydroxybutyrate (GHB), a central nervous system (CNS) depressant, is easily synthesized and has become popular among young people. It has a short half-life and is difficult to interpret analytically because it is also endogenously produced. LeBeau[157] recommends that a urine drug screen be performed because it allows a long window for detection of various drugs and metabolites. In all rape victims, urine and blood should be collected.

The presence of sperm provides evidence of sexual contact within the previous 72 hours. Live, motile sperm are detected by using a saline wet mount of a freshly collected specimen. The sperm remains mobile in the vagina of a living victim, for 1–6 hours, with a mean of 2–3 hours.[156] The mouth is a particularly hostile environment making identification of motile sperm unlikely. After ejaculation, the sperm begin to degenerate. The tail is lost after approximately 16 hours in the cervicovaginal area and after approximately 6 hours in the rectum. After the

TABLE VIII-2

LABORATORY EVIDENCE FROM SEXUALLY ABUSED

Skin:

Moist swab of dried secretions for sperm analysis, secretor substance, DNA fingerprinting. Look for trace evidence. Photograph and imprint bite marks. Moist swab for secretor substance and DNA fingerprints.

Clothes:

Cut out a portion which appears to contain seminal material. Use Wood's light to highlight. Also, cut out portion for negative control. Test for sperm analysis, secretor substance, DNA fingerprints. Look for trace evidence.

Fingernails:

Scrape and clip nails for foreign blood, hairs and skin. Place materials from each finger in separate containers.

Pubic Hair:

Comb for foreign hair. Pull pubic hair and scalp hair for comparison.

Mouth:

Swab anterior areas for sperm, acid phosphatase and P30 glycoprotein. Make smears and stain for sperm. Obtain saliva control. Culture for gonococcus.

Perianal region and anal canal:

Swab for sperm, acid phosphatase and P30 glycoprotein. Make smears and stain for sperm. Culture for gonococcus.

Vagina and cervix:

Swab for sperm. Make smears and stain.

Vaginal aspirate:

Test for sperm motility, acid phosphatase, P30 glycoprotein, secretor substance, DNA fingerprints and Trichomonas. Culture for gonococcus, Chlamydia trachomatis, human papilloma virus (HPV).

Blood:

Place in screwtop containers. Store at 4°C. Test for blood type, drug analysis, DNA fingerprinting, syphilis and HIV serology and pregnancy.

Gastric material:

Test for ingested sedatives, medications, poisons, etc.

Cultures for gonococcus, Chlamydia trachomatis

Autopsy: Culture all vaginal or genital discharges and vagina fluid

Living patients:

Prepubertal girls: culture: mouth, anus, vagina or vaginal oriface, urethra

Pubertal girls: culture: mouth, anus, vagina, cervix

Boys: culture: mouth, anus, urethra

Urethral cultures from prepubertal girls and boys

Urine:

Test for pregnancy, toxicology.

Convey all samples by chain of custody procedures.

up to 6 hours.[158,159] In the postmortem specimen the average interval for sperm identification in the vagina is 23–38 hours, and in the rectum it is 12–28 hours.[160] Dry specimens from any site are stable, and sperm may be detected in stains on clothing for 12 months or longer.

Acid phosphatase is present in many body fluids, including vaginal secretions. It is present in high quantities in male seminal ejaculates (130–1,800 international units per liter), but in low concentrations (less than 50 international units per liter) in vaginal fluid.[141] Thus, an elevated acid phosphatase concentration supports a determination of penetration and ejaculation. Acid phosphatase levels remain elevated in the vagina for 8 hours, decrease during the next 12 hours, and return to normal within 48 hours.[156] Collins documents average postmortem intervals for acid phosphatase in the vagina as 30 hours; rectum 35 hours; and mouth 33 hours.[160] In some cases, acid phosphatase levels return to normal within 3 hours, and one-half of the specimens will have undetectable concentrations within 24 hours.[141]

The absence of sperm, but presence of elevated acid phosphatase or p30 glycoprotein in vaginal fluid or on skin, or clothes implies that the assailant may be aspermic. Aspermia may be due to elective vasectomy, sexual dysfunction, lack of ejaculation during the assault or disease, such as alcoholic cirrhosis which causes hyperestrinism and atrophy of the seminiferous tubules. Urination, defecation, douching, use of oral contraceptives, or bathing by the victim will decrease the likelihood of obtaining positive results. Prepubertal girls have decreased cervical mucus which shortens survival time of sperm.[161]

P30 glycoprotein[146,155] is a more sensitive indicator of seminal fluid. The ELISA technique can detect glycoprotein in concentrations as low as 4 nanograms per milliliter. P30 glycoprotein declines to undetectable levels within 48 hours after ejaculation, so its presence indicates recent intercourse. Recently a prostate specific antigen (PSA) membrane test has been utilized for rapid screening analysis of p30 glycoprotein,[162] however, one must be cautious when interpreting the results. A negative result with the PSA mem-

tail is lost, the sperm head can still be seen, however, it needs to be distinguished from naked nuclei and yeast. After consensual intercourse, cervicovaginal smears are usually positive for sperm for 48 to 72 hours, but have been reported for as long as 10 days. Anorectal smears are typically positive up to 24 hours and oral smears brane test may indicate the absence of the antigen, antigen below the level of detection, or excess antigen in the sample. Therefore, a dilution of the sample to at least 1:100 should be used to evaluate the presence of excess antigen whenever there is a negative result.

DNA analysis has become a valuable tool in cases of sexual assault. Sperm, blood, hair root and/or tissue from the perpetrator found on the victim's body are all utilized as resource material for analysis. The sensitivity and accuracy of DNA analysis, demands that the procedures be done with careful attention to source identification, collection and analytic technique, quality assurance, and proper chain of custody.[163] DNA has been used to determine the innocence of accused persons in many circumstances.

Child Neglect

Up to 60% of reports made to child protective services involve allegations of neglect.[21,22] Although most neglected children show no external evidence of physical abuse, all have symptoms of failure to thrive. Failure to thrive may result from neglect, accident, or inherent organic disease, thus each case should be fully evaluated to determine the correct etiology. Evaluation of 100 cases of failure to thrive, 70% were associated with non-organic causes and 30% were associated with underlying organic conditions.[2] In the non-organic group, approximately 50% of the cases were due to neglectful or psychological causes and 20% were accidental, due to inadvertent poor feeding techniques or formula preparation.

Accidental failure to thrive is usually corrected by counseling and changes of formula or feeding technique. Organic failure to thrive has multiple causes. These include central nervous system abnormalities; sequelae of nervous system infection; gastrointestinal diseases, such as malabsorption, cystic fibrosis, celiac disease, liver disease, severe gastroesophageal reflux; cleft palate; lung, heart, and kidney disease; chronic systemic infection; malignancy; immunodeficiency disease; chromosomal disorders; and congenital syndromes.

If alive when first seen, the child should be hospitalized for a minimum of one week and given a trial of unlimited feedings of a diet appropriate for age. If the child gains approximately one pound per week, failure to thrive by neglect is presumed.

Review of the family background and home conditions usually reveals that a child expiring as a result of overt neglect is the last-born of a family averaging six to seven children. Birth out of wedlock is common, and the socioeconomic level of the home is usually low (Fig. VIII-37). In most cases, neglected children are less than 2 years of age.

Trained social workers and investigators frequently make reference in their reports to filthy homes, wherein they describe the odor of urine, feces (both human and animal), and infestation by insects, particularly roaches and flies. Baby food supplies are often minimal with sparse quantities of the necessities. In some instances, the homes are considered unfit for human habitation. Interviews often indicate a pattern of long-standing dereliction with no apparent regard for the children's welfare. Another indication of lack of parental concern for the offspring may be found in the child's medical records. Frequently, well-baby appointments are not kept and the infants are not afforded medical treatment when ill.

Physical examination of these infants demonstrates a significant decrease in the subcutaneous fat and loss of skin turgor. The skin hangs loosely over the bones of the extremities and is often depressed around the bony structures of the face (Fig. VIII-38). The abdomen is often sunken, and the ribs unusually prominent.

Infrequent changing of diapers and bedding is often manifested by severe diaper rash and weeping, malodorous denudation of the skin of the genitalia and perineum. However, a neglected child may not have diaper rash, as diapers may not have been used. Diaper rash, when present for an extended duration, may cause severe scarring, skin hypopigmentation and pock-like lesions secondary to infected sores (Fig. VIII-39a–b).

Such infants during the terminal period of their lives usually present an extremely low state of metabolism associated with marked diminution in respiratory rate, low body temperature, and vascular collapse. These children often are presented with the story that the baby was put to

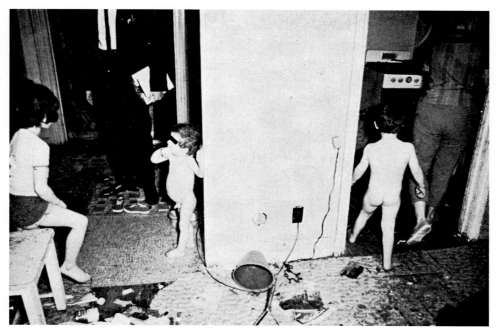

FIGURE VIII-37. Typical home environment of a neglected child. Note absence of clothing on preschool children, presence of soiled food containers, fecal matter, papers, etc. on the floor, and state of disrepair of the home and furniture.

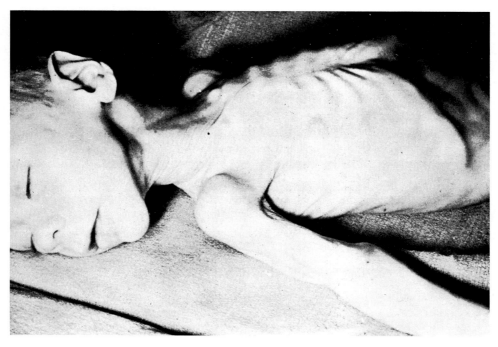

FIGURE VIII-38. Four-month-old child with complete absence of fatty tissue on the face, neck and trunk and relative increased in front-to-back diameter of the chest. Note the absence of a rachitic rosary, but other children may show this lesion.

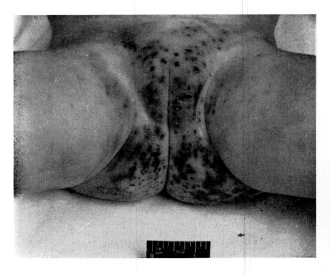
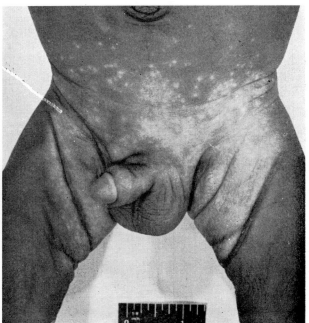

FIGURE VIII-39a–b. (a) Ten-month-old child with pock-like diaper rash. This extent of diaper rash is common and indicates neglect. (b) Punctate and confluent residual scars of earlier diaper rash.

bed well the evening before and later found extremely sick or dead for no explained reason.

The weights of neglected infants at the time of death may vary from as low as 35 to 90% of the expected weight, except for isolated instances in which death resulted from neglect apart from food deprivation.

Autopsy reveals depletion of fat, not only of the subcutaneous tissue, but within the internal fatty deposits. The stomach and intestine usually contain little or no recently digested food, although there may be terminal fecal impaction. Dehydration is characterized by sunken periorbital skin, sunken cheeks, loss of skin turgor and a dehydration pattern upon chemical analysis of the ocular fluid.

The poor general state of health of such infants represents a significant predisposing factor for the development of medical complications that eventually lead to death. Most common among these are bronchopneumonia, sepsis associated with cellulitis, otitis media, laryngotracheobronchitis, and urinary tract infection. Undiagnosed congenital or acquired diseases that could contribute to starvation and emaciation are rare. Nevertheless, cystic fibrosis, celiac disease, and possibly more obscure pancreatic exocrine disorders must be excluded.

Exhaustive chemical analyses in most neglected infants have failed to reveal any evidence of lead or other exogenous poisons or drugs, except for two known instances of methemoglobinemia associated with exposure to sodium nitrate. There are reported instances of children maintained in clinical semicoma or coma by extended use of tranquilizers or barbiturates.

If the medical examiner/coroner determines that abuse or neglect was a factor in the infant's death, the conclusions must be conveyed to law enforcement, child welfare agencies and the courts in a clear, concise, and well-reasoned manner.

PSYCHOLOGICAL AND EMOTIONAL ABUSE

Psychological abuse is difficult to define, in part, because it includes acts of commission (physical and sexual abuse) and acts of omission (neglect). The reader is referred to a review on this subject by Brassert and Hardy.[164] They define psychological maltreatment as *"a repeated pattern of caregiver behavior or extreme incident(s) that convey to children that they are worthless, flawed, unloved, and unwanted."* The authors prefer the term psychological rather than emotional maltreatment because it seems to better incorporate the cognitive, effective, and interpersonal conditions that are the primary components of this form of child abuse and neglect. Six forms of pyschological maltreatment are described: (1) spurning, (2) threatening, (3) isolating, (4) exploiting or corrupting, (5) denying emotional responsiveness, and (6) unwarranted denial of mental health care, medical care, or education.[164] Some authors include family violence as an additional form.

The incidence of psychological maltreatment is not well documented, partly because the criteria for its identification are poorly defined and because it often remains unreported to child protective agencies. Only 5–7% of cases come to the attention of authorities. Psychological maltreatment is almost always a component of physical and/or sexual abuse and neglect.

Diagnostic clues, in addition to the presence of physical and sexual abuse and neglect, include severe emotional distress in the child, a high level of tension in the household, frequent fighting between the parents, repeated rejection of the child, and repeated life-threatening statements made to the child. Verbal aggression and verbal abuse by the parents contribute to poor child development and may cause the child difficulty in controlling his or her own aggression.

Therapy requires resolution of the physical/sexual abuse and neglect and active intervention so that the child's emotional needs are met. Home visitor programs, parent education, and parent support groups are effective at improving the quality of the home situation.

REFERENCES

1. Child Abuse Prevention and Treatment Act (PL 93-247) 42 USCS Section 5106(4), 1988.
2. Schmitt, B.D., and Krugman, R.D.: Abusive and neglect of children. In Behrman, R.E., Vaughn, V.C., III, and Nelson, W.E. (eds.). *Nelson textbook of pediatrics,* 14th ed. Philadelphia: W.B. Saunders, 1992, pp. 78–83.
3. Leventhal, J.M.: The challenges of recognizing child abuse. *JAMA, 281:* 657–659, 1999.
4. Adelson, L.: Pedicide revisited. *Am J. Forensic Med Pathol., 12:* 16–26, 1991.
5. Jenny, C., and Hymel, K.P.: Analysis of missed cases of abusive head trauma. *JAMA, 281:* 621–626, 1999.
6. Herman-Giddens, M.E., Brown, G., Verbiest, S., et al.: Underascertainment of child abuse mortality in the United States. *JAMA, 282:* 463–467, 1999.
7. Kairys, S.W.: Comment. In *Yearbook of Pediatrics 2000.* Stockman, J.A., III, ed. St. Louis: Mosby Yearbook, 2001, p. 137.
8. Asser, S.M., and Swan, R.: Child fatalities from religion-motivated medical neglect. *Pediatrics, 101:* 625–629, 1998.
9. Ewigman, B., Kivlahan, C., et al.: The Missouri Child Fatality Study: Underreporting of maltreatment fatalities among children younger than five years of age, 1983 through 1986. *Pediatrics, 91:* 330–337, 1993.
10. Handy, T.C., Nichols, G.R., et al.: Repeat visitors to a pediatric forensic medicine program. *J Forensic Sci, 41* (5): 841–844, 1996.
11. Hanzlick, R., Combs, D., et al.: Death investigation in the United States, 1990: A survey of statutes, systems, and educational requirements. *J Forensic Sci, 38:* 628–632, 1993.
12. Landeros v. Flood, 17 Cal 3d 399, 131 Cal Rptr 69, 551 P2d 389 (1976): 73ALR 4th (782).
13. State v. Adams, 89 N.M. 737, 557 P2d 586 (1976); Pope v. State, 294 Md 309, 396 A2d 1054 (1979); distinguish State v. Williquette 370 NW 2d 282 (1985).
14. Daubert v Merrill Dow Pharmaceuticals Inc. 509 US 579, June 18, 1993 and Kuhmo Tire Co. LTD, et al v Carmichael, et al. 526 US 1998, March 23, 1999, No. 97–1709.
15. Risinger, D.M., et al. The Daubert implication of observer effects in forensic science. *California Law Review,* Jan 2002, 1–56.
16. Kaplan, S.R., Granik, L.A.: *Child fatality investigative procedures manual.* Chicago: American Bar Association, 1991.
17. Granik, L.A., Durfee, N., and Wells, S.J.: *Child death review teams: A manual for design and implementation.* Chicago: American Bar Association, 1991.
18. Guidelines for Death Scene Investigation of Sudden Unexplained Infant Deaths. Interagency Panel on Sudden Infant Death Syndrome, June 21, 1996, *Morbidity and Mortality Weekly Report,* Volume 45, # RR-10. Superintendent of Documents, U.S. Government Printing Office, Washington, D.C.

19. Wagner, G.N.: Crime scene investigation in child abuse cases. *Am J Forensic Med Pathol., 7:* 94–99, 1986.

20. Adelson, L.: The battering child. *JAMA, 22:* 159–161, 1972.

21. Winsaw, L.S.: Child maltreatment. In McMillan, J.A., DeAngelis, C.D., Feigin, R.D., and Warshaw, J.B. *Oski's pediatrics principles and practice,* 3rd edition. Philadelphia: Lippincott, Williams & Wilkins, 1999.

22. Johnson, C.F.: Abuse and neglect of children. In Behrman, R.E., Kliegman, R.M., and Jenson, H.B. *Nelson textbook of pediatrics,* 16th edition, Philadelphia: W.B. Saunders Co., 2000.

23. Merten, D.F., Radkowski, M.A., and Leonidas, J.C. The abused child: A radiological reappraisal. *Radiology, 146:* 37–38, 1983.

24. Kleinman, P.K.: Postmortem Imaging. In Kleinman, P.K. *Diagnostic imaging of child abuse,* 2nd ed. St. Louis, MO: Mosby, Inc., 1998, pp. 242–246.

25. Kleinman, P.K., Marks, S.C., and Blackbourne, B. The metaphyseal lesion in abused infants: A radiologic-histologic study. *Am J Radiol, 146:* 895–905, 1986.

26. Plunkett, J., and Plunkett, M.: Physiologic periosteal changes in infancy. *Am J Forensic Med Pathol, 21:* 213–216, 2000.

27. Brogdon, B.G.: Child abuse, radiology of abuse. In Brogdon, B.G. (ed.), *Forensic radiology.* Boca Raton, FL: CRC Press, 1998, pp. 282–314.

28. Gunther, W.M., Symes, S.A., et al.: Characteristics of child abuse by anteroposterior manual compression versus cardiopulmonary resuscitation. *Am J Forensic Med Pathol, 21:* 5–10, 2000.

29. Feldman, K.W., and Brewer, D.K.: Child abuse, cardiopulmonary resuscitation, and rib fractures. *Pediatrics, 73:* 339–342, 1984.

30. Belfer et al.: Use of the skeletal survey in the evaluation of child maltreatment. *American Journal of Emergency Medicine,* March 2001.

31. Norman, M.G., Smialek, J.E., Newman, D.E., and Horembola, E.J.: The postmortem examination on the abused child. *Perspectives Pediatr Pathol, 8:* 313–343, 1984.

32. Dalton, H.J., Slavis, T., Helfer, R.E., et al.: Undiagnosed abuse in children younger than 3 years with femoral fracture. *Am J Dis Child, 144:* 875–878, 1990.

33. Kanda, M., Thomas, J.N., and Lloyd, D.W.: The role of forensic evidence in child abuse and neglect. *Am J Forensic Med Pathol, 6:* 7–15, 1985.

34. Brill, P.W., Winchester, P., and Kleinman, P.K.: Differential diagnosis I: Diseases simulating abuse. In Kleinman P.K. (ed.), *Diagnostic imaging of child abuse,* 2nd ed. St. Louis, MO: Mosby Inc., 1998, pp. 178–196.

35. Kleinman, P.K., and Kwon, D.S.: Differential diagnosis, IV, normal variants. In Kleinman, P.K. (ed.), *Diagnostic imaging of child abuse,* 2nd ed. St. Louis, MO: Mosby, Inc. 1998, pp. 225–236.

36. Anderson, W., and Hudson, R.: Self inflicted bite marks in battered child syndrome. *J For Sciences, 7:* 71, 1976.

37. McCann, J., Reay, D., et. al.: Postmortem perianal findings in children. *Am J Forensic Med Pathol, 17:* 289–298, 1996.

38. Stephens, B.G.: Forensic interpretation of blood in the anus. *Am J Forensic Med Pathol, 21:* 93–96, 2000.

39. Wilson, E.F.: Estimation of the age of cutaneous contusions in child abuse. *Pediatrics, 60:* 750–752, 1977.

40. Atwal, G.S., Rutty, G.N., et al.: Bruising in non-accidental head injured children: A retrospective study of the prevalence, distribution and pathological associations in 24 cases. *Forensic Sci Int, 96:* 215–230, 1998.

41. Robertson, I. and Mansfield, R.A.: Ante-mortem and postmortem bruises of the skin. *J For Med, 4:* 1–10, 1957.

42. Raekallio, J.: Estimation of time in forensic biology and pathology. *Am J Forensic Med Pathol, 1:* 213–218, 1980.

43. Robertson, I., and Hodge, P.R.: Histopathology of healing abrasions. *J For Sci, 1:* 1725, 1972.

44. Hanzlick, R.: Book review of: The estimation of the time since death in the early postmortem period by Henssge, C., Knight, B., et al. Little, Brown & Co. Boston, MA (1995). *Arch Pathol Lab Med, 121:* 652, 1997.

45. Case, M.E., Graham, M.A., Handy, T.C., Jentzen, J.M., and Monteleone, J.A.: Position paper on fatal abusive head injuries in infants and young children. *Am J Forensic Med and Pathol, 22:* 112–122, 2001.

46. Shaken baby syndrome: Rotational cranial injuries-technical report. American Academy of Pediatrics, Committee on Child Abuse and Neglect. *Pediatrics, 108:* 206–210, 2001.

47. Caffey, J.: The whiplash shaken infant syndrome: Manual shaking by the extremities with whiplash induced intracranial and intraocular bleeding. *Pediatrics, 54:* 396–403, 1974.

48. Caffey, J.: On the theory and practice of shaking in infants. *Am J Dis Child, 124:* 161–169, 1972.

49. Duhaime, A.C., Gennarelli, T.A., et al.: The shaken baby syndrome: A clinical, pathological and biomedical study. *J Neurosurg, 66:* 409–415, 1987.

50. Ommaya, A.K., Corrao, P., and Letcher, F.S.: Head injury in the chimpanzee: Biomechanics of traumatic unconsciousness. *J Neurotrauma, 12:* 527–546, 1995.

51. Kirschner, R.H.: The pathology of child abuse. In Helfer, M.E., Kempe, R.S., Krugman, R.D. (eds.), *The battered child,* 5th ed. Chicago: University of Chicago Press, 1997, pp. 248–295.

52. Kirschner, R.H., and Wilson, H.L.: Fatal child abuse; The pathologist's perspective. In Reece, R.M. (ed.), *Child abuse, medical diagnosis and management.* Baltimore: William and Wilkins, 1996, pp. 325–357.

53. Gilliland, M.G.F., and Folberg, R.: Shaken babies— Some have no impact injury. *J Forensic Sci, 41:* 114–116, 1996.

54. Krous, H.F., and Byard R.W.: Shaken infant syndrome: Selected controversies. *Pediatric and Developmental Pathology, 2:* 497–498, 1999.

55. Byard, R.W., et al.: Shaken-impact syndrome and lucidity. *Lancet, 355:* 758, 2000.

56. Cohle, S.D., Foster, A., and Cottingham, S.L.: Shaken baby syndrome. (Letter) *Am J Forensic Med Pathol, 21:* 198–199, 2000.

57. McCormick, W.F.: Pathology of closed head injury. In Wilkins, R.H., and Rengachary, S.S., (eds.), *Neurosurgery,* Vol. II, 2nd edition. New York: McGraw-Hill, 1996, pp. 2639–2666.

58. Duhaime, A.C., Alario, A.J., et al. Head injury in very young children: Mechanisms, injury types and ophthalmologic findings in 100 hospitalized patients younger than 2 years of age. *Pediatrics, 90:* 179–185, 1992.

59. Conway, E.E., Jr.: Nonaccidental head injury in infants: The shaken baby syndrome revisited. *Pediatric Annals, 27:* 677–690, 1998.

60. Budenz, D.L., Farber, M.G., et al.: Ocular and optic nerve hemorrhages in abused infants with intracranial injuries. *Ophthalm, 101:* 559–525, 1994.

61. Marcus, D.M., and Albert, D.M.: Recognizing child abuse. *Arch Ophthalmol, 100:* 766–767, 1992.

62. Elner, S.G., Elner, V.M., Arnall, M., and Albert, D.M.: Ocular and associated systemic findings in suspected child abuse. *Arch Ophthalmol, 108:* 1094–1101, 1990.

63. Feldman, K.W.: Evaluation of physical abuse. In Helfer, M.E., Kempe, R.S., and Krugmon, R.D. (eds.), *The battered child,* 5th ed., Chicago: University of Chicago Press, 1997, pp. 175–220.

64. Plunkett, J.: Sudden death in an infant caused by rupture of a basilar artery aneurysm. *Am J Forensic Med Pathol, 20* (1): 45–47, 1999.

65. Prahlow, J.A., Bushing, E.J, and Barnard, J.J.: Death due to a ruptured berry aneurysm in a 3.5 year old child. *Am J Forensic Med Pathol, 19:* 391–394, 1998.

66. Ommaya, A.K., and Yarnell, P.: Subdural hematoma after whiplash injury. *Lancet, 294:* 237, 1969.

67. Gennarelli, T.A., and Thibault, L.E.: Biomechanics of acute subdural hematoma. *J Trauma, 22:* 680–886, 1982.

68. Krauland, W., Mallach, H.J., Missoni, L., and Spitz, W.U.: Subdurale Blutungen aus isolierten Verletzungen von Schlagadern an der Hirnoberfläche durch stumpfe Gewalt. *Virchows Arch Path Anat, 336:* 87–98, 1962.

69. Plunkett, J.: Fatal pediatric head injuries caused by short-distance falls. *Am J Forensic Med Pathol, 22:* 1–12, 2001.

70. Lee, K.S., Bae, J.W., Doh, J.W., et al. Origin of chronic subdural hematoma and relation to traumatic subdural lesions: Review. *Brain Injury, 12:* 901–910, 1998.

71. Dias, M.S., Backstrom, J., Falk, M., and Li, V.: Serial radiography in the infant shaken impact syndrome. *Pediatr Neurosurg, 29:* 77–85, 1998.

72. Swift, D.M., and McBride, L.: Chronic subdural hematoma in children. *Neurosurg Clin N Am, 11:* 439–446, 2000.

73. Chen, T.J., and Kuo, T.: Giant intracranial Masson's hemangioma. *Arch Pathol Lab Med, 108:* 555–556, 1984.

74. Miller, L.R.: Giant intracranial Masson's hemagioma versus chronic subdural hematoma. *Arch Pathol Lab Med, 109:* 6–7, 1984.

75. Hulka, F., Mullins, R.J., and Frank, E.H.: Blunt brain injury activates the coagulation process. *Arch Surg, 131:* 923–928, 1996.

76. Hymel, K.P., Abshire, T.C., Luckey, D.W., and Jenny C.: Coagulopathy in pediatric abusive head trauma. *Pediatrics, 99:* 371–371, 1997.

77. Feldman, K.W., Bethel, R., et al: The cause of infant and toddler subdural hemorrhage: A prospective study. *Pediatrics, 108:* 636–646, 2001.

78. Denny-Brown, D., Russell, W.R.: Experimental cerebral concussion. *Brain, 64:* 93–164, 1941.

79. Adams, J.H., Doyle, D., Ford, I., et al. Diffuse axonal injury in head injury: Definition, diagnosis and grading. *Histopathology, 15:* 49–59, 1989.

80. Duhaime, A.C., Christian, C.W., et al.: Nonaccidental head injury in infants—The "shaken-baby syndrome." *N Engl J Med, 338:* 1822–1829, 1998.

81. Willman, K.Y., Bank, D.E., et al. Restricting the time of injury in fatal inflicted head injuries. *Child Abuse Negl, 21:* 929–940, 1997.

82. Johnson, D.L., Bogl, D., and Baule, R.: Role of apena in non-accidental head injury. *Pediatr Neurosurg, 23:* 305–310, 1995.

83. Atkinson, J.D.D.: The neglected pre-hospital phase of head injury: Apnea and catecholamine surge. *Mayo Clin Proc, 75:* 37–47, 2000.

84. Geddes, J.F., Vowles, G.H., Hackshaw, A.K., et al.: Neuropathology of inflicted head injury in children: II. Microscopic brain injury in infants. *Brain, 124* (7): 1299–1306, 2001.

85. Calder, I.M., Hill, I., and Scholtz, C.L.: Primary brain injury in non-accidental injury. *J Clin Pathol, 37:* 1095–1100, 1984.

86. Gleckman, A.M., and Bell, M.D.: Diffuse axonal injury in infants with nonaccidental craniocerebral trauma: Enhanced detection by beta-amyloid precursor protein immunohistochemical staining. *Arch Path Lab Med, 123:* 146–151, 1999.

87. Gleckman, A.M., and Evans, R.J.: Optic nerve damage in shaken baby syndrome: Detection by beta-amyloid precursor protein immunohistochemistry. *Arch Path Lab Med, 124:* 251–256, 2000.

88. Geddes, J.F., Hackshaw, A.K., Vowles, G.H., et al. Neuropathology of inflicted head injury in children: I. Patterns of brain damage. *Brain, 124* (7): 1290–1298, 2001.

89. Hymel, K.P., Bandak, F.A., Parlington, M.D., and Winston, K.R.: Abusive head trauma? A biomechanics-based approach. *Child Maltreatment, 3:* 116–128, 1998.

90. Naoumenko, J., and Feigin, I.: A stable silver solution for axon staining in paraffin sections. *J Neuropath and Exp Neurol, 26:* 669–673, 1967.

91. Voules, I., Scholtz, C.L., and Cameron, J.M. Diffuse axonal injury in early infancy. *Clin Pathol, 108:* 185–189, 1987.

92. Shannon, P., Smith, C.R., et al.: Axonal injury and the neuropathy of shaken baby syndrome. *ACTA Neuropathologica, 95:* 625–631, 1998.

93. Lindenberg, R., and Freytag, E.: Morphology of brain lesions from blunt trauma in early infancy. *Arch Pathol, 87:* 298, 1968.

94. Bruce, D., Alvai, A., Bilaniuk, L., et al.: Diffuse cerebral swelling following head injuries in children: The syndrome of malignant brain edema. *J Neurosurg, 18:* 482–494, 1981.

95. Popp, A.J., Feustel, P.J., and Kimbelberg, H.K.: Pathophysiology of traumatic brain injury. In Wilkins, R.H. and Rengachary, S.S. (eds.), *Neurosurgery, Vol. II,* 2nd ed. New York: McGraw-Hill, 1996, pp. 2623–2637.

96. Lehman, R.A.W., Krupin, T., and Podos, S.M.: Experimental effect of intracranial hypertension upon intraocular pressure. *J Neurosurg, 36:* 60–66, 1972.

97. Goetting, M.G., and Sowa, B.: Retinal hemorrhage after cardiopulmonary resuscitation in children: An etiologic reevaluation. *Pediatrics, 85:* 585–588, 1990.

98. Christian, C.W., Taylor, A.A., et al.: Retinal hemorrhages caused by accidental household trauma. *J Pediatr, 135:* 125–127, 1999.

99. Gilliland, M.G.F., and Luckenbach, M.W.: Are retinal hemorrhages found after resuscitation attempts? *Am J Forensic Med Pathol, 14:* 187–192, 1993.

100. Wilbur, L.S. Abusive head injury. *APSAC Advisor, 7:* 16–19, 1994.

101. Wilbur, L.S. Magnetic resonance imaging evaluation of neonates with retinal hemorrhages. *Pediatrics, 89:* 332–333, 1992.

102. Johnson, D.L, Braun, D., and Friendly, D. Accidental head trauma and retinal hemorrhage. *Neurosurg, 33:* 231–234, 1993.

103. Odom, A., Christ, E., et al.: Prevalence of retinal hemorrhages in pediatric patients after in-hospital cardiopulmonary resuscitation: A prospective study. *Pediatrics, 99* (6): E3, 1997.

104. Kanter, R.D.: Retinal hemorrhage after cardiopulmonary resuscitation or child abuse. *J Pediatr, 108:* 430–432, 1986.

105. Emerson, M.V., Pieramici, D.J., Stoessel, K.M., et al. Incidence and rate of disappearance of retinal hemorrhage in newborns. *Ophthalmology, 108:* 36–39, 2001.

106. Gilliland, M.G.F., Luckenbach, M.W., et al.: The medicolegal implications of detecting hemosiderin in the eyes of children who are suspected of being abused. *Arch Ophthalmol, 109:* 321–322, 1991.

107. Parsons, M.A., and Start, R.D. Necropsy techniques in ophthalmic pathology. *Journal of Clinical Pathology,* May 2001.

108. Margulies, S.S., and Thibault, K.L.: Infant skull and suture properties: Measurements and implications for mechanisms of pediatric brain injury. *J Biomech Eng, 122:* 364–371, 2000.

109. Thibault, K.L., and Margulies, S.S.: Age-dependent material properties of the porcine cerebrum: Effect on pediatric inertial head injury criteria. *J Biomech, 31:* 1119–1126, 1998.

110. Williams, R.A.: Injuries in infants and small children resulting from witnessed and corroborated free falls. *J Trauma, 3:* 1350–1351, 1991.

111. Chadwick, D.L., Chin, S., Salerno, C., Landsverk, J., and Kitchen, L.: Deaths from falls in children: How far is fatal? *J Trauma, 31:* 1353–1355, 1991.

112. Spivack, B.: Fatal pediatric head injuries caused by short distance falls: Letter to the editor. *Am J For Med and Pathol, 22* (3): 332–336, 2001.

113. Nitnityongskul, P., and Anderson, L.D.: The likelihood of injuries when children fall out of bed. *J Pediatr Orthop, 7:* 184–186, 1987.

114. Lyons, J.L, and Oates, R.K. Falling out of bed: A relatively benign occurrence. *Pediatrics, 92:* 125–127, 1993.

115. Snoek, J.W., Minderhoud, J.M., and Wilmink, J.T.: Delayed deterioration following mild head injury in children. *Brain, 107:* 15–36, 1984.

116. Gilliland, M.G.F.: Interval duration between injury and severe symptoms in nonaccidental head trauma in infants and young children. *J Forensic Sci, 43* (3): 723–725, 1998.

117. Kim, K.A., Wang, M.Y., Griffith, P.M., Summers, S., and Levy, M.L.: Analysis of pediatric head injury from falls. *Neurosurg Focus, 8* (1): Article 3, 2000.

118. Towbin, A., Sudden infant death related to spinal trauma. *Lancet, 2:* 940–942, 1967.

119. Gennarelli, T.A., and Meaney, D.F.: Mechanisms of primary head injury. In Wilkins, R.H., and Rengachary, S.S. (eds.), *Neurosurgery, Vol. II,* 2nd ed. New York: McGraw-Hill, 1996; pp. 2611–2621.

120. Hutchins, K.D., and Natarajan, G.A.: Blunt impact abdominal injury in child abuse. Check Sample FP00-5 (FP-256). *Amer Soc Clin Path,* 53–67, 2000.

121. Price, E.A., Rush, L.R., Perper, J.A., and Bell, M.D. Cardiopulmonary resuscitation-related injuries and homicidal blunt abdominal trauma in children. *Am J Forensic Med Pathol, 21:* 307–310, 2000.

122. Spitz, D.J.: Unrecognized fatal liver injury caused by a bicycle handlebar. *Am J of Emerg Med, 17* (3): 244, 1999.

123. Kleinman, P.K. Visceral trauma. In Kleinman, P.K. (ed.), *Diagnostic imaging of child abuse,* 2nd ed. St. Louis, MO: Mosby, 1998, pp. 248–284.

124. Cooper, A., Floyd, T., Barlow, B., et al.: Major blunt abdominal trauma due to child abuse. *J Trauma, 28:* 1483–1487, 1998.

125. Brown, S.L., Elder, J.S., and Spirnak, P.: Are pediatric patients more susceptible to major renal injury from blunt trauma? A comparable study. *J Urol, 160* (1): 139–140, 1998.

126. Cohle, S.D., Hawley, D.A., Berg, K.K., et al.: Homicidal cardiac lacerations in children. *J Forensic Sci, 40:* 212–218, 1995.

127. Denton, J.S., and Kalelkar, M.B.: Homicidal commotio cordis in children. *J Forensic Sci, 45:* 734–735, 2000.

128. Link, M.S., Wang, P.J., Pandian, N.G., et al: An experimental model of sudden death due to low energy chest waves (commotio cordis). *N Eng J Med, 338:* 1805–1811, 1998.

129. Zumwalt, R.E., and Fanizza-Orphanos A.M.: Dating of healing rib fractures in fatal child abuse. *Advances in Pathology and Laboratory Medicine, 3:* 193–205, 1990.

130. Gunther, W.M., Symes, S.A., and Berryman, H.E.: Characteristics of child abuse by anteroposterior manual compression versus cardiopulmonary resuscitation. *Am J For Med and Pathol, 21* (1): 5–10, 2000.

131. Schullinger, J.N.: *Forensic histopathology.* New York: Springer-Verlag, 1984.

132. Dressler, D., and Hozid, J.: Thermal injury and child abuse: The medical evidence dilemma. *J of Burn Care and Rehabilitation,* March/April, 2001.

133. Pickering, D.: Salicylate poisoning as a manifestation of the battered child syndrome. *Am J Dis Child, 130:* 675, 1976

134. Smialek, J.E., Monforte, J.R., Aronow, R., and Spitz, W.U.: Methadone deaths in children: A continuing problem. *JAMA, 238:* 2516, 1977.

135. Zumwalt, G.J., and Hirsch, C.S.: Subtle fatal child abuse. *Hum Pathol, 11:* 167–174, 1980.

136. Nichols, G.R., II., Corey, T.S., and Davis G.J.: Non-fracture-associated fatal fat absorption in a case of child abuse. *J Forensic Sci, 35:* 493–499, 1990.

137. Kaplan, J.A., and Fossum, R.M.: Patterns of facial resuscitation injury in infancy. *Am J Forensic Med Pathol, 15:* 187–191, 1994.

138. Rosenberg, D.A.: Munchausen's syndrome by proxy. In Helfer, M.E., Kempe, R.S., and Krugman, R.D. (eds.), *The battered child,* 5th ed. Chicago: University of Chicago Press, 1997, pp. 413–430.

139. Rosenberg, D.A.: Munchausen's syndrome by proxy. In Reece, R.M. (ed.), *Child abuse, medical diagnosis and management.* Baltimore: Williams & Wilkins, 1996, pp. 266–278.

140. Kempe, C.H.: Sexual abuse, another hidden pediatric problem. *Pediatrics, 62:* 382, 1978.

141. Finkel, M.A., and DeJong, A.R.: Medical findings in child sexual abuse. In Reece, R.M. (ed.), *Child abuse, medical diagnosis and management.* Boston: Williams & Wilkins, 1996, pp. 185–247.

142. Madison, A.B., Feldman-Winter, L., et al.: Consensual adolescent sexual activity with adult partners-conflict between confidentiality and physician reporting requirements under child abuse laws. *Pediatrics, 107* (2): e16, 2001.

143. Krugman, R.D.: Physical and sexual abuse in ambulatory pediatrics. In Green, M., and Haggerty, R.V. (eds.), *Pediatric Diagnosis,* 4th ed. Philadelphia: W.B. Saunders, 1990, pp. 504–507.

144. Schmitt, B.D., and Krugman, R.D.: *Incest.* In Behrman, R.E., Vaughan, V.C., III, and Nelson, W.E. (eds.), *Nelson textbook of pediatrics,* 14th ed. Philadelphia: W.B. Saunders, 1992, pp. 81–83.

145. Gordon, I.B.: Sexual misuse in children and adolescents. In Behrman, R.E., Vaughan, V.C., III, and Nelson, W.E. (eds.), *Nelson textbook of pediatrics,* 13th ed. Philadelphia: W.B. Saunders, 1987, pp. 1174–1175.

146. Woodling, B.A. and Kossoris, P.D.: Sexual misuse: Rape, molestation and incest. *Pediatrics Clinics of North America, 28:* 481–499, 1981.

147. De Jong, A.R., and Rose, M.: Legal proof of child sexual abuse in the absence of physical evidence. *Pediatrics, 88:* 506–511, 1991.

148. Lauritsen, A.K., Meldgaard, K., et al.: Medical examination of sexually abused children: Medico-legal value. *J Forensic Sci, 45* (1): 115–117, 2000.

149. Reichert, S.K.: Medical evaluation of the sexually abused child. In Helfer, M.E., Kempe, R.S., and Krugman, R.D. (eds.), *The battered child,* 5th ed. Chicago: University of Chicago Press, 1997, pp. 313–328.

150. McCann, J., et al.: Genital findings in prepubertal girls selected for non-abuse: A descriptive study. *Pediatrics, 86:* 428, 1990.

151. Gardner, J.J.: Descriptive study of genital variation in healthy, non-abused premenarchal girls. *J Pediatr, 120:* 251–257, 1992.

152. Bays, J.: Conditions mistaken for child sexual abuse. In Reece, R.M. (ed.), *Child abuse, medical diagnosis and management.* Baltimore: Williams and Wilkins, 1996, pp. 396–402.

153. Berenson, A.B.: Appearance of the hymen at birth and one year of age: A longitudinal study. *Pediatrics, 91:* 820–825, 1993.

154. McCann, J., et al.: Perianal findings in prepubertal children selected for non-abuse. *Child Abuse Negl, 13:* 179, 1989.

155. Sensabaugh, G.F.: Isolation and characterization of a semen-specific protein from human seminal plasma. *J Forensic Sci, 23:* 106–115, 1978.

156. Ricci, L.R., and Hoffman, S.A.: Prostatic acid phosphatase and sperm in the post-coital vagina. *Ann Emerg Med, 11:* 530–534, 1982.

157. LeBeau, M., Andollo, W., et al.: Recommendations for toxicological investigations of drug-facilitated sexual assaults. *J Forensic Sci, 44:* 227–230, 1999.

158. Willott, G.M., and Allard, J.E.: Spermatozoa-their persistence after sexual intercourse. *Forensic Sci Int, 19:* 135–154, 1982.

159. Enos, W.F., and Beyer, J.C.: Spermatozoa in the anal canal and rectum and in the oral cavity of female rape victims. *J Forensic Sci, 23:* 231–233, 1978.

160. Collins, K.A., and Bennett, A.T.: Persistence of spermatozoa and prostatic acid phosphatase in specimens from deceased individuals over varied postmortem intervals. *Am J Forensic Med Pathol, 22:* 228–232, 2001.

161. Ludwig, S., and Kronberg, A.E.: Child abuse: A medical reference. New York: Churchhill Livingsone, 1992, pp. 275–278.

162. Hochmeister, M.N., Budowle, B., et al.: Evaluation of prostate-specific antigen (PSA) membrane test assays

for the forensic identification of seminal fluid. *J Forensic Sci, 44:* 1057–1060, 1999.

163. Lander, E.S.: DNA fingerprinting on trial. *Nature, 339:* 501, 1987.

164. Brassard, M.R., and Hardy, D.B.: Psychological maltreatment. In Helfer, M.E., Kempe, R.S., and Krugman, R.D. (eds.), *The battered child,* 5th ed. Chicago: University of Chicago Press, 1997, pp. 392–412.

Part 3

THE DIFFERENTIAL DIAGNOSIS OF CHILD ABUSE

MARVIN S. PLATT AND LISA KOHLER

SUDDEN UNEXPLAINED, accidental, and natural deaths need to be distinguished from child abuse. The entities to be considered include:
1. Sudden Infant Death Syndrome (SIDS)
2. Natural Diseases
    a. Metabolic Diseases
    b. Bone Diseases
    c. Coagulation and Hematological Disorders
    d. Congenital Malformations
3. *Non-Abusive* Injuries
4. Accidental Deaths

SUDDEN INFANT DEATH SYNDROME (SIDS)

Introduction

SIDS was defined by the National Institute of Child Health and Human Development in 1989 as: *The sudden death of an infant under one year of age which remains unexplained after a thorough case investigation, including (1) performance of a complete autopsy which fails to demonstrate an adequate cause of death; (2) an examination of the death scene which reveals no evidence of an unnatural cause of death; and (3) a review of the maternal and infant clinical histories which reveal no conditions which might have caused the death.** Cases failing to meet the standards of this definition, including those without a postmortem examination should not be diagnosed as SIDS. The 1989, National Institute of Health conference considers unresolved cases as those for which the history, investigation, or autopsy reveals evidence that places death outside the SIDS category, but does not adequately explain the cause of death. Examples of this subgroup include suspected, but unproven, abuse, neglect or accidental suffocation; episodes of vomiting or diarrhea in the 24 hours prior to death without pathologic evidence of infection; unreliable information regarding the death; minimal bronchopneumonia which is insufficient to cause death; and a history of maternal drug abuse.[1]

In 2001, the Committee on Child Abuse and Neglect of the American Academy of Pediatrics[2] advised that an infant's death could be ruled as SIDS when all of the following are true: (1) a complete autopsy is performed, (2) there is no gross or microscopic evidence of trauma or significant disease, (3) there is no evidence of acute or remote trauma on skeletal survey, (4) other causes of death are adequately ruled out including meningitis, sepsis, aspiration, pneumonia, myocarditis, abdominal trauma, dehydration, fluid and electrolyte imbalance, significant congenital malformations, inborn metabolic disorders, carbon monoxide toxicity, drowning and burns, (5) there is no evidence of acute alcohol or drug intoxication or medication use, and (6) a thorough death scene investigation and review of the clinical history are negative. According to this committee, a diagnosis of SIDS should be avoided in children who are found to have an isolated remote rib fracture or who have recently taken prescription medication. One must assume that therapeutic concentrations of acetaminophen or other such medications admittedly given to the child by the caretaker may permit consideration of a SIDS determination by the forensic pathologist.

Although a variety of criteria exist to help standardize the diagnosis of SIDS, there is much subjectivity when evaluating these cases and

---

* At a recent conference, SIDS was redefined and stratified into four subgroups. See Krous, H.F., et al. *Pediatrics, 114:* 234–238, 2004.

there is no accepted understanding as to what SIDS really means. Medical examiners will often interpret the evidence associated with a suspected SIDS death differently and come to different conclusions. For these reasons, there is no uniformity when it comes to making a diagnosis of SIDS.

SIDS is the leading cause of postneonatal mortality in the United States accounting for approximately one-third of all such deaths.[3] In 1988, 5,476 infants succumbed to SIDS representing a rate of 1.4 deaths per 1,000 live births making SIDS the second most common cause of infant death in the United States. SIDS was the leading cause of death among black infants. It was reported to be the cause of death in 12.8% of deaths that involved black infants, representing a rate of 2.26 per 1,000 live births.[4] Since the American Academy of Pediatrics has recommended changes in sleep patterns, including the *Back to Sleep* campaign, the SIDS rate has decreased an average of 5.6% per year; and in 1994, 4,073 infants expired from SIDS, a rate of 1.03 per 1,000 births.[3] Although the data indicate a decrease in the SIDS rate, the lack of uniformity in the way these cases are evaluated must be taken into account before definite conclusions can be made. The way death certificates are signed may be at least partly responsible for the decrease in the SIDS rate. What is classified as SIDS by one medical examiner, may be classified as accidental suffocation associated with inappropriate bedding or overlay by another.

The limitation of one year of age recognizes the fact that most cases of SIDS occur in children between 1 and 6 months of age. The incidence of SIDS follows a bell-shaped curve with the peak between 2 and 4 months of age. SIDS is uncommon in children less than one month or greater than 6 months of age. Approximately 90% of SIDS deaths occur before the age of 6 months.[2]

SIDS is suspected when a previously healthy infant, usually younger than 6 months, is found dead in bed, prompting an urgent call for emergency assistance. Often the baby is fed just before being placed in bed to sleep. No outcry is heard, and the baby is usually found in the position in which he or she had been placed. The episodes typically occur at night or in the early morning. Cardiorespiratory resuscitation attempts may be made by emergency personnel, however, despite resuscitative measures, the child is pronounced dead. There may be serosanguineous, watery, frothy, or mucoid discharge coming from the nose and mouth. Skin mottling and postmortem lividity in the dependent portions of the infant body are commonly found.[2]

Despite extensive research, the etiology of SIDS is not known and thus remains a diagnosis of exclusion. The current popular theory is that of ineffective respiration and chronic hypoxia, in part, related to faulty maturation of the central nervous system. It has been suggested that laryngeal chemo-reflex apnea or obstructive sleep apnea may be factors in some of these cases.[5,6] Elevated levels of vitreous humor hypoxanthine;[7] thickening of the small pulmonary artery walls due to hypertrophy and hyperplasia;[8] brain stem gliosis; abnormal receptor sites in the external arcuate nucleus and the ventral medulla;[9,10] petechial hemorrhages in the thymus, pleurae, and epicardium;[11-13] and extramedullary hematopoiesis in the liver[8] provide evidence to support hypoxia as the mechanism of death. Unfortunately, these findings are non-specific and not all of these studies have been replicated. More recently, Kemp and Thach have supported this theory.[14-17] They maintain that prone sleeping promotes the accumulation of carbon dioxide in a microenvironment around the baby's face resulting in apneic episodes. Cases associated with co-sleeping adults or constriction and confinement of small infants by soft and inappropriate mattresses or bedding further support a hypoxia mechanism.[18-20] Antenatal and postnatal smoking by the mother or a smoker in the household is associated with a higher incidence of SIDS.[21] Cardiac arrhythmias account for a small percentage of cases. A prolonged QT interval (long QT syndrome) has not been accepted as a common cause of SIDS,[22-24] but may account for 3–5% of cases.[25-27] Gastrointestinal reflux (GER) was once thought to be a cause of SIDS, but remains unproven.[28,29]

In recent years, national campaigns aimed at reducing prone position sleeping during infancy have dramatically decreased the incidence of SIDS in the United States and worldwide.[3,15,29] Many of these educational campaigns have also emphasized prompt evaluation and treatment of sick infants, appropriate immunizations, breast feeding, and the avoidance of overheating and co-sleeping with adults. They have also recommended the avoidance of gestational or postnatal passive smoke exposure and use of inappropriate bedding, including adult comforters or excessive sheets and pillows.[18,19,30–33]

Occasionally a physician will see an infant that is said to have had an apparent life-threatening event (ALTE) which, in the past, was referred to as *a near miss or aborted SIDS*. This is an episode in which an infant becomes apneic for a short period of time, but begins to breathe either spontaneously or with stimulation. Recently, well-validated reports of child abuse and infanticide perpetrated by suffocation and masqueraded as apparent life-threatening events or SIDS have appeared in the medical literature.[2] The differentiation between SIDS and homicidal smothering is a critical diagnostic decision. When there are other infants or children in the family who experience such "apneic episodes," conditions to be excluded include abuse, metabolic defects,[34,35] respiratory malfunction[5,36] and obstructive sleep apnea.[6] However, there are certain situations that should raise the suspicion of suffocation.[2,4] These include the death of a child older than 6 months, previously unexpected or unexplained deaths of one or more siblings, simultaneous or nearly simultaneous death of twins,[37,38] previous death of an infant while under the care of the same person, a scene investigation that is suspicious, conflicting or inconsistent statements made by the caregiver(s), a caregiver with mental illness and/or a physical examination of the infant which shows abrasions on the nose or around the mouth, bruises of the lips and frenulum and/or pinpoint hemorrhages (petechiae) in the conjunctivae or on the eyelids.

The Workup

A thorough investigation is a requirement in every case of suspected SIDS. The present defi-nition requires medical examiners and investigators to undertake a well-constructed plan to properly evaluate all of the evidence.

The elements of this plan include the following:
- Scene investigation
- Prenatal care and birth records
- Medical records (well and sick baby visits)
- Family history (including siblings and parents)
- Full body radiographs and special radiographic techniques if deemed necessary
- Complete autopsy (including gross and microscopic examinations)
- Clinical pathological studies (including microbiology and toxicology)
- Expedited communications with the parents, family physicians, and state agencies
- Review by locally-based infant death review teams

Initial Management

Most sudden infant deaths occur at home. The parents are in shock, bewildered, and distressed. Parents who are innocent of blame in their child's death often feel responsible and imagine ways in which they might have contributed to or prevented the tragedy. The appropriate professional response to any child death must be compassionate, empathic, supportive, and non-accusatory. Inadvertent comments, as well as necessary questioning by medical personnel and investigators are likely to cause additional stress.[2]

Personnel on the first response team should be trained to make observations at the scene including the position of the infant, marks on the body, body temperature, degree of rigor and livor, type of bed or crib, amount and position of clothing and bedding, room temperature, type of ventilation and heating, and reaction of the caregivers. Paramedics and emergency department personnel should be trained to recognize postmortem artifacts such as anal and vaginal dilatation, and skin discoloration from lividity, in order to distinguish these entities from abusive injuries.

It is reasonable to allow the parents to see and hold the infant once death has been pronounced. Information is available to help families address the many issues that require attention, including grief counseling, funeral arrangements, religious support and the reaction of surviving siblings.

Scene Investigation

Scene investigation in a case of suspected SIDS is important, as it may uncover evidence in support of an accidental death or abuse. Utilization of a standard investigation form is most helpful. We have found that the Sudden Unexpected Infant Death Reporting Investigation Form (SUIDRF) meets that need. Offices may choose to modify the elements of the form, and/or place the responses in their own computer database. The elements of this form are listed in Table VIII-3. The complete form is available from the Centers of Disease Control.

Although a complete autopsy is essential when investigating sudden deaths in infancy, a scene investigation is crucial in determining environmental hazards that may be present at the time of death. Defective cribs, beds, mattresses, cradles,[39] and improper bedding are the most common sources of accidental suffocation deaths in infants. A bed or crib with widely placed bed slates or side rails can cause accidental suffocation if the infant gets caught between the side rails and the bed (see Fig. XIV-12 a). Soft mattresses, large pillows, polystyrene bead-filled cushions, faulty waterbeds, sheepskin bedding, beanbag cushions, or plastic sheets can obstruct the baby's airway.[15,30-32,40] Toys, pacifiers, and bed connections must be examined, since some of these contain parts which may become dislodged, and aspirated.[32] Dangerous sleeping practices which include sharing of beds by adults and children (co-sleeping) should be addressed.[41] Individuals under the influence of alcohol or sedative medications are at particular risk of overlay.[29] If the death occurs while at day care, the sleeping arrangements at the day care center need to be addressed.[42] The misuse of commercially prepared anti-SIDS devices should be considered.[43]

When a child is found unresponsive, the body is almost always moved from its original position, either by the caregiver or by rescue personnel.

For this reason, the person who first finds the child should be interviewed to gain an understanding of the exact location where the baby was found and the position of the body at the time of discovery. This information may render evidence to support a determination of suffocation or positional asphyxia.[44] In most cases, the infant is transported from the scene to a local hospital where death is pronounced. In all infant deaths, paramedics and emergency room personnel should be interviewed since they are privy to important findings such as rigidity, lividity, body temperature, skin lesions, and caregiver responses. A rectal temperature taken by emergency room personnel may provide additional information.

Even if the child's body is no longer at the scene, a scene investigation by medical examiner personnel should still be conducted. The scene investigation should occur as soon as possible as important findings may be transient, including environmental hypothermia or hyperthermia.[45,46] Some infants sleep with multiple siblings who may harbor infection. The home may be poorly kept so as to suggest economic circumstances which compromise adequate nutrition or care, although the latter circumstances account for a relatively small portion of infant deaths.

Clinical History

The clinical history of a child dying of SIDS often reveals that the child was in good health, or that the child had non-specific symptoms including nasal congestion, occasional loose stools or vomiting. It is now recognized that a recent DPT immunization is not a cause of SIDS. Other epidemiological factors seen in SIDS cases are noted in Table VIII-4. Some of these are child oriented, others are family oriented, but none are predictive of an individual SIDS case. SIDS in siblings is said to be 2–3 times greater than in the general population, however, Peterson[47] has shown using controlled studies, that the incidence is not higher. Thus, the occurrence of recurrent SIDS in a household or simultaneous deaths in twins should raise serious suspicion of child abuse. Although some twin deaths may be

TABLE VIII-3

SUDDEN UNEXPLAINED INFANT DEATH INVESTIGATION FORM–(SUIDIRF*): ELEMENTS

Demographics:
Name   Age   D.O.B.   SSN
Address   Race   Sex   Ethnicity
Police Report

I. Circumstance of Death:
ME/C notified
NOK notified
Scene address
Condition of infant
Events before death
Discovery
Arrival   Transport   Hosp.
Pronounced   Scene/EMS/ED/Surg/Inpt
Injury?
Infant when found: Alive? First response: EMS, Police
Where died. Home; outside; vehicle; witnessed

II. Basic Medical Information: Physician   Medical Records
Labor/Delivery
Maternal illness/complications of pregnancy
Birth defects
Birth weight   Single/twin/etc.
Hospitalization
ER past 2 weeks
Allergies
Growth/weight gain
Exposure to contagious disease
Illness past 2 weeks
Lethargy, crying/48 hours
Appetite/48 hours
Sx; Fever, vomiting, diarrhea, apnea/cyanosis.
Breastfed/when
Vaccinations/72 hours
Injury before
Diet- Breast, formula, solids
Medications
ED visits   Meds/Resus/Tx's/Fluids

III. Household/Environment:
Time of house visit
Evidence of alc, drugs
Physical or mental illness
Police reports/calls
CPS involved?
Prev-child abuse

III. Household/Environment (continued)
Odors, fumes, paint
Damp/molds
Pets
Dwelling: Water, rooms
Family: Language
Income, assistance/adults/children
Smokes
Marital
Education
Employment

IV. Infant and Environment:
In crib/bed/ other
Position placed/found; back, stomach, side.
Face/nose up/down/side
Blanket/covers
Sleeping surface
Other items in crib
PM change   Rigor/Vigor/Temp
Heat/cooling sources:
Items collected: Bottle, formula, meds, diaper, clothes, pacifier, bedding, apnea monitor.

V. Interview with (Name/Date/Time/Phone/Relationship to infant;)
Mother
Father
Caregiver/usual
Caregiver/last
Last witness
First responder
EMS
Police

Medical Record Review
Physician Review
Social/SIDS Agency referral

Scene:
Doll reenactment
Scene diagram
Body diagram

VI. Preliminary Summary:
Notes to pathologist
Preliminary COD Presumed SIDS? Suspect

VII. Case Disposition:
Case disposition–declined? Brought in
Body disposition: Brought in   Release FH
Transporter
Investigator
Supplemental:
a)   Scene diagram
North ↑ (Direction)
Windows/door
Furniture location
Crib location
Body location
Heater/cooler location
Check for: gas furnace
electric furnace
forced air
steam/hot water
electric baseboard
Thermostat reading/setting
Room temp.
Outside temp.
b)   Baby Diagram
Ant/post, Lat. face; genitals
Drainage/discharge
Marks/bruises
Location: diagnostic or therapeutic devices
Lividity
Pressure marks
Temp. of body/site where taken

* Complete form is available from Center of Disease Control or MMWR. CDC may revise the SUIDIRF guidelines in 2005.

related to premature twin births,[48] there is concern that some of these deaths may be due to environmental factors such as overheating,[29,46,47] neglect, household drug abuse, faulty water beds, or suffocation.[2,29] Hanzlick and Graham[37] cite cases wherein suffocation was highly suspect in simultaneous deaths in twins. Koehler et al.[49] reviewed 41 cases of simultaneous sudden infant death syndrome (SSIDS) reported in the world literature between 1900 and 1998 and concluded that before a diagnosis of SSIDS is made, certain criteria should be met. These include: (1) each death fits the same criteria as used in single deaths attributed to SIDS, (2) the infants must be either monozygotic or dizygotic twins, and (3) simultaneous implies that the deaths occurred within 24 hours of each other. Of the 41 cases reviewed, only 12 met all three criteria. Essentially, the likelihood of SSIDS is extremely remote.

Radiology

Full body radiograms may yield findings which support a determination of abuse. A *baby-gram* on an adult-sized film is inadequate and should be avoided. Kleinman[50] and Brogdon[51] recommend multiple x-rays covering the infant's entire body. A child may sustain a clavicular fracture during vaginal delivery, making dating of the fracture in relationship to the age of the child very important. The merits and procedures used in the radiographic work-up of these cases are addressed in greater depth in *Part 2* of this chapter.

Autopsy

In all suspected cases of SIDS, a complete autopsy with toxicology and microscopic examination is necessary. Early studies showed that of 100 infants found dead in bed, approximately 80 to 85% were SIDS. About 15% of the deaths were found to be secondary to abuse, infection, or accident. Perrot[52] showed that in approximately 60% of infant deaths, SIDS was the most appropriate diagnosis, whereas in 40% of cases,

TABLE VIII-4

EPIDEMIOLOGICAL FACTS RELATING TO SIDS

Maternal:
  Young
  Unmarried
  Low socioeconomic group
  History of smoking
  History of drug abuse (opiates, methadone, cocaine)
  Minority group
  Overcrowded home
  Inadequate prenatal care
Infant:
  Premature
  Low birth weight
  Male sex
  Multiple births
  Brain and skeletal growth retardation
  Age 2–4 months
  Prone position

an alternative diagnosis was evident. More recently, Mitchell et al.[53] showed that a more thorough clinical history review, death scene investigation and autopsy examination resulted in increased diagnosis of accidental asphyxia due to unsafe sleeping environments. In another study, Mitchell et al.[54] demonstrated that the more thorough the investigation of a possible SIDS death, the greater likelihood of finding a cause of death other than SIDS.

Several autopsy protocols have been recommended. We suggest that the reader review the ones listed below and choose the one most applicable for their forensic office.

- 1983 Armed Forces Institute of Pathology Perinatal Autopsy Manual[55]
- Australian protocol[56]
- International standardized autopsy for sudden unexpected infant death[57]

The gross autopsy examination may reveal a small amount bloody-tinged fluid or foam in or around the nose and mouth. This may stain the bedclothes and bedding and suggest abuse, but is most often due to terminal pulmonary edema and congestion. However, the presence of injuries to the face, lips, or mouth or a history of previous ALTE should raise the suspicion of death by intentional suffocation. Whether resuscitation was attempted is important since resuscitative measures may cause abrasions and scratches on the face and chest.

Mongolian spots on the back and buttocks of dark-skinned infants and mottled discoloration of the face due to postmortem lividity should not be mistaken for bruises. Mongolian spots are common in black, Asian, and Hispanic babies and occasionally in white infants. Mongolian spots appear as variably sized, blue-gray discolorations of irregular shape. Skin lesions associated with hematologic, infectious, congenital, or metabolic disease, as well as lesions related to accidental injury or Folk cultural therapy (see below) should be distinguished from abuse. These conditions are listed in Table VIII-5. Impetigo, a superficial infection of the skin caused by streptococcus or staphylococcus, primarily affects infants and children. The lesions appear as blisters and can rupture leaving red circular ulcers. A common mistake is to misdiagnose impetigo for cigarette burns. The lesions of impetigo are typically superficial, occur in clusters and heal completely with antibiotic therapy.[58] Postmortem ant or roach bites may resemble scratches or fingernail marks and should not be construed as evidence of abuse (Fig. VIII-40). Prominent horizontal neck creases or furrows may incorrectly suggest strangulation, however, this is a normal postmortem finding in infants. (see Fig. VIII-33).

Full-term infants are usually well nourished and well developed, while premature or neglected infants usually lag behind on the growth curves. The external examination of an infant's body should therefore include body length (crown to heel), body weight, head, chest and abdominal circumferences, state of development and nutrition, state of hydration, presence of anomalies or malformations, and evidence of injury and treatment. The height and weight should be plotted on an infant growth chart to ascertain the percentile.

The internal examination usually reveals numerous petechial hemorrhages on the surface of the thymus gland. Pleural and epicardial petechiae may also be found.[11] Intrathoracic petechiae are seen in approximately 80% of SIDS cases, but are not a pathognomonic finding and cannot be used to determine the terminal position of the infant.[11-13] Non-specific

TABLE VIII-5
CONDITIONS MISTAKEN FOR CHILD ABUSE

Skin:
Mongolian spots
Capillary hemangiomas
Allergic periorbital edema
Bruising or bleeding due to: leukemia, ITP, hemophilia, coagulation disorders, platelet disorders, vitamin K deficiency of prematures and cystic fibrosis, DIC, Ehler-Danlos, vasculitis, Henoch-Schonlein
Burns/scalding; Epidermolysis bullosa
Erythema multiformae
Contact dermatitis; phytodermatitis
Congenital indifference to pain
Hair tourniquets on fingers, toes, penis
Folk therapies: spoon rubbing, cupping, moxibustion, coining

Intracranial hemorrhage, retinal hemorrhage:
Newborn vaginal delivery
Vitamin K deficiency
Cerebral aneurysms/arteriovenous malformations
Intrathoracic/intracranial hypertension
Child walker injuries on stair wells

Metabolic Diseases:
Insulin dependent diabetes mellitus
Adrenal hypoplasia
Congenital adrenal hyperplasia
Reyes syndrome
Fatty acid beta oxidation defects
Carnitine palmitoyl transferase beta deficiency
Median chain acyl Co A dehydrogenase deficiency (MCAD)
Long chain acyl CoA dehydrogenase deficiency
Short chain acyl Co A dehydrogenase deficiency
3 Hydroxy-3 methyl glutaric aciduria
Defects of glyconeogenesis, glycogenolysis, pyruvate oxidation
Oxidative phosphorylation
Lysosomal disorders
Peroxisomal disorders

Bone Lesions:
Rickets or scurvy
Congenital syphilis
Copper deficiency after hyperalimentation
Osteogenesis imperfecta (especially Type IV)
Birth injuries
Child walker injuries on stair wells
Caffey's disease
Osteomyelitis
Prematurity (bone mineral deficiency, parental nutrition)
Methotrexate osteoporosis
Hypervitaminosis A
Hypophosphatasia
Subperiosteal new bone formation of long bones (physiologic)
Menkes kinky hair syndrome (copper deficiency)
Osteopetrosis
Seizure induced fractures
Congenital indifference to pain
Premature's prostaglandin therapy induced periostitis
Homocystinuria

Failure to thrive:
Above metabolic diseases
Dysmorphism/cytogenetic abnormalities.
Organ anomalies: Congenital heart, renal liver, pulmonary defects.
Renal tubular defects

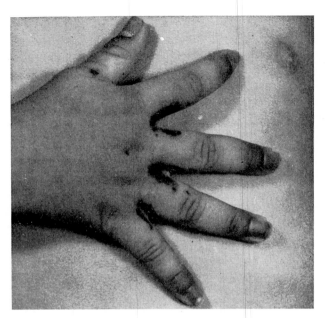

Figure VIII -40. Postmortem roach bites in webs of the fingers, as well as on the face and left arm of this infant, misinterpreted as scratches, led to the diagnosis of child abuse in the hospital emergency room. The cause of death was SIDS.

autopsy findings include an enlarged thymus gland and visceral congestion. Milk may be inhaled into the airways during the dying and CPR process and is not indicative of true aspiration.[5] The importance of certain autopsy findings should be considered when evaluating a case. Incidental findings should not be construed as a factor in the death. Mild upper respiratory tract infection or otitis media may be found, but are generally not considered a likely cause of death. Atrial and ventricular septal defects are not the cause of death unless there is a concurrent severe anomaly with ventricular hypertrophy and congestive heart failure. Significant congenital heart defects are usually found at birth or within the first month of life. It is rare for an undiagnosed congenital heart defect to cause sudden death in a child who is several months of age. The brain is usually congested and may show variable degrees of edema. The infant brain is soft and difficult to examine, it is therefore good practice to cut the brain after at least two weeks of formalin fixation.

It is recommended that multiple microscopic sections be taken so that each organ system can be evaluated. Lung sections which reveal severe pulmonary hemorrhage, abundant alveolar macrophages,[59] or the presence of alveolar pigmented macrophages[60] should be stained with Prussian blue to highlight iron. Approximately 5–10% of sudden unexpected infant deaths under 1 year of age show impressive pulmonary hemosiderosis. The etiology of pulmonary hemosiderosis remains unexplained, but is occasionally seen in association with asphyxia,[61-65] or the presence of certain types of fungus contaminants in the environment.[66,67] Until the issue of infantile pulmonary hemosiderosis is clarified and depending on the circumstances surrounding the death, the manner of death in such cases is best ruled as undetermined.

Paraffin embedded tissue may also be used should immunohistochemical studies be desired at a later time. Portions of heart, lung, liver, kidney, and brain can be frozen and serve as a source of tissue for future genetic, toxicological and metabolic studies. If metabolic disease is suspected, cultures of skin fibroblasts may be helpful for biochemical and genetic testing.

Clinical Pathological Studies

In all infant deaths, body fluids and samples of solid organs should be retained for toxicologic testing. These include tubes of blood, urine, vitreous, bile, gastric contents, liver and brain. Other solid organs can be collected if deemed necessary.

Blood: Sterile blood samples should be submitted in aerobic and anaerobic culture bottles. Additional blood should be collected in tubes with EDTA (purple top), sodium fluoride (gray top) and without preservative (red top). A portion of whole blood should be centrifuged and plasma and/or serum frozen at –20° C (preferably –70° C). It is unclear whether fetal hemoglobin is elevated in SIDS,[68,69] thus we do not perform hemoglobin electrophoresis except in cases where sickle cell disease is a possible factor in the death.

Urine: All available urine should be collected and subsequently refrigerated or frozen. When the bladder is empty, a bladder or renal pelvis wash with 5–10 mL of sterile distilled water or a swab of the mucosa may occasionally be a valuable specimen. Drops of urine may be placed on a urine strip to ascertain the presence of hyperglycemia or ketones. Laboratory testing using urine will help in the diagnosis of metabolic diseases, as well as identify drugs and poisons.

Vitreous: Vitreous fluid is a good alternative specimen for drug testing when urine is unavailable. Vitreous may be used to analyze for hyponatremia of cystic fibrosis[70] and hypernatremia, hyperchloremia, and elevated urea nitrogen in dehydration or electrolyte imbalance. In renal failure, the vitreous creatinine is elevated.

Microbiology: Blood from the heart or great vessels, lung tissue or swab (from each lung), spleen, and any inflammatory lesions should be cultured. Although the merit of autopsy bacterial cultures has been debated, the presence of a single organism may support a diagnosis of sepsis or determine the organism associated with pneumonia. Using sterile equipment decreases the degree of contamination. Viral cultures may be taken, however, the results are usually negative. The results should only be used in conjunction with a clinical diagnosis of a viral infection or to provide supportive evidence of a specific viral infection when viral inclusions are found during microscopic examination. Occasionally, viral culture may clarify the cause of inflammation in the heart or lungs and further characterize nonspecific viral inclusions as being related to herpes, CMV, adenovirus, etc. We also obtain a nasal swab for respiratory syncytial viral antigen. Samples may be submitted for polymerase chain reaction (PCR) to enhance a diagnosis of human herpes virus 6 infection.[71]

Cerebrospinal fluid: The cerebrospinal fluid in cases of SIDS may reveal postmortem-derived round cells.[72] Sections of brain in these circumstances show no inflammation, and cultures are negative. Thus, postmortem round cell pleocytosis must not be misinterpreted as meningitis. Spinal fluid should be collected using sterile technique via lumbar puncture or directly from the brain after opening the skull. If the culture of the spinal fluid yields a significant bacterium, sections of the brain should be re-examined and gram stained for organisms.

Bile: Bile should be collected by direct aspiration from the gallbladder and subsequently refrigerated or frozen. Fatty acid oxidative metabolic disorders are more easily identified by analysis of bile.[34,35]

Toxicology: Samples of blood, urine, gastric contents, kidney, liver, brain, bile, and vitreous should be collected in all cases of suspected SIDS to rule out the possibility of drug toxicity or poisoning. If the infant was treated in a hospital prior to death, the first urine specimen and blood taken at admission should be analyzed. Toxic agents and metabolic disease products are best found in these samples because they are not diluted by treatment.

Special studies: If facilities are available, portions of tissue may be placed in glutaraldehyde for electron microscopy to identify viral, lysosomal or peroxisomal residues. Samples are best if obtained within 1 to 2 hours postmortem, but can be collected up to 4–6 hours after death. Samples used for biochemical studies should be frozen at –70° C. If metabolic studies may be necessary it is good practice to collect and store portions of frozen liver, urine, kidney, and brain.

Expedited Communications

As mentioned previously, cases of fatal child abuse should be reported to the police and to appropriate state child protective services as defined by state law.

If the case is one of sudden infant death syndrome, the child's physician should be advised as soon as possible. Many pathologists can make a preliminary judgment from the gross examination and advise the physician, law enforcement agency, and family, however, some pathologists prefer to wait for microscopic sections and culture findings before making a determination of SIDS. Once the death is determined to be SIDS, the child's family should receive communication including the cause of death and important findings, in addition to information about SIDS. The parents should be provided with information about SIDS and given the telephone number of the local SIDS support group. SIDS should be depicted as a natural, unpredictable and unpreventable condition. Parents need support, personal insights, reference materials, information, and counseling. The National SIDS Foundation, International Guild for Infant Survival and the SIDS Alliance serve as excellent resources.

Child Fatality Review Teams

In many states, multidisciplinary teams have been established to review child fatalities.[73-75] The review committee should include a child welfare/child protective services social worker, a law enforcement officer, a public health officer, a medical examiner or coroner, a pediatrician with expertise in child maltreatment, a forensic pathologist, a pediatric pathologist, and a local prosecutor. Sharing of data among agencies helps insure that the deaths attributable to child abuse are not missed and that surviving and subsequent siblings are protected. Some child fatality teams routinely review infant deaths attributable to apparent SIDS. Periodic review by these committees has shown that abuse has been missed by physicians, radiologists, emergency room personnel, and pediatricians. The findings of the Missouri Infant Mortality Committee, addressed in *Part 2,* is of interest in this matter.[75]

NATURAL DISEASES

Natural disease causing death should be distinguished from SIDS. Many of these diseases are described in Table VIII-6.[96-112] Metabolic and congenital diseases are listed in Table VIII-5.

Diseases involving the *cardiovascular system* include myocarditis, usually of viral origin, aortic stenosis, congenital heart disease, and anomalous coronary arteries. Although rare, fibromas of the heart, histiocytic cardiomyopathy, rhabdomyoma, left ventricular hypoplastic syndrome, and endocardial fibroelastosis may be seen in the first three months of life. DiGeorge syndrome may be associated with an aberrant vascular outflow tract, immunodeficiency and hypocalcemia. Fatty acid oxidative metabolic defects may cause fatty infiltration of the heart.

Respiratory disease: Acute bronchopneumonia may be present without any clinical manifestations. Premature children who have had a prolonged hospitalization secondary to bronchopulmonary dysplasia may later expire with catecholamine induced bi-ventricular hypertrophy. Choanal atresia, macroglossia, and micrognathic syndromes may cause respiratory compromise from airway obstruction.

Gastrointestinal system: Children may acquire viral and bacterial intestinal infections and die rapidly of dehydration. Under certain circumstances, fatal dehydration may develop in hours. Although persistent diarrhea may be seen, some children may have few bowel movements, but their gut is distended with watery feces and toxins. Salmonella sepsis, without diarrhea, has been associated with sudden death. Culture of the intestinal contents may reveal enteroviruses or significant bacterial pathogens. Rotavirus can be diagnosed by tests based on immunologic procedures. Dehydration can also be caused by abuse when water is deprived or excess salt is ingested. Scene investigation and vitreous electrolyte studies are helpful in such cases. Clostridium botulinum infection has rarely caused sudden death. More commonly the child presents with muscular weakness prompting a test to identify the botulinum toxin. E. coli induced hemolytic uremic syndrome (HUS) may cause renal failure and central nervous system hemorrhage. Fatty acid metabolic defects cause microvesicular changes in the liver (see below). Agonal intussusception is a postmortem artifact and is not a cause of death. Bonafide intussusception should show intestinal wall hemorrhage, inflammation, and necrosis. Volvulus may be caused by a mesenteric cyst or congenital band. Perforation of the small bowel may follow acute appendicitis, or complications of necrotizing

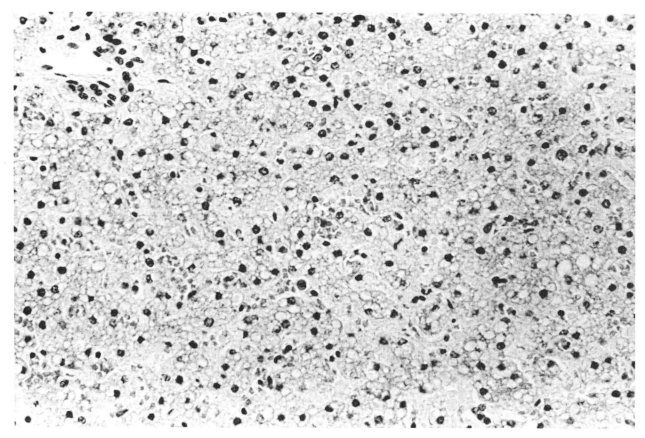

Figure VIII -41. Finely dispersed fat droplets as seen in liver cells of infants with inborn errors of oxidative metabolism of fatty acids and Reye's Syndrome. Note that the nuclei tend to be central. Oil red O stain of frozen sections.

VIII-5). These conditions may be inherited or acquired. The inherited diseases include osteogenesis imperfecta and copper deficiency (kinky hair disease/Menkes syndrome). The acquired diseases include syphilis, rickets, scurvy, osteomalacia, infantile cortical hyperostosis (Caffey disease), vitamin A intoxication and congenital indifference to pain.[89] The latter condition is not a bone disorder, but rather a rare neurologic disease which is associated with fractures because of the inability to perceive pain. Radiographic features in the shafts of long bones, skull, and pelvis, in areas outside of fracture sites, often suggest systemic bone disease.

Osteogenesis imperfecta (OI) or *brittle bone disease* exists as a heterogeneous group of inherited collagen disorders associated with reduced bone density. The bone fragility is due to abnormal Type I collagen, the protein that forms the bone matrix, before the bone is mineralized. Osteogenesis imperfecta is usually diagnosed by family history, physical examination and radiographic findings.[90] OI can usually be diagnosed using a collagen analysis, however, this type of testing is not necessary in most cases. Biochemical testing of collagen in cases of OI is positive in 85% of cases, meaning 15% of OI patients have a normal collagen test.

OI Type I is the most common form and accounts for 80% of cases. It is almost always associated with blue sclerae, but has less severe skeletal manifestations than the other types. Type IB is characterized by tooth deformity (dentinogenesis imperfecta). Type II is extremely severe and usually results in death in the perinatal period. Type III is less severe than Type II, and is associated with progressive bowing deformity, blue sclerae, deafness and dentinogenesis imperfecta. Type IV is a milder form of the disease that is variable in severity and may not become manifest until later in childhood. Type IV is usually not associated with blue sclerae. Signs and symptoms of Type IV include joint hypermobility, early onset deafness and a family history of OI. Some patients with OI Types I and IV have abnormal x-rays, but most do not. The osteopenia of OI results from the long periods of immobilization used to treat fractures. A diagnosis of OI does not preclude a diagnosis of child abuse. Knight[91] reported an infant with OI who was physically abused. The diagnosis of abuse was based on the distribution of the bruises on the head and neck.

Bone fractures may also be seen in homocystinuria which causes osteoporosis and in hypophosphatasia which may resemble rickets. Premature infants who are not given vitamin C or D are prone to scurvy or rickets, respectively.

A child with scurvy may present with diffuse ecchymoses and painful, swollen limbs. Radiographic features include metaphyseal irregularity and fracture, periosteal hemorrhage and bone with a ground glass appearance. A dense ring of sclerotic bone surrounding a hyperlucent epiphysis (Wimberger line) is specific for scurvy. The metaphyseal injuries are similar to those found in abuse, however, the atrophy is more generalized with thin cortices and osteopenia.[92]

Rickets is caused by a lack of vitamin D. Milk fortified with vitamin D makes this condition very rare in the United States. Rickets is more common than scurvy, especially among premature infants. Infants maintained on total parenteral nutrition (TPN) have an increased risk of rickets because of insufficient calcium and phosphorus. Radiographic features include metaphyseal irregularity, periosteal reaction and generalized demineralization of bone. With advanced rickets, the serum calcium and phosphorus levels are low and the alkaline phophatase is elevated.[92]

Coagulation and Hematologic Defects

Parents of abused children usually claim that their child bruises easily, and although coagulation defects are rare in children, the possibility of a bleeding disorder should be considered in certain situations (see Tables VIII-5 and VIII-6).

Coagulation defects are seen in Factor VIII and IX deficiencies and von Willebrand's disease. Family history and coagulation studies, if the patient is alive, help classify the disorder.[93,94] Parents and siblings should also be studied.

Thrombocytopenia, a decrease in the number of platelets, may be associated with several disorders. When the platelet count decreases below 20,000 mm,[3] spontaneous bleeding in the skin and mucus membranes may occur. One condition associated with a low platelet count to the point that bleeding may occur is idiopathic thrombocytopenia purpura (ITP). This condition causes destruction of platelets usually following a viral illness. Other conditions that may lead to bruising secondary to low platelets include various tumors, including leukemia and neuroblastoma. Leukemia can be diagnosed from blood, lymph node, spleen, and bone marrow smears, as well as microscopic sections of bone marrow. Immunohistochemical and chromosome studies may further aid in the specific classification. The immune-mediated thrombocytopenias are usually viral or drug induced. Peripheral blood, bone marrow smears, and clinical history lead to the diagnosis. Antiplatelet antibodies may be identified in the sera.

Infectious mononucleosis is usually associated with splenic enlargement and rarely with rupture of the spleen, which may be misinterpreted as abuse. Sections of lymph nodes and spleen show plasma cells and reactive lymphocytes. The presence of Epstein-Barr viral antibodies helps in the diagnosis.

The bleeding associated with coagulation and hematological defects differs from that seen in child abuse. With coagulation and hematological disorders, the bleeding may be intracranial or involve the gastrointestinal system or skin. The skin hemorrhage is often diffuse and does not show a pattern so often seen in abuse. It should be remembered that children with coagulation and hematological disorders may still be abused making it necessary to thoroughly evaluate each case.

Genetic conditions that may be associated with extensive bruising include Ehlers-Danlos syndrome (EDS) and von Willebrand disease. EDS is due to abnormal collagen and is characterized by hyperextensible joints and blood vessel fragility, leading to easy bruising. Von Willebrand disease is due to an abnormality in a blood protein called von Willebrand factor. The protein is either defective or not produced in sufficient quantities. The most common symptoms include nose bleeds, bleeding from gums, heavy periods and easy bruising. According to Harrison, VWD is the most common inherited bleeding disorder occurring in as many as 1 in 800 to 1000 individuals.[113]

Congenital Malformations

Children with undiagnosed brain, lung, heart, or kidney malformations sometimes die suddenly and unexpectedly. The malformation must be shown to compromise organ function and induce cardiorespiratory arrest. Sudden unexpected death may result from endocardial fibroelastosis, fibroma of the heart, hypoplastic left heart syndrome, anomalies of the aortic arch and coronary arteries, and hemangioma of the trachea (see Table VIII-6). Norman[70] and Weissgold[78] documented a sudden infant death from a ruptured cerebral arteriovenous malformation, and Plunkett[76] and Prahlow[77] described childhood deaths related to aneurysms of the brain. The subarachnoid hemorrhage which arises in these entities should not be confused with that seen in shaken baby (impact) syndrome.

Non-Abusive Injuries

Several folk medicine remedies used for treatment of childhood illnesses have the appearance of abusive injuries. Some such remedies include cupping, coining and spooning, all of which are dermabrasion techniques used to *draw-out* illness.

Cupping is practiced primarily by Mexican and Eastern European immigrants. A cup partially filled with alcohol is ignited. The cup is then inverted and placed on the skin. As it cools, suction is created between the cup and skin which causes a characteristic circular ecchymosis as the cup is removed. The process is repeated in all areas of discomfort.[58]

Coining is practiced in Southeast Asia as a treatment for fever, chills and headache. This folk remedy consists of massaging the back or chest with oil and then vigorously rubbing the area using the edge of a coin until petechiae or purpura are visible. The lesions heal spontaneously usually without complication.[58]

Spooning is practiced in China and is similar to coining, except that the body is scratched with a porcelain spoon until ecchymotic lesions appear.[58]

ACCIDENTAL DEATHS

Distinguishing accidental deaths from death secondary to child abuse or intentional acts of violence is obviously critical. Unsafe sleeping circumstances invite accidental deaths in infants. For this reason, the child's sleeping arrangements should be a primary focus of any investigation dealing with sudden death in an infant. Any defective items uncovered during the investigation should be reported to the Consumer Product Safety Commission. When infants die from accidental drowning, the scene examination and statements made by the caregiver are important. Infants or children who drown in bathtubs should immediately raise suspicion of abuse or neglect. Death may be caused by accidental fires rather than arson/homicide. In fire deaths, postmortem carbon monoxide, i.e., the carboxyhemoglobin saturation, is usually elevated and the infant should have soot in the respiratory tract. A negative carboxyhemoglobin level and no evidence of soot inhalation indicates the child was dead prior to the fire and should raise suspicion of foul play.

Children have been known to independently ingest medications left unsecured in the home, and siblings, as well as parents, have accidentally overdosed infants on various medications. One child died from isopropyl alcohol intoxication when the mother used the alcohol to treat the child's burns.[95] These cases should be reported to the National Association of Medical Examiner's Toxicology Center (E-mail: www.thename.org) as well as local authorities.

Infants have died from aspiration of various objects and food. Aspiration usually causes death from obstruction of the airway, however, depending on what is aspirated or swallowed the esophagus or airway may be perforated. Rarely,

a sharp object may perforate the heart or great vessels. Commonly aspirated foods include pieces of hot dog, grapes and nuts.

Iatrogenic deaths may be due to incorrect anesthesia or anesthetic-induced toxic reactions. Airway obstruction, cardiac arrhythmias, fluid and electrolyte imbalance, and pneumothorax, following bronchial lavage have been noted.

Hyperthermia may be caused by excessive clothes or bedding, misuse of heaters, or leaving infants and small children in closed automobiles in the summer.

REFERENCES

1. Willinger, M., James, L.S., Catz, C., et al.: Defining the sudden infant death syndrome (SIDS). *Pediatric Pathology, 11:* 677–684, 1991.

2. Distinguishing sudden infant death syndrome from child abuse fatalities. *American Academy of Pediatrics. Pediatrics, 107:* 437–441, 2001.

3. Centers for Disease Control (CDC). Sudden infant death syndrome–United States, 1983–1994. October 11, 1996, Vol. 45 No. 40 pp. 859–863.

4. Reece, R.M.: Fatal child abuse and sudden infant death syndrome. In Reece, R.M. (ed.), *Child abuse, medical diagnosis and management.* Baltimore: Williams and Wilkins, 1996, pp. 107–137.

5. Thach, B.T.: Sudden infant death syndrome: Can gastroesophageal reflux cause sudden infant death? *Am J Med, 108* (4A): 144S–148S, 2000.

6. McNamara, F., and Sullivan, C.E.: Obstructive sleep apnea in infants: Relation to family history of sudden infant death syndrome, apparent life-threatening events, and obstructive sleep apnea. *J Pediatr, 136:* 318–323, 2000.

7. Rognum, T.O., and Saugstad, O.D.: Hypoxanthine levels in vitreous humor evidence of hypoxia in most infants who died of SIDS. *Pediatrics, 87:* 306–310, 1991.

8. Valdes-Dapena, M.A.: The sudden infant death syndrome and perinatal deaths. In Froede, R.C. (ed.), *Handbook of forensic pathology.* Northfield, IL: College of American Pathologists, 1990, pp. 92–95.

9. Gilson, T.P., Balko, M.G., et al.: Morphologic variations of the external arcuate nucleus in infants dying of SIDS: A preliminary report. *J Forensic Sci, 39:* 1076–1083, 1994.

10. Panigraphy, A., Filiano, J. et al: Decreased serotonergic receptor binding in rhombic lip derived regions of the medulla oblongata in the sudden infant death syndrome. *J Neuropatholo Exp Neurol, 59:* 377–384, 2000.

11. Beckwith, J.B.: Intrathoracic petechial hemorrhage: A clue to the mechanism of sudden infant death syndrome? *Annals of New York Academy of Science, 533:* 17–47, 1988.

12. Krous, H.F., and Nadeau, J.M.: Intrathoracic petechiae in sudden infant death syndrome. *Pediatric and Developmental Pathology, 4:* 160–166, 2001.

13. Krous, H.F., and Nadeau, J.M.: Neck extension and rotation in sudden infant death syndrome. *Pediatric and Developmental Pathology, 4:* 154–159, 2001.

14. Kemp, J.S., Livne, M., et al.: Softness and potential to cause rebreathing: Differences in bedding used by infants at high and low risk for sudden infant death syndrome. *J Pediatr, 132:* 234–239, 1988.

15. Kemp, J.S., Nelson, V.E., et al.: Physical properties of bedding that may increase risk of sudden infant death syndrome in prone-sleeping infants. *Pediatr Res, 36:* 7–11, 1994.

16. Thach, B.T.: Sleep, sleep position, and the sudden infant death syndrome: To sleep or not to sleep? That is the question. *J Pediatr, 138:* 793–795, 2001.

17. Horne, R.S.C., Ferens, D., et al: The prone sleeping position impairs arousability in term infants. *J Pediatr, 138:* 811–816, 2001.

18. Kemp, J.S., Unger, B., et al.: Unsafe sleep practices and an analysis of bed sharing among infants dying suddenly and unexpectedly. *Pediatrics, 106* (3): e41, 2000.

19. Thogmartin, J.R., Siebert, C.F., et al.: Sleep position and bed-sharing in sudden infant deaths: An examination of autopsy findings. *J Pediatr, 138:* 212–217, 2001.

20. American Academy of Pediatrics Task Force on Infant Position and SIDS: Does bed sharing affect the risk of SIDS? *Pediatrics, 100:* 724–727, 1997.

21. Wisborg, K., Kesmodel, U., et al.: A prospective study of smoking during pregnancy and SIDS. *Arch Dis Child, 83:* 203–206, 2000.

22. Lucey, J.F. Comments. *Pediatrics, 103:* 812, 1999.

23. Prolongation of the QT interval and sudden infant death syndrome. *N Engl J Med, 339:* 1161–1163, 1998.

24. Arad-Cohen, N., Cohen, A., and Tirosk, E.: The relationship between gastroesophageal reflux and apnea in infants. *J Pediatr, 137:* 321–326, 2000.

25. Schwartz, P.J., Prior, S.G., et al.: A molecular link between the sudden infant death syndrome and the long-QT syndrome. *N Eng J Med, 343:* 262–267, 2000.

26. Ackerman, M.S., Tester, D.J., and Driscoll, D.J.: Molecular autopsy of sudden unexplained death in the young. *Am J Forensic Med and Pathol, 22:* 105–111, 2001.

27. Ackerman, M.J., Siu, B.L., Sturner, W.Q., et al: Postmortem molecular analysis of SCN5A defects in sudden infant death. *JAMA, 286:* 2264–2269, 2001.

28. Byard, R.W., Moore, L.: Gastroesophageal reflux and sudden infant death syndrome. *Pediatric Pathology, 13:* 53–57, 1993.

29. American Academy of Pediatrics: Task Force of Infant Sleep Position and Sudden Infant Death Syndrome. Changing Concepts of Sudden Infant Death Syndrome: Implications for Infant Sleeping Environment and Sleep Position. *Pediatrics,* 650–655, 2000.

30. Thach, B.T.: Sudden infant death syndrome: Old causes rediscovered? *N Engl J Med, 315:* 126–128, 1986.

31. Kemp, J.S., and Thack, B.T.: Sudden death in infants sleeping on polystyrene-filled cushions. *N Engl J Med, 324:* 1858–1864, 1991.

32. Gilbert-Barnes, E.F., Hegstrand, L., Chandra, S., et al.: Hazards of mattresses, beds, and bedding in deaths in infants. *Am J Forensic Med Pathol, 12:* 27–32, 1991.

33. Paris, C.A., Remler, R., Daling, J.R.: Risk factors for sudden infant death syndrome: Changes associated with sleep position recommendations. *J Pediatr, 139:* 771–777, 2001.

34. Boles, R.G., Buck, E.A., et al.: Retrospective biochemical screening of fatty acid oxidation disorders in postmortem livers of 418 cases of sudden death in the first year of life. *J Ped, 132:* 924–933, 1998.

35. Cederbaum, S.D.: SIDS and disorders of fatty acid oxidation: Where do we go from here? *J Pediatr, 132:* 913–914, 1998.

36. Oren, J., Kelly, D.H., and Shannon, D.C.: Long-term follow-up of children with congenital central hypoventilation syndrome. *Pediatrics, 80:* 375–380, 1987.

37. Hanzlick, R., and Graham, M.A.: *Forensic pathology in criminal cases,* 2nd ed. Lexis Publishing, 2000.

38. Feldman K.W.: Evaluation of physical abuse. In Helfer, M.E., Kempe, R.S., Krugman, R.D. (eds.), *The battered child,* 5th ed. Chicago: University of Chicago Press, 1997, pp. 175–220.

39. Moore, L., Bourne, A.J., et al.: Unexpected infant death in association with suspended rocking cradles. *Am J Forensic Med Pathol, 16:* 177–180, 1995.

40. Smialek, J.E., Smialek, P.Z., and Spitz, W.U.: Accidental bed deaths in infants. *Clin Pediatr, 17:* 17–32, 1977.

41. Collins, K.A.: Death by overlaying and wedging A 15-year retrospective study. *Am J Forensic Med and Pathol, 22:* 155–159, 2001.

42. Moon, R.Y., Patel, K.M., et al.: Sudden infant death syndrome in child care settings. *Pediatrics, 106:* 295–300, 2000.

43. Mallak, C.T., Milch, K.S., et al.: A deadly anti-SIDS device. *Am J Forensic Med Pathol, 21:* 79–82, 2000.

44. Guntheroth, W.G., and Spiers, P.S.: Sleeping prone and the risk of sudden infant death syndrome. *JAMA, 267:* 359–362, 1992.

45. Stanton, A.N.: Overheating and cot death. *Lancet, 2:* 1199–1201, 1984.

46. Guntheroth, W.G., and Spiers, P.S.: Thermal stress in sudden infant death. Is there an ambiguity with the rebreathing hypothesis? *Pediatrics, 107:* 693–698, 2001.

47. Peterson, D.R., Sabotta, E.E., and Daling, J.R.: Infant mortality among subsequent siblings of infants who died of sudden infant death syndrome. *J Pediatr, 108:* 911–914, 1986.

48. Smialek, J.E.: Simultaneous sudden infant death syndrome in twins. *Pediatrics, 77:* 816–821, 1986.

49. Koehler, S.A., Ladham, S., et al.: Simultaneous sudden infant death syndrome. A proposed definition and worldwide review of cases. *Am J Forensic Med Pathol, 22:* 23–32, 2001.

50. Kleinman, P.K.: *Diagnostic imaging of child abuse,* 2nd edition. St. Louis, MO: Mosby, Inc., 1998.

51. Brogdon, B.G.: *Forensic radiology.* Boca Raton, FL: CRC Press, 1998, pp. 281–314.

52. Perrot, L.J., and Naworjczyk, S.: Non-natural death masquerading as sudden infant death syndrome. *Am J Forensic Med Pathol, 9:* 105–111, 1988.

53. Mitchell, E., Krous, H.F., et al.: An analysis of the usefulness of specific stages in the pathologic investigation of sudden infant death. *Am J Forensic Med Pathol, 21:* 395–400, 2000.

54. Mitchell, E., Krous, H.F., et al.: Changing trends in the diagnosis of sudden infant death. *Am J Forensic Med Pathol, 21:* 311–314, 2000.

55. Valdes-Dapena, M., and Huff, D.: *Perinatal autopsy manual.* Washington, D.C.: Armed Forces Institute of Pathology, October, 1983, pp. 68–71.

56. Byard, R.W.: Autopsy protocols and information. In Byard, R.W., and Cohle, S.D. (eds.), *Sudden death in infancy, childhood, and adolescent.* Cambridge University Press, 1994, pp. 498–520.

57. Krous, H.F.: Instruction and reference manual for the international standardized autopsy for sudden unexpected infant death. *J Sudden Infant Death Syndrome Infant Mortal, 1:* 203–246, 1996.

58. Stewart, G.M., and Rosenberg, N.M.: Conditions mistaken for child abuse: Part II. *Pediatric Emergency Care, 12* (3): 217–221, 1996.

59. Delaney, K., Hanzlick, R., et al.: Pulmonary macrophage counts in deceased infants. *Am J Forensic Med Pathol, 21:* 315–318, 2000.

60. Hanzlick, R., and Delaney, K.: Pulmonary hemosiderin in deceased infants. *Am J Forensic Med Pathol, 21:* 319–322, 2000.

61. Yukawa, N., et al.: Intra-alveolar hemorrhage in sudden infant death syndrome. *J Clin Path, 52:* 581–587, 1999.

62. Dorandeu, A., Peri, G., et al.: Histological demonstration of haemosiderin deposits in lungs and livers from victims of chronic physical child abuse. *Int J Legal Med, 112:* 280–286, 1999.

63. Becroft, D.M.O., Lockett, B.K.: Intra-alveolar pulmonary siderophages in sudden infant deaths. *Pathology, 29:* 60–63, 1997.

64. Stewart, S., and Fawcett, J.: Interstitial hemosiderin in the lungs of sudden infant death syndrome. *J Pathol, 145:* 53–58, 1985.

65. Byard, R.W., Telfer, S.S., and Beal, S.M.: Assessment of pulmonary and intrathymic hemosiderin deposition in sudden infant death syndrome. *Ped Pathol and Lab Med, 17:* 275–282, 1997.

66. U.S. Centers for Disease Control and Prevention. Update: pulmonary hemorrhage/hemosiderosis among infants–Cleveland, Ohio, 1993–1996. *MMWR, Morbid Mortal Wkly Rep, 46:* 33–35, 1997.

67. Availability of case definition for acute idiopathic pulmonary hemorrhage in infants. *MMWR, Morbid Mortal Wkly Rep, 50:* 494–495, 2001.

68. Giulian, G.G., Gilbert, E., and Moss, R.L.: Elevated fetal hemoglobin levels in sudden infant death syndrome. *N Engl J Med, 316:* 1122–1126, 1987.

69. Zielke, H.R., Meny, R.G., O'Brien, M.J., and Smialek, J.E.: Normal fetal hemoglobin levels in sudden infant death syndrome. *N Engl J Med, 321:* 1359–1364, 1989.

70. Norman, M.G., Smialek, J.E., Neuman, D.E., and Horembala, E.J.: The postmortem examination on the abused child. *Perspectives in Pediatric Pathology, 8:* 313–343, 1984.

71. Hoang, M.P., Ross, K.F., et al.: Human Herpesvirus-6 and sudden death in infancy: Report of a case and review of the literature. *J Forensic Sci, 44* (2): 432–437, 1999.

72. Platt, M.S., McClure, S., and Clarke, R.: Postmortem cerebrospinal fluid pleocytosis. *Am J Forensic Med Pathol, 10:* 209–212, 1989.

73. Granik, L.A., Durfee, N., and Wells, S.J.: Child Death Review Teams: A manual for design and implementation. Chicago: American Bar Association, 1991.

74. Kaplan, S.R., and Granik, L.A.: Child Fatality Investigative Procedures Manual. Chicago: American Bar Association, 1991.

75. Ewigman, B., Kivlahan, C., and Land, G.: The Missouri child fatality study. *Pediatrics, al:* 330–337, 1993.

76. Plunkett, J.: Sudden death in an infant caused by rupture of a basilar artery aneurysm. *Am J Forensic Med Pathol, 20* (1): 45–47, 1999.

77. Prahlow, J.A., Rushing, E.J., and Barnard, J.J.: Death due to a ruptured berry aneurysm in a 3.5-year-old child. *Am J Forensic Med Pathol, 19:* 391–394, 1998.

78. Weissgold, D.J., Budenz, D.L., Hood, I., and Rorke, L.B.: Ruptured vascular malformation masquerading as battered/shaken baby syndrome: A nearly tragic mistake. *Surv Ophthalmol, 39:* 509–512, 1995.

79. Nyhan, W.L.: Abnormalities of fatty acid oxidation. *N Engl J Med, 319:* 1344–1346, 1988.

80. Bennett, M.J., Hale, D.E., Coates, P.M., et al.: Postmortem recognition of fatty acid oxidation disorders. *Pediatric Pathology, 11:* 365–370, 1991.

81. Byard, R.W., and Cohle, S.D.: *Sudden death in infancy, childhood, and adolescent.* Cambridge University Press, 1994.

82. Zinn, A.: Genetic disorders that mimic child abuse or sudden infant death syndrome. In Reece, R.M. (ed.), *Child abuse, medical diagnosis, and management.* Baltimore: Williams and Wilkins, 1996, pp. 404–429.

83. Stanley, C.A.: Disorders of mitochondrial fatty acid oxidation. In Behrman, R.E., Kliegman, R.M., and Jenson, H.B. (eds.), *Nelson textbook of pediatrics,* 16th ed., Philadelphia: W.B. Saunders, 2000; pp. 377–380.

84. McMillan, J.A., DeAngelis, C.D., Feigin, R.D., and Warshaw, J.B.: *Oski's pediatrics,* 3rd edition. Philadelphia: Lippincott Williams & Wilkins, 1999.

85. Harpey, J.P., Charpentier, C., Coude, M., et al.: Sudden infant death syndrome and multiple Acyl-Coenzyme A dehydrogenase deficiency. *J Pediatr, 110:* 881–884, 1987.

86. Rinaldo, P., O'Shea, J.J., Coates, P.M., et al.: Medium chain Acyl Co A dehydrogenase deficiency. *N Engl J Med, 319:* 1308–1310, 1988.

87. Ding, J.H., Roe, C.R., Iafolla, A.K., et al.: Medium chain acyl coenzyme A dehydrogenase deficiency and sudden infant death. *N Engl J Med, 325:* 61–62, 1991.

88. Rinaldo, P., Stanley, C.A., et al.: Sudden neonatal death in carnitine transporter deficiency. *J Pediatr, 131:* 304–305, 1997.

89. Spencer, J.A., and Grieve, D.K.: Congenital indifference to pain mistaken for non-accidental injury. The *British Journal of Radiology, 63:* 308–310, 1990.

90. Dehner, L.P.: *Pediatric surgical pathology,* 2nd ed. Baltimore: Williams and Wilkins, 1987, pp. 18–19, 946–947.

91. Knight, D.J., and Bennet, G.C.: Non-accidental injury in osteogenesis imperfecta. *J Ped Orthopaedics, 10:* 542–544, 1990.

92. Stewart, G.M., and Rosenberg, N.M.: Conditions mistaken for child abuse: Part I. *Pediatric Emergency Care, 12* (2); 116–121, 1996.

93. Behrman, R.E., Vaughn, V.C., III, and Nelson, W.E., (eds.): *Nelson textbook of pediatrics,* 14th ed. Philadelphia: W.B. Saunders, 1992, pp. 1275–1277.

94. Bays, J.: Conditions mistaken for child abuse. In Reece, R.M. (ed.), *Child abuse, medical diagnosis and management.* Williams and Wilkins, 1996, pp. 358–385.

95. Russo, S., Taff, M.L., Mirchandani, H.G., and Spitz, W.U.: Scald burns complicated by isopropyl intoxication. *Am J Forensic Med Pathol, 7:* 81–83, 1986.

96. Stocker, J.T., and Dehner, L.P.: *Pediatric pathology.* J.B. Lippincott, 1992, p. 982.

97. Hutchins, K.D., Dickson, D., et al.: Sudden death in a child due to an intrathoracic paraganglioma. *Am J Forensic Med Path, 20:* 338–342, 1999.

98. Meissner, C., Minnasch, P., et al: Sudden unexpected infant death due to fibroma of the heart. *J Forensic Sci, 45* (3):731–733, 2000.

99. Ruszkiewicz, A.R., and Vernon-Roberts, E.: Sudden death in an infant due to histiocytoid cardiomyopathy. *Am J Forensic Med Path, 16:* 74–80, 1995.

100. Little, D., and Wilkins, B.: Hemorrhagic shock and encephalopathy syndrome. *Am J Forensic Med Path, 18:* 79–83, 1997.

101. Kanthan, R., Moyana, T., and Nyssen, J.: Asplenia as a cause of sudden unexpected death in childhood. Am *J Forensic Med Path, 20:* 57–59, 1999.

102. Hermann, M.E., Mileusnic, D., et al.: Sudden death in an 8-week-old infant with Beckwith-Wiedemann syndrome. *Am J Forensic Med Path, 21:* 276–280, 2000.

103. Chhanabhai, M., Avis, S.P., and Hutton, C.J.: Congenital diaphragmatic hernia. *Am J Forensic Med Path, 16:* 27–29, 1995.

104. Byard, R.W.: Mechanisms of sudden death and autopsy findings in patients with Arnold-Chiari malformation and ventriculoatrial catheters. *Am J Forensic Med Path, 17:* 260–263, 1996.

105. Nields, H., Kessler, S., et al.: Steptococcal toxic shock syndrome presenting as suspected child abuse. *Am J Forensic Med Path, 19:* 93–97, 1998.

106. Herrmann, M.A., Doursa, M.K., and Edwards, W.D.: Sudden infant death with anomalous origin of the left coronary artery. *Am J Forensic Med Path, 13:* 191–195, 1992.

107. Lalu, K., Karhunen, P.J., and Rautiainen, P.: Sudden and unexpected death of a 6-month-old baby with silent heart failure due to anomalous origin of the left coronary artery from the pulmonary artery. *Am J Forensic Med Path, 13:* 196–198, 1992.

108. Wong, S.W., and Gardner, V.: Sudden death in children due to mesenteric defect and mesenteric cyst. *Am J Forensic Med Path, 13:* 214–216, 1992.

109. Lipsett, J., et al.: Anomalous coronary arteries: A multicenter pediatric autopsy study. *Pediatr Pathol, 14:* 287–300, 1994.

110. Perper, J.A., and Ahdab-Barmada, M.: Fatty liver, encephalopathy, and sudden unexpected death in early childhood due to medium-chain acyl-coenzyme A dehydrogenase deficiency. *Am J Forensic Med Path, 13:* 329–334, 1992.

111. Byard, R.W., and Moore, L.: Sudden and unexpected death in childhood due to a colloid cyst of the third ventricle. *J Forensic Sci, 38:* 210–213, 1993.

112. Prahlow, J.A., and Teot, L.A.: Histiocytoid cardiomyopathy: Case report and literature review. *J Forensic Sci, 38:* 1427–1435, 1993.

113. *Harrison's Principles of Internal Medicine,* 14th edition, editors, Anthony S. Fauci, et al. McGraw-Hill, 1998.

Chapter IX

TRAUMA AND DISEASE

Vernard I. Adams, Mark A. Flomenbaum, and Charles S. Hirsch

An important proportion of all deaths that occur following a traumatic episode will raise questions of interpretation of the cause of death because of the concurrent presence of a disease process. When trauma and disease are present simultaneously, the following questions can be anticipated: (a) Was the traumatic event wholly and solely responsible for the death? (b) Did the death result from the combined effects of trauma and disease? (c) Was the death in fact due solely to disease, and should the trauma be excluded as a factor in causation of the death?

The evaluation of deaths involving considerations of disease and injury requires the highest degree of analytical skill. It is appropriate, then, to place our discussion of medicolegal evaluations and the approach to case analysis within a chapter, the theme of which is the interaction of trauma and disease. Because the interaction of disease and injury in the dying process is expressed in terms of sequential and confluent chains of physiological events, the analysis of such cases requires a rigorous consideration of mechanisms of death, which in turn depends on evaluations of terminal circumstances and autopsy findings. Therefore, the discussions of mechanisms of death and the role of the autopsy in the overall investigation form the backbone of this chapter and are augmented by definitions and discussions of the concepts of cause and manner of death.

The cause-of-death opinion must be expressed in such a way that the public is served well and fairly. The consumers of such opinions comprise attorneys involved in criminal, probate, tort, and administrative proceedings; the vital statistics bureaus of the local, state and federal governments; the insurance industry; health care professionals and families of the deceased. Consequently, we have included discussions of death certificates, formation of and foundation for opinion, and the needs of some of the consumers.

MANNER OF DEATH

The need to assign responsibility for human deaths is without doubt older than history and has found expression in both religious and judicial language. From a religious perspective, deaths could be classified as acts of God, comprising deaths caused by natural disease and accidental violence, and acts of human beings, comprising suicide and homicides. This four-part classification scheme, minus the references to a supreme being, persists as the classification used for vital statistics registration in contemporary times. For modern administrative usage, the manners of death can be defined as follows:

Natural: Death caused *exclusively* by disease.

Accident: Death caused by violent means, not due to an intentional or criminal act by another person. Traffic fatalities are an exception to the latter part of our definition, because we classify them as accidents for vital statistical purposes regardless of the potential criminal responsibility that may arise from the incident.

Suicide: Death caused by an act of the decedent with the intent to kill himself.

Homicide: Death at the hand of another person. For practical purposes, we suggest that in most instances this can be refined to include

436

deaths due to the hostile or illegal act of another person.

The term *undetermined* is used when a reasonable classification cannot be made.

When medical examiners or coroners indicate a manner of death on a death certificate, they are not making a ruling despite what the press may report. They are merely rendering an opinion to the vital statistics bureaus of their jurisdictions as to how the death should be statistically coded by the bureau. A ruling may indeed emanate from a coroner's inquest, in those jurisdictions which have them, but it is not necessarily binding in the adjudication of civil or criminal matters. In other words, the determination of manner of death by a medical examiner is an administrative function.

Manner-of-death determination is not always a predictable, routine function. The definitions used above will generate a variety of usages, depending on how the words disease, violence and intentional act are defined. Some usages derive purely from long-established custom.

The following remarks and examples serve to further define and explain the process of determining manner of death.

Natural

Disease is considered to include chronic environmental insults such as habitual excessive ingestion of alcohol, inhalation of asbestos or chronic sequelae of drug abuse such as AIDS or endocarditis. Acute environmental insults are considered as being violent unless they represent infections by microorganisms. Thus, deaths due to alcoholic liver disease, asbestosis, mesothelioma and tuberculosis are natural. Envenomation by snakes and insects or an unintentional drug overdose are considered accidental. The impossibility of constructing a perfectly consistent manner-of-death classification is illustrated by acute ethanol intoxication. When such a fatality is a consequence of chronic alcoholism, the National Center for Health Statistics regards the intoxication as an acute exacerbation of a chronic disease and the death is classified as natural. When fatal acute ethanol intoxication is due to

experimental drinking by a teenager, it is accidental.[1]

Similarly, an acute dislocation of the spine is considered an injury, whereas degenerative changes resulting from a lifetime of mechanical wear and tear are considered to be disease. Haddon speculated that the apparent logical flaws in our current distinctions between *injury* and *disease* result from the words having been defined in a time when diseases were not understood, but acute injuries were clearly understood to be results of defined causes.[2]

Accident

This category excludes deaths in which there is an intent to do harm. Most non-traffic accidental fatalities result from human negligence, the elements, or natural disasters. A large proportion of accidental deaths in any western jurisdiction will be represented by road traffic fatalities. Only rarely is a motor vehicle used deliberately with the intent to do harm. When such usage results in death, the death is classified as a homicide or a suicide for vital statistics purposes. There are numerous traffic fatalities in which prosecutors bring charges of vehicular homicide against the responsible operator. This is most frequently done when the operator is chemically impaired or leaves the scene of an accident. Such deaths are still classified as accidents on death certificates. The common but erroneous practice of certifying these deaths as homicides is prematurely judgmental on the part of the medical examiner and results in the state registrar having to reclassify the manner of death for coding purposes.

Suicide

This is self-murder and requires a determination, with reasonable medical certainty, that the person's lethal act was intentionally inflicted. When suicide is strongly suspected, but reasonable certainty is absent, the death can be classified as manner *undetermined*. If suicide is merely a suspicion, the presumption favors classification as accident.

Homicide

In contrast to the category of suicide, the demonstration of intent to kill is not necessary for a determination of homicide. The certifier is not required to differentiate murder from manslaughter or justifiable homicide. With the possible exception of situations involving long guns used for hunting or any firearm used on a practice range, a determination of accident for a firearm death should be infrequent.

Complications of Therapy

Deaths due to a physician's act of omission are generally regarded as due to the underlying disease or trauma and are so classified. Deaths due to diagnostic maneuvers or therapy represent acts of commission and can pose some difficulty in classification. By convention, deaths caused by physicians are classified as homicides only if there is demonstrable intent to kill or if there is gross and wanton disregard for the safety of the patient. We use the following guidelines.

Generally, an untreated patient dies of complications of disease, whereas a treated patient dies of complications of disease, complications of therapy, or a combination of the two. In contemporary times, most ill persons seek treatment. Therefore, deaths due to complications of treatment are frequent and should not be automatically classified as unnatural deaths. If the risk of treatment is comparable to the risk of disease, the death is classified as natural. In other words, if the underlying disease has the potential to cause death, or if the therapeutic procedure is risky, with an anticipated fatal outcome in some instances, then the death is natural. For example, patients who undergo heart surgery and cannot be weaned from extracorporeal circulation are not rare. Certifying such deaths as anything other than natural does a disservice to competent thoracic surgeons.

If the risk of death is almost entirely attributable to the procedure, certification of the death as accidental or as a therapeutic complication may be warranted. For example, if a man with no cardiovascular or pulmonary disease suffers a fatal adverse reaction to general anesthesia for an elective inguinal herniorrhaphy, certification of the death *inguinal hernia, natural* raises more questions than it answers. In New York City, whose Health Department registrar permits the use of *therapeutic complication* as a manner of death, we would certify the manner as *therapeutic complication*.

If the death is entirely due to an obvious gross mishap, we use the term *accident*. For example, we would classify an intraoperative death due to perforation of a common iliac artery during a lumbar laminectomy as an accident.

The classification *therapeutic complication* as a manner of death is not accepted by most state registrars. In such jurisdictions, the choice of terms is between natural and accident. In choosing which term to use one must be careful not to imply the occurrence of malpractice when there is none, nor to give the appearance of covering up malpractice when it is obvious. In the hypothetical case of the adverse reaction to anesthesia cited above, we would certify the death as natural, if the choice of therapeutic complication were not an option. In this instance, the cause-of-death opinion tells the entire story. The *natural* certification will not hinder any action for malpractice, whereas an *accidental* certification might invite a suit where none had been contemplated. We wish to discourage the use of the term *therapeutic misadventure,* since it is inflammatory.

In any event, the state registrar of vital statistics will often ignore the certifier's manner of death and code the manner according to local practice, using the information supplied to the cause.

Intoxication by Drugs

In some medicolegal jurisdictions, deaths due to drug abuse are routinely certified as *unclassified*. The reasons given for such a practice are: (1) homicidal injection by another person cannot be excluded, (2) sale of a *hot* packet of drugs with the intent to kill cannot be excluded, and (3) suicide cannot be excluded, because chronic substance abusers are self-destructive. As nearly as we can determine, the practice of leaving the manner unclassified originated decades ago and was based more on the inability to quantitate blood morphine in that era.

We cannot endorse this practice for the following reasons: (1) Homicidal injection and homicide by sale of a *hot shot* are theoretical, speculative possibilities. In our experience, persons in the drug subculture are not subtle when they wish to kill; they use firearms, knives, or other more efficient lethal instruments to insure that their murderous intent is fulfilled. Furthermore, given the increasing purity of street drugs, the term *hot shot* has become increasingly meaningless. (2) In the absence of demonstrable suicidal intent, the presumption always favors accident in spite of voluntary indulgence in a self-destructive lifestyle. For example, we know of no medical examiner who advocates classifying the lung cancer deaths of cigarette smokers as suicides. Use of unclassified as the manner of death causes unnecessary delay and expense in settling insurance claims, because the insurer has no clue as to the manner of death. Therefore, we classify drug intoxications as suicide or homicide, when the evidence supports it, and as accident when there is no other history than chronic substance abuse.

Intentional Cessation of Life-Saving Therapy

All mentally competent adults have the right to refuse or discontinue medical treatment. We do not classify such deaths as suicides.

Manner of Death—Concluding Remarks

Because the manner of death as certified by the medical examiner or coroner is not binding on any party, one may reasonably ask why the medical examiner should bother to certify a manner at all. There are several practical benefits. First, the vital statistics registrar needs the information for coding purposes. As mentioned elsewhere in this chapter, the registrar may code a manner differently from the manner specified by the certifier, but this is rare when the medical examiner certifies according to the guidelines issued by the registrar.

Insurance companies, which are bound only by the language in their insurance policies, often rely on death certificate information for the numerous claims on policies whose values are too low to justify the expense of an independent investigation.

Police agencies and state attorneys often use the medical examiner's manner of death for internal administrative purposes. For instance, police departments often use the certification of natural causes, suicide and accident to close cases in which no arrest is made. District attorneys, even though they believe no indictment is warranted in a particular case, will often present to the grand jury any death certified as homicide by the medical examiner.

Interestingly, a medical examiner's classification of manner of death will usually not be made known to grand or trial juries, since, for purposes of criminal trials, the determination of manner of death is the province of the jury.

When the third edition of this book was published, objections to a manner of death certification came most often from families of suicides. The objection may be on the basis of the perceived stigma attached to suicidal deaths or on a financial basis. Many whole life insurance policies have a suicide exclusion clause which denies payment if suicide occurs in the first year or two of the policy. Many term life insurance policies never outlive a suicide exclusion clause.

With the recent popularity of inexpensive accidental life insurance policies, the most frequent objections now arise from certification of a natural manner of death for a decedent whose next-of-kin hold a term insurance policy that pays only for accidental death.

CAUSE OF DEATH

The term *cause of death* means different things to different people. For the purposes of forensic medicine, vital statistics and the law, the cause of death is the original underlying medical condition which *initiates* the lethal chain of events culminating in death.[3,4] In the absence of a wrongful death action, the legal synonym for *original,* as used above is *proximate.* However, attorneys customarily reserve the term *proximate cause of death* for a negligent act alleged to have caused or contributed to death. In a traffic fatality the underlying medical cause of death might be a laceration of the aorta, while the proximate cause of death in the eyes of the plaintiff attorney is negligent engineering design of a mechanical system. The medical condition, as used above, is a disease or an injury, not a complication or secondary physiological derangement. Diseases and injuries competent to be listed as proximate causes of death should be etiologically specific. Most are found in the *International Classification of Diseases.*[6]

Immediate causes of death are complications and sequelae of the underlying cause. There may be one or more immediate causes, and they may occur over a prolonged interval, but none absolves the underlying cause of its ultimate responsibility. When the interval between proximate cause and death is brief and there is a simple complication, the cause-and-effect linkage remains obvious. For example, a 30-year-old woman is rendered comatose by a head injury and dies four days later with bilateral confluent bronchopneumonia. Her bronchopneumonia is the immediate cause of death, and the proximate cause of death is the blunt impact to the head with brain contusions. When the interval increases and the complications multiply, there exists an opportunity to focus on the complications and lose sight of the proximate cause. For example, a 20-year-old man sustains an open comminuted

tibial fracture in a motorcycle accident. He develops chronic osteomyelitis with a draining sinus that persists for many years. Ultimately, a squamous cell carcinoma develops in the draining sinus, and he dies from metastatic squamous cell carcinoma. In spite of an interval of 20 years or more between injury and death, the fractured tibia sustained in the motorcycle accident is the proximate cause of death.

For administrative medicolegal purposes, we advocate strict linkage of proximate cause to a determination of manner of death, regardless of the practical consequences from a law enforcement or criminal justice perspective. For example, a 25-year-old man is rendered quadriplegic by a gunshot wound of the neck that perforates his vertebral column and spinal cord. Because of his spinal cord injury, over the next 15 years he develops chronic urinary cystitis and multiple episodes of pyelonephritis progressing to bilateral chronic pyelonephritis with renal insufficiency. Ultimately, he dies from urinary sepsis and renal failure. The gunshot wound is the proximate cause of death, and the manner of death is homicide. If the shooting occurred in a state that has a *year and a day rule,* the assailant could not be prosecuted for homicide. However, this prosecutorial stricture is irrelevant to a medicolegal determination of homicide. Likewise, police officers may be chagrined when they receive a report of a homicidal death stemming from a 15-year-old injury. The case may be impossible for them to investigate and will leave an unsolved homicide on their books. That statistical consequence cannot influence the judgment of the medical examiner, who is charged with the responsibility to determine the manner of death.

MECHANISM OF DEATH

In formulating a cause-of-death opinion, the medical examiner must consider plausible physiological chains of events which could connect the cause of death to the moment when vital functions cease and death occurs. In the parlance of medical death investigation, such physiological scenarios are *mechanisms.*[4] Although mecha-

nisms do not usually appear as part of the cause-of-death opinions rendered on death certificates or on autopsy reports, the formulation of mechanism-of-death opinions can be as important as the formulation of cause-of-death and manner-of-death opinions. It is only by considering plausible mechanisms of death that one places the causes of death in the context of time and sequence.

In some cases, the cause of death is not readily apparent but the mechanism is reasonably obvious. When the mechanism is known, it helps in determining the cause of death. In other instances, it is the mechanism that is inferred from the cause and circumstances. In either event, simultaneous consideration of cause and mechanism serves to improve the rigor of the mental processes involved in formulating opinions in the course of medicolegal death investigations.

In "Sudden and Unexpected Death due to Natural Causes in Adults," we discussed the heart and central nervous system as electrical entities, focused on the pertinent anatomy and physiology, and touched upon a few mechanisms of death for purposes of clarity. Natural mechanisms of death were discussed under pertinent disease headings. In the following section, we list and discuss physiologic derangements operative in both natural and violent deaths. In keeping with the purpose of this chapter, which is to clarify the potential relationships of the contributions of trauma and disease to individual deaths, we have organized the mechanisms by physical rather than physiological terms, and we have emphasized the mechanisms of violent deaths.

Electrical Disturbances of the Heart and Central Nervous System

The physiological derangements leading to death can be simple and few, or numerous, complex and sequential. The final, or occasionally the only, mechanism almost always involves malfunction of the electrochemical intercellular communications of the heart, central nervous system or both. Electrical irritability of the heart generates ventricular arrhythmia, and electrical irritability of the brain finds expression as seizures. Electrical depression of the heart, for example, by global hypoxia or the effects of drugs or vagotonicity, finds lethal expression as bradyrhythmias degenerating to idioventricular complexes without effective pump activity (electromechanical dissociation). Cerebral electrical depression, caused for example by cerebral hypoxia or

depressant drugs, leads to respiratory arrest. Virtually all the mechanisms that are discussed below find their final expression in electrical excitation or depression of the heart or central nervous system.

Exogenous Electrical Disturbances of the Heart and Nervous System

The physiological derangements caused by electrocution vary depending on the magnitude of electron flow, that is, the amperage, and on whether the system for distributing electricity uses alternating or direct current.[7] The heart is susceptible to the development of ventricular fibrillation when alternating current passes through it during the vulnerable phase of depolarization. Direct current and alternating current of high amperage produce tetany of skeletal muscles and the heart. Spontaneous resumption of sinus rhythm is possible after cessation of direct current electrocution.[8] Although the neural effects of electroconvulsive therapy are well known, the possible lethal effects of electrical current on the brain are poorly described in comparison to the cardiac effects.

Conversion of Impulsive Mechanical Energy (Impact) to Electrical Energy

With blunt impact to any part of the body, the transferred energy is conserved as mechanical energy to some degree, with the production of motion of the stricken member, and part of the transferred energy is absorbed as harmonic oscillations which are dampened out and converted to heat. A small part of the imparted kinetic energy may be converted to electrical impulses. The medical term for the functional consequence of this phenomenon is *concussion*. Concussion can involve the brain, spinal cord or heart, and it can be lethal. Cardiac concussion can induce immediately lethal ventricular fibrillation or asystole. Concussion of the brain or spinal cord can paralyze respiration or produce surges or autonomic current flow to the heart, with the same result. By definition, a concussion does not require demonstrable cerebral, spinal cord or cardiac pathology.

Evidence of blunt impacts to the head, internal derangements of the neck, or impacts to the chest are, however, helpful in deducing the occurrence of concussion.

Non-Impact Pressure Gradients in Vital Sensitive Areas

Subarachnoid hemorrhages so voluminous as to constitute hematomas can be produced by ruptured aneurysms of cerebral arteries or by blunt impact trauma. Ventricular cardiac arrhythmias have been clinically documented in surviving patients with ruptured cerebral aneurysms. Instantaneous death from subarachnoid hematomas most likely involves fatal autonomic discharge to the heart, induced by the bloody tamponade of the brain stem and hypothalamus. A plausible alternative mechanism which is not mutually exclusive involves spasm of the cerebral arteries serving the brain stem and hypothalamus. Those persons who do not experience instantaneous death can develop respiratory arrest from pressure on the brain stem.

Cardiac tamponade can be produced by cardiovascular trauma, dissecting aortic aneurysms and ruptured myocardial infarcts. The mechanism of death involves mechanical interference with the filling of the cardiac chambers, and thereby of forward circulation. Cardiac hypoxia develops concomitantly as effective central blood flow diminishes. Victims of cardiac tamponade often demonstrate bradyrhythmias with electromechanical dissociation now referred to as pulseless electrical activity, similar to the findings with thrombo- or air-embolism to the pulmonary circulation.

Another form of pressure gradient occurs with herniation of the brain, which accompanies the edematous swelling caused by brain tumors, strokes, contusions, and diffuse axonal damage from blunt impact. Before the era of mechanical ventilation, the mechanism of death was often failure of the medullary respiratory centers. When ventilation is maintained mechanically, these patients survive the risk of respiratory arrest but are then at risk of pneumonia, bleeding gastric stress ulcers, and cardiac arrest from cerebral hypertension involving the vasomotor centers.

Exogenous Chemical Interference with Electrochemical Cellular Communication

Ethanol can induce cardiac arrhythmias directly as a cardiac irritant. Various drugs interfere with synaptic transmission in autonomic ganglia or skeletal muscles. Curare, and its purified derivative D-tubocurarine, competitively block acetylcholine receptors in the neuromuscular end-plates of skeletal muscle and can produce diaphragmatic paralysis and hypoxic death in persons not mechanically ventilated.

Other drugs exert excitatory or depressant actions in the central nervous system. Central nervous excitation can induce lethal seizures. As examples, isoniazid, theophylline, and cocaine in toxic doses can induce seizures. Numerous neuroleptic drugs induce central nervous system depression, leading to diminished tidal volume and frequency, with the risk of pneumonia, or to complete respiratory arrest. Heroin is an example. Phenothiazines, tricyclic anti-depressants, monoamine oxidase inhibitors, anti-arrhythmic drugs and cocaine can induce lethal cardiac arrhythmias.

Thermal Disturbances of Physiology

Hyperthermia can occur with environmental exposure, malignant hyperthermia, neuroleptic malignant syndrome and as a complication of cocaine or phencyclidine intoxication. In the case of heat stroke with dehydration, the mechanism of death can involve cardiac arrhythmias, seizures or hypovolemic shock with tachycardia and eventual circulatory collapse. *Hypothermia* usually occurs with environmental exposure. The mechanism of death often involves depressed myocardial conduction, with the emergence of an ectopic pacemaker followed by ventricular fibrillation.

Obstruction or Diversion of Central Blood Circulation

Diversion of effective blood volume occurs with exsanguination, acute neurogenic shock and anaphylaxis. When one-third of the blood volume is lost rapidly, shock ensues. Death results from a rapid 50% blood loss, when physical failure to fill capacitance vessels and the aorta results in inadequate coronary perfusion.

Clinically, neurogenic shock can mimic exsanguination. In neurogenic shock, disordered agonal autonomic discharges result in redistribution of blood, possibly to the skeleton, leaving the capacitance vessels and the heart empty. At autopsy, the heart and great vessels are collapsed and nearly devoid of blood, the organs are pale and the musculature is not congested.[9] Neurogenic shock most often results from blunt impact to the head with concussion or mechanical injury somewhere between the third cerebral ventricle and the mid-cervical spinal cord.

Anaphylactic shock ensues when histamine released from mast cell degranulation results in a voluminous shift of fluid from plasma to extravascular interstitial tissues.

Obstruction of central blood circulation occurs with cardiac tamponade, cardiac thromboembolism, pulmonary thromboembolism, and venous (cardiac) air embolism. In these instances, venous blood is effectively dammed behind the heart, and little or no blood is propelled through the lungs to be oxygenated. The heart suffers hypoxia and, typically, a bradyrhythmia without a peripheral pulse then degenerates to an agonal idioventricular tracing. Obstruction to central circulation can also occur when the chest is severely compressed by external mechanical means.

Obstruction of Arterial Blood Supply to Heart and Central Nervous System

Coronary arterial flow can be obstructed not only by thrombi in cases of coronary atherosclerosis but by thromboemboli, in cases of endocarditis of the mitral or aortic valves, gas emboli in cases involving SCUBA diving or open heart surgery, and fat emboli in victims of blunt trauma. The resulting coronary insufficiency, regional myocardial ischemia and arrhythmias are similar to those observed with arteriosclerotic heart disease.

Identical thrombotic and embolic processes can involve the cerebral arteries. When the involved arteries are branches of the internal carotid, stroke is the usual outcome. When the involved vessel is a vertebral artery, not only stroke but sudden death from brain stem ischemia is possible.

External compression of the neck can obstruct carotid blood flow, leading to sudden death or cerebral infarction. Lesser degrees of compression can obstruct venous return, which in turn obstructs capillary flow and produces congestion and passive hyperemia in both the brain stem and cerebrum. The vertebral arteries are relatively protected from compression.

Mechanical Interference with Respiration

Mechanical interference with respiration can occur at any of several levels. Compression of the neck, as for example in strangulation or hanging, externally constricts the trachea or the larynx or simply pushes the tongue back so that it obstructs the pharynx. Mechanical occlusion of the nose and mouth, as in suffocation, can occur by the direct effect of a hand or tape or by the slower accumulation of saliva in a porous gag.

Postural asphyxia, known also as positional asphyxia, occurs when the head and neck are turned or situated so as to obstruct the upper airway, and the reflex drive to right the head is dulled by intoxication, concussion, or neurologic disease.

External compression of the chest, termed *pressing* by seventeenth century Salem jurists, is called traumatic asphyxia by forensic pathologists when ventilation is lethally prevented. This usually occurs with industrial accidents or with shade-tree mechanics whose portable automobile jacks fail.

Internal occlusion of the airways, that is, choking, can be caused by inhaled foreign bodies or food. An expression of caution is in order concerning the overdiagnosis of choking on food and the incomplete evaluation of death due to aspiration of food. A neurologically intact, sober adult is at no appreciable risk of choking on a bolus of food. Such accidental deaths occur in persons who are intoxicated or who have a variety of neurological disorders that impair their gagging, choking, and swallowing reflexes. Some psychiatric patients have a tendency to rapidly ingest unmasticated food or foreign bodies and to choke in the process. Absent any of the foregoing abnormalities or an intoxication, it is rare for an adult to choke to death. Therefore, in the evaluation of a fatality due to choking, the pathologist should always consider the choking as no more than the immediate cause of death and operate under the assumption that the case study is incomplete until the underlying cause of death is identified.

Precisely the same reasoning extends to the evaluation of aspiration pneumonia; it always requires an underlying explanation. Experienced medical examiners rarely accept at face value a clinical diagnosis of aspiration as an immediate cause of death, because such clinical diagnoses are usually incorrect. All too often a treating physician fails to identify as an agonal phenomenon the regurgitation and aspiration of vomitus in a person dying from heart disease, abnormalities of the central nervous system, or an intoxication. Such persons do not die from aspiration of vomitus; they aspirate vomitus because they are dying. Furthermore, the pathologist must not overinterpret the peripheral location of foreign material in the lungs as an indication of forceful and clinically meaningful aspiration of vomitus. Once vomitus makes its way into the larynx or trachea, attempted resuscitation can move the material deep into the lungs. If artificial ventilation is sufficiently forceful to expand the lungs, it also can move meat and potatoes to the peripheral airways.

Pneumothorax kills by preventing oxygenation of blood flowing through the lung on the affected side. The hypoxemia produced by the resulting shunt may be tolerated briefly by a young person with a healthy heart, or not at all by an elderly person or someone with a diseased heart. Pneumothoraces are sometimes occasioned by subclavian catheterization, traumatic intubation, high ventilation pressures, lacerations of lungs, and spontaneous rupture of subpleural blebs.

Flail chest results when rib and sternal fractures are numerous enough to permit a portion of the thoracic cage to move paradoxically inward with inspiration, thus preventing the development of adequate intrathoracic negative inspiratory pressures. Hypoxemia ensues.

Flail diaphragm is more properly described as pleuroperitoneal fistula and is the condition in which a defect of the diaphragm permits communication between a pleural space and the peritoneal space. It is sometimes accompanied by herniation of abdominal viscera into the chest. Such diaphragmatic hernias can cause pulmonary atelectasis.

Inhalation of a small amount of liquid is termed aspiration. Pool water, beverages, vomitus and blood from airway trauma can all be inhaled. Agonal vomit fouling is discussed above. Deleterious effects, when present, are due to chemical irritation more than to occlusion. Inhalation of a medium consisting only of liquid occurs during submersion; drowning is discussed in detail elsewhere in this book.

In all of the foregoing forms of respiratory impairment, hypoxemia is the common mechanism, although other mechanisms may be operative.

Chemical Interference with Oxygen Metabolism

The simplest form of chemical interference with oxygen metabolism is depletion of oxygen from the inspired gas mixture. This can occur in pilots at high altitude without supplemental oxygen, in SCUBA divers who use old tanks which consume oxygen by incorporating it into rust, and in SCUBA divers and anesthetized patients who are victims of wrongly filled or labeled tanks.

Caves and manholes can have unacceptably low oxygen pressures, owing to displacement by carbon dioxide and other gaseous products of plant metabolism or decomposition. Drowning involves breathing an oxygen-poor medium.

Carbon monoxide reversibly binds to hemoglobin and is discussed elsewhere. Cyanide poisons the mitochondrial cytochromes and is discussed elsewhere as well.

Shock

Neurogenic, hypovolemic and anaphylactic shock are mentioned above. Septic shock produces leaky capillaries and pre-capillary arterioles as well as depressed myocardial contractility. In refractory septic shock, administered intravenous fluids are in essence pumped by the heart into extravascular spaces, so that patients maintained with pressor therapy can develop striking body edema. Shock following generalized hypoxemia, now frequently seen in persons resuscitated from cardiac arrest, shares some similarities with septic shock. The common feature of all forms of shock is inadequate functional tissue perfusion, usually manifested by arterial hypotension.

Effects of Resuscitation

In the process of analyzing the mechanisms operative in a death involving attempted resuscitation, one must decide whether the operative mechanisms are relevant to the dying process, to the resuscitation effort, or to both. For instance, the finding of an endotracheal tube in the esophagus is of no medical import in a victim of atlanto-occipital dislocation who experiences instantaneous death. Similarly, the presence of tension pneumothoraces in a person with a lacerated thoracic aorta is relevant to the efficiency of artificial ventilation but represents a postmortem phenomenon with no bearing on the mechanism of death. In making these kinds of analyses, autopsy-derived information must be correlated with sequential, time-based data available from rescue personnel. Such data must be pursued vigorously, since memories fade rapidly, and the written reports filed by rescue personnel contain information mainly of administrative interest to the ambulance company.

A 74-year-old woman with hypertension left her restaurant table. Shortly thereafter, she was found without vital signs at the bottom of the stairs leading to the restroom. The autopsy revealed a scalp laceration and internal derangement of the C1-C2 cervical articulation, with fracture of the dens and softening of the spinal cord. The heart was not hypertrophied but had a 90% obstruction of the anterior descending artery and calcification of the mitral annulus. Since both heart disease and high neck injury can result in instantaneous death, follow-up investigation was requested. A witness was found who had observed the decedent slump at the top of the stairs and fall unconscious. Based on the implicit probability that the collapse at the top of the stairs was due to an irreversible ventricular arrhythmia, death was certified as being due to atherosclerotic heart disease. An alternative but unlikely mechanism, reversible cardiac syncope followed by lethal neck trauma, would result in a violent cause-of-death opinion.

A 28-year-old woman was a passenger in an automobile involved in a frontal crash. Fourteen minutes after the crash, rescue workers found her without vital signs in the rear passenger area. Resuscitation efforts were fruitless and she was pronounced dead at the hospital. The autopsy revealed a non-displaced frontal sinus fracture, a few rib fractures with parietal pleural lacerations and a 100 mL hemothorax, pulmonary contusions, subcapsular liver hematomas, and a splenic laceration with a 550 mL hemoperitoneum. The brain had no contusions, and there was no neck injury. The conjunctivae had petechiae and a column of edema froth filled the airways. Her mechanical injuries were insufficient to explain the loss of vital signs in less than 14 minutes.

The fireman who was the first to respond was questioned. He stated that the decedent was found with her legs and buttocks in the rear seat. Her upper torso and head were on the floor pan. The front and rear seats were jammed close together, causing the head to be angulated toward the chest. The cause of death was then listed as concussion and postural asphyxia due to blunt impact to the head.

THE ROLE OF THE AUTOPSY IN THE FORMULATION OF CAUSE-OF-DEATH OPINIONS

The pathologist who searches for recent pathological alterations to explain every death is doomed to failure. An insistence on an *anatomic cause of death* is the hallmark of a pathologist who thinks exclusively as a morphologist and not as a physician. To reiterate the discussion in "Sudden and Unexpected Death due to Natural Causes," death is a functional event, not an anatomical event. A misconception prevalent outside the medical community, and surprisingly common within the medical community, is the notion that the cause of death is always revealed by structural changes detected at autopsy. This view was held by nineteenth century European pathologists, who believed that they could accurately divine antemortem physiological events by interpreting autopsy observations in a vacuum. The notion has been propagated by subsequent generations of disciples and trainees.

Using this system to its perverse extreme, a pathologist, unburdened by background information of any sort, performs an autopsy. If he finds an anatomic lesion which is sufficient in his mind to cause death, he opines that the lesion is the cause of death, if no evidence to the contrary is provided. The fallacy of this system is illustrated by the following hypothetical cases, which have identical autopsy findings but different circumstances and histories.

Assume that the autopsy reveals arteriosclerotic heart disease with high-grade obstructive coronary atheromas in multiple epicardial arteries, no coronary thrombi, no marks of injury, and congestion of organs. Without knowledge of the circumstances and with no background information, the pathologist with a morphological orientation opines that death was caused by arteriosclerotic heart disease and speculates that the lethal mechanism was coronary spasm with regional ventricular ischemia and ventricular fibrillation. The fallacy of this approach is evident when one considers that *all four of the following histories fit the foregoing autopsy findings.*

Scenario A. A 65-year-old man has a failing business, expresses the wish to die in order to solve his problems, and walks into the ocean. His body is found hours later.

Scenario B. A 65-year-old locksmith, while drilling holes for locks in a wet basement, suddenly screams. He puts the drill down, walks to the far side of the basement, and collapses without vital signs, 20 feet from the drill.

Scenario C. A 65-year-old jeweler has been recently widowed. He tells his children that life isn't worth living any more. He is found dead in his easy chair with a glass containing a residue of a colored beverage nearby.

Scenario D. A 65-year-old man collapses lifeless in the bathroom 30 minutes after transplanting a rose bush.

The last example is the only one of the four in which the morphology-oriented pathologist would be correct.

The death in Scenario A is a suicidal drowning. Drowning is a functional event and leaves no specific autopsy findings.

The death in Scenario B is an electrocution. One hundred ten volt electrocution leaves electrical burns only if the resistance of the skin is high enough that heat sufficient to burn is generated.

Jewelers routinely use cyanide to clean jewelry and are knowledgeable concerning its poisonous effects. Therefore, in Scenario C, the presumption initially favors cyanide poisoning.

The correct approach to evaluating deaths will have a familiar ring to all physicians. In clinical medicine, it is axiomatic that the physician first takes a history, then performs a physical examination, and lastly orders laboratory tests. During this sequence, the physician is forming hypotheses, testing them, refining them and rejecting some of them. The physical examination is focused to confirm or refute hypotheses developed during the taking of the history. The laboratory tests are selected to confirm or refute hypotheses still under consideration at the conclusion of the physical examination.

The mental processes involved in correctly determining the cause of death are identical. The autopsy in reality is a battery of laboratory tests which must be interpreted in the light of historical information.

A good medical examiner first considers the medical history, social history, and terminal circumstances and then forms hypotheses.[10] If no single hypothesis is particularly supported by the background information, more information is probably required. At some point, enough information is available to perform an autopsy that focuses on the questions that need to be answered. At the conclusion of the autopsy, one hypothesis may be confirmed and an opinion is issued. Or, the hypotheses may be refuted, in which case further background information or further autopsy studies may be necessary. At all times, there is a dynamic feedback loop in which historical information is tested against the autopsy, and autopsy findings are evaluated in light of historical information. The operational evidence of this mental feedback loop is the presence of the medical examiner at the death scene investigation and the presence of the detective at the autopsy.

We will apply this approach to the four hypothetical scenarios. In Scenario A, the leading hypothesis is suicidal drowning. The investigation should focus on evaluating other possible risk factors for drowning such as high surf, treacherous currents, cold water temperature, and inability to swim. The autopsy is expected to show any age-related diseases with which the subject was co-existing and the non-specific changes associated with submersion. After these inquiries, if no alternative hypotheses arise, the original hypothesis acquires a sufficient degree of probability to become opinion.

In Scenario B, the investigational hypothesis was electrocution. In this case, the important autopsy is the one conducted on the drill, which is expected to show a current leakage into the casing. The autopsy on the decedent is expected to show any pre-existing disease. The likelihood of finding electrical burns is approximately 50%. In other words, the autopsy on the decedent is not a good laboratory test for low voltage electrocution.

Scenario C involves a depressed jeweler. The scene investigation should focus on impounding the beverage container for later toxicological testing and a search for a can of cyanide eggs on the premises. At the autopsy, the information most pivotal to further directing the investigation will be yielded by summoning a person from the office staff who is known to be able to smell cyanide vapor. The autopsy may or may not show oral or gastric mucosal burns and may show pink livor mortis.

The man in Scenario D died in a setting which strongly suggested sudden ventricular fibrillation due to natural cardiac disease. If the man died at home in the presence of his family, the likelihood of a natural death is so overwhelming that many jurisdictions would forego the autopsy. If the man was on the job as an employee of a landscaping contractor, an autopsy may be done to answer anticipated later questions with more certainty.

In only a small minority of death investigations do the autopsy findings alone provide the necessary foundation for a cause-of-death opinion. This small group of fatalities is distinguished by the fact that the mechanism of death is structurally demonstrable. For example, exsanguination or hemopericardium with tamponade leaves no room for doubt.

In contrast, the majority of death investigations involve lethal mechanisms which are func-

tional derangements and which are not structurally demonstrable. In these instances, the degree of certainty with which the pathological findings translate into a cause of death depends on the nature of the available background information. For example, in Scenario D, ventricular fibrillation can be inferred from the totality of the case information but not from the autopsy alone.

In other instances, the positive autopsy findings do not translate into cause-of-death opinions but served only to exclude possible scenarios in which the opinion rests on circumstantial, historical or non-autopsy laboratory data. Scenarios A, B, and C, described above, illustrate this group of deaths.

To formulate the concepts involved in using autopsy observations as part of the foundation for cause-of-death opinions, we use the following five-part classification of autopsy findings.[11] In classes I, II, and III, the autopsy findings are inclusionary, with the greatest inclusionary value being in class I and the least in class III. In classes III, IV, and V, the autopsy findings are exclusionary, and are solely exclusionary in classes IV and V.

CLASS I. The autopsy findings are inconsistent with continued life and were not produced by resuscitation efforts. Therefore, the cause of death is identified by pathological findings with absolute certainty. Class I fatalities are those in which the lethal mechanism is structurally demonstrable or inferred irrefutably. In medicolegal autopsies on persons who die from natural causes, a small minority, approximately 5% of cases, fall into this class. Most of them result from ruptured myocardial infarcts, ruptured aneurysms, obstructive intracardiac or pulmonary thromboemboli, and lesions of the brain stem. Typical hypertensive spontaneous intracerebral hemorrhages fall into class I, but atypically located intracerebral hemorrhages in non-hypertensive persons, such as those produced by cocaine intoxication, would not fall into class I.

Before moving to class II, we must emphasize again that only approximately 5% of natural deaths in a medicolegal autopsy population will have class I findings. Consequently, in approximately 95% of deaths due to disease, the pathologist must consider non-autopsy information in the medicolegal evaluation of the fatalities.

CLASS II. In natural deaths, this class is defined by the presence of a disease with lethal potential, sufficiently advanced that any competent pathologist will recognize the findings as capable of causing the death. However, the absence of complications that promote the pathological findings to class I requires that the pathologist take into consideration the history, the circumstances surrounding the death and often the toxicological data before reaching a conclusion about the cause of death. The large majority of natural deaths in medicolegal autopsies are class II fatalities.

The violent counterpart of class II is best exemplified by deaths due to various forms of cervical compression, in which the compressive agent has been removed by the assailant. For example, in deaths due to manual and ligature strangulation and other forms of external compression of the neck, at autopsy one can demonstrate neither an interference with cerebral circulation by compression of arteries or veins in the neck nor airway obstruction. The possibility of a lethal mechanism mediated by carotid sinus stimulation from cervical compression usually is impossible to prove and difficult to exclude. Therefore, the autopsy evaluation of deaths due to cervical compression is far more difficult than the interpretation of findings in a person who sustains a knife through the heart or a bullet through the brain.

CLASS III. In natural deaths, this class is defined as marginal pathology, ordinarily regarded as insufficient to cause death, combined with a compelling history and the exclusion of other causes. For example, a customarily sedentary, 50-year-old man is witnessed to drop dead after running one mile in an attempt at physical conditioning. The autopsy discloses atheromas in his coronary arteries with no focus of more than 60% luminal stenosis, a normal weight heart, moderate obesity, and no other functionally important abnormality. Toxicological testing is negative. Histopathological study of the heart, including the conducting system, fails to reveal myocarditis or any other pathological change.

Most pathologists would be reluctant to attribute death to the moderate coronary atherosclerosis described in this example. However, the autopsy exclusion of other causes and the witnessed sudden death under natural circumstances lead to the conclusion that a ventricular arrhythmia was the fatal mechanism. The negative anatomical and toxicological studies clearly focus responsibility for his death on the cardiac disease, with unaccustomed physical exertion as the lethal trigger, that is, the operative transient risk factor.

The importance of class III lies in the conceptual model, not in the number of deaths involved, because class III fatalities are infrequent. This class exemplifies the potential for dominance of history and circumstances over pathological findings. In the preceding example, moderate coronary atherosclerosis, in the face of unaccustomed physical exertion, was the most reasonable conclusion as to the cause of death. In contrast, similar or more advanced coronary atherosclerosis is seen commonly as an incidental finding in many persons who die from causes unrelated to heart disease. Pathologists will be comfortable with the class III model only when they see the autopsy as part of an entire case study and not as a substitute for a competent investigation.

CLASS IV. This class of deaths is defined as a lethal lesion which is not structurally demonstrable. The diagnosis is made on the basis of history and the exclusion of other causes. Epilepsy is the most frequent disease in this class, and low-voltage electrocution is a frequent injury responsible for violent deaths in this class. The autopsy serves to exclude reasonably possible alternatives. Paradoxical as it may seem, the autopsy, by revealing nothing else, raises the degree of certainty.

CLASS V. This class comprises deaths in which the cause of death is undetermined following investigation, autopsy and toxicological examination. The importance of this class lies in the recognition of its existence, not in the number of instances encountered.

The proportion of autopsies in which the cause of death eludes detection is determined by the efficiency of case investigation, the skill of the pathologist, the expertise of support in the toxicology laboratory, the selection of cases for autopsy, and the inclusion or exclusion of sudden infant death syndrome fatalities in the statistics on undetermined cause of death. Changes in these variables will alter the proportion of undetermined causes but will not eliminate this class entirely. Stated another way, excellent pathologists working in an optimal medicolegal environment with superb investigators and supported by state-of-the-art toxicological services will occasionally encounter cases in which their collective best efforts fail to identify the cause of death.

This class of deaths is neither more nor less than a recognition of the limitations of our science and the inability of morphologic and toxicologic studies to demonstrate functional derangements. The pathologist should bear in mind that a class V autopsy is not a wasted effort. Even in these frustrating instances, the negative anatomical and chemical examinations have considerable value in excluding injuries or poisons that may have been alleged to have caused or played some part in the death. The possible presence and participation of infectious, cancerous, occupational, and other diseases are also eliminated from consideration. The result is that although the pathologist cannot establish the cause of death, he can rule out many possibilities that have been conjectured erroneously as having some role in the death.

What constitutes a complete autopsy? In many pathology training programs, a complete autopsy is administratively defined as one in which microscopic slides are prepared from a prescribed number of organs. This definition may be useful for internal administrative purposes in training programs, but it is inadequate for autopsies in the public arena. The best contemporary definition of a complete autopsy is an autopsy which answers all the anticipated later questions. The ability to anticipate later questions depends on past experience and training. With this definition, equally complete autopsies may vary greatly in extent. As a minimum standard, it can be stated that an autopsy that does not include gross examination of the cranial contents, neck, chest, and abdominal and pelvic organs is inadequate

for medicolegal work. For example, sudden unexpected deaths due to ruptured cerebral aneurysms or due to choking on food may present in exactly the same manner as deaths due to arteriosclerotic heart disease. The finding, early in an autopsy, of severe arteriosclerotic heart disease does not warrant concluding that the subject was immune to cerebral aneurysms or choking and is therefore not an acceptable reason to omit the examination of the head and neck. A class II diagnosis in the chest does not rule out a class I diagnosis in the head.

The Death Certificate

The death certificate is one of several government documents which record changes in the civil status of citizens. Births, marriages, stillbirths and deaths are recorded by several levels of government. Death certificates are first filed with either a town or county official, depending upon the custom of each state. That official usually carries the title of clerk or registrar. Local officials then file the certificates with a state agency responsible for compilation of vital statistics and maintenance of vital records. Statistical summaries and much of the information on individual certificates are forwarded to federal health agencies.

The oldest tradition of governmental vital record keeping in the world is in the Commonwealth of Massachusetts, where the colonial laws have required the town clerks to maintain records since 1639. The anti-ecclesiastical Puritan colonists had been previously accustomed in England to a requirement dating back to 1538 that parish clergy maintain records of christenings, marriages and burials. Secondary compilation at the state level began in 1841, again in Massachusetts.[11]

Birth, marriage, and death certificates identify a citizen not only by date of birth and address but also by place of birth and parents' name. Parents' occupations are listed on birth certificates and the occupation of the decedent is on the death certificate. The linkage to parents' and spouses' records and to prior civil records of the citizen permits tracing of records for legal or genealogical purposes. All three types of certificates are filed by persons who are not generally government officials but who are professionally licensed by the state. These *de facto* agents of the town and state comprise physicians in the case of birth, stillborn and death certificates; the clergy and the judiciary in the case of marriage certificates; and funeral directors in the case of death certificates. Identifying information on birth, marriage and death certificates is respectively provided by parents, the subjects themselves, and a person designated on the certificate as an informant, who is usually the person contracting with the funeral director.

The death certificate differs from birth and marriage certificates in three important respects. It records a *cause* for the change in civil status, it records a *manner* of death, and it is always put to an *immediate non-archival use.* The non-archival function of the death certificate is to generate or to directly function as a burial permit. Without a burial permit, a body cannot be legally disposed of by burial, cremation, or shipment out of state.

Individual death certificates are used by numerous individuals and agencies. Genealogists, probate lawyers, issuers of burial permits, cemeteries and crematories are primarily concerned with three items: the fact that death occurred, the date the death occurred and the identity of the deceased. Insurance companies and workmen's compensation boards are additionally interested in the manner and to a lesser extent the cause of death. The most important item on a death certificate is the simple fact that the death has occurred, thereby altering the civil status of the person.

In the small print above the physician's signature, most death certificates indicate that the cause and manner of death are *opinions* when certification is by a medical examiner or coroner. In the case of private attending physicians a lesser degree of certainty is required; the operative phrase is *to the best of my knowledge* rather than *in my opinion.*

No insurance company, religious authority, state's or district attorney, judge, jury or individual party is bound by the opinions expressed on the death certificate. The registrar of vital statistics in most states is empowered to enter causes and manners of death under his or her own authority and to exercise editorial discretion in the process of coding causes and manners. As a matter of routine practice, when a medical examiner office functions with a reputation for consistency, reliability and competence, insurance companies, district attorneys and police investigators will generally rely heavily on the medical examiner's opinion.

A death certificate can be issued without listing a cause or manner, provided that a final certificate is later filed listing a cause and manner. With this procedure, the initial certificate, listing the cause and manner as pending further study, functions as or generates a burial permit without delay.

The formats for the death certificates used in the 50 states are based on recommendations from the federal government, first promulgated in 1900 by the Census Office, and later by the National Vital Statistics Division of the Public Health Service, Department of Health, Education and Welfare.[12,13] The federal guidelines in turn have been based on recommendations from an international conference of persons concerned with public health, medical demography and vital statistics, which meets every ten years. It was not until 1948 that a satisfactory statistical definition of the cause of death evolved. Prior to that time, registrars confronted by a multiplicity of diseases on a certificate used confusing and contradictory rules to select the one disease to be coded as the cause of death. In 1948, the Sixth Decennial International Revision Conference agreed that vital statisticians should code the *underlying* cause of death. This was defined as: *(a) the disease or injury which initiated the train of morbid events leading directly to death, or (b) the circumstances of the accident or violence which produced the fatal injury.* The conference went on to design the modern death certificate format, which for the first time required separate entries for cause, manner and circumstances of death, and on which the condition to be coded was always the bottom entry in Part 1.[3]

With this format, the physician is allowed four spaces for the cause-of-death opinion. Three of the spaces, designated as Part 1, are allotted for the primary cause of death. Only one, the top space, line 1a, need to be used. The lower two, lines 1b and 1c, are available for causes which must be described as a logical chain of events and are preceded by the connecting words *due to or as a consequence of.* Part 2 is the fourth space and is for diseases or injuries which significantly contribute to death but are not complications of, causes of, or related to the cause listed in Part 1.

The manner of death must be specified as natural, accident, suicide, homicide or undetermined. Some jurisdictions permit the use of *therapeutic complication* as the manner of death in fatalities due to complications of diagnostic and therapeutic procedures. There is no need for mixed manners of death, such as *natural-accident* in an elderly person with serious chronic disease and a fractured femur. *The presence of an injury dominates the manner-of-death determination.* Deaths are classified as natural when they are caused exclusively by disease. If an injury of any sort causes or contributes to death, the manner of death cannot be natural. It makes no difference whether the injury is listed in Part 1 or Part 2 of the death certificate; the listing of an injury anywhere on a death certificate precludes classification of the death as natural.

In cases where the manner of death is other than natural, the certificate requires a simple explanation of circumstances. In some instances, the circumstantial summary is necessary to make sense of the cause and manner of death. For instance, *blunt impact head trauma* as a cause, coupled with *accident* as a manner, requires an explanation of how the injury occurred, for example, *passenger in a single auto crash.* In other cases, for example, *gunshot wound of head; suicide,* the entry *deceased shot himself* merely states explicitly what is implicit in the cause and manner. Accompanying the space for the description of circumstances are spaces to list the date, time, place and location where the injury was sustained and a check-off box to indicate whether or not the injury was sustained at work. Since the injury often occurs at a time and place different from the time and place of death, these entries permit a researcher to find investigative reports from police agencies distant from the place of death.

In our experience, the rigidity of the format promotes brevity and clarity of thinking and reduces extraneous verbiage. We offer the following additional guidelines for using the death certificate format as an instrument of communication to maximum effect.

1. Because only one underlying cause of death is allowed in Part 1, which has three lines, but any number of conditions can be listed in the one space allotted for Part 2, the format might at first glance seem unduly cramped. Unused spaces on the physician's part of the certificate can be borrowed to accommodate entries too long for the designated box. For example, if Part 1 has an entry only in line 1a, the headings for lines 1b and 1c can be stricken out to accommodate a wordy entry in Part 2 or a necessarily lengthy description of how the injury occurred.

2. Part 2 should be used sparingly. Part 2 should list only those conditions which make a physiological contribution to death, and it should never serve as a repository for fascinating or medically interesting findings which do not contribute to death. We particularly discourage the routine listing in Part 2 of any malignancy discovered at autopsy, unless the tumor contributed to death. Such a practice is misleading for vital statistical purposes, and it can result in the denial of accidental death benefits to a deserving family when an insurance policy requires that an injury be the sole and only cause of death in order to qualify for payment.

3. If available information is sparse but not so meager that an *undetermined* cause of death is in order, the term *probable* can be used before the cause-of-death opinion to convey the idea that the degree of certainty is not great, and the opinion can be changed by information made available in the future.

4. There is no way to specify whether a Part 2 entry is of major or minor contributory importance. Prosecuting attorneys and criminal defense lawyers tend to regard Part 2 as being of minor importance, whereas insurance companies will magnify the importance of any entry in Part 2 which will reduce the payout to insured individuals.

Thus, for example, in the case of a homicide in which stab wounds and strangulation both contributed in a major way to the lethal train of events, or in which we wanted to reserve our opinion as to which cause was major and which was minor, we would place both on line 1a. This represents a deliberate misobservance of the rule which permits only one underlying cause to be entered in Part 1. We justify this type of certification on two grounds. First, the needs of the vital statistics bureau must be subordinate to the needs of the criminal justice system. Second, prudent forensic practice dictates that the wording of the cause-of-death opinion on the autopsy report and the certificate should be identical.

5. Cause-of-death opinions should never be restricted to anatomic diagnoses. Furthermore, when diagnoses not derived from the autopsy are used, it is not only unnecessary but bad practice to use modifiers such as *clinical* or *anamnestic* on the certificate, although the same terms will probably appear on the list of diagnoses in the corresponding autopsy report.

6. Mechanisms of death should be used sparingly in the cause-of-death section. Their use will usually be for the purpose of improving communication to the user agencies other than the vital statistics bureaus and to individuals. Thus, in the case of an elderly person who sustains pelvic fractures and no other important injuries in a traffic accident, the certificate might appropriately read: Pelvic fractures with hemorrhage due to blunt impact on torso.

The use of *pelvic fractures* alone would tend to leave the reader wondering why the person died.

Opinion, Probability, Possibility, and Speculation

In medicine, absolute diagnostic certainty is the exception rather than the rule. Proof *beyond a shadow of a doubt* is a concept derived from written and televised fiction dealing with the law. In reality, the law demands lesser degrees of proof. In criminal proceedings, conclusions are based on a reasonable degree of certainty. In other words, the conclusion is beyond any *reasonable* doubt. This is the highest degree of certainty demanded of physicians testifying as expert witnesses in court. The operative term is *reasonable degree of medical certainty.*

Rather than dealing in possibilities and certainties, the medical examiner deals with probabilities. There are several degrees of probability. The highest level of probability is absolute certainty or certainty beyond a possible doubt, where the likelihood is 100%. In order to render an opinion with certainty beyond a possible doubt, one must hold that every other imaginable contingency is impossible.

Next is a reasonable degree of certainty. *Reasonable degree* has no numerical probability definition, except that it far exceeds 50%. Reasonable certainty is that degree of assurance that a reasonable person relies upon in his most important business. For instance, the operation of a motor vehicle on the streets and highways entails a real risk of crash, but the risk is usually so small that the driver is reasonably certain that he will not crash. The same person might avoid driving during a hurricane, because he would not be reasonably certain of safe passage.

The next highest degree of certainty is a *preponderance of evidence.* This is the standard used in civil court proceedings. It essentially means *more likely than not,* and permits reasonable doubts. *More likely than not* may be defined as *probable,* or having a likelihood exceeding 50%. This is the standard required by vital statistics bureaus for opinions expressed on death certificates. Any contingency having a greater than 50% likelihood is probable because no other contingency can have as great a likelihood. Physicians must understand that the statistical definition of *probable* used in medical research applies only to data numerous enough to permit statistical analysis. A p value of less than .05 or .03 merely indicates that the likelihood of a difference between two data sets being due to chance is 5% or 3%. This is an incorrect and inappropriate standard to require when rendering a medicolegal opinion in a single death, because a single datum is not amenable to statistical analysis.

The knowledge that their opinions will be used in legal forums requiring a higher degree of certainty than probable causes most medical examiners to use a higher degree from the outset on death certificates for homicides, suicides and negligent accidents. The higher standard may be met by requiring a greater factual data base or by using brevity and broadly defined terms in their opinions.

Probabilities of less than 50% fall into one of two categories. Reasonable possibilities have a probability of less than 50% and may be discussed in courtroom proceedings. Speculation involves possibilities which are so remote that they have no basis in reason. Speculation is not permitted in most criminal proceedings. When an attorney asks if something is conceivable or possible, one may answer *yes* if it is a reasonable possibility. If it is not a reasonable possibility, one can so answer and then decline to speculate. To say that something is possible or conceivable means only that the hypothesis does not defy the laws of nature; such a standard has negligible evidential importance.

Quasi-judicial proceedings, such as workmen's compensation hearings, may not require even the degree of certainty required in civil court. The establishment of a reasonable possibility may be sufficient for such proceedings, in which the presumption ordinarily favors the worker.

In summary, the degree of certainty required for a medical opinion depends on the foreseeable actions and claims that will rest on those opinions. Criminal prosecutions require reasonable medical certainty; therefore, demonstration of a reasonable doubt is all that is required to avoid a criminal conviction. Various civil actions require proof by the lesser certainty of preponderance of the evidence.

Medical opinions are conclusions based on facts. Some facts, such as gross or microscopic autopsy findings, generally do not change. Other facts, especially those derived from witness accounts, do change. Opinions are based on the facts and findings as they are known at the time the opinion is formulated. If the facts which form the foundation for the opinion change, the opinion can and often will change.

Complications of Therapy

The frequency with which complications of therapy appear in a given medicolegal practice depends on whether such deaths are considered to be of public or private interest. Before the widespread adoption of peer review committees and mortality conferences, it was natural for hospital deaths from therapeutic complications to be investigated by the medical examiner or coroner. Now, practices vary. Some medical examiners pursue all therapeutic complications; others accept only those which are deemed to be of public interest and avoid those in which the outcome is of interest only to the next of kin, the provider of care and the insurance industry. As a practical matter, therapeutic and diagnostic complications are more likely to be reported and investigated by a medicolegal official when the injury includes an act of commission rather than an act of omission and when the injury is anatomic rather than pharmacologic or physiologic. The bias is formalized in some jurisdictions by a requirement specifying that operative or anesthetic deaths must be reported to the medical examiner or coroner. The discussion which follows is, likewise, focused on procedures.

Investigations of deaths occurring during anesthesia often require the medical examiner to enlist the aid of a consultant anesthesiologist. In such investigations, the autopsy serves as a laboratory test for only some of the items on the list of differential diagnoses. These items include pulmonary air- or thromboembolism, airway edema, and misplaced catheters and tubes. Examination of equipment and medical records and interviews of witnesses provide the bulk of investigative findings in most cases.

The investigation of deaths associated with advanced cardiopulmonary resuscitation less often requires specialized consultants, unless the error is one of omission, such as failure to infuse adequate volumes of plasma expanders. The investigation of these deaths is simplified if the central venous catheters and artificial airways can be left in place until their positions can be documented during the internal phase of the autopsy. In the case of deaths occurring during insertion of central venous catheters, the pathologist should do an evaluation for air emboli in the right side of the heart.

Arterial air embolism can occur with lung biopsies and with open heart surgery involving the left chambers. The diagnosis is usually based on the medical history, with autopsy exclusion of reasonable alternatives.

Pneumothorax will not be missed if the autopsy pathologist routinely looks for it. A supine posteroanterior radiograph will not reliably demonstrate a small pneumothorax to the viewing pathologist, because the bubble is parallel to the chest field. The time-honored technique of flooding the exposed chest wall with water, after reflection of the skin, followed by pleural puncture, is effective. The drawback of this technique is that it is too cumbersome to use except in a suspected case of pneumothorax. Therefore unsuspected cases are not detected. We find it practical in every autopsy, as a matter of routine, to simply scrape intercostal muscle from between two anterior ribs, thereby converting the parietal pleura into a window through which one visualizes the lobular pattern of pulmonary pleura, the red blood of a hemothorax, or the patternless blackness indicating a pneumothorax.

The possibility of electrocution from indwelling catheters has been addressed in the anesthesia literature.[6] Because there is virtually no resistance between the catheter and the heart, such electrocution can occur with extremely small stray currents induced by faulty equipment, remote from the patient, which is plugged into a different outlet on the same circuit. The patient need only complete a circuit by touching a grounded object such as a bedside radio. This risk is vastly reduced in the operating room by the use of circuits which have no electrical reference to ordinary ground potential. In other words, no circuit is completed by touching objects which are in electrical continuity with the neutral line of the current supply to the building. This electrical independence is accomplished by the use of transformers to generate current circuits which are isolated from household circuits. The investigation of possible electrocution involving central vascular catheters or in the operating suite will require the services of a hospital-based electrical engineer in most cases.

The certification of deaths from therapeutic complications is discussed elsewhere in this chapter.

COEXISTENCE OF TRAUMA AND DISEASE–CONSEQUENCE OR COINCIDENCE

The victims of sudden natural death may sustain non-contributory injury incident to agonal episodes in which they collapse and fall without being able to protect themselves. If the fall takes place on a hard surface, cutaneous abrasions, contusions and lacerations may be sustained that suggest that trauma is somehow involved in the deaths. This is especially true if the decedent falls down a flight of stairs or from an elevated position. The correlation of terminal circumstances and anatomic findings is essential to disclose the role, if any, played by trauma in such a death.

On the other hand, natural diseases do create situations that can lead to fatal injury. Epileptics can drown as a result of a seizure; the patient with Meniere's disease can fall from a height during an episode of nausea and dizziness; and the cardiac patient can incur fatal injury from an automobile accident that results from his losing consciousness during an attack of cardiac syncope as he drives along the highway.

The potential interplay of trauma and natural disease in causing or contributing to death can give rise to even more complex and perplexing situations. If a victim dies of injury shortly after being hurt or at some considerably later time from a continuous chain of complicating events, there is no problem as to the manner of death. However, knotty questions may arise when there is a symptom-free interval between apparent recovery from trauma and death from well-documented natural disease. If justice is to be done, the casual or contributory effect of the injury to death must be accurately evaluated. For example, granted that the victim died of a myocardial infarct secondary to arteriosclerotic heart disease, what weight, if any, should be given to the leg fractured at work two weeks prior to the fatal

TABLE IX-1

PHASES		HUMAN	VEHICLES AND EQUIPMENT	PHYSICAL ENVIRONMENT	SOCIO-ECONOMIC ENVIRONMENT
	PRE-EVENT				
	EVENT				
	POST-EVENT				
	LOSSES	DAMAGE TO PEOPLE	DAMAGE TO VEHICLES & EQUIP.	DAMAGE TO PHYSICAL ENVIRONMENT	DAMAGE TO SOCIETY

episode? Such questions require circumspect and objective assessment of all data based on consideration of mechanisms of death and risk factors for natural and unnatural events, before one can offer a sound and fair opinion as to the contributory role of trauma in causing death.

Risk Factors for Accidental Events

The late Dr. William Haddon developed for epidemiological purposes the matrix method of analyzing factors involved in the production of accidents.[2] The same matrix analysis also serves the purposes of medicolegal death investigation.[14] Haddon divided the factors into human, mechanical, environmental and socioeconomic categories, and by sequence into pre-event, event, and post-event categories. A matrix of 12 cells or categories of factors is created (Table IX-1). Human, mechanical, environmental and socioeconomic losses are then tabulated by the epidemiologist. The medical examiner is concerned with the human losses, measured by extent of medical injury, and with risk factors for the occurrence of the accidental event, which are labeled pre-event factors. For a traffic crash fatality, the possible factors are numerous and occur in every matrix cell. A few examples follow. Pre-crash human risk factors would include alcohol

intoxication, cardiac syncope and natural death at the wheel. Post-crash human factors would include the number and severity of injuries. Pre-crash physical environmental factors would include the presence of ice on the road, fog and obscure traffic signals. Crash-phase mechanical factors would include the presence or absence of air bags, collapsible steering columns, and the mass of each vehicle. In traffic fatality investigations, the identification of human factors is a function of the medical investigation *and* the police investigation, as in the determination of syncope based on witness accounts of a driver slumped at the wheel before a crash. Road traffic crashes, drownings, SCUBA accidents, falls, and industrial accidents all lend themselves well to this type of analysis.

Pre-Event Human Risk Factors vs. Contributory Causes of Death

When forming a cause-of-death opinion involving the potential interplay of disease and trauma, it is essential to distinguish between pre-event human risk factors and the diseases or intoxications which contribute to death. The distinction depends on appreciating the difference between the chain of medical events culminating in death and the chain of human, mechanical, environmental and social events culminating in the traumatic incident.

With deaths in which the pre-event risk factors are limited in number and knowable in their entirety, it is useful, permissible and a part of effective communication to list on the death certificate, as contributory causes of death, the human factors, if they are medically codeable conditions. Other factors can be listed in the *how injury occurred* section of the death certificate. For example, when epileptics drown in bathtubs, without sustaining head injuries, the only pertinent risk factors are the seizure disorder, representing a pre-event human risk factor, the seizure, representing the event phase human factor, and the watery environment, representing the event phase environmental factor. In this situation, it makes sense to certify the death as drowning due to the seizure disorder.

However, when the number of risk factors for an accidental event is large and their delineation is a function of the extent of the investigation, and when there are multiple participating persons in the event, it is a poor practice to single out human risk factors identified by the pathologist for inclusion as contributory causes of death. For instance, a pathologist may determine that a decedent in a two-car crash was intoxicated and list ethanol intoxication as a contributory cause of death. Months later, after traffic safety consultants, reconstruction experts, engineers and mechanics have studied the crash, it may be determined that the surviving driver had defective brakes or made an improper turn or that a traffic signal was obscured or faulty. The frequently flawed logic of listing human risk factors as contributory causes is revealed if a person other than the decedent is at fault because of intoxication. It would be absurd to list the intoxication of another person as a contributory cause on the decedent's certificate of death.

Therefore, with traffic crashes, it is not customary or even correct practice to list alcohol intoxication as a contributory cause of death, unless the concentration of alcohol is so high that it contributes to cardiac instability, respiratory depression or postural asphyxia and thereby forms a direct link in the medical chain of events leading to death.

In summary, we advocate listing risk factors as contributory or underlying causes of death in two circumstances. The first is when the risk factor physiologically contributes to death (e.g., marked ethanol intoxication in a person who dies from postural asphyxia). The second is when the evaluation of the fatality makes no sense without the explanation provided by the risk factor (e.g., submersion in a bathtub of a person who has epilepsy).

Since police interest in non-traffic accidents tends to be minimal if there is no evidence of criminal wrongdoing, the quality of investigation in those accidents will directly reflect the interest and input of the medical examiner. The matrix approach to case analysis can be effectively used to focus the investigation and to suggest to the police or lay investigators productive lines of inquiry. For example, deaths involving bodies found in water, not all of which represent drownings, can involve a few or many possible risk factors of human, mechanical, environmental and socioeconomic types.

The autopsy can reveal evidence of disease, injury or intoxication which can be implicated as a risk factor for drowning. However, in most drownings, exclusive of SCUBA deaths, the risk factors are environmental (choppy seas, high wind, undertow, currents, cold water, underwater snags) or socioeconomic (poor swimming ability owing to lack of swimming lessons). One human risk factor which is revealed only by questioning of witnesses, friends or family is deliberate hyperventilation preceding underwater swimming. The discovery of this risk factor can explain drowning deaths which involve competent young swimmers in shallow, calm water.

If a violent cause of death *can* stand alone on the death certificate without a contributory natural condition, then it should do so. If the effect of the disease is merely to hasten certain death from injury, it generally should not be listed as a contributory cause. For example, if a person commits suicide by diversion of exhaust fumes into an automobile and is found dead with the ignition on, the engine cold, and the fuel tank empty, we would not list severe arteriosclerotic heart disease as a contributory cause because of a blood carboxyhemoglobin concentration substantially less than the usual 70 to 80%. We would certify the death as carbon monoxide poisoning with no contributory natural disease.

The preceding discussion has focused on disease and intoxication as risk factors in traumatic deaths. The following sections deals with risk factors in deaths largely due to disease.

Natural Risk Factors for Disease Events

Transient risk factors are the events which are responsible for lowering the threshold for ventricular fibrillation or increasing cardiac irritability. Common transient risk factors include rage; fear; the anniversary of a spouse's death; the times before and after micturition, defecation and sexual intercourse; heavy meals; mental stress and physical exertion.

Traumatic Risk Factors for Disease Events

When the transient risk factor is a codeable medical injury or emotional stress occasioned by the direct threat of a crime, the manner of death is no longer natural, and the transient risk factor must become a contributory or proximate cause of death for the cause-of-death opinion to make sense.

For example, if a person with longstanding arteriosclerotic heart disease falls and fractures his femoral neck, undergoes open reduction and fixation under general anesthesia, sustains a myocardial infarct and dies, the death is accidental. In this instance, a chronic disease is the lethal substrate, and the mechanical injury is the lethal trigger.

Or, consider the elderly woman whose handbag is seized and stolen. Without being physically touched by the robbers, she collapses and dies on the spot. The autopsy discloses arteriosclerotic heart disease. In this situation the heart disease is the lethal substrate and the stress of the robbery, with its implied physical threat, is the lethal trigger. The cause of death can reasonably be certified as arteriosclerotic heart disease, with a contributory cause of emotional stress. The manner of death is homicide. To complete the story, the *how injury occurred* section can indicate that the deceased was the victim of a robbery.

Homicide by Heart Attack

Davis has published guidelines for certifying homicides by heart attack which have found general acceptance by medical examiners and courts. These guidelines require that (a) the crime be of such a nature, that, if physical injury had ensued, a homicide charge would be supported; (b) the victim realize an implicit threat to his or her safety; (c) the circumstances be of an obvious emotional nature; (d) the cardiac arrhythmia and collapse occur during the criminal act or in the ensuing emotional response period and (e) that chronic heart disease be demonstrable.[15]

Natural Death at Work

Workmen's compensation boards frequently may be involved with claims arising from natural deaths said to be precipitated by the physical or emotional stress of work. If it can be satisfactorily shown in a given case that the transient risk factor acting as the lethal trigger mechanism was work-related stress, then compensation may be awarded.

A satisfactory cause-and-effect relationship is ordinarily based on the temporal relationship between the putative risk factor and the onset of the fatal episode. That onset may be defined as the occurrence of a lethal ventricular arrhythmia or of the onset of angina in instances of myocardial infarction. In these situations, since the manner of death remains natural and the transient risk factor is not a codeable disease or injury, the responsible stress does not appear in the cause-of-death opinion on the certificate.

Medicolegal Masquerades

In this final section we discuss trauma which mimics disease and disease which mimics trauma. One manner of death frequently masquerades as another. This is especially true when an entire fatal episode transpires so quickly that it is not possible to establish either the cause or the manner of death with sufficient certainty or precision to allay suspicion and to eliminate violence as a factor.

Deaths from natural causes often occur so rapidly or under such circumstances as to suggest erroneously that violence has somehow been involved. Unless one establishes the true manner of such a death, the police may be put into the impossible position of trying to find a nonexistent murderer; the deceased may be unfairly stigmatized as having committed suicide, followed by the voiding of life insurance policies or the withholding of religious burial rites; or a double indemnity accidental death benefit may be wrongly awarded.

A married couple was heard scuffling and arguing in their apartment about the wife's excessive drinking. A door slammed, and the husband was seen leaving the house. Several hours later, neighbors found the woman dead in a pool of blood. Her face, arms and trunk bore multiple recent and fading bruises. The husband was found and immediately taken into custody by the police on suspicion of homicide. The autopsy revealed no evidence of injury. The blood at the scene was the result of hemoptysis from ruptured esophageal varies, secondary to alcoholic liver cirrhosis. This death, which had presented itself originally as a homicidal assault, was thus demonstrated to have arisen from a totally different, non-criminal causation. The husband was released immediately.

In another case, the driver of a speeding automobile that ran into a tree was dead when he was removed from the wreckage. He had multiple bilateral rib fractures, a fractured sternum, and lacerations of the heart, lungs and liver, accompanied by no internal bleeding. Severe coronary atherosclerosis and a healed myocardial infarct were also present. It was concluded that death had occurred as a result of natural disease prior to the violent impact, and that death had caused the accident.

The converse of the preceding proposition is equally true. Persons may be murdered, commit suicide, or die as a result of accidental injuries, in such a fashion that when studied casually the circumstances lend themselves to the mistaken impression that death was due to natural disease. This erroneous conclusion becomes even more plausible where the decedent has a history of some disease with lethal potential. The presence of previously diagnosed, far-advanced natural disease affords no guarantee that violence played no part in the death.

When a physician is called to the scene of death of a stranger or even one of his patients, he should approach the body and his responsibilities with a healthy suspicion that the obvious or the expected may not have happened. Too often there is a naive presumption of natural death.

Rapid or delayed deaths can result from violence which produces little or no external evidence of injury. The variety of such concealed or latent trauma is quite broad.

Fatal electric shock can occur with only a minute and readily overlooked electrical burn to indicate the nature of the agent responsible for death. Indeed, when death is caused by passage of a 110-volt alternating current, visible cutaneous injuries are present in only approximately half of the victims,[7] despite the fact that the electrical disturbance was sufficiently potent to cause ventricular fibrillation.

Fatal blunt head trauma can occur with no externally visible injury of the scalp, especially when the decedent has a full head of hair or is wearing a hat. Likewise, blunt force applied over a broad area of the trunk can create lethal abdominal and thoracic injuries without the telltale presence of external bruises or abrasions. Many deaths from poison provide the most striking examples of fatal violence that kills without creating external or internal anatomical evidence of injury.

A fifty-seven-year-old woman with known disseminated cancer of the breast, who had been slowly failing, was unexpectedly found dead one morning. The autopsy revealed that the cancer had spread to her lungs, liver, lymph nodes and vertebrae. Chemical analyses of her blood and viscera demonstrated large concentrations of a sedative. Interrogation of the family revealed that a suicide note had been discarded in an attempt to conceal the true nature of her death. As in deaths due to combinations of trauma and disease, the correct approach is to consider the totality of investigative and laboratory data and to mentally organize the data by mechanism-oriented analysis.

In conclusion, we emphasize that the competent medicolegal evaluation of death requires a systematic consideration of all available data and cannot be focused exclusively on the autopsy. The information must include accounts of the decedent's history and descriptions of the fatal environment and circumstances surrounding death and is optimally provided by *primary* sources. Reliance upon information related by treating physicians is an invitation to error, because the information may be secondhand and somewhat distorted before it comes to the treating physician. Further distortion often is added by the clinician in transmitting the information to the pathologist, because the specifics of the transmittal may be colored by the physician's interpretation of everything he knows about the decedent. Physicians usually communicate in the abbreviated language of diagnoses, which are the equivalent of editorials, when what the pathologist really needs is the objective news. The autopsy and the toxicological studies should be regarded as a battery of postmortem laboratory tests that in most instances cannot be interpreted independent of historical considerations. Pathologists will make fewer medicolegal blunders if they do not attempt to use the autopsy as a substitute for a case investigation.

REFERENCES

1. *Medical Examiner's and Coroner's Handbook on Death Registration and Fetal Death Reporting.* DHEW Publication No (PHS) 1110, US Dept of Health and Human Services, Public Health Service, National Center for Health Statistics, Oct. 1987.
2. Haddon, W., Jr. (Insurance Institute for Highway Safety): Advances in the epidemiology of injuries as a basis for public policy. Public Health Reports, Vol. 95, Sept–Oct 1980, pp. 411–421.
3. *Medical Certification of Cause of Death: Instructions for Physicians on Use of International Form of Medical Certificate of Cause of Death.* World Health Organization. Geneva, 1958.
4. Adelson, L.: *The Pathology of Homicide.* Springfield, IL: Charles C Thomas, 1974, pp. 15–17.
5. 22 A Am Jur 2d, §48, §49, §50.
6. U.S. Department of Health and Human Services: *International Classification of Diseases, 9th revision, 3rd ed., Clinical Modification,* volumes 1, 2, and 3. Practice Management Information Corporation, Los Angeles, 1989.
7. Leonard, P.F.: Characteristics of electrical hazards. *Anesth Anal, 51:* 797–809, 1972.
8. Wright, R.K., and Davis, J.H.: The investigation of electrical deaths: A report of 220 fatalities. *J Forensic Sci, 25:* 514–521, 1980.
9. Hirsch, C.S., and Zumwalt, R.S.: The empty heart sign. *Am J Forensic Med Pathol, 7:* 112–114, 1986.
10. Wright, R.K., and Wetli, C.V.: A guide to the forensic autopsy–Conceptual aspects. *Pathol Annual,* 16:273-288, 1981.
11. Adelson, L.: No anatomic cause of death. *Conn State Med J, 18:* 732, 1954.
12. "History and Organization of the Vital Statistics System," Chapter 1 of *Vital Statistics of the United States,* Washington D.C., United States Department of Health, Education and Welfare; Public Health Service; National Vital Statistics Division, Vol. I, pp. 2–19, 1950.
13. Wilbur, C.L.: *Manual of the International List of Causes of Death, Based on The Second Decennial Revision by the International Commission, Paris, July 1 to 3, 1909.* United State Department of Commerce, Bureau of the Census, Washington, D.C., Government Printing Office, 1913.
14. Davis, J.H.: Automobile death investigation and prevention programs. In: Curran, W.J., McGarry, A.L., and Petty, C.S., eds. *Modern legal medicine, psychiatry and forensic science.* Philadelphia: F.A. Davis Co., 1980, pp. 307–337.
15. Davis, J.H.: Can sudden cardiac death be murder? *J Forensic Sci, 23:* 384–387, 1978.

Chapter X

BLUNT FORCE INJURY

WERNER U. SPITZ

A SHARP OBJECT, such as a knife or a broken piece of glass, cuts and divides the tissues as it penetrates. In contrast, a wound produced by blunt impact tears, shears and crushes. Falls, or blows with a blunt instrument, such as a hammer, brick, bat, fist or pipe, typically result in blunt force injury. Blunt trauma crushes, causing bleeding into the traumatized area, i.e., a bruise, due to tearing of small arteries and veins in the depth of the wound from which blood is literally impregnated into the area tissues. Bruising surrounding cuts and stab wounds is unlikely, unless the hilt or handle of the knife, or the fist of the assailant holding it, abut the skin. Blunt force is probably the single most common type of trauma.

The skin manifestations of blunt trauma differ depending on the force, location of the injury, and the nature of the impact. When injuries caused by blunt trauma are patterned, they may depict the outline, shape, even the structure, consistency or other characteristics of the weapon, or parts of the weapon (Figs. X-1a–b and X-2). The pattern may allow matching of the injury with the object that caused it (Figs. X-3 to X-8). In this regard, analysis of blunt force trauma is especially challenging.

Three basic types of injury are recognized: (a) contusion, (b) abrasion, (c) laceration. Skeletal injuries, i.e., fractures, represent a separate entity, also discussed below.

CONTUSION

A contusion (bruise) signifies hemorrhage into the skin, tissues under the skin or organs. The severity of a bruise is largely dependent on the intensity and location of the impact. Other factors include age and the physical condition of the victim. Older people bruise more easily, presumably due to greater capillary fragility. People with cirrhosis and other liver diseases, or those on blood thinner medication bruise excessively due to interference with blood clotting mechanisms. The half-life time of Coumadin exceeds 2.5 days, which means that some bleeding may continue for an extended period. A slap, as with an open hand or the likes of an air bag, deploying in a motor vehicle crash, often causes a red, swollen mark on the skin, which when viewed closely, consists of numerous tiny hemorrhages from ruptured capillaries. Such clusters of small hemorrhages, occasionally resembling petechiae, should not be interpreted as a manifestation of

asphyxiation. Severe internal injuries may exist in the absence of external evidence of trauma. A contusion is usually the result of a blow or squeeze that crushes the tissues and ruptures blood vessels, but does not break the skin. A *black eye* following a fistfight, scalp hemorrhage from a fall and a *black and blue mark* after an arm is grabbed or squeezed or pinched too firmly are some examples.

A fresh pinch would consist of two round or semicircular areas of bruising in close proximity to each other. With time these bruises may merge, as they spread as part of the healing process, resulting in a single larger bruised area. In the case of an impact, consideration must be given to the fact, that early on only the area of contact is bruised. With time, the bruise spreads and may diffuse any pattern it had initially. The bruise also changes color which may alter initial injury characteristics.

460

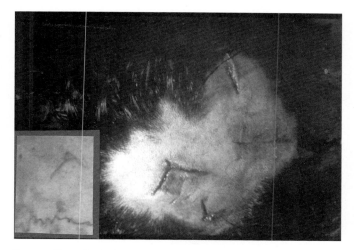

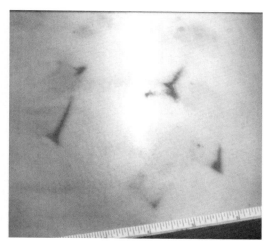

FIGURE X-1a–b. Scalp and skull showing well defined, right angled, straight injuries (lacerations and bruises) which suggest a sharp edged, rectangular metal instrument. A wooden instrument with similar shape would be less likely to indent the skull (insert) with as sharp an outline as shown. It was later learned that the back of a hatchet was the weapon used. Figure X-1b shows the outline.

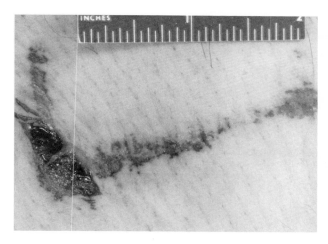

FIGURE X-3. Four parallel scratches made by a fork. A second-degree burn under the ear in conjunction with the fork markings indicates torture. Death was caused by head injuries sustained in a beating.

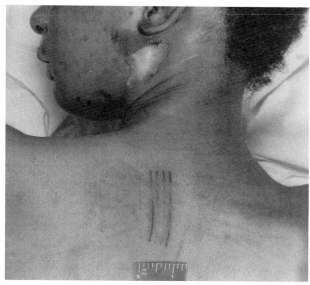

FIGURE X-2. Blow with a 2x4 on the center of the abdomen. The edges of the piece of lumber abraded the skin, while its corner sank into the skin, causing a well-defined laceration.

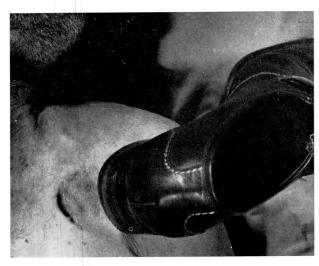

FIGURE X-4. Semicircular abrasion and contusion produced by the heel of a shoe.

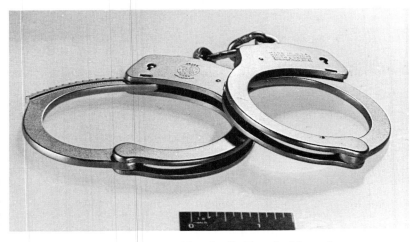

FIGURE X-5a. Typical handcuffs. Note double tracks.

Some bruises are patterned because of their shape and the image they portray, others are patterned due to their location, distribution and relationship to one another. Recognition of the pattern may help in reconstructing the circumstances of injury. The circular bruise of a steering wheel on the chest of a driver or tire marks on a pedestrian who was run over by an automobile are familiar examples.

Also known are the two, parallel, train track-like lines of bruising that result from a blow with a smooth pipe or stick. The skin between the lines remains uninjured because blood that is shed from torn vessels under the skin is displaced sideways by the pressure of the blow (Figs. X-9 and X-10a–b). The same results from the strike of a fast tennis or baseball which causes a circular bruise with a pale center. A rough textured weapon such as a piece of lumber may cause parallel abrasions on the skin, with or without bruising. Horseshoe-shaped, double-lined bruises sometimes seen in cases of child abuse are caused by whipping with a looped electric or phone cord, or other flexible object, such as a

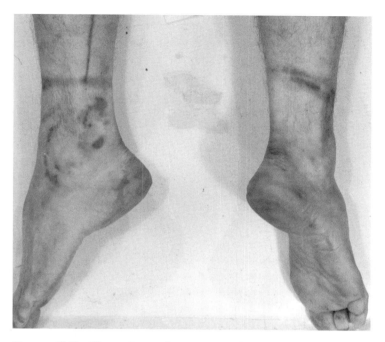

FIGURE X-5b. Circumferential contusions of the legs due to binding. Restraint marks are usually more pronounced on the outer surfaces of the wrists and ankles.

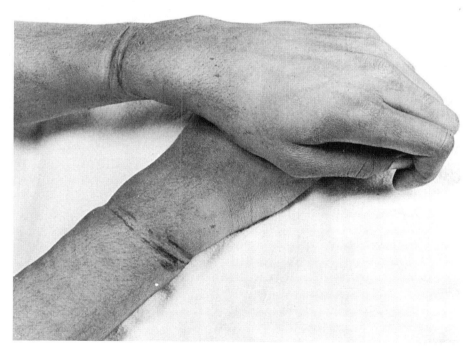

FIGURE X-5c. Typical train track-like, handcuff marks of the wrists. Incision often shows subcutaneous bruising more pronounced on the ulnar side.

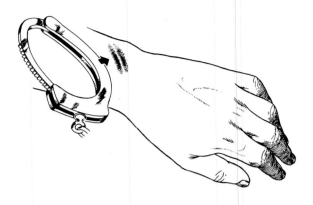

FIGURE X-6. Hasty application of handcuffs sometimes led to misuse. The oblique markings are the result of striking the wrist with the stationary portion of the handcuffs instead of the hinged section.

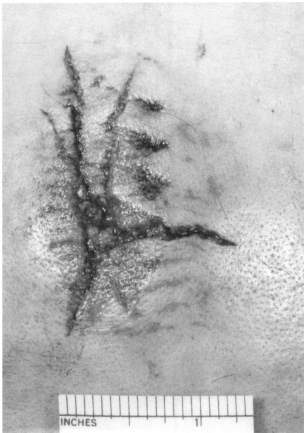

FIGURE X-8. Bald top of the head showing a distinct pattern of horizontal parallel equidistant bruises and vertical, also equidistant perforations on the right side. The area of intimate contact between the weapon and the skin is the dark center of the injury from which fine long splits radiate in different directions. The pattern in this injury can be matched with a weapon. Note that due to the curvature of the head only a partial pattern of the weapon is present.

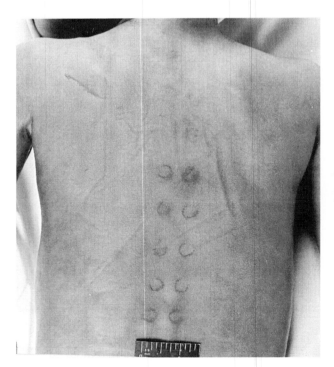

FIGURE X-7. Beating with a belt. The circular bruises are from double belt holes.

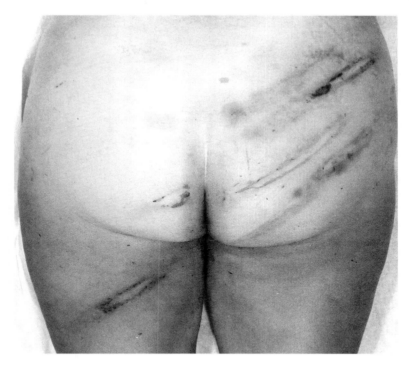

FIGURE X-9. Injuries inflicted with a baton. Two parallel linear bruises are caused by each impact.

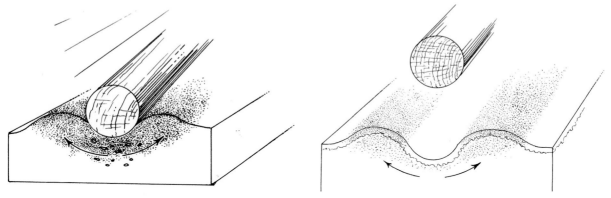

FIGURE X-10a–b. Diagrams showing train track-like bruises inflicted with a stick or rod. The area of contact with the stick is dented. Blood shed from torn superficial veins is displaced sideways (arrows). The gap between the bruised lines corresponds to the width of the weapon.

wire coat hanger. The weave pattern of certain types of clothing pressed against the skin often shows up as uniformly spaced pinpoint size dots from knots in the fabric, and the pattern of intertwining threads or cords may sometimes be identified in the case of an injury by a rope. When a regular household extension cord is used for beating, the mark may depict the image of the two insulated wires. A flexible whip adapts to the contour of the body, and will wrap itself around, causing a continuous welt on the front and back of the victim.

Clusters of pinpoint hemorrhages sometimes occur adjacent to tight straps as in someone strapped on a gurney or in a restraining chair. Occasionally, such pinpoint hemorrhages occur under tourniquets or tight elastic bandages.

It is always advantageous to use a magnifying glass when viewing injuries.

A young man came to a Los Angeles hospital ER complaining of injury of his right leg. The leg was painful and did show some swelling and faint red discoloration, however not in any comparison to what was observed when he returned the next day when he had more pain and more swelling and prominent parallel linear bruises on the leg. He now claimed he had been struck by police officers using batons. A law suit was filed against the police. Close examination of photographs a year later showed the bruised lines to correspond to overlapping turns of the ace bandages which had been placed on his leg at the first ER visit and typical, clusters of pinpoint hemorrhages and the imprinted weave pattern of the wrappings were also recognizable (Fig. X-11).

Computer produced overlays or transparencies have been successfully used for comparing injuries with patterned designs, such as a slap mark on a child's face or stomping injuries. However, such injuries may also be recognized by just looking, discerning, and studying the injury for its pattern. To enable *retaining* and revisiting the injury days later, photographs are advantageous. It is amazing how much additional detail one sees on a photograph by repeated viewing. Slap marks on the face show swelling caused by edema and reddish discoloration with occasional clusters of pinpoint hemorrhages which become observable within minutes. Sometimes parallel finger imprints of the slapping hand are also recognizable.

Stomping may display the sole or heel pattern of the assailant's shoe (Figs. X-12a–b and X-13). The other side of the face will depict the patterned imprint of the floor or ground (Fig. X-14). Bruising caused by stomping are especially prominent over bony prominences and careful dissection of such areas will show crushed subcutaneous fat.

Repeated minor blows to the head, inflicted in a close timely relationship, are likely to be cumulative in their effect, even if struck in different locations. The skin in areas of injury may appear undamaged, or focally bruised, but bruises are likely to occur in the underlying scalp. If a blow to the head is severe enough to break the skin,

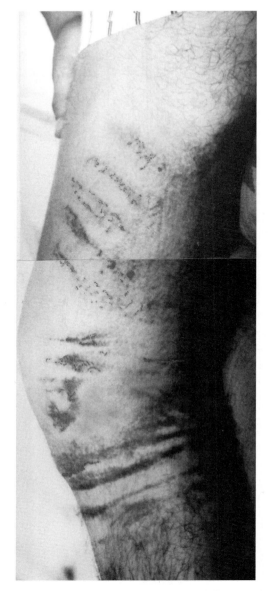

FIGURE X-11. Patterned linear bruises and clusters of pinpoint hemorrhages caused by an ace bandage wrapped too tight due to swelling of the leg.

regardless of depth or extent, dazing of the senses may be expected. Disorientation, confusion, even unconsciousness is likely to occur. In more severe cases resulting in death, the brain is usually swollen and may show evidence of tonsillar and internal herniation. Cortical contusions, subdural and subarachnoid hemorrhage and other gross manifestations of traumatic brain injury, such as pinpoint hemorrhages in the white matter

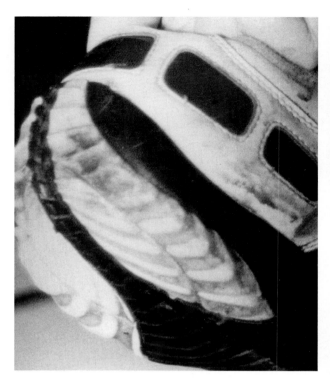

FIGURE X-12a–b. Heel of an athletic shoe (a) used for stomping with characteristic marks on the chest (b). The bruises of the face and a fractured nose were sustained in the preceding altercation.

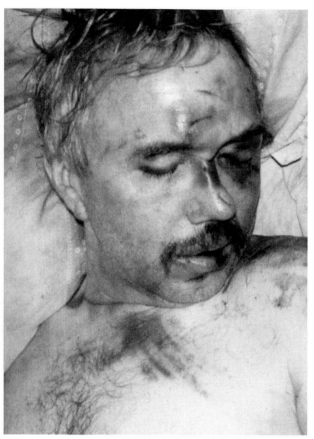

are other associated findings. The posterior end of the corpus callosum, the internal capsule and the cerebral peduncles are particularly sensitive to diffuse axonal injury (DAI). However, at least fifteen hours of post injury survival are needed to enable documentation of characteristic DAI findings, such as swollen, varicose or dystrophic axons, on routine hematoxylin and eosin stained sections. A recently developed immunostain, β-amyloid precursor protein (BAPP), although not specific for axons injured by trauma, (staining axons in proximity of infarcts) reduces the critical post injury survival time to 2 hours to detect injured axons. After 30 days' survival no BAPP staining may be expected.[1,2]

A karate chop with the side of an outstretched hand causes an elongated rectangular bruise, 1 to 1-1/2 inches wide. In evaluating such injury, consideration must be given to other causative mechanisms. A similar rectangular bruise may result from a kick with the side of a boot. A pat-

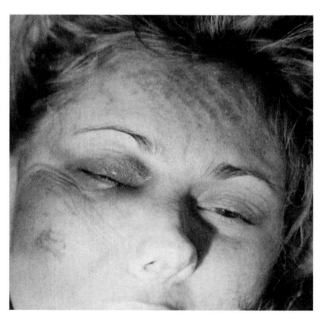

FIGURE X-13. Typical sole pattern of a shoe on the forehead and the right cheek bone with deformity of the nose due to fracture. Blood from the site of fracture seeped into the right eye socket and the lids.

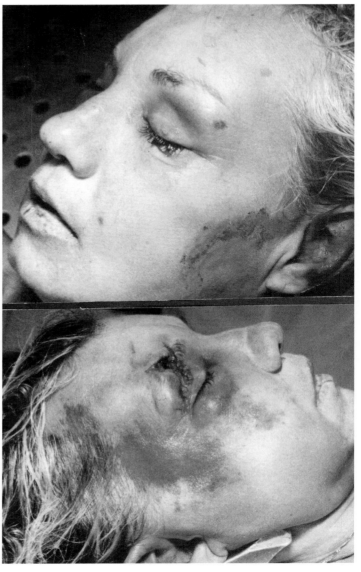

FIGURE X-14. The nude body of a middle-aged woman was found raped and bound at the wrist and ankles on a tile floor. Her head was covered with a plastic bag. *(Top)* Her face had been stomped on the left side *(upside)* which shows minimal surface bruising. *(Bottom)* The right side *(downside)* of her face was against the tile and shows extensive abrasion, extending over most of the right side of the face with a laceration over the supraorbital ridge. Note that the downside is significantly more damaged than the upside. This is a characteristic of stomping when the body is crushed against the hard surface.

tern in the bruise, may correspond to irregularities caused by wear, the tread design in the side of the sole, the imprint of stitches, or lace loops. In the head, such a blow may be fatal due to concussion, in the chest, the heart may be sent into ventricular fibrillation, with or without externally manifested injury (Fig. X-15). A sharp blow to the front of the neck may lacerate the airway and fracture laryngeal cartilages (Fig. X-16). A karate chop will cause this type of injury, but so will a kick to this area or an impact on the neck of an unrestrained driver on the top of the steering wheel, in a head-on collision. Death due to asphyxiation results from airway obstruction by swelling, hemorrhage or displacement, unless promptly relieved. In the nape of the neck, such blows may be instantaneously fatal due to injury of the medulla. A sharp chop to the side of the neck may cause subarachnoid hemorrhage, presumably related to a sudden surge of the blood pressure due to stimulation of the carotid body or laceration of the vertebral artery.

Kicks to the hairy scalp, even with a tennis shoe, may be fatal. Instant death may result from head trauma without significant brain swelling or microscopic changes.

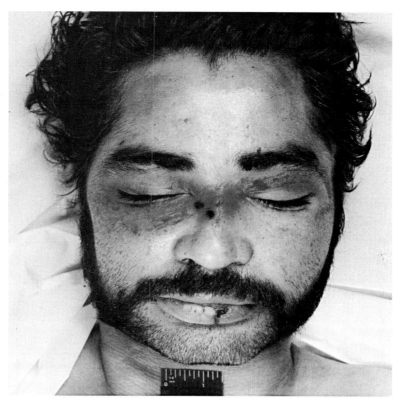

FIGURE X-15. Karate chop across the face. The nose and right maxillary bone were fractured. Death was instantaneous as a result of concussion.

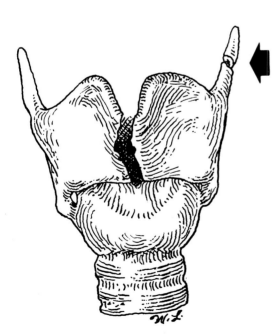

FIGURE X-16. Karate chop across the neck often causes a vertical fracture running down from the thyroid prominence and/or fracture of one or both superior horns (arrow).

Tearing of the basilar artery sometimes results from kicking of the head, especially in cases of alcoholic intoxication. Although kicking is likely to cause minimal external injuries, often not exceeding dime-size, deep organ damage may be severe and kicks with leather shoes or boots may fracture the skull or ribs.

Contostavlos described a case of instantaneous collapse and death due to subarachnoid hemorrhage caused by laceration of a vertebral artery as a result of a blow with a cue stick at the level of the mandibular angle, behind the ear. This injury is often associated with fracture of the transverse process of the first vertebra. Contostavlos suggests that the vertebral arteries be examined in all cases of subarachnoid hemorrhage with a history of possible trauma in the absence of an anatomic abnormality.[3] Postmortem angiography to demonstrate the source of hemorrhage is undoubtedly advantageous.

A kick or an energetic blow with a fist to this strategic location may have the same result. The procedure for evaluating the vertebral arteries is described in Chapter XXV.

Strategic areas should be explored in autopsies of individuals who died while incarcerated or in police custody. This involves incisions in both shoulders, elbows, wrists, ankles and a long vertical incision of the back down to the buttocks. All incisions should be undermined to allow for maximal exposure. The scalp should be reflected down to the nape of the neck, or lower. This procedure will document any injuries in areas of susceptibility.

Bruises are sometimes confined to deep tissues, especially if caused by a blow with a wide and smooth object or involving an area of the body protected by heavy clothes or dense hair. Such hemorrhage may gravitate along fascial planes to adjoining areas, giving the impression that the injury occurred at the place at which the hemorrhage becomes apparent (Fig. X-17). The *Battle sign,* where blood from a basilar skull fracture percolates behind and below the ear to the area of the mastoid process, is one such example. The actual site of injury must at all times be ascertained at autopsy. A fractured jaw is frequently followed by *gravity shifting* of the hemor-

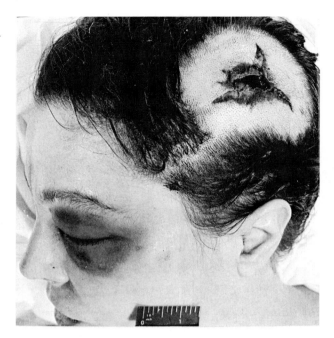

FIGURE X-17. Blow to the left side of the head. The hemorrhage of the left eyelids is by seepage and does not represent an independent injury.

rhage into the neck, simulating neck trauma. Fracture of the posterior pelvis may result in extensive bleeding into the extra-peritoneal space. Several pints of blood may be lost into the abdominal wall and pelvis in this way. Death may result from blood loss, with no evidence of external injuries and absent autopsy findings, unless specific attention is focused on these areas.

An elderly woman slipped and fell in her bathroom at home and was admitted to the hospital for evaluation. She gradually developed ischemic bowel disease and died 18 hours after admission. Autopsy revealed vast hemorrhage into the abdominal and pelvic walls, down the fascial planes into the thigh and buttock. X-ray examination showed an undisplaced posterior pelvic fracture.

Gravity shifting of blood into the occipital area of the scalp is common following survival of temporal or parietal scalp injury or a surgical procedure in these areas. This makes it difficult or impossible to determine whether there was an independent injury to the back of the head. However, if an area of crushed and disrupted tissue is identified at autopsy, this is the site of impact.

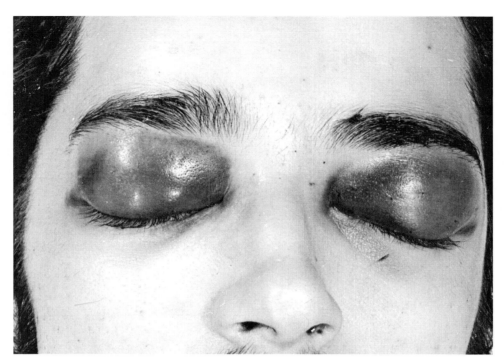

FIGURE X-18. Injury of the back of the head, which caused *contre coup* fractures of the roofs of the eye sockets and raccoon eyes.

Hemorrhages in the soft tissues around the eyes and in the eyelids, so-called *spectacle hematomas* or *raccoon eyes* (Fig. X-18), often suggests fracture of the base of the skull. Sometimes orbital hemorrhages and raccoon eyes occur as a result of falling on the back of the head, causing rebounding of the frontal lobes of the brain and fractures of the roofs of the eye sockets. Less frequent and not associated with any fractures, such hemorrhages may also follow blunt impact to the forehead that jolts the eyeballs out of their sockets, causing tears of small orbital blood vessels. If hemorrhage is limited to one side, the term *monocle hematoma* is sometimes used. Injury around the eyes may not become apparent for several hours, sometimes days, unless the body lies face down and the blood seeps downward by gravity (Fig. X-19). Hemorrhage in the eyelids, which simulates injury during life, is sometimes seen after the eyes have been harvested by tissue banks. In cases of suspected child abuse, turning the body overnight and reexamining it the next day, is always advantageous. To distinguish a genuine bruise from blood which accumulated as a result of seepage, microscopic examination may be required. Such examination of a bruise will show crushing of the tissue and homogeneous infiltration of blood into all layers of the skin, as opposed to blood limited to fascial planes.

Blood seepage proceeds along tissue planes, whether in the face or elsewhere. Seepage of blood from an injury to the forehead will run down into the eye socket on the same side, causing what will look like a *black eye*. However, if bleeding at the original source continues for a day or two, as is common in individuals on blood thinner therapy, including aspirin, the hemorrhage may cross over to the other side, causing bilateral periocular hematomas, i.e., *two black eyes*. This does not require a basilar skull fracture.

A 75-year-old male on aspirin therapy fell down several steps and sustained a half inch laceration of the right side of the forehead. The next day there was right periorbital hemorrhage. On the third day, the hemorrhage spread to the left side with a sharply demarcated horizontal subcutaneous bruise over the bridge of the nose (Fig. X-20a–b).

A 2-year-old child presented to the ER with bruising and severe swelling of the face, more prominent on the left side. There was also left middle-ear hemorrhage with rupture of

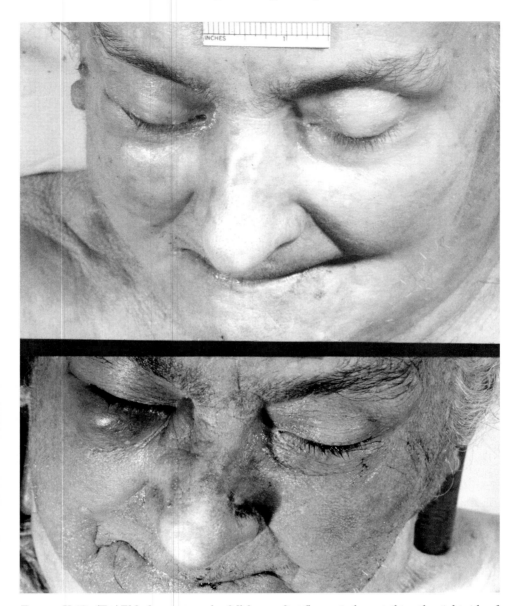

FIGURE X-19. *(Top)* Elderly woman who fell from a first floor window, striking the right side of her forehead. No periocular hemorrhage was noted when the body was first viewed six hours after death. *(Bottom)* Same woman after the body lay face down overnight. The hemorrhage in the right lower eyelid was the result of seepage from the forehead. No intracranial injury was noted at autopsy. The dusky color of the face is due to postmortem lividity.

the tympanic membrane. The next day a greenish-blue band of contusion was noted across the bridge of the nose and poorly defined, diffuse greenish-blue discoloration and swelling became apparent on the right cheek. The child had been violently slapped across the left side of the face. The bruising and swelling on the right side were the result of blood migration.

Bruises are sometimes seen in areas of livor mortis on the upper arms or shoulders of over-weight individuals without evidence of trauma elsewhere on the body. These hemorrhages are produced by tearing of veins in the skin when the body is lifted for removal from the scene (Fig. X-21). In an individual who survives an injury, a deep bruise may not become apparent on the skin until several days following the trauma. When ultimately, the bruise appears it may be

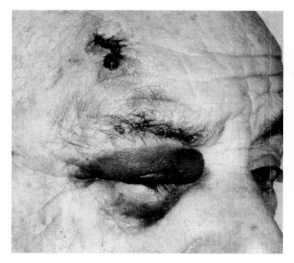
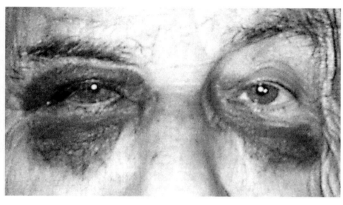

FIGURE X-20a–b. (a) Hemorrhage around the right eye after 2 days. No discoloration over the bridge of the nose and no hemorrhage on the left side. (b) On the third day, hemorrhage on both sides connecting over the bridge of the nose.

discolored, possibly green, yellow or brown, depending on the time which elapsed since injury. If death occurs before the bruise has had time to appear on the surface, only incision of the area will disclose the presence of injury. Embalming may enhance the appearance of a bruise on the body surface. Fluids injected into the arterial system in the process of embalming move the blood column, causing blood to seep out of previously torn vessels.

The color of a bruise changes with time from light bluish-red to dark purple, green, yellow and brown. A bruise heals from the periphery toward its center and vice versa. Thus, a discolored bruise with pale center is likely to be several days old. During this period the overall size of the bruise has become smaller. The change of color may be used as a guide for aging the bruise. In broad terms it may be said that the light bluish-red discoloration usually becomes noticeable after a few hours; until that time slight swelling may be all that is evident externally. The change to dark purple occurs roughly within a week, at the end of which greenish yellow and later brown discoloration appear. Disappearance of a bruise may be expected within two weeks to one month. This, however, depends on numerous factors, including the dimensions of the bruise, its depth and efficiency of the local circulation.

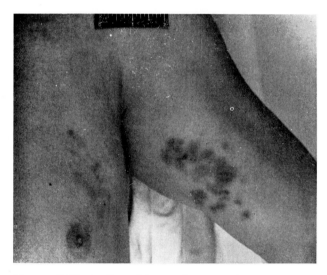

FIGURE X-21. Artifactual hemorrhages on the inner aspect of the arm produced by seepage of blood from small veins torn when the body was lifted for the purpose of removal.

The age and skin color of the individual are also important considerations. Caution is warranted when estimating the time of injury based on the color of a bruise. The bluish discoloration sometimes seen on the palm side at the base of the thumb, which is the thenar eminence, and the lateral dorsal side of the foot in fair, thin skinned, mostly female individuals, is from the color of the underlying muscle, not from bruising.

Microscopic examination for aging of a bruise is considerably more reliable and should be employed whenever more accurate evaluation is required. Perivascular neutrophils appear within 3–4 hours and peak in 1–3 days. Macrophages peak in 16–24 hours and hemosiderin within macrophages may be seen as early as 24 hours after injury. Hematoidin is also intracellular, but does not appear before several days or a week. Hematoidin is deposited as amorphous yellow granules or sheaves of crystals. Unlike hemosiderin, it does not react with potassium ferrocyanide and hydrochloric acid (Prussian blue).

Bruises of different ages, that is of various colors, located predominately over joints and other protuberant, frequently traumatized areas of the body are often encountered in alcoholics. Such injuries are usually due to repeated falls and bumping into objects, such as furniture. The head is also injured quite frequently and subdural hemorrhage may well be the cause of death.

Any head injury may be associated with subdural hemorrhage. This is more common in alcoholics with brain atrophy who loose balance and fall frequently. The increased volume of the subdural space that results from brain atrophy causes excessive exposure of the *bridging veins* between the dura and the arachnoid membrane on the brain surface. These vessels are the usual source of subdural bleeding. Increased tension on the *bridging veins* renders them especially susceptible to tearing as a result of minor trauma. The increased volume of the subdural space is often associated with larger than usual subdural hematomas. Fatal subdural bleeding may take hours to develop before intracranial pressure rises to the point of compressing the vital structures in the medulla. It is therefore common to find an alcoholic dead following a head injury sustained the preceding day. Unless an autopsy is performed the death may appear to be due to natural causes.

Chemical analysis of a subdural hematoma may reflect alcohol or drug intoxication at the time of injury, but exact blood alcohol or drug levels are not determinable. Because the brain reacts to injury by swelling, which starts at the time of injury and continues until the subdural space is obliterated and the bridging veins collapse, subdural hemorrhage may be delayed until brain swelling diminishes as a result of treatment or subsides spontaneously over a period of several hours. During this interval alcohol and drugs, especially those with a short half-life time, such as cocaine, may be partly metabolized or eliminated from the peripheral blood.

Arterial subdural hemorrhage is rare. It originates from small arachnoidal arteries sheared as a result of a tangential, i.e., grazing blow to the head. Such bleeding is significantly more rapid, therefore more lethal than the usual subdural hemorrhage of venous origin.[4]

At autopsy, many alcoholics are found to have advanced fatty infiltration of the liver and/or cirrhosis, either of which may be associated with impaired blood clotting (Fig. X-22a–b). This leads to easy bruising and extensive hemorrhage from relatively minor trauma. Pools of blood, blood-soaked clothes and walls smeared with blood frequently suggest murder; however, the explanation of many of these scenes is the terminal confusion of the alcoholic victim. Multiple injuries of different ages so often observed in alcoholics are indicative of repetitive trauma (Fig. X-23).

Fatal bleeding from minor injuries sometimes occurs in conditions other than alcoholism. Blood diseases associated with clotting defects and anticoagulant therapy also give rise to excessive hemorrhage. Investigation, including review of the medical history, is required in such cases.

A relatively common injury known for causing extensive bleeding in the absence of underlying disease is a tear of the eyebrow, such as frequently seen in boxers. The origin of such bleeding is from small arteries that are crushed on the bony ridge above the eye socket. Medical attention to stitch or cauterize the arterial branch is usually required to halt the bleeding, and many boxing matches have been stopped for just this reason. Face and scalp wounds generally tend to bleed more profusely than similar injuries elsewhere (Figs. X-24 and X-25).

Elderly people often have superficial hemorrhages in the skin following trivial injury, especially on the forearms, due to particular age-linked fragility of small blood vessels and skin atrophy. While technically these are contusions,

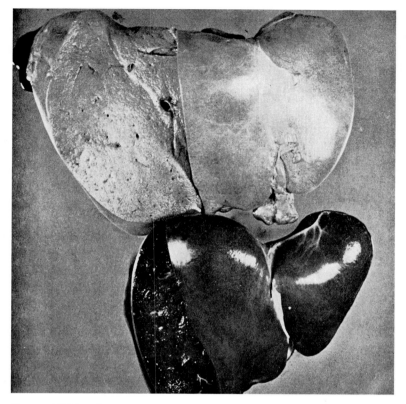

FIGURE X-22a. Comparison of a fatty liver of an alcoholic (above) with a normal liver (below).

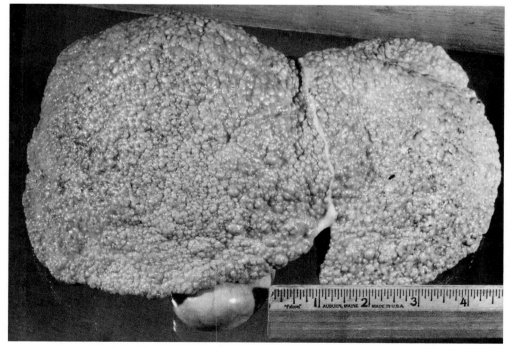

FIGURE X-22b. Rock-hard cirrhotic liver of a chronic alcoholic.

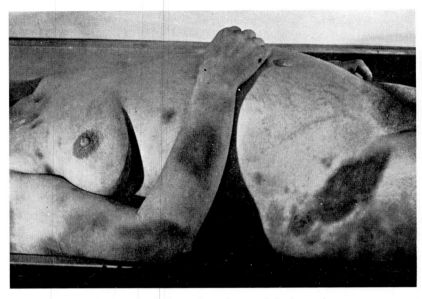

FIGURE X-23. Chronic alcoholic with cirrhosis of the liver showing numerous bruises of various ages over the entire body, but particularly involving protuberant areas. Death was due to subdural hemorrhage.

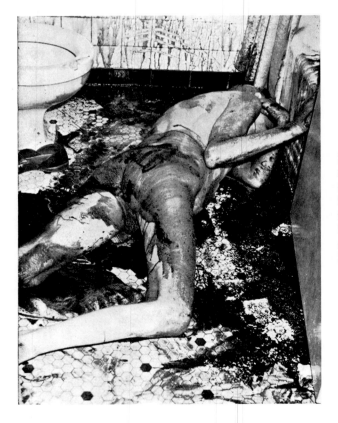

FIGURE X-24. This seventy-one-year-old man with history of hypertension and arteriosclerotic heart disease fell, striking his head on the bathtub. He sustained a superficial 3/4 in. laceration above the eyebrow and a 1/2 in. laceration at the outer angle of the eye. No other injuries were noted. A heart attack apparently caused the fall, and the subsequent confusion and excitement explain the findings at the scene. Note the extensive blood loss. No blood alcohol.

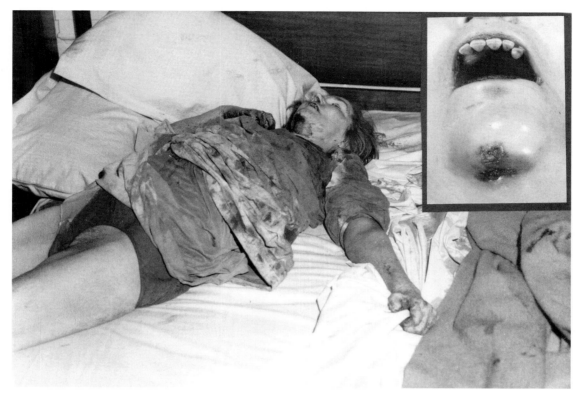

FIGURE X-25. Elderly woman found dead in her apartment. Her clothes were soaked with blood, and blood-stains and smears were present throughout the room and on the walls. There was a bloody screwdriver on the windowsill. The window was slightly raised, and the lower part of the frame was likewise smeared with blood. Postmortem examination showed far advanced nutritional changes of the liver resulting from chronic alcoholism. The only injury found at autopsy was a laceration of the chin *(insert)*. This was initially believed to be a stab wound inflicted with the screwdriver. Postmortem examination, however, showed this to be a superficial abraded tear due to a fall. The screwdriver was apparently used to pry open the window in search of help. Her blood alcohol concentration was 0.32%.

for practical purposes they are considered spontaneous (Fig. X-26). Physical abuse of the elderly often involves various types of trauma involving different areas of the body, including the head. More commonly such injuries are inflicted over an extended period of time. It is essential that they be adequately documented and recorded and the appropriate agencies notified.

Bleeding from open wounds is more extensive and bruises are larger than usual in all forms of asphyxial deaths, drug intoxications, electrocution and drowning, due to intense congestion associated with these conditions.

Fair-haired, often overweight individuals, of North European descent tend to bruise more readily than the general population.

Blunt trauma can be fatal without external or internal evidence of injury. Thus, a sudden forceful blow to the chest in the area of the heart may cause instantaneous cardiac arrest *without* demonstrable damage to the chest wall or the heart. Arrhythmia of the heartbeat is presumed to be the causative mechanism of this phenomenon, known as concussion of the heart or commotio cordis. Similarly, cardiac arrest is sometimes reversed by a forceful thump on the chest, as practiced in cardiopulmonary resuscitation. Steering wheel impact in an automobile driver may cause this type of *cardiac concussion*. We have seen a similar instance where a middle-aged worker in a factory was struck in the chest by a broken-off piece of a grinding wheel. He collapsed instanta-

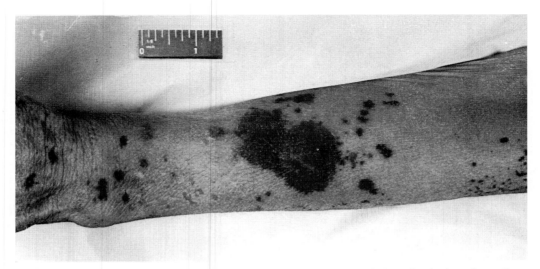

FIGURE X-26. Spontaneous skin hemorrhages as often observed in elderly individuals with capillary fragility.

neously and died within minutes. The skin over the chest plate was abraded by the impact, but there was no evidence of internal injury (Fig. X-27a–b). Another case was that of a 16-year-old who was struck during practice in the center of his chest by a hockey puck, collapsed and was DOA at a nearby hospital. Microscopic, perivascular hemorrhages in the heart muscle may sometimes be observed.

Occasionally, severe injuries occur to players and spectators during baseball games. Swung by a major league player, the end of a baseball bat can reach in excess of 60 mph and a home-run swing will generate a force as high as 8,000 lbs at the time of impact with the ball.[5] Occasionally, nonpenetrating blunt trauma of the chest causes bruising of the heart muscle or the epicardium, laceration of heart valves, rupture of a papillary muscle and more infrequently, laceration or thrombosis of a coronary artery resulting in myocardial infarction.

ABRASION

An abrasion is a scrape with removal of the superficial layers of the skin. More infrequently, an abrasion may involve the subcutaneous tissues and rarely muscle, even bone. In a pedestrian who was struck and dragged by an automobile, the hip joint was *shaved or planed down* into the acetabulum as a result of scraping on the road. Tissue paper-like, wrinkled, whitish gray flaps of epidermis, the outer layer of the skin, may remain attached to one side of the abraded area, indicating the direction in which the scraping occurred (Fig. X-28a-c).

Drying of the area causes the initial pink of the exposed surface to turn pale, yellow-brown, then dark brown, even black. Abrasions may therefore be overlooked on first inspection of a body. When a body is recovered from water, injuries may remain unnoticed until drying occurs. The same hold true for a body covered with wet clothes.

During life abraded skin oozes serum, then becomes scabbed. A scab may drop off after about one week leaving a mildly pale whitish-pink, shiny sunken area which gradually disappears after an additional period of 1–2 weeks. Deeper abrasions bleed and ultimately scar.

Depending on the mechanism of abrasion it may be called a *graze*, such as when a bullet sideswipes the body, a *scratch* when caused by a sharp edge or fingernails, or a *brush burn*, if caused by

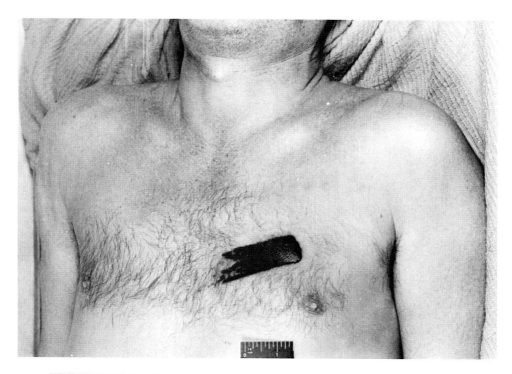

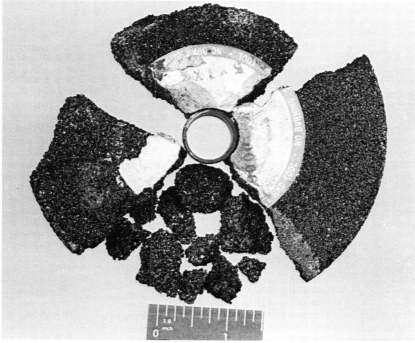

Figure X-27a–b. Worker in a tool and die shop who was struck by a broken chunk of a grinding wheel. The skin on the chest was abraded in the area of impact. The blow caused instantaneous ventricular fibrillation followed by death within a few minutes.

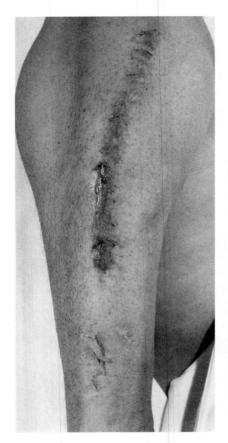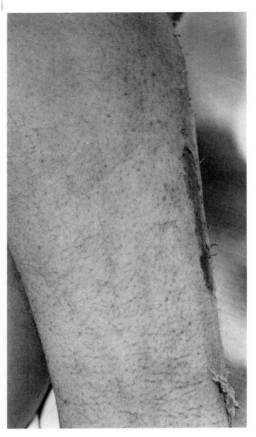

FIGURE X-28a–b. Abrasion of the forearm from the wrist toward the elbow as shown by suspended fragments of epidermis. This occurred as a result of scraping of the arm along the edge of the ulna against the sharp edge of a piece of furniture. The same would occur along the shin.

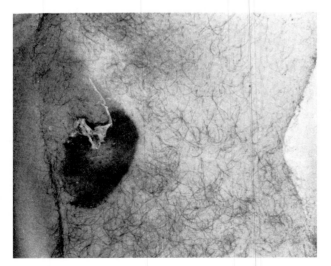

FIGURE X-28c. Dry, dark brown scrape of the knee. Flaps of epidermis attached to the upper edge of the wound, indicate the direction in which the scraping occurred.

the frictional force of rubbing against a rough surface as in dragging on the ground (Figs. X-29a–b and X-30).

A scratch, especially when dry and dark brown, may resemble a burn. A dry linear scratch may resemble an injury caused by the sharp edge of a hot blade. Microscopic examination is sometimes required to establish the true nature of the wound.

Rope burns are caused by friction of the rope against the skin. The rope need not be rough. While considerable heat may be generated by such friction, causing a second degree burn, it is more likely that friction causes blisters mechanically by expressing tissue fluids into the upper layers of the skin. A rope burn would thus be another form of abrasion (Fig. X-31a–b).

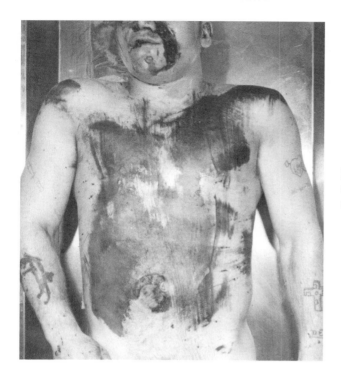

FIGURE X-29a. Unrestrained driver thrown from his vehicle as a result of a collision and received brush burn injuries by scraping on the road surface.

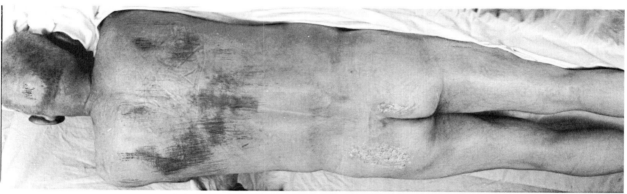

FIGURE X-29b. Victim of homicide dragged away from the scene to hide the body. Brush burns are noted on protuberant areas of the back and the occipital area of the scalp.

Abrasions are also caused by handcuffs, binding and tying. In all such cases, the skin should be incised under the restraint in search of hemorrhage. Where wrists or ankles have been restrained incisions should be made over the bony prominences which is where subcutaneous hemorrhages are more likely to be found, rather than on the front or back surfaces. Undermining such cuts with the use of a scalpel broadens the examined area with no additional disruption. The presence of hemorrhage indicates that the

victim was alive and struggling when being restrained and may suggest that the cuffs were too tight. Conversely, the absence of hemorrhage does not imply that the individual was dead. Certain types of ligatures are more apt to cause hemorrhage than others. A clothesline or electric cord is more likely to bruise skin than wide tape, a towel or smooth articles of clothing. Denim, as in certain types of blue jeans, is abrasive.

It is frequently difficult to distinguish between an abrasion sustained during life and one that

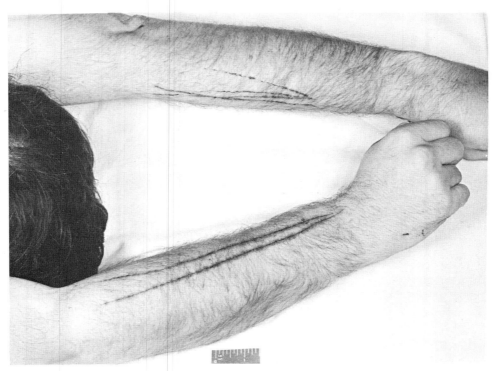

FIGURE X-30. Scrapes of the forearms with sharp and pointed object.

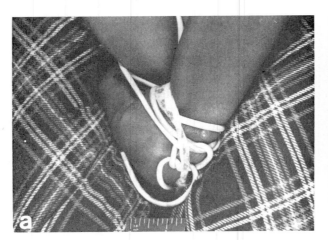
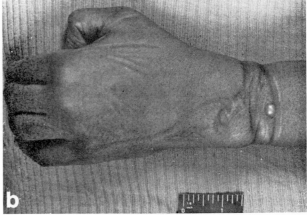

FIGURE X-31a–b. (a) Tight binding with smooth nylon clothesline. (b) Rope burns with blister formation caused by twisting of the forearm and pinching of the skin by the binding. Also note the dark discoloration of the hand compared to the skin above the binding due to obstruction of the venous return.

occurred after death. Bleeding into the surrounding tissues does not usually occur due to the superficial nature of an abrasion, unless the scraping is associated with a direct, forceful impact. Hemorrhage into the surrounding tissue typically indicates that the victim was alive at the time of injury. Brush burns for instance sustained by scraping along a road surface and extending over vast areas of the body, usually show no underlying bleeding. *Bleeding by gravity* may be seen in areas of livor mortis due to blood vessels torn after death. It may be difficult to distinguish this type of *bleeding* from genuine antemortem injury. Whereas, such bruises are unlikely to be extensive, a pint or more of blood may trickle from an open wound situated in a dependent area of a dead body. Liver diseases, certain blood clotting defects and therapeutic blood thinner medication will enhance such postmortem blood loss.

Noticeable healing begins soon after injury. The reaction of the body to an injury generally permits a rough estimate of the age of a wound. A fresh abrasion is moist, leaking serum for a day or two before it is gradually covered by a crust or scab under which the healing proceeds until complete. Some red blood cells may be trapped within the scab. The duration of the healing process depends on the extent of the injury, the presence of secondary infection and repeated trauma to the same area.

Abrasions are often characteristically patterned providing information regarding the nature of the force (Fig. X-32). A fall to the ground or a hard blow to the body with a flat object may cause an abrasion matching the weave pattern of the clothing worn by the victim. This is especially true with coarse fabrics. Zippers give a very distinct image (Fig. X-33). Scraping on a wooden surface may show irregularly spaced, parallel scratches which correspond to the grain pattern in the wood. An impact with a textured object, such as a rough board or a threaded pipe may also cause a patterned injury (Figs. X-34 to X-39). We have seen the pattern of the wood grain of a baseball bat imprinted in the skin in a case of bludgeoning.

An elderly man who was found unconscious on a sidewalk was DOA at a local hospital. At autopsy the cause of death was determined to be an acute myocardial infarction. The cause of injuries on the left side of the face was not resolved until scene investigation showed the pattern to be the result of striking gravel (Fig. X-40 a-b).

Gravel may cause a dense distribution of irregular abrasions or a more subtle pattern of sparsely scattered similar abrasions. Of course, the dimensions of each individual injury depends on the size of the rocks and whether this was a stationary impact or if there was movement. In the latter case, the abrasions are elongated and wavy, sometimes overlapping as a

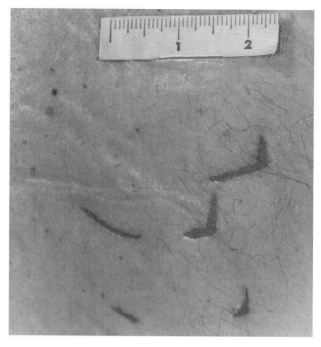

FIGURE X-32. Ninety-degree angled abrasions caused by blows with a 2 X 4. The corners of the board caused the injuries. Any board with straight corners would do the same.

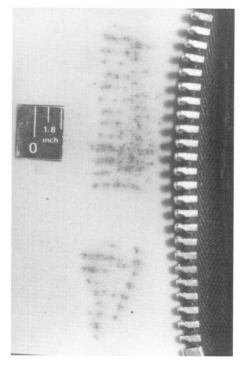

FIGURE X-33. Patterned abrasion of a zipper sustained when the clothes were grabbed during an altercation.

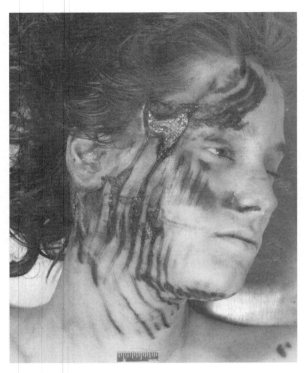

FIGURE X-34. Fourteen-year-old spectator at a stadium stampeded to death when the moving stairway on which she was standing came to a sudden halt causing her to fall. The face and neck show the pattern of the escalator tread.

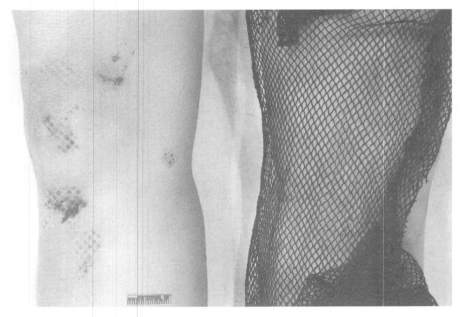

FIGURE X-35. Young woman pedestrian who was struck by an automobile and survived three days. At autopsy it was first thought that she had been run over by a motorcycle because of the peculiarly patterned abrasions on her knee and leg. Investigation revealed that the pattern was caused by the imprint of her stocking.

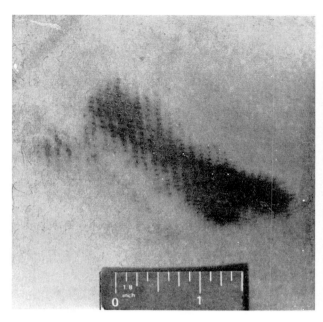

FIGURE X-36a. Superficial scrape (abrasion) showing a pattern of parallel vertical lines consisting of dots produced by the knots in the weave pattern of the shirt worn by the deceased. Such an injury must not be mistaken for a brush burn in which the pattern is usually finer and not as regular. Only a fabric's weave pattern would produce the regularly spaced dots.

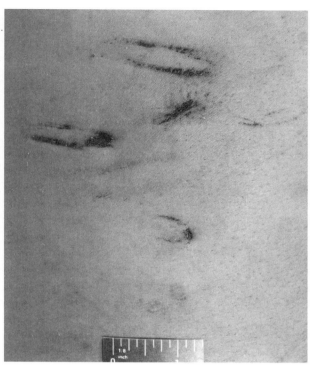

FIGURE X-36b. Subtle fabric weave pattern indicating that clothes were worn during beating with a pipe. The top injuries show the pattern better.

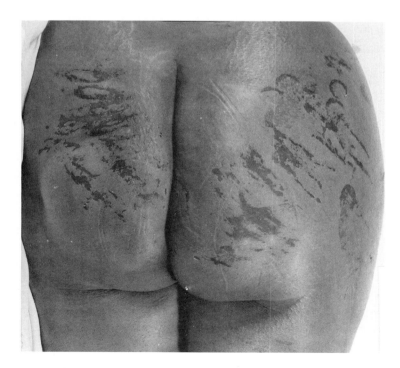

FIGURE X-37. Beating with hammer. The parallel abrasions are produced by the handle which due to the force of impact and obesity of the deceased sunk well into the tissues. The circular and semicircular injuries are the imprints of the head of the tool.

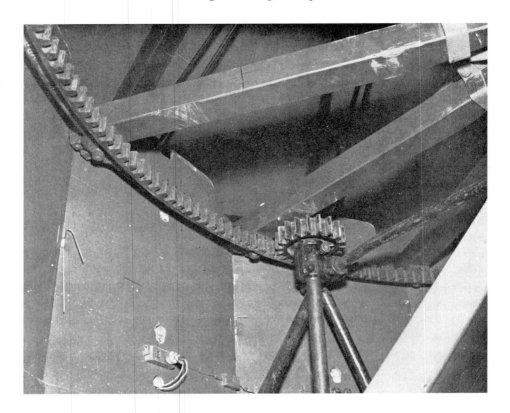

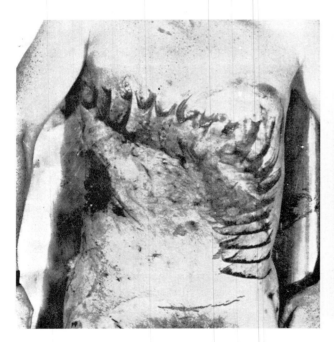

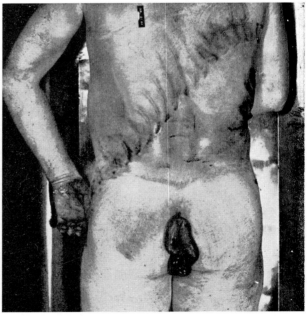

FIGURE X-38a–c. (a) Gears of a merry-go-round. The clothes of the operator were caught in the gears, and pulled him in. (b) Imprint of the gears on the chest and abdomen. Just above the pubic hair and in the right groin are superficial tears which are due to overstretching. (c) Rear view. Bowel prolapse due to perineal tear as a result of immense pressure on the abdomen. This sometimes occurs when individuals are run over by motor vehicles. The perineum is the area of least resistance.

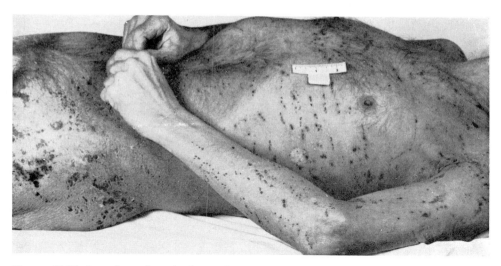

FIGURE X-39. Scratch marks spread over the entire body in an alcoholic due to flea infestation. Irritation of the skin leads to scratching, infection and crusting. The crusts on the chest are situated along the ribs, on the hip they are clustered, and on the arm and forearm the scratch marks suggest a vertical pattern. The patterns correspond to the normal and usual way people scratch themselves.

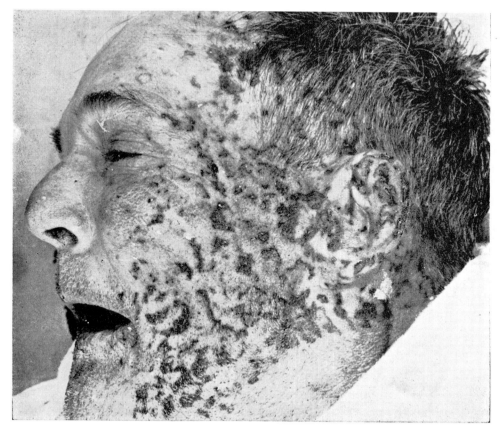

FIGURE X-40a. Patterned abrasions from impact on gravel. Note the irregular outline of each of the injuries and their superficiality. Protuberance of the lower jaw protects the neck.

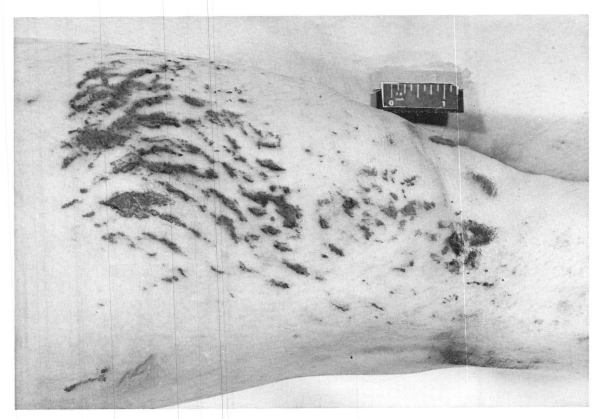

FIGURE X-40b. Irregular, wavy, parallel abrasions from rolling on gravel.

result of rolling, as opposed to each injury showing the outline of the stone imprinted in the skin. Rarely, a stone may be embedded, but frequently there is dust or sand on the body surface. Only examination of the scene will establish compatibility of the injuries with the terrain (Fig. X-41a–b).

Although, not a pattern in the true sense of the word, crawling causes a pattern by way of location and distribution of the injuries. Bruises and abrasions will be apparent primarily on the bony prominences of the elbows, knees and shin areas. The bruises are diffuse, many times over large

areas. Abrasions correspond to the irregularities of the surface on which the crawling occurs and may closely resemble those sustained by impact on gravel. Many of the abrasions are confluent and deep and obviously sustained during life as shown by the extent of underlying hemorrhage. Crawling on rough ice or frozen ground causes similar, but often more pronounced and extensive injuries (Fig. X-42a–b).

Skin slippage as in decomposition, second-degree burns or prolonged immersion in water may render identification of an abrasion difficult or impossible.

LACERATION

A laceration is a tear produced by blunt trauma. Typical lacerations occur in the head due to the underlying supportive skull. The force of the impact and its direction determine the appear-

ance and depth of the wound along with associated injuries, such as fractures. Undermining of the edges of a laceration indicates the direction in which an impact occurred (Fig. X-43). Equal

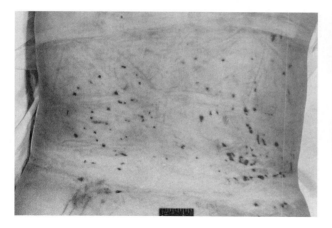

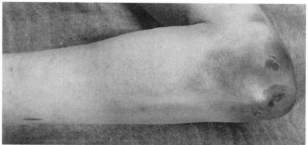

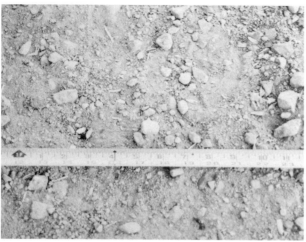

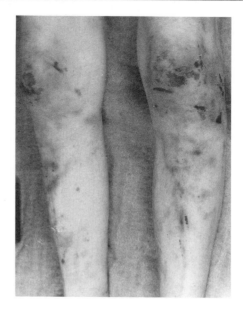

FIGURE X-41a–b. (a) Fall from the eighth floor of an apartment building. The scattered irregular discreet abrasions of gravel in a sparse pattern. (b) Gravel comprised of stones of different sizes. This type of gravel would not cause a pattern as shown in Figure X-41(a).

FIGURE X-42a–b. Crawling injuries. Note the extent of bruising and abrasions which resemble those from gravel.

undermining on all sides suggests a perpendicular force.

Two types of lacerations are common: Those due to a perpendicular blow and those caused by a glancing blow. Perpendicular blows are caused by objects such as a hammer, pipe or bottle (Figs. X-44 to X-49), or as is frequently sustained when falling to the ground (Figs. X-50 to X-60a–b). A glancing blow may tear only the skin, or if deeper may separate the skin and subcutaneous tissues from the underlying muscle fascia, creating a gaping and profusely bleeding wound. Anytime the skin is not torn by the impact incision

will reveal a subcutaneous pocket filled with blood and crushed fat (see Chapter XVII).

The shape of a laceration produced by striking the head on a flat surface will differ depending on the location of the impact. Such laceration may be straight, semicircular or star-shaped, due to the different curvatures of the skull, the amount of subcutaneous tissue in the particular area and other factors.

A young man who had been arrested for drunk and disorderly conduct, and placed in the back of a police car, struck his head repeatedly on the plexiglass divider between the front and rear seats. He sustained a one-inch diameter, concave, semicircular laceration on his upper forehead, at the hairline with a two-inch diameter underlying bruise. The injury was photographically documented.

Following his release the next day, he filed a complaint that he had been struck with a police baton. The injury

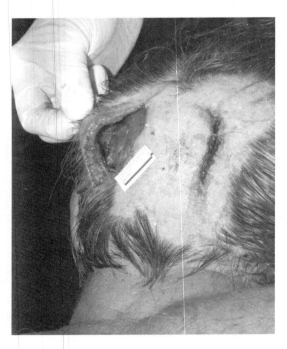

FIGURE X-43. Undermined laceration. The subcutaneous *pocket* which becomes apparent when the skin is lifted indicates the direction of the impact (right to left).

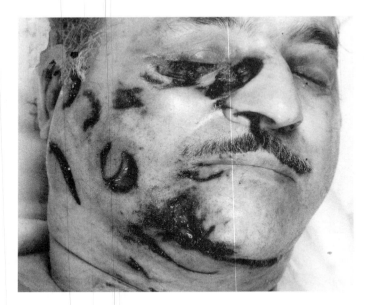

FIGURE X-44. Crescent-shaped lacerations from impacts with the round end of a hammer. Note that injuries of the eye, nose and chin are also hammer blows but appear different. In identifying the weapon, it is necessary to recognize patterns and realize that different areas of the body react differently to trauma. Areas with underlying bone, folds and recessed areas will distort the pattern.

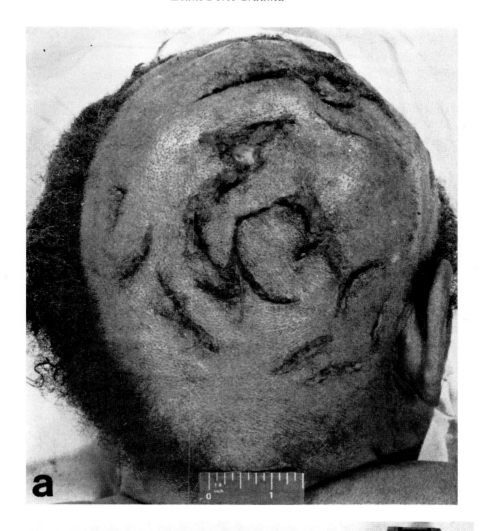

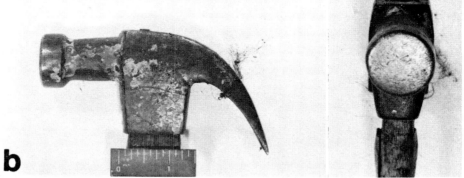

FIGURE X-45a–b. (a) Semicircular tears of the scalp due to blows with the round end of a claw hammer. (b) The victim's hair is on the hammer. Completion of the circle of the scalp wounds indicates the diameter of the round end of the hammer, thus its weight.

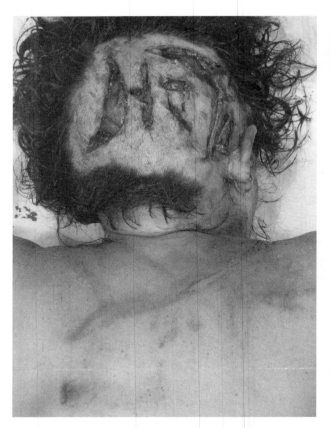

FIGURE X-46. Numerous lacerations on the back of the head, when considered in conjunction with the elongated bruises on the back, suggest that a pipe was used. The diameter may be represented in the bruise at the bottom of the picture which shows the imprint of the end of the pipe.

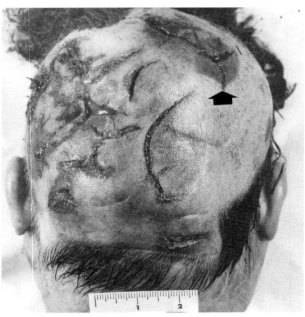

FIGURE X-47. Multiple injuries caused by a hexagonal side of a hammer. The hexagonal shape is shown in abrasion indicated with the *arrow*. The central lacerations of the two adjacent wounds are splits. The large curvy linear split in the center back shows the abraded rectangular impact at its lower end. Many of the remaining injuries, although complex, do show the typical abrasions of the weapon contact.

FIGURE X-48. Injuries caused by both sides of a claw hammer. Note the overlapping of the injuries produced with the claw end. The use of a magnifying glass when viewing the original pictures showed the weave pattern of the clothes the victim was wearing when he was struck in all of the injuries.

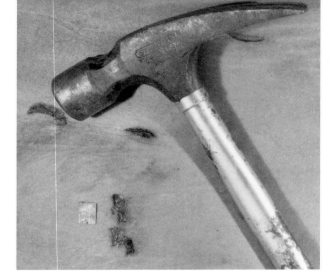

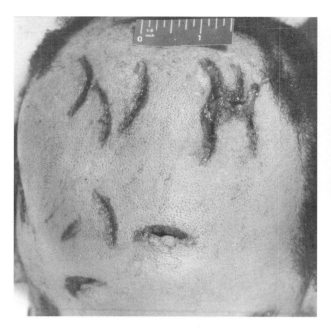

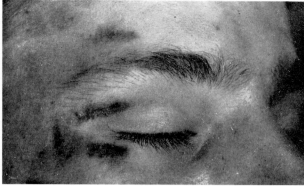

FIGURE X-50. Injury sustained in a fall: superficial abrasion above the eyebrow and outlining the outer rim of the eye socket. Many times the side of the nose is also scraped. A fall to one side of the face would place all three locations on one plane.

FIGURE X-49. Blows with the edge of a wooden mallet. Note that the edges of the injuries are just a little more ragged, less defined, more abraded than those caused by a hammer. A metal hammer usually has a sharper edge, thus the wound edges would be less abraded.

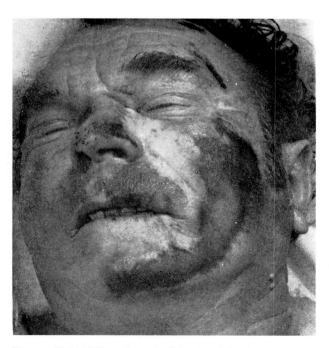

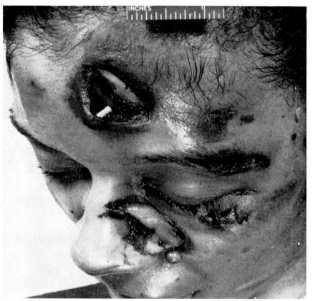

FIGURE X-52. Middle-aged woman who was found raped and beaten in the basement of an abandoned house. A lamp and a broken bottle caused her injuries. The tear on the forehead is propped open showing undermining of the edges. The edges of the wound are abraded and ragged. This wound was probably made by the heavy lamp base. The cut on the left side of the nose was produced by the jagged ends of the broken bottle; it showed no marginal abrasion, no undermining and smooth edges. The tear in the left eyebrow, the abrasion immediately above it and the abrasion and tear below the eye were sustained when she fell.

FIGURE X-51. Fall, striking the left side of the face on a concrete surface. The protuberant parts in the areas of impact, i.e., the chin, left side of the lower jaw, left cheek, left side of forehead at the outer end of the eyebrow, and left side of the nose and lip, are abraded. The paler area within the abrasion on the cheek is due to the abundance of soft tissues in that location and the absence of underlying bone.

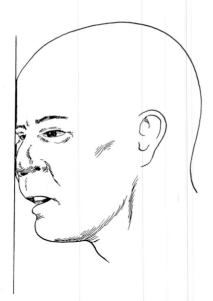

FIGURE X-53. Diagram showing protuberant parts of the face in contact with a flat surface. These are the areas often injured in a fall. Note, the nose is pushed to the left.

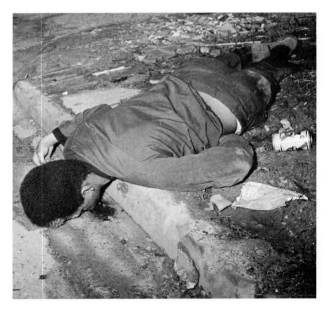

FIGURE X-54. Shot in the back of the head, protuberant parts of the central portion of the face making contact with the flat surface of the pavement. These areas are often injured in an unmitigated fall.

FIGURE X-55. A full face forward fall, striking the forehead, the bridge and the tip of the nose. The forehead is lacerated at the midline, which is the most protuberant part in that position. The skin is scraped in the middle of the forehead and the injury extends above the right eyebrow. The tip of the nose gave way on impact, permitting the bridge of the nose to make contact.

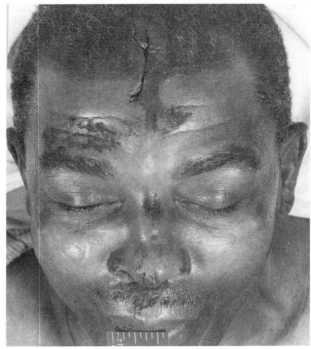

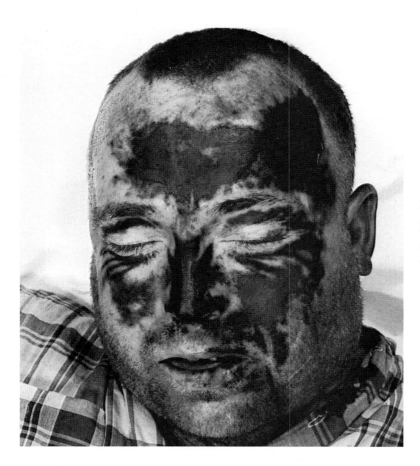

FIGURE X-56. Lineman who fell to the ground from a utility pole as a result of electrocution. His face was abraded by impact on the ground. Note the eyelids, creases and other recessed areas are intact.

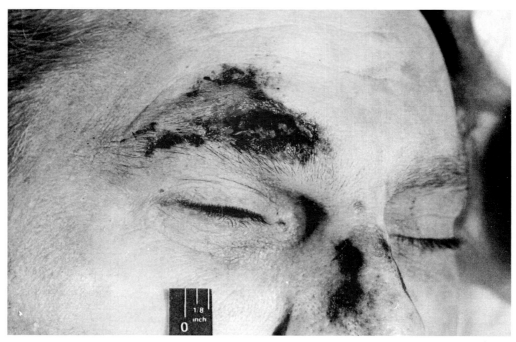

FIGURE X-57. Laceration of the forehead above the eyebrow is often due to a fall. Note the injury of the right side of the nose, which is in the same plane as that of the forehead.

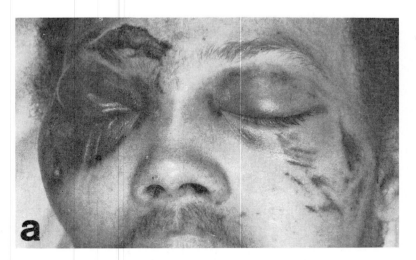

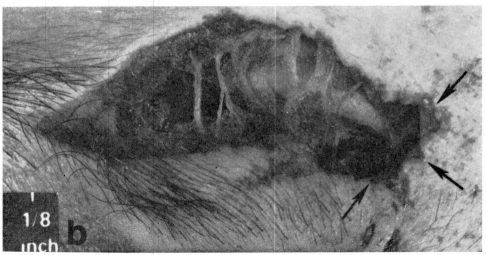

FIGURE X-58a–b. (a) Multiple injuries of various shapes and severity; some suggest a pattern, others are irregular and nondescript. The right black eye was caused by seepage of blood under the skin. (b) The tear above the eyebrow (close-up) was caused by a blow above and to the right of the bridge of the nose, at which place the wound edges are typically abraded (arrows). From here, the skin split with nonabraded, jagged edges connected by tissue bridges.

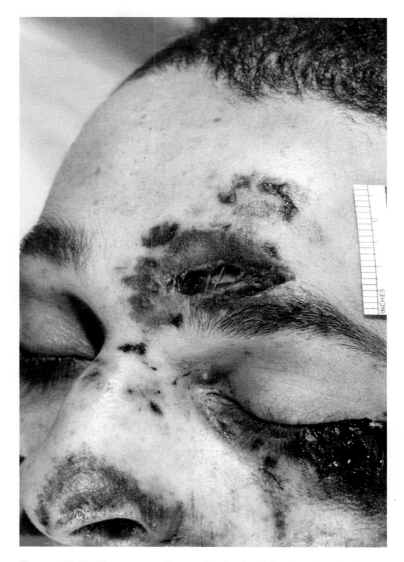

FIGURE X-59. Young man shot in the back of the head while fleeing police. He fell to the pavement. The injuries shown were sustained in the fall and involved the facial prominences. Note the delicate tissue bridges, undermining and the marginal abrasion of the laceration above the eyebrow. The area of abrasion corresponds to the area of contact with the pavement. The protected contents of the eye socket are not damaged. The combination of a bruise, abrasion or laceration of the forehead, temple (near the eye) and the side of the nose on the same side indicates a fall.

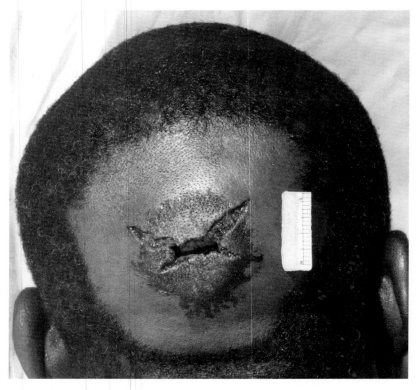

FIGURE X-60a. Star-shaped tear of the posterior scalp due to a fall on pavement while heavily intoxicated. The circular abrasion surrounding the tear represents the area of contact. Separation of the edges of the wound disclosed multiple tissue bridges and undermining, extending under the abraded area.

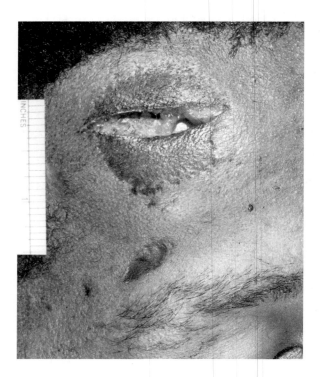

FIGURE X-60b. Forward fall striking the right side of the forehead. Note the distribution of injuries: Frontal protuberance showing circular undermined abrasion with central split laceration and abrasions above the eyebrow and below the eye.

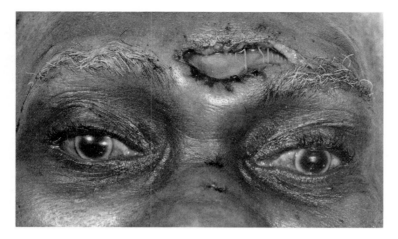

FIGURE X-61a. Elderly man who collapsed to the ground as a result of a heart attack. The laceration of the forehead is due to the fall. The wound edges are abraded and delicate whitish-gray strands of tissue (nerves, blood vessels, collagen, etc.) extend between the edges. The lower edge of the laceration is elevated from the underlying bone (undermined). Tissue bridges can be subtle and may be missed without careful examination. Wound edges may need to be gently separated manually.

could indeed have been caused by a strike with a baton, however, he was observed striking his head in the vehicle and recreation of the event with similar results, convinced the Board of Review of the false nature of the complaint. For recreation, stamp ink was placed on the forehead of a human skull, then imprinted on a sheet of white paper. This produced a pattern compatible with the normal curvature of the skull and the semicircular laceration of the complainant.

In the contact area, the edges of such laceration are characteristically undermined due to the crushing and shearing force against the bone. Between opposing edges of the wound run multiple delicate threads of tissue consisting of nerves, elastic and connective tissue fibers and blood vessels, collectively known as *tissue bridges* (see Figs. X-58a–b, X-59, and X-61a). Tissue bridges are especially abundant in splits which extend from the area of contact. Splits are not abraded or undermined. They result from dissipation of residual energy which extends from the area of contact, similarly to what happens with a ripe watermelon which splits into multiple pieces upon falling to the ground. Tissue bridges become apparent when the edges of the wound are gently separated manually. The presence of tissue bridges invariably distinguishes blunt from sharp trauma, i.e., a blow from a cut.

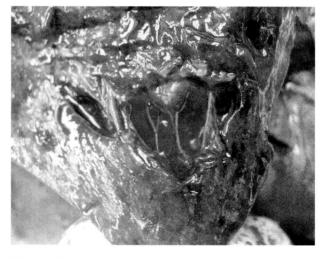

FIGURE X-61b. Driver of automobile with crushed chest. The lung shows a laceration with tissue bridges.

The skin is not the only tissue which shows *bridging*. Internal organs, more commonly the lungs and heart, may also show lacerations with evidence of bridging, confirming the crushing nature of the injuries (X-61b). Liver, kidney, pancreas and spleen do not usually show bridging, presumably due to the limited amount, or absence of interstitial tissues.

Pistol whipping is an all-encompassing term not necessarily limited to firearms. Injuries identical to pistol whipping may be inflicted with the back end of the handle of a knife.

Lacerations from pistol whipping are predominately located on the head (Figs. X-62 to X-66). These injuries are typical yet often misunderstood. Usually only a part of the weapon, often a corner, strikes the skin causing a central abraded depression from which splits with typical tissue bridges radiate. The shape and dimensions of the abrasion display those of the impacting surface. Sometimes a pattern may be recognized within the abrasion. The tissue underlying the split skin is not crushed and therefore not bruised. Any blood which may come from torn superficial vessels in the edges of a split runs outward and does not permeate the tissue. Consequently, the extent of bruising associated with pistol whipping and other blows with rounded, cornered or pointed weapons may be quite limited. In the case of a corner impact, crushing of the skin is so focal that bruising may be absent. The force of the blow may cause underlying fracture, however, sometimes only the outer layer of the skull is focally dented while a larger defect occurs in the inner surface. The energy of the impact spreads through the brain in a funnel shape. It would not

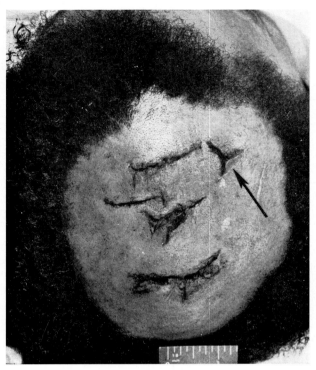

FIGURE X-62. Irregular and ragged lacerations of the scalp caused by pistol-whipping. The triangular-shaped wound (arrow) was caused by a pointed corner of the weapon, which produced the center of the wound; the three radiating tears were caused by splitting of the skin. The four parallel horizontal injuries were likely produced by the blunt edge of the pistol handle. The underlying skull was fractured.

FIGURE X-63. Three pistol whipping injuries. Note that the injuries run in parallel. The subtle bruises to the right and left of the injuries may have been caused by other parts of the weapon.

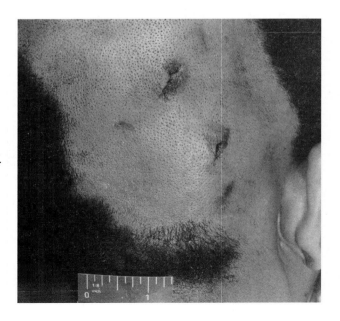

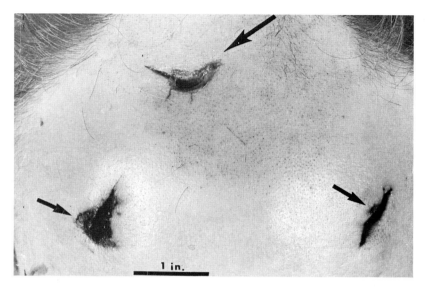

FIGURE X-64a. Pistol whipping injuries likely caused by a corner of the grip. The abraded areas (arrows) are points of contact with the weapon. All three impacts show a pattern. Extension of the lacerations is the result of skin splitting.

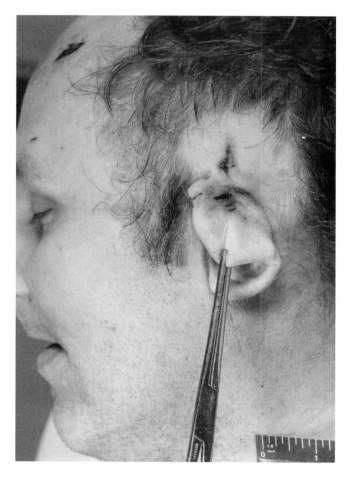

FIGURE X-64b. Pistol whipping showing ragged laceration of the back of the ear and adjacent scalp with pattern evident. This can be matched to the weapon.

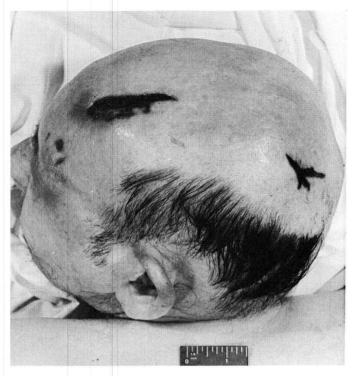

FIGURE X-65. Pistol whipping. Different areas of the weapon cause injuries of different shapes.

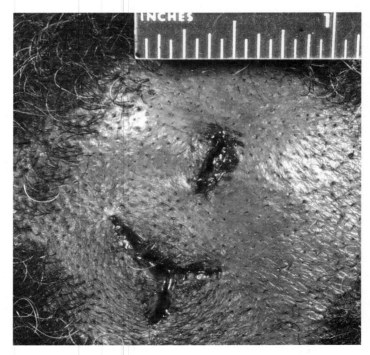

FIGURE X-66. Pistol whipping. The lower triangular laceration shows no abrasion suggesting that a corner impacted. The upper injury shows a semicircular abrasion on the right edge.

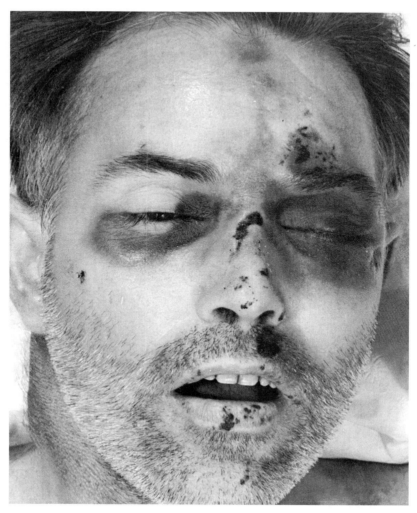

FIGURE X-67. Injuries sustained in a fist fight, recessed as well as protuberant areas are injured. The clusters of abrasions above the medial left eyebrow, the tip of the nose and the lower lip resulted from a fall onto a gravelly road.

be unusual for a forceful focal impact to spread through the entire brain, causing severe dazing or loss of consciousness.

A superficial, horizontal split measuring 3/4–1 inch in length in one or both of the upper eyelids sometimes occurs in cases of prolonged swelling. Such swelling is brought on by edema or hemorrhage and causes thinning of the skin due to stretching and necrosis. This condition may be seen in falls on the back of the head with rebound fractures of the orbital roofs resulting in seepage of blood into the eyelids. In contrast to this type of splitting of the eyelid, a fist blow to the eye frequently lacerates the skin of the cheek along the lower outline of the eye socket, as a result of crushing of the skin between the fist and the boney ridge. Additionally, a fist blow to the eye often causes extensive subconjunctival and scleral hemorrhage. The entire front of the eye may be red and laceration of the eye, though uncommon, may be seen on occasion. Air bag deployment in a car crash may cause similar injury.

Blows to the face, especially fist blows, may injure both protuberant and recessed areas (Figs. X-67 to X-69). Injuries sustained by falling on a flat surface, such as the floor, are generally located on the protuberant parts of the body, i.e., over

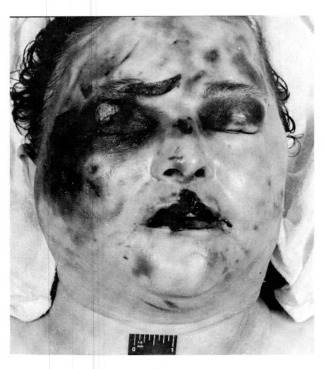

FIGURE X-68. Fist fight. Note the multitude of injuries involving protuberant as well as recessed areas.

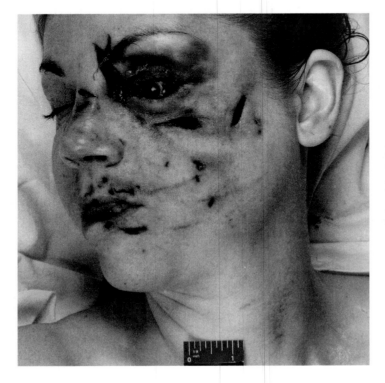

FIGURE X-69. The skin of the left upper eyelid was crushed against the rim of the eye socket and split. All the injuries of the left eye area could have been produced by a single fist blow. The parallel abraded lines, continued with deeper abrasions above and below the mouth suggest a pattern.

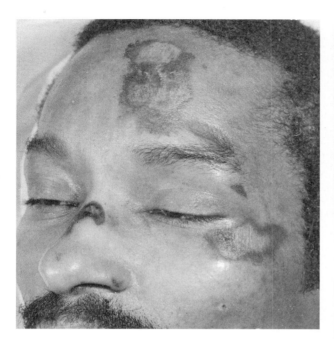

FIGURE X-70. Injuries sustained in a fall. The protuberant areas are involved showing vertical parallel deeper linear scratches from the cement surface.

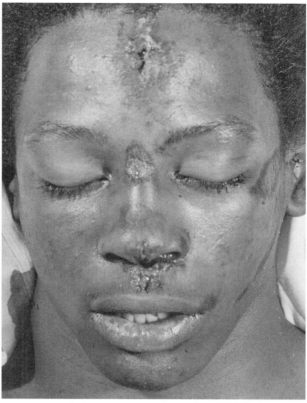

FIGURE X-71. Full face unmitigated fall. All areas of contact are abraded.

bony prominences (Figs. X-70 to X-71). Thus, in a fall, the eye and eyelids are typically spared, while the skin over the outer and upper rim of the eye socket is commonly abraded or torn, depending on the severity of the impact. The skin over the cheekbones and the lower jaw is also commonly injured in a fall. An unmitigated fall from an upright position usually results in extensive lacerations and fractures. Some of the fractures result directly from the impact, others from fractured bone piercing the skin from within.

In the case of a fall on the back of the head the abraded scalp surface many times is circular and circumscribes the laceration (see Fig. X-60a–b). The abraded area is crushed and often detached from the skull, i.e., undermined. The soft tissues over a broad area under the scalp are infiltrated with blood and a *pocket* produced by the undermining contains liquid blood and crushed fat. In contrast, a blow with a narrow, blunt object, such as the edge of an angle iron or a crowbar, produces a linear tear with finely abraded edges and minimal undermining limited to the area of contact with the impacting surface or no undermining at all (Figs. X-72 to X-76). A ball-peen

hammer would fall into the same category (Fig. X-77).

Foreign bodies such as fragments of glass, chips of paint, or gravel are sometimes found in a laceration. The finding of foreign material in a wound may be invaluable in the case of a hit-and-run traffic accident. It is therefore good practice to examine surgically debrided skin from trauma cases for trace evidence when indicated. The use of a dissecting microscope is advantageous for this purpose.

A severe blunt impact may cause minimal external evidence of injury, however internal injuries may be catastrophic. A sudden sharp turn of a bicycle may cause a blow to the abdomen by the handlebar which can tear the liver or spleen and result in massive internal bleeding (Fig. X-78).[6] A kick or punch in the upper abdomen may crush the pancreas[7] causing spillage of digestive enzymes and pancreatitis, or injure the small intestine and cause death

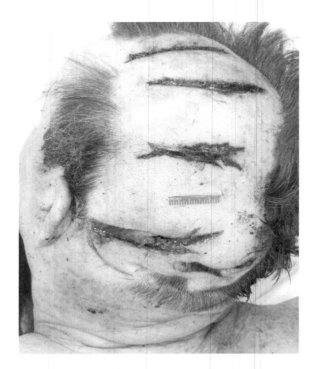

FIGURE X-72. Night watchman stuck with a crowbar during a robbery. Note the linear shape of the injuries and the V-shaped extensions from each end. These extension tears result from bursting or splitting of the skin due to crushing between the weapon and the bone in the central segment of the wound.

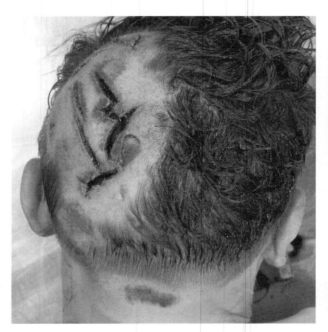

FIGURE X-73. Struck by unidentified weapon. Several of the lacerations have straight abraded edges. The width of the abraded skin, after the wound edges are approximated, represents the approximate dimension of the weapon in the area of contact. The well demarcated bruise in the nape of the neck also shows the width of the weapon.

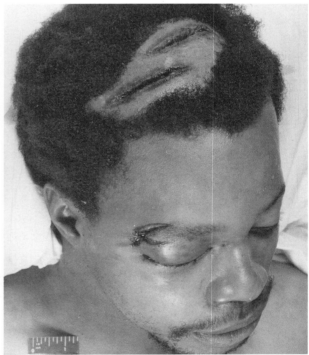

FIGURE X-74. The abraded margins of two parallel scalp wounds are easily visible. Re-approximation of the wound edges indicates the area of contact with the weapon.

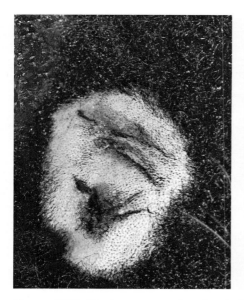 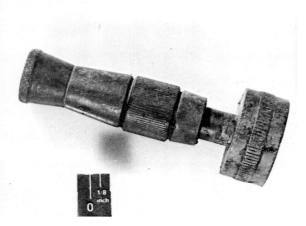

FIGURE X-75. Head injuries produced with the brass hose nozzle shown on the right. The areas of contact are abraded. The skin is torn and split beyond the abraded areas. One would not select this tool as having caused these injuries, however considering that the abraded edges conform to areas of contact, the weapon is consistent.

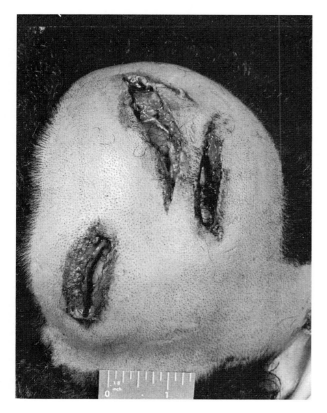

FIGURE X-76. Injuries of the head produced with a pipe. The diameter of the pipe corresponds to the width of the injuries, after approximation of the edges to counteract gaping.

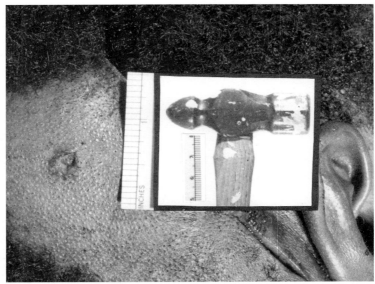

FIGURE X-77. Impact with peen end of a ball-peen hammer (insert) behind the ear. The injury shows a circular laceration surrounded by abrasion which at first site suggests a bullet wound.

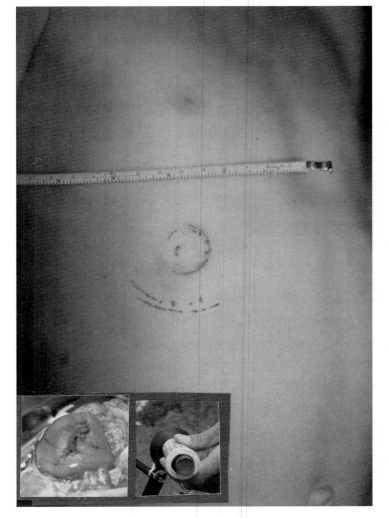

FIGURE X-78. Young boy riding a bicycle on a rural road turned sharply to the right, when a vehicle came toward him, striking a tree stump buried in tall grass. As he turned the cycle, he slammed the exposed end of the handlebar (insert–right) into his right abdominal quadrant. The picture shows the bruised imprint of the grip end of the handlebar on the skin. He died from bleeding from a torn liver (insert–left).

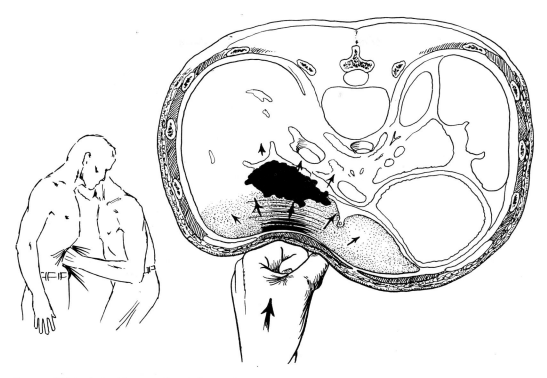

FIGURE X-79. A fist blow to the abdominal area often reveals no external evidence of injury, despite extensive damage to underlying organs.

within a few days from peritonitis. Injury to the abdominal wall is seldom visible in any of these examples (Fig. X-79). The lack of external evidence of trauma in the case of injury to the pancreas may make a causal relationship between a blow and the death difficult to prove, particularly in the absence of witnesses and because pancreatitis occurs spontaneously, frequently in alcoholics and in people with gallstones. Tears of the liver caused by a flat impact to the right upper abdomen are commonly located close to the hepatic ligament, due to the fact that fixation of any part of an organ makes it more vulnerable to blunt trauma. Similarly the aorta tears most frequently at the ligamentum arteriosum.

A glancing blow to the right upper abdominal quadrant sometimes separates the liver capsule from the underlying liver tissue. Bleeding beneath the capsule, so-called subcapsular hemorrhage may rupture into the abdominal cavity. Such rupture of the liver capsule may take several days to develop. Subcapsular liver hemorrhage in newborns during delivery was relatively common prior to improved obstetrical care. The mecha-

nism of this injury is crushing and shearing forces applied to the newborn's abdomen during passage through the birth canal (Fig. X-80a–b). Death due to massive abdominal bleeding often resulted two or three days after delivery. Potter[8] describes a similar injury to newborns if the upper abdomen is grasped too firmly during delivery and Stahl relates having seen battered children with lacerations of the liver due to the same mechanism. Tearing of the liver in an infant is sometimes associated with death caused by shaking.

Injuries due to crushing may cause deep damage with tearing of muscles and fractures. On the body surface, i.e., on the skin, crushing injuries are sometimes manifested by typical tears of the epidermis, unless the crushing is severe in which case full thickness tears result. Superficial overstretching injuries create an image suggestive of stretch marks with densely distributed parallel, intertwining defects. When one or several of these superficial tears is subjected to an increasing load, the elasticity of the skin will eventually be overcome and at that time vast lacerations occur (Fig. X-81).

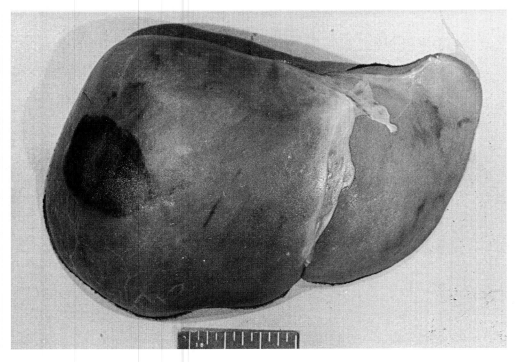

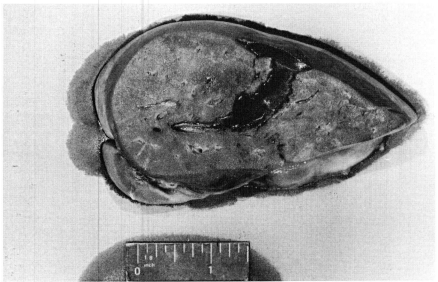

FIGURE X-80a–b. (a) Subcapsular hemorrhage and torn liver and of a newborn sustained during delivery. (b) As seen on the cross section.

SKELETAL INJURIES

Just as distinctive trauma of the body surface and certain types of internal organ damage may permit determining a particular method of violence, similar information may be derived from injuries of the bony skeleton. The skull is especially amenable to this type of assessment. Although the skull is largely resistant to fractures due to its shape, its bony elasticity and its con-

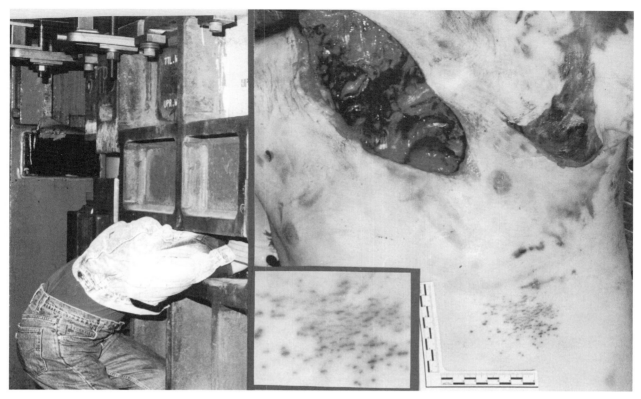

FIGURE X-81. Worker in a stamping plant who was crushed in a press *(left)*. The major pressure was exerted on the upper chest and shoulder girdle, causing vast deep bilateral lacerations exposing the fractured rib cage *(right)*. The pressure in this area caused overstretching injuries below, next to the ruler *(see enlarged insert center)*. Additional discussion and illustrations may be found in the traffic chapter, since overstretching skin injuries frequently occur in pedestrian accidents.

struction in a number of resilient arches, when fractures do occur the fracture lines tend to conform to characteristic patterns. We have seen depressed skull fractures in numerous cases and the following are a few examples: A fall on the sharp corner of a piece of furniture, an impact with the pointed edge of a rock, a blow with a hammer, and an impact with the grab handle on the A-pillar of an automobile, as may occur in an unrestrained occupant in a frontal collision. Sometimes only a single piece of bone is driven inward corresponding to the outline of the impacting surface. A punch used to cut out various shapes may be used as an analogy.

In the publicized case of Jon Benét Ramsey, the 6-year-old girl found murdered at her parents' residence in Boulder, Colorado, there was a perfectly rectangular depressed right parietal skull fracture. Soft tissues of the galea still held in place one side of the knocked out piece of bone. The underlying brain was extensively bruised and the entire brain was swollen. A 3-cell mag flashlight, found on the kitchen counter of the home is consistent with the murder weapon. The head of a 3-cell mag flashlight sunk perfectly into a recreated bony defect, illustrating that the skull, as a membranous bone, accurately keeps the shape of the penetrating object (Fig. X-82).

Rarely, only the inner bony layer at the site of impact may fracture leaving the outer table intact (Fig. X-83a–b). The mechanism of this type of fracture can be compared to the breaking of a *plaster* ceiling when the floor above is hit with the end of a broomstick. The loose plug of bone may push down on the brain and on x-ray resemble a foreign object or a calcified falx of the dura. Such injuries have been known to occur due to pistol whipping, a blow with the corner of a hand-held two-way radio or an object of similar shape.

More frequently, by far, are depressed skull fractures, where the bone fragments still attached at one edge, are bent inward, often in the shape

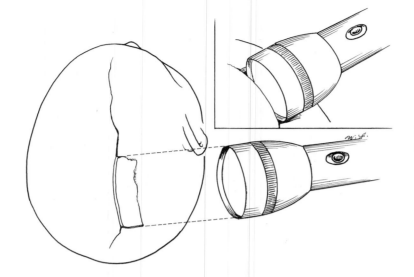

FIGURE X-82. The defect in the skull corresponds to the dimensions of the weapon.

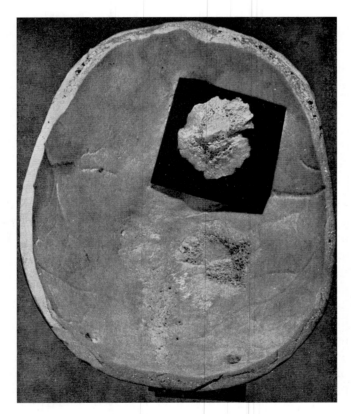

FIGURE X-83a. Experimental fracture of the inner layer of the skull produced by a blow on the outer surface with the flat end of a small hammer. The outer table of the bone is intact, while a *plug* is broken out of the inner table.

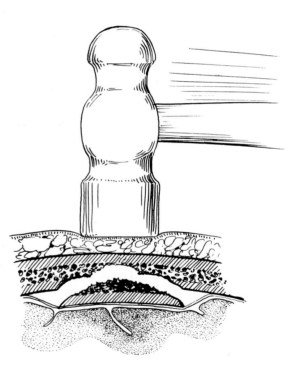

FIGURE X-83b. Diagram showing the mechanism causing the fracture shown in Figure X-83a.

of a funnel. Invariably, anytime a depressed skull fracture occurs, something penetrated, although, due to its elasticity, the skin may remain intact (Figs. X-84 to X-85).

The dismembered, decomposed remains of a recently divorced young woman were found in a remote rural area. The only injury discovered at autopsy consisted of a depressed skull fracture behind the ear. The fracture was roughly circular and depressed down to a central point which showed black discoloration with a metallic sheen. The police were informed that a heavy metallic object with a sharp corner caused this injury.

The ex-husband was a suspect and a hardware store receipt was found during a search of his residence. The police took the receipt to the store and discovered that a wood splitting wedge had been purchased the day before the murder although, the house had no fireplace. The sharp corner of the wedge fit perfectly into the bony defect (Fig. X-86).

Forty-three-year-old construction worker was struck on the head by a falling brick. The top of the skull was fractured in a pattern of concentric ripples. The depressed center of the fracture is the site of the actual impact by a corner of the brick (Fig. X-87).

In contrast, a fall on a flat surface resulting in a fractured skull shows one or several fracture lines radiating in different directions from the area of impact, but depression of bone fragments is unlikely to occur. However, it needs to be understood that a single large piece of bone may be pushed inward, i.e., depressed, by a fall on a

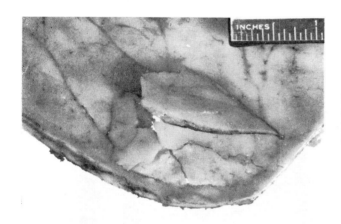

FIGURE X-84. Internal view of a depressed skull fracture caused by a fall on a sharp corner of a piece of furniture. Note the inward displacement of the bone fragments in a funnel shape.

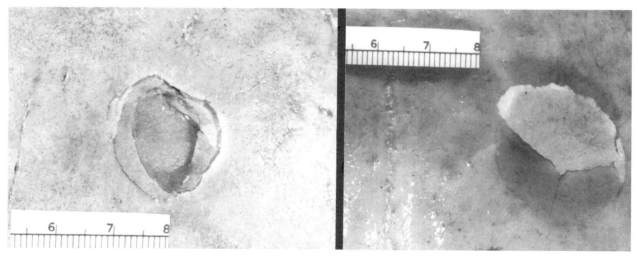

FIGURE X-85. External view (left) and internal view (right) of an experimentally produced depressed fracture of the skull using a ball-peen hammer.

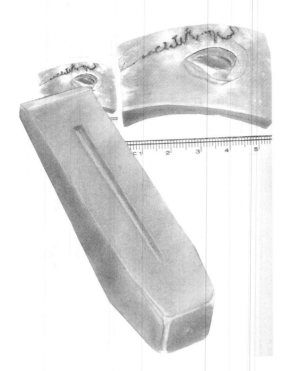

FIGURE X-86. Sharp corner of wood splitting wedge which caused a depressed skull fracture. Note, the indented area of contact in the center of the fracture and the ripple effect on the surrounding bone.

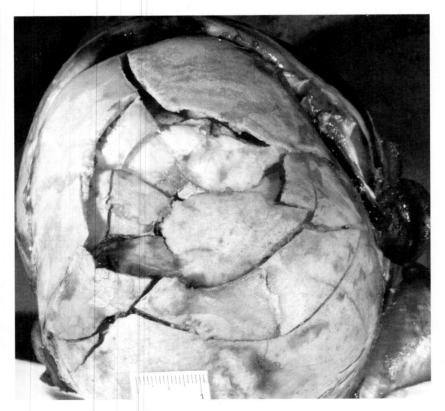

FIGURE X-87. Well-pronounced ripple effect surrounding a focal point of contact by the corner of a brick which fell from a height at a construction site.

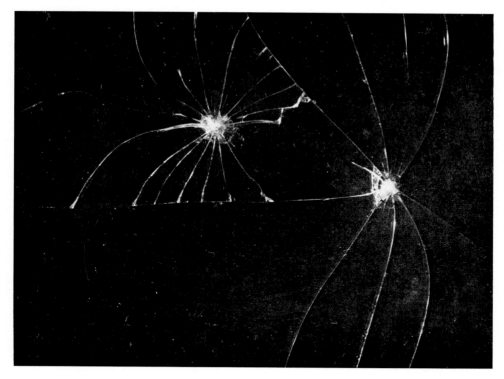

FIGURE X-88. Piece of glass showing two impacts, each with radiating cracks. The cracks indicate that the blow on the right was made first. The cracks radiating from the blow on the left are arrested by those already present due to the first blow on the right.

flat surface merely as a result of impact on a curved area of the skull. Such fractures show no fragmentation, do not have a central depression and except for being circular are usually devoid of pattern. The scalp indicates the site of impact by an extensive bruise surrounding an area of crushed tissue and hemorrhage may sometimes be noted in the underlying spongy layer of the bone. In the case of a blow followed by a fall, fracture lines resulting from the fall are arrested by those produced by the blow. The same is true of two blows, and it may be possible to determine which of the two was inflicted first. Cracks in a pane of glass illustrate this sequence (Fig. X-88). In general, it may be said that an injury to the head sustained as a result of a fall is more likely located in the level of the *brim of the hat*, while an injury resulting from a blow is usually situated above this level. In cases of bludgeoning, bone fragments are often extensively displaced so that evaluation and interpretation of

the injuries is impossible without prior reconstruction as discussed in Chapter XXV.

The changes in the skull correspond to contusions in the brain (*as described in* Chapter XIX) and should be considered together for proper interpretation. A fall on the back of the head or a blow to the top of the head frequently causes independent fractures of the orbital roofs, particularly in elderly individuals. These fractures may be comminuted and sometimes depressed, but they are not usually evident at autopsy unless the overlying dura mater is removed. Such fractures result from the *contre coup* of the orbital lobes of the brain on these paper-thin bony surfaces (Fig. X-89). Cortical contusions in the orbital gyri, including the olfactory bulbs, and also in the temporal poles are frequent. Orbital roof fractures may also be seen as a result of sudden violent increase in intracranial pressure, as in suicidal gunshot wounds of the head where the weapon is fired in contact with the skin. The sud-

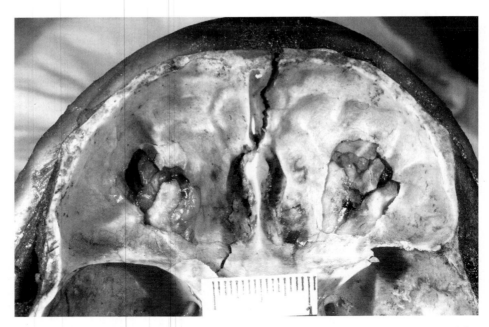

FIGURE X-89. Front half of the base of the skull showing bilateral depressed fractures of the orbital roofs as a result of impact by a falling brick on the top of the head transmitted by the frontal lobes of the brain *(contre coup fractures)*. The same *contre coup fractures* sometimes occur in falls on the back of the head.

den release of gases inside the skull is the major cause of these fractures.

If the victim survives for several hours or longer, hemorrhages associated with orbital roof fractures are often seen around the eyes and in the eyelids due to bleeding into the soft tissues of the eye sockets. This condition is sometimes referred to as *raccoon eyes* or *spectacle hematomas*. Such hemorrhages must not be interpreted as evidence of independent blows. Other times, hemorrhage around an eye resembling a *black eye* may result from blood seepage along tissue planes from bruises situated in the forehead or elsewhere, depending on the position of the head (as described in connection with Figs. X-17 and X-20a–b earlier in this Chapter).

Stomping of the head often causes fragmentation of the facial skeleton (Fig. X-90) and aspiration of blood and may be fatal as a result of brain injury. Breathing usually continues for some time, causing a fine spray of blood onto objects nearby. The pattern of the sole of the shoe sometimes leaves a bruised outline on the victim's skin (see Fig. X-12a–b). The pattern may be faint, requiring repeated viewing and study. Since the body is not usually available for longer than one or two days, it is recommended that photographs be taken. The side opposite the stomped side is usually abraded by contact with whatever surface the victim is lying on, predominantly over bony prominences of the skeletal contour. Of the two, the side which was stomped (the up-side) usually displays the lesser degree of injury as compared to the side against the ground (the down-side) (Fig. X-91a–b). Typically, the down-side displays the particular pattern of the surface in contact with the skin, such as cement, gravel, grass, wood, etc. Recognition of the pattern may be of considerable significance if the body was subsequently dumped elsewhere. In infants and small children there often is separation of individual skull bones with bruised brain tissue squeezed out between adjacent overlapping bone pieces. Yet, there is minimal disfigurement due to resilience and flexibility of the young bony structures. There may even be no skull fractures at all.

Sometimes it is difficult to distinguish between a case of stomping and a body that was run over

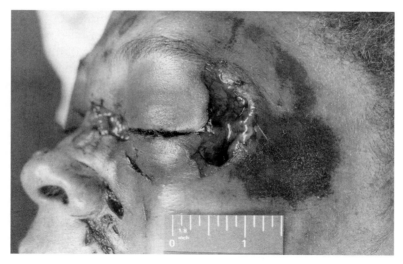

FIGURE X-90. Witnessed stomping of an elderly woman. The left side of the face was against the pavement. The injuries of the temple consist of abrasions and a vertical laceration. The latter is situated over the outer rim of the eye socket with extension tears on each end. The abrasion shows the outline of the temple and adjacent forehead. The facial bones were fragmented. The lacerations on the nose, below the eye and next to the left nostril are from bone fragments.

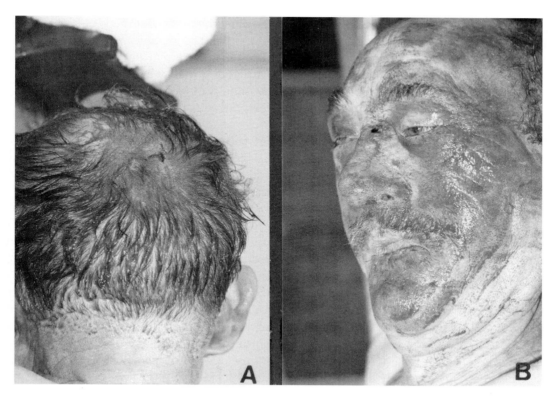

FIGURE X-91a–b. Stomping on the back of the head (upside). Note the insignificant appearing laceration in the area of the cowlick (A). The face was extensively abraded (B) as a result of impact against the pavement. A deep laceration caused by the shattered nose bone was situated at the bridge of the nose. The interior of the lower lip was extensively bruised and torn and the lower jaw was fractured on both sides.

by a motor vehicle. Of course, the presence of tire marks on the up-side is invaluable. An individual who was on the ground perhaps after being struck by an automobile, and is then run over by a second vehicle, may have his clothes pulled in the direction of travel. The rear wheel may run over the head imprinting tire marks on the clothes. Tire marks on the hairy scalp would be unlikely. It must be recognized that the skull is not necessarily always fractured by being run over, even in an adult.

Although not absolute, three principal types of fractures of the base of the skull are recognized, depending on the direction and location of the impacting force (Fig. X-92a–c):

1. *Longitudinal* (front-to-back) fracture divides the base of the skull into two halves (right and left). This may occur as a result of blunt impact either on the face, forehead, back of the head or in situations causing front-to-back (and vice versa) crushing.

2. *Transverse* (or side-to-side) fracture divides the base of the skull into a front and rear half. This type of fracture occurs from impact on either side of the head or as a result of side-to-side compression. Thus, it may be said that fracture lines of the base of the skull run in the same direction as the force. The fracture line drawn on the diagram is simplified. The fracture usually runs in the petrous portion of the temporal bones through the sella turcica, sometimes avulsing the pituitary gland. Blood exuding from both ears in cases of head injury suggests this type of fracture. This is by far the most common fracture of the base of the skull. Sometimes fracture lines radiate from the transverse fracture, and extend into the orbital roofs with evidence of periorbital hemorrhage and/or the ethmoid plate causing extensive nasal bleeding. Fracture through the sella causes profuse aspiration of blood. In children and young persons in whom the sutures between skull bones are still open, fractures need not occur due to separation of the sutures and considerable latitude in displacement of the bones.

Another common mechanism of this type of fracture, (sometimes referred to as *hinge fracture,* because of the independent movement of the front and rear halves of the base of the skull) is a

sharp blow or impact on the chin, as in a fall on concrete or other hard surface. This transmits the energy to the base of the skull by way of the rami of the lower jaw and the temporomandibular joints. The injury on the chin need not exceed an abrasion or superficial laceration the size of a coin (Fig. X-93).

3. *Ring fracture,* of the base of the skull separates the rim of the foramen magnum from the remainder of the base. This type of fracture occurs in a fall from a height when the victim lands on his feet or buttocks driving the skull downward onto the vertebral column. The mechanism of this fracture may be compared to seating of the head of a hammer on the handle by pounding the opposite end of the handle on the floor.

In a fall from a height, the leg bones, i.e., the tibias, are sometimes driven through the soles of the feet (Fig. X-94). Severing of major blood vessels at the base of the heart and small parallel horizontal tears of the inner lining of the carotid arteries are due to overstretching which results from the heart's continued inertia after the body has struck the ground. The heart may be driven through the pericardial sac and the diaphragm. In a young man who jumped from the roof of a thirteen-floor apartment building, landing on his feet, the intact heart was found among intestinal loops within the abdomen. It had been sheared off at its base about one-and-a-half inches above the aortic valve. Bursting of the heart and exposure of its ventricles is also known to occur in this type of fall.

Many times the aorta is partially torn or severed at the ligamentum arteriosum which is the point of fixation of this vessel. It is important to recognize that a severed aorta results in instantaneous arrest of circulation, absence of blood flow to the brain and absence of bruising in other areas of injury. However, in cases where there is severe crushing of the body even with a severed aorta there may still be some bruising in areas of injury due to the fact that crushing forces move the blood column and may result in what appears to be hemorrhage in a remote injury. The blood column is incompressible, no different than water. Consequently, a crushed chest may

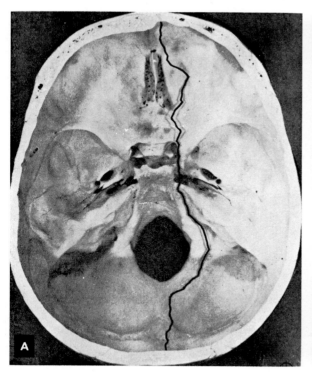

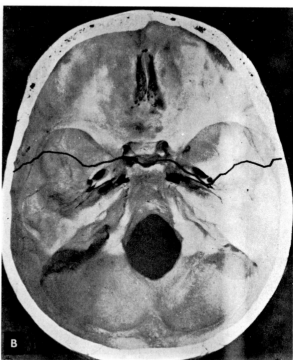

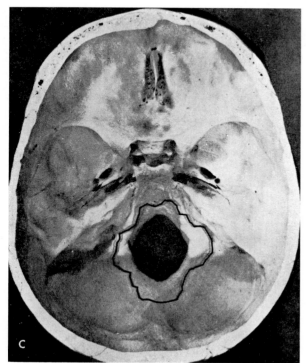

FIGURE X-92a–c. (a) Longitudinal fracture of the base of the skull, dividing it into two halves. (b) Simplified diagram of transverse, so-called *hinge* fracture of the base of the skull. (c) Ring fracture of the base of the skull.

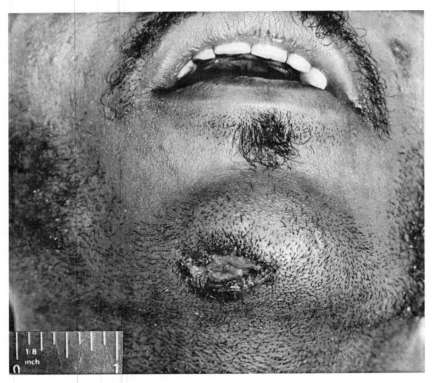

FIGURE X-93. Young man who struck his chin in a partially mitigated fall. A transverse, *hinge-type* fracture was observed at autopsy.

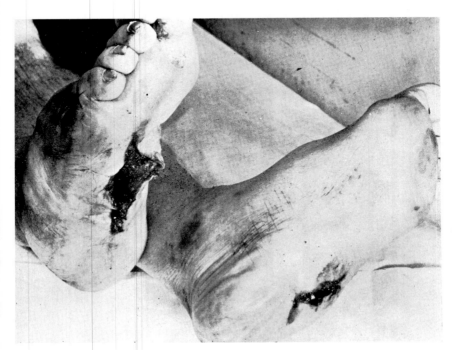

FIGURE X-94. Window washer fell on his feet from the tenth floor of an office building. The tibias were driven through the feet into the soles of the shoes. The right foot shows a large deformity and hemorrhage of the back of the foot presumably caused by the talus driven forward by the impact. A ring fracture was noted around the foramen magnum.

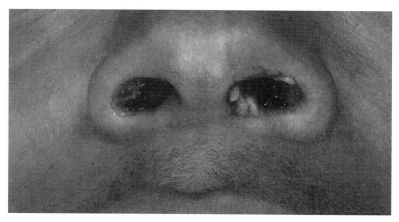

Figure X-95. Brain tissue in the left nostril due to extensive fractures of the base of the skull sustained in a motorcycle accident. There were no external head injuries. Occasionally, brain tissue will exude from the ears.

result in hemorrhage surrounding a fractured ankle, even if the aorta was severed.

Autopsy findings in a victim of an accidental or suicidal fall from a height may be indistinguishable from a homicidal fall where the victim was deliberately pushed or thrown off a roof or out of a window.

The body of a young woman was found some 50 feet under one of the large rocks in Yosemite National Park. Her husband claimed she had fallen accidentally. However, in an accidental fall, the body would have landed directly under the rock and not 8 feet out. Upon questioning, the husband confessed to pushing her.

The type of injuries differs depending on the area of the body which impacted with the ground and the consistency of the surface which was struck. Thus, impact on cement pavement may be expected to be more devastating than an impact on grass, bushes or a canvas awning. Impact on gravel leaves typical markings on the skin (see Fig. X-41a–b). The majority of adults who fall from heights sustain severe internal injuries and skeletal fractures with comparatively little external damage. In infants and toddlers, fractures are unusual in falls from levels of less than ten feet due to the relative resilience of their young skeletons. Thus, in young children, tears of the lung causing pneumothorax and pleural hemorrhage may occur in the absence of rib fractures and severe brain injury may be seen with an intact skull. Shearing off of other organs, specifically the lungs, spleen and kidneys occurs at points of suspension. The liver typically tears along the falciform ligament hepatis which attaches it to the diaphragm. The root of the mesentery, which suspends the bowel, may also tear.

Bleeding from the ears, nose or mouth following closed head injury suggests fracture of the base of the skull. Brain tissue may exude through these apertures, even in the absence of external evidence of injury (Fig. X-95). A fracture of the base of the skull involving the sella turcica provides direct communication between the cranial cavity and the airway through the sphenoid sinus situated above the posterior palate. This permits the passage of blood from the base of the skull into the airways. Hexagonal, sharply delineated subpleural areas of aspirated blood indicate that death was not instantaneous. Respiration must have continued for even a small quantity of blood to be inhaled.

Numerous other fractures that are characteristic of the mechanism of injury are well documented, particularly in the orthopedic and surgical literature. Colles' fracture, which is a fracture of the distal end of the radius, occurs frequently from a fall on the outstretched hand. A Colles' fracture in someone who was struck on the head before falling indicates that the individual was conscious and tried to mitigate the fall with his hand, prior to striking the ground.

Another common injury is fracture of the calcaneus. It is generally due to a fall from height when the victim lands on one or both heels. The height does not need to be great and in older individuals such injury may occur in a fall from four or five feet or less. In falls from a greater height other skeletal injuries, particularly compression fractures of the vertebrae, are frequently observed. Stepping onto an improperly secured manhole may cause the lid to flip into a vertical position. Such a fall may result in severe injuries by impact of the perineum on the upright lid, resulting in laceration of the scrotum, testicular injuries, fractures of the pelvis and laceration of the urethra.

Fractures of the sacroiliac joints may occur as a result of a fall on the buttocks. In older people, the space between the articular surfaces of these joints is increased allowing for significant movement. Dislocation, with or without fracture of a sacroiliac joint is often associated with fracture of the pubic ramus on the opposite side or separation of the pubic symphysis. Autopsy diagnosis of fracture of a sacroiliac joint should be made only after removal of the soft tissues from the area and direct viewing.

Fracture of the pelvic ring and sacrum is also referred to as an *open book fracture*. This is an anteroposterior compression injury of the pelvis and occurs in a frontal impact such as in a pedestrian or occupant of a motor vehicle who is thrown against the dashboard and sometimes in a motorcyclist propelled against the gas tank of his cycle. The pubic symphysis is disrupted and the sacroiliac ligaments are torn, causing the pelvis to open like a book, hence the name of the fracture.

Vertical shear injuries of the pelvis result from axial loading as in a fall from a height. Such fractures include busting of the acetabulum by impact of the femoral head. The same type of fracture sometimes occurs in a driver of a motor vehicle involved in a head-on collision, where application of brakes causes transmission of energy directly up the outstretched leg. In rare instances, knee impact on the dashboard may also cause acetabular perforations.

Assessment of the degree of osteoporosis at autopsy is helpful in evaluating skeletal fractures in the elderly. The procedure for such assessment is separation of the intercostal muscles using a scalpel and manual fracture of a rib. In cases of advanced demineralization, the rib snaps easily with a sound similar to breaking cardboard. In the absence of significant osteoporosis deliberate fracture of a rib is difficult.

Fractures of metacarpal bones can occur as a result of a punch or a fall on a clenched fist.

Some fractures do not lend themselves to easy interpretation of mechanism.

A partly decomposed and frozen body of a young woman was found in a field in the rear of an abandoned brick factory about three months after she had disappeared. A perfectly circular, centrally depressed fracture two inches in diameter was found in the left temple. The overlying skin was mostly mummified but revealed no open wounds. At autopsy the pathologist was unable to determine what could have caused the fracture. The police had evolved the theory that the murder had taken place in a different location since no evidence of bleeding was detected where the body was found.

Experimentation showed that an identical fracture could be produced by a blow with the corner of a brick. The impact did not break the skin indicating that bleeding had not necessarily occurred if a brick was the murder weapon (Fig. X-96 a-b).

In another case, a young woman's body was found face down on the ground and partially disrobed in an alley. Sexual assault was suspected. Autopsy was negative, but dissection of the neck by posterior approach showed dislocation of the atlanto-occipital joints with intracapsular hemorrhage and C-1 bruising and swelling of the cord. This led to the determination of homicide by forceful rotation of the head.

Experimental sled crashes using cadavers report typical patterns and mechanisms of skeletal injuries characteristic of certain types of trauma. We have found that some of these fractures are highly unusual and question their occurrence in real life. One vertebral fracture described in cadavers of sled crashes is a transverse fracture of the second cervical vertebra due to whiplash movement of the head (Fig. X-97). This injury resembles Chance's[9] fracture, which usually involves the lumbar spine and is most often associated with lap seat belts. However, the fractures we have observed in the C-spines of restrained motor vehicle crash victims were typically of the non-transverse type.

In assessing total blood loss in cases of blunt trauma involving closed skeletal fractures, the

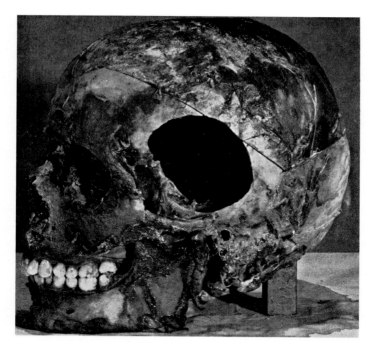

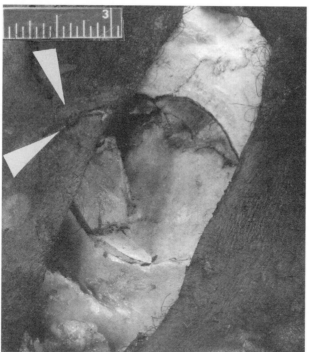

FIGURE X-96a–b. (a) Circular depressed fracture of the left temple. Very little bleeding was noted in the soft tissues surrounding the defect in the bone. An important aspect of the investigation pertained to the weapon used to cause this injury. (b) Experimentally produced fracture of the left temple produced by impact with the corner of a brick. The point of impact in the skin, which moved to the left after incision, is indicated by the arrow. There was no perforation of the skin and had this person lived, the amount of external bleeding from this injury would have been minimal.

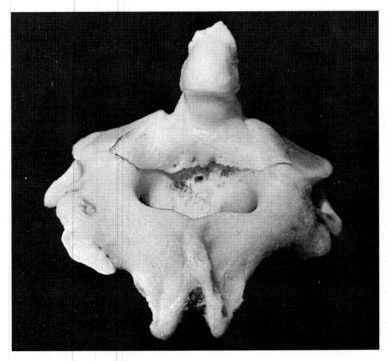

FIGURE X-97. Bizarre fracture of C-2 in a restrained cadaver used as a driver of a car in a sled experiment.

following estimates may be applicable to some of the major bones:

- Humerus   10 ounces
- Ulna & Radius   5–6 ounces
- Femur   40 ounces
- Tibia & Fibula   20 ounces
- Pelvis   45 ounces

Fat Embolism

An infrequent cause of death complicating injury is fat embolism which signifies the presence of fat droplets in the bloodstream. The large network of lung capillaries makes them the ideal tissue for detection of fat embolism. Fat embolism occurs in all varieties of blunt force trauma. Thus, no fat emboli may be expected in the lungs of a stabbing victim unless the perpetrator's fist crushed the victim's skin as the entire blade was thrust into the victim's body. The most common injuries which cause fat embolism are: (a) skeletal fractures, predominately of the femur, vertebrae and pelvis, due to their abundant marrow content and (b) crushing and tearing injuries of subcutaneous fat.

Studies have shown that the incidence of fat embolism following skeletal fractures is almost 100%. But, any blunt trauma severe enough to cause even localized crushing of fat cells is likely to result in fat droplets appearing in alveolar capillaries in lung sections. According to Mudd et al. soft tissue injury is the primary cause of pulmonary fat embolism.[10] The finding of fat in lung capillaries may be used as evidence that the blood circulation was functional at the time of injury. Thus, it is obvious that most cases of posttraumatic fat embolism are not fatal. Estimates of the amount of embolic fat necessary to produce death in adults range from 12 to 120 mL.

Shrinkage of tissues, as in postmortem charring of the body, may cause fat to be moved into blood vessels and produce a picture identical to that of fat embolism. In a decomposed body, fat droplets from merged chylomicrons and large pools of liquefied fat derived from fat cells in the tissues may be found in the blood. The presence of fat in the bloodstream is also frequently associated with surgical procedures, particularly orthopedic surgery and operations involving adipose tissue. Interestingly, fat embolism occurs infrequently following liposuction. A further source of fat and bone marrow elements in lung capillaries is fractures of the ribs and sternum which may occur during resuscitative efforts. Cardiopulmonary resuscitation is probably the most common cause of pulmonary fat embolism seen at autopsy. Quantitatively, such fat in the bloodstream cannot be equated with pulmonary fat emboli that cause death. Fat droplets in the blood may be seen in certain non-traumatic conditions such as diabetes mellitus, sickle cell crisis, pancreatitis, a variety of infectious diseases, following blood transfusions, carbon tetrachloride and phosphorus poisoning and in fatty infiltration of the liver as often seen in alcoholics.

There is some controversy regarding the origin of embolic fat and two main views currently prevail:

1. The classical mechanical theory holds that fat embolism is due to the entrance of crushed fat, bone marrow and even bone spicules into traumatized vascular channels at the site of an injury.
2. According to the physical-chemical theory most of the intravascular fat is derived from lipids normally present in the plasma. Following trauma, alteration of the normal plasma colloidal dispersion of chylomicrons causes coalescence of chylomicrons to form larger fat droplets. The high cholesterol content of some embolic fat globules, as described by LeQuire et al.,[11] substantiates that the circulating fat is not solely derived from stationary fat depots.

Much research has been directed toward the resolution of this controversy, and while the argument remains unresolved important information has been gained concerning the changes that occur in the physical properties and coagulation of blood following trauma. Indeed, an attractive theory postulates that the state of shock which follows trauma results in certain physical-chemical changes in the blood which are further influenced by sudden mobilization of storage fat for energy purposes to combat shock. This mobilized fat acts as a trigger to disturb the equilibrium of fat normally suspended in the circulating blood leading to formation of large globules of visible fat.

Only a few expulsive heartbeats are required to move a droplet of fat from anywhere in the body into the pulmonary circulation. The presence of intravascular fat globules in the lungs does not necessarily preclude *instantaneous* death considering that the heart may continue to beat for some time after respiration and other vital functions have ceased. Obviously, fat embolism cannot be expected if the heart is severed from the great vessels. Systemic fat embolism develops when fat globules are forced through the lung capillaries and arteriovenous anastomoses into the pulmonary veins. The pulmonary vascular tree is an efficient filter. Two or three days after an injury systemic fat embolism usually becomes apparent. This gives rise to a characteristic clinical picture. Depending on severity, symptoms of central nervous system involvement include restlessness, delirium, or drowsiness progressing to coma, seizures, and generalized brain edema. According to Harrison,[12] about half the patients have retinal and conjunctival punctate hemorrhages or visible fat in retinal vessels. Petechiae may be observed on the chest around the armpits and above the collar bones. Occult blood and sometimes fat occur in the urine if the kidneys are involved. Coma and death may occur suddenly due to involvement of vital centers in the brain or following embolization to the heart muscle and damage of the conduction system. At autopsy, cerebral fat embolism is manifested by numerous pinpoint hemorrhages predominately in the white matter due to capillary occlusion by fat globules.

The question of whether death can result from fat embolism in the lungs has not been resolved. Some suggest this is unlikely.[11,13,14] In our opinion fatal pulmonary fat embolism alone is uncommon. Indeed, one study has shown the incidence of pulmonary fat embolism associated with clinical manifestations and recovery to be 99.2 percent.[15] However, a large amount of fat dispersed in the lungs in some crushing injuries and massive pulmonary edema in such cases certainly tend to support that pulmonary fat embolism which precipitates pulmonary edema may well play a role in causing *wet lung syndrome*. It has been postulated that this may represent an important factor in death from shock following trauma.

On rare occasions fat embolism has been demonstrated in *decompression sickness* (caisson disease), in too rapid ascent to high altitudes without a functional pressurized cabin or under simulated flight conditions in decompression chambers.[16] In divers, fat embolism has also been documented in conjunction with the general picture of caisson disease. In both instances, death due to systemic fat embolism may occur within a few hours.

The salient gross anatomical findings in death from systemic fat embolism are pinpoint hemorrhages in the skin and conjunctivae. In the skin, the purpura is conspicuous on the shoulders, predominantly around the armpits. In the brain, pinpoint hemorrhages are scattered throughout the white matter. In the lungs, the findings are nonspecific and consist essentially of edema and congestion. Individual pinpoint hemorrhages may be noted on the surface of the kidneys and throughout the cortex. Microscopically, fat embolism is readily demonstrated in frozen sections stained with any of the conventional fat stains. In hematoxylin-eosin-stained paraffin sections fat embolism may still be recognized as small hollow intravascular spaces from which the fat has been dissolved by xylene. These are especially prominent in the alveolar capillaries of the lungs and the renal glomeruli.

Air Embolism

Autopsy demonstration of air embolism has been discussed in Chapter XXV. In addition to the usual sources and mechanisms of air embolism, open head trauma and exposure of dural sinuses may also cause the presence of air in the right side of the heart. Even in cases of severely destructive craniocerebral trauma, cardiac action usually continues for several minutes allowing for air drainage into the heart. We have seen large amounts of air in the right side of the heart in shotgun blast cases involving the head and Adams, et al.[17,18] described similar findings in cases of blunt force cranial-cerebral injuries.

In a traffic accident, if the question arises whether the driver in a motor vehicle crashed as a result of his death, as from a heart attack or stroke, the presence of a large quantity of air in the right side of the heart, i.e., air embolism, would rule out that circulation had ceased prior to the crash. Air in the right ventricle or atrium may be documented by x-ray.

Intravascular air has also been described as a complication of open neck injury, obstetric procedures, chest trauma and decompression sickness, as seen in divers. Air bubbles in the circulatory system mix with blood to form froth which acts as thrombi, causing ischemic changes in tissues. Myocardial infarction, necrotic foci in the spinal cord and stroke occur in severe cases. No reliable figures are available regarding the quantity of air capable of causing death in man.

Animal experiments have also given variable results. In dogs, 7.5 mL of air per kg of body weight rapidly injected intravenously produced death in all tested animals. This would be the equivalent to 525 mL in a 70-kg man. The rapidity with which air reaches the heart would appear to be the determining factor. One report relates to a case of a 60-year-old physician who injected herself intravenously with 80 mL of air in an attempt to commit suicide and survived with no evidence of permanent damage.

Injuries by Medical Treatment and Resuscitation

Injuries during medical treatment may be mistaken for manifestations of abuse or assault. We have observed parallel, linear, horizontal marks on the face and neck thought to be finger imprints as a result of slapping, but actually were due to irritation by elastic straps and adhesive tape used to secure an endotracheal or tracheostomy tube. Similar markings can occur as a result of tightly applied bandages.

Fractures of the sternum and ribs are common due to cardiopulmonary resuscitation. The sternum fractures through the middle of the sternal body or at the junction of the body and manubrium. Hemorrhage often infiltrates the soft tissues in the area of the fracture as CPR may either produce some pumping action or reactivate the spontaneous heart beat for a short time. Fractures

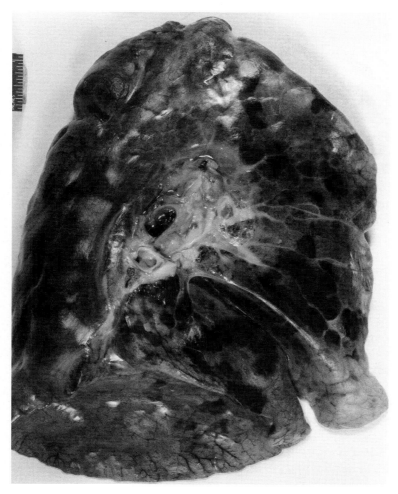

FIGURE X-98. Lung: Foci of aspirated blood. The blood originated in the mouth.

may be associated with tears in the lungs and release of free air, causing subcutaneous emphysema and pneumothorax. Contusions in the lungs may cause foci of parenchymal and subpleural aspirated blood, away from the contused areas. Aspirated blood appears as hemorrhagic hexagonal foci and can be differentiated from a contusion. Aspirated blood distant from a pulmonary contusion occurs as a result of respiratory movements which can move the blood to any area of the lung, including the lung on the opposite side (Fig. X-98). Hemorrhages in the heart muscle, bleeding into the pleural cavities and tears of the liver may also occur as complications of resuscitative efforts. Liver tears result from direct manipulation as by pushing and pulling on the hepatic ligaments and the diaphragm. More infrequently, the spleen may be lacerated due to the same mechanism. The pericardial sac may contain blood as a result of intracardiac injections, such as epinephrine. At autopsy, several ounces of blood may be found in the pericardial cavity if a branch of a coronary artery was punctured. It behooves the pathologist to check the chest wall for needle tracks. Distinguishing between injuries due to resuscitation and those resulting from an assault may be difficult in the absence of a detailed account from the ambulance or rescue squad or the hospital emergency room or intensive care unit, particularly since both sets of injuries commonly occur a short while prior to death (Figs. X-99 to X-100).

Crushing of the chest, as occurs when the victim is run over by an automobile, usually causes extensive damage to all structures involved. In children, however, the ribs may not be fractured due to their marked resiliency. The heart is usually torn because the blood it contains is incompressible. It is believed that the heart is especially susceptible to rupture when full, as at the end of the diastolic phase. Bursting of the heart may result from a violent blow to the chest, as may be caused by steering wheel impact in an automobile collision. Bursting of the heart as a result of a fist blow has been observed, but is quite rare. Stomping or kneading of the chest with a knee may bruise or lacerate the heart. Under no circumstances, will a simple fall do the same, even in a child.

As a general proposition, if the area of impact is small, the force required to cause severe damage to underlying tissues and organs is less.

Tears of the heart more often involve the right ventricle. The right ventricle is thinner than the left and is located between the sternum and the vertebral column. Thus, a load on the chest or back will crush the right side of the heart between two hard surfaces. The left ventricle more often ruptures spontaneously due to acute myocardial infarction. A two-inch laceration of the left ventricular wall of the heart was observed in the driver of a motor vehicle, as a result of steering wheel impact. The body of the sternum was fractured horizontally. One of the sharp edges of the fracture was driven into the heart. There was no evidence of crushing of the surrounding heart muscle. Four hundred mL of fluid and clotted blood were noted in the pericardial sac. A tear of the heart wall causes bleeding into the pericardial sac. The amount of blood in the pericardial sac required to cause cardiac tamponade, i.e., heart standstill, depends on the rapidity with which blood accumulates. The amount of blood found in the pericardial sac in fatal stabbings or shootings is usually 10 to 12 oz. (approximately 280 to 340 mL), but considerably more blood may accumulate, depending on length of survival and in cases in which the aorta is perforated.

Certain abdominal injuries have been described earlier in this chapter. Other abdomi-

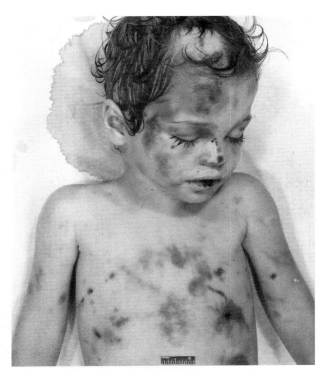

FIGURE X-99. Three-year-old child who was brought to the hospital unconscious following an alleged fall in the bathroom in which he struck his head on the tub. Oxygen and CPR were administered. The injuries suggested a battered child. Subsequent investigation, which extended to two hospitals, the ambulance crew that transported the child, and the parents, indicated that the history of a fall as given by the parents was correct. The child had struck the right side of his forehead and right temple. All remaining injuries had resulted from attempted resuscitation and remained unnoticed until drying. Abrasions are colorless or light pink when they first occur. They gradually turn yellow, brown, and dark brown as oozing ceases and drying sets in. Consequently, none of the health care providers noticed abrasions until later when the medical examiner received the body.

nal injuries include bursting of hollow organs as a result of blunt trauma. As in the case of the heart, a full stomach is more likely to rupture due to the hydrostatic effect. Of particular significance is rupture of the stomach or the small intestine as a result of a forceful unexpected abdominal blow. The unexpectedness of such a blow is associated with relaxed abdominal wall musculature. The abdominal skin and the abdominal wall often show no evidence of injury. The colon bursts infrequently. The urinary bladder is more often torn as the result of piercing by a sharp fragment of fractured pelvic

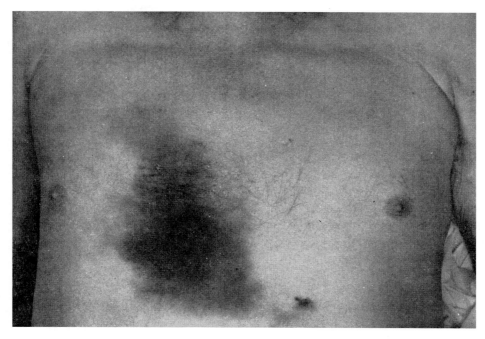

FIGURE X-100. Bruises of the chest wall due to improperly administered CPR. Note that the bruises are on the right, more commonly, the bruises are in the middle or on the left overlying the heart.

bone rather than by an explosive type of bursting as in the case of the stomach or small bowel.

INJURIES FROM BITING

Injuries due to biting are rare. Human bites seldom cause tears of the skin and far more frequently result in semicircular or crescentic patterned abrasions with underlying soft tissue hemorrhage and crushing. Bites are especially painful due to crushing. Injuries from biting often have sexual overtones. They are usually located on or about the genitalia and the female breasts. Bites on an assailant may occasionally be observed as a result of self defense. Identification of a suspect by comparing his or her bite pattern with marks left on the victim may be done, but not without caution and awareness of limitations (Fig. X-101). The skin may be twisted or distorted during the act of biting causing changes in the pattern and changes in the teeth may have occurred between the time of commission of the assault and apprehension of the suspect. Expert dental consultation is advisable (see Chapter VI).

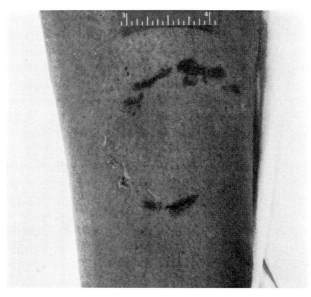

FIGURE X-101. Arm of a man who was bitten during an argument. The imprint on the skin suggests an incomplete denture, although the assailant had all his teeth.

Animal bites are recognizable by their patterns (Fig. X-102a–c). The number and depth of individual injuries reflects the number and length of

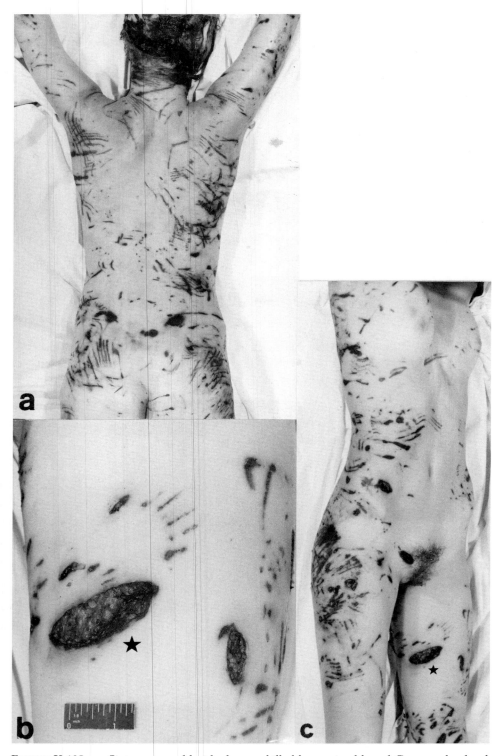

FIGURE X-102a–c. Sixteen-year-old girl who was killed by a mixed breed German shepherd dog. (a) The patterned injuries on her back and buttocks are bite and claw marks. (b and c) The oblique, parallel scratches were produced by the teeth of the upper jaw. Some of the deeper injuries resemble stab wounds (stars).

the teeth. The distance between adjacent injuries, particularly those made by the incisors and canines, may permit identification of the species. An attacking dog usually tears his prey extensively. Due to the length and sharpness of a dog's canines, individual punctures may resemble stab wounds.

A growing number of severe injuries by pit bull terriers and other dogs has recently been reported and in some instances infants, children and even adults have been killed.

Postmortem mutilation of the human body by animals has been mentioned in Chapters III and IV. Such mutilation may proceed to dismemberment if dogs or other carnivorous animals are involved. Decapitation and removal of the head or other parts of the body from the scene by animals may suggest foul play. Both antemortem and postmortem injuries by wolves and bears have been reported.

REFERENCES

1. Gleckman, A.M., and Evans, R.J.: Optic nerve damage in shaken baby syndrome: Detection by β-amyloid precursor protein immunohistochemistry. *Arch Pathol Lab Med, 124* (February): 251–256, 2000.
2. Geddes, J.F., Whitwell, H.L., and Graham, D.I.: Traumatic axonal injury: Practical issues for diagnosis in medicolegal cases. *Neuropathology and Applied Neurobiology, 26,* 105–116, 2000.
3. Contostavols, D.L.: Massive subarachnoid hemorrhage due to laceration of the vertebral artery associated with fracture of the transverse process of the atlas. *J Forensic Sci, 16:* 50–56, 1971.
4. Krauland, W., Mallach, H.J., Missoni, L., and Spitz, W.U.: Subdurale Blutungen aus isolierten Verletzungen von Schlagadern an der Hirnoberfläche durch stumpfe Gewalt. *Virchows Arch Path Anat, 336:* 87–98, 1962.
5. Adair, R.K.: *The physics of baseball.* New York: Harper and Row, 1990.
6. Spitz, DJ. Unrecognized fatal liver injury caused by a bicycle handlebar. *American Journal of Emergency Medicine, 17:* 3, 244, May 1999.
7. Spitz, W.U.: Hemorrhagic pancreatitis following a kick in the abdomen. *J Forensic Med, 12:* 105, 1965.
8. Potter, E.L.: *Pathology of the fetus and newborn.* Chicago: Year Bk Med, 1953, 336.
9. Chance, G.Q.: Note on a type of flexi-on fracture of the spine. *Brit J Radiol, 21:* 452–453, 1948.
10. Mudd, K.L., Hunt, A., Matherly, R.C., Goldsmith, L.J., Campbell, F.R., Nichols, G.R., and Rink, R.D.: Analysis of pulmonary fat embolism in blunt force fatalities. *J Trauma, 48 (4):* 711–715, 2000.
11. LeQuire, V.S., Shapiro, J.L., LeQuire, C.B., Coob, C.A., Jr., and Fleet, W.F., Jr.: A study on the pathogenesis of fat embolism based on human necropsy material and animal experiments. *Am J Pathol, 35:* 999, 1959.
12. Fauci, A.S., et al. (editors): *Harrison's principles of internal medicine,* 14th edition. New York: McGraw Hill, 1998.
13. Sevitt, S.: *Fat embolism.* London: Butterworth, 1962.
14. Simpson, K.: Fat embolism. *J. Forensic Med, 6:* 19, 1959.
15. Wilson, J.V., and Salisbury, C.V.: Fat embolism in war surgery. *Brit J Surg, 31:* 384, 1944.
16. Mason, J.K.: *Aviation accident pathology.* London: Butterworth, 1962, p. 165.
17. Adams, V., and Guidi, C.: Venous air embolism in homicidal blunt impact head trauma. *American J Forensic Med Pathol 22* (3): 322–326, 2001.
18. Adams, V.I., and Hirsch, C.S.: Venous air embolism from head and neck wounds. *Arch Pathol Med, 113:* 498–502, 1989.

Chapter XI

SHARP FORCE INJURY

Werner U. Spitz

CUTTING AND STABBING

CUTTING AND STABBING injuries are second only to gunfire as a means of homicide in the United States. Yet, review of 25 years of English language literature on the subject of sharp force injury adds remarkably little to this topic. Sharp force covers a vast array of injuries produced with sharp objects capable of cutting or stabbing or both. Thus, a hand may be cut while opening a metal can with a handheld opener, the broken windshield of an automobile may produce distinctive cuts in certain types of traffic crashes, the door and rear windows of an automobile may produce a typical pattern of superficial cuts known as *dicing;* a shard of plate glass may cause a deep accidental cut in someone who falls through a window, or it may be used as a lethal weapon for the purpose of stabbing, we have even seen or heard of paper cuts. A large amount of relevant information can be gained from precise analysis of a cut or stab wound.

A *cut (or incised wound)* results whenever a sharp-edged object is drawn over the skin with sufficient pressure to produce an injury that is longer than it is deep. For example, a sharp knife, a razor blade or a piece of glass or china could cause a typical cut. The wound edges may be straight or jagged, depending on the shape of the cutting object, but they are never abraded or undermined. These features distinguish an injury caused by a sharp object from one caused by blunt impact, as from a hammer or a rock. Blunt force produces a tear or laceration.

A distinctive characteristic of an injury produced by a sharp instrument is the absence of small, thin delicate *bridges of soft tissue* between the sides of the stab wound or cut. A sharp object cuts and divides as it penetrates, whereas a blunt impact, such as a blow crushes and tears, often sparing small blood vessels, nerves and strands of connective tissue (Fig. XI-1a–b).

Typically, lacerations have abraded edges. A laceration in which abrasion of the edges is limited to one area is likely to be the result of splitting of the skin, where the abraded part represents the area of contact (Fig. XI-2). The shape of the abrasion suggests the shape of the impacting surface. This may be compared to a watermelon dropped on a hard floor, where the area of contact with the floor is abraded and crushed, while sharp, unabraded, straight splits may extend from this area in different directions.

It is important to distinguish between a laceration at the site of contact, where the lacerated edges are abraded and the underlying tissue crushed, bruised and possibly undermined, from a split, which shows none of the above indicated characteristics of a blunt injury. Splits are common in the head due to the support given the scalp by the underlying skull. Usually, the splits run in the direction of the force. Thus, a forceful blow from behind on the back of the head with a metal pipe will likely extend the original laceration with splits running forward or rearward or both, originating at the site of the original injury, but lacking marginal abrasion, undermining, even bruising. A split which arises at the same distance from the site of contact represents a separate, independent impact. A depressed skull fracture may tear the scalp from within, also resulting in an unabraded scalp wound, resembling a split or cut. Great care must be taken in clearly distinguishing a split from sharp force injury.

A *stab wound* results from penetration of a pointed or thin tapered instrument into the depth of the body, causing a wound that is deeper than

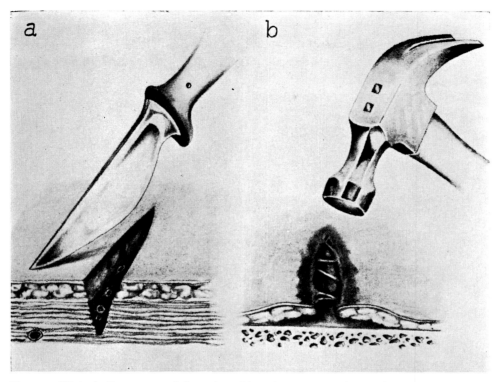

FIGURES XI-1a–b. Distinction of sharp from blunt force injury. The cut shows straight, clean, non-abraded edges (a), compared to the abraded and irregular undermined margins of the laceration (b). Also, note the thin and delicate bridges of soft tissue within the laceration.

its length on the skin. The thrust of a knife, for example, produces such an injury. As in a cut, the edges of a stab wound are sharp, straight and not undermined. The lack of crushing and tearing associated with sharp force injury is the reason why the skin around a stab wound is usually devoid of bruising. Bruising in proximity of a stab wound, is likely to be caused by impact of the fist that held the weapon (Figs. XI-3 and XI-4). An exception is the occasional bruise around a stab wound or cut situated in a dependent area, i.e., an area of livor mortis, or a stab wound or cut traumatized by CPR.

There is no abrasion of the edges of a stab wound, except when blunt parts of the knife, such as the handle or hilt abut the skin (Fig. XI-5). Abrasion or bruising of the edges of a stab wound therefore suggests that the entire blade had penetrated the body, particularly if clothing made of coarse fabric intervened between the handle of the weapon and the skin. Course fabric, such as denim, accentuates the blow. It is

essential in cases where a *hilt mark* or suspected *hilt mark* is found on the skin that the suspected knife, if available, be examined by the pathologist who performs the autopsy. Compatibility of the shape of the abrasion in proximity of the stab wound with the actual handle of the knife can be determined. However, unless the blade penetrates the body at a 90-degree angle, all sides of the hilt may not equally abut the skin (Fig. XI-6a–c). Consequently, if the blade strikes in a downward direction, the hilt mark is observed above the stab wound; if the blade is directed upward, the mark is below the wound. The same is true if the weapon is thrust sideways (Figs. XI-7a–c and XI-8a–b).

A patterned abrasion at the sharp end of a stab wound, which corresponds to the cutting side of the blade, is likely to be produced by the thicker, hinge portion of a pocket knife (Fig. XI-9a–c). A *one-to-one* photograph of the hilt or hinge surface of the blade, taken from the tip of the knife toward the handle, will illustrate the similarity

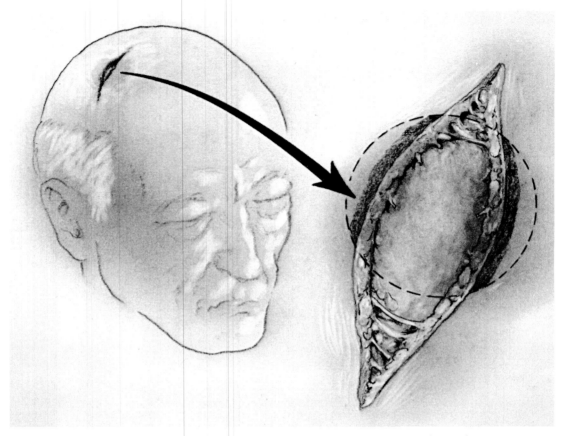

FIGURE XI-2. Laceration. The area of contact with the impacting force is abraded (circled). The extensions of the laceration on both sides (outside of the circled area) result from splitting of the skin. Tissue bridges are more noticeable in areas of splitting. Tissue bridges distinguish a laceration from a cut. Splitting occurs more often in head injuries. Splits are incomplete lacerations.

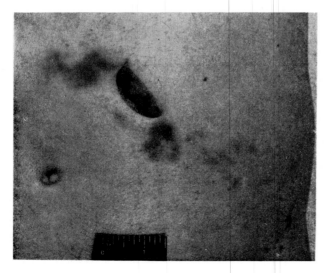

FIGURE XI-3. Bruising adjacent to an abdominal stab wound caused by impact of the fist holding the knife against the skin.

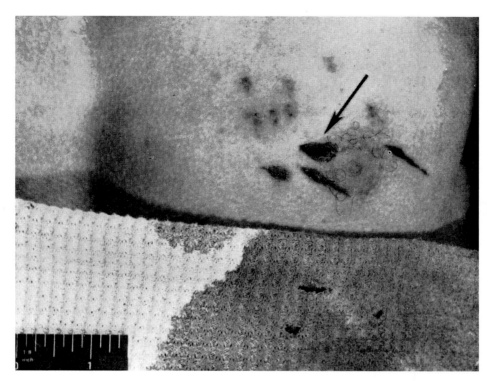

FIGURE XI-4. Stab wound (arrow) and three superficial cuts around the left nipple. The bruises above and to the right of the nipple depict the weave pattern of the T-shirt and were caused by impact of the fist holding the knife.

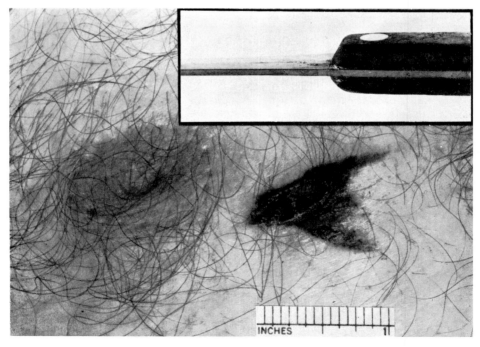

FIGURE XI-5. Stab wound of chest. The dovetail-like abrasion of the margins is due to impact of the handle of the knife (insert).

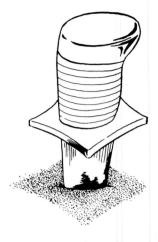
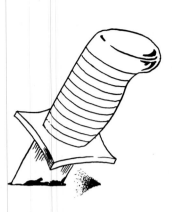

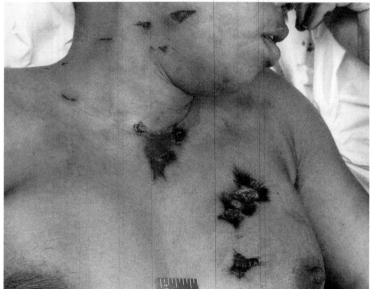

FIGURE XI-6a–c. (a) Hilt marks. (b) Multiple stab wounds of the chest. Shape of wounds varies with angle of impact. Select the most typical appearing wound for comparison. (c) Same weapon used in figure b.

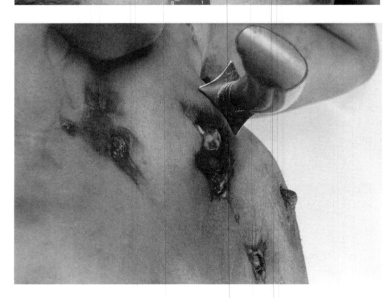

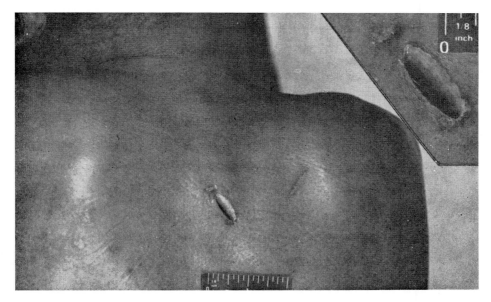

FIGURE XI-7a. Stab wound with hunting knife. Because of the downward thrust, only the upper edge of the plate between the blade and handle abraded the skin.

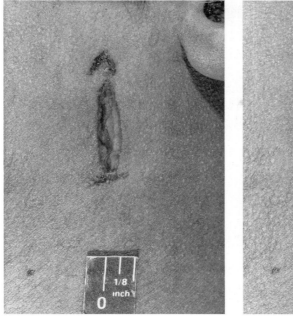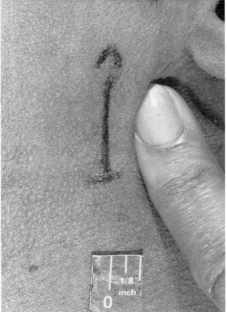

FIGURE XI-7b. Stab wound of the left cheek with distinctive imprint of handle. The pressure by the finger on the right against the side of the wound helps restore the wound's dimensions. It would certainly be possible to identify a suspected knife by comparison with this injury.

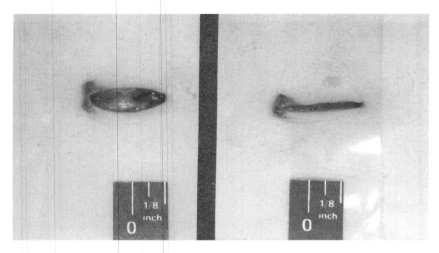

FIGURE XI-7c. Stab wound with evidence of downward thrust and distinctive handle or hilt mark. (The wound on the right has been realigned and taped, more accurately representing its dimensions.)

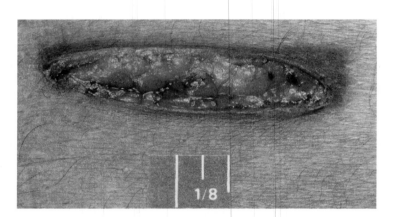

FIGURE XI-8a. Rectangular, hilt mark over the upper edge of a stab wound. The thrust of the knife was downward. The dimensions of the plate can be measured on the photograph for comparison with a weapon.

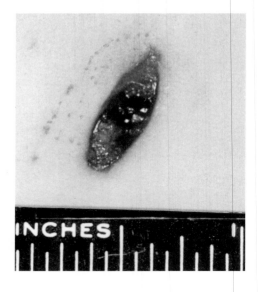

FIGURE XI-8b. Hilt marks may be subtle and may be missed without careful examination.

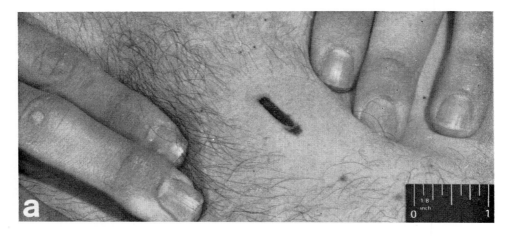

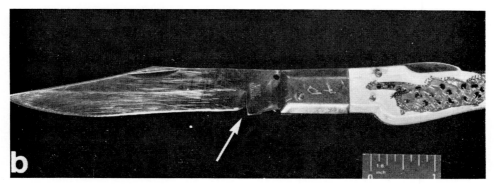

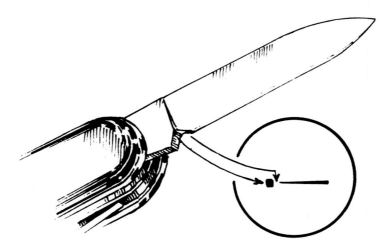

FIGURE XI-9a–c. (a) Stab wound of the chest with a folding pocket knife. The edges of the injury are approximated to counteract gaping produced by the inherent elasticity of the skin. The upper end of the wound corresponds to the spine of the blade. (b–c) The lower end of the wound shows a patterned abrasion caused by impact against the hinge portion of the blade (arrows). The patterned abraded area is separated from the stab wound as a result of the notch between the cutting edge of the blade and the hinge portion.

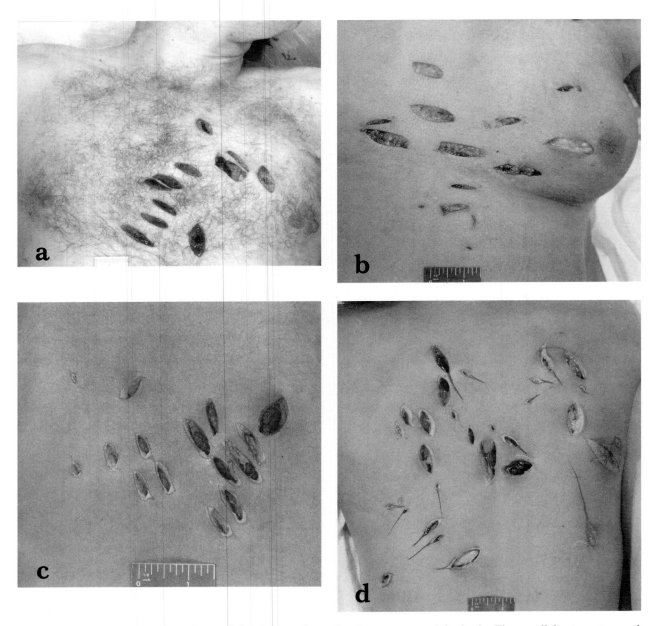

FIGURE XI-10a–d. Multiple, mostly parallel stab wounds confined to one area of the body. The parallel orientation and *scratch-like extensions* from some of the wounds, support the rapidity in which the wounds were inflicted.

between a particular knife and the wound. Another method to document this evidence is by application of stamp ink to the knife surface in question, then stabbing a piece of paper mounted on cardboard (for support). These are good exhibits for use at trial.

Examination of a cut or stab wound frequently permits determination of the manner in which the injury was inflicted. A stab wound generally suggests a homicidal assault. The amount of blood lost at the scene is often minimal, since bleeding may be mostly internal. Multiple stab wounds, most or all penetrating internal organs, are usually indicative of homicide (Fig. XI-10a–e).

Cuts or slashes on the upper extremities, especially the forearms and hands, are referred to as *defense wounds*. These are sustained when the vic-

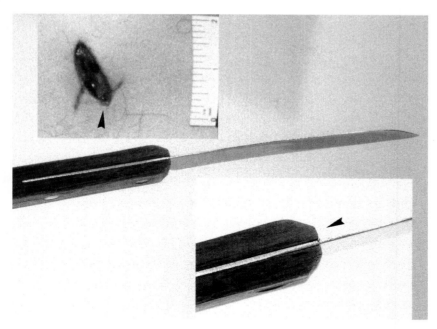

FIGURE XI-10e. In the case of a single wound, the cause of these superficial extension cuts is not as obvious. Here the two *scratches* occurred, one when the blade entered, the other at the time of withdrawal. Note the imprint of the handle shown by the arrowhead.

tim raises his or her arms or grabs the blade in an effort to protect the face or chest by warding off the assailant's weapon (Figs. XI-11a–b to XI-14a–b). Such *defense wounds* must be distinguished from offensive cuts of the assailant's hand sustained when the hand holding the knife slips off the bloodied handle onto the blade. Depending on how the knife was being held, such cuts occur predominately on the under side of the index finger (Fig. XI-15). Wooden handles of old kitchen knives and one piece all-metal knives are particularly conducive to this type of injury.

Cuts and stab wounds may be found on the lower extremities if the victim was laying on the ground and used his or her legs for defense. Such injuries are more common in female victims and suggest sexual assault (Fig. XI-16). *Vaginal, oral and rectal smears* should be prepared to determine the presence of *spermatozoa,* and swabs from these areas should be submitted for *blood typing* or preferably, for *DNA testing.* Absence of defense wounds may suggest that the victim was incapacitated or unconscious or was being held, or tied.

Postmortem examination in such cases should include incisions in the arms, wrists and ankles to detect possible bruises caused by restraint. To avoid unnecessary mutilation it suffices to place a single vertical cut in each of the bicipital regions of the arms, a horizontal cut in each shoulder, a vertical cut of the radial and ulnar regions of each wrist and the internal and external malleoli of the ankles. Each cut is then undermined for more extensive subcutaneous exploration.

Besides cuts on the extremities sustained in attempted self-defense, certain other injuries on the body indicate that a struggle had taken place.

Superficial cuts in a horizontal, vertical or large circular pattern on the chest, abdomen, or face, indicate wielding of the knife in front of the victim (Fig. XI-17a–c). Interruptions in the pattern are caused by movement of the victim and/or the assailant. Skips in the pattern may be caused by bony ridges, tendons, or if a dull weapon was used over areas of loose, thin, atrophic skin, such as the back of the hand in an elderly victim (Fig. XI-18a–c).

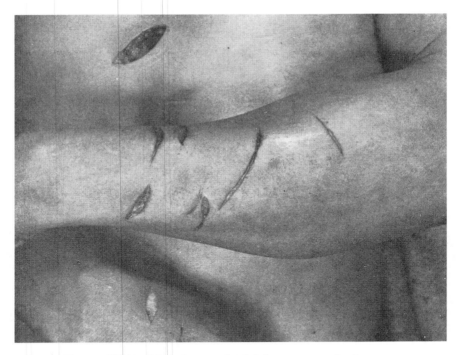

FIGURE XI-11a. Multiple superficial defense cuts on the forearm.

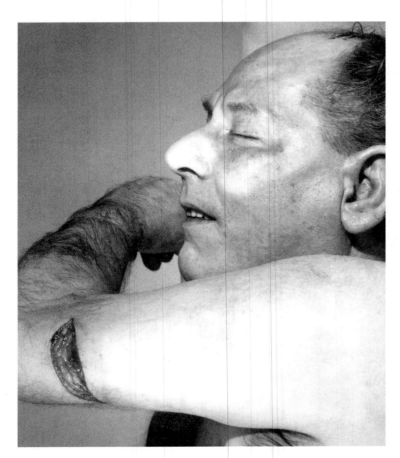

FIGURE XI-11b. Defense wound of arm. The cause of death was a stab wound of the chest.

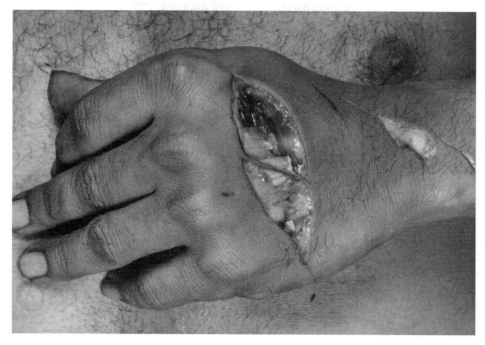

FIGURE XI-12. Defense wounds on back of hand and wrist. The bridge of skin separating the wound across the back of the hand indicates two separate cuts. Two extensor tendons are severed.

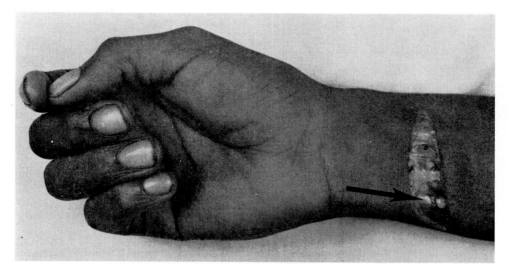

FIGURE XI-13. Defense cut of the wrist. A tendon is severed (arrow). Severed tendons and major nerves are disabling and should be noted in the records.

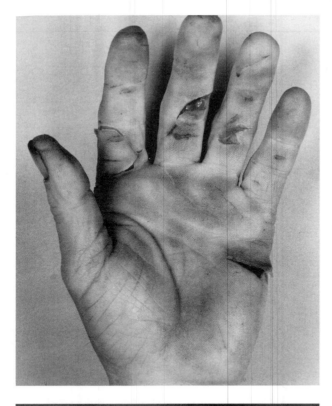

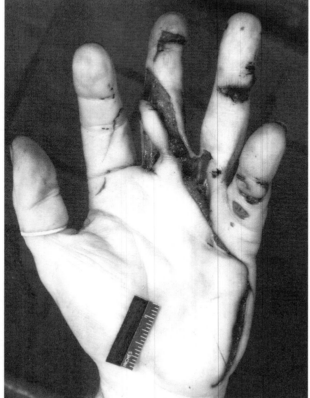

FIGURE XI-14a–b. (a) Defense wounds of the hands. (b) Attempt to grab the knife. Tendons and major blood vessels are severed.

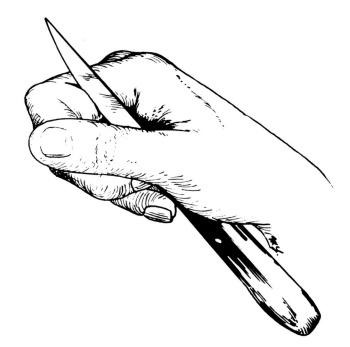

FIGURE XI-15. Cuts incurred by the assailant's hand slipping onto the blade.

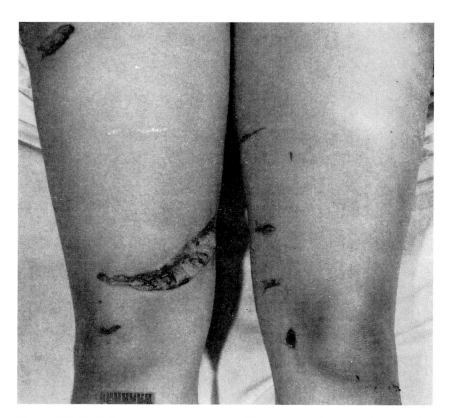

FIGURE XI-16. Defense wounds on knees and legs suggest victim was lying on the ground during the attack. Such injuries tend to support a sexual motive.

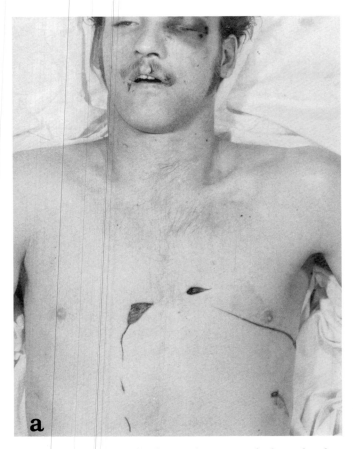

a

FIGURE XI-17a-c. Young man involved in an altercation which escalated into the use of a knife. A wielded knife caused the circular array (b) of the injuries. The injury pattern begins on the right side, just above the scale, continues up and to the left and terminates in the fatal stab wound (c). Complete insertion of the blade and impact of the hand holding the knife against the rib cage accounts for the bruising and scraping below the wound. Approximation of the sides of the stab wound shows the blunt edge caused by the spine of the blade (arrow).

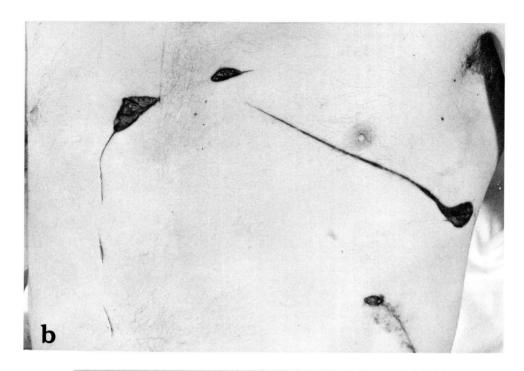

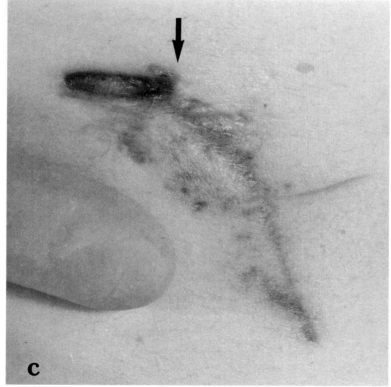

FIGURE XI-17b–c.

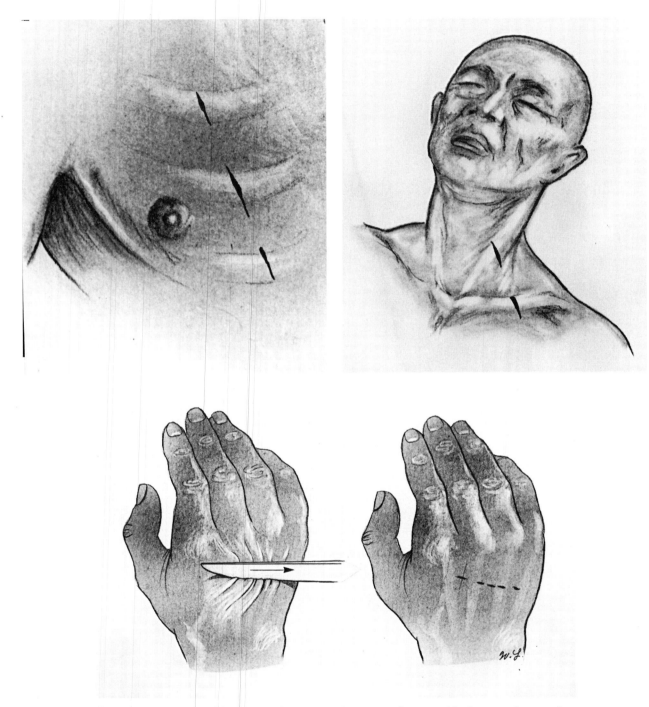

FIGURE XI-18a–c. Straight skips in the pattern of a cut may be caused by boney ridges, under-lying tendons, or the use of a dull blade.

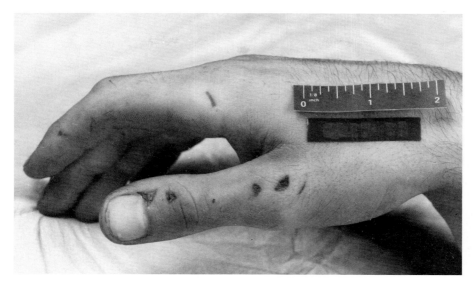

FIGURE XI-19. Fingernail marks resembling gouges.

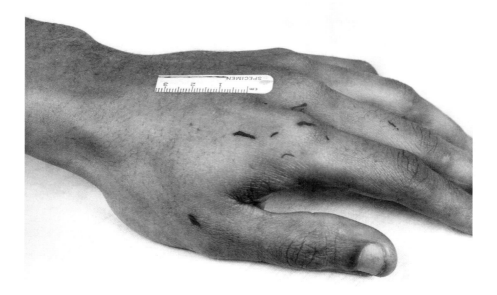

FIGURE XI-20. Typically curved fingernail marks.

Fingernail marks (Figs. XI-19 to XI-22), bruises and abrasions often produced by tugging and rubbing of clothing (Figs. XI-23 to XI-25) are frequently observed in victims of cutting and stabbing. Fingernails and clothes often leave telltale patterns. Recognition of such injuries is imperative. For example, in the case of a struggle for the weapon, fingernail marks, bruises and scratches on the victim's body may lend support to a defendant's claim that he or she stabbed the deceased in self-defense.

In an attack from the rear, where the assailant holds the victim around the face or neck, *fingernail marks* on the assailant's forearm and hand are often caused by the victim's frenzied attempt to remove the grip (Fig. XI-26).

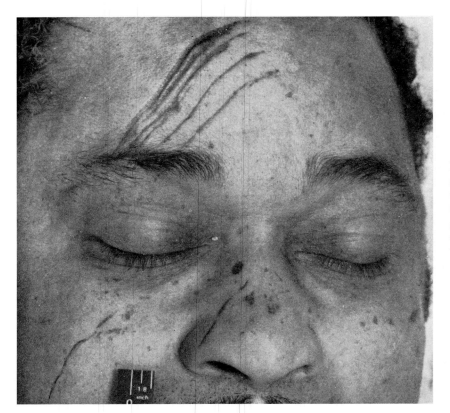

FIGURE XI-21. Different types of fingernails marks: Curved impressions on the right cheek and right side of the nose, gouges on the nose and grouped scratches by all five fingers on the forehead. The cause of death was multiple stab wounds.

FIGURE XI-22. Stab wound of chest (arrow). Multiple fingernail marks, suggesting an attack by someone of equal or less strength.

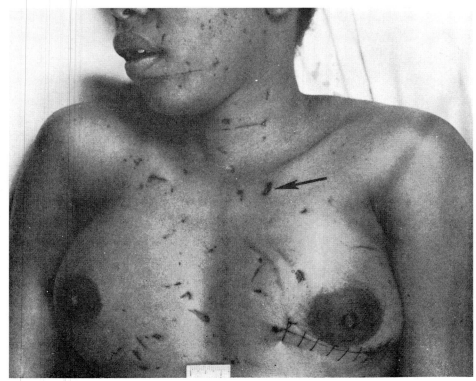

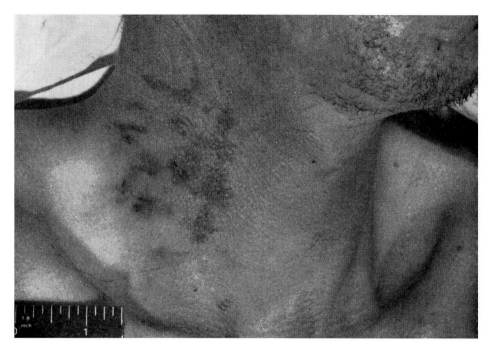

FIGURE XI-23. Bruising of neck during a struggle over knife. The pattern suggests knuckles.

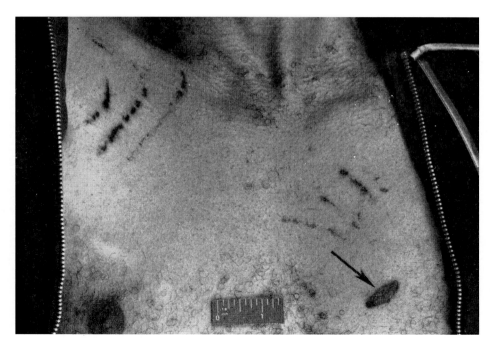

FIGURE XI-24. Patterned abrasions on both sides of chest caused by zipper.

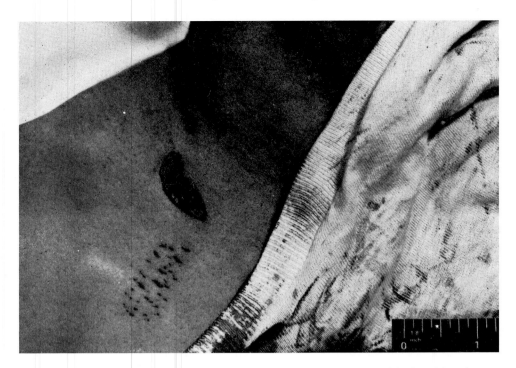

FIGURE XI-25. Patterned abrasions below stab wound caused by ribbed neckband.

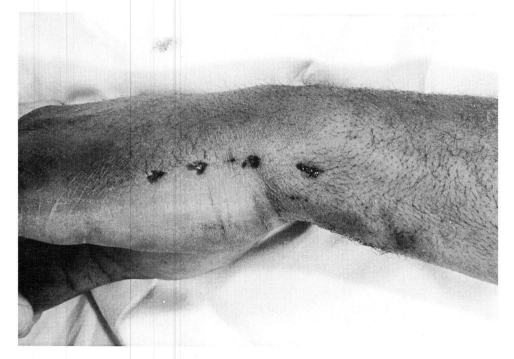

FIGURE XI-26. Gouges produced by fingernails. Common location injured on an assailant when the victim held from behind struggles to break the hold. Note bruises and abrasions on wrist.

Fingernail marks are most often located on the hands and wrists and less frequently on the face, neck and chest (see Fig. XI-22). Whereas, fingernail marks may manifest themselves in different ways, they usually consist of superficial, curved and irregularly shaped defects of the outermost layers of the skin (see Figs. XI-19 to XI-22). Fingernail marks often resemble scratches and are frequently referred to as such. Gouges, which correspond in size to fingernail tips are also encountered occasionally. When fresh and moist, fingernail marks are yellow pink and may not be recognizable. After a few hours, when oozing has stopped and drying has set in, they become dark brown, even black. In a case of death by strangulation, where the body was out in heavy rain, fingernail marks may not be apparent until the body is thoroughly dried. Drying is best achieved by dabbing (not rubbing) with a soft absorbent cloth or paper towel, followed by exposure to air. If the assailant's nails are long, fingernail marks may resemble small cuts which perforate the entire thickness of the skin. The extent of injury to the soft tissues under fingernail marks varies from slight bruising, barely recognizable with the naked eye, too deep and more extensive bleeding. Artificial, acrylic, fingernails are especially hard and sturdy, capable of inflicting injury with less chance of breakage.

Fingernail clippings are routinely collected in cases following physical assault. Although by no means always positive, (success rate estimated at up to 25%), fingernail clippings from the victim should be retained for laboratory analysis to determine the presence of assailant's skin, blood, hair, fibers and DNA evidence in all cases of suspected physical confrontation. By the same token, if available, fingernail clippings from a suspect may also be revealing. Experiments to determine the success rate of this procedure question its value.[1] In spite of the controversy, we believe fingernail clippings should be kept, if for no reason other than completeness.

Self-inflicted stab wounds are uncommon. When they occur, such injuries are usually multiple and superficial, although one or two may penetrate a vital organ, and result in death from blood loss (Fig. XI-27). Needless to say, self-inflicted injuries must be situated in accessible areas of the body. Suicidal stabbings are frequently accompanied by superficial, hesitation-type cuts predominately situated in the wrists and front of the neck, less commonly in the bend of the elbows or on the ankles. Single or grouped superficial stab wounds below the chin are more likely the result of taunting in a case of homicide.

The appearance of suicidal cuts is usually characteristic: they are multiple and parallel of variable depth whose edges commonly reveal several sharp angles, as if resulting from *sawing* of the skin, with repeated tentative incisions at the same location (Figs. XI-28 to XI-30a–b). Frequently numerous superficial, parallel cuts and scratches indicate repeated trials before the build-up of sufficient courage for the final deep gash that severs major blood vessels or exposes the trachea or larynx (Fig. XI-31). Such superficial cuts, or evidence of *sawing,* are referred to as *hesitation wounds* or *hesitation marks*. These cuts are mostly straight because sharp knives and razor blades are used. Suicidal cuts with a straight razor are unusual, except in older individuals, due to the decreased popularity of this type of shaving device. Occasionally, suicidal cuts are jagged and irregular, as when a piece of broken glass was used (Fig. XI-32).

Hesitation cuts on the front (palm side) of the wrists are usually horizontal. Vertical cuts are distinctly rare. Hesitation cuts in right-handed individuals usually involve the left wrist and vice versa.

The appearance of suicidal cuts may be misleading. Frequently they appear considerably deeper than they are (see Figs. XI-28 and XI-33), and because estimation of the amount of blood at the scene is usually deceiving, dissection of the wounds to ascertain their depth is well advised. Death may have been due to a cause other than exsanguination (Figs. XI-34 and XI-35).

It is important to realize that deep wounds usually involve arteries. Even cuts of small arteries cause extensive, pulsating, spurting hemorrhage. More superficial injuries usually involve veins which lack pressure, therefore bleed slowly, and are unlikely to cause significant blood loss. For example, suicidal cuts of the wrists which are

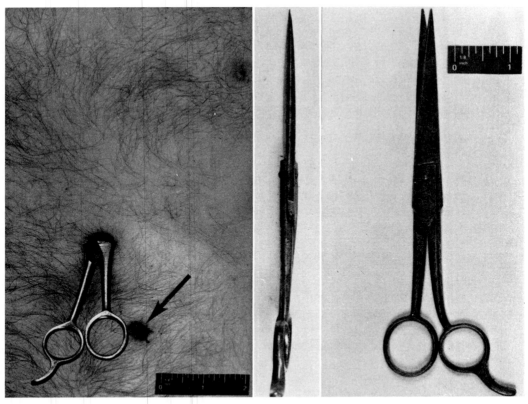

FIGURE XI-27. Elderly barber died of a self-inflicted stab wound of the chest. The shears penetrated the heart. In the lower wound (arrow) the skin is barely perforated and is probably the result of hesitation. The undisturbed scene, recent depression and history of suicide attempts, substantiates death by suicide. No other injuries were noted on the body. The edges of both injuries are abraded and may be mistaken for bullet wounds.

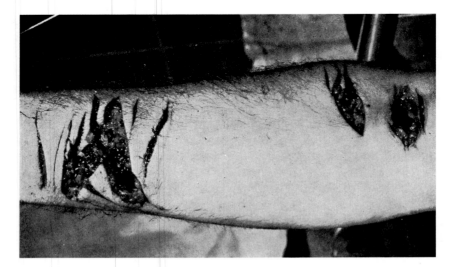

FIGURE XI-28. Multiple hesitation cuts of forearm by razor blade. Autopsy showed that none extends beyond the fat layer under the skin and no major blood vessels were involved. This individual stabbed himself with a pair of scissors in the chest and right temple and used a razor blade to slash his throat. Only the combined bleeding resulted in sufficient blood loss to cause death. He was still alive when found and uttered, "God will hate me for this."

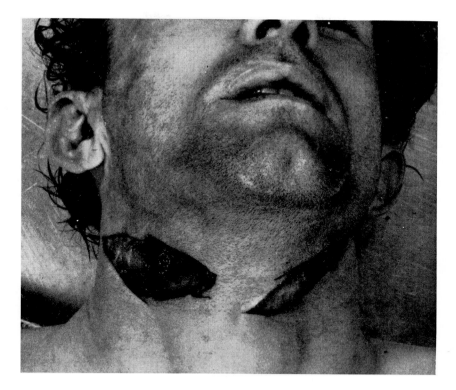

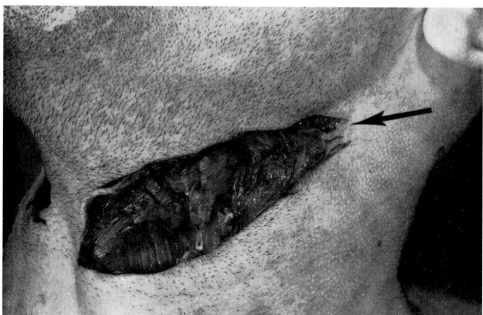

FIGURE XI-29. Suicidal wounds of the neck. Hesitation cuts are indicated by arrow.

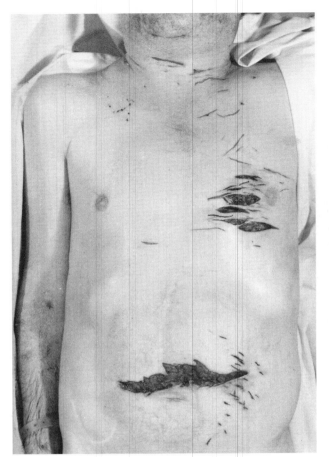

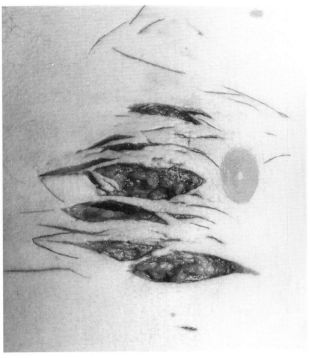

FIGURE XI-30a–b. (a) Death was caused by a single stab wound to the heart. All other injuries are superficial cuts. (b) Closeup of left chest.

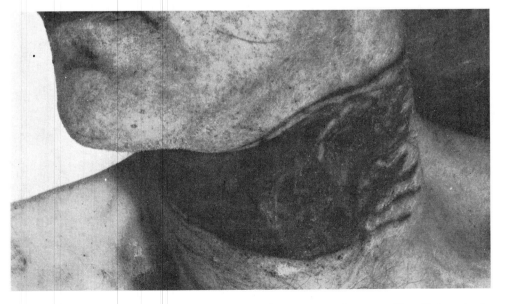

FIGURE XI-31. Suicide by multiple cuts of throat, showing typical sawing effect. Only a single cut was deep and involved the airway, causing inhalation of blood and death by suffocation.

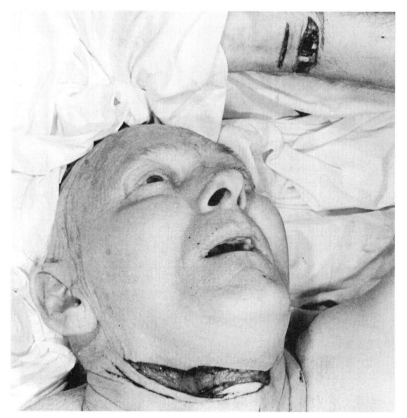

FIGURE XI-32. Cuts on neck and wrist made with a broken drinking glass. Note jagged lower edge of gaping neck wound. A tendon in the left wrist is severed. The victim was a cancer patient in a hospital.

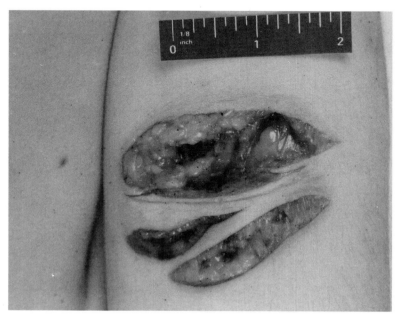

FIGURE XI-33. Suicidal cuts with evidence of hesitation.

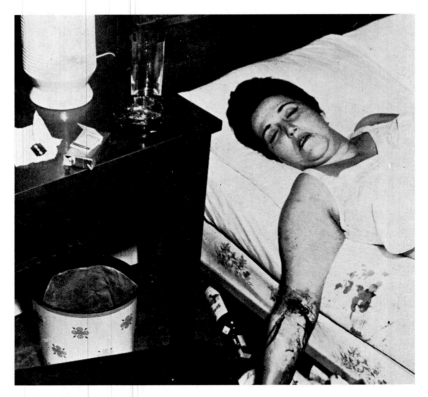

FIGURE XI-34. Thirty-two-year-old woman found dead in a motel room. She had checked into the motel twenty-four hours earlier with a male companion. There was very little blood at the scene. Autopsy showed only one severed medium-sized superficial vein of the right arm bend. The cause of death was acute alcohol intoxication, with a blood alcohol level of 0.45%. A blanket was neatly folded under the arm, apparently to absorb the expected bleeding, and the bloodstained razor blade was placed on a handkerchief on the dresser.

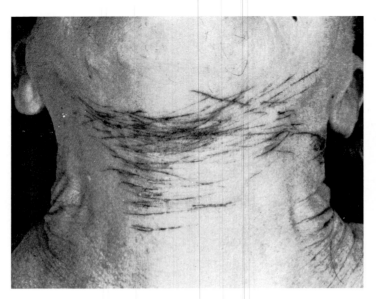

FIGURE XI-35. Attempted suicide of a seventy-five year old woman. Numerous superficial parallel cuts of throat inflicted with a razor blade. The injuries resemble linear scratches. Death was due to arteriosclerotic heart disease, apparently associated with the emotional stress of the attempt to terminate her life.

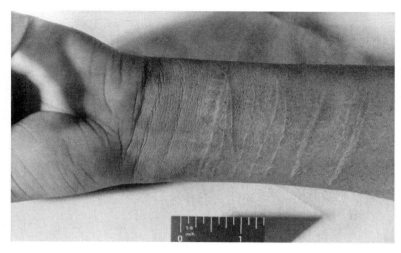

FIGURE XI-36. Linear, mostly transverse and parallel scars on the wrist due to previous suicide attempts. The wounds show evidence of surgical suturing.

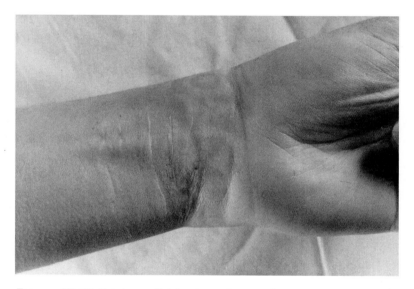

FIGURE XI-37. Faint parallel horizontal scars due to previous suicide attempt.

often superficial are not likely to bleed heavily, except when submerged in warm water which causes vasodilatation and prevents clotting. The likelihood of an artery to stop bleeding spontaneously as a result of clotting is improbable.

Deep, sometimes mutilating wounds in atypical locations, such as the back of the knees, should be carefully examined for the presence of hesitation cuts. Such evidence would suggest that the wounds were self-inflicted. We have seen such injuries in individuals who feigned assault for the purpose of collecting compensation.

Horizontal linear scars on the inner wrists are always suspect of one or more previous suicide attempts (Figs. XI-36 to XI-38). Such scars may be single, subtle and faint requiring some stretching of the skin and good lighting to be recognized. Stretching of the skin is best accomplished by bending the hand backward. Where no cause of death is apparent, suspicion of drug overdose

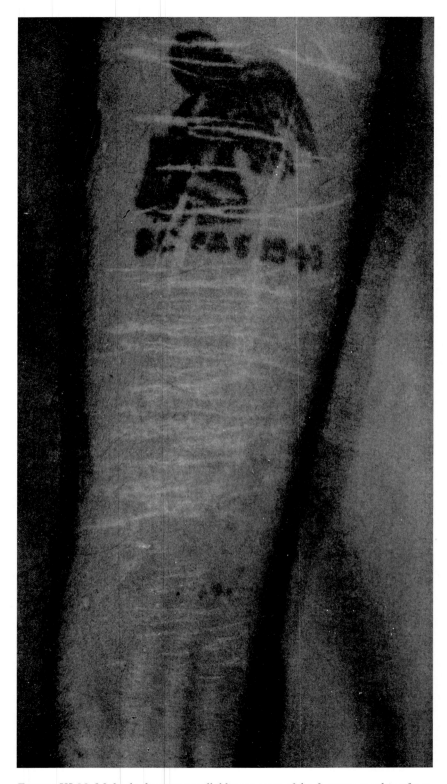

FIGURE XI-38. Multiple discrete parallel linear scars of the forearm resulting from superficial cuts. This number of scars is distinctly unusual.

is warranted and a thorough investigation of the scene and circumstances of the death, in conjunction with toxicological analysis of body fluids or tissues, should be undertaken. Suicide attempts are frequently repeated until successful. Such attempts may extend over many years. A variety of means may be employed by the same individual on one or successive occasions.

A twenty-seven-year-old male with a history of repeated episodes of depression jumped out of a fifth floor window after razor blade cuts of his wrists and throat failed to produce the desired effect.

In another case, a forty-two-year-old woman was found in her bathtub with her head submerged in bloody water. Her wrists, ankles and neck showed hesitation cuts. There was a star-shaped bullet wound in her forehead. The weapon had been fired with the muzzle in contact with the skin. At autopsy, a .38 caliber bullet was recovered from the brain. In addition, she had ingested a fatal dose of sleeping pills.

Deep and mutilating, widely gaping cuts such as slash wounds are fortunately rare in suicides. When they occur, they indicate determination and the definitive nature of the act (Fig. XI-39). More commonly, such wounds occur in homicides. The sweeping manner and malicious intent with which these injuries are inflicted are usually apparent. The finding of defense wounds or evidence of restraint indicates the manner of death as homicide. In questionable cases, the presence of defense wounds and injuries indicative of a struggle distinguishes a homicidal from a suicidal cut of the neck. Of course, the presence of hesitation cuts is equally significant.

Although it may be impossible to establish whether a slash across the front of the neck runs from right to left or vice versa, a short superficial or scratch-like tail usually indicates the terminal segment of the wound while a superficial gradually deepening, longer cut suggests the location where the wound began. Most homicidal throat slashings are produced with the assailant behind the victim (Fig. XI-40). In this position, a slash of the neck would run from left to right, if the assailant is right-handed, and in the opposite direction, if he is left-handed. The spray of blood at the scene, in a semicircular distribution in front of the victim also, supports the position of the assailant behind the victim. Several parallel superficial cuts, above and below the deep, gaping, fatal slash are the result of the victim's desperate attempts to get away and do not necessarily suggest torture. A parallel orientation of such cuts or stab wounds, further supports that the victim was being forcefully held, with the head and neck immobilized, to produce this geometric pattern (Fig. XI-41). Exceptions to this occur if the assailant is markedly intoxicated or demented (Fig. XI-42). A slash of the neck usually causes death from blood loss. Death from inhalation of blood or air embolism is infrequent.

Multiple uniformly deep, parallel stab wounds clustered in one area of the body, commonly the chest or back, are usually the result of rapid thrusts and overkill. Such murders commonly suggest a crime of passion with sexual overtones, jealousy, or profound hate (Figs. XI-43a–b to XI-44a–b). Emotionally driven killings stand out from random killings by their excesses and mutilation.

Conflicting expert testimony was obtained in the civil trial of O.J. Simpson in regards to certain wounds on his left hand. By way of background, the body of O.J. Simpson's ex-wife, Nicole was found with her throat slashed, on the ground, near the front gate of her residence. The body of her friend, Ronald Goldman, was found a few feet away with multiple stab wounds. O.J. Simpson's intact left leather glove was on the ground midway between the bodies and Nicole's acrylic fingernail tips had blood on them.

A total of eleven gouges, linear scratches and superficial semicircular wounds, all consistent with fingernail marks, were documented on the back of Mr. Simpson's left hand and fingers, inflicted by Nicole as she was being held from behind, fighting for her life.

The frenzy and rapidity with which such wounds are inflicted often precludes complete withdrawal of the weapon between stabs, resulting in a linear scratch on the skin preceding actual penetration and sometimes a superficial trailing tail on withdrawal, before the next stab. These scratches may be long or short and usually extend from either end of the skin wound, although they may connect with either side of the wound, depending on whether the weapon was being twisted at the time.

Self-inflicted cuts in different areas of the body, sometimes seen in individuals trying to avoid prosecution, may be identified by their superfi-

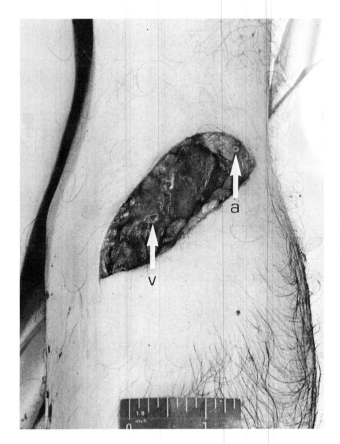

FIGURE XI-39. A single, suicidal cut of the elbow crease of the left arm, inflicted with a razor blade. A severed artery (a) and vein (v) are recognizable. The cause of death was blood loss. The absence of hesitation cuts coupled with the depth of the wound indicate determination.

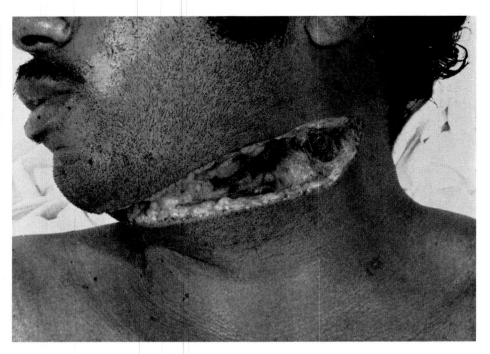

FIGURE XI-40. Homicidal slashing of throat.

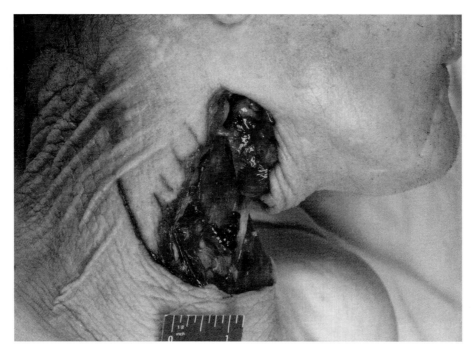

FIGURE XI-41. Mutilating slash of throat indicating presence of multiple cuts and attempted restraint.

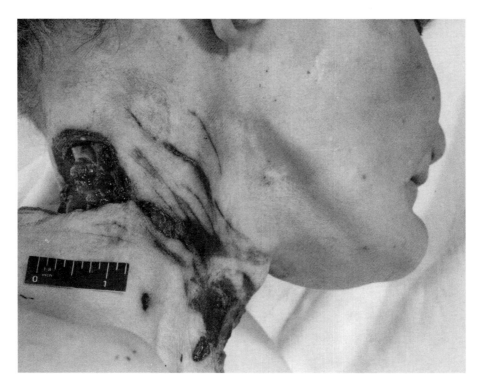

FIGURE XI-42. Irregular mutilating cuts of the front and back of the neck. This murder occurred in a nursing home for the mentally ill.

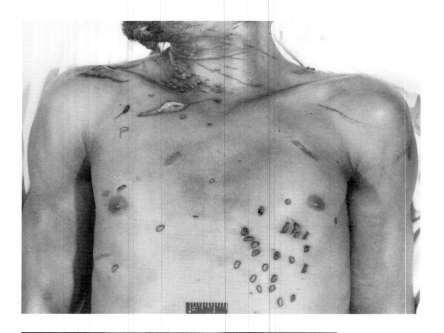

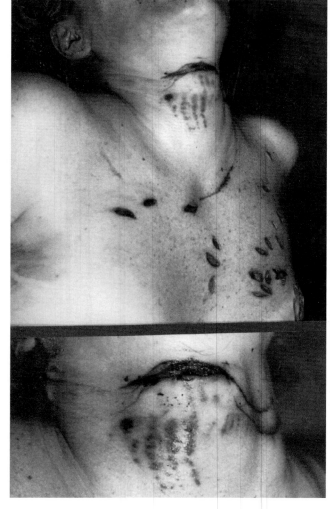

FIGURE XI-43a–b. (a) Sexually motivated murder: Numerous screwdriver stab wounds predominately over the left side of the chest and multiple superficial razor cuts of the neck. (b) Multiple stab wounds on the chest and attempted slashing of the neck. The patterned vertical bruises are caused by pressure of the assailant's arm against a turtleneck sweater. Close inspection reveals individual knots within the weave pattern.

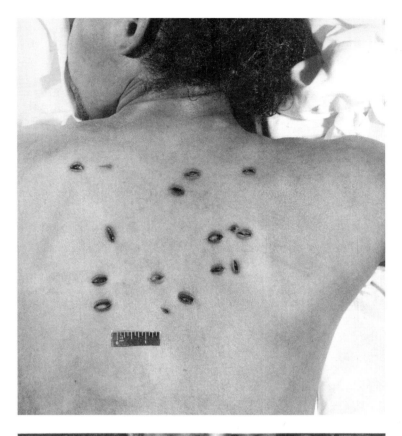

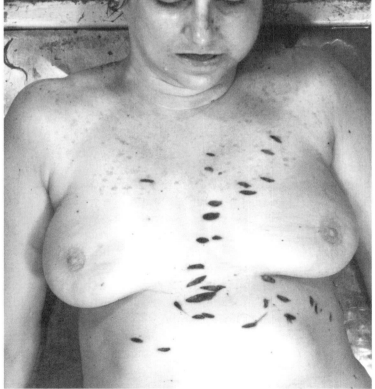

FIGURE XI-44a–b. (a) Numerous abraded stab wounds centered in upper back. A screwdriver was the weapon. (b) Multiple clustered stab wounds. The majority of the wounds run parallel suggesting that the victim was immobilized.

ciality, all or most of the wounds of the same depth, their directions consistent with whether the individual is right- or left-handed and often many of the wounds run parallel to each other. Depending on dexterity more wounds are seen on the left side of the body in a right-handed individual. Obviously, there are no self-inflicted cuts or stab wounds in areas beyond reach.

Superficial injuries such as jabs with a knife or other sharp instrument, cuts, cigarette or lighter burns, or evidence of beating are sometimes used as means of torture. The cause of death is usually readily recognizable in such cases. An *execution-style,* point-blank gunshot wound in the head or blows on the head with a heavy object, such as, a hammer, are common. Such deaths are often associated with the illicit drug traffic (Figs. XI-45 to XI-49).

Background information, including study of the circumstances surrounding the death and the scene where the body was found, is essential in all these situations. Interpretation of the injuries alone may be misleading. The cuts on the neck shown in Figure XI-46, could be interpreted as hesitation cuts, and the picture could have been further complicated by other indications of suicide, as, for example, a contact shot of the temple or a fall from a height.

IDENTIFICATION OF THE WEAPON AND DIRECTION OF THE WOUND TRACK

It is relatively uncommon that an assailant is apprehended while in possession of the murder weapon. Rarely is the knife left at the scene. Sometimes the blade breaks off and is lodged in the wound (Fig. XI-50a–b). Occasionally, only the tip of the blade is broken off, as a result of striking bone. X-ray examination of a stab wound may locate such fragments, which can be matched with a suspected knife by use of a comparison microscope. Metal fragments embedded in bone must be removed with utmost care so as not to damage any markings or add artefacts. Larger pieces may contain fingerprints. To remove portions of the blade the bone is sawed on the opposite side, deep enough to enable cracking the bone by hand, freeing the fragment. In the majority of cases, however, identification of a weapon is based on postmortem examination of the wounds.

Although a knife that was used in a stabbing may appear to be clean, it is likely that blood will be detectable on chemical analysis, unless the knife was rinsed and deliberately cleaned. Chemical analysis for the detection of blood is extremely sensitive, unlikely to miss even minute amounts. In situations where there is no blood apparent on the knife, removal of the grip and testing under the handle is often successful.

Serrated blades cause stab wounds and cuts which are indistinguishable from such wounds produced with ordinary knives. Only when the blade scrapes the skin surface sideways, will the serrations appear as sharp, parallel, linear scratches. The distance between the scratches on the skin corresponds to the distance between the serrations on the blade (Figs. XI-51a–b to XI-52a–b).

Serrated knives are available in a variety of types, depending on their intended use. Each type of blade will cause a distinct wound (Fig. XI-53). Serrated blades with double serrations cause parallel scratches in the skin if scraped lightly, but twice as many scratches, half as distant from each other, if more pressure is applied to the blade (Bottom blade on Figure XI-53).

A stab wound with scissors, screwdriver or another elongated, thick and dull object can be distinguished from one produced with a knife. The edges of a knife wound are sharp and non-abraded, as contrasted with the edges of a wound caused by scissors or screwdriver which are scraped during penetration by the dull surface of the weapon (Figs XI-54a–c to XI-57).

Due to its blunt tip a Phillips screwdriver will require much more force to perforate the skin compared to a regular screwdriver. A Phillips screwdriver with a very prominent bit sometimes produces a distinct cross-shaped perforation presumably due to the cutting effect of the bit's tip. In an attempted stabbing where no penetration

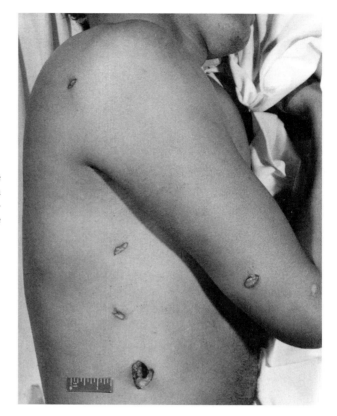

FIGURE XI-45. Knife wounds in a straight vertical line. The arm wound would probably also fit into the vertical pattern if aligned. The totality of the injuries suggest a trapped victim. All wounds are superficial except the bottom one which entered the peritoneum.

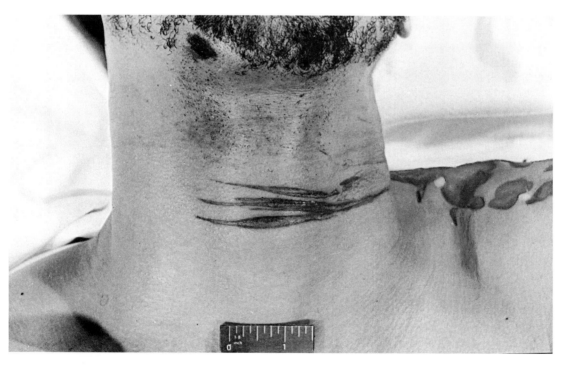

FIGURE XI-46. Parallel superficial cuts of neck and burns of left shoulder showing soot deposit in one area as a means of torture. The dismembered body was found wrapped in plastic bags in a city dumpster. Death was due to multiple hammer blows of the head.

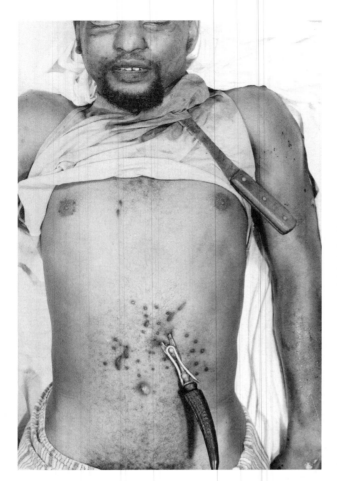

FIGURE XI-47a–c. (a–b) Paired circular puncture wounds produced with meat fork shown (c). The edges of each injury are abraded due to the thickness of the prongs. Above and to the left of the navel, two injuries show complete penetration with laceration by the bridge between the prongs. None of the abdominal wounds are immediately fatal.

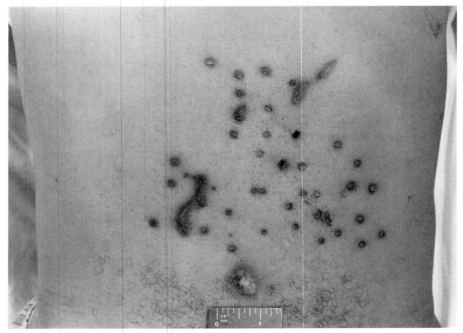

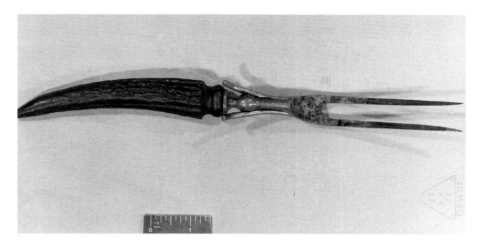

FIGURE XI-47c.

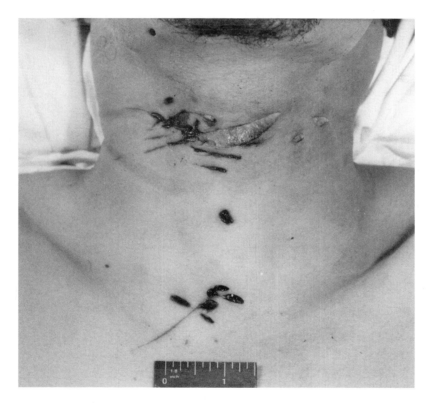

FIGURE XI-48. Superficial torture stab wounds and cuts with a small knife. Cause of death was a stab wound of the heart.

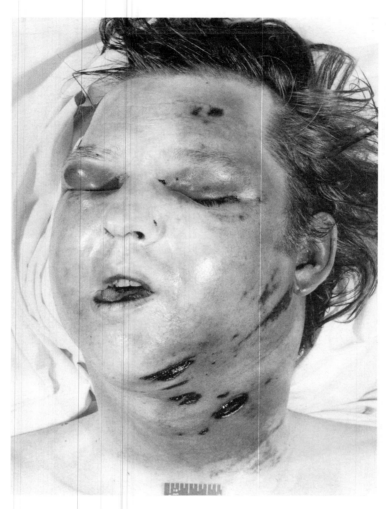

FIGURE XI-49. Multiple superficial stab wounds and cuts of face and neck. Cause of death was a gunshot in the back of the head.

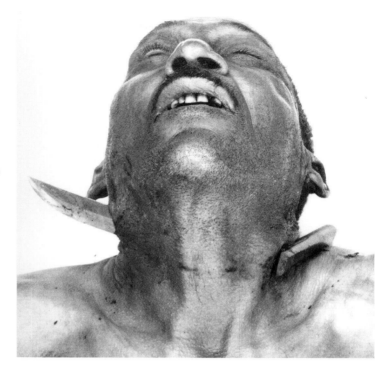

FIGURE XI-50a. Homicide. Entire knife left in wound. Handle of knife was bent over.

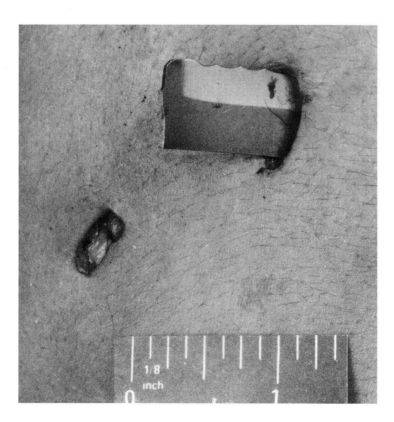

FIGURE XI-50b. Serrated blade which broke off at handle. The broken edge can be matched with remaining portion of the knife. Note that the wound with the blade is much larger than the wound below. Also, the shape of the second wound is different due to the contractility of the skin after withdrawal of the blade.

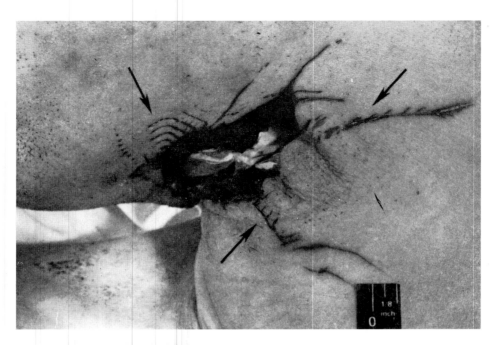

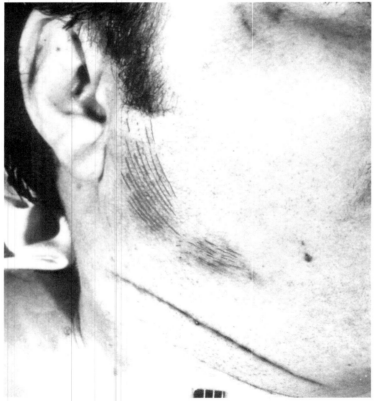

FIGURE XI-51a–b. (a) Homicidal slashing of throat with a serrated knife. The patterned parallel scratches (arrows) were produced by the serrated edge and permit identification of the type of weapon used. (b) Serrations of knife depicted in equidistant parallel lines on the face of a stalking victim.

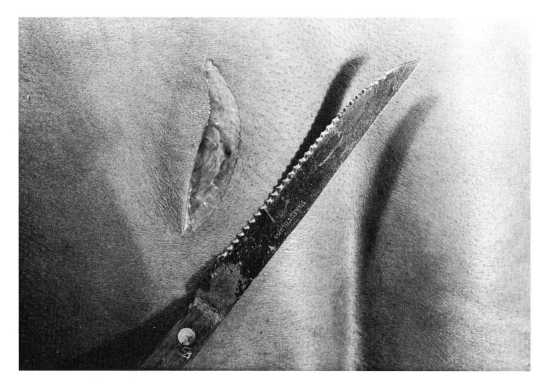

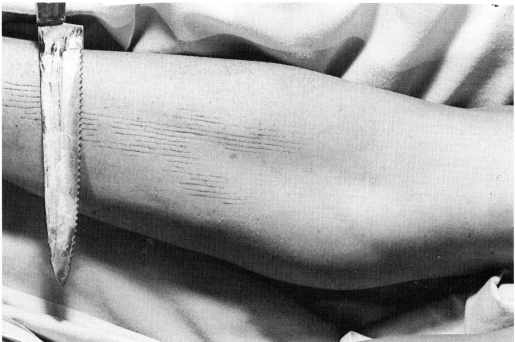

FIGURE XI-52a–b. (a) Stab wound showing absence of serrations on the wound edges. (b) Sharp, parallel, linear scratches corresponding to the distances between the serrations.

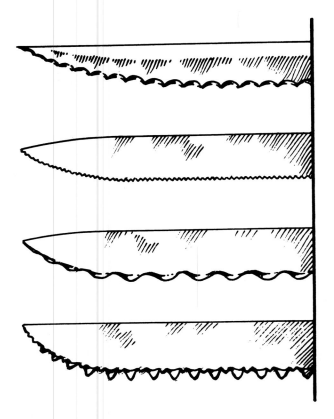

FIGURE XI-53. Different types of serrated blades are available.

has occurred the cross-shaped configuration may be recognizable on the skin, representing the actual dimensions of the tool. Thick, blunt-edged blades, such as bayonets, often cause cross-shaped wounds as a result of the same mechanism. A pointed target arrow will produce an entrance wound virtually indistinguishable from a gunshot wound.

The pattern or distribution of wounds may also suggest a specific type of instrument. In the case of stab wounds with a two-pronged fork, such as a barbecue or meat fork, the distance between the two punctures in the skin depends on the angle of stabbing (Figs. XI-58 to XI-60). If the meat fork was perpendicular to the skin, the distance between the punctures is representative of the distance between the prongs. If, however, the fork was held at an acute angle, the wounds are likely to be further apart. The edges of such stab wounds are usually abraded (see Fig. XI-60).

The most consistent feature of stab wounds caused with open scissors is a pair of wounds with one wound above and somewhat oblique to the other (Figs. XI-61a–b to XI-63). As in the case of wounds produced with a two-pronged fork, the distance between the two wounds differs depending on the angle of stabbing. Obviously, the distance between the scissor blades is variable unless the scissors are locked in position (Fig. XI-64). The edges of wounds produced with scissors are scraped because of the width of the blades. In the case of closed scissors a protuberant screw or rivet holding the blades may mark the skin in close proximity of the stab wound (see Fig. XI-54a–c).

Broken beer and wine bottles are sometimes used as weapons. Such injuries are usually irregular or semicircular, ragged and jagged; their edges are sharp and not abraded. Their depths may vary, but they seldom penetrate a body cavity (Fig. XI-65a–b). Wounds suspected of being

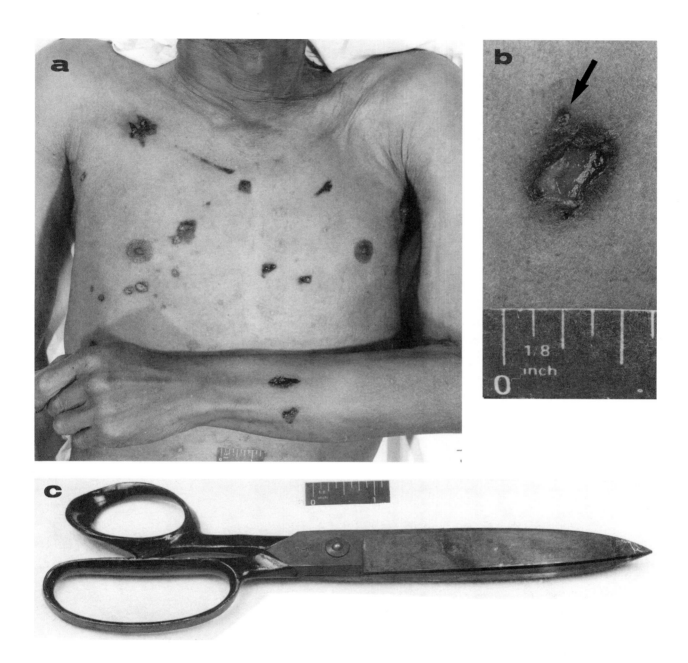

FIGURE XI-54a–c. Stab wounds produced with closed shears. The wound in Figure b has maintained the rectangular shape, which corresponds to the cross-section of the closed blades. The wound edges are abraded. The small circular defect at the top left of the wound (arrow) was produced by the screw lock. Several of the other stab wounds exhibit the same finding.

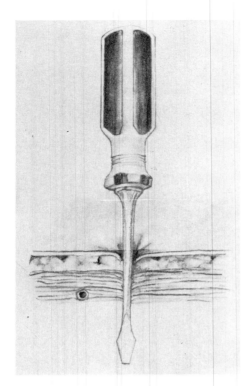

FIGURE XI-55. Scraping of the edges of the stab wound along the surface of a blunt weapon produces marginal abrasion.

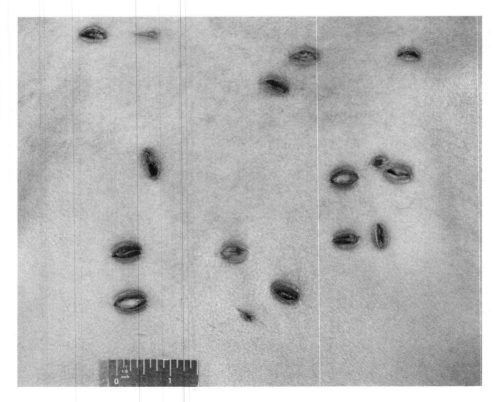

FIGURE XI-56. Clustered screwdriver wounds with abraded edges darkened by drying. The large number of wounds in one location represents *overkill*, suggestive of a crime of passion.

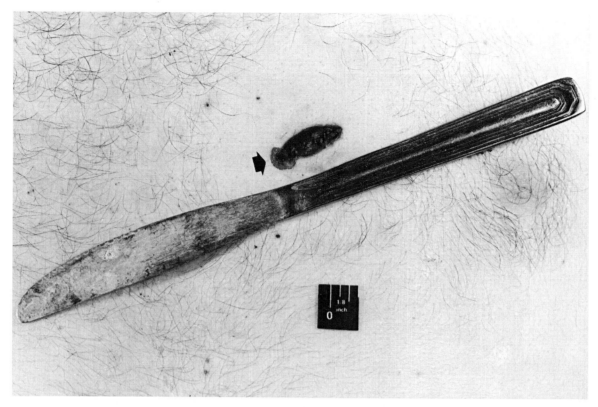

FIGURE XI-57. Stab wound with a table knife. A portion of the handle penetrated the skin, causing the half moon shaped abrasion (arrow).

FIGURE XI-58. Stab wounds with a meat or barbecue fork are paired, and their edges are abraded. The distance between the wounds may differ, depending on the angle of stabbing.

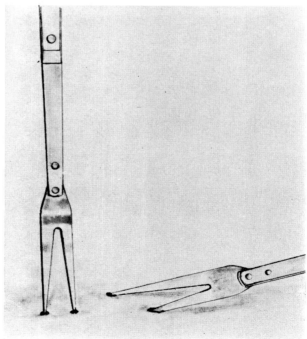

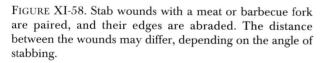

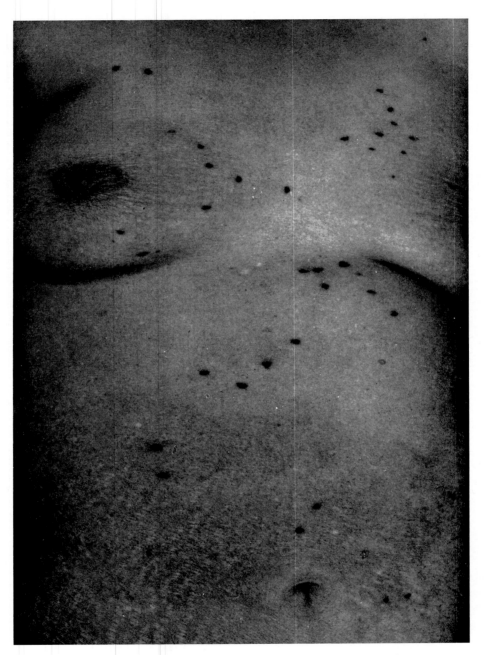

FIGURE XI-59. Multiple paired punctures from a barbecue fork.

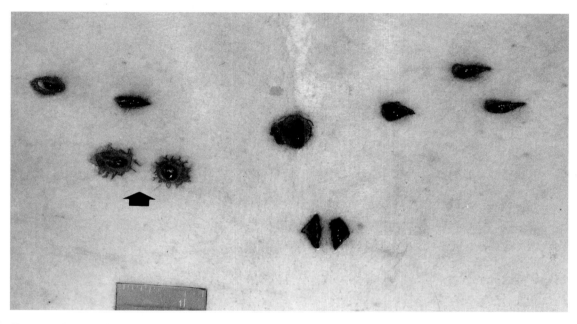

FIGURE XI-60. Multiple stab wounds of the back in an elderly woman during a robbery. The weapon was probably a carving fork, as suggested by the grouping in pairs of many of the injuries and their depths. The two wounds on the left (arrow), show a pattern of peripheral radiation presumably caused by the clothing being pushed into the wound by the weapon.

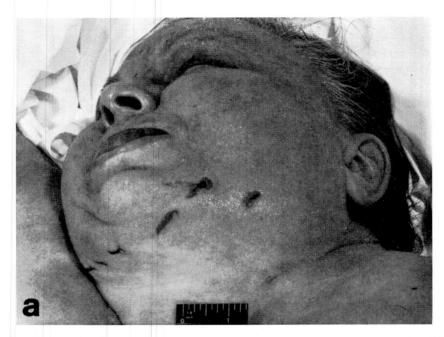

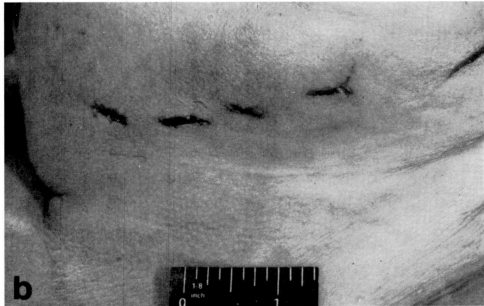

FIGURE XI-61a–b. (a) Stab wounds of the lower jaw inflicted with a pair of semi-opened pointed scissors. (b) The wounds are jagged and slightly abraded. In addition to being paired, one wound is always above and oblique to the other.

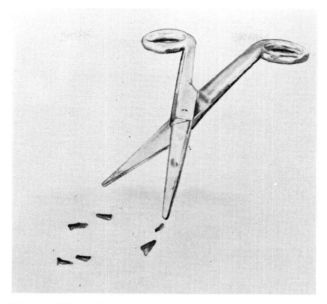

FIGURE XI-62. Characteristic stab wounds with scissors are paired, often abraded injuries. Each wound is oblique and above the other.

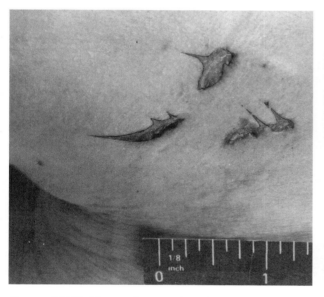

FIGURE XI-63. Four stab wounds with semi-open barber shears. The bottom edge of all wounds has a tongue of intact skin protruding into the wound indicating that each consists of two cuts, one by each blade. The scratch like extensions, all in the same direction, are caused by the pointed ends scraping the skin on rapid withdrawal.

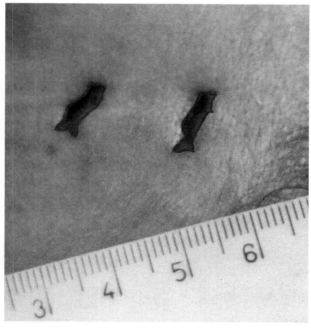

FIGURE XI-64. Wounds produced with closed shears are rectangular. The irregularity of the left edge of each wound on the photograph is caused by the screw or rivet securing the blades.

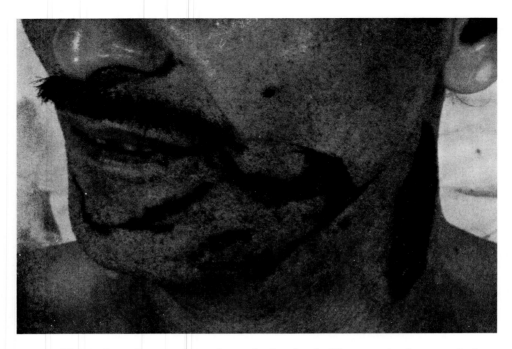

FIGURE XI-65a. Irregular jagged cuts from a broken bottle. The wounds often contain fragments of broken glass.

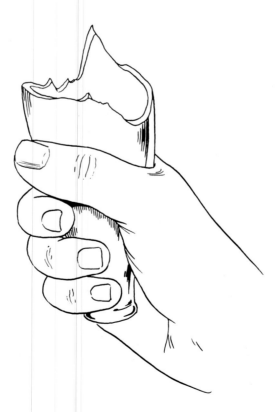

FIGURE XI-65b. Broken bottle used as weapon.

caused with broken bottles should be carefully inspected. If glass fragments are found inside cuts or on the surrounding skin or clothes, they should be preserved for possible later use as evidence. Glass slivers may be analyzed and their chemical composition compared with that of a given bottle. Cuts inflicted with broken bottles are usually located on the face, neck and chest. Cuts on the hands and forearms may represent defense wounds. Small, superficial, scratch-like cuts by glass splinters in the area of bottle wounds may resemble fingernail marks.

Another characteristic injury is a wound from a blow with a *chopping instrument* (Figs. XI-66 to XI-70). Meat cleavers, axes and machetes fall into this category. These are gaping, ominous appearing wounds, often showing fine abrasion of the edges. The width of these abrasions depends on the thickness of the blade and may reflect on depth of penetration. Typical chopping injuries to underlying bone are common.

Depending on the thickness and sharpness of the blade and the presence of underlying bone, the wound edges may be bruised due to some element of crushing. Markings on the edges of the cut bony surface are sometimes caused by irregularities on the blade. Such markings can be matched with the edge of a suspected weapon.

Rough spots on knife blades or chopping tools, such as nicks on the cutting edge and rusted and eroded areas, the screw or rivet holding the blades of a pair of scissors, a knife with a fish scaler, etc. may transfer fibers from a garment to another location on the same victim or to another victims's clothes or wounds. Body hair may be transferred in the same way.

Due to their rigidity, bone and cartilage maintain the dimensions and shape of a stab wound better than skin or other soft tissues (Fig. XI-71). The temporal bone of the skull will probably best display the dimensions of the weapon.

A homicidal stab wound is rarely inflicted without some simultaneous cutting. The knife is likely to be pulled upward or downward during entry or withdrawal, or the victim may move rearward or sideways, thereby causing an injury that is longer than the widest part of the blade (Figs. XI-72 and XI-73a–b). However, the width

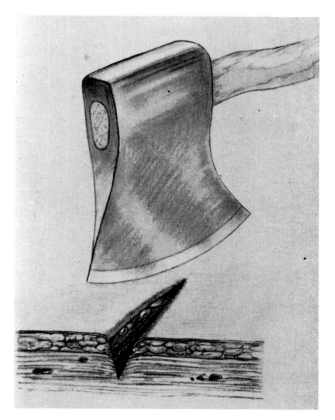

FIGURE XI-66. An axe causes a sharp cut with fine abrasion of the wound edges due to the thickness of the blade.

of the back or spine of the blade, i.e., its thickness, is *retained* in the wound. Realignment, while slightly twisting the edges of the wound, may be necessary in order to document the thickness of the blade. Abrasion of the upper layer of the skin (epidermis) by the blunt spine of the blade enables accurate recreation of its thickness. This will allow distinction of one knife from another, provided the thickness of their spines is sufficiently different (Figs. XI-74 to XI-76a–d). In the case of very thin blades, it may be necessary to use a magnifying lens and optimal lighting to identify the blunt and abraded edge of the wound (Fig. XI-77a–b). Obviously, the thicker the spine of the blade the easier it is to recognize. Also, a dry wound will show the thickness of the blade's spine as a dark brown, even black rectangle, while in an oozing injury or one wet from rain, the area in question may not be recognizable.

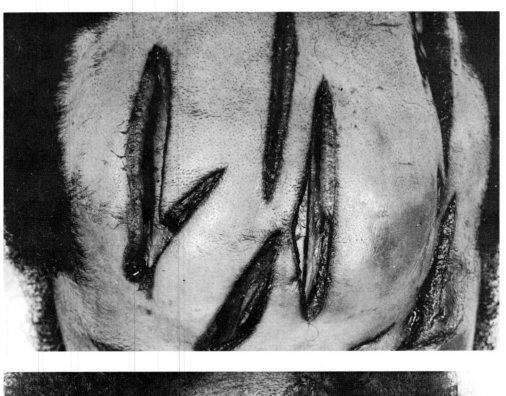

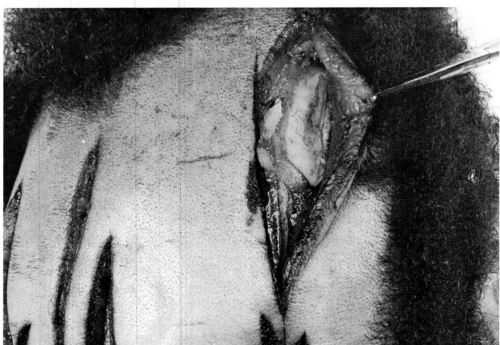

FIGURE XI-67a–b. An axe or machete causes a sharp, well-defined cut, distinguishable from a knife wound by fine abrasion of the edges. Underlying skull would be cut.

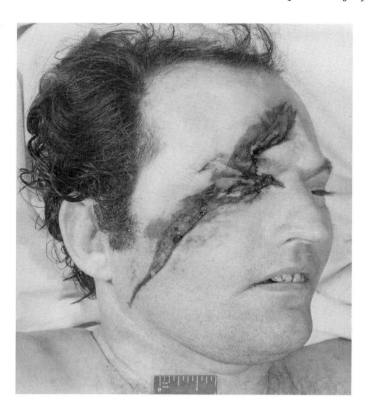

FIGURE XI-68. Chop wound: The abrasion along the posterior edge of the wound suggests that the direction of the blow was from back to front.

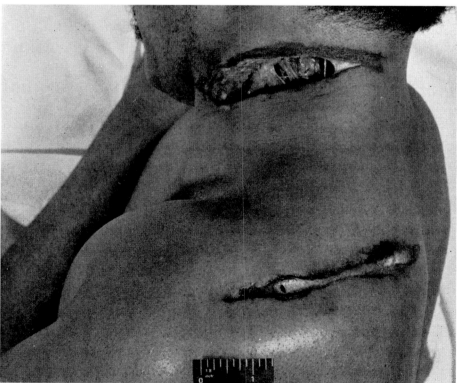

FIGURE XI-69. Injuries caused by the propeller of a small plane sustained during attempts to start the engine. The wound edges are sharp, as in a cut, but are abraded due to the thickness of the blades. Injuries such as these are referred to as chop wounds.

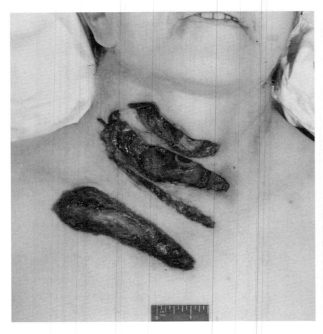

FIGURE XI-70. Deep parallel chop wounds produced by the spinning propeller of a boat.

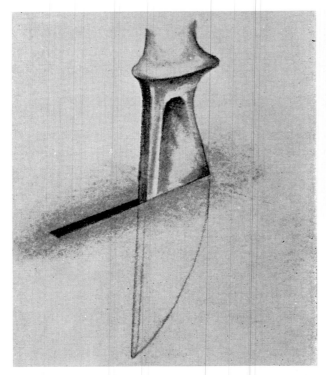

FIGURE XI-72. Stab wounds are often a combination of stabbing and cutting. The length of the wound in the skin is therefore not necessarily indicative of the width of the blade.

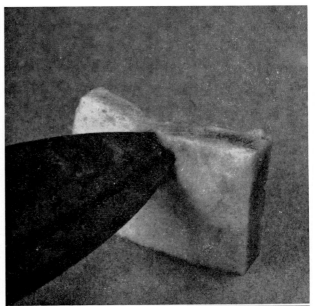

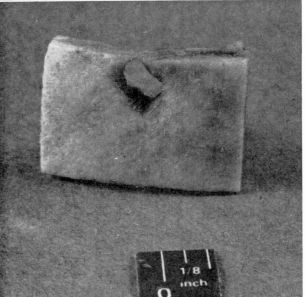

FIGURE XI-71. Rectangular defect in the skull produced with shears.

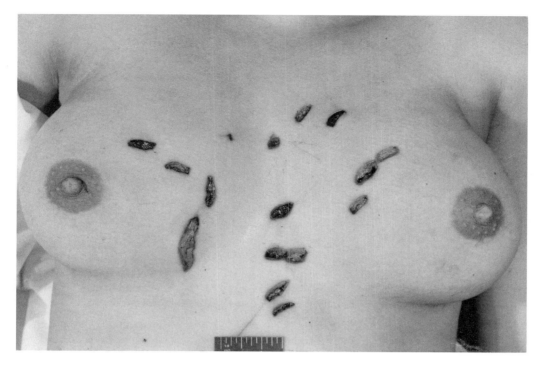

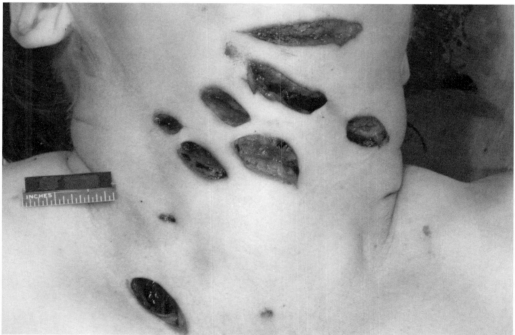

FIGURE XI-73a–b. While the stab wounds are of different dimensions, they were all inflicted with the same knife.

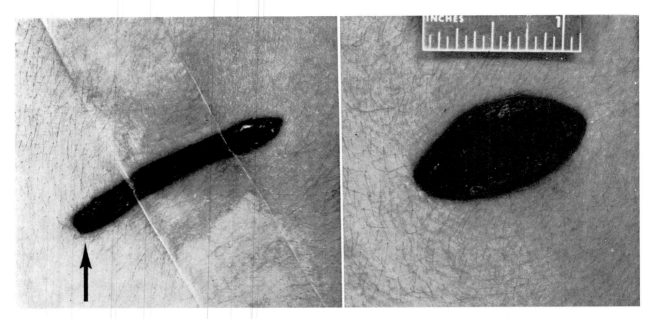

FIGURE XI-74. Stab wound of chest: On the right the injury is gaping and boat-shaped; on the left it is reconstructed with adhesive tape, indicating the thickness of the blade (arrow). The wound on the left is considerably longer.

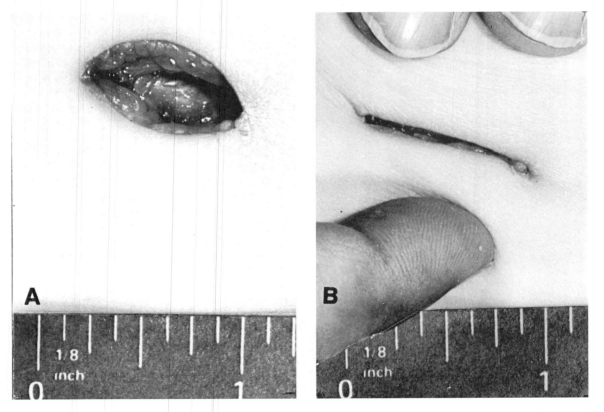

FIGURE XI-75a–b. Reconstruction of a stab wound to show thickness of blade. Approximation of the wound edges shows the stab wound to be narrower and longer. Only when the wound is reconstructed, as in B, can the rectangular spine of the blade be recognized. The spine of the blade which is a blunt object scrapes the epidermis and the area darkens as it dries.

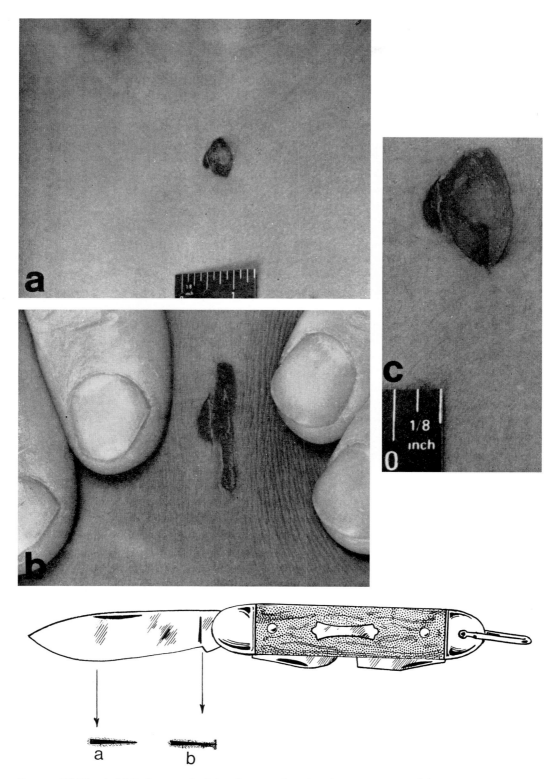

FIGURE XI-76a–d. (a) Stab wound of the chest produced with a pocket knife (d). A half-moon-shaped mark caused by the handle can be seen on the left side of the injury. (b) After approximation of the edges, the wound appears significantly longer, and (c) the back of the blade may be recognized at the upper end. (Parts b and c are reproduced in the same scale.) (d) Small pocket knife used to inflict the wound shown in a–c. Note the half-moon-shape casing of the hinge part of the handle.

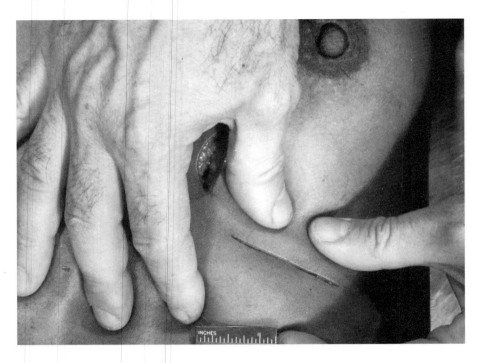

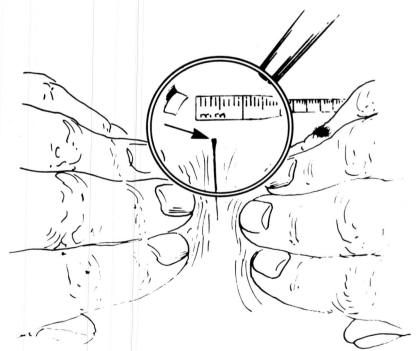

FIGURE XI-77a–b. Alignment of the wound and use of a magnifying glass permit identification of the blunt end of the stab wound not otherwise recognizable.

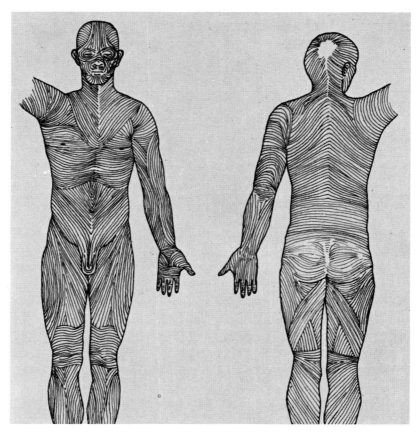

FIGURE XI-78. Cleavage lines of Langer.

A stab wound with two sharp angles is often instinctively thought to have been caused by a double-edged stiletto. However, realignment readily shows most of these wounds to be due to conventional, thin, but nevertheless, single-edged blades. The use of double-edged blades is very rare.

Stab wounds and deep cuts will either remain slit or boat-shaped with two acute angles or gape open, depending on their locations and their orientation with respect to the so-called *cleavage lines of Langer*. These are lines of tension that are determined by the direction of the elastic and collagenous fibers in the skin. Their locations and pathways are well established (Fig. XI-78). The elastic fibers in the skin are situated in the dermis, therefore a cut must be deep to gape.

The cleavage lines correspond to the creases of the body surface. Surgeons are well aware of the directions of the cleavage lines in the various regions of the body. An incision parallel to these lines heals with a fine linear scar, whereas an incision across the lines may result in an unsightly scar and considerable deformity.

A stab wound that severs the elastic fibers by cutting through the cleavage lines will gape, whereas one that runs parallel to these lines will remain slit or wedge-shaped and represent, with considerable accuracy, the dimensions of the blade with which it was inflicted. In attempting to *restore* a knife wound it may be necessary to return the skin to its original condition before it was divided. The edges of the wound may be manually approximated, or they may be held together with transparent adhesive tape (see Fig. XI-74). The new dimensions of the stab wound should be recorded and the restored injury photographed, with scale, for later use as evidence. The dimensions of the gaping wound serve no useful purpose.

In a stab wound which has dried and lost pliability, placing a wet paper towel on the wound for 20–30 minutes, or longer if necessary, then working a moisturizing cream into the wound edges may soften them to enable alignment and recognition of wound characteristics. The edges of a large tangential cut may shrink and curl, then dry and darken giving the erroneous impression of a chop wound by a machete or an axe (Fig. XI-79).

Restoration or reconstruction of a stab wound often shows the resulting slit to be considerably longer than the original oval-shaped wound. This may be of significance to counter a possible later claim that the suggested knife could not have produced a stab wound of such small dimensions.

Strangely shaped wounds, such as A or V-shaped (sometimes S or C), may be interpreted as resulting from two separate stabs in the same location. Whereas, realignment and restoration of the wound edges does occasionally verify the double nature of such a stab wound (Fig. XI-80a–b), in most instances the unusual shape results from stabbing followed by simultaneous twisting and cutting (Figs. XI-81 and XI-82a–e). During the process of stabbing there is considerable relative movement between the individuals involved in the struggle. Following the thrust of the knife, the victim may stumble and fall, causing the blade to be twisted in his body, or the assailant may twist the blade during withdrawal, simultaneously, cutting the skin. Countless possibilities exist, all capable of causing atypically-shaped stab wounds, the interpretation of which is frequently difficult and challenging.

Double wound tracks are rare and difficult to document, except in the presence of two or more tracks running in different directions, wound tracks through facial bones or the temporal squame and in the case of multiple exits, as sometimes seen in stab wounds of limbs or the chest wall. It must be remembered that stab wounds, however devastating are not usually immediately incapacitating, thus the fight goes on and movement of the individuals and weapon(s) continues.

A stab wound through a crease or fold in the skin, such as through a sagging abdomen or

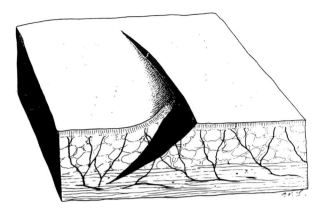

FIGURE XI-79. Cut in skin with curled up, dried and discolored edge.

female breast, a wound in the crease of the arm pit or groin in proximity of the scrotum, are likely to result in an atypical injury (Fig. XI-83). A stab wound with a knife in such a location may appear round and be mistaken for a gunshot. Slit-shaped stab wounds may be round when in or near a crease and a wound produced with a weapon having a triangular shaft, such as a file, may lose its true identity, unless properly realigned and repositioned. It is necessary to straighten the skin to eliminate the crease in order to view and accurately evaluate the characteristics of such a wound. Similarly, atypical cuts occur in creases, pleats and folds of garments. Examination of the clothes may shed light on the peculiar shape of a particular stab wound.

Ice picks produce puncture wounds resembling small caliber bullet wounds (Fig. XI-84). When situated under one or both collarbones, such injuries may resemble hospital-placed hypodermic needle marks (Fig. XI-85). A small pocketknife may cause similar injuries (Fig. XI-86). An exit bullet wound may resemble a knife wound if the bullet is fragmented or flattened by prior impact on bone. Fragments of bone shattered by a bullet may also leave the body, producing wounds that suggest stabbing.

The sharpened end of a wire coat hanger is sometimes used as a weapon by inmates in prison fights. Such injuries are indistinguishable from wounds made with ice picks and are just as

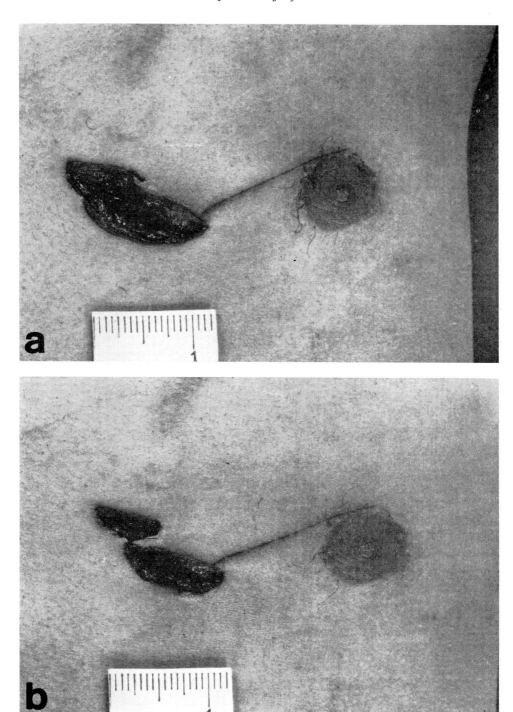

FIGURE XI-80a–b. Alignment of wound (a) showed it to consist of two stab wounds.

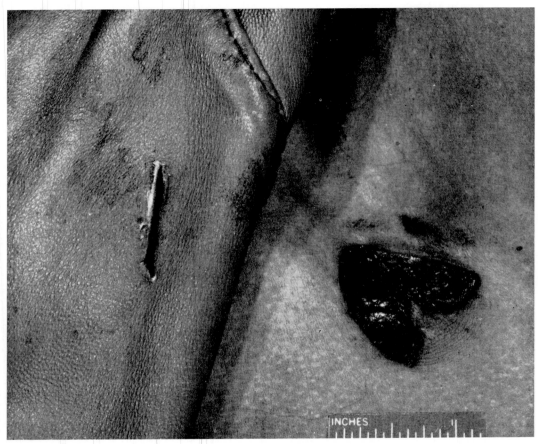

FIGURE XI-81. Stab wound below the right collarbone. The jacket shows a single slit, while the skin suggests two stab wounds. Twisting of the knife through the loose vinyl jacket produced this A-shaped injury.

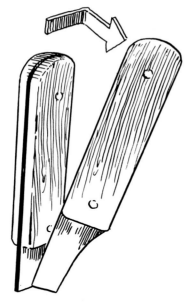

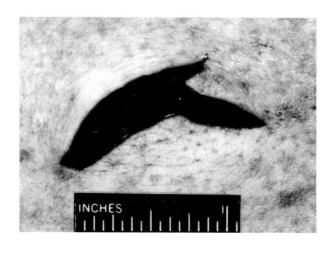

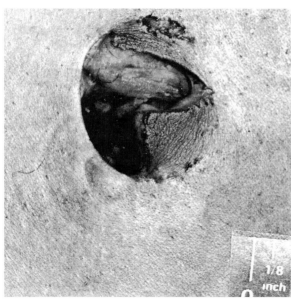

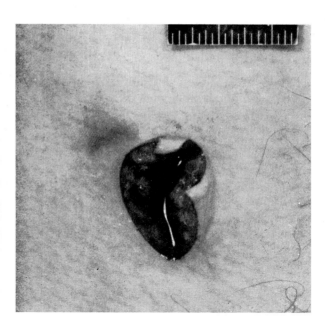

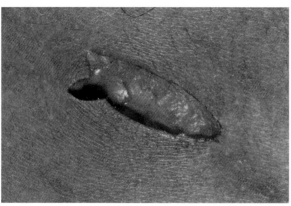

FIGURE XI-82a–e. Odd shaped wounds are produced by twisting of the knife while in the body. This can result by twisting of the hand holding the knife or movement of the victim.

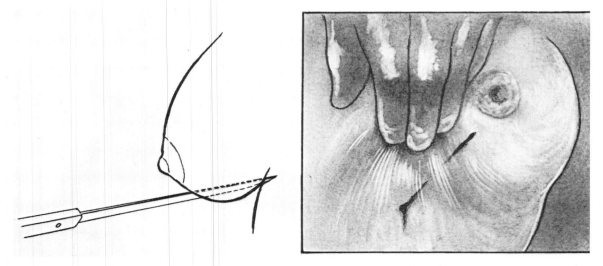

FIGURE XI-83. Atypical injury caused by a stab wound through a crease or fold of skin. It is necessary to straighten the skin to eliminate the crease in order to view and accurately evaluate the characteristics of such a wound. Both wounds were produced by a single stab.

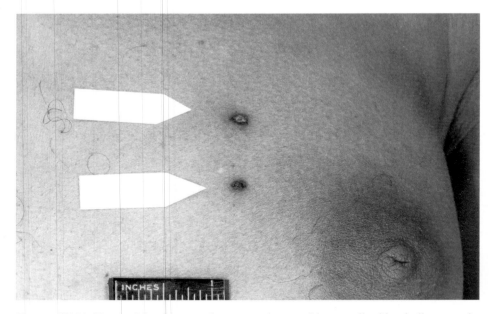

FIGURE XI-84. Homicidal stabbing with an ice pick, resembling small caliber bullet wounds.

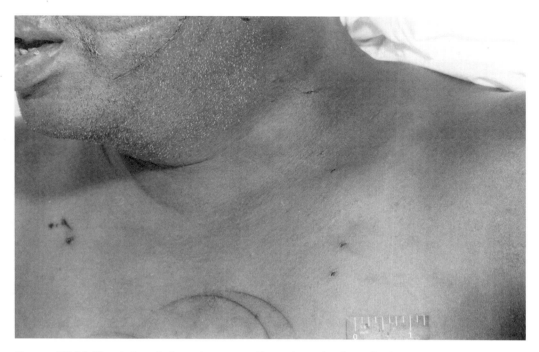

FIGURE XI-85. Hospital made hypodermic needle marks under the collar bones. Also note the defibrillator marks on the chest.

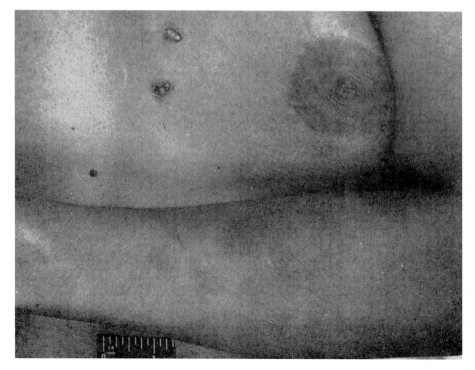

FIGURE XI-86. Two stab wounds in the chest by a small pocketknife. The initial police report was of a shooting.

devastating. The existence of such wounds, usually located in either side of the lower rib cage, may not be apparent for a day or two when bleeding and infection, become symptomatic.

Occasionally, such injuries occur outside of prison. A 44-year-old woman collapsed in a bar, believed to have overdosed on *street* drugs. On undressing the body, a 1/8" apparent wound track was noted in the left groin. Autopsy revealed massive hemorrhage in the pelvic soft tissues and muscles of the thigh originating from a deep stab wound from an ice pick-type weapon which perforated the iliac artery.

The wedge-like shape of a knife wound is often retained and recognizable in serosal planes and muscle fasciae. The pleural surfaces, liver and kidney capsules, the pericardial sac and the peritoneal lining of the abdominal wall are common examples. Accurate measurements of the dimensions of injuries in these areas are often helpful in attempts to assess the size and shape of the weapon in question and may reflect the thickness of a given blade with considerable accuracy.

The depth of a stab wound does not depend on the length of the blade alone. Actually, the depth of a knife wound may exceed the length of the blade that caused it. This is primarily due to *denting* or the *give* of the body surface as a result of the thrust of the fist holding the knife (Fig. XI-87). While such denting occurs more commonly in wounds of the abdomen, it also occurs in stab wounds of the chest and back, since the rib cage has considerable resilience, particularly in young individuals. Expansion and retraction of the chest during breathing must also be considered. We have seen stab wounds with a depth of six to seven inches produced by four-inch pocketknives.

The amount of force required to inflict a stab wound is frequently subject of inquiry. Whereas, the quantitation of such force is subjective and variable, less than two pounds of pressure is required to penetrate skin, if the knife is forcefully thrust and the tip of the blade is sharp and pointed. Whether the wound track passes through bone or cartilage must also be taken into account. Similarly, the type of bone involved and its thickness are equally important factors, as are the age and stature of the victim. Usually however-

er, once the tip of the blade has passed beyond the skin, the amount of force needed to penetrate inner organs is minimal. Consequently, the same, or a very similar amount of force is required to inflict a deep or shallow stab wound. Despite the ease of penetration, the author finds absurd the assertion sometimes held by the defense in criminal trials whereby the victim fell on the knife, casually held by the defendant.

Injection into the stab wound of dyes or radiopaque material to enable viewing of the wound track by x-ray has been attempted and claimed by some to be advantageous.[2,3] In our experience this procedure is seldom successful and frequently gives rise to false results. We do not use it.

As a general proposition, deep exploration of a knife wound may be a tedious procedure. A wound track through skeletal muscle, such as the thigh or shoulder usually lacks evidence of bleeding, due to the relatively small number and caliber of blood vessels. Wound tracks in the chest and abdomen are determined more by repositioning of the organs and aligning the injuries to conform with their locations while the victim was upright rather than by pursuit of the trail of hemorrhage.

Pain associated with stab wounds bears no relationship to the depth or severity of such an injury. Only the skin has nerve terminals sensitive to all varieties of pain, including crushing, burning, sharp and blunt injury and gunfire. Whereas, most internal organs are sensitive to crushing and stretching, they lack nerve endings stimulated by cutting and stabbing. A stab wound of the liver may remain painless for hours, even days, until deep hemorrhage causes stretching of the liver capsule. A stab wound of the heart, kidney, spleen, mesentery and bowel is painless. Discomfort, pain and fear of impending doom may be caused by bleeding, later onset of swelling and infection, but not as a result of penetration of the organ. Cuts are often more painful than stab wounds because larger areas of skin are involved.

The direction of a knife wound can only be determined at autopsy by meticulous dissection of the wound track. The indiscriminate and ran-

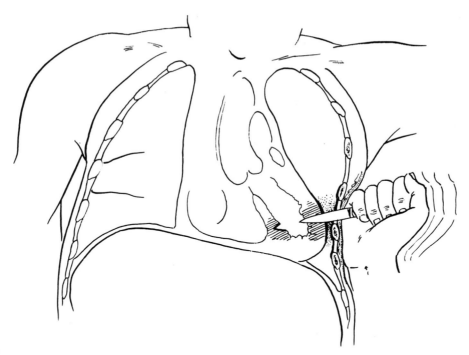

FIGURE XI-87. Denting due to thrust of the fist against the chest. The same occurs in the abdominal area.

dom probing of a knife wound is usually misleading. Probing a stab wound with a finger should be avoided at all times and probes should only be passed under direct vision. Probing prior to opening the body may invalidate the results by producing artifacts. After withdrawal of the blade, the wound track tends to close by expansion of the tissues along the weapon's pathway. The probe may then easily pass between tissue planes or within the musculature, producing a false track.

Organs tend to hang several inches lower in an upright position. Movement of the chest and diaphragm must also be considered. When evaluating the direction of a wound track, allowance must be made for the fact that the body is lying flat on the autopsy table.

Excision of a stab wound with its surrounding skin for the purpose of preservation of the specimen by freezing, or by tacking the specimen onto a board and chemically fixing it for later use as evidence is both impractical and serves no useful purpose. Removal of a flap of skin from the body alters tone and pliability of the tissue, and fixa-

tion adds further artifacts. Photographs at a 90° angle, particularly close-ups with a scale included in the frame, adequate description of location of the injury in relation to certain body landmarks, including its dimensions after restoration, will usually suffice.

The clothing in a case of cutting or stabbing should be thoroughly examined, and unusual findings associated with the injury should be recorded. If wet, it is best to dry the clothing to prevent mildew and deterioration and preserve each item in a separate paper bag, appropriately labeled for later examination by the crime laboratory and use as evidence. It is advantageous that the clothing be removed from the victim without cutting or tearing. The shape of a cut in the fabric may aid in explaining the mechanism of injury and complement the examination of the wound regarding the weapon involved. Leather, vinyl and other synthetics often maintain the shape of a cut with an excellent degree of accuracy.

Individuals contemplating suicide often remove their clothing from the area intended to be injured.

Just as bulletproof vests protect against a wide range of gun ammunition, stab-resistant body armor is now becoming a standard item of equipment for police officers in the United Kingdom. While these vests allow penetration of the pointed tip of a blade, they are resistant to cutting.

COMPLICATIONS OF CUTTING AND STABBING INJURIES

The main complications of cutting and stabbing injuries are (a) blood loss, (b) asphyxiation due to inhalation of blood, (c) air embolism, (d) pneumothorax, (e) infection.

Blood loss (exsanguination) is by far the most common cause of death from cutting and stabbing. Bleeding is mainly into body cavities, since the outer parts of the wound track frequently close after withdrawal of the weapon. The amount of blood at the scene of injury may be minimal, unless the extremities, the head or neck are involved. The amount of outward bleeding also depends on whether the wound is situated in a dependent area of the body, in which case it is likely that outward spillage is of much greater volume.

TIMING OF STAB WOUNDS

In cases of multiple stab wounds and cuts, pathologists often opine that one or the other injury occurred after death. Such determinations are usually based on the small amount of bleeding, or no bleeding at all, at the site of injury. Assessment of when a wound was inflicted in relation to the time of death by the amount of hemorrhage is neither accurate nor reliable. For example, in the case of a transected aorta, blood flow to areas distal to the transection is interrupted and only seepage of blood by gravity is still likely after such injury. Seepage of blood continues for several hours after death, until all blood from area arteries and veins has drained. A pint of blood or more may seep into a body cavity from a major artery or vein. It must be emphasized however, that even in the absence of other injuries, a stab wound or gunshot wound through the thigh, arm, back, or buttock often leaves little or no trail of hemorrhage in the skeletal muscles.

An interesting twist of the O.J. Simpson civil trial was the testimony of a defense expert, whereby the double murder took at least 20 minutes to accomplish. No consideration was given to the fact that Ronald Goldman's first stab wound was the one to his left flank, which practically severed his aorta resulting in massive retroperitoneal bleeding, loss of blood pressure, reduced consciousness and rapid collapse. Consequently, the two stab wounds in the right side of his chest, both penetrating the lung, resulted in only 200 mL of blood in the chest cavity.

The cut of the aorta clearly shortened the duration of the assault to less than one minute, enabling Mr. Simpson to make it back to his home, clean up and get to the airport in time for his scheduled flight to Chicago.

Physical activity of varying degree and duration may be expected in fatal stabbing cases, even if the heart, major blood vessels or the lungs are involved.[3] Review of case histories and the relevant literature on the subject illustrates dramatically the great extent of activity that an individual may perform following fatal wounding:

A thirty-seven-year-old man was stabbed in the chest with a butcher knife. Following the injury he got into his automobile and drove four city blocks; he then lost control of the vehicle and crashed into a parked car. He proceeded to the hospital on foot and died in the emergency room about twenty minutes after the injury. At autopsy there was a 1/4 inch slit-like cut in the right ventricle of the heart. There were 1-1/2 quarts (approximately 1400 mL) of blood in the left pleural cavity and in the pericardial sac.

A twenty-three-year-old man was stabbed with a kitchen knife, walked and staggered a distance of 358 feet and died at the hospital a few minutes after arrival. A 1/4 inch wound in the left ventricle of the heart and the aorta caused internal bleeding of nearly two quarts (1900 mL).

A twenty-five-year-old man was stabbed with a kitchen knife, causing severance of his left subclavian artery and vein. Following the injury the victim ran four city blocks and collapsed. He died at the hospital one hour later. The total blood loss was estimated at about three quarts (2800 mL).

Disability of victims of fatal gunshot injuries appears to be more rapid than in those fatally wounded by sharp weapons.

Asphyxiation due to blood inhalation may result from a cut or a stab wound in the neck area, exposing the larynx or trachea. A stab wound in the lung may cause spreading of hemorrhage to both lungs through the tracheobronchial tree. Death due to asphyxiation is usually rapid, often associated with choking and sometimes convulsions due to obstruction of the air passages and reduction of the breathing surface of the lungs.

Air embolism is usually the result of a cut or stab wound of the neck that exposes and penetrates one of the larger veins. Due to the negative pressure in veins, air is *sucked* into the vessels. When mixed with blood, air causes foam to be formed, which produces a valve lock in the heart. Death from massive air embolism is usually sudden and rapid. The victim gasps once or twice and collapses.

Pneumothorax, or air in the pleural cavity, occurs when a penetrating wound in the chest voids the normally present subatmospheric pressure in the pleural space. Such a wound is usually accompanied by hemorrhage. The term *hemopneumothorax* is therefore more appropriate. The presence of air and blood in the chest cavity may compress the lung and push the chest organs, to the opposite side (tension pneumothorax). Tension pneumothorax occurs when a check valve mechanism in a penetrating wound of the chest wall permits air to enter the pleural cavity, but not to leave. Such an injury represents a potentially fatal medical emergency by compromising heart and lung function.

Infection of a stab wound or a cut is a late complication that may take days or weeks to develop. It is a rare cause of death, except in stab wounds of the abdomen, in which bowel contents are spilled into the peritoneal cavity causing peritonitis or the neck, where an abscess may cause sepsis, erode a major blood vessel, or compress the airway.

DISMEMBERMENT

Disposal of a homicide victim by dismemberment is rare, but individual cases are on record in most major medicolegal departments. Postmortem dismemberment is usually readily recognizable as such. The edges of the injuries are dry and lack evidence of bleeding. The joints may be disarticulated, without fracture or the use of an axe or saw may be evident from examination of the bones.

Disarticulation, especially involving the cervical spine, may be suggestive of a perpetrator with some knowledge of anatomy. The use of an axe may be evident from fragmentation of the severed edges of long bones (Fig. XI-88). In contrast, skull, ribs and pelvis which are membranous bones are cut, not fragmented, by an axe or meat cleaver (Fig. XI-89). Parallel, horizontal or oblique furrows in the bone surface are caused by slipping of the saw blade prior to establishing a rut. Slipping of the blade over the surface of the bone produces equidistant, parallel grooves or ruts by the teeth of the blade. Similar to those pro-

duced on the skin by a serrated blade. Such pattern on the bone may assist in identifying the particular saw used (Fig. XI-90a–d).

A chain saw works on a different principle. A chain saw cuts bone and generates bone dust more coarse than that produced by a conventional saw. An axe or machete is more likely to fragment the bone rather than producing clean, smooth cuts. Identification of the utensil used for *postmortem mutilation* is important in the interpretation of such murders. Postmortem dismemberment is often performed for easier disposal of the body.

The meticulously disarticulated and dismembered remains of a young woman were found in plastic bags in several commercial suburban dumpsters. The husband, with an engineering degree, claimed his wife had committed suicide following a domestic argument. He dismembered and dumped the remains to hide the death.

Several, superficial stab wounds below the woman's chin, interpreted to have been caused by taunting, a deep stab wound in the back, beyond her reach, and superficial slashes in the face, indicative of a fight, led to the determination of homicide as the manner of death. The husband

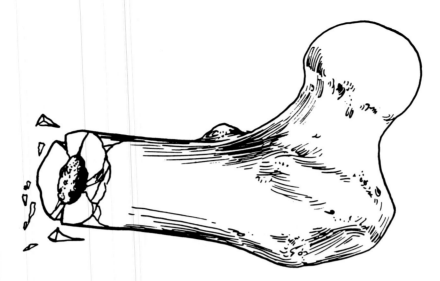

FIGURE XI-88. The use of an axe may be evident from fragmentation of the severed edges of long bones.

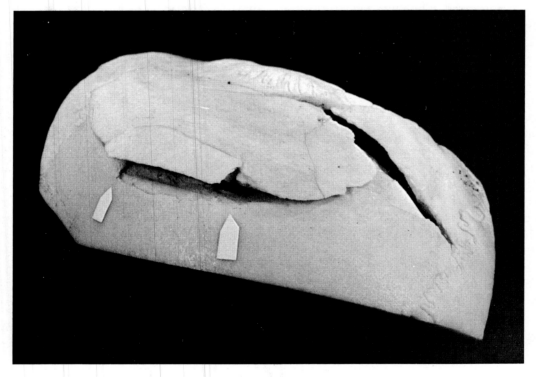

FIGURE XI-89. Skull cut by a meat cleaver.

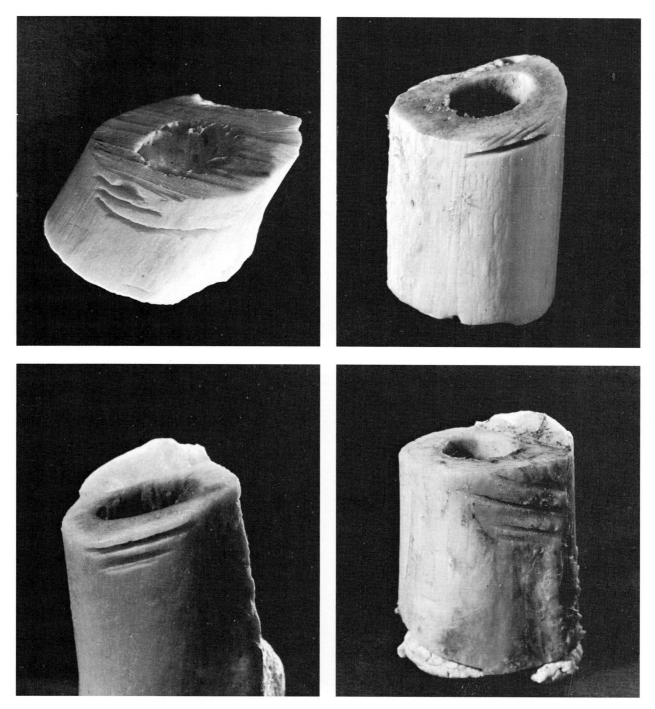

FIGURE XI-90a–d. Skipping of saw blade on bone surface prior to establishing depth. The width of the ruts corresponds to the thickness of the saw blade.

had a deep, horizontal cut across his index finger where his hand had slipped off the bloody old wooden handle of the kitchen knife he had used.

Identification of a knife or chopping weapon, such as a meat cleaver or an axe can be made by tool mark comparison of injured bone with a sus-pected weapon. This method of weapon identifi-cation is sometimes successful in head wounds, especially if tangential. The principle is the same as that which is applied to identification of a ser-rated knife in the case of a skin wound or a saw if bone is injured.

OTHER SHARP FORCE INJURIES

In falls through plate glass, areas most often injured are the groin, armpit and neck and death results from hemorrhage due to severed major arteries (Figs. XI-91 and XI-92). Cuts and stab wounds sustained in this way may closely resemble homicidal type injuries. However, careful examination of such wounds reveals dif-ferent depths ranging from small superficial cuts to deep, mutilating stab wounds and slashes. Tiny superficial scratch-like marks, resembling fingernail marks, usually straight, but in differ-ent orientations are often present. Bruising is usually lacking unless there was a blunt force component.

It is good practice to search for glass slivers in the depth of the wounds.

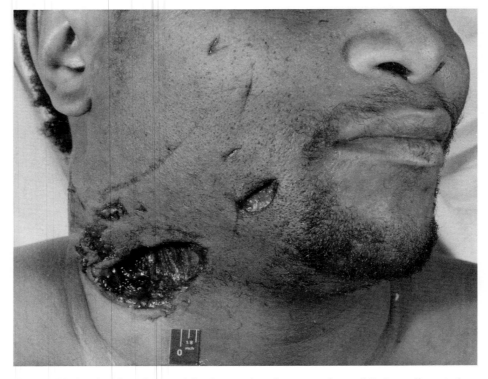

FIGURE XI-91. Accidental cuts of the face and neck sustained in a fall through a window while intoxicated. The injuries are deep, sharp and in the absence of other circumstantial findings, are hard to distinguish from homicidal cuts.

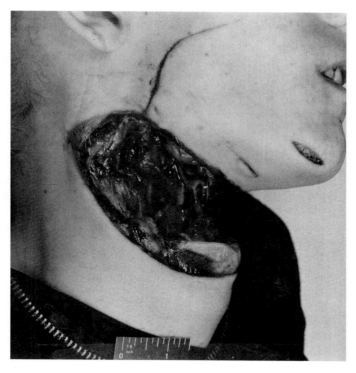

FIGURE XI-92. Fall through plate glass window. Note the similarity with a homicidal injury.

Tempered glass has replaced the use of plate glass in sliding doors, shop windows, shower stalls, etc. and has dramatically reduced the number of fatalities caused by such injuries.

Other sharp force injuries include those produced by the propeller of a boat or ship. Such injuries resemble large cuts or chopping wounds. These wounds are usually multiple and parallel because of the rapid spinning of the propeller. The location and orientation of the cuts suggest the position and activity of the individual in the water.

The body of a decapitated woman was found on the bottom of a busy waterway. The head was a few feet away. Numerous, parallel cuts from the boat's propeller blades were noted on her face and chest and several cuts were situated on her arm. When the arm was raised at autopsy, it became apparent that the parallel orientation of the cuts on the arm aligned with those of the face and chest, compatible with backstroke swimming when struck.

In another boating mishap, a young lady partying and drinking with friends, claimed she had been struck by the turning propeller as she descended into the water. The injury to her leg was a reverse S-shaped gash which ran from the thigh to the calf, consistent with her slipping off the boat, striking a stationary propeller (Fig. XI-93).

In reconstructing these injuries, we have found it beneficial to compare the boat's propeller with the wounds by actually holding the propeller against a body.

The question of pre- or postmortem occurrence of such wounds in a body recovered from water is often difficult due to *leaching* of blood from the tissues. Submersion of less than 24 hours in warm water suffices to simulate postmortem occurrence of an open wound sustained during life. Bloody infiltration of tissues at the site of an injury is probably the most valuable criterion that the injury was sustained during life. The nature of the injuries, their extent and locations may suggest pre- versus postmortem occurrence and exclude homicide with subsequent disposal of the body to simulate drowning.

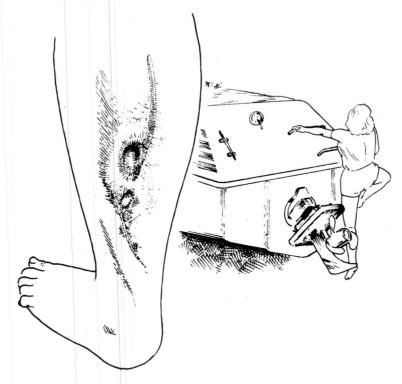

FIGURE XI-93. The injury depicts the parts of the propeller and indicates that the propeller was not spinning. The illustration was drawn from a color photograph.

REFERENCES

1. Cina, S.J.: The tale of the nail: Does it yield relevant DNA evidence? *Forensic Med Sci Select, 1* (3): 1–3, 2000.
2. Rabinowitsch, A.: Medico-legal conclusions on the form of the knife used, based on the shape of the stab wounds produced. *J. Forensic Med, 6:* 160, 1959.
3. Mueller, B.: *Gerichliche Medizin*. Berlin: Springer, 1953, p. 275.
4. Spitz, W.U., Petty, C.S., and Fisher, R.S.: Physical activity until collapse following fatal injury by firearms and sharp pointed weapons. *J Forensic Sci, 6:* 290, 1961.

Chapter XII

INJURY BY GUNFIRE

General Introduction

FIREARMS ARE INVOLVED in approximately two-thirds of all homicides in the United States. Handguns, i.e., automatic pistols and revolvers, are used in the majority of cases. Rifles and shotguns are used far less commonly.[1] Complete and accurate interpretation of firearm wounds is mandatory for effective prosecution. Because of the many similarities between handguns and rifle wounds, they will be considered together as gunshot wounds. Shotgun wounds will discussed separately.

Part 1

GUNSHOT WOUNDS

WERNER U. SPITZ

The following are essentials which can be derived from the external examination of a gunshot wound:
• range of fire
• direction of fire

RANGE OF FIRE

Accurate assessment of the range of fire requires test firing of the gun with the type of ammunition that was used in the shooting. Since gunpowder particles which hit the body at close range penetrate the skin, causing small, superficial wounds, it is advisable that skin be used for the test target shot. Fresh pigskin usually fills the need. Even though the test shot will appear somewhat different than that on live skin, the overall pattern of gunsmoke is comparable. Basic criteria exist that permit a general estimate of a muzzle-to-target distance by examination of a bullet wound.

While on the subject of test shots, when assessing size and shape of bullet wounds in bone,

attempts to duplicate an existing wound by test firing into dry bony specimens may not always yield reliable data.

When a firearm is discharged, smoke containing abundant soot and gunpowder is ejected from the muzzle along with the bullet (Fig. XII-1). These deposits that occur around the bullet holes in cases of close-range fire are referred to as smudging and tattooing or stippling. It is the diameter of spread and the density of these deposits which permit assessment of the range of fire (Fig. XII-2a–b).

Thorough examination of the victim's clothes is imperative to ascertain the presence of gunpowder and soot around a bullet hole. When the

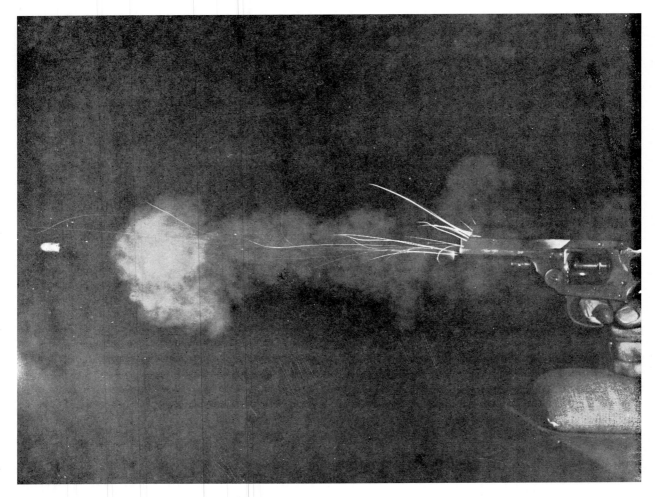

FIGURE XII-1. Gunsmoke ejected from the muzzle of a revolver. The light streaks are glowing particles of gunpowder. The bullet is seen on the left. (Courtesy: Donald M. Flohr, H. P. White Laboratories, Bel Air, Maryland.)

clothes are light in color, soiling by soot and gunpowder are easily recognizable. However, when the clothes are dark or blood soaked, identification of powder residue may not be as simple. Chemical identification of gunpowder residue has proven valuable for clothing items and occasionally for skin, when grains seen on the target are not identifiable as gunpowder by naked-eye examination or the use of a large, preferably illuminated, magnifying lens.

Combing of hair with a fine tooth comb has been used successfully to gather organic gunshot residue resulting from incomplete combustion of smokeless gunpowder. Such test results are valuable when estimating distance of fire in shots involving the head.[2]

Identification of gunpowder residue is feasible by scanning electron microscopy (SEM). Alternative, but less likely methods of identification are atomic absorption, and thin-layer chromatography. The terminology most often used to describe the range of fire is as follows:

- *contact shot,* when the weapon is fired with the muzzle in contact with the body,
- *close-range shot,* when gunsmoke is deposited on the target,

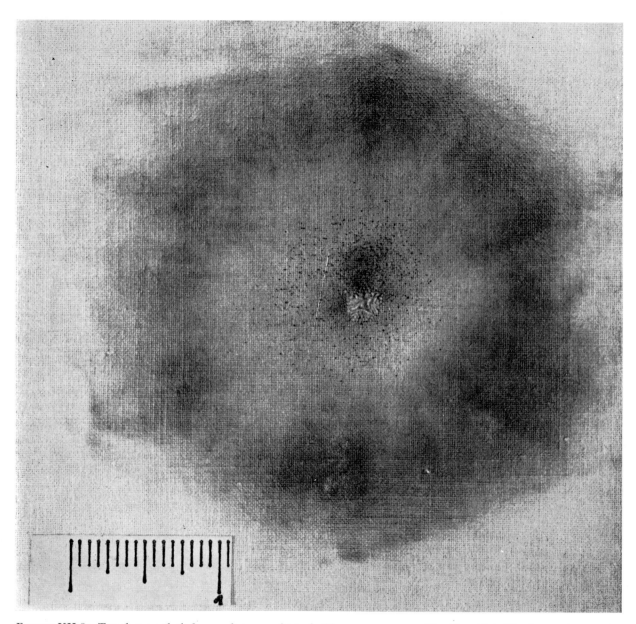

FIGURE XII-2a. Test shot on cloth from a distance of 1 inch. The weapon was a .22 caliber Colt Woodsman Automatic, the ammunition .22 caliber Western Super X-Long Rifle. Note, densely scattered gunpowder around the bullet hole. Soot is spread over a 3-1/2 to 4 inch diameter.

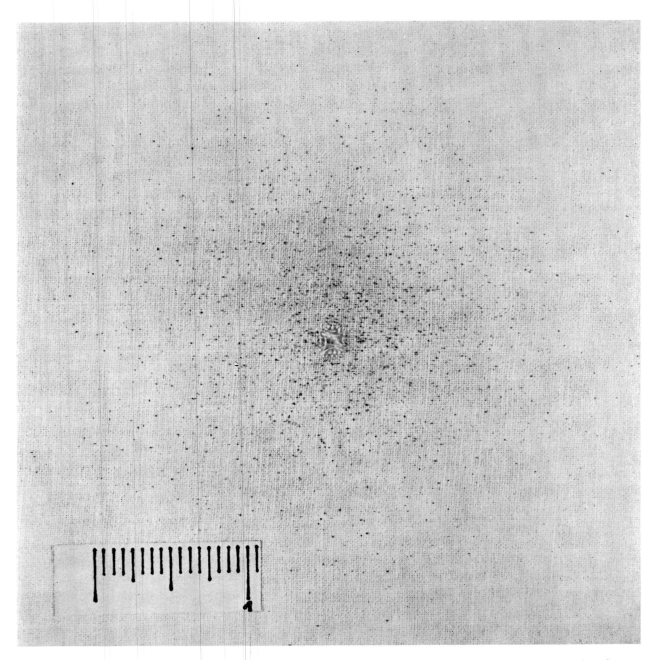

FIGURE XII-2b. Same weapon and ammunition at 6 inches, muzzle-to-target distance, practically no soot reaches the target. Gunpowder spreads over a 3 to 4 inch diameter.

• *distant shot,* when the muzzle to target distance exceeds the limits in which gunsmoke is identifiable on the target.

Contact Shots

When a gun is fired with the muzzle against a clothed part of the body, the bullet hole in the fabric touching the muzzle is sometimes surrounded by a flat ring, which corresponds to the profile of the muzzle. This ring is caused by the heated barrel, similar to an iron pressing cloth. The loose and frayed fibers of fabric in the center of the bullet hole are usually turned outward, away from the body, as a result of the expanding gases returning through the defect. Commonly, these fibers are blackened by gunsmoke and in the case of synthetic fabrics, the edges may be melted. Soot, in varying amounts, is also deposited around the bullet hole, depending on how tightly the gun was held against the body (Fig. XII-3).

Although deposits of gunsmoke on clothing frequently remain unrecognized if the clothes are blood soaked, the inner surface of the garment may show abundant deposits of gunsmoke, even if none were noted on the outside. This results from spreading of smoke between the skin and the clothing by the muzzle blast and is observed especially if the shot passed through several layers of fabric. The same occurs if the shot was fired through a pocket. Each layer is blackened individually on both sides of the fabric, while the wound in the skin may be devoid of gunpowder or soot.

In the absence of clothing intervening between the muzzle and the skin, all the gunsmoke enters the wound, although, a small amount may be deposited on the wound edges, particularly, if contact with the muzzle was loose (Fig. XII-4). Thus, in the case of a shot fired with a gun pressed against the skin, no gunpowder will be deposited on the skin around the bullet wound. Exception to this rule is the use of some poor quality handguns where gunpowder particles may be spewed on the target from a loosely fitting cylinder. Small fragments of lead shaved

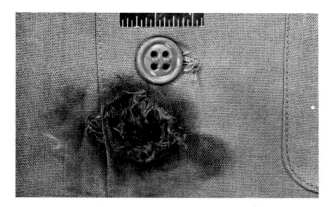

FIGURE XII-3. Contact shot of upper abdomen. Soot around the bullet hole in the shirt. The fibers of the fabric are turned outward by the expanding gases returning through the hole.

from the bullet by a loose cylinder may also reach the target in similar fashion.[3]

The likelihood of soot or gunpowder in tissues near the exit wound is remote, even if the gun was pressed tightly against the body. Although, if the shot involved a thin area of the body, such as a hand or in the case of a tangential shot in the neck or arm, some gunpowder, even soot may be found.

Careful handling and layerwise dissection of contact and near contact bullet wounds is required to reveal fine granules of burned and unburned gunpowder and deposits of black soot in the depth of the wound. Incorrect handling of a wound may cause the mistaken impression of a distant shot. This may mean the difference between a self-inflicted bullet wound and involvement of another party. In the case of a contact shot of the head with a revolver or a semiautomatic pistol, the wound is frequently star-shaped due to tears that radiate from the sides of the wound. These tears are caused by the blast effect that follows the sudden release of gases into a confined area, between the skin and underlying bone (Figs. XII-5 and XII-6). A *pocket* under the skin, containing blood mixed with gunpowder, is formed by separation of the tissues. Additionally, stretch mark-like tears confined to the epidermis further indicate the tremendous pressure within the pocket (Figs. XII-7 and XII-8a–b).

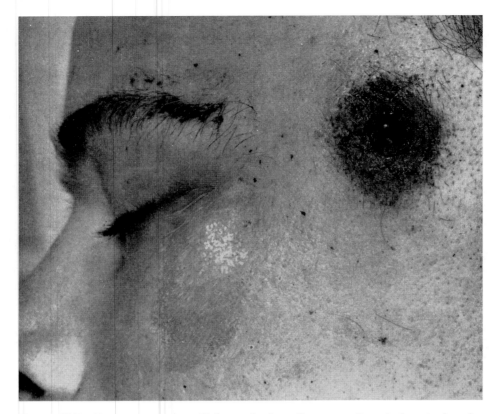

FIGURE XII-4. Loose contact shot of left temple. A small amount of soot is deposited on the wound edges.

Soot may also be deposited on the bone around the bullet hole (Fig. XII-9). An ideal procedure to document this soot is to incise the periosteum around the defect at twelve, three, six and nine o'clock, then raise the periosteum using dissecting forceps. If the surface is soiled with blood, gentle blotting of the area using a moist, then dry paper towel usually reveals the blackened edges of the hole in the bone. The deposit of soot must not be mistaken for lead rubbed off on the bone by the passing bullet. Close examination of the defect in the bone usually shows the soot distributed circumferentially, in contrast to a localized area occupied by the lead (Figs. XII-10 and XII-11); additionally, the metallic sheen of a fragment of lead is usually recognizable. Even in cases of prolonged survival, deposits of soot on the bone may be identified for a considerable time. We have observed soot on the temporal bone of a young woman who survived three months after she shot herself in an attempted sui-

cide. Frequently, soot is pushed deeper into the wound, and faint gray or black discoloration may be noted on the inner surface of the skull around the bullet hole and on the dura mater.

Small, irregular fragments of bone from the bullet hole in the skull are sometimes carried by the missile deep into the brain tissue. Sometimes the fragments are circular and their diameter corresponds to the caliber of the bullet which knocked them out. Such pieces of bone become secondary missiles. Recovery of these bone fragments is important in cases where a contact shot is suspected, yet, no soot was identified on the skin or the subjacent tissues. The fragments should be rinsed under cold water to remove blood and to disclose the presence or absence of soot deposits. Often these fragments will bear the signature of the lead (non-jacketed) bullet, namely punctate deposits of lead which should not be mistaken for soot. Small pieces of fabric from the victim's clothing are occasionally carried into the wound

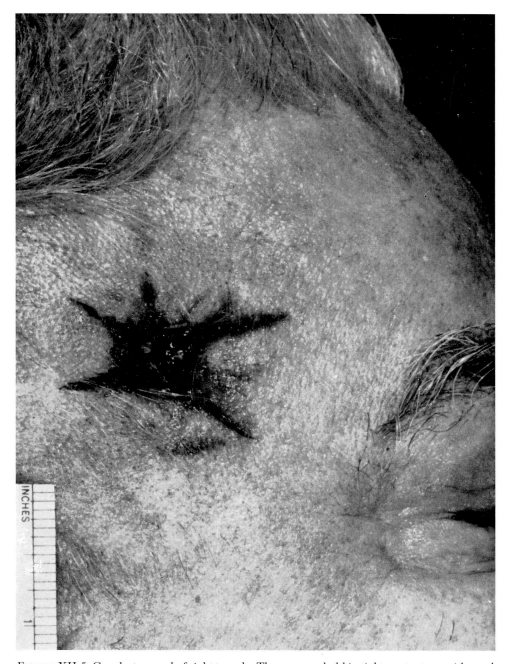

FIGURE XII-5. Gunshot wound of right temple. The gun was held in tight contact, as evidenced by the star-shaped wound and the absence of gunsmoke on the wound edges. All the gunsmoke entered the bullet wound. The small, horizontal abrasion under the bullet wound represents a partial muzzle imprint.

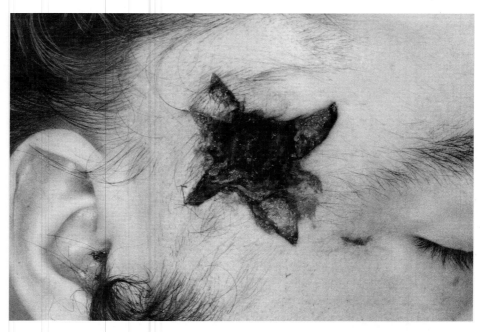

FIGURE XII-6. Tight contact, star-shaped wound of right temple with .38 caliber automatic pistol. The semicircular injury at 4 o'clock and the upward curved abrasion at the bottom of the eyebrow are imprints of the weapon's guide pin and housing.

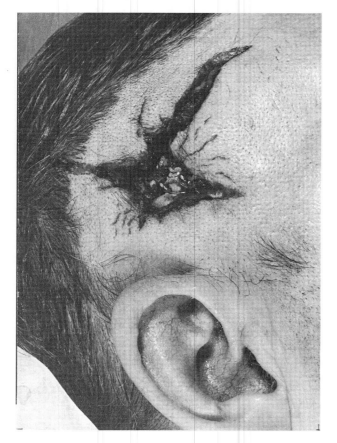

FIGURE XII-7. Tight contact wound showing marginal epidermal tears and full thickness lacerations, both due to overstretching of the skin by muzzle gases.

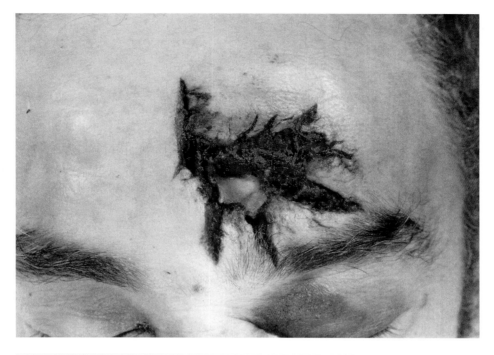

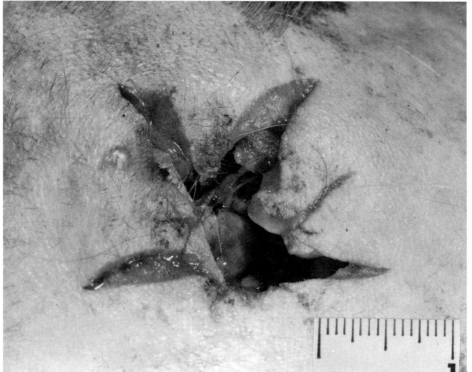

FIGURE XII-8a–b. Pressure contact with marginal superficial and full thickness tears.

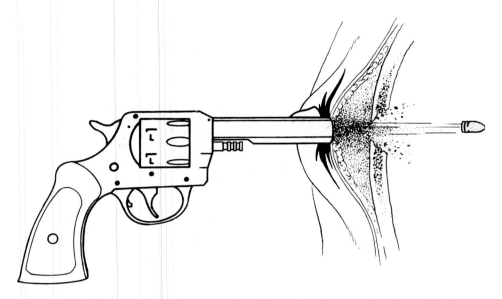

FIGURE XII-9. Mechanism of tight contact shot. The pocket between the skin and the bone is filled with gas, soot and gunpowder. No gunsmoke is deposited on the skin. The wound edges are split by the force of the expanding gases.

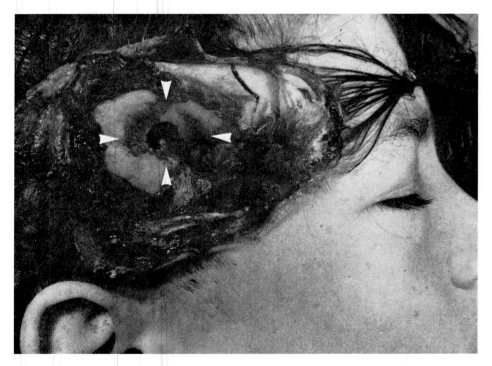

FIGURE XII-10. Soot is frequently deposited on the bone underlying a contact bullet wound. The presence of soot can usually be demonstrated after removal of the soft tissues. Care must be taken in stripping the periosteum. Gunsmoke is often deposited on the bone after the periosteum has been elevated by gas pressure.

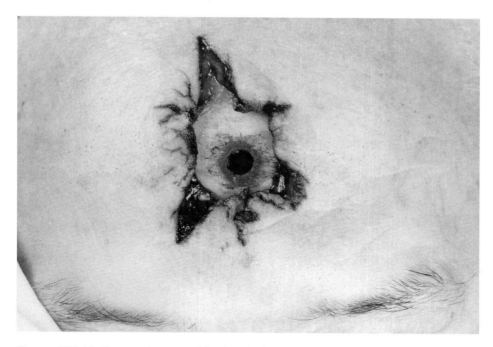

FIGURE XII-11. Contact shot in mid-forehead. The wound edges are torn by the blow back and soot is deposited on the bone around the bullet hole. The weapon was a .25 caliber pistol.

by the bullet, regardless of the range of fire. Such fabric, if dark or blood soiled, may resemble soot, and its presence in a wound has led to the mistaken determination of a contact shot. Microscopic examination of suspicious fragments may be required to ascertain their true nature.

Fracture lines often radiate from the circular defect caused by the bullet, particularly in the case of *pressure contact* shots. Undoubtedly, the mechanism of these fractures is the tremendous sudden expansion resulting from the muzzle blast. Independent fractures of the orbital roofs due to the same mechanism are frequently observed in contact shots of the head, particularly in elderly individuals in whom these bony plates are thin and fragile. The dura mater over the orbits is usually intact and must be removed in order to visualize these fractures. Care must be taken when stripping the dura not to create artifactual fractures of the orbital roofs. True fractures of the orbital roofs cause hemorrhage into the soft tissues around the eyes, which develop into *raccoon eyes,* if the victim survives (Fig. XII-12). With some high-powered ammunition, the destructive effect is often magnified (Fig. XII-13a–b).

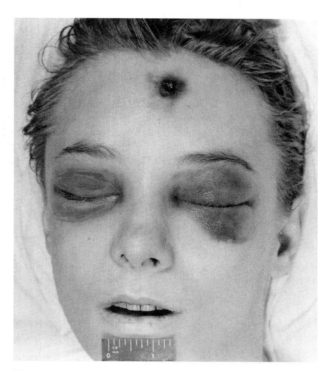

FIGURE XII-12. *Racoon eyes* due to fractures of the roofs of the eye sockets caused by increased pressure within the skull.

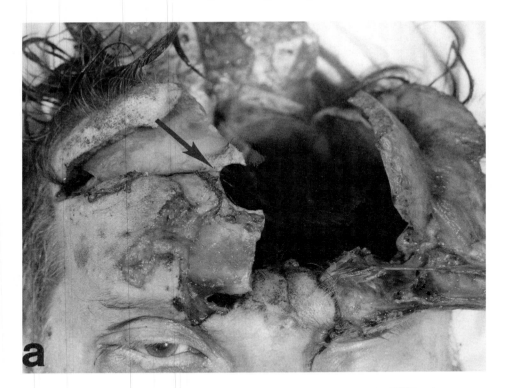

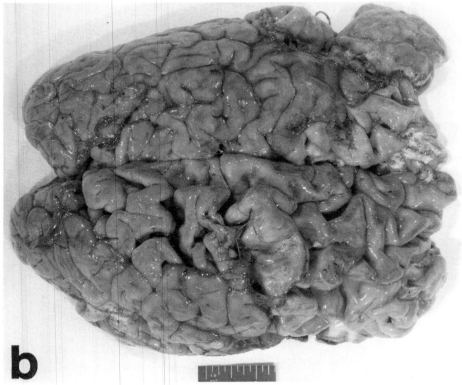

FIGURE XII-13a–b. Tight contact shot with .357 magnum (arrow). The top of the head is split open (a). The slightly damaged brain (b) was ejected from the skull by the muzzle gases and was found 6 feet from the body. Even if no soot had been found on the edges of the wound, the nature of this injury indicates close contact firing.

Fractures of the orbital roofs were described in the autopsy of President Abraham Lincoln, although the shot was not fired at contact range. Lincoln was shot in the back of the head at close range with a Derringer pistol firing a 1/2 inch lead ball. It appears likely that the increase of intracranial pressure which resulted from hemorrhage and brain swelling, as well as the large caliber of the missile caused the orbital roof fractures. A comprehensive discussion of the medical aspects of the assassination of Abraham Lincoln was published by Gilmore.[4]

In the case of a high-powered rifle, the amount of gas generated by the blast is so large that a shot fired in contact with the head causes extensive destruction (Figs. XII-14 to XII-16). Facial features are frequently distorted beyond recognition. Discharge of a high-powered rifle into the mouth or below the chin is associated with tremendous overexpansion of the soft tissues of the head and massive fractures of the skull. This causes vertical tears of the skin in front of the ears and along the creases on either side of the mouth and nose, as well as the inner angles of the eyes. The presence of such tears suggests the location of the entrance wound. Destruction is often so extensive that identification of the entrance wound may be possible only by finding the muzzle imprint on the skin, or evidence of soot and gunpowder on a fragment of bone. Identification of gunsmoke may be further compounded by widespread tissue scattering. Restoration of the skull by replacement of the bone fragments to determine the direction of the shot by direction of the beveling is helpful and is performed as outlined in Chapter XXV. Also, the skin is often torn to such an extent that the location of the entrance wound blends into the tears. Under such circumstances, the center, from which the tears emanate are likely to reappear when the flaps of skin are replaced and stitched together, revealing at least some of the criteria consistent with the entrance wound such as, abraded edges and possibly soot or gunpowder (Fig. XII-17a–b). A shot in the back of the head is usually suspicious of homicide, while a shot in the temple, under the chin or in the mouth often suggests suicide.

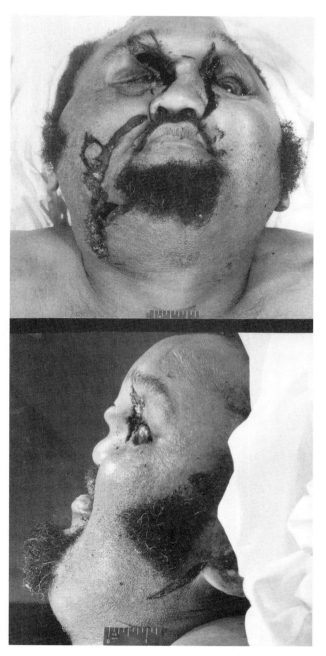

FIGURE XII-14. High-powered rifle shot in mouth. Gaping exit wound in the back of the head. The facial skeleton is fractured and caved in. Tears at the inner angles of the eyes and in front of the ears are due to blowout from overstretching.

The muzzle blast of a gun fired in contact with a body and the negative pressure in the barrel following discharge may cause blood, hair and

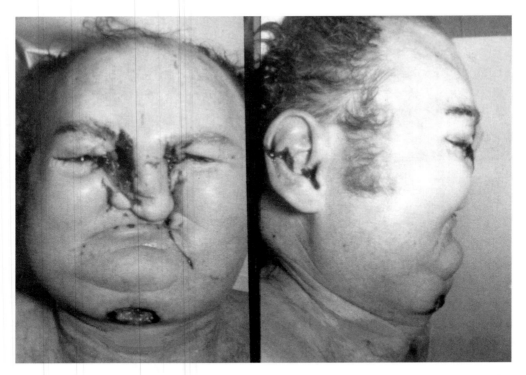

FIGURE XII-15. Rifle shot below the chin. Fragmentation of the facial skeleton; tears on both sides of the nose.

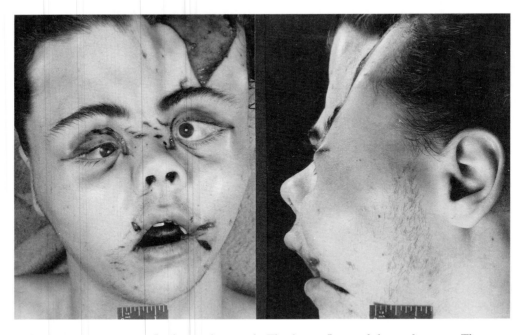

FIGURE XII-16. .30-30 rifle shot in the mouth. The face is flattened due to fractures. The tears at the corners of the mouth, the bridge of the nose and the eyelids are due to gas pressure within the skull.

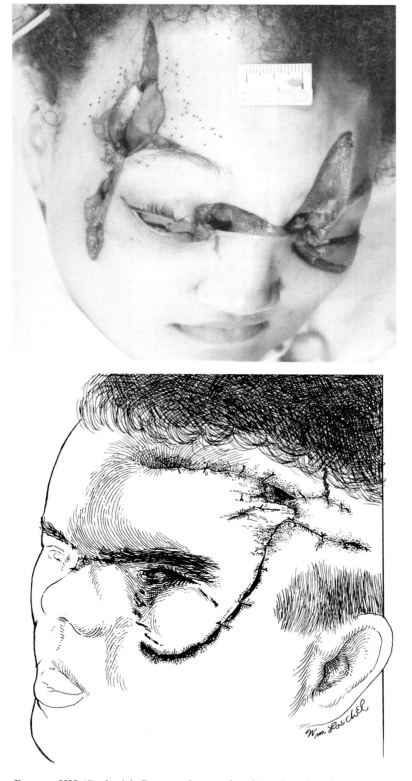

FIGURE XII-17a–b. (a) Gunpowder on the skin identifies the entrance wound. (b) After stitching the injury, the entrance wound became apparent.

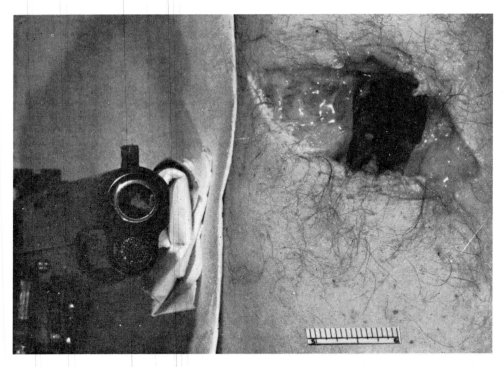

FIGURE XII-18. Contact shot with .45 caliber, blank cartridge. Note, fat tissue in the barrel.

fragments of tissue and fabric to be found several inches inside the barrel (Fig. XII-18). We have seen blood and tissue inside a six-inch barrel of a revolver, near the cylinder, following a contact shot. An imprint of the muzzle profile on the skin around a bullet wound or adjacent to it is due to the recoil of the gun and the muzzle blast (Figs. XII-19 to XII-22). The imprint of the muzzle on the skin is not limited to contact bullet wounds of the head area; the same imprint may be observed in contact shots in other parts of the body (Fig. XII-23).

Near-contact between the muzzle and the skin will provide for escape of gases when the gun is fired, with resulting dispersion of the muzzle blast. The characteristic features of such a shot are consequently somewhat modified. The blast effect is not as pronounced as in the case of tight contact, and splitting of the wound edges does not usually occur. Fractures of the skull radiating from the bullet hole are observed only rarely. The bright yellow flame, which extends from the muzzle at the time of discharge, scorches clothing and adjacent skin and singes hair up to a distance of several inches (Fig. XII-24). A large amount of soot is deposited on the target, but relatively little gunpowder may be scattered on the surface. Most of the gunpowder is propelled into the bullet wound (Fig. XII-25).

Evidence of scorching is noted on microscopic examination of near-contact bullet wounds. A comprehensive microscopic study of dermal gunshot wounds was described by Lester Adelson,[5] and more recently by Werner Janssen[6] and Vincent DiMaio.[7]

Carbon monoxide in gunsmoke can transform hemoglobin and myoglobin into carboxyhemoglobin and carboxymyoglobin. A cherry-red color of the muscle under a contact bullet wound may suggest the presence of carbon monoxide but, perforation of the lung, as by a stab wound or a distant gunshot, may also cause a bright red discoloration of the musculature around the site of injury. This, however, results from perfusion of the area by oxygenated blood not from exposure to carbon monoxide. The cherry-red discol-

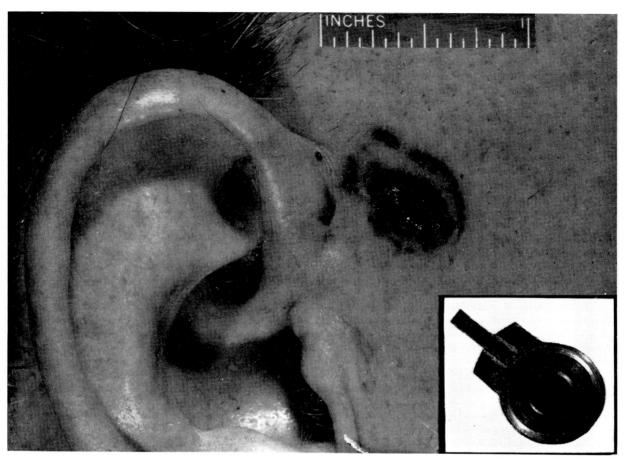

FIGURE XII-19. Suicidal shot of right temple. Patterned abrasion around the bullet wound corresponds to the contour of the muzzle profile shown in the insert. The weapon was a .22 caliber, Ruger, semiautomatic pistol.

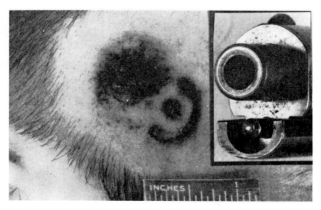

FIGURE XII-20. Contact shot of the right temple. Patterned injury caused by housing frame and recoil spring guide.

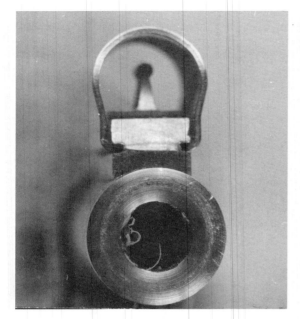

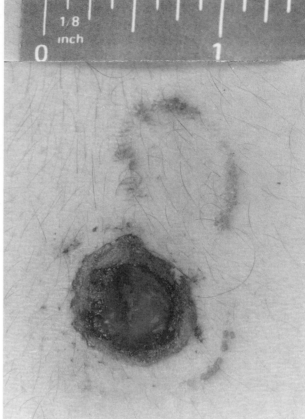

FIGURE XII-21. Hair and tissue in the muzzle due to blow back and imprint of site above the contact wound. The abrasions between 4 and 5 o'clock and 10 and 12 o'clock are from muzzle impact.

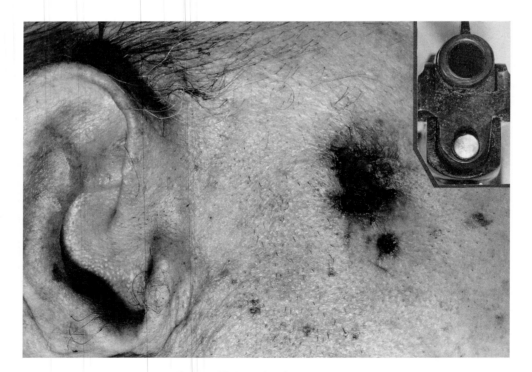

FIGURE XII-22. Guide pin imprint.

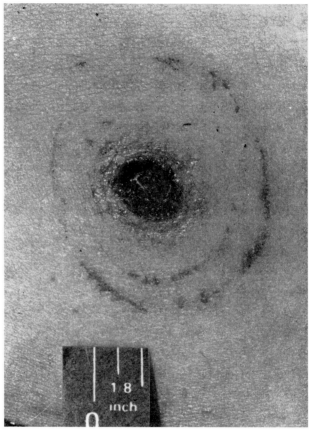

FIGURE XII-23. Muzzle imprint of .22 caliber rifle on abdominal skin. The absence of soot on the surface suggests pressure contact shot. The edges of the bullet wound are not torn because of ample space for gas expansion inside the abdominal cavity.

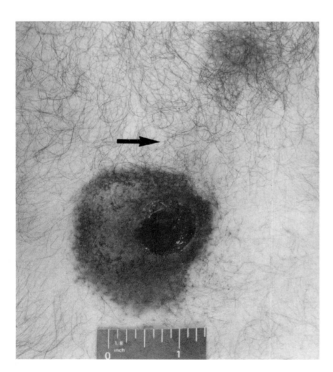

FIGURE XII-24. Scorched skin by the muzzle flame. Hair is singed and gunpowder is scattered in the area that is burnt. The direction of the shot is as shown by the arrow.

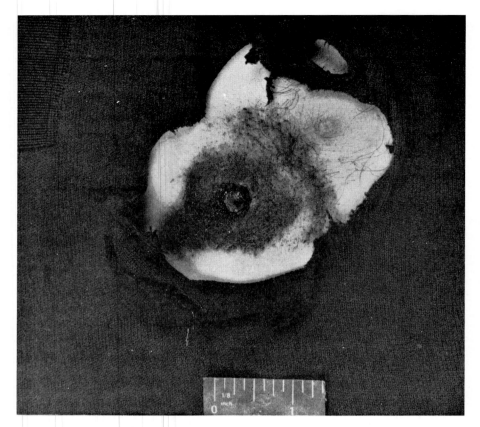

FIGURE XII-25. Near-contact shot of chest. Synthetic fabric of the shirt is scorched. The skin is superficially burned around the bullet wound, and the hairs in the area are singed. Few specks of gunpowder are scattered on the skin surface.

oration of the muscle by oxyhemoglobin is temporary and will revert to the original brownish red color with time.

Close-Range Shots

A close-range shot is one that is fired from a distance at which gunpowder residue, as well as particles of primer and small fragments of metal from the bullet, may be identified around a bullet hole (Figs. XII-26 to XII-30).

On naked-eye examination, these particles are indistinguishable from one another. The diameter and density of the pattern of particles on the target are useful in evaluating the distance of fire. Patterns vary widely with different guns and types of ammunition. For most handguns, demonstrable residues on skin are found at firing distances of 18 to 24 inches. With rifles, this may reach several feet. At greater distance, the small particles of gunpowder that are emitted from the barrel at the time of firing lack the inertia required to reach the target. As mentioned earlier, the approximate distance from which a close-range shot was fired can be evaluated only by test firing the particular weapon, using the same type of ammunition as that used in the shooting case under consideration.

A frequent source of error in evaluating the distance from which a gun was fired is the comparison of test patterns on white paper or cloth with the pattern of the wound on skin. Scattered specks of gunpowder are certainly not as conspicuous on skin as they are on a smooth white background such as cloth or paper. This discrepancy should be considered, especially when test patterns of shots fired from a distance exceeding a few inches are evaluated.

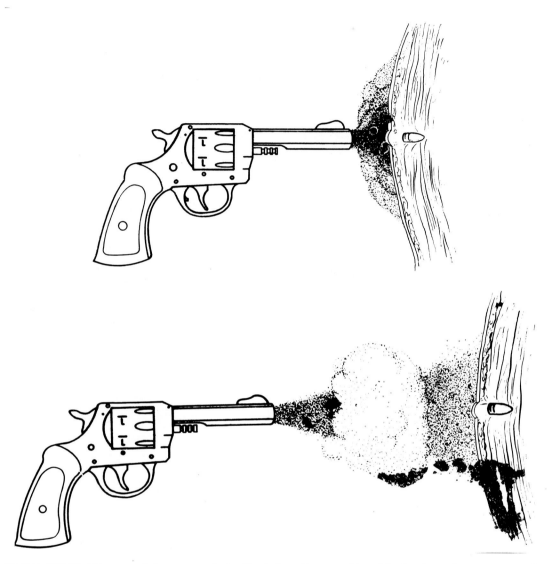

FIGURE XII-26. Diagram of close-range shots: (Top): At a distance of 1 to 2 inches from the target, particles of gunpowder are centered around the bullet hole, while waves of soot disperse over a much wider area (see Figure XII-2a). (Bottom): As the muzzle-to-target distance increases, the dispersion of particles increases in diameter, while the density of particle scattering decreases. At a distance of 6 or 7 inches, abundant gunpowder and little if any soot are deposited on the target (see Fig. XII-2b.)

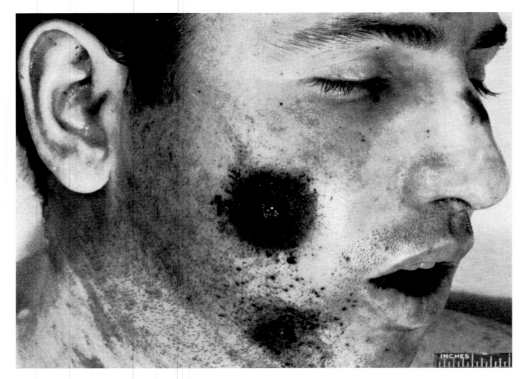

FIGURE XII-27. Two shots of the right side of the face. The upper shows abundant soot and very little gunpowder. This shot was fired at near-contact. The lower shot is surrounded by a small amount of soot, while particles of gunpowder are scattered over a diameter of about 2 inches. This shot was fired from a distance of a few inches.

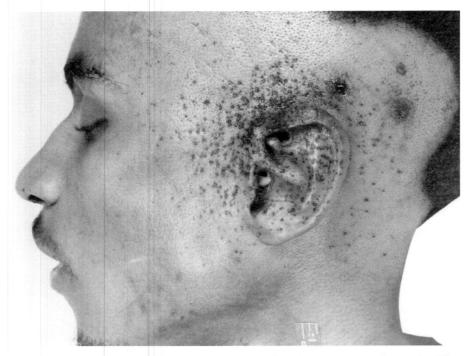

FIGURE XII-28. Grouping of multiple close range shots for execution style murder. The hair behind the ear was shaved. Head hair in an area of shooting is best combed with a fine tooth comb which is then submitted for GSR testing.

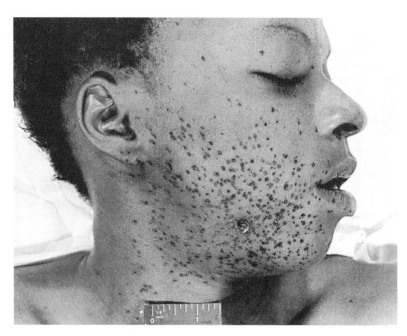

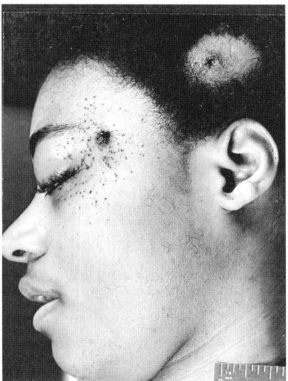

FIGURE XII-29a–b. (a) Close-range, gunshot with .25 caliber pistol using Western ammunition loaded with ball powder. Ball powder causes typical punched-out, pock-mark-like injuries. In determining the diameter of spread, the main bulk of gunpowder should be considered for comparison with test shots. (b): Close-range shot at the angle of the eye with .22 caliber revolver. The shot above the ear may have been fired at contact, but any soot or gunpowder would have been filtered out by the hair and marginal tears are not usually seen with .22 caliber ammunition, even in the head.

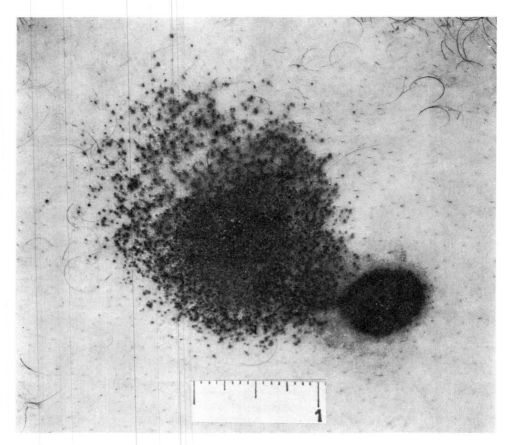

FIGURE XII-30. Young man who committed suicide by shooting himself in the chest. The bullet wound on the right is surrounded by a well-demarcated ring of soot, and the wound margins are scorched. This injury was inflicted at near-contact. The adjacent injury (left) is surrounded by densely scattered powder stipples, with a small amount of soot in the immediate vicinity. This injury was inflicted at close range (2 to 3 inches), as determined by test firing. (Ruger revolver, .22 caliber magnum ammunition.)

The length of the barrel of a firearm has considerable bearing on the diameter of the pattern of gunsmoke deposited on the target. For example, a snub-nosed revolver with a 2-inch barrel spreads gunsmoke over a considerably larger area than a pistol having a 6- or 8-inch barrel, fired from the same distance and employing the same type of ammunition (Fig. XII-31). A rule of thumb for handguns is that gunpowder residue may be identified by naked-eye examination of the target at a distance double the length of the barrel.[8] Barrel length is considered from the cylinder to the muzzle.

Gunpowder residue is usually distributed circumferentially, more or less equally, around a bullet hole. When more residue is noted on one side of the target than the other, the weapon is likely to have been fired at a shallow angle. Powder residue is more densely scattered and extends over a larger area on the side from which the shot was fired. The same applies to the outer garment (Fig. XII-32a–b).

A gun firing different ammunition from various manufacturers will produce different powder residue patterns. This is due to gunpowder peculiarities, such as the use of *ball* or *flake* powder, and other manufacturing characteristics. The powder charge in some *magnum*-labeled handgun ammunition is significantly larger than that in ordinary ammunition of the same caliber. This

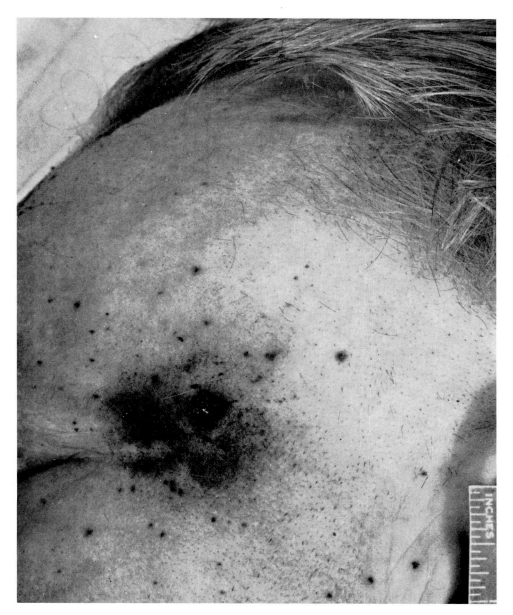

FIGURE XII-31. Close-range shot of left temple. The weapon was not recovered, but a .38 caliber non-jacketed bullet was found in the brain. Note the soot centered around the bullet wound, while gunpowder particles are scattered over a diameter of close to 3 inches. The relative distribution of soot and gunpowder around this injury suggests that a short-barreled gun had been used. Test shots confirmed this assumption. A pattern similar to that in this photograph was obtained with a snub-nosed, 2 inch barrel, .38 caliber Special, firing matching ammunition.

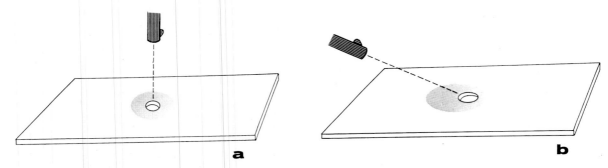

FIGURE XII-32a–b. Gunpowder residue is usually distributed circumferentially, more or less equally, around a bullet hole. When more residue is noted on one side, the weapon is likely to have been fired at a shallow angle. Powder residue is more densely scattered and extends over a larger area on the side from which the shot was fired.

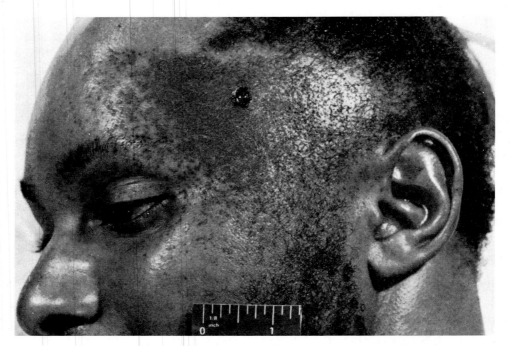

FIGURE XII-33. Close-range shot of left temple with .357 magnum. The gunpowder particles in the skin in proximity of the bullet wound are so densely scattered that there is no undamaged intervening skin, giving the impression that the area was abraded. The lack of gunpowder stippling along a straight edge above the wound is due to a hat.

difference can be observed when such a cartridge has been discharged at close range. The spread of stippling on the skin extends over a larger diameter, and the density of powder flecks is significantly greater than that produced by ordinary ammunition (Figs. XII-33 to XII-36).

Generally speaking, as the distance between the muzzle and the target increases, the pattern of particles on the target increases in diameter and the density of particle dispersion decreases. In handguns, at distances up to 6 or 7 inches from the muzzle, abundant gunpowder and diminishing amounts of soot are deposited on the target.

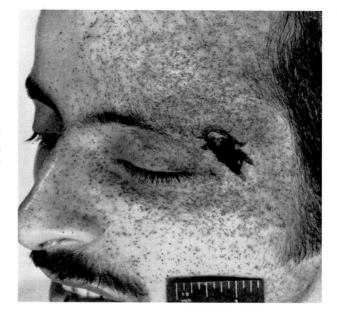

FIGURE XII-34. Close-range shot. The abundance and density of gunpowder suggests that a round with a magnum load was used. When no missile is recovered, this information may be of significance.

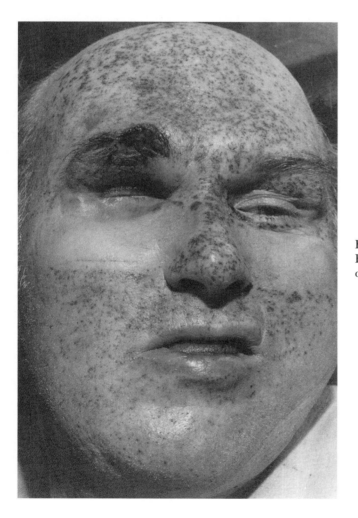

Figure XII-35. Large quantity of apparent ball powder. Entrance wound is in the right eyebrow. Glasses filtered out the stippling.

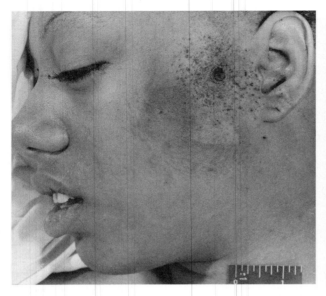

FIGURE XII-36. Homicidal close-range shot in front of the left ear. Gunpowder stippling and soot deposit around the injury were partially filtered out by what is believed to have been an earring.

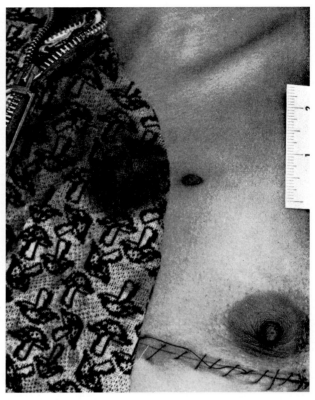

FIGURE XII-37. Suicidal contact shot of the left side of the chest. All evidence of contact-range firing is on the dress, where abundant soot is noted around the bullet hole. Any soot that may have been present in the bullet wound or on the surrounding skin was cleansed at the hospital.

On a human body, no soot can usually be identified in shots fired from a distance greater than 6 or 7 inches. In close-range shots of the head, dense hair may filter out powder particles entirely. This obviously interferes with attempts to evaluate the distance from which a shot was fired. It may be possible to identify gunpowder particles on hair using neutron activation analysis or chemical tests, as outlined earlier in this chapter.

Clothing may also filter out soot and gunpowder particles so that none may be seen on the skin (Figs. XII-37 to XII-39). However, cotton and polyester T-shirts allow gunpowder particles to pass freely, causing small holes in the fabric. The victim's clothing must, therefore, be removed and handled carefully to prevent dislodging of loose particles. Measurement of the spread of particles on the target is necessary for subsequent comparison with test shot patterns to evaluate the range of fire. Obviously, a hand held in front of the face in a defensive motion would also filter out gunsmoke. The presence of gunsmoke alone on a part of the body, as may occur during a struggle for the gun, sometimes enables reconstruction of the position of the victim at the time of the shooting (Figs. XII-40a–b and XII-41).

The terms *tattooing, powder stippling* and *powder burns* are often used to describe the dispersed grains of gunpowder and primer around a bullet wound. The term *fouling* is reserved for small fragments of metal derived from the bullet. Particles that are ejected from the barrel of the gun can usually be identified on the skin without difficulty. Such particles are embedded in the superficial layers of the skin and cannot be removed by wiping or even shaving of the area. Examination of particles embedded in the skin may permit identification of the type of gunpowder used in the ammunition, and identify it as lead shaving or other material. Each particle produces a small superficial wound. In case of survival, evidence of powder stippling becomes more noticeable after a day or two, when each wound is surrounded by a red halo indicative of

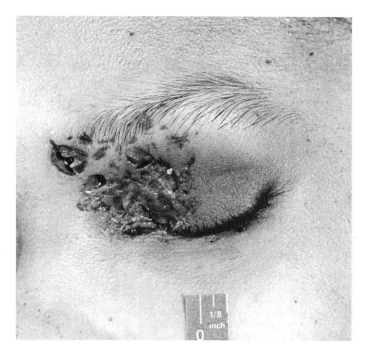

FIGURE XII-38. Wound by a .22 caliber bullet with entrance at the inner end of the eyebrow. The bullet fragmented the eyeglasses and all remaining wounds are due to the shattered lens. The shot was allegedly fired at close range. The wound does not permit assessment of range of fire.

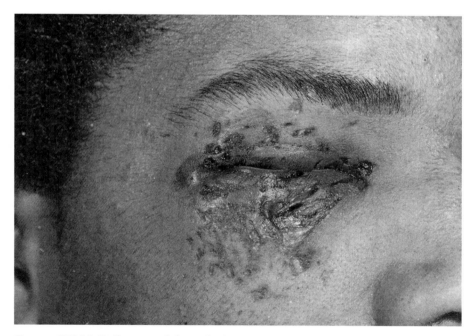

FIGURE XII-39. Bullet wound through glasses at the inner angle of the eye. No apparent presence of gunpowder stippling, but definitive determination of range of fire is not feasible.

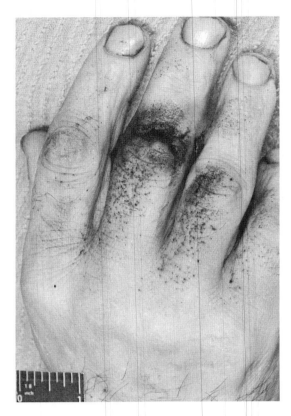

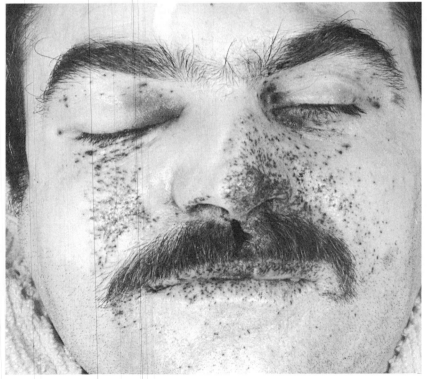

FIGURE XII-40a–b. Holdup: The right middle finger shows a close-range gunshot wound (a). The bullet wound of reentry is in the center of the upper lip (b). The victim held his hand in front of his face in protection.

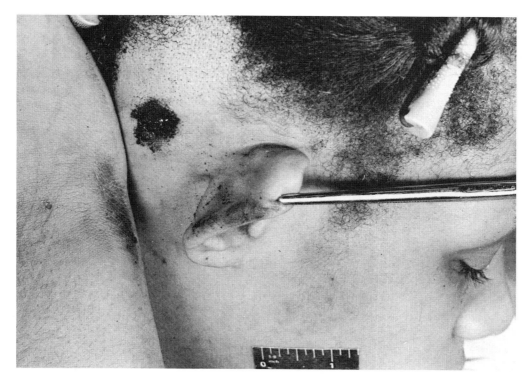

FIGURE XII-41. Near contact shot behind right ear. The presence of soot on the forearm suggests that the victim held her forearm against the side of her head.

inflammation which is part of the normal healing process (Fig. XII-42). This is in contrast to soot, which is situated on the skin surface and is easily removed by wiping and improper handling.

Silencers mounted on firearms to muffle the sound of discharge significantly reduce the amount of gunsmoke ejected from the muzzle. Silencers extend the length of the barrel and can absorb some or most of the powder residue. Hence, the use of a silencer may cause misinterpretation of the distance from which a gun was fired. According to FBI reports, powder residue on clothing or on a body may be entirely absent if weapons equipped with certain types of silencers were used. The .22 caliber is the only production-model handgun that can be effectively silenced. This may account for the large number of *execution-style* murders in which .22 caliber automatic pistols are used.

A cushion placed on the victim's body to act as a silencer will effectively filter out gunpowder and soot, while significantly muffling the sound of the discharge. Fibers of fabric and cushion stuffing are sometimes lodged in the wound track. Such items and the imprint of a coarsely woven fabric may occasionally be embedded in a lead bullet.

Pseudo-tattooing is a term used to describe *tattooing* produced by something other than gunpowder. For example, postmortem insect bites, spattered grease burns, superficial pinpoint size wounds from fragmented glass (especially tempered glass from side and rear automobile windows), and from slivers of wood (where someone was shot through a door), have all been mistaken for evidence of close-range fire. DiMaio also described scarred needle marks on both sides of a bullet wound from surgical stitches as resembling *pseudo-tattooing*. In general however, gen-

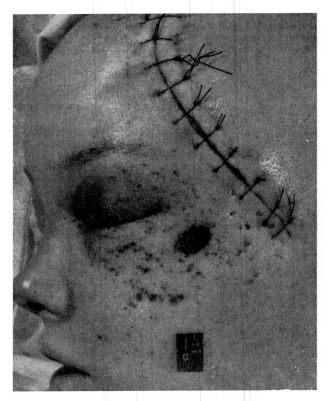

FIGURE XII-42. Homicidal through-and-through shot of the head. The victim survived for twenty-four hours. Unlike the soot, which was cleaned away prior to surgery, gunpowder stippling is still present and more prominent due to onset of healing process.

uine *tattooing* by grains of gunpowder is readily recognizable by the experienced observer.

Distant Shot

A distant shot is one that is fired from a distance at which gunsmoke will no longer reach the target. In the case of most handguns, this distance exceeds 18 inches depending again on the weapon and the type of ammunition that were used. In the absence of gunsmoke around a bullet hole, no distinction with respect to distance can be made between one distant shot and another. Consequently, the appearance of a bullet wound inflicted from a distance of 6 feet does not differ from one inflicted from 16 or 60 feet. In evaluating a bullet wound, consideration must be given to any intermediary target which may

account for the absence of gunpowder residue around the injury. For example, a shot fired through a door from a distance of a few inches, wounding a person on the other side, will produce an injury that lacks all evidence of close-range firing due to retention of powder residue around the hole in the door.

In the case of a high-powered rifle, the external appearance of the entrance wound does not materially differ from that of a gunshot wound inflicted with a handgun or an ordinary rifle (Fig. XII-43). However, internal destruction is considerably more severe. Due to the high velocity of the missile, the soft tissues collapse into a temporary cavity produced by a vacuum created in the wake of the bullet. This cavity is visible on x-ray and microscopic examination shows disruption of the tissue and hemorrhage in the area of cavitation. The skull, including the base, is often shattered, and in solid organs such as the liver, the wound track may exceed 3 or 4 inches in diameter (Figs. XII-44 and XII-45). We have observed large, gaping tears of the heart where the wound track passed through the chest, but did not directly involve the heart. The diameter of the temporary cavity depends in great part on the kinetic energy of the bullet. It is the location of the temporary cavity with respect to vital organs that produces varying degrees of incapacitation.

The exit wound of a high-powered rifle shot is frequently large and ragged and quite out of proportion to exit wounds produced by other types of firearms, as discussed later in this chapter (Fig. XII-46a–b). If no bullet is recovered and the weapon is unknown, the extent of external and internal damage may suggest that a high-powered rifle had been used.

The body of a sixteen-year-old boy was found in a wooded area. An entrance bullet wound that measured 1/4 inch in diameter was noted in the back of his head (see Fig. XII-43), and a large, gaping exit wound was located in the center of the forehead. The entire skull was shattered.

Subsequent investigation disclosed that the boy had been accidentally shot with a .35 caliber Remington high-powered rifle while deer-hunting.

High-powered rifle ammunition is known to fragment upon striking a firm target, spraying a large area with shrapnel. The fragments of an

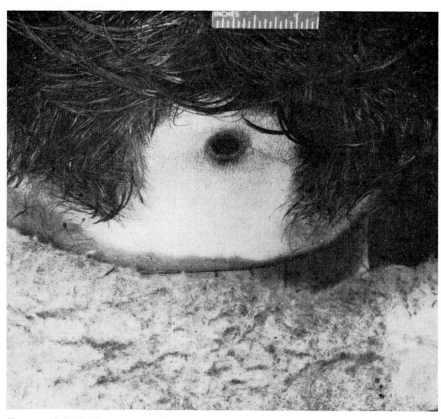

FIGURE XII-43. Hunting accident involving a high-powered rifle. A bullet wound of entrance is located in the back of the head.

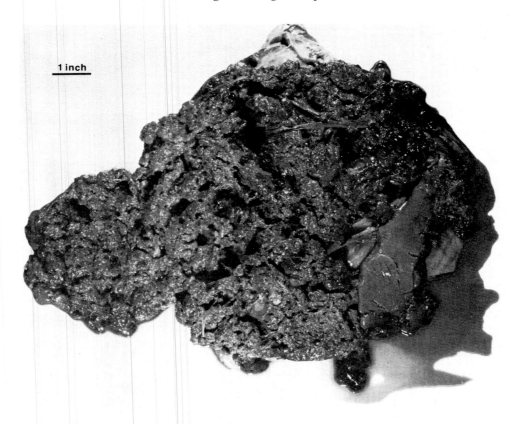

FIGURE XII-44. Disintegration of the liver due to a shot from a .30-30 rifle fired from a distance of 20 feet. In a through-and-through shot the extent of injury would suggest a high-powered weapon.

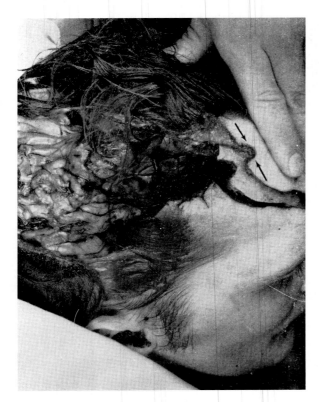

FIGURE XII-45. Shot from a .30-30 rifle, fired from a distance of about 60 feet. The wound of entrance is indicated by arrows.

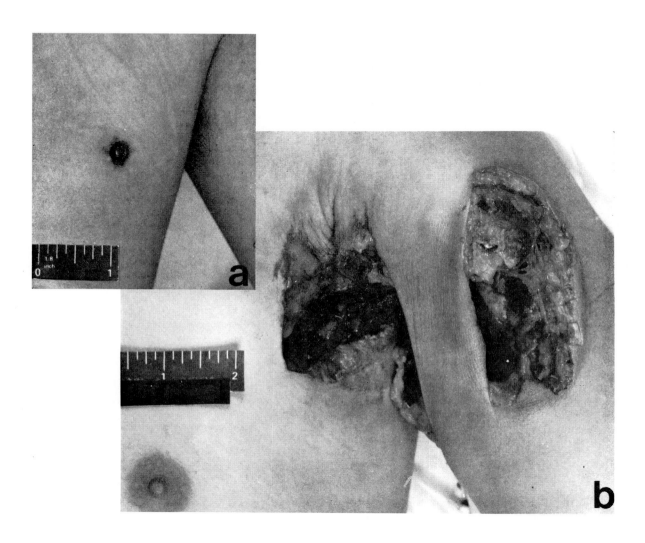

FIGURE XII-46a–b. Gunshot wound with a .308 Winchester high-powered rifle. (a) The entrance wound is in the right side of the back. (b) The exit wounds are through the left chest and arm. The shot was fired from a distance of 25 to 30 feet.

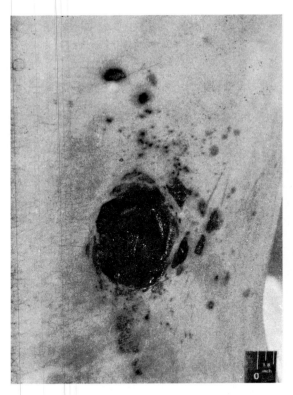

FIGURE XII-47. A .30-06 shot through the door of an automobile. The bullet disintegrated, and numerous fragments of different sizes struck the passenger.

exploded bullet may be so small and numerous as to simulate a shotgun wound, gunpowder stippling or both. Small superficial perforations of the skin produced by fragments from the original target may significantly compound the wound pattern (Figs. XII-47 to XII-49a–b).

DIRECTION OF FIRE

The direction of fire may be derived from the relationship of entrance to exit wounds, although internal deviation of the bullet, as by impact on bone, must be considered. For this purpose it is essential that the wound of entry be distinguished from the wound of exit.

A point frequently overlooked in comparing entrance and exit wounds is that approximation of the edges of an entrance wound usually retains a small central defect, i.e., a missing area of skin, while the exit, re-establishes the skin's integrity.

The characteristic feature of a bullet wound of entrance is circumferential marginal abrasion regardless of the distance from which the shot was fired (Fig. XII-50). This abrasion results from scraping of the wound edges on the shaft of the bullet as it perforates the skin. A wound by a round-tipped arrow or a stab wound with a screwdriver would cause an identical injury.

As in the case of abrasions in general, the abrasion around an entrance bullet wound darkens as it dries, becoming more conspicuous with time. The abrasion is circular and of uniform width if the bullet strikes the body at a right angle. Under such circumstances, the scraping by the bullet is equal on all sides of the wound.

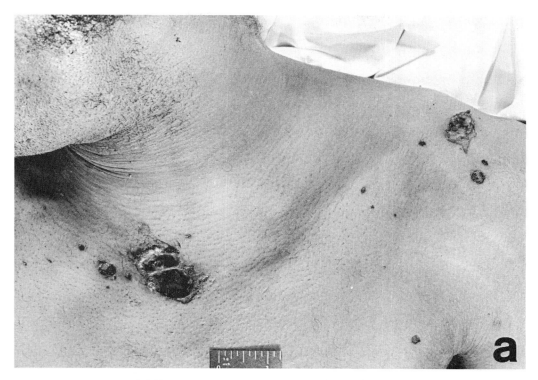

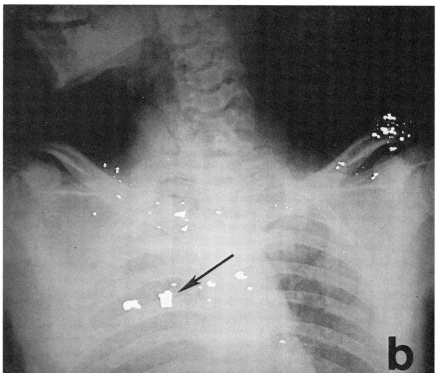

FIGURE XII-48a–b. Man struck by shrapnel from a .30 caliber rifle bullet which fragmented when it passed through a screen door (a). The x-ray shows the metal fragments (b).

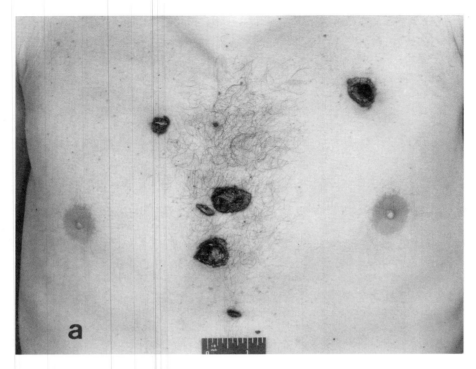

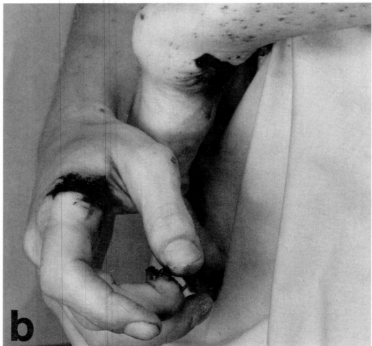

FIGURE XII-49a–b. Close range, multiple penetrating wounds in the chest (a) caused by a .44 caliber non-jacketed slug which fragmented upon striking the deceased's wrist and hand (b). The left wrist shows gunpowder stippling. The presence of small pieces of lead, sometimes no larger than a pinhead, in some of the chest wounds indicates that the missile broke apart after hitting the extremities.

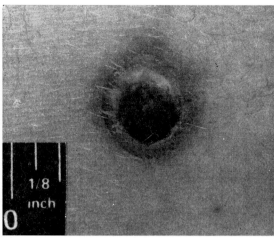

FIGURE XII-50. Characteristic circumferential marginal abrasion of an entrance bullet wound. The abrasion is dark as a result of drying.

However, if the bullet strikes at an angle, the wound itself may be round, but the marginal abrasion is oval, due to the wide inferior surface of the bullet scraping the skin (Figs. XII-51a–b to XII-54a–b).

The length of the abrasion depends on the angle at which the bullet struck. A grazing shot thus produces a superficial shallow wound with marginal abrasion and small superficial tears extending diagonally from the furrow in the direction of the traveling missile, giving the wound the appearance of a narrow, upside down, fir tree (Fig. XII-55a–b). If the bullet strikes at a very shallow angle, a grazing shot may cause an abrasion of the approximate width of the bullet, without tearing the skin. When an entry bullet wound involves a crease, especially in the face, it may not show the typical characteristics of marginal abrasion when the skin is pulled and straightened. A pattern of bruises is sometimes produced by a bullet traveling under creased skin (Fig. XII-56).

Irregular and occasionally patterned abrasions around an entrance bullet wound are sometimes produced by stiff and coarse articles of clothing as the missile pushes the fabric ahead before perforating (Figs. XII-57 to XII-58). Thus, a bullet which strikes a solid object, such as a key or coin in a pocket, is likely to cause an entrance wound with torn and atypically abraded edges (Fig. XII-59). Such abrasions are sometimes quite large and may extend beyond the confines of the mar-

ginal abrasion. We have seen a case in which a bullet went through the center of a pen in the breast pocket of the victim and made a near perfect abraded outline of the top and bottom halves of the pen on the skin. Careful examination of the clothing will usually enable proper interpretation of such a wound (Fig. XII-60).

Marginal abrasion of an exit wound is rare, and when present may confuse even the experienced examiner. It occurs when a firm object such as a belt, necktie or brassiere is pressed against the body at the site of the exiting bullet or if the body is leaning against a hard surface such as a wall, floor or pavement. In such cases, the exiting bullet crushes the skin against the hard surface, abrading the skin immediately around or adjacent to the exit wound. Occasionally, if the hard surface against which the body is leaning is patterned, or the weave pattern of overlying clothing is prominent, this pattern may be imprinted into the skin in the area crushed by the bullet. Abraded exit wounds are sometimes referred to as *shored* (Figs. XII-61a–b to XII-67a–b).

Much of the controversy surrounding the assassination of President John F. Kennedy is based on misinterpretation of the wound in the front of his neck as an entrance bullet wound. Conspiracy proponents hold that the President was shot from the front, as well as the rear. In reality, both bullets which struck JFK, struck from the rear, hitting the back of his right shoulder and his head.

The wound in the front of JFK's neck was circumferentially abraded, resembling an entrance wound to inexperienced examiners at the autopsy. The marginal abrasion of

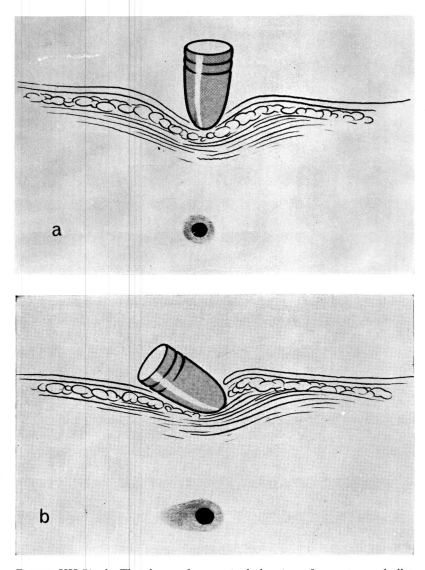

FIGURE XII-51a–b. The shape of a marginal abrasion of an entrance bullet wound is dependent on the angle of entry. (a) Perpendicular shot. (b) Tangential shot.

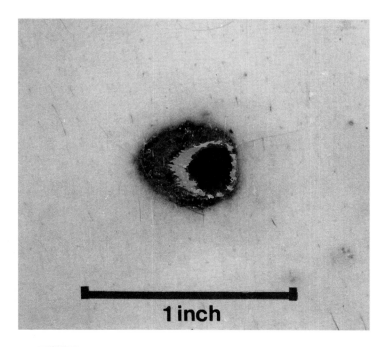

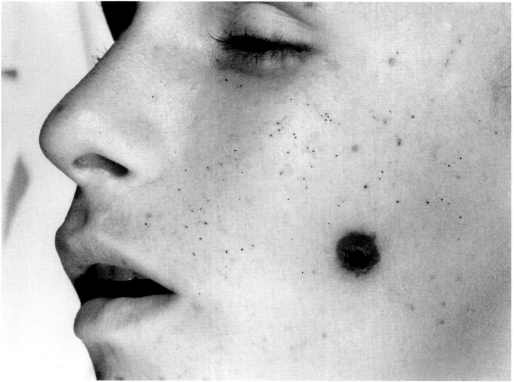

Figure XII-52a–b. (a) Tangential (left to right on photograph) gunshot wound of chest, from a distance of several feet. (b) Close-range shot with gunpowder stippling mostly above the wound and a wider upper margin of the wound (9 to 3 o'clock).

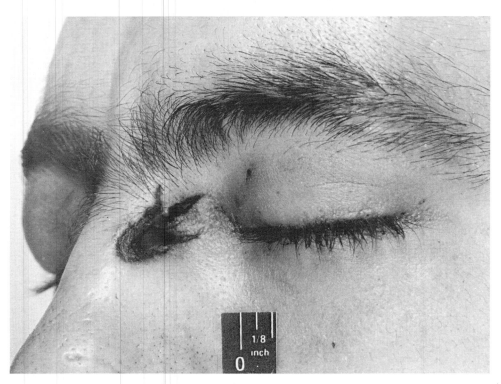

FIGURE XII-53. A bullet wound to the bridge of the nose where there is little subcutaneous tissue, often causes a *crowfoot*-like wound.

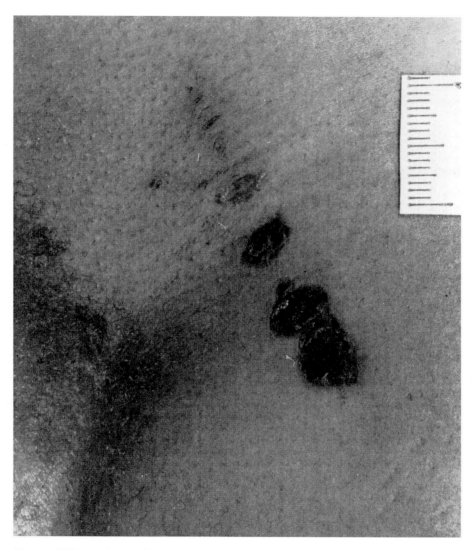

FIGURE XII-54a. Single shot of the left groin, simulating several bullet wounds due to skin folds. The lowest wound is the primary entrance wound, showing a wide abrasion, which indicates the upward pathway of the bullet. The bullet then exited and reentered several times before proceeding into the abdominal cavity.

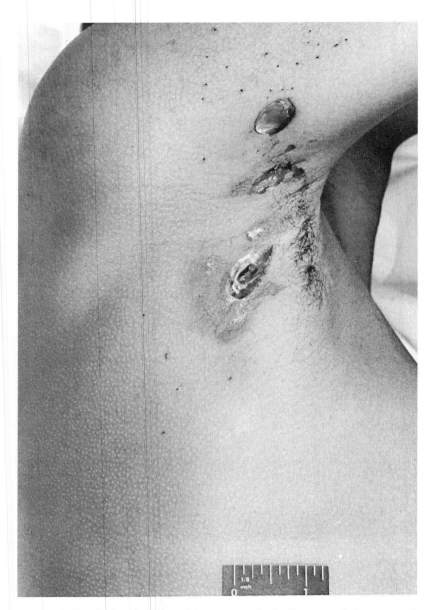

FIGURE XII-54b. Similar shot of the armpit; the bullet entered the arm and shows powder stippling.

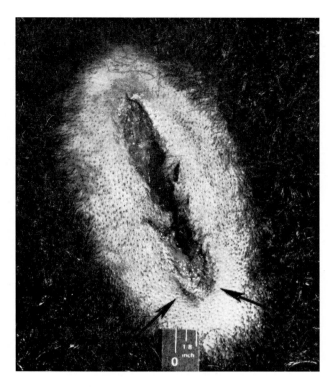

FIGURE XII-55a–b. (a) Grazing bullet wound of the head. The actual entrance wound is indicated by arrows. (b) Grazing bullet wound, the direction is shown by the arrow.

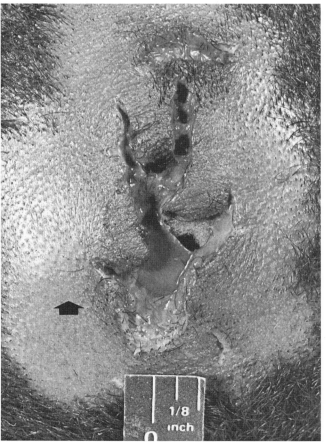

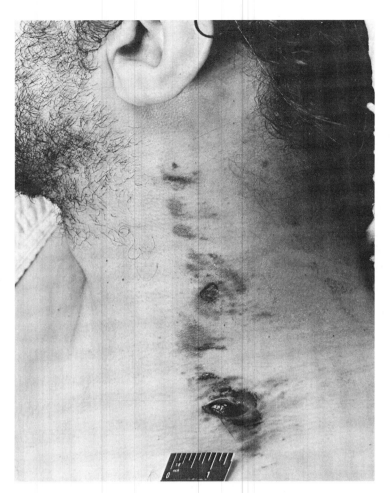

FIGURE XII-56. Patterned bruises corresponding to skin creases caused by the bullet passing just under the skin. The entrance wound is situated above the scale.

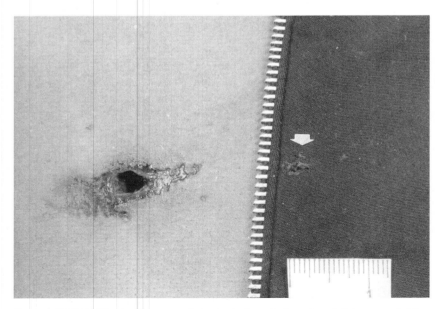

FIGURE XII-57. The bullet entered through the windbreaker (white arrow). The irregular abrasion adjacent to the bullet wound was caused by the zipper, which vibrated against the skin.

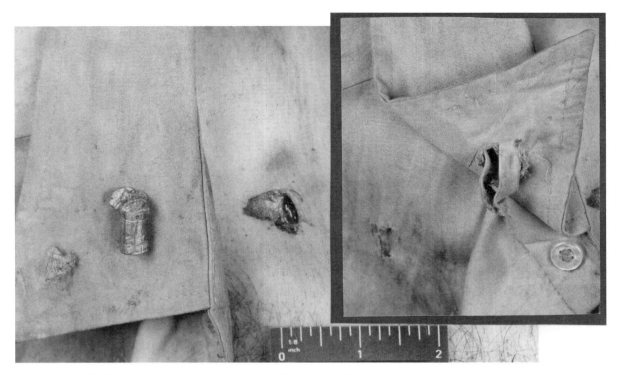

FIGURE XII-58. Shot in the right collarbone area. The shirt collar has been turned (insert) showing the material dragged into the wound by the bullet, indicating the direction of travel and causing an irregular abrasion on the left side of the injury.

FIGURE XII-59. Unusually shaped entrance bullet wound in the thigh (insert). The slug hit a brass key in the deceased's pocket and split into three fragments.

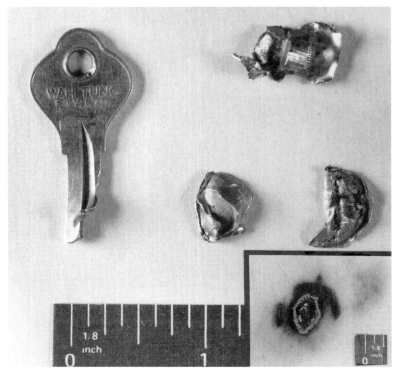

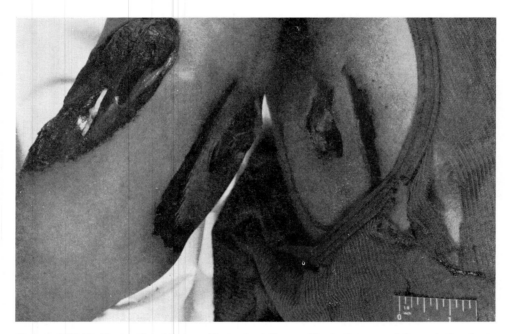

FIGURE XII-60. Shot with a Mauser rifle in the left arm. The bullet passed through the chest, exited on the right side (depicted), reentered and exited through the right arm. The humerus was shattered. Note that the band of the undershirt, with some of its weave pattern, abraded the skin around the exit wound of the chest and the reentry wound of the arm. This was caused by the percussive effect of the passing missile. The size of the injury is suggestive of a high-powered weapon.

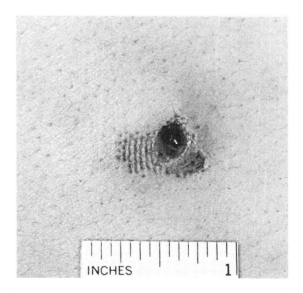

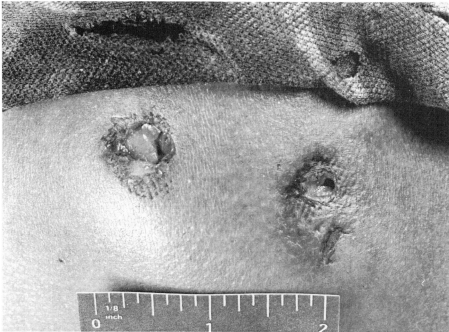

FIGURE XII-61a–b. (a) Exit wounds on back. Patterned marginal abrasion by clothes. The victim was leaning against a wall when he was shot in the chest. The skin was crushed between the missile and the wall. A .38 caliber slug was removed from under this injury. (b) Exit wounds depict the weave pattern of the overlying clothes.

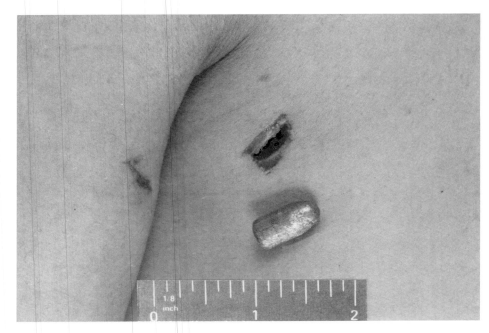

FIGURE XII-62. Shored exit wound.

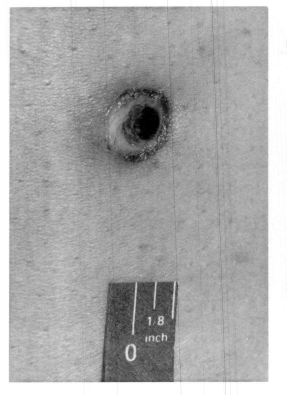

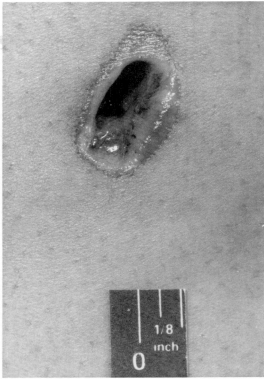

FIGURE XII-63. Entrance wound on left, shored exit on the right with weave pattern, especially noticeable on the top.

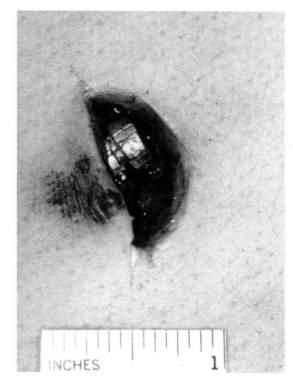

FIGURE XII-64. Incision shows a bullet under the skin. Note, the weave pattern from clothing.

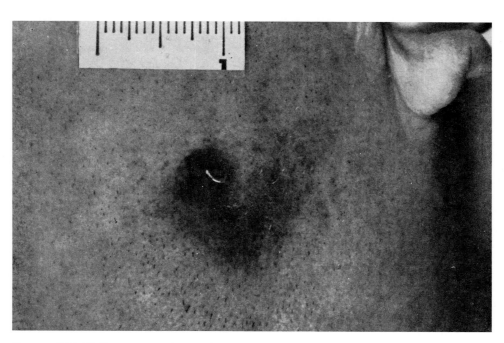

FIGURE XII-65. Execution-style murder. The victim was laying face down with the cheek against the cement floor. The entrance wound was a contact shot under the lower jaw on the opposite side. A jacketed .32 caliber slug is seen in the wound. The abrasion around the wound was caused by crushing of the skin against the floor by the exiting bullet. The percussive effect produced by the exiting slug accounts for the large area of abraded skin.

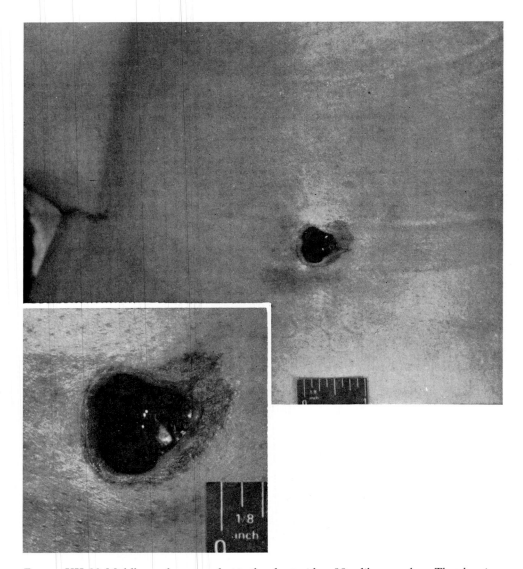

FIGURE XII-66. Middle-aged woman shot in the chest with a .38 caliber revolver. The abrasion of the exit wound in the back resulted from crushing of the skin between the slug and the band of the brassiere. The insert shows a closeup.

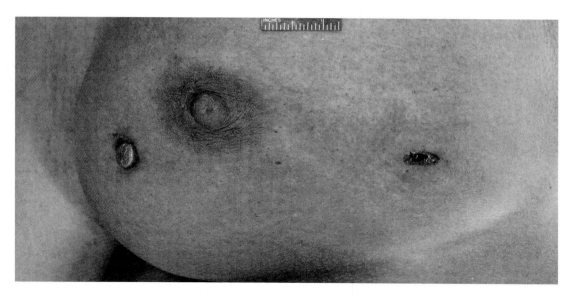

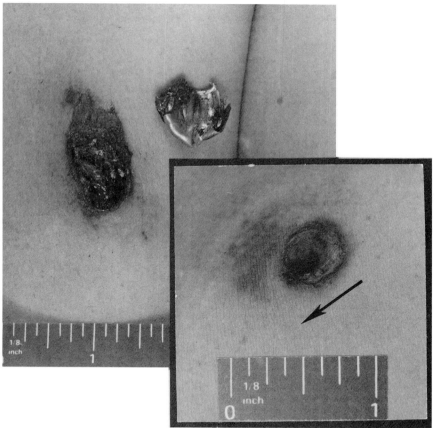

FIGURE XII-67a–b. (a) Exiting .22 caliber bullet stopped by brassiere. The head of the bullet is flattened and shows the fabric imprint. (b) Shored partial exit. The brass jacket was trapped in the wound. The entrance wound is depicted in the insert, the direction of fire is shown by the arrow.

this wound was caused by tearing of the bullet through the left side of the President's tie, adjacent to the knot.

If the President had been struck in a crossfire, i.e., the wound in the back of the shoulder and also the one in the front of the neck were both entrance wounds, there would have been two bullets in his body or two exit wounds. No bullets were recovered and none were seen on x-ray examination. Also, no additional injuries were found at autopsy.

Sometimes, when the body is on the ground, especially on a hard solid surface such as, concrete, the bullet fragments when exiting, spewing small pieces of metal which scrape the skin in the direction of the shot.

Bullets sometimes use up their energy passing through the body and stop short of perforating the skin. Occasionally, the bullet can be seen, but more often felt laying just under the skin (Fig. XII-68).

The use of an embalmers button for sealing holes in a body, whether gunshot wounds, stab wounds or incisions such as those made for insertion of the embalmer's trocar, will cause any of these holes in the skin to resemble entrance bullet wounds. The button is screwed into the skin and as it is tightened, the rim at the base scrapes the epidermis while converting the hole into a circular wound with an abraded edge (Fig. XII-69).

Dirt and lubricant from the gun barrel and bullet and metal rubbed off from the bullet surface may be deposited on the edges of a bullet hole in clothing (Figs. XII-70 to XII-73). This phenomenon may be observed with both jacketed and non-jacketed bullets. The black deposit is particularly conspicuous on a light-colored garment, and should not be mistaken for soot. The *ring of dirt,* as it is called, is sharply outlined and appears as if it were printed on the fabric. Soot, by contrast, is dark in the center and fades toward the periphery. In questionable cases, laboratory examination will resolve the problem. The *ring of dirt* is not recognizable on skin, and any suggestion that the dark edge of a bullet wound may have been caused by dirt or lubricant or, for that matter, by the heat of the bullet, is in error. The fired bullet is warm at best and certainly unable to cause a burn of flesh at a distance beyond that of the muzzle flame.

The frayed edges of a bullet hole in a garment follow the path of the bullet, depending on the

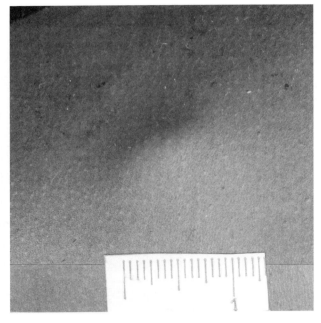

FIGURE XII-68. Slug under the skin.

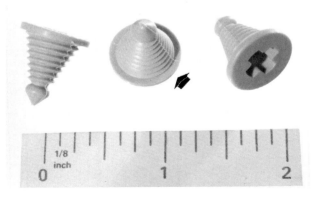

FIGURE XII-69. Embalmer buttons showing the rim (arrow) which abrades the wound edges.

type of fabric (Fig. XII-74 a-b). This may be helpful in distinguishing an entrance from an exit wound in questionable cases.

As mentioned earlier in this chapter, pieces of fabric may be carried into the entrance wound. It is rare, that such pieces are carried through the wound and deposited at the exit, except if the shot involves a thin part of the body, such as a hand, or in case of a grazing shot.

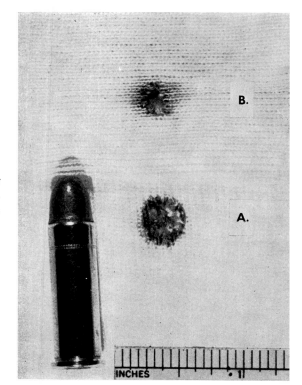

FIGURE XII-70. *Ring of dirt* produced by test firing a .38 caliber bullet into a white garment. (a) Outer surface; (b) Inner surface. The *ring of dirt* may be mistaken for soot due to close-range firing.

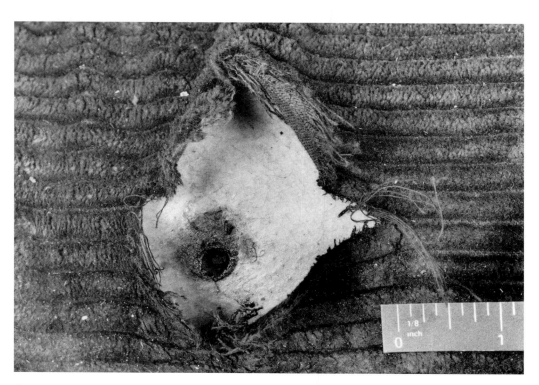

FIGURE XII-71. Contact shot of the chest. The tear in the garment is large and the fibers of the fabric are turned outward by the expanding gases returning through the hole.

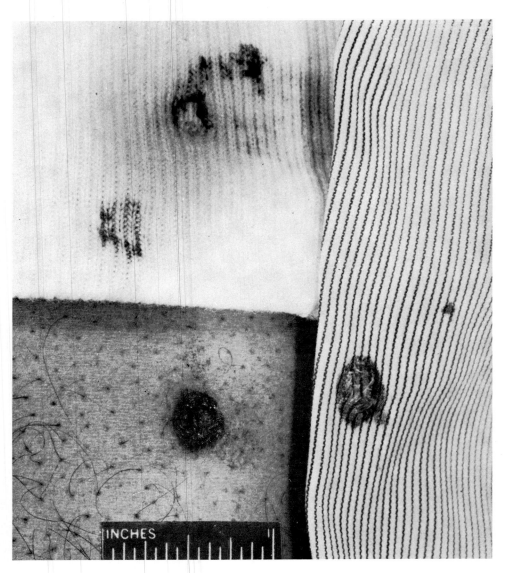

FIGURE XII-72. *Ring of dirt* in the shirt of a homicide victim who was shot in the abdominal area from a distance of about 15 feet. Also, depicted is the entrance wound in the skin.

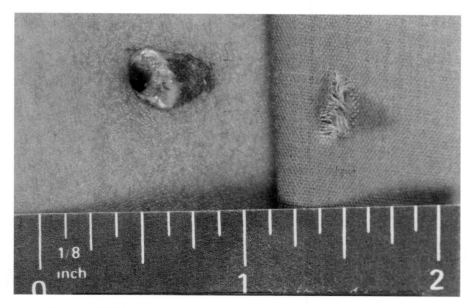

FIGURE XII-73. Bullet wipe on the garment over an exiting bullet wound.

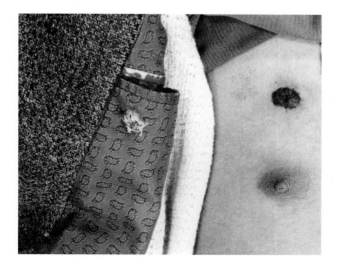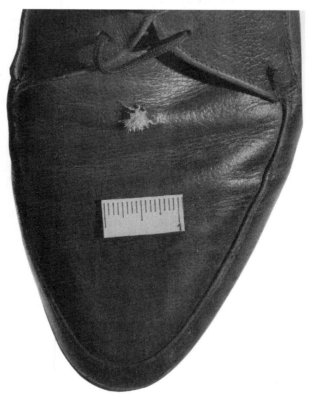

FIGURE XII-74a–b. The frayed edges of the bullet holes in the jacket and shoe point in the direction of the wound track. This finding may be important when distinguishing an entrance from an exit wound.

Whereas, bullet wounds of entrance usually conform to a set pattern, exit wounds may vary considerably in size and appearance. A bullet wound of entry is often smaller than the caliber of the bullet, while the exit wound is frequently larger. The skin is stretched by the penetrating bullet, and it returns to its former dimensions and shape after the bullet has passed, accounting for a small entrance wound. Consequently, assessment of the caliber of a bullet based on the diameter of the entrance wound is speculative and inadvisable (Fig. XII-75a–b).

In the case of an exit wound, tissues, including bone, are often pushed ahead by the bullet, causing a larger defect. Added to this is the *tumbling* effect of the bullet, which results from the resistance of the tissues as it passes through the body. Obviously, if the bullet exits sideways a larger wound results (Fig. XII-76). Slit-like exit wounds are occasionally encountered. They are attributed to deformity of the bullet, usually caused by impact on bone. An exit wound of a fragment of bone may also be slit-like, while the bullet remains in the body (Fig. XII-77a). Such wounds are mostly seen on the head and over the shoulders. Care must be taken not to mistake such wounds for stab wounds (Fig. XII-77b–c).

In an experimental animal series, non-deforming missiles (steel spheres) with high impact velocity were found to cause smaller exit than entrance bony defects.[9]

Exit wounds of the head are frequently star-shaped, resembling contact entrance wounds, except for the absence of marginal abrasion and gunsmoke in the depth of the wound (Fig. XII-78).

A bullet which changes course as a result of striking a solid surface is known as a *ricochet*. The edges of a wound caused by a *ricochet* are usually abraded, the same as any other entrance wound. If a *ricochet bullet* has been markedly deformed, the resulting wound may be large and of a bizarre shape (Fig. XII-79).[10] Occasionally, the bullet is flattened to resemble the blade of a knife. When this happens, the injury may resemble a stab wound and show no marginal abrasion. Reentry bullet wounds are usually atypical. For example, a bullet which strikes an arm held against the chest, exits and reenters the chest is

likely to cause an atypical exit on the arm and an atypical reentry on the chest. The reentry wound is unusually large, peculiarly abraded and ragged as a result of *tumbling* and also due to the percussive effect of the limb against the area of reentry (Figs. XII-80 to XII-82). Recognition of reentry wounds is essential for proper interpretation of the position of the victim and other significant conclusions (Fig. XII-83).

Occasionally, in a shallow shot to the top of the head, an entrance and exit wound are located within one or two inches of each other, and at autopsy, a wound track under the skin is found to connect the two injuries (Fig. XII-84). When this occurs, it is usually due to separation of a fragment of lead from the bullet during its passage through the bone (Fig. XII-85). The separated fragment proceeds under the skin until it exits or remains lodged between the skull and the scalp, while the major portion of the bullet enters the brain rarely exiting in a different location. The missile involved in this type of occurrence is usually a small caliber and never a jacketed bullet.

Bullets sometimes disintegrate upon impact on bone. In the head, many metal fragments may be found scattered in the brain and, on x-ray film, occasionally resemble a shotgun injury. More commonly, the wound track produced by the missile after striking or grazing bone is outlined on an x-ray film by a deposit of *metallic snow* (Fig. XII-86a–b). This consists of punctate particles of metal scattered along some distance of the wound track, indicating the direction of the shot, as particle dispersion is wider in the direction of travel.

X-ray films taken during the autopsy of President John F. Kennedy indicate a fine metallic snow in the lower right neck area, suggesting that a lateral vertebral process was fractured by the jacketed rifle bullet.

The so-called *pristine bullet* was undoubtedly responsible for this snow. This bullet, which struck both Kennedy and Governor Connally, was in fact, severely squeezed and reports that this missile was intact are based on a published photograph which depicts the undamaged side of this bullet.

Contact shots fired into the back of the head suggest *execution-style* murder (Fig. XII-87a–c). We have observed four such shots in one individual. None of the .22 caliber slugs penetrated the bone, but were found flattened against the

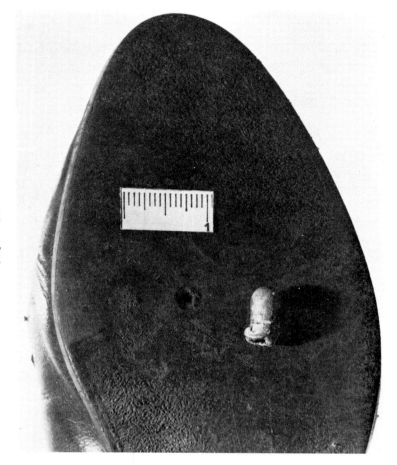

FIGURE XII-75a. The caliber of a bullet cannot be determined by the size of the defect in the garment or the skin. This .38 caliber bullet passed through the hole in the rubber sole of this shoe. The elasticity of the rubber provides for the discrepancy in size. Note the *marginal abrasion* surrounding the defect in the sole of the shoe.

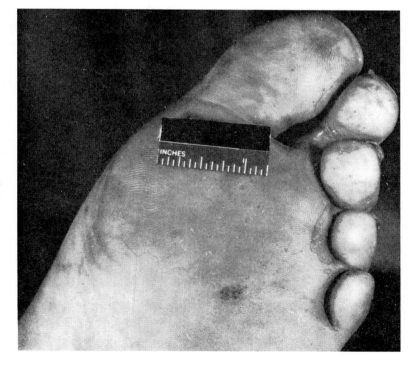

FIGURE XII-75b. The small wound in the sole of the foot was caused by the same bullet (.38 caliber). The spots around the bullet wound are dry blood. The slug was found in the exit wound on the dorsum of the foot.

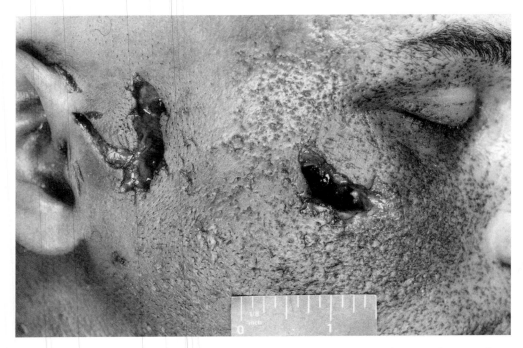

FIGURE XII-76. Close-range shot of the right cheek with large amount of surrounding stippling. The wound in front of the ear is from an exiting bullet and the surrounding epidermal tears, as well as the large tear on the left are from overstretching. The bullet was likely tumbling.

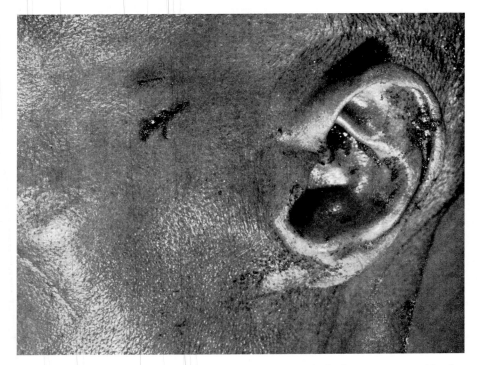

FIGURE XII-77a. Two exit wounds. It cannot be determined which one was caused by the bullet and which by a fragment of bone. A complete, but deformed .38 caliber slug was recovered from a wall.

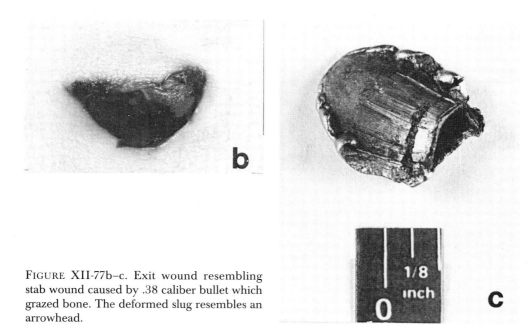

FIGURE XII-77b–c. Exit wound resembling stab wound caused by .38 caliber bullet which grazed bone. The deformed slug resembles an arrowhead.

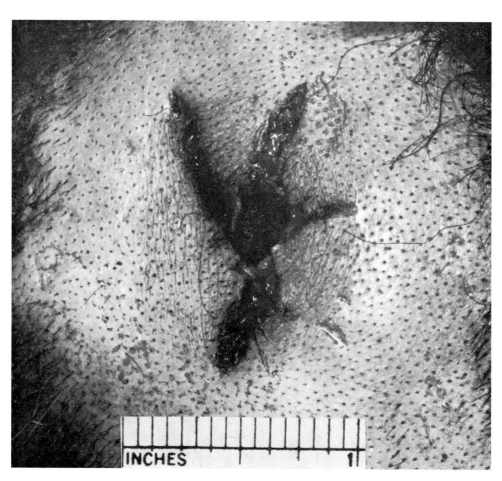

FIGURE XII-78. Exit wound on the top of the head. Note the absence of marginal abrasion. The bullet entered through the left eye.

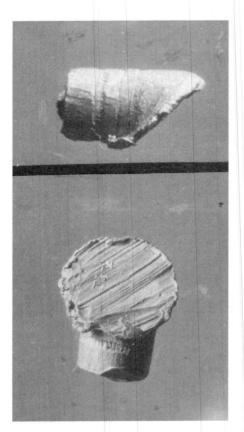

FIGURE XII-79. Lead bullet which struck cement, flattened and shows typical parallel ridges. The bullet ricocheted and caused a bizarre wound.

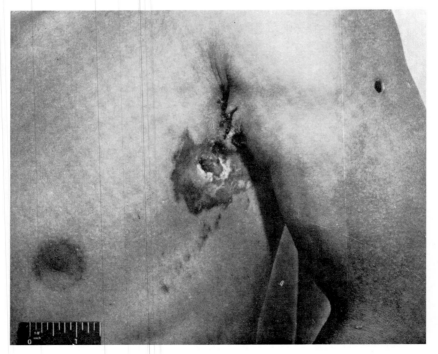

FIGURE XII-80. Entrance bullet wound on the outer surface of the left arm. The high-powered, .30 caliber rifle slug passed through the arm, fractured the bone and reentered the chest at the armpit. The reentry wound is ragged, unusually shaped and irregularly abraded. The peculiar wound is due to the percussion of the arm against the chest.

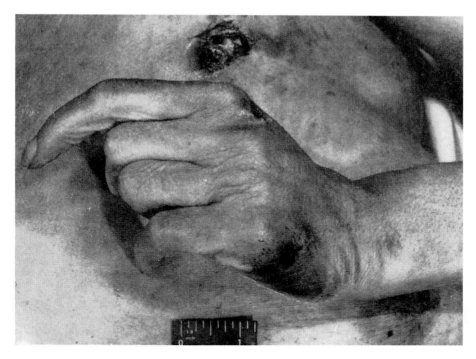

FIGURE XII-81. Close-range shot of the left hand, showing soot and gunpowder stippling. The .38 Special slug exited at the knuckle of the index finger and reentered the chest. The reentry is large and unusually abraded.

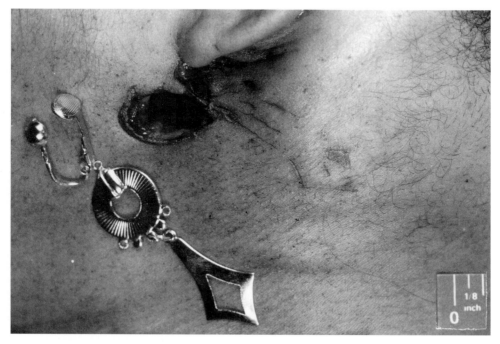

FIGURE XII-82. Entrance bullet wound below the ear. Note the imprint of the undamaged earring as a result of percussion generated by the entering slug.

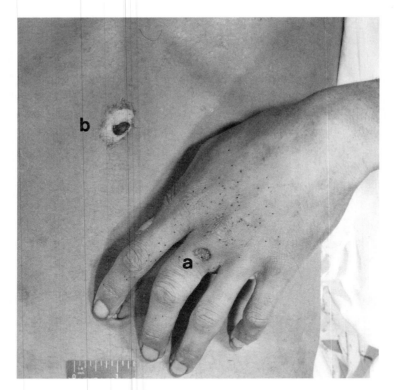

FIGURE XII-83. Close-range gunshot wound with powder stippling through the left middle finger (a) with fracture and reentry into the upper abdomen. The reentry wound (b) shows atypical marginal abrasion.

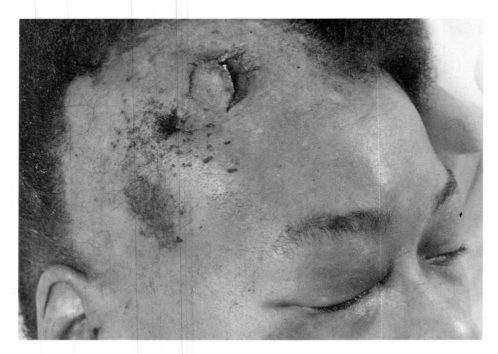

FIGURE XII-84. Close range shot of the head. The major portion of the bullet exited at the raised flap, while a fragment of lead entered the brain.

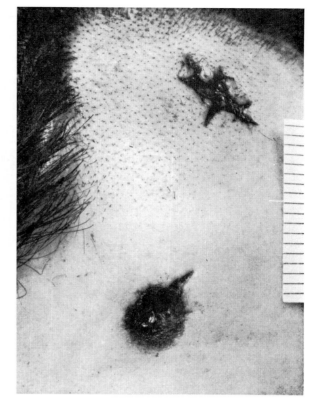

FIGURE XII-85. Entrance wound of the forehead. A fragment of the slug was *shaved off* as it penetrated the bone. The fragment proceeded under the skin exiting an inch or two above the entrance wound. The shot was fired from a distance of several feet, and the weapon was a .38 caliber Colt. Each division of the scale in the photograph equals 1/16 inch.

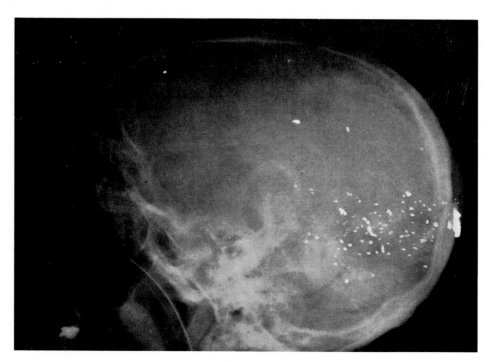

FIGURE XII-86a. A .22 caliber shot into the back of the head. The major fragment of the lead slug is situated on the outer surface of the occipital bone. The remainder of the missile fragmented, and *metallic snow* is scattered along the wound track in the brain.

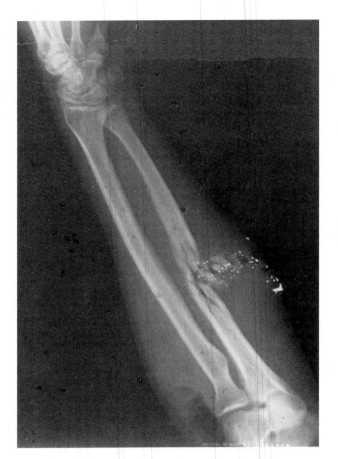

FIGURE XII-86b. Small caliber bullet, which struck an arm, fractured the left ulna and fragmented into *snow*.

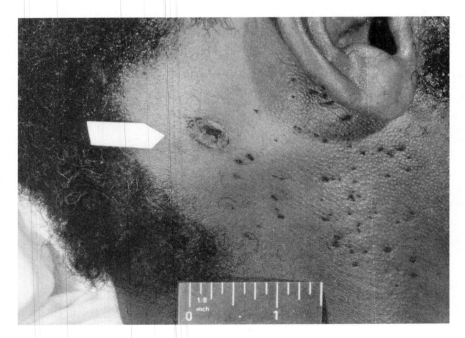

FIGURE XII-87a. Execution style shot behind the ear at close range.

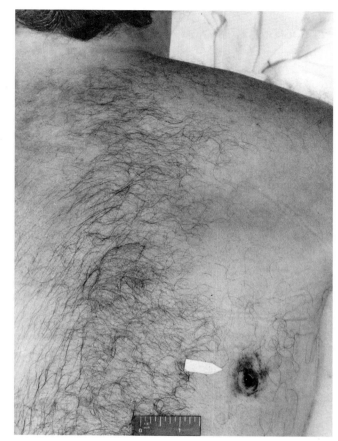

FIGURE XII-87b. Contact shot in the side of the back, stickup style.

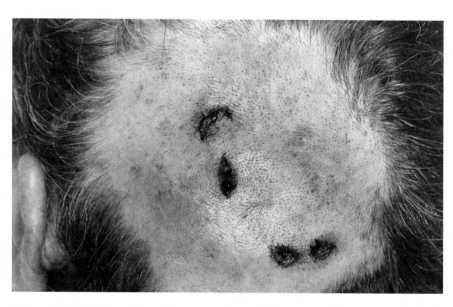

FIGURE XII-87c. Execution-style contact shots with corresponding exits in the back of the head. Death was due to the concussive effect of the contact shots.

outer surface of the skull. Death was concluded to be due to brain injury caused by the concussive effect of the impacts. Such a finding suggests defective, possibly old, ammunition where corrosion between the cartridge case and the bullet allowed for escape of gases and reduced the rounds efficiency (Fig. XII-88). In another case a .22 caliber slug fragmented on striking the occipital bone. The major fragment of lead remained under the scalp, while *metallic snow* was found scattered along the wound track in the brain (see Fig. XII-86 a). Frangible bullets, used in shooting galleries and cattle stunning, have been described as giving a similar picture.[11]

Sometimes the jacket of a bullet separates from the core upon impact on a firm object, such as a button, a coin, a key in the pocket, or bone. In such cases, the jacket and the core each assume separate paths. Whereas, the core may leave the body, the jacket very seldom does (Fig. XII-89a–b). Although fragments of the jacket may break off, in our experience the major portion of the jacket of a bullet remains in the body and should be recovered. Recovery of the jacket is of particular importance for identification of the weapon, as it carries the rifling marks of the barrel.

When a jacketed bullet strikes an adult long bone, often the femur or humerus, the bullet becomes deformed and the jacket is torn, which frequently results in separation of the jacket from the core. The jacket is often entangled in the soft tissues among the bone fragments due to its deformity and ragged edges, the core proceeds independently.

In the case of a gunshot wound of the head, the direction of fire may be readily apparent from the appearance of the bullet holes in the skull. An entrance hole is beveled inward; the defect on the inner surface of the bone is larger than that on the outer surface. An exit hole in the skull is beveled outward; it is larger on the outer than on the inner surface of the bone and may be justly referred to as crater shaped (Fig. XII-90). The same phenomenon may be observed in a plate glass window struck by a BB pellet. Asymmetry of the beveling may aid in assessing the angle of fire. Symmetrical beveling on all sides

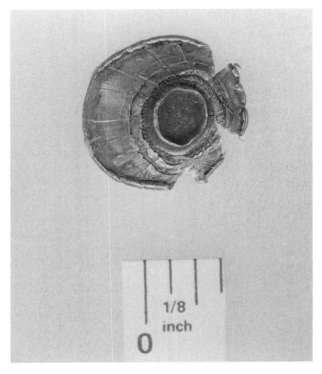

FIGURE XII-88. Old corroded .22 caliber ammunition flattened when it struck the skull's surface.

usually indicates that the bullet struck the skull head on.

Thin parts of the skull, such as facial bones and the temporal squame, do not bevel. Neither do teeth. The latter shatter with no predictability as to the direction of the impacting force. In the case of a suicidal shot into the mouth, the presence of soot on the inner, i.e., the lingual surface of teeth, even if the teeth are blown out of the mouth and are scattered outside the body, may indicate the location and direction of the shot. Ribs, sternum and pelvis also do not bevel. Direction of fire is determined by *snow* and/or bone fragment spread.

A bullet fired perpendicularly to the skull is unlikely to be deflected from its intended course. However, if the bullet strikes the head at a shallow angle, or in an area of significant curvature, at least some deflection of the bullet's trajectory may be expected. Occasionally, such deflection results in a wound track which runs under the skin, as the bullet follows the curvature of the

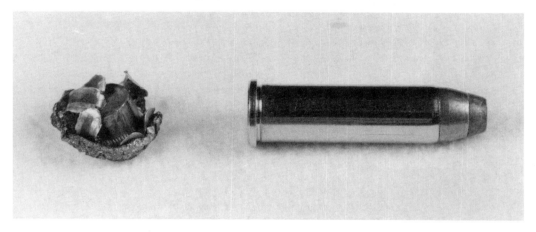

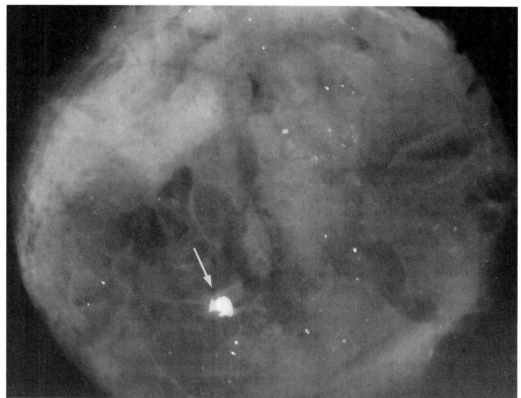

FIGURE XII-89a–b. (a) Deformed mushroomed Smith and Wesson .38 caliber special hollow point (left). Note the peeled pack petals often trapped in tissues. Jackets rarely leave the body. The actual round is displayed on the right. (b) Viscera bag containing the internal organs after autopsy shows a bullet jacket (arrow).

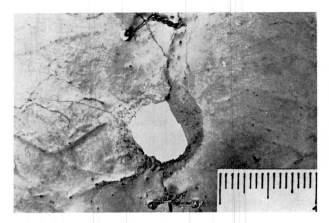

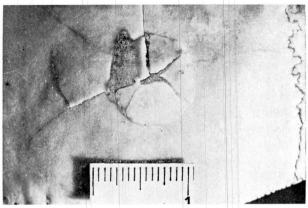

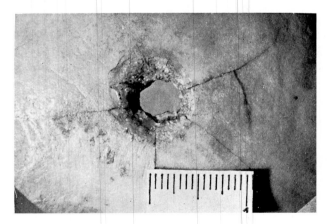

FIGURE XII-90. *Upper:* Internal surface of the skull, showing inward beveling of the defect in the bone under the entrance wound. *Middle:* Outer surface of the skull, to show the mechanism of outward beveling at the exit. Note the raised bone fragments by the exiting bullet. The actual hole is shown in the lower photograph. *Lower:* Outer surface of the skull, showing outward beveling of the exit defect.

bone. The bullet may eventually exit without having penetrated the skull. Similarly, a bullet that has penetrated the skull may travel as above, along the inner surface of the bone, and remain lodged within the skull having caused little or no damage to the brain. In the same way, a bullet which strikes a rib at a shallow angle may pass under the skin, partly encircling the chest, and possibly exiting on the opposite side, without having penetrated the chest cavities. A tight garment worn over the area of a subcutaneous wound track may cause an abrasion of the skin outlining the path of the bullet, as the skin is being pushed by the bullet against the garment.

A shot fired at a curved part of the head at a shallow angle, i.e., a tangential shot, often causes a typically inward-beveled entrance hole adjacent to an outward-beveled exit hole, producing a *keyhole*-shaped defect in the skull (Figs. XII-91a–c to XII-95). A fragment of the slug may be *shaved off* by the bone at the entrance hole and penetrate the brain. The skin shows the presence of an entrance wound as well as, a bullet wound of exit. Fractures of the orbital roofs, as a result of the transmitted shock wave, are occasionally seen in cases of *keyhole* type wounds involving the top of the head or forehead. Eyelid hemorrhage on the same side may result from seepage, especially in cases of survival. Occasionally, in contact shots of the head, the same entrance hole in the skull is beveled both inward and outward, due to chipping of the outer layer of the bone around the defect by the forceful return of gases through the bullet hole or by the twisting force of the rotating bullet (Fig. XII-96). Other parts of the skeleton may also suggest the direction of fire by the inward displacement of bone fragments adjacent to the entrance wound, in contrast to outward displacement of the fragments near the exit. Ribs and pelvis are common areas in which this occurs.

The pathologist is often asked to evaluate positions of the shooter and victim using wound tracts through the victim's body. Witness statements and findings at the scene must be correlated with wound tracts. Otherwise, the pathologist is in the predicament illustrated in Fig. XII-97a–b where a horizontal shot through

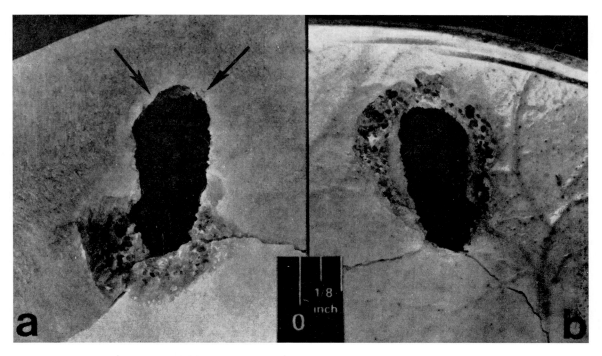

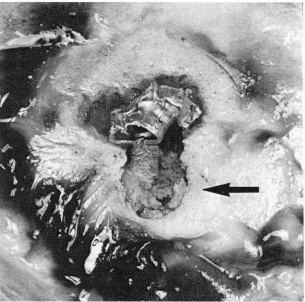

FIGURE XII-91a–c. Keyhole-shaped defect in the parietal bone of the skull due to a tangential gunshot. Figures (a) and (b) are the outer and inner surfaces of the bone respectively. The entrance of the slug is marked by the inward beveled part of the keyhole (arrows); the exit, at the lower part of the defect, is beveled outward. (c) .38 caliber bullet causing a keyhole defect. The bullet entered and depressed the bone at the lower end of the fracture (arrow). The picture illustrates the mechanism of keyholing.

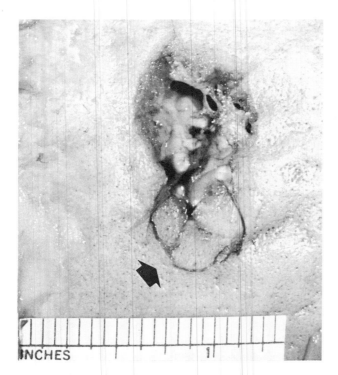

FIGURE XII-92. Circular depressed fracture (arrow), caused by the shallow strike of a bullet. The bullet traveled on the bone, split, one part entering the skull, the major portion did not penetrate. Note top half of the fracture is beveled outward, as a typical exit.

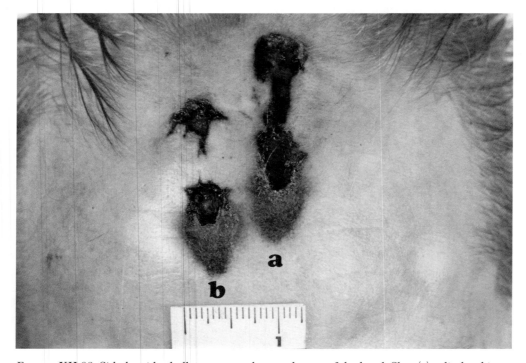

FIGURE XII-93. Side-by-side shallow contact shots at the top of the head. Shot (a) split the skin as it traveled posteriorly and exited. This was a suicide and shot (a) may be considered a hesitation wound. Shot (b) was also fired at a shallow angle, but less than shot (a). The bullet of shot (b) traveled under the skin, split, one part exited, the other penetrated the brain.

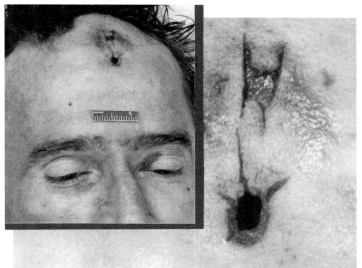

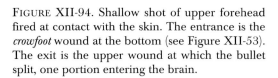

FIGURE XII-94. Shallow shot of upper forehead fired at contact with the skin. The entrance is the *crowfoot* wound at the bottom (see Figure XII-53). The exit is the upper wound at which the bullet split, one portion entering the brain.

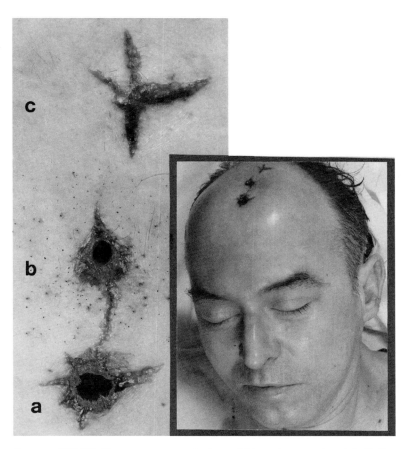

FIGURE XII-95. Two entry wounds (a and b); exit wound at (c). Bullet wound (a) was a contact shot, part of this bullet proceeded forward as shown by the connecting split between wounds (a and b), the major portion of this bullet proceeded to (c) and exited. Wound (b) was inflicted at close range as shown by stippling. The shot was slightly forward, the entire bullet entered the skull.

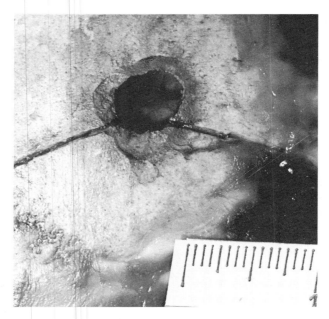

FIGURE XII-96. Contact shot of the back of the head showing outward beveling of the bone. Soot is deposited on the
edges of the defect.

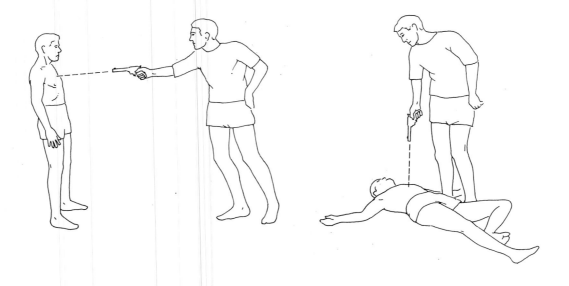

FIGURE XII-97a–b. Diagram depicting direction of wound track with victim standing or lying on the ground.

the chest may have been inflicted with the victim upright or lying on his back. With regards to limbs, it should be feasible to align the wound track (Figs. XII-98 and XII-99).

Homicide, Suicide, or Accident

Distinction between homicide, suicide, or accident may be difficult and sometimes impossible, yet it is the first question asked by the investigator in every death involving a shooting. Certain criteria are used by pathologists to define the manner of death within reasonable degree of medical certainty. Among these, evaluation of the range of fire is of utmost importance. It is obvious that a distant shot could not have been self-inflicted in the absence of a contraption specifically designed for this purpose. The presence of gunpowder stippling, soot, or both around a bullet wound are consequently of great significance. In the absence of recognizable gunpowder residue, sensitive laboratory analyses may turn up findings missed by naked-eye examination. Examination of the clothing over the gunshot wound area should be included in the search for powder residue, particularly as this may be the only site to yield a positive result. It should be emphasized that gunpowder is by no means always found inside of contact bullet wounds. For instance, a contact shot of the heart area may be devoid of identifiable powder residue due to the fact that the pow-

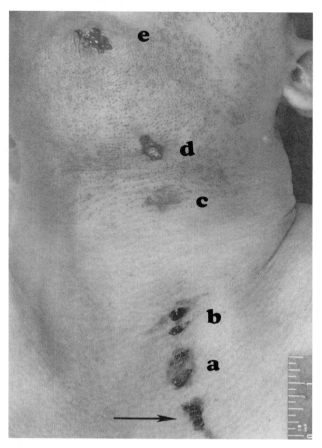

FIGURE XII-98. Bullet wound in the upper chest which entered at the *arrow* and traveled upward under the skin. The double wounds at (a) and (b) are due to creases. A bruise is noted at (c) and a partial exit at (d) was the result of striking the jaw with the major portion of the bullet exiting at (e).

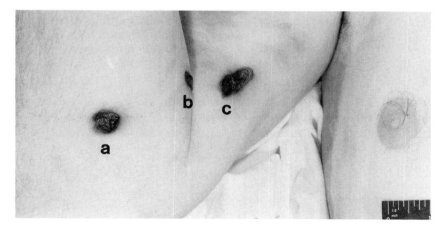

FIGURE XII-99. Alignment of bullet wounds: (a) is entrance; (b) is exit; (c) is reentry.

der is spread and partly washed out of the wound by extensive bleeding as long as the heart is pumping. In such cases, gunsmoke may still be detectable on the inner surface of the garment, as indicated earlier in this chapter. In the case of close-range shots, where gunpowder is expected to be scattered on the target, it is interesting to note that clothing of a body drenched in decomposition fluids may completely lose any evidence of gunpowder; hence, estimation of the range of fire based on the presence of powder residue may not be feasible.

In the case of a gunshot that was survived and surgically debrided, microscopic examination may reveal the presence of gunpowder, amorphous particles of soot and possibly heat coagulation in tissue fragments that were excised. Such findings would indicate a contact or near-contact shot and for practical purposes, eliminate the likelihood of an accidental discharge, as by dropping the weapon on the floor. An autopsy on an individual who has undergone such surgery is unlikely to reveal information regarding the distance of fire and often, the manner of death. Consequently, it is recommended that the pathologist performing the autopsy obtain the tissues removed at surgery or slides of same for his own examination.

A gunshot wound in an area of the body not accessible to the victim, or one that is accessible with difficulty, e.g., in the back of the head, or between the shoulder blades, is always suspicious of homicide. The vast majority of suicidal shots are in the temple, heart, forehead and mouth. Among these, the temple area is used most frequently.

Right-handed individuals are more likely to shoot themselves in the right side of the head, but a contact shot of the right temple does not necessarily imply that the victim was right-handed. We have observed many times where a right-handed individual shot himself in the left temple and vice versa. Why? Probably no one knows! Suicide is usually an irrational act which a rational individual would be unlikely to understand.

Gunsmoke deposits on the hand that fired the gun are sometimes seen (Figs. XII-100 and XII-101a–c). This gunsmoke originates in part from the blow back associated with the muzzle blast, as well as from loose fittings in the frame of the weapon. Thus, revolvers, especially if poorly constructed, such as notorious *Saturday night specials,* are more likely to deposit gunsmoke on the firing hand than pistols of good quality. With rifles and shotguns in good condition, it is very unlikely that identifiable gunsmoke will be found on the hand that pulled the trigger. Different firearms tend to deposit gunsmoke in different patterns. This may be useful in determining whether a bullet wound was self-inflicted. Laboratory experiments involving handguns have shown that the index finger, thumb and connecting web area of the shooting hand are most likely to be contaminated with gunshot residue. Occasionally, gunsmoke deposits are noted on both hands, especially on the one that was used to steady the weapon while the other pulled or pushed the trigger.

Black grease deposits, pinch marks, cuts or scrapes are sometimes seen on hands which handle automatic or semiautomatic handguns. These injuries are found predominately in the area of the web of the thumb. They can occur when pulling the slide back to load the chamber or when the weapon is fired and the expansion of gases forces the slide rearward (Fig. XII-102a–d).

A twenty-four-year-old woman was found in her bedroom wedged between the bed and dresser. On the bed were male undershorts smeared with blood. Near the body on the floor was a male shoe print pointing away from the body. A .38 caliber Colt revolver was in her left hand, the index finger in the trigger guard. A near-contact gunshot wound was present on the right cheek (Fig. XII-102a–b). On the palm of the left hand, just below the index finger, were two, parallel, 1/4-inch long, pinch marks surrounded by faint brownish discoloration due to gunsmoke (Fig. XII-102c). The fired cartridge in the cylinder of the revolver was at six o'clock. The weapon was clean, apparently freshly oiled.

The boyfriend, a gun collector, free on probation, was seen driving away from the house after a shot was heard, and he was not apprehended until late that night. He stated that they had had an argument following which she shot herself. He took the weapon from the pool of blood on the floor and wiped the blood on a pair of shorts. When it occurred to him that possession of the gun might incriminate him in a murder charge, he cleaned and oiled the weapon, then placed it back into her hand. His statement sounded credible. When the cocked gun was held in the

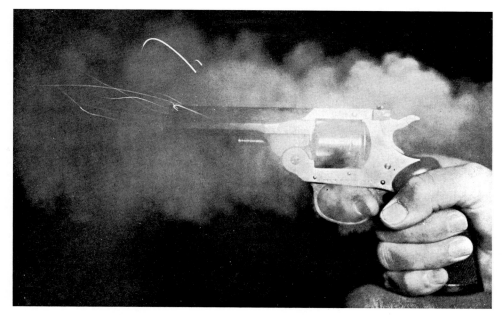

FIGURE XII-100. Cloud of gunsmoke engulfing the hand. The presence of gunsmoke and its distribution on the hand are important for the determination of whether a bullet wound was self-inflicted. The light streaks emerging from the muzzle are glowing particles of gunpowder. (Courtesy: Donald M. Flohr, H. P. White Laboratories, Bel Air, Maryland)

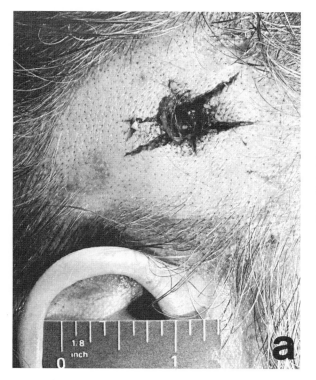

FIGURE XII-101a–c. Suicidal shot of the right temple with a .38 caliber snub-nosed revolver by a left-handed individual. The right thumb was used to push the trigger, while the left arm was passed over the head and the hand was used to steady the barrel. The soot distribution indicates how the gun was held.

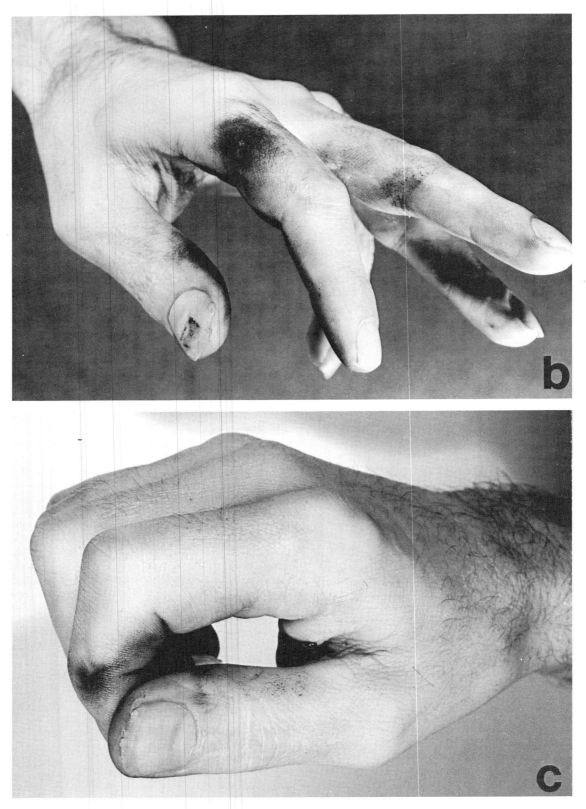

FIGURE XII-101b–c

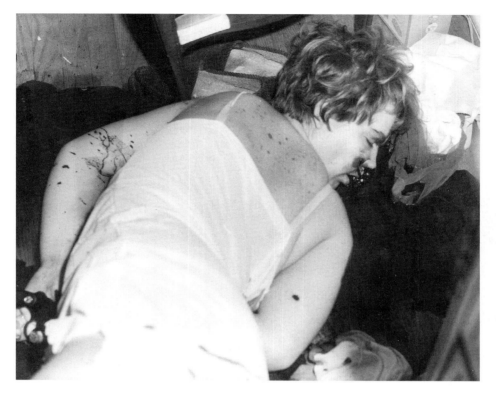

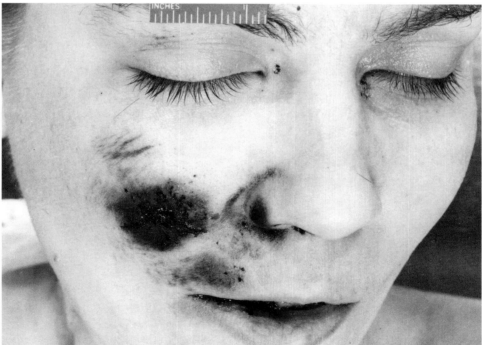

Figure XII-102a–d. (a) The body of the victim wedged between bed and dresser. A .38 caliber Colt revolver is noted in her left hand; the index finger is in the trigger guard. The right cheek displays a near-contact wound. (b) Closeup of a near-contact bullet wound of the right cheek.

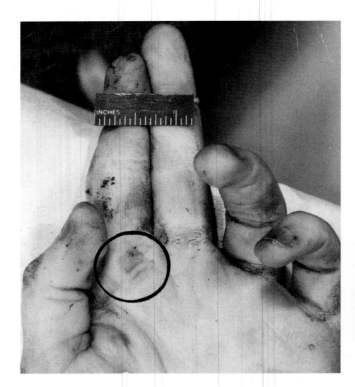

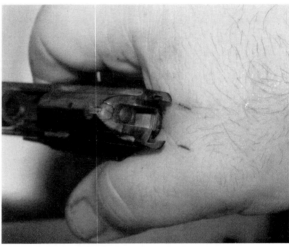

FIGURE XII-102c–d. (c) Two parallel 1/4-inch-long *pinch marks* surrounded by faint brownish discoloration from gunsmoke on the palm of the left hand. The hand had been used to steady the weapon when it was fired. (d) Suicidal intraoral shot using a semiautomatic Beretta 950 BS. Parallel abrasions by the downward projecting rails of the slide. The finding puts the gun in the hand of the shooter at the moment of firing. *(Courtesy of Stuart L. Dawson, M.D., Suffolk County Medical Examiner's Office, New York.)*

right hand with the thumb pulling the trigger and the muzzle pointing toward one's own cheek and the left hand placed over the cylinder to steady the weapon, the downing hammer inflicted a pinch of the same appearance and in the same location as on the left hand of the deceased.

Gunsmoke and tiny particles of primer material, gunsmoke residue (GSR), are expelled from the front of the gun and also leak from the open back of the cylinder in revolvers and when the chamber opens and the cartridge is ejected in automatics.

Gunsmoke deposits on hands obscured by extensive blood soiling can be identified by gentle rinsing of the hand under running cold water. Cold water which dissolves dried blood without

scrubbing, will not wash away oily gunsmoke residue.

Despite serious limitations in testing, hands suspected of having fired a gun should be examined for gunshot residue (GSR). GSR persists for approximately six hours, but is lost if the hands are washed. Fingerprinting should be delayed until after samples for GSR analysis have been obtained.

Different tests, such as the paraffin for nitrates, neutron activation analysis, flameless atomic absorption spectroscopy have been used in the past and abandoned due to false positives and other limitations. Currently, scanning electron microscopy or SEM is the preferred method of

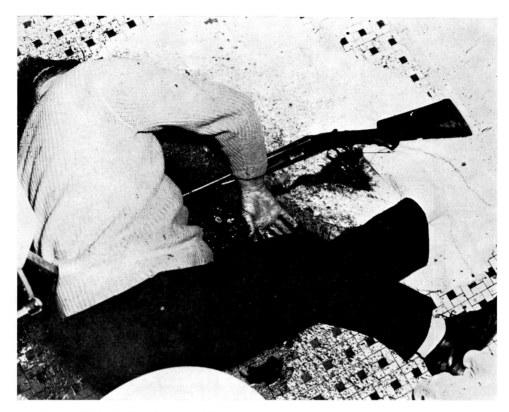

FIGURE XII-103. Suicidal shot of the chest. A coat hanger was used to pull the trigger.

GSR evaluation. The hands or clothes are swabbed, then the swabs are sent to the crime laboratory for analysis. The SEM provides high magnification to detect GSR particles and is equipped with an x-ray analyzer used to confirm elements present in the sample. However, SEM is expensive, requires a special environment and specially trained scientists, consequently, few law enforcement agencies own their own equipment requiring the use of outside laboratories.

The presence of GSR does not prove someone fired a gun, the absence of GSR does not prove they did not. There are too many factors, such as, improper collection techniques and washing of hands, including false positives which caused some laboratories, such as the Michigan State Police Forensic Laboratories, to discontinue GSR analysis.

In the case of suicide by rifle fire, the victim may be in practically any position to fire the gun. Nevertheless, depending on the position in which the victim is found, it is sometimes neces-sary to verify whether he was capable of reaching the trigger. Measurement of the victim's arm length may yield the required information. We have seen cases where individuals have used a toe, stick, or coat hanger to pull or push the trig-ger. These methods are not uncommon (Figs. XII-103 and XII-104).

Multiple bullet wounds invariably arouse sus-picion of homicide. However, in certain cases suicide must also be considered. Multiple suici-dal shots commonly involve the same general area of the body. It is unusual to find the shots scattered.

A forty-three-year-old man addressed a suicide note to his wife before shooting himself three times (Fig. XII-105). A superficial graze was noted in the forehead, another bul-let pierced both cheeks and a gunshot of the right temple (no doubt the third by chronological order) proved lethal by penetration of the brain.

Any attempt to establish the sequence of shots must take into consideration the degree of inca-pacity that results from each shot. This will

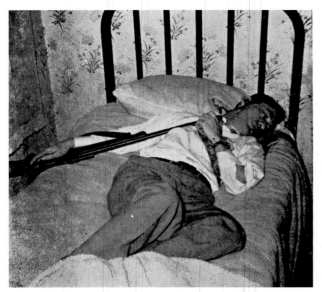

FIGURE XII-104. The length of the victim's arm is important when determining whether he could have fired the weapon himself.

enable the examiner to determine which was the fatal shot and allow conclusions regarding the physical activity of the victim following the other shots. In the case of the man mentioned earlier, one may wonder whether the graze of the forehead and the shot of the cheek were *hesitation shots* similar to hesitation cuts outlined in Chapter XI.

In another case, a seventy-two-year-old man used a .25 caliber pistol and fired three contact shots into his chest (Fig. XII-106a–b). The incident occurred in the bathroom. After the shooting, he walked into the bedroom and laid down on his bed. The body was discovered the next day. At autopsy, it was found that all three shots had perforated the heart.

Occasionally, in gunshots of the head, it may be possible to ascertain the sequence of shots by the pattern of fracture lines that radiate from each defect. The fractures that extend from the second bullet hole are arrested by those that

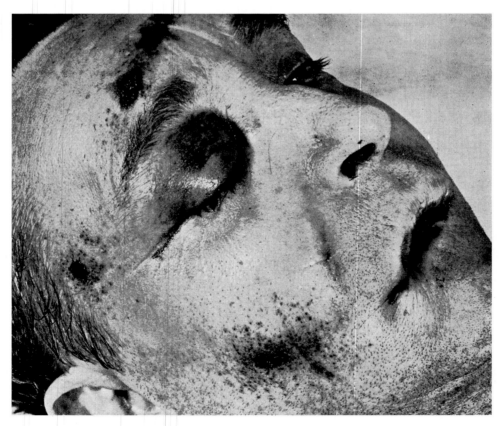

FIGURE XII-105. Suicide with three close-range shots: graze of the forehead, through-and-through bullet wound of the cheeks, not involving vital organs, and fatal shot of the right temple.

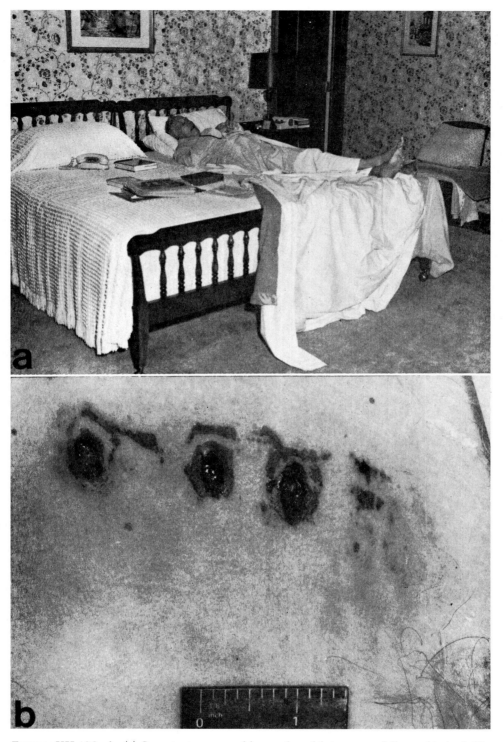

FIGURE XII-106a–b. (a) Seventy-two-year old man found lying peacefully on his bed. No bleeding was noted anywhere. The pistol and cartridge cases were in the bathroom, seen with the door open. (b) Three contact shots in the left side of the chest above the nipple. Each injury shows the muzzle imprint.

originated from the first (Fig. XII-107a–b). This is in keeping with characteristics of breaking plate glass and of fractures of the skull due to blunt trauma as outlined in Chapter X.

Another point in distinguishing homicide from suicide is the observation that individuals sometimes remove their clothing from the area they intend to shoot. Thus, an open shirt is not unusual in suicidal shots of the heart area. Some dispute this statement and consider removal of clothes in suicides to be a myth based on old misconceptions.[12]

Location of the gun is often a point of contention in determining whether a death is a suicide. A study of 498 suicides over a thirteen-year period found that 69% of the time, the gun was on the body, touching the body, or within 12 inches of the body. Further, in 24% of the cases the gun remained in the hand of the deceased.[13]

An accidental gunshot can be distinguished from a homicidal or suicidal injury only by the circumstances that surround the incident. It is the duty of the pathologist to confirm or dispute the account that was given of the incident, based on his findings at the postmortem examination of the victim, i.e., to prove whether the injury is consistent with the manner in which it was said to have occurred. The availability of photographs and diagrams of the scene is helpful, but personal viewing of the scene gives a better perspective (Fig. XII-108).

Russian roulette is termed *accidental* by many pathologists. This is a betting game in which the players take turns holding a revolver loaded with a single round, the position of which in the cylinder is unknown, to their temple and pull the trigger. It is our contention that these deaths are suicides due to the obvious significant element of deliberate self-destruction.

Ricochet

A ricochet is a missile that has deviated from its course by striking an intermediary object. Such missiles are commonly deformed. The degree of deformity varies depending on the texture of the bullets, the angle of impact and the consistency of the object which is struck. Jacket-ed bullets have a greater ricochet potential than non-jacketed ones. When striking a body, a ricochet bullet seldom exits.

The path of a ricochet is unpredictable, although in the case of a ricochet on a body of water, the angle of incidence equals the angle of reflection. The missile penetrates the water for a short distance. The same may occur with a shot fired at a block of hard wood or ice. An injury by ricochet cannot usually be inflicted intentionally. These missiles are, therefore, of considerable legal significance.

Experimentation with .38 special, jacketed hollow-point bullets, fired at tempered glass automobile windows, indicated severe deflection, particularly if the window was angled inward. Also, separation of the bullet jacket from the core was observed in approximately half of the test firings with this type of ammunition.[14]

It is important in the case of a suspected ricochet that the missile be examined for possible foreign inclusions originating from the intermediary target. Such inclusions are common in lead bullets because of metal softness. Sensitive analyses are available to identify these substances.

An entrance wound produced by a ricochet is not necessarily different from that produced by an ordinary bullet, although it may be larger and assume a bizarre shape, due to deformity and tumbling of the missile.

A twenty-two-year-old woman who witnessed an argument between her husband and two men suddenly slumped over dead when the husband fired his gun at the men (Fig. XII-109a). At postmortem examination, she had an injury in mid-forehead, resembling a typical contact gunshot wound, except for the absence of gunsmoke (Fig. XII-109b). The weapon used was a 9 mm Luger with corresponding ammunition. The husband was found guilty of murder despite his claim that he had not fired in the direction of his wife.

Puzzled by the absence of soot and gunpowder in and about the bullet wound, close-range firing seemed doubtful, and the possibility of a ricochet was entertained. Test firing of the same gun with matching ammunition was carried out at contact with the skin as well as, from a distance of 7 to 9 feet. Injuries bearing some similarity to the wound of the deceased could be obtained only when the bullets were inverted in their cartridge cases, thus striking the target base first (Fig. XII-109c–d). These results suggested that the woman may have been struck by a deformed bullet, namely a ricochet. When the luger bullets were fired as manufactured, the injuries that resulted had the expected appearance.

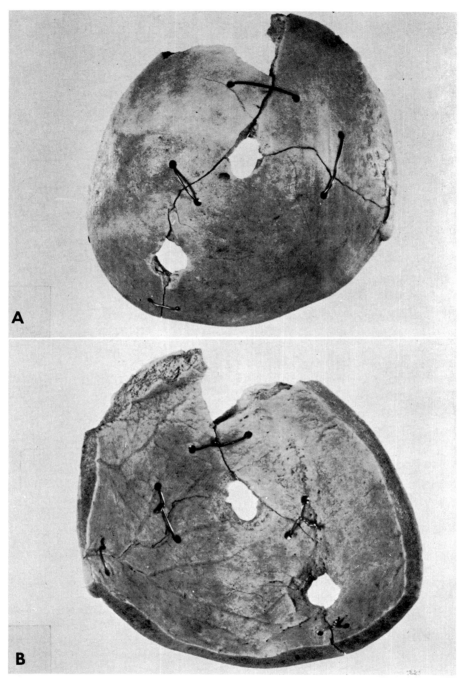

FIGURE XII-107a–b. Exterior (a) and interior (b) aspects of the skullcap with two experimental entrance holes. The pattern of the fracture lines which radiate from the holes and the interrupted beveling of the upper defect indicate that the lower wound must have been inflicted first.

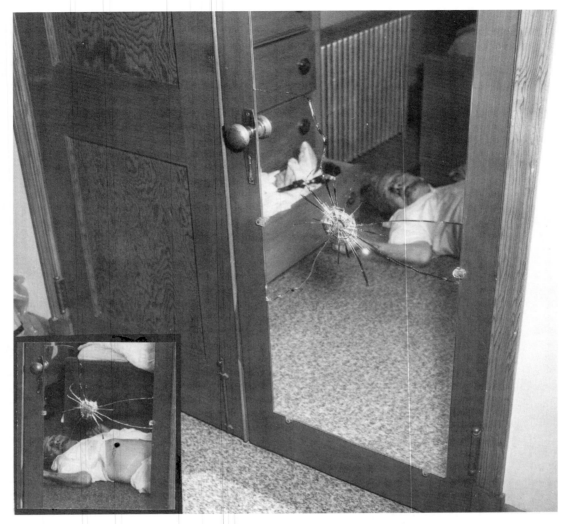

FIGURE XII-108. Suicidal shot in the right chest (insert). The gun is in the open lower dresser drawer. The gunshot in the mirror is a practice shot. Practice or warning shots sometimes precede suicidal shots.

On the basis of this new experimental evidence, the trial was reopened and the case was dismissed.[10]

In another case, an eighteen-year-old boy was found dead beside a narrow path in a forest. He had a bullet wound of the groin, and autopsy showed that death had resulted from blood loss due to laceration of the iliac artery and vein. A lead bullet was recovered from the soft tissues of the pelvis.

Meanwhile, a friend of the victim surrendered to the police, claiming that the death of his friend was accidental. They had been playing *chicken,* a game of courage, the object of which is to avoid taking cover while shots are fired by the other player. He had definitely not shot at his friend, but admitted shooting in the same direction when suddenly his friend collapsed and was dead a short time later.

At this point the bullet that had been removed from the victim was examined. The tip of the bullet was flattened on one side, and the base bore the imprint of the weave pattern of the victim's trousers. A few threads of the fabric were actually trapped in the lead. It was thus evident, that the bullet struck the victim base-first after it had apparently glanced off one of the trees between the two players. The flattened tip of the bullet and numerous grazes in the bark of the trees in that section of the forest supported this version and criminal charges were dropped.

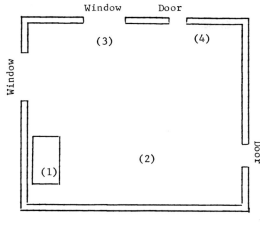

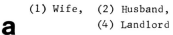

(1) Wife, (2) Husband, (3) Lover
(4) Landlord

a

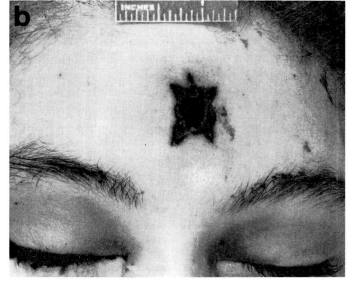

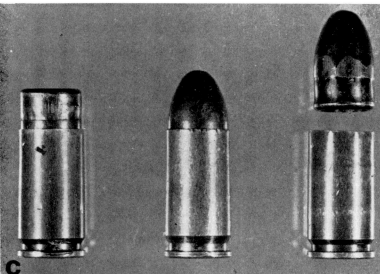

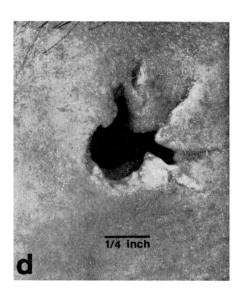

1/4 inch

FIGURE XII-109a–d. *Ricochet*. (a) Layout of the room and position of the parties. (b) Entrance bullet wound in the forehead of the victim resembling a contact shot, but showing no presence of soot or gunpowder. (c) The bullet in the center is original Luger ammunition. A slug inverted in the cartridge case is displayed on the left. (d) Injury bearing similarity to the bullet wound of the victim is obtained by a test shot from a distance of 9 feet using Luger ammunition with inverted slug. (Figures XII-109a–d reproduced from Spitz, W. U.: *Rikoschett- oder Kontaktscussverletzung. Dtsch Z Ges Gerichtl Med, 66:*153, 1969. Courtesy of Bergmann Verlag, Heidelberg.)

PHYSICAL ACTIVITY FOLLOWING FATAL INJURY BY GUNFIRE

Contrary to popular belief, physical activity of a person who is fatally shot does not necessarily cease immediately following injury. Missile wounds of the brain are common exceptions, because unconsciousness sets in rapidly. A bullet that severs the neck segment of the spinal cord causes immediate collapse due to quadriplegia or paraplegia, depending on the level of spinal cord injury. Death is instantaneous if the medulla oblongata is involved.

A study conducted of 111 homicidal firearm and stabbing cases, to determine the duration and type of activity of the victims before they collapsed, was published by Spitz et al. in 1961.[15] Gunshot wounds of the heart and lung are often associated with extended activity until blood loss causes shock, followed by death. Many fatally injured attempt to reach help. Some crawl, run or use the phone.

One thirty-nine-year-old man, who was shot in the chest with a .32 caliber pistol, ran seven city blocks before he collapsed and died two hours later at the hospital. Autopsy of

the victim showed severed intercostal vessels and a wound tract through the right lung. There was 1 quart (approx. 900 mL) of blood in the pleural cavity in addition to a large amount of blood at the scene.

A thirty-one-year-old man was shot in the chest with a .38 caliber bullet. He was witnessed crawling 55 feet following the injury, then collapsed. He died a few minutes later. Autopsy showed that the wound track passed through the left lung and heart, resulting in hemorrhage into the chest cavity and massive hemopericardium.

In general, capability to act is shorter in shooting than in stabbing victims. Whereas, gunshot wounds cause a hole, the edges of a stab wound tend to close together after the knife is withdrawn.

PAIN AND GUNSHOT WOUNDS

Pain following a gunshot wound is limited to the skin. Internal organs usually lack the type of pain receptors present in the skin and thus are significantly less sensitive.

The lung tissue feels no pain. However, the pleura, which lines the lung, is sensitive to friction against the chest wall. For instance, chest pain in pleurisy is the result of rubbing of the visceral pleura, which lines the lung surface, against the parietal pleura lining the chest wall. Cutting, stabbing, shooting, burning, or tearing of the lung would cause no pain.

Liver tissue is insensitive, but swelling of the liver, as in hepatitis, causes pain by stretching of the liver capsule. The same is true of gallstones which stretch the bile ducts. Thus, an impacted stone in a bile duct may cause extreme pain, but cutting or cauterizing or crushing such a duct will remain painless. Similarly, the intestines hurt as a

result of stretching, as by gas, however are insensitive to other types of trauma. Cautery for the removal of polyps during colonoscopy causes no pain.

The brain lacks pain receptors, as do the heart, kidney, pancreas and other organs. The pain of kidney stones is the result of ureter distension, similar to that caused by gallstones.

Governor Connally shot through the chest, right wrist and left thigh, as he was seated in front of President John Kennedy in the limousine when the President was assassinated, displays no reaction when first shot on photographs of the motorcade.

The assassination attempts on President Ronald Reagan and Pope John Paul II illustrate these facts clearly. Neither realized that they had been shot, until so told by others.

DIVERSE CHARACTERISTICS OF LESS COMMON AMMUNITION AND THEIR EFFECTS

Many types of ammunition are available. Most are conventional varieties that produce known patterns of injury. Occasionally, however, gunshot wounds are observed that exhibit unusual characteristics.[16]

Frangible Bullets

Frangible bullets, .22 caliber ammunition, have been used for years in shooting galleries and to stun cattle. The bullet is manufactured of bonded powdered lead or iron. It disintegrates on striking the target; consequently, frangible bullets do not ricochet. Frangible bullets manufactured today have advanced performance characteristics, i.e., reduced hazard/no ricochet, controlled fragmentation, higher accuracy and velocity and are therefore used by police departments for target practice.

Graham et al.[11] reported a death due to a self-inflicted gunshot of the head involving a frangible bullet. These authors conducted experiments with this type of ammunition to determine its disintegrating and penetrating characteristics, and the suitability of such bullets for comparison microscope identification. They concluded that penetration of the skull occurs at distances from 0.5 to 36 inches.

Location and recovery of the bullet fragments are greatly facilitated by the use of x-rays. Due to the extent of fragmentation and mutilation, these bullets are generally unsuitable for microscopic matching.

Birdshot

Birdshot is available in a variety of calibers and loads. The more commonly used cartridges are .22 and .38 caliber. Birdshot is considered low-powered and is used for pest control. The .22 cartridge is loaded with approximately 150 pellets of No. 12 shot. At 20 yards the pellets will barely penetrate thin cardboard. At close range, however, birdshot can be extremely dangerous. DiMaio and Spitz[17] observed a victim of homicide with a shot of the head involving this type of ammunition. The distance from which the fatal shot had been fired was unknown, and test shots were carried out in an attempt to establish the penetration power and wounding characteristics of this ammunition at various distances. The victim had been shot through the temple. X-ray showed numerous metallic pellets scattered throughout the brain.

The dispersion pattern of the pellets in the body cannot be applied to estimation of the range of fire, as demonstrated by Breitenecker et al.[18] Considerable dispersion of the shot within the body occurs if the majority of the pellets

strike the target together. This dispersion is the result of deflection of the pellets by striking each other at the time of penetration of the target (so-called *billiard ball* effect). The same phenomenon occurs in the case of shotgun injuries, discussed in *Part 2*.

Test firings indicated that in the homicide in question the gun had been fired from a distance of less that 6 inches. The possibility of a contact shot should always be ruled out.

Piggyback Bullet

A *piggyback* or tandem bullet is one that results from the discharge of a second bullet while the first is still inside the barrel. A *piggyback* bullet is thus a projectile composed of two independent bullets, where one is pushed into the rear of the other. The projectile weighs double or nearly double the weight of an ordinary bullet of the same caliber. As in the case of any bullet, parts of this projectile may be chipped off as it penetrates the target. The occurrence of a *piggyback* bullet is rare, but when it happens is usually associated with faulty ammunition or a defective firearm.

The body of a fifteen-year-old youth was found in the basement of a vacant house. A gunshot wound, which indicated no evidence of close-range fire, was noted in his chest. The bullet had passed through the lungs and heart, and a relatively well-preserved .38 caliber lead bullet weighing 140.2 grain was recovered from under the skin of the chest wall on the opposite side. A second bullet wound was noted in the inner angle of the right eye. This injury was surrounded by an abundant amount of gunpowder and soot. A large irregular missile weighing 266.5 grain was found in the center of the brain (Fig. XII-110). From the appearance of this missile it was evident that two bullets had been joined together at the time of discharge. A defective .38 caliber revolver was later recovered and associated with this homicide.

Another instance where two bullets are discharged simultaneously may occur with Saturday night specials, usually .22 caliber. One bullet is discharged through the barrel while the second is ejected from the cylinder. In close shots, wounds are seen in such cases, usually side by side (Fig. XII-111). Not so with distance shots. Often the bullet which discharges from the cylinder is shaved off by the frame of the weapon.

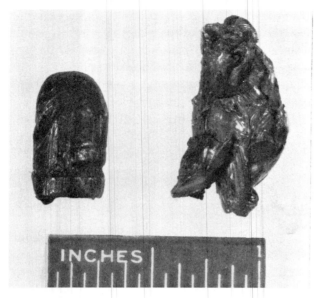

FIGURE XII-110. Well-preserved .38 caliber missile recovered from the chest of the victim (left) and *piggyback* bullet recovered from his brain (right).

Blank Cartridges

A blank cartridge is one with primer, gunpowder and wadding, but without a bullet. It contains a faster-burning propellant than an ordinary cartridge of the same caliber. Due to the considerable noise produced by this ammunition, it is used for starter pistols, signals, etc. Smokeless powder has largely replaced black powder in blank cartridges. Smokeless powder produces a larger amount of gas than black powder; consequently, blanks loaded with smokeless powder produce larger injuries. Experiments indicate that distant shots with blank cartridges are harmless; however, at a 1 inch distance significant tears of the skin and underlying tissues are observed regularly. At contact with the skin using .38 and .45 caliber blanks, devastating wounds are produced due to the large amount of

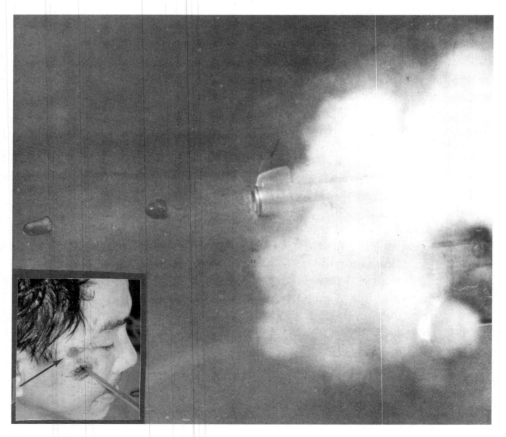

FIGURE XII-111. Test firing of a ramshackle revolver simultaneously ejecting two bullets. A similar weapon caused two side-by-side bullet wounds as shown in the insert. Note the lower wound on the cheek is a contact shot and would have come from the barrel while the one by the eye was from the shaved bullet which came from the cylinder.

gas generated by the exploding gunpowder. These wounds measure up to 3 by 2 inches and 2-1/2 inches in depth. A contact shot to the head with a blank cartridge can be fatal as a result of penetration of the skull and the concussive effect on the brain produced by sudden release of gases under tremendous pressure.

Stud Guns (Nail Guns)

Stud guns are firearm-like tools used in construction work for firing metal studs into steel, wood, or concrete. An interchangeable breech plug enables a choice of calibers, depending on the power required for adequate penetration. Calibers usually range from .22 to .38. Due to their marked penetration power, injuries by stud guns are severe. The size and shape of the stud and its tendency to tumble and ricochet are other features that cause atypical and larger wounds than those produced by ordinary bullets. The trajectory of these missiles are unpredictable and matching of the missile to the gun is not feasible.

A series of test shots into human cadavers indicates the destructive capacity of this tool.[19] The shots were fired at close and distant ranges using .22 caliber cartridges. At 27 inches, 6 feet and 9 feet studs struck the body sideways. Marginal abrasion of the wound in the skin was absent. The studs passed through the entire body and then penetrated a wooden block. At 3 inches, a wound in a thigh was a gaping circular defect measuring one inch in diameter. A shot of the forehead from this distance fractured the skull extensively. The stud exited posteriorly then penetrated a wooden block to a depth of several inches.

Zip Guns

Zip guns are usually homemade handguns which fire a single shot. Such weapons are dangerous to use and provide little or no accuracy and reliability. Some are crude to the point of consisting of a tube and some improvised type of firing device.

The use of zip guns is rare. The appearance of wounds produced by zip gun fire depends largely on the type of missile that is used and may be indistinguishable from a wound made by any ordinary bullet.

Ball Powder

Ball powder is a variety of smokeless gunpowder in which the grains are spheres rather than flakes or cylinders (Fig. XII-112). A non-jacketed bullet fired from a cartridge loaded with ball powder shows typical small indentations resembling *pockmarks* on its exposed lead base. These are due to the explosion in the cartridge at the time of discharge, which, by increasing the pressure in the cartridge, imprints the spherical grains of gunpowder on the soft lead bullet. There is considerable significance to ball powder, as it is mainly used in Winchester-Western ammunition. Since most ammunition is not loaded with ball powder, it is important, for exclusion purposes, to determine when such powder is used.

THE AUTOPSY

In addition to general information that is applicable to every autopsy report, the autopsy of a victim of gunfire should include at least the following observations:
• description of clothing
• pertinent findings regarding bullet wounds
• cause of death
• toxicological and serological analyses

The autopsy file should also include an adequate police report with a concise description of the scene. Appropriate sketches and photographs of the scene are desirable. Further guidelines

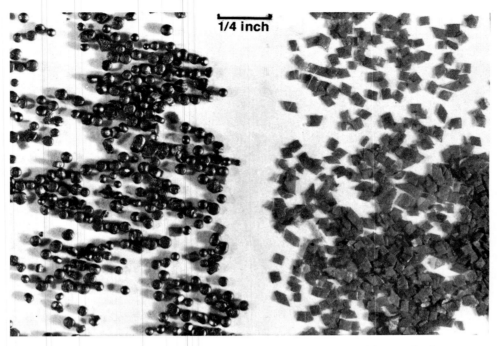

FIGURE XII-112. Two kinds of gunpowder. Left: Ball powder. Right: Flake powder (more commonly used).

concerning the medicolegal autopsy and different techniques of the postmortem examination are outlined in Chapters XXIV and XXV.

Description of Clothing

The body is to be disrobed with care. The clothing should not be torn or cut, and the examiner must be alert to the possibility of finding bullets among the clothing items. List all items and their condition and the extent of bloodstaining. The number and location of bullet holes should be recorded. It usually suffices to describe the number of bullet holes in the outer garment and to add that the bullet holes in the remaining items correspond in location to those already mentioned. The location of bullet holes in clothes is described in relation to the distance from the collar, seams, pockets, etc. Several holes may result from a single bullet due to creases and folds in the garment, simulating more than one shot.

Observe any evidence of close-range firing. Measure the extent of soot and gunpowder distribution, and note the density of powder stippling. This will enable subsequent comparison with test shot patterns for evaluation of the distance from which the weapon was fired. Record the size of the bullet hole in the garment. Mention whether the fibers of the fabric are frayed inward or outward; this may aid in determining the direction of the shot, particularly if other criteria are uncertain. Remember that blow back, in the case of a contact or near-contact shot, may cause fibers to be turned outward. Photography of pertinent findings is often helpful but does not replace a good description.

The clothing should be retained for subsequent examination by the police crime laboratory and a receipt must be obtained when handing over the items. If soiled with blood or otherwise wet, the clothes should be dried before storage. The pathologist must observe that his part in maintaining the chain of custody is preserved at all times.

Pertinent Findings Regarding Bullet Wounds

Number entrance and exit wounds and grazes, naming them accordingly. Lengthy descriptions tend to confuse. In the case of multiple gunshot wounds, it is advisable that a number be assigned to each wound, disregarding whether it was caused by entry or exit of a bullet.

The location of each wound should be described in relation to its distance from the top of the head (or the sole of the foot) and from the midline of the body, as well as from a recognized and relatively fixed landmark, e.g., "in the abdomen, 31 inches below the top of the head, 4 inches to the right of the midline and 6 inches below the umbilicus is located an entrance bullet wound. . . ." A diagram or a photograph showing the location of the numbered wounds is helpful. Following a close search for the presence of gunsmoke, hairy areas such as the scalp should be shaved to insure adequate documentation on a photograph.

One of the gravest errors made during the autopsy of President John F. Kennedy was the fact that the back of the head was never shaved. Thus, to this day, speculation and innuendoes persist regarding the exact location of the wound, and some even claim that this shot came from the front or the grassy knoll, at the right side of the President's motorcade, suggesting a conspiracy by at least two assassins (Fig. XII-113).

It is advisable that, the wound in the skin and the wound track through the body be recorded in the same section of the report entitled *Evidence of Injury*. Description of the injuries in this sequence will facilitate future recall and enable rapid reference. Two separate paragraphs are helpful.

External Evidence of Injury

Include any features of the bullet wound that distinguish it as an entrance or an exit wound. Describe the shape of the wound, such as stellate, round, oval, slit-like or jagged. Record the width of the marginal abrasion, particularly if it is oval, as in the case of a shot that strikes the body at an angle. Measure the wound and the diameter of powder residue deposits. Because of the considerable significance of the spread of soot and powder stippling on the body surface for estimating the range of fire, bodies should not be fingerprinted before the autopsy to avoid any possible contamination by fingerprint ink. If the distance from which a shot was fired is unknown and the presence of gunpowder inside the bullet wound is suspected, excision of the wound for microscopic examination is advisable. However, a bullet wound must never be excised until its description and measurements have been recorded and the autopsy has been completed. Because elastic fibers of the skin are severed during excision of the wound, neither dimensions nor the exact appearance of the wound can be preserved for adequate evaluation.

In gunshot wounds of the face, small slivers of tissue for microscopy can be obtained from the edges of a bullet wound without undue disfigurement.

Probing of wound tracks to establish direction of shot must be done with great care to avoid creating false pathways when inserting and guiding the probe within the tissues. The ideal probe is 12 inches long, with a knobby end about 3/16 inches in diameter. A small diameter probe is advantageous even for large caliber bullet wounds. A chrome-plated or polished metal probe will slide through a wound track, requiring minimal or no pushing. Vigorous pushing causes artefactual tracks, except in bone (Fig. XII-114).

When decomposition sets in, wound analysis is often difficult and maggot infestation of the body further complicates bullet wound interpretation. Maggots infesting a particular area on the body suggests the presence of an open wound in that location. Maggots feed on blood and soft tissues and seek shelter under the skin. Thus, a bullet wound is an ideal location (Fig. XII-115). Whenever, maggots are present, the wound is likely to be altered to the point of destroying evidence of direction of fire, i.e., entrance versus exit, and the distance of fire. In fact, as decomposition progresses, the bullet wound may become unrecognizable. The prosector should be aware of any underlying bone damage, and if present the direction of dispersion of bone fragments. X-ray may be revealing.

Internal Evidence of Injury

Describe the wound track in anatomical order. The path of the bullet is best documented by fol-

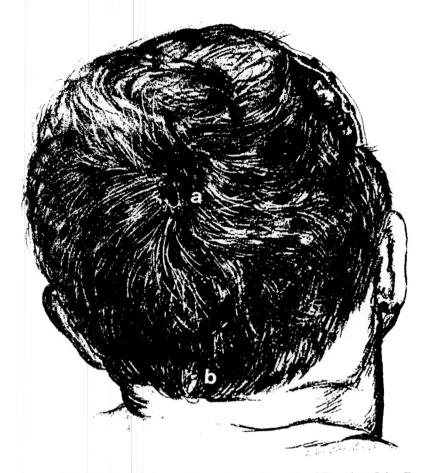

FIGURE XII-113. An artist's rendition of a photograph of President John F. Kennedy's head taken during the autopsy. What appears to be an entrance bullet wound is noted in the area of the cowlick. A small fragment suggestive of brain tissue is located closer to the nape of the neck. Comparison of the two areas certainly supports that the upper is the entrance wound. When one considers that the brain reacts to injury by swelling, it is understandable that brain tissue would have exuded from the entrance wound and spilled downward *(William E. Loechel, Medical Illustrator)*.

lowing the track of hemorrhage through the organs before their removal from the body. This will usually obviate the need for x-rays for locating the bullet. However, wound tracks through skeletal muscles are usually not associated with major bleeding and require a careful dissection technique.

Finally, a description of the missile path through the body should be given in relation to the planes of the body, e.g., "the wound track passes from front to back, from left to right, and slightly downward. . . ." Angular estimates of the wound track to the horizontal, vertical and sagittal planes of the body are also useful in completing the description.

In the absence of an exit wound, it is often rewarding to palpate the body opposite the wound of entrance in an attempt to locate the bullet under the skin. If the bullet is felt in this manner, it may be removed through a small incision and the location described. Such incision is best placed to the side of the area suspected of containing the bullet to avoid damaging the missile.

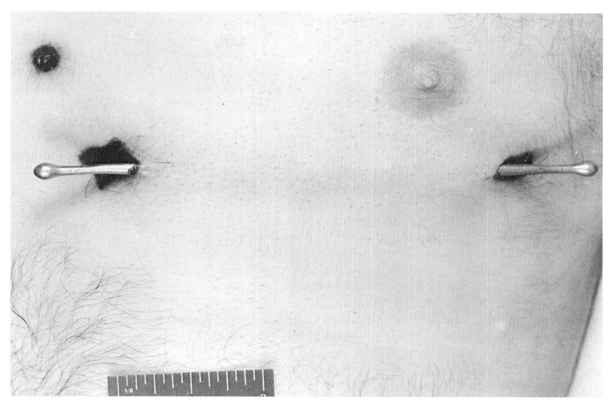

FIGURE XII-114. Probe used to show path of subcutaneous wound track.

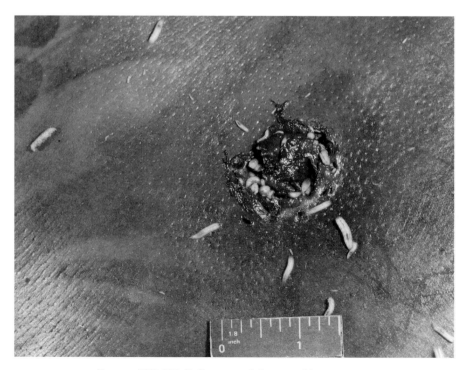

FIGURE XII-115. Bullet wound destroyed by maggots.

Handling the bullet with forceps or hemostats will destroy the features required for matching the missile with a particular firearm. Meticulous care to avoid scratching the bullet must be taken when removing a bullet from bone. Excision of the segment of bone containing the bullet, followed by manual bending and prying of the specimen, often releases the missile without actually handling it. All bullets and as many bullet fragments as possible should be recovered for subsequent firearm identification.

Occasionally, a bullet penetrates a hollow viscus and the wound track is interrupted. For example, a bullet in the stomach may be moved into the intestines while peristalsis continues. A bullet that penetrates the aorta may be transported with the bloodstream anywhere in the body. This is referred to as a *bullet embolism*. A wound track may also be interrupted by surgical procedures and as a result of healing, in cases of prolonged survival. Obviously, the use of x-ray in such situations is an invaluable time saver. An explanation in the autopsy report of the reasons for discontinuity of the wound track is advantageous.

Whenever a bullet is found, its appearance should be described accurately: intact, deformed or fragmented, lead or jacketed and the caliber, if known or small (.22), medium (.25 and .32) and large (.38, 9 mm, .357, .44, .45). The bullet should be marked for subsequent identification. The initials of the prosector are used ordinarily, but the case number or the initials of the victim serve the same purpose. The base of the bullet, or any other area which is devoid of identifying characteristics, is usually chosen for such marking. Photography of a bullet for later identification at trial is an excellent procedure.

Each bullet should be preserved in a separate envelope stating the name of the victim, date and number of the autopsy and location of the bullet, as well as the name of the prosector. Bullets placed together in the same container will rub against each other and cause damage, unless individually wrapped.

X-rays are sometimes used for assessing the caliber of a bullet, particularly in living patients if surgical removal of the missile is not clinically indicated. It must be remembered, that the dimensions of the bullet on the film represent a shadow, therefore, the image is larger than the actual dimensions of the bullet. Magnification and vagueness are increased the further the object is removed from the recording plane (Fig. XII-116). Anteroposterior and lateral roentgenograms are therefore mandatory. Even with such x-ray films, the exact caliber of a bullet remains speculative. Peculiar characteristics of a bullet, such as its shape and the presence of cannelures, are identifiable features.

The use of x-ray is of considerable value in the case of skeletonized remains. Bone fractures may be due to blunt injury or postmortem mutilation by animals. A fracture may also be caused by a perforating bullet. X-ray films of bullet tracks through bones may reveal the presence of minute scattered fragments of metal in fracture areas. The composition of these fragments may be analyzed and compared to that of projectiles found among the remains or at the scene, in the vicinity of the remains.

The skeletonized remains of a young male were found in a remote area of a public park. The upper half of the skeleton was resting on a wooden board to which was caked a cluster of approximately fifteen shotgun pellets. A .38 caliber lead bullet was found in the neck area, resting on one of the vertebrae. No fractures were noted in that region. Three ribs overlying the heart area showed fractures, and one rib had a track through it which measured the size of the lead pellets that were found behind the body.

X-ray of the skeleton showed minute metallic deposits along the rib fractures (Fig. XII-117). Analytical comparisons of this metal with the shotgun pellets showed an identical composition, indicating that the fractures were caused by the shotgun pellets and that death was due to a shotgun blast of the left side of the chest.

The .38 caliber bullet could not be associated with a particular injury, since no metallic deposits from this bullet could be identified in any of the bones. This bullet might have been present in the victim following a previous shooting incident.

Cause of Death

Hemorrhage is by far the most common cause of death in victims of gunfire. Depending on the organ or blood vessels involved, death from bleeding usually occurs within a few minutes to several hours. In gunshots of the abdomen with

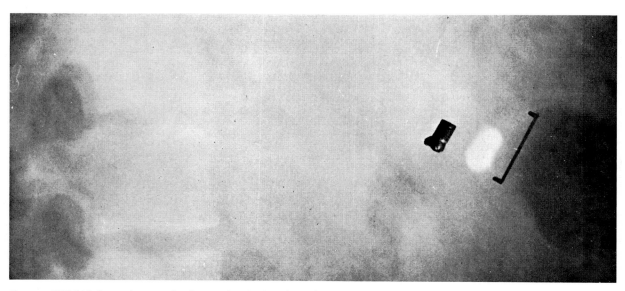

FIGURE XII-116. Lateral x-ray, displaying the shadow (white) of a .22 caliber bullet in a homicide victim. The bullet was located under the skin of the left side of the chest. After the autopsy, the bullet was placed on the x-ray film adjacent to its shadow and photographed to show the discrepancy in size. The line on the right is a 1 inch scale.

several days' survival, infection is the prevalent cause of death. Peritonitis develops due to leakage of contents from the perforated intestines into the abdominal cavity. Death from peritonitis may not occur until months after the injury.

Pneumonia develops frequently in cases of prolonged prostration and is especially common in gunshot wounds of the head with extended unconsciousness. Pulmonary embolism is a less frequent complication of injury by gunfire. This usually results from migrating blood clots which originate in the calves as a result of prolonged bed rest or if the extremity is immobilized due to fracture. Other complications of gunshot wounds occur, but because of their relative rarity they will not be listed.

Toxicological and Serological Analyses

Analyses should include determination of blood alcohol concentrations of the victim and his blood type/DNA. Comprehensive drug screening is of unquestionable advantage. Blood typing or DNA testing may furnish additional circumstantial information relating bloodstains found at a crime scene to the victim. The finding of a different blood type in stains would positively eliminate the victim as a source of this blood. In the case of several hours' survival, urine alcohol and drug determination may shed light on possible intoxication at the time of the incident (see Chapter XXIII).

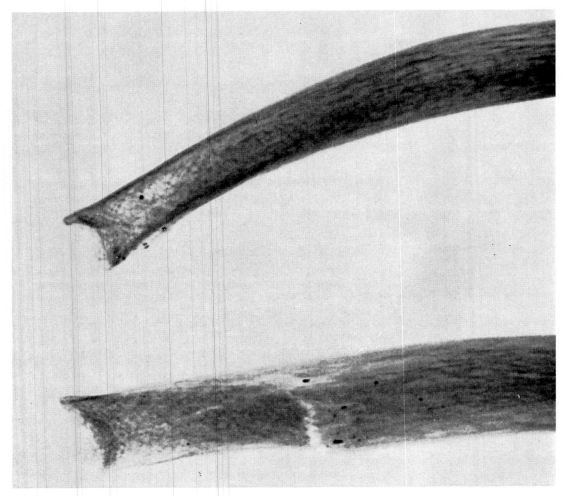

FIGURE XII-117. X-ray of ribs of an individual who was killed by a shotgun blast. Minute fragments of lead are deposited in the ribs along pellets' pathways.

REFERENCES

1. Federal Bureau of Investigation Uniform Crime Reports, 2002.
2. MacCrehan, W.A., Layman, M.J., and Secl, J.D.: Hair combing to collect organic gunshot residues (OGSR). *Forensic Sci Int, 135:* 167–173, 2003.
3. Schmidt-Orndorff, H.S., Reitz, J.A., and Spitz, W.U.: Peculiarities of certain .22 caliber revolvers (Saturday night specials). *J Forensic Sci, 19* (1): 48, 1974.
4. Gilmore, H. R.: Medical aspects of the assassination of Abraham Lincoln. *Proc R Soc Med, 47:* 103, 1954.
5. Adelson, L.: A microscopic study of dermal gunshot wounds. *Am J Clin Pathol, 35:* 393, 1961.
6. Janssen, W.: *Forensic histopathology.* Translated by S. Forster. Berlin: Springer-Verlag, 1984.
7. DiMaio, V.J.M.: *Gunshot wounds,* 2nd edition. New York: CRC Press, 1999.
8. Sellier, K.: *Schusswaffen und Schusswirkungen.* Lubeck, Schmidt-Romhild, 1969, p. 44.
9. Light, F.W.J.: Gunshot wounds of entrance and exit in experimental animals. *J Trauma, 3:* 120–128, 1963.

10. Spitz, W.U.: Rikoschett-oder Kontaktschussverletzung. *Dtsch Z Ges Gerichtl Med, 66:* 153, 1969.

11. Graham, J.W., Petty, C.S., Flohr, D.M., and Peterson, W.E.: Forensic aspects of frangible bullets. *J Forensic Sci, 11:* 507, 1966.

12. Davis, J.H.: Bodies found in the water. *Am J Forensic Med Path, 7:* 291–297, 1986.

13. Garavaglia, J.C., and Talkington, B.: Weapon location following suicidal gunshot wounds. *Am J Forensic Med Path, 20* (1): 1–5, 1999.

14. Thornton, J.: The effect of tempered glass on bullet trajectory. *Assoc of Firearms and Tool Mark Examiners, AFTE, 15* (3): 29, 1983.

15. Spitz, W.U., Petty, C.S., and Fisher, R.S.: Physical activity until collapse following fatal injury by firearms and sharp weapons. *J Forensic Sci, 6:* 290, 1961.

16. DiMaio, V.J.M., and Spitz, W.U.: Variations in wounding due to unusual firearms and recently available ammunition. *J Forensic Sci, 17:* 377, 1972.

17. DiMaio, V.J.M., and Spitz, W.U.: Injury by birdshot. *J Forensic Sci, 15:* 396, 1970.

18. Breitenecker, R., and Senior, W.: Shotgun patterns. I. An experimental study on the influence of intermediate targets. *J Forensic Sci, 12:* 193, 1967.

19. Spitz, W.U., and Wilhelm, R.M.: Stud gun injuries. *J Forensic Med, 17:* 5, 1970.

Part 2

SHOTGUN WOUNDS

WERNER U. SPITZ

HOTGUNS OR SCATTER GUNS were developed as an alternate to the single-missile rifle or handgun in order to enable the shooter to spray a wide area with shot and thus kill birds and other small animals too difficult to hit with single-missile weapons. As the popularity of shotguns grew, ammunition was developed for larger game. The use of shotguns on humans is common, and indeed, special improvisations, such as the *sawed-off* shotgun, attest to their effectiveness.

The inherent differences in these weapons and their ammunition are reflected in the typical wounds which they cause. Nevertheless, reconstruction of range and direction of shotgun fire is similar to that of single-missile weapons.

Shotgun ammunition is diverse; the prime difference is in the multiplicity of missiles which vary from 1, as in the rifled slug, through 9 to 12 in 00 buckshot, to as many as 270 in the 12 gauge No. 9 birdshot. The number of the shot is the diameter of the individual lead pellets. Thus, the diameter of No. 9 birdshot is .08 inches. The diameter of 00 buckshot is .33 inches, which is similar to that of a .32 caliber bullet.

The gauge of a shotgun indicates the inside diameter of its bore. It is an antiquated measure defined as the number of lead balls, each of the diameter of the bore, together weighing one pound. Thus, for a 12-gauge barrel, a lead ball would weigh 1/12 pound or 1-1/3 ounces. This measure is still used in all, except the .410 shotgun, .410 reflects the bore of the barrel as measured in inches. The 12-gauge is by far the most used and, with a variable choke, is the most versatile shotgun available.

The smooth bore of a shotgun may be of uniform diameter, as in *cylinder bore* weapons, or it may be narrowed at the muzzle to a lesser or greater degree, as in *medium* and *full choke* guns. The degree of choke obviously modifies the spread of pellets and governs the size of the shot pattern at a given distance from the muzzle. The

choke of a gun barrel is usually expressed in shot percentages that fall within a 30-inch circle at 40 yards:

65%–75% . . . . .full choke
55%–65% . . . . .modified
45%–55% . . . . .improved cylinder
35%–45% . . . . .cylinder bore

Whereas, shotguns have their own characteristics, in conducting test firing to determine range of fire, it is significantly more important to use the identical ammunition than the same weapon.

Contact and Near-Contact Shotgun Wounds

The characteristics already described for small arms fire, particularly those of close-range shots, are also observed in shotgun wounds, except that the injury pattern of the latter is significantly more extensive and devastating as compared to wounds caused with conventional handguns. In general, it may be said that at close range, the destructive force of a shotgun compares with that of a high-power rifle.

The typical contact range shotgun wound in areas except the head, measures the approximate diameter of the barrel. Marginal abrasion of the wound, similar to that of a single bullet gunshot wound is observed as the shot penetrates the body in a conglomerate mass (Figs. XII-118a–b to XII-122). The wound edges are blackened by gun smoke. Inside the wound abundant soot and gunpowder may be recognized by granularity of the tissues, resembling scattered fine sea sand. In the heart area, massive hemorrhage may have *washed out* most powder residue. In the abdomen, omental fat, or rarely a loop of small bowel may protrude through the wound. Cherry-red discoloration of the skin and underlying muscle surrounding a chest wound may be due to carbon monoxide from the yellow flame of the muzzle blast, but more likely is the result of oxyhemo-

Injury by Gunfire   707

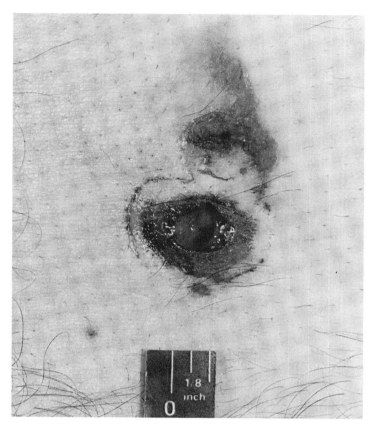
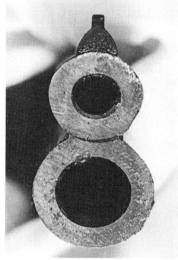

FIGURES XII-118a–b. (a) Contact shot with sawed-off, over and under, rifle shotgun combination. (b) The shotgun part was discharged, the rifle was not. The right side of the shotgun wound shows short, parallel, horizontal, equidistant lines which represent saw marks on the end of the barrel.

FIGURE XII-119. Double-barrel shotgun wounds inflicted at contact range. Each of the wounds represents the gauge of the muzzle (12 gauge).

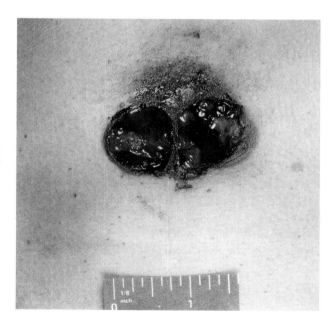

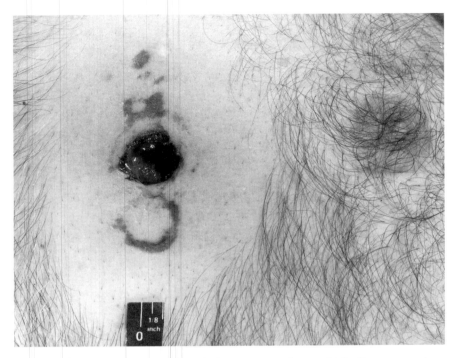

FIGURE XII-120. Muzzle imprint with distinctive markings which allow comparison with weapon.

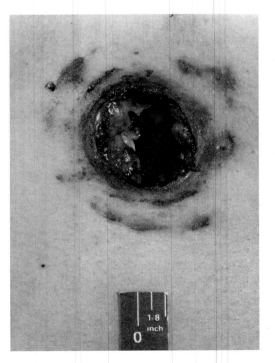

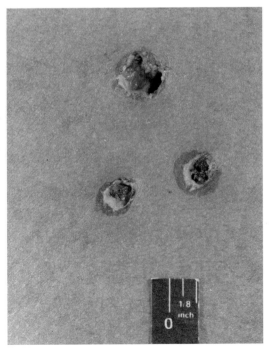

FIGURE XII-121. Contact shot with 12 gauge shotgun showing muzzle imprint and abundant soot within the wound. The three wounds on the right are *shored* exits of 00 buck (32 caliber) pellets.

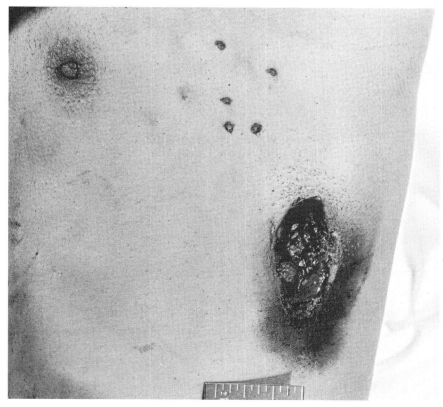

FIGURE XII-122. Near-contact .410 shot in the left side of the chest showing abundant soot and gunpowder at the lower edge and stippling at the upper edge. Five pellets exited and numerous pellets were found under the skin. This is a stickup-type injury.

globin, due to the presence of arterial blood from injury of the lung or the left side of the heart. Analyses of the carboxyhemoglobin content in these tissues have shown a concentration not exceeding 15%. Cherry-red discoloration of carboxyhemoglobin is usually not observable at this low level. Tissues around contact abdominal shotgun wounds often display a brownish hue, presumably due to intestinal gases.

In the head, contact shotgun wounds are devastating (Figs. XII-123 and XII-124). The restricted space for gas expansion causes fragmentation of the skull and vast lacerations of the soft tissues. The contour of the head is often destroyed and facial features are unrecognizable due to extensive mutilation.

The point of muzzle contact or entry wound, may be difficult to locate, especially if the muzzle had been placed in the mouth or under the chin. In all cases involving the head, bone and soft tis-

sues may be scattered over a wide area and the entire brain may be eviscerated and often shredded. It is essential that all bone fragments be obtained and re-assembled in order to locate the wound of entry. Superficial and deep tears of the face, specifically the inner angles of the eyes, the sides of the nose and mouth and in front of the ears, are the result of overstretching of the skin by a tremendous increase of intracranial pressure created by the large quantity of gases *injected* into the head (Figs. XII-125 and XII-126).

At autopsy, it is often possible to determine which fractures were the result of gas expansion versus those caused by the direct impact of pellets. Fractures situated in areas where pellets did not reach, often including the facial skeleton would be explosive fractures from gases.

At loose contact, there is considerable scorching and soot and powder residue soiling on the target surrounding the entry wound (Fig. XII-

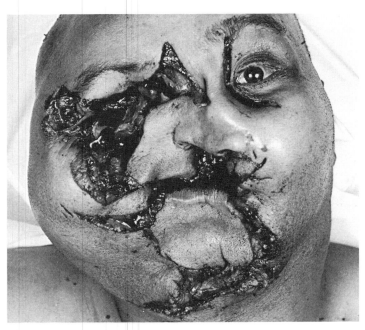

FIGURE XII-123. 12 gauge shotgun blast at contact range under the chin. The tears at the inner angles of the eyes and the sides of the mouth are the result of massive expansion of the head caused by the gases of the discharge. On both cheeks are noted a few, stretchmark-like epidermal tears.

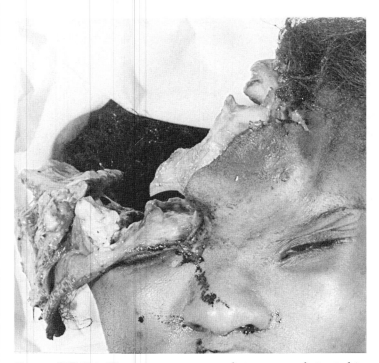

FIGURE XII-124. 12 gauge, near-contact shotgun wound situated in the center of the forehead. Soot is noted on the skin. The brain was shredded and only small portions of the brain stem and cerebellum were left within the cranium. No pellets or wad were recovered from inside the head.

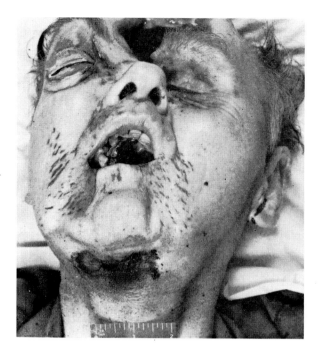

FIGURE XII-125. Contact shot, using 12 gauge shotgun with No. 6 shot, below the chin. The facial skeleton is fragmented, and tears caused by overstretching are noted on both sides of the mouth and the inner angles of the eyes. The shot partly exited from the top of the head.

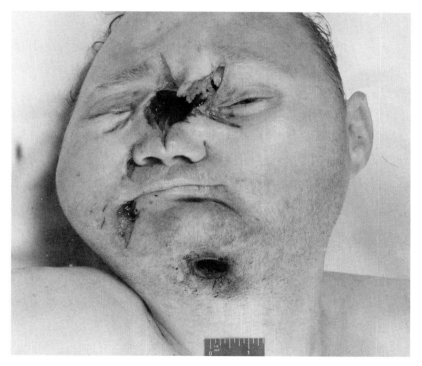

FIGURE XII-126. Contact shotgun wound below the chin. Overstretching tears on the right side of the mouth and under both eyes. The wound in the nose was a partial exit. The face is deformed as a result of fragmentation of the skull, mostly from the gases.

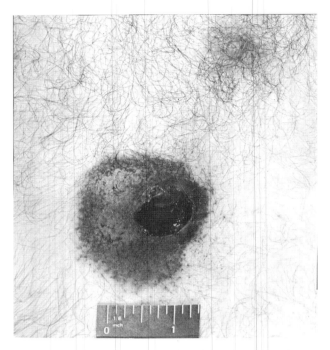

FIGURE XII-127. Near-contact shot showing soot and gunpowder deposit, as well as singeing of the skin and hair. The direction of shot is from left to right as depicted.

127). The shotgun muzzle flame is large and intense and the fact that clothes do not usually catch on fire in shots fired from a distance of a few inches, within the reach of the muzzle flame, is to a greater extent due to the reduced flammability of present-day fabrics rather than gunpowder characteristics.

Annular abrasions surrounding a shotgun entry wound at a distance of up to 1 inch are the result of *blow back* which stretches the skin around the wound (Fig. XII-128). Similar and often larger patterned abrasions may be seen occasionally in distant shots due to elevation of the skin against tight articles of overlying clothes by the mass of pellets (Figs. XII-129 to XII-131).

Close-Range Shotgun Wounds

The discharge of a shotgun will likely reach the target as a single mass when fired from a distance of 4 to 5 feet. At this distance, the shot will usually penetrate through a round defect which can measure the size of the barrel up to a two-inch diameter. The margins of such wounds, in addition to showing abrasion, are apt to display scalloping, due to spreading of some peripheral lead pellets. In gunner's terminology, this phenomenon is often described as a *cookie cutter* pattern (Figs. XII-132a–b to XII-135a–b).

Beyond this range, the diameter of the wound increases, as the load begins to fan out and stray pellets penetrate independently, away from the main entry. The minimal distance for the spread of pellets to occur is variable. It may be 3 or 4 feet with some sawed-off shotguns (Fig. XII-136), but tends to be 6 feet (Fig. XII-137) or more with a cylinder bore barrel and as great as 18 feet with a full choke shotgun.

To make a substantial difference in target pattern, a shotgun would have to be sawed off to a barrel length of 9 to 10 inches. Police departments often use 18 or 20 inch barrel lengths for easier and faster handling. Regular hunting shotguns have barrel lengths varying from 28 to 36 inches.

At distances up to 4 or 5 feet, the average shotgun will deposit considerable powder and some soot and smoke soiling on the clothing or skin.

Irregular and patterned abrasions are occasionally seen in the immediate vicinity of the wound. These are caused by the abrasive effect of clothing on the stretched skin during penetration of the mass of pellets. Such abrasions are more frequently observed in wounds caused by rifled slugs, when the bulk of lead pushes the clothing forward into the wound. Obviously, rough fabrics tend to have a more abrasive effect (Figs. XII-138a–b to XII-140).

Most shotgun wounds are inflicted at contact and close range. Distance shots are far less frequent. When shotguns are used in robberies, many shootings involve a shot to the side of the chest. This is the same type of injury and location seen in *stickups* (Figs. XII-141 and XII-142).

Defense wounds may be observed in shotgun injuries as with any other type of violence (Fig. XII-143).

In the case of multiple shots, it is important to determine the approximate distance of fire for each and if possible, the sequence of the shots (Fig. XII-144).

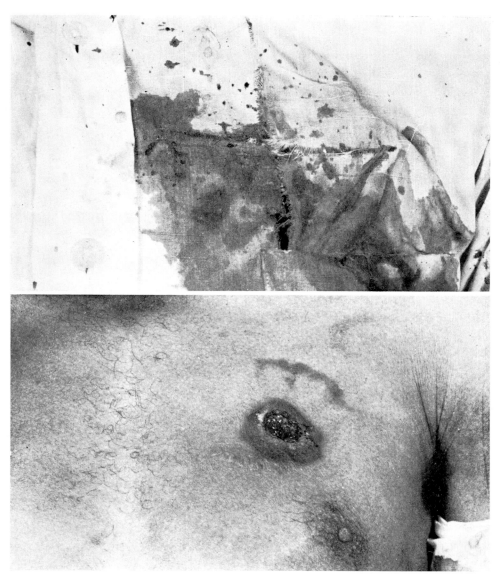

FIGURE XII-128. Contact wound with 12 gauge shotgun. Note that no fabric of the shirt is missing, even though it is torn. The muzzle was placed under the shirt, between the buttons. The tears were caused by *blow back*. The abraded area above the wound was due to stretching of the skin by *blow back* and gases expanding under the skin.

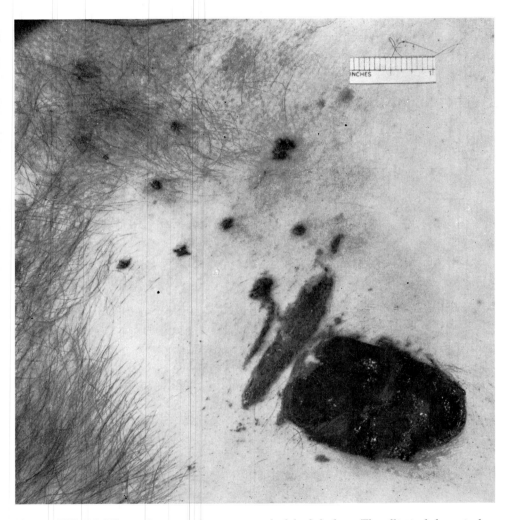

FIGURE XII-129. Elliptical contact shotgun wound of the left chest. The elliptical shape is due
to the direction of the shot from below, upwards and to the right. The linear abrasions and due
to stretching of the skin and a ball-point pen in the pocket, as blow back of gases occurred. The
discrete perforations are due to exiting shot ricocheting from the main mass of pellets. *(See later
in this chapter.)*

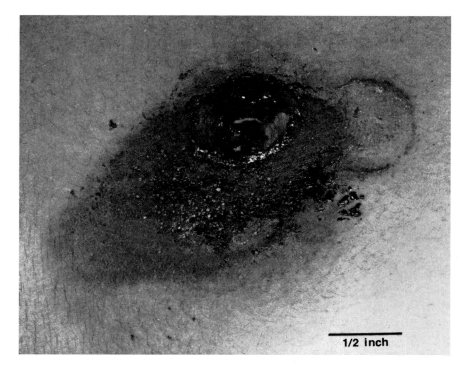

FIGURE XII-130. Self-inflicted shotgun wound of the chest. Muzzle imprint of a double-barrel 20 gauge shotgun fired at loose contact. Only the left barrel was discharged. The muzzle imprint of the right barrel is due to *blow back* as the gases expanded under the skin.

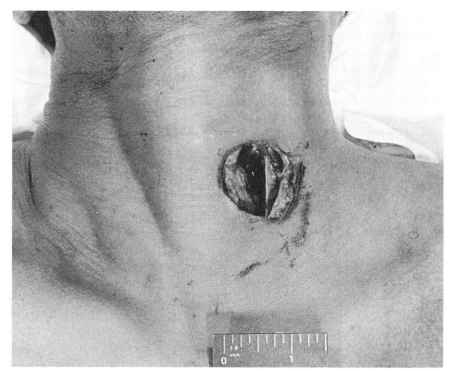

FIGURE XII-131. Shotgun blast of the neck. The abrasions near the wound are the result of elevation of the skin against tight overlying clothes.

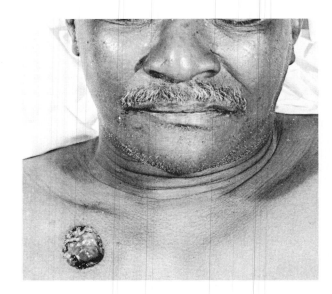

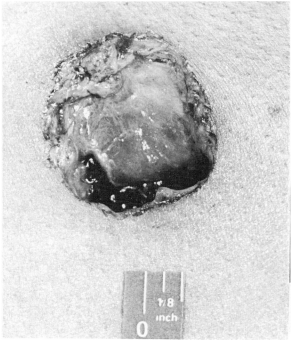

FIGURE XII-132a–b. Shotgun wounds showing cookie cutter pattern.

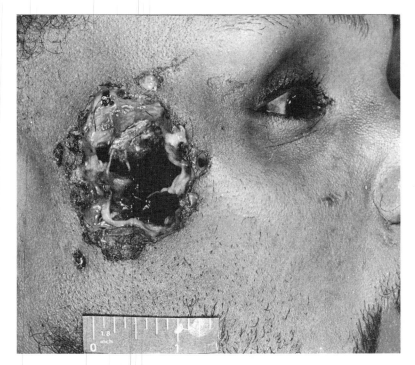

FIGURE XII-133. Cookie cutter pattern of temple with early separation of birdshot.

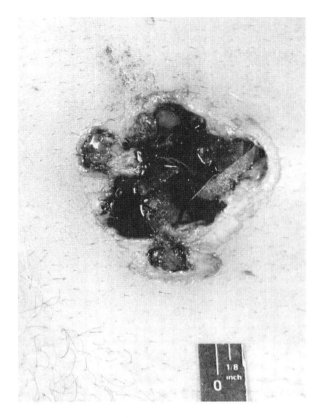

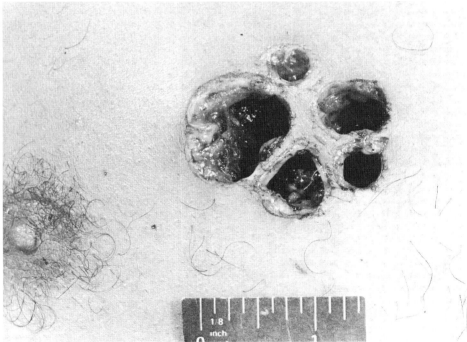

FIGURE XII-134a–b. (a) Bunched 00 buckshot showing wound with cookie cutter pattern. Shot was fired from a distance of 3 to 4 feet. (b) Same individual shot with same ammunition from slightly greater distance. The pellets were separating causing multiple wounds.

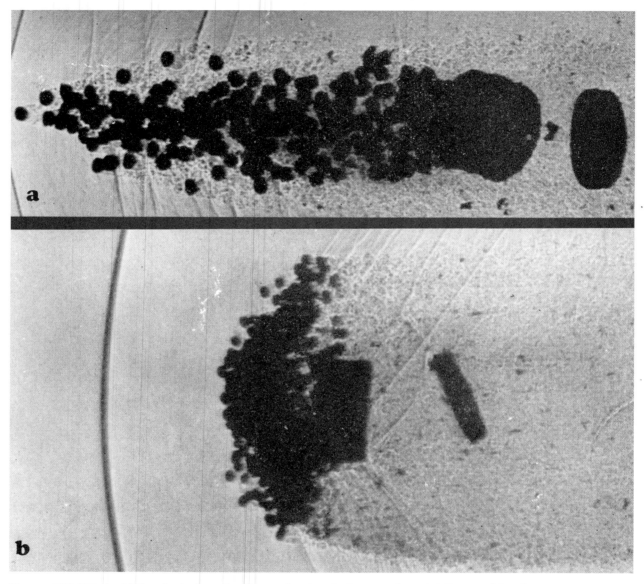

FIGURE XII-135a–b. (a) Bunched, aligned pellets early after discharge with wad following. (b) Pellets are beginning to spread out, but are still tightly bunched, six feet after discharge from a long-barreled shotgun with medium choke. Pellets would cause a cookie cutter pattern. Wad is still following.

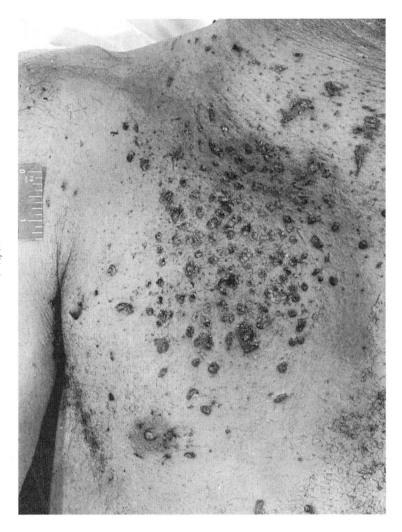

FIGURE XII-136. *Sawed-off* shotgun with barrel length of 10 inches fired from a distance of about 3 feet. Note the pellet wounds intermixed with gunpowder stippling.

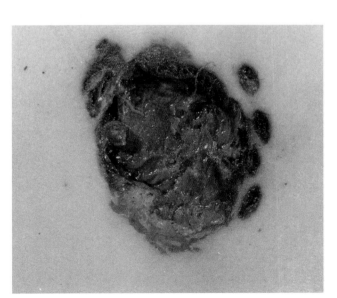

FIGURE XII-137. Wound showing early separation of pellets caused by a regular shotgun with medium choke at about six feet.

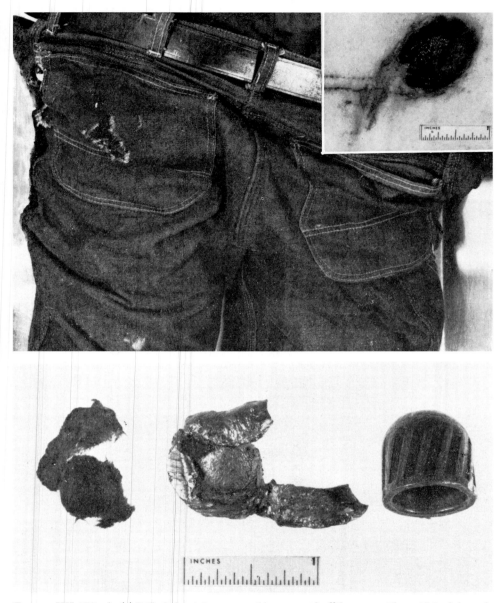

FIGURE XII-138a–b. (a) Rifled slug injury caused by a *sawed-off* shotgun with an 18 inch barrel, fired from a distance of 40 feet. Note the pocket seam of the denim pants imprinted on the skin (insert). Compare with Figure XII-139, which shows a similar pattern. (b) Same case as shown in Figure XII-138(a). Deformed slug (center) and wadding (left) removed from the body. An intact rifled slug is shown on the right for comparison.

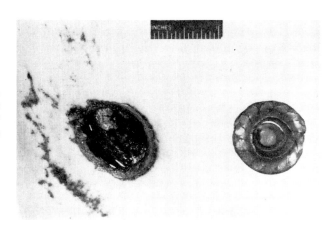

FIGURE XII-139. Rifled slug injury by a 12 gauge shotgun, fired from a distance of 100 feet. Note the characteristic marginal abrasion, but there is also an unusual annular abrasion and contusion of the skin, due to impact of the leather jacket, which was stretched by the penetrating slug.

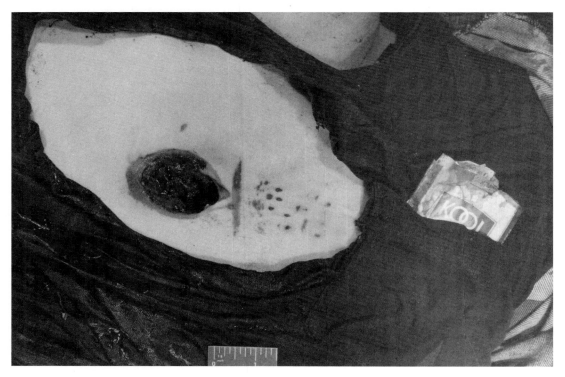

FIGURE XII-140. Birdshot injury with exit wounds. The vertical abrasion between the entrance and exits was caused by elevation of the skin against the pack of cigarettes.

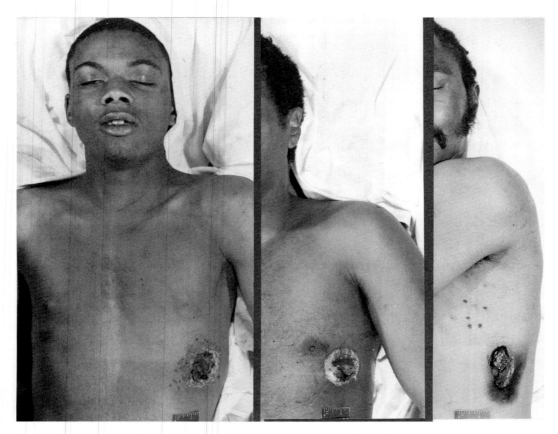

FIGURE XII-141. Examples of *stickup-type* injuries: near-contact on the *right* with exit wounds; from a distance of 5 or 6 feet, *center;* from 10 feet, *left*.

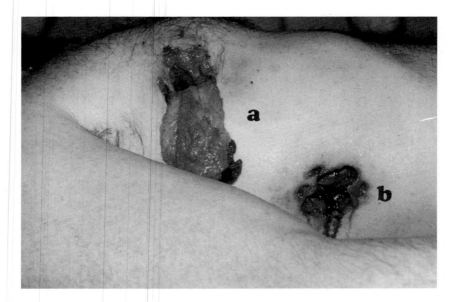

FIGURE XII-142. Two 00 Buck shotgun wounds inflicted in rapid succession. Injury (a) was inflicted first. Internal tissues were pushed out of (a) when the second shot (b) was fired. Both wounds are *stickup-type*.

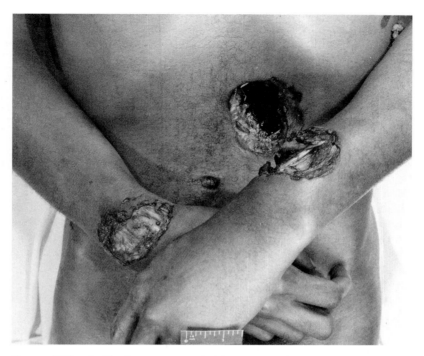

FIGURE XII-143. The forearms were held in front of the body for defense.

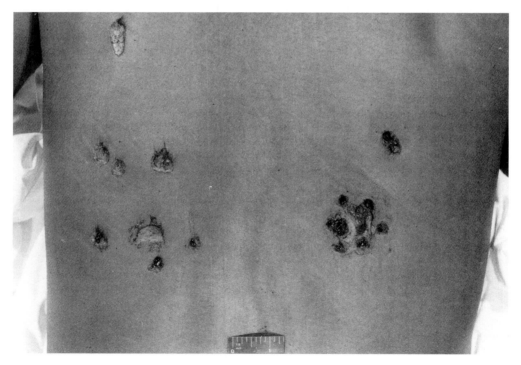

FIGURE XII-144. Two shotgun wounds. The injury on the right was inflicted from a closer range than the injury on the left. It would seem logical that both injuries were sustained as the victim was collapsing and bent forward to account for the stray single pellet above each wound.

Distant Shotgun Wounds

The pattern made by a shotgun from a distance of over a few feet varies with the choke, length of barrel, powder load, size of shot and gauge of the gun and is further modified by varying designs of the inner liner within the shotgun shell (Figs. XII-145 and XII-146). For example, the Remington power piston and post wad, the Winchester AA trap and skeet shot shell and the Winchester winwad are all variants of devices built into the shell itself that will modify the pattern. In general, these are devices designed to improve the pattern by reducing the number of stray pellets and by compressing the pattern into a tighter circle, but some have the opposite effect.

With small shot individual pellets penetrating the skin produce round wounds with narrow marginal abrasion (Figs. XII-147 to XII-154); in the case of buckshot, the individual wounds closely resemble bullet wounds (Figs. XII-155 and XII-156a–b). A rifled slug represents the largest bullet fired by any conventional low

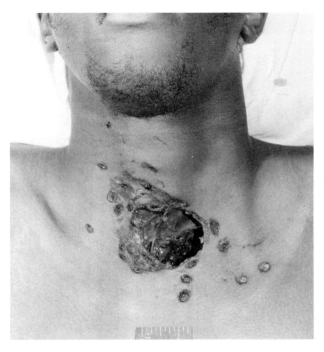

FIGURE XII-145. Shotgun wound showing early spread. The weapon was a 12 gauge shotgun, cylinder bore, loaded with No. 6 shot and fired from a distance of approximately 8 to 10 feet.

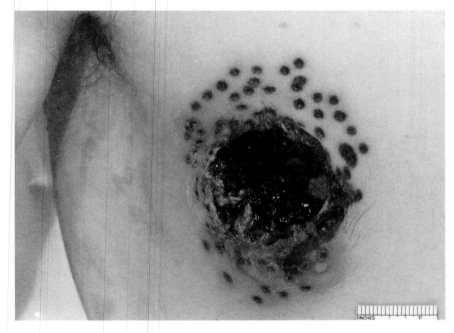

FIGURE XII-146. Injury by a 12 gauge pump action shotgun and No. 5 shot from a distance of 10 to 12 feet.

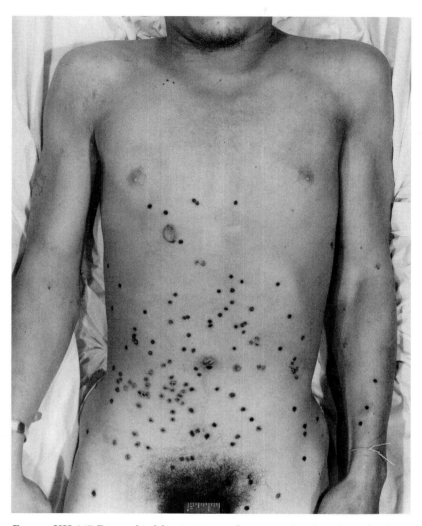

FIGURE XII-147. Distant birdshot injuries and imprint of wad on the right chest.

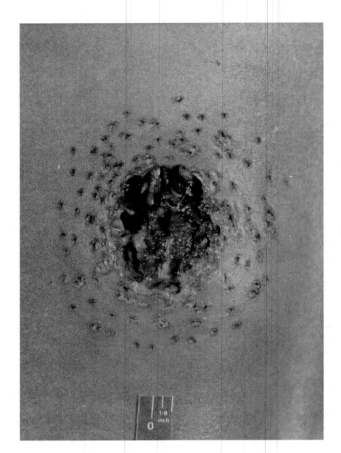

FIGURE XII-148

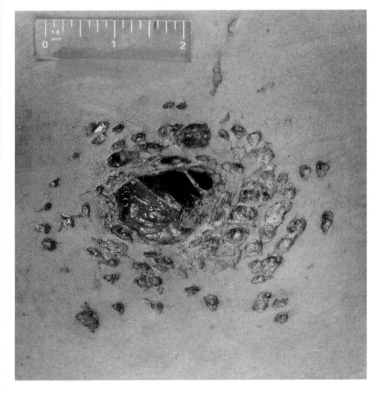

FIGURE XII-149. Two shots fired from a distance of 15 to 20 feet. The wads are deep within the wounds.

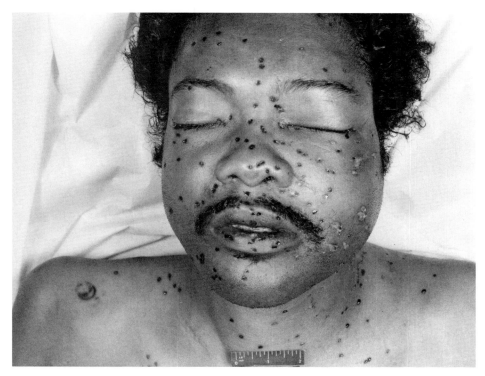

FIGURE XII-150. Birdshot injuries with wad imprint on the right shoulder.

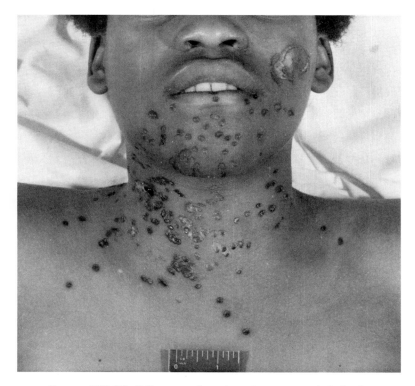

FIGURE XII-151. Pellet wounds with wad imprint on left cheek.

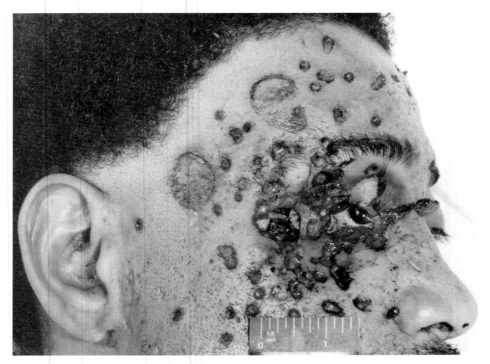

FIGURE XII-152. Clustered pellet wounds with two wad imprints.

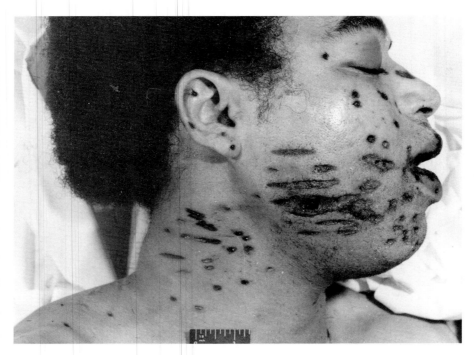

FIGURE XII-153. Grazing pellet wounds of the right cheek.

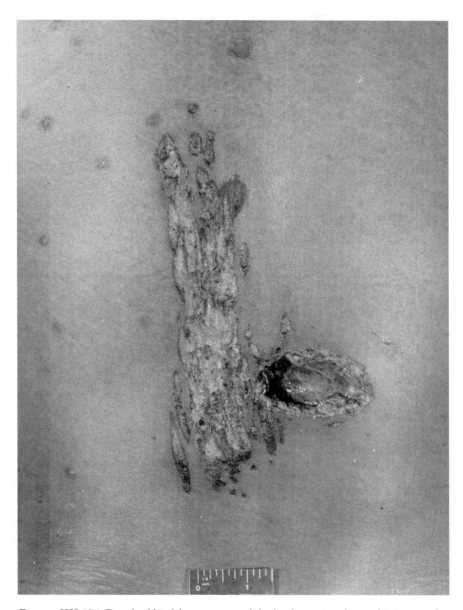

FIGURE XII-154. Bunched birdshot penetrated the back causing the oval injury on the right. Discreet pellets from this shot are spread under the skin on the left, obviously a shallow shot *(billiard ball effect, see later in this chapter),* as also suggested by the oval shape of the entrance. Distance of fire, probably around 5 to 6 feet. A second shot grazed the skin as the body was collapsing probably due to the first shot which severed the spine. It would appear that both shots were fired from the same or similar distance.

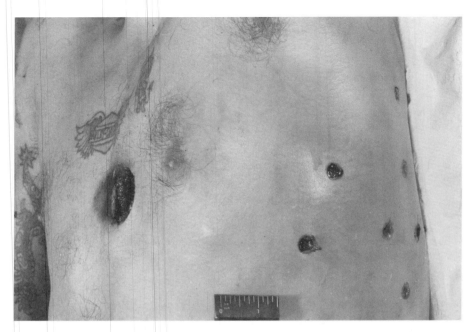

FIGURE XII-155. Contact shot of left side of chest, with 12 gauge shotgun and 00 buck. Note seven exit wounds, two wounds are not shown. The exit wounds resemble gunshots.

velocity weapon available outside of military channels.

In addition to holes in the skin made by entering shot, the target frequently shows larger circular or elliptical contused and abraded areas, due to impact of the shotgun wadding. A wad may cause a typical injury as illustrated in Figures XII-147, XII-150 to XII-152 and XII-156a–b, up to a distance of 50 feet. However, whereas a wad may penetrate the body, it will only do so if bunched pellets create the opening, i.e., a wound large enough to accommodate the wad. Thus, occasionally a wad may be found lodged in the opening (Figs. XII-157 and XII-158a–d). At ranges in excess of 10 or 12 feet, the wad is unlikely to penetrate the body. It is important that the wad be recovered whenever possible, since its diameter corresponds to the gauge of the gun and will disclose the manufacturer of the particular ammunition. Plastic wads retain their shape and diameter within the body, but old type felt and cardboard wads soak up blood and body fluids and swell, often causing the diameter to be altered.

For the purpose of identification, cup wads of .410 ammunition have 3 petals as compared to 4 with other gauges. The petals of such plastic wads may mark the skin around the entry wound at close range. Sometimes, in the case of a sawed-off shotgun or a mutilated muzzle, possibly caused by previous dropping of the gun, irregularities or rough edges of the muzzle may be transferred to the wad, such irregularities may assist in identifying a particular weapon.

A rule of thumb for estimating distance of fire for birdshot injuries is: Measure the largest cluster of wounds in inches, multiply the finding by 3 to obtain the number of feet from which the weapon was fired. This is assuming that the shot encountered no intermediary target.

Patterns of Shotgun Wounding

Suicidal shotgun wounds are nearly always fired at contact or very close range, since the length of the barrel and the length of the victim's arm do not allow for true distant firing. Occasionally, suicidal shots are inflicted using a stick or a string to pull or push the trigger. Rarely, the weapon is discharged by the use of a big toe. Removal of a shoe, sock, or cutting the sock to

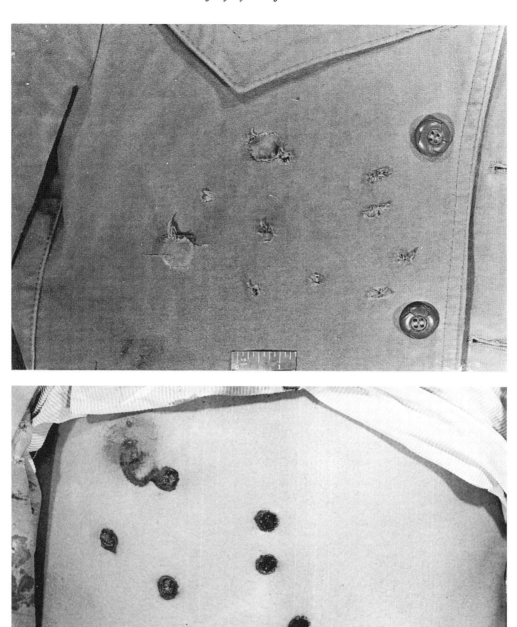

FIGURE XII-156a–b. (a) Coat of victim shown in Figure IX-156 (b) depicting pellet wounds and two circular impacts by wads. (b) Distant 00 buckshot wounds. Wad injury is noted below the nipple. Nine individual pellet wounds indicate the entire load struck the victim.

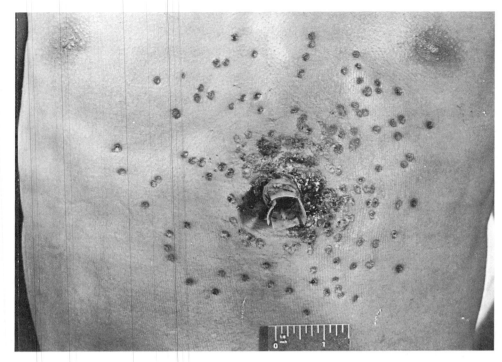

FIGURE XII-157. Sawed-off shotgun injury. The weapon was fired from a distance of 15 feet. The wad partially penetrated the chest.

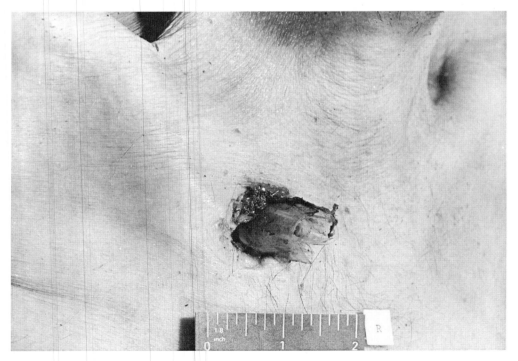

FIGURE XII-158a. Plastic liner protruding from the wound inflicted at close range. The collar bone stopped the liner from penetrating in its entirety.

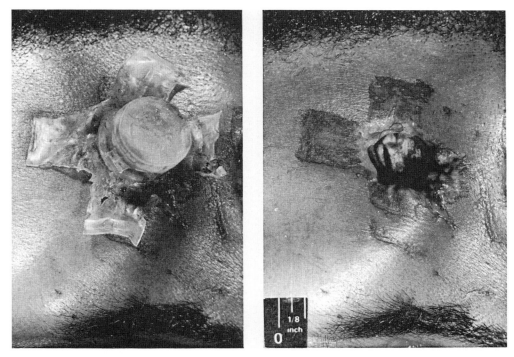

FIGURE XII-158b. Shot with 12 gauge shotgun. Four petals of the plastic wad are imprinted on the skin.

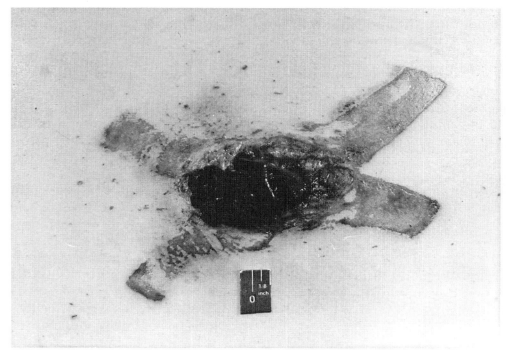

FIGURE XII-158c. X-shaped imprint of plastic wad. The wound was inflicted from an angle which accounts for the oversize of the right petal imprints. *(Courtesy, Jason D. Brown, St. Clair Shores Police Department, Michigan).*

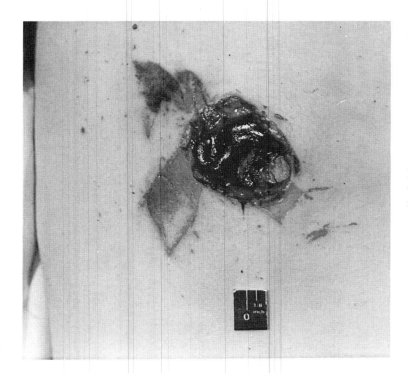

Figure XII-158d. Peculiar abrasions are sometimes seen in the vicinity of shotgun wounds from wad impacts.

expose the big toe, is likely to be important in ruling out an accidental manner of shooting. Placement of the shotgun muzzle in the mouth causes tremendous destruction of the head. A shot in the mouth is usually indicative of suicide.

Accidental shotgun wounding shows many variants, principally related to carelessness in handling the weapon. Determination of the range of fire is critical in such cases, provided the shotgun and the ammunition that was used to inflict the wound are available for test firing.

A twenty-four-year-old man had reportedly committed suicide by shooting himself in the head. Investigation revealed that there had been an altercation between the deceased and his landlord. Examination of the wound indicated that it had been inflicted from a distance of several feet, excluding the likelihood of suicide.

The weapon, an old single-shot 12-gauge shotgun, was test fired using the same ammunition as in the case under consideration (No. 6 shot). The test shot from a distance of 10 feet, closely resembled the pattern of the wound of the victim, indicating that the deceased was shot from approximately that distance. The landlord was charged with murder and confessed to the crime (Fig. XII-159a–c).

Whenever there is allegation of accidental shooting in an attempt to mask a homicide, test firing at different ranges will produce a target pattern similar in size and density to that of the victim. This enables evaluation of the circumstances of the incident and testing of the suspect's alibi.

In attempting to determine the range of fire in decomposed, burned, or otherwise mutilated remains where the skin pattern is not readily identifiable, x-ray examination may be of assistance, but results must be interpreted with caution. At close range, small pellets, such as birdshot, reach the body in a single mass, the pellets strike one another as they penetrate. They then spray out in a wide pattern as they continue on into the body.[1,2] This produces a wide dispersion of the shot and may lead to significant overestimation of the range of fire. The same occurs if the shot strikes any other primary target, such as a door or window, before reaching the victim. The phenomenon may be compared to billiard balls hit at the break by the cue ball and is appropriately termed the *billiard ball ricochet effect*. Only when the range of fire is such that the pellets are spread out before striking the target will final shot dispersion, as shown by x-ray, yield a true picture of the range of fire (Figs. XII-160a–d to XII–164).

In contact shots of the head, the opposite inner surface of the skull often shows small round black

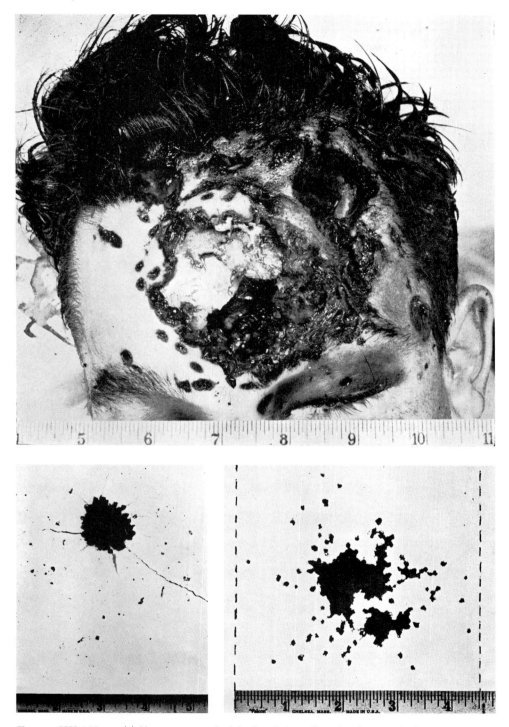

FIGURE XII-159a–c. (a) Shotgun wound of the head, first alleged to be suicide. Diameter of the wound is approximately 4 1/2 inches. (b) Pattern at 3 feet is 1 3/8 inch diameter, ruling out suicide in the absence of a contraption. (c) Pattern at 10 feet is similar to that of the deceased, who was shot from the doorway of his bedroom in which he was asleep.

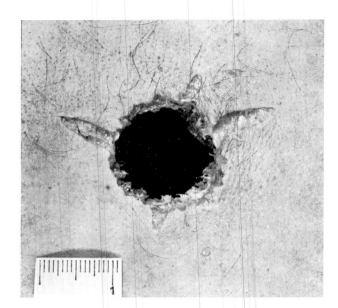

FIGURE XII-160a–d. Experimentally produced billiard ball ricochet effect, with 12 gauge shotgun loaded with No. 6 shot. Note the different skin wounds (a and c), but almost identical x-ray patterns of shot spread in the body (b and d). (a) Wound inflicted from a distance of 4 feet, shows the scalloped *cookie cutter* pattern, but almost identical x-ray patterns of shot. The stellate shape of the wound is not usually seen in shotgun injuries inflicted from this distance. It is attributed to congealed fat under the skin due to refrigeration. (b) X-ray of shot pattern associated with the wound in Figure IX-160 (a).

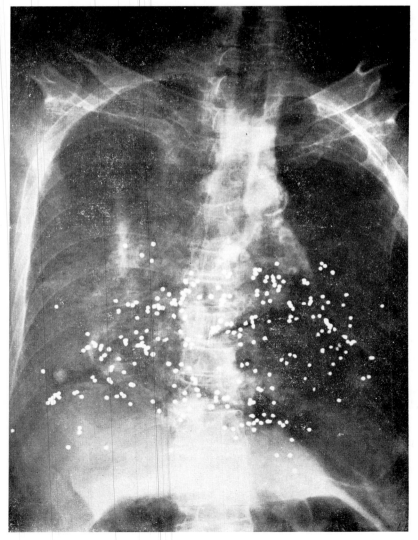

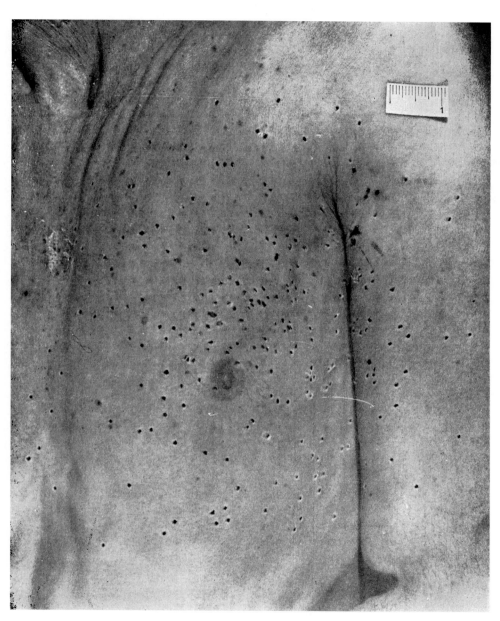

FIGURE XII-160c. Wound inflicted from a distance of 16 feet.

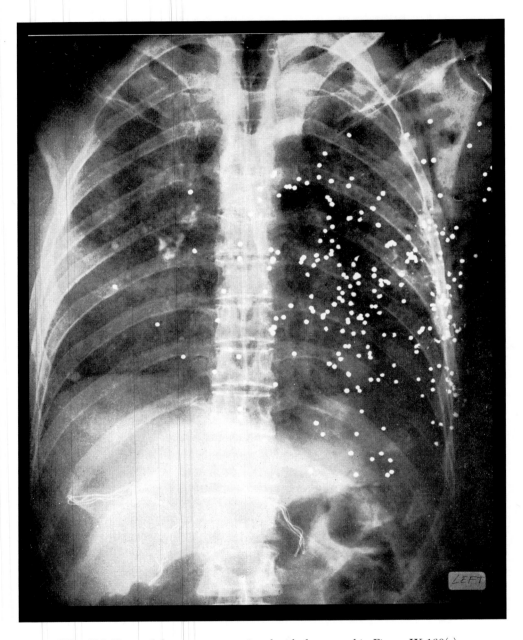

Figure XII-160d. X-ray of shot pattern associated with the wound in Figure IX-160(c).

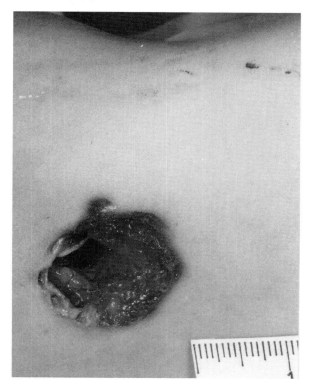

FIGURE XII-161a–b. (a) Homicidal shotgun wound of right shoulder from a distance of 4 to 5 feet with a 12 gauge shotgun and No. 6 shot. The bunched shot struck the body, producing a single wound with scalloped edges (*cookie cutter* wound). (b) The x-ray shows wide dispersion of the shot.

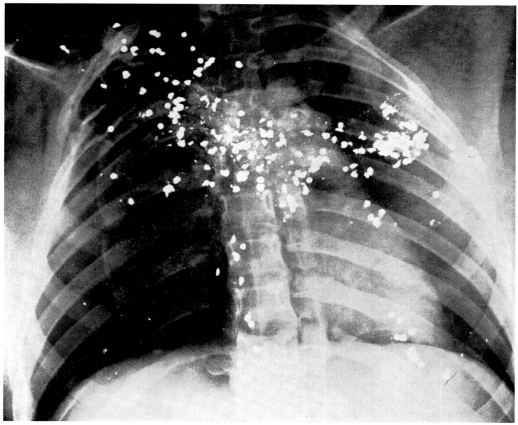

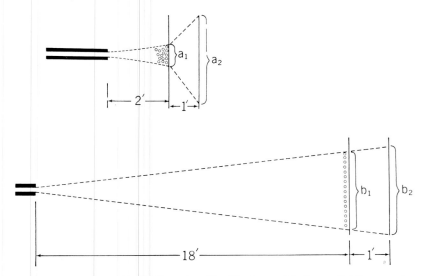

FIGURE XII-162. *Billiard ball ricochet effect.* The heavy black parallel lines on the left represent the shotgun barrel. At close range the pellets are bunched, and as they strike the primary target (a_1) the leading pellets are slowed and are hit by the following pellets, causing them to veer off in a wide pattern as billiard balls do when hit at the break by the cue ball. At greater distances, the shot are spread out and (a_2) may show the same spread as (b_2).

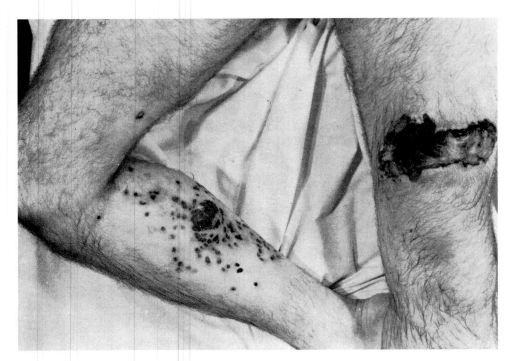

FIGURE XII-163. Shot fired from a distance of about 5 feet, grazed the left thigh, causing the shot to scatter over a wide area, as indicated by the wounding pattern on the right leg.

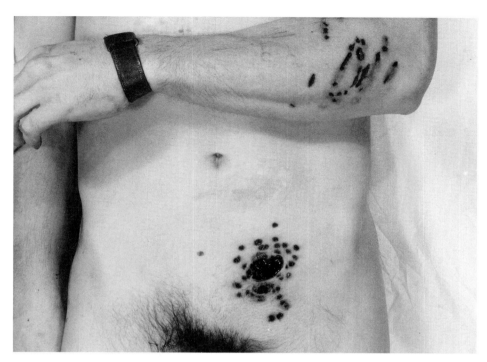

FIGURE XII-164. Grazing defensive wound on left forearm may be the same shot which penetrated above the pubis, if the arm was in very close proximity to the abdomen. If the arm was further away, it would seem likely that these are two separate shots considering that more scattering of pellets would have occurred after striking the primary target in the arm.

imprints of lead scattered over an area of 4 to 5 inches (Fig. XII-165). The wide area covered by these imprints is the result of dispersion of the pellets by ricocheting off each other at the entry into the skull. When the shotgun wound of entrance is difficult to locate because of extensive mutilation and scattering of tissues over a large area, the finding of a fragment of bone with these imprints will suggest the direction and range of fire.

The *billiard ball* effect may not occur with old shotgun cartridges. Corroded pellets often adhere to each other and may not separate upon striking an intermediary target. This would change the pattern of injury and lead to considerable variance in estimating the range of fire. The *billiard ball* effect also does not usually apply to 00 buck shot because of its larger mass.

Shotgun Exit Wounds

Shotgun exit wounds are uncommon even in contact or close-range shots, except if the shot involves the head or if the victim is very thin. In head shots, the entire head may be shattered and all pellets and the wad may exit. Even if the wad exits, it is often entangled in hair. The entire load of pellets and the wad may also exit if the shot is tangential, striking the body at a sharp angle, involving a limited amount of tissue and no major bony structures (Figs. XII-166 and XII-167). Large shot sizes, especially 00 buck, are likely to pass through the body somewhat more frequently due to their greater mass and energy as compared to bird shot (Figs. XII-168 to XII-170). More common is the accumulation of large numbers of shot under the skin opposite the entry wound (Fig. XII-171). As with single missile weapons, a shotgun load fired at close range may exit and re-enter the body as depicted in Figure XII-172.

Survivability of Shotgun Wounds

As with small arms fire, shotgun wounds, particularly when relatively small shot are used, are

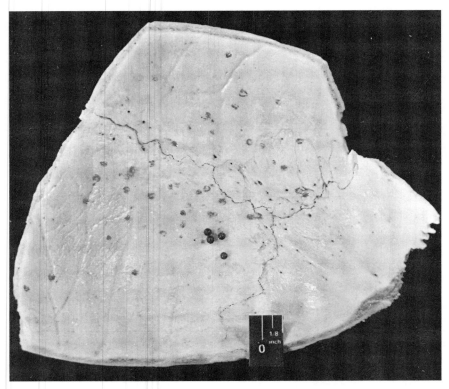

FIGURE XII-165. Inner view of the vault of the skull in a contact shot of the opposite temple. Note the wide scattering of pellet imprints.

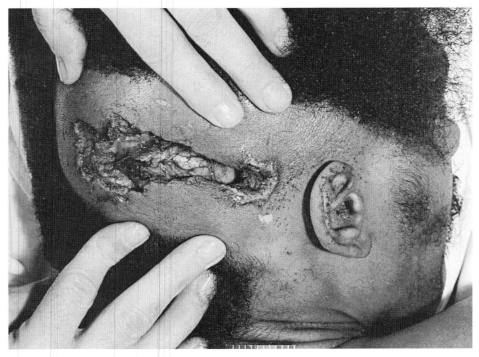

FIGURE XII-166. Close-range, grazing wound behind the right ear showing gunpowder stippling on and around the ear. The wound edges are held together to show the path. No pellets or wads were recovered from the injury.

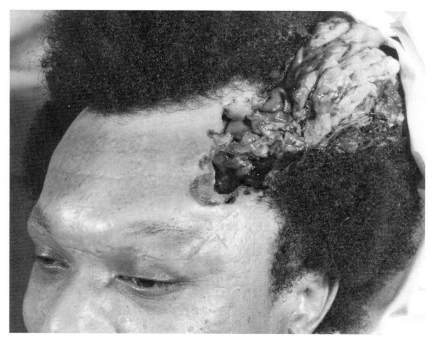

FIGURE XII-167. Entrance shotgun wound showing early spread of pellets grazing the left side of the head. The skull is fragmented and lacerated brain matter protrudes from the defect.

FIGURE XII-168. Contact shot of neck, no load remained in the body. The gases which emanated from the muzzle caused blowout tears from over distention between the entrance and exit wounds. These are comprised of the large vertical tear and several small superficial linear tears all running in parallel.

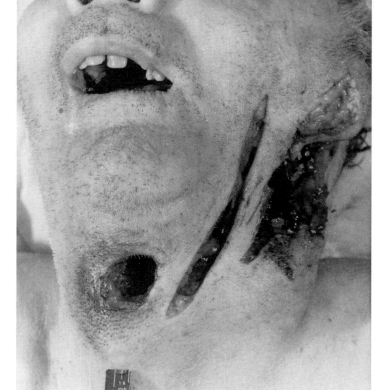

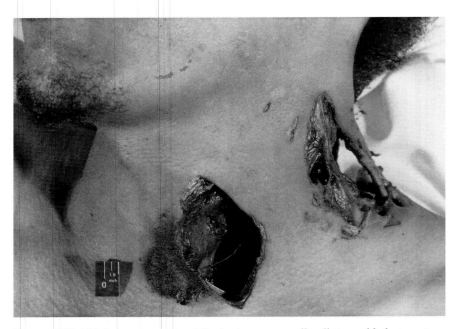

FIGURE XII-169. In narrow parts of the body, even small pellets are likely to exit as is the wad. This is especially true in the case of contact shots where the gases push the load ahead and out.

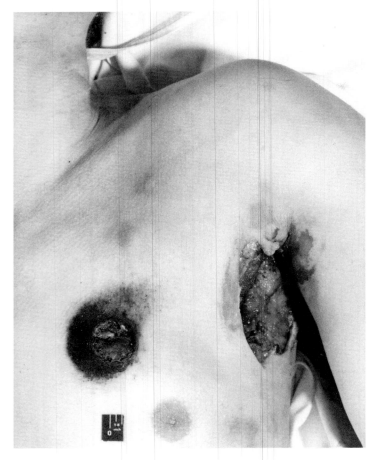

FIGURE XII-170. Contact shot above the nipple. The full load exited from the left side of the chest and armpit.

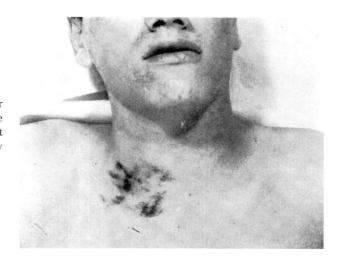

FIGURE XII-171. Shotgun wound between the shoulder blades, with a 12 gauge shotgun, No. 4 shot, from a distance of approximately 2 feet. The injury shown includes exit wounds of two pellets and extensive bruising of the skin by shot that failed to break the skin.

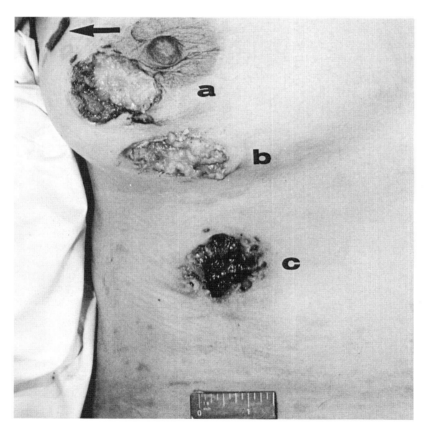

FIGURE XII-172. Single entrance wound (arrow). The shot separated, exiting at (a) and (b). Pellets exiting wound (b) re-entered the body at injury (c).

quite variable in their effect upon the victim. At contact or close range the blast effect, as well as shot damage, may cause major destruction. In fact, death can be caused by the blast effect alone, using *blank* shells, if the range of fire is under one or two feet. At greater ranges, where only a few shot reach the victim, the injury may be insignificant or there may be considerable delay in the development of blood loss to cause collapse.

A fifty-five-year-old man was rabbit hunting with a friend when he was shot from approximately 20 feet with a 12-gauge shotgun, cylinder bore, loaded with No. 5 shot. Only three of the shot struck the body; one of these produced an insignificant skin wound, but the two others penetrated the back and perforated the aorta in the abdominal area. The individual realized he was injured and started to walk to the nearest road, where his friend meanwhile had gone to pick up their car. He did succeed in walking more than 1000 yards and was able to get into the car by himself, but upon arrival at the hospital 20 minutes later he was dead. He died as a result of blood loss into the retroperitoneal area caused by the two perforating wounds of the aorta made by the birdshot.

The ability to walk more than 1000 yards while fatally wounded is remarkable. This case further illustrates that a fatal shotgun injury can occur with small shot, even from a relatively great distance.

Beanbag Ammunition

The police beanbag ammunition, sometimes used in riot control, is the latest alternative to deadly force. It has gained widespread popularity. It consists of a synthetic fabric bag filled with 40 grams of No. 9 lead shot and is fired from a shotgun. The recommended range of fire is 30 to 90 feet and a *close range* round has a recommended range of 9 to 45 feet.

The bag is designed to unfold, so that its' largest surface impacts the body. The bag fired a distance of 30 feet delivers a kinetic energy of nearly double that of a major league fastball.

While beanbags are considered non-lethal, deaths have occurred and internal injuries are common. It would seem that the severity of injury caused by beanbag ammunition has been vastly underestimated.[3] In fact, in a recent case in Portland, Oregon (*Marshall* vs *City of Portland*) a Federal District judge determined that the use of beanbag ammunition does constitute lethal force.

REFERENCES

1. Breitenecker, R., and Senior, W.J.: Shotgun patterns. I. An experimental study on the influence of intermediate targets. *J Forensic Sci, 12:* 193, 1967.
2. Breitenecker, R.: Shotgun wound patterns. *Am J Clin Pathol, 52:* 258, 1969.
3. de Brito, D., Challoner, K.R., Sehgal, A., and Mallon, W.: The injury pattern of a new law enforcement weapon: The police bean bag. *Ann Emerg Med, 38:* 4, 383–390, 2001.

Chapter XIII

THERMAL INJURIES

Werner U. Spitz

Thermal burns remain a prominent cause of injury and death. Approximately 8,000 fire-related deaths occur in the United States each year.

Chances of survival following burn injuries largely depend on the severity and extent of the burns, the age of the victim and the timeliness of specialized medical care. With recent advances in the care of burns, an expected 50% mortality rate has been reported to have improved to 98% for children and 72% for adults.[1] The very young and the elderly are particularly vulnerable to lethal complications.

Burns are commonly classified according to the depth of tissue destruction:

1. First-degree burns are superficial. They show the early manifestations of inflammation, i.e., red discoloration and increased local skin temperature due to congestion, swelling of the area caused by edema and pain which results from stretching of the skin and stimulation of nerve endings. Blisters do not form, but peeling may follow. On a dead body, the red discoloration rapidly fades and may not be recognizable at postmortem examination. When circulation ceases with death, blood from congested areas settles by gravity into dependent areas. Swelling may diminish as a result of diffusion into surrounding tissues. A mild sunburn may be considered a first degree burn.

2. Second-degree burns typically show blisters. The upper layers of the skin are destroyed (Figs. XIII-1 and XIII-2). Healing takes place from the edges and from small epithelial remnants. Nevertheless, scarring sometimes follows.

3. Third-degree burns involve the entire thickness of the skin and are referred to as full thickness burns. Both epidermis and dermis are damaged. Pain is usually absent because nerve endings in the skin are destroyed. Healing is from the edges of the injury, and scarring is the rule. Skin grafting is usually necessary.

4. More severe thermal injury is charring. Complete destruction of skin and underlying tissues, often including bone, is referred to as a fourth-degree burn.

The extent of burns should be specified. It is conveniently estimated using the *rule of nines* (Fig. XIII-3a–b). In infants, the head area accounts for 18% of the body surface and each lower extremity is estimated at 13.5%. The remaining body surface is the same as that of an adult.

The severity of burn injuries depends directly on the intensity of the heat and duration of exposure. Fire temperatures differ considerably, depending on the materials that are burning. Some chemical fires rapidly reach several thousand degrees. Ordinary house fires range from about 900° to 1200° F (500°–650° C) and seldom exceed 1300° F. It is unlikely that the body of an adult will burn so completely in a house fire as to leave no trace (Figs. XIII-4a–b). Disposal of a victim of homicide by setting fire to a building is, therefore, usually unsuccessful.

For the purpose of illustration, cremation in a gas-fired chamber requires 1-1/2 to 2 hours at 1600–1800° F to reduce an average built adult body to *ashes*. To obtain bone dust, bone pieces would need to be pulverized (Figs. XIII-5a–b). Cremation of an elderly individual with osteoporosis will proceed at a significantly faster rate at the same or lower temperature.

The bodies of two badly burned women were recovered following a house fire. The unburned body of a man was found in a part of the house that was not damaged by the flames. Subsequent investigation of the circumstances showed that all three had been drinking when an argument developed, during which the man stabbed the women and attempted to dispose of their bodies by setting fire to the premises. The man then went to sleep in another part of the

Medicolegal Investigation of Death

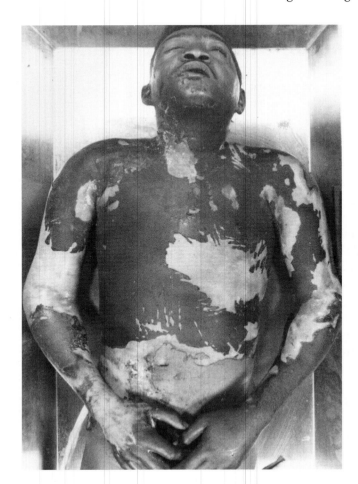

FIGURE XIII-1. The pale areas are denuded of the epidermal covering, thus second-degree burns.

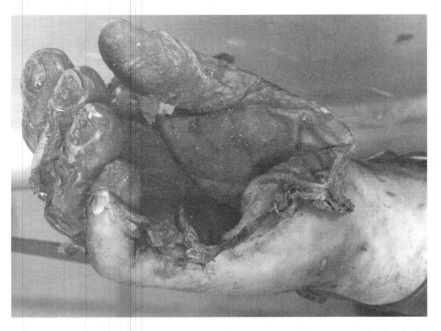

FIGURE XIII-2. Second-degree burn of the hand. The epidermis is markedly thicker in the hand and rolls when separated.

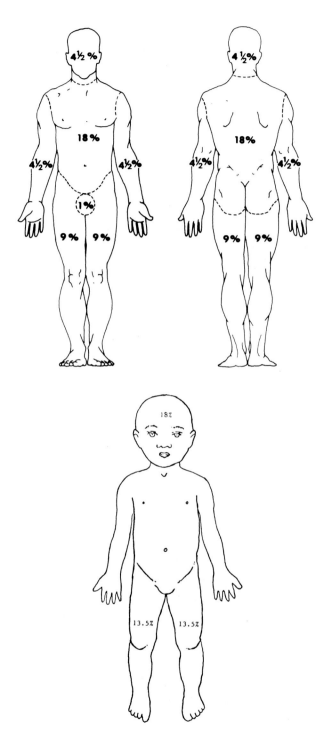

FIGURE XIII-3a–b. Adult's and infant's body surface expressed as percentages using the *rule of nines*.

house, but succumbed to inhalation of carbon monoxide with a blood saturation of carboxyhemoglobin (COHb) of 65%. He also had a blood alcohol concentration of 0.28%. The two women were likewise markedly intoxicated. Autopsies revealed that both had died of multiple stab wounds before the fire started, as evidenced by negative carboxyhemoglobin in blood specimens.

By contrast, the body of a child, in the first few years of life, may be reduced to a few ounces of ashes in a relatively short time by a fire that would not similarly affect the body of an adult.

The charred body of an adult was found in the rubble of a burned-down log cabin. Anthropologic studies and dental records identified the remains as those of a thirty-two-year-old woman who was known to have lived at that location with her three-year-old daughter. No remains of the child could be recovered after a thorough search. A death certificate was ultimately issued after a court determined that the child had perished in the fire.

The body of a newborn child can be incinerated in an ordinary stove in less than two hours.[2]

Obesity and clothes contribute to faster and more complete destruction of a body in a fire. After burning through the skin, the heat exposes body fat, which then continues to burn independently. According to Icove and DeHaan the flames produced by combustion of body fat will generate a temperature of 1475–1650° F, which will enhance disintegration of the remains.[3] Clothes act as a wick, providing for more complete combustion. However, tight articles of clothing, such as belts, shoes and socks preserve underlying skin in the early stages of a fire by excluding air, according to the dictum *"where there is no oxygen there can be no fire."* Of course, ultimately such articles of clothing will also burn. On the other hand, metal objects on the body, such as buttons, belt buckles, chains, and watches, will conduct heat and cause patterned burns which may be observed where charring does not occur.

In a ravaging house fire a body is usually extensively charred in less than 20 minutes. A body in a fully developed fire in an automobile will undergo superficial charring in a similar time span. For the purpose of comparison, it has been said that timber (pine) is charred to a depth of one-half inch after exposure for the same duration, i.e., the rule of 1 inch (2.54 cm) in 45 min-

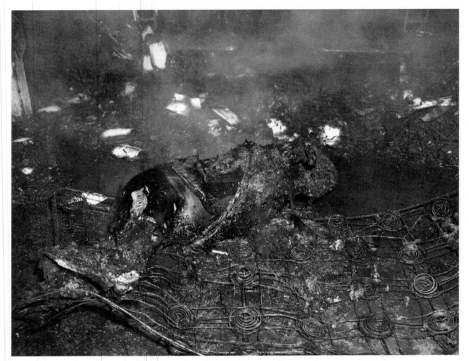

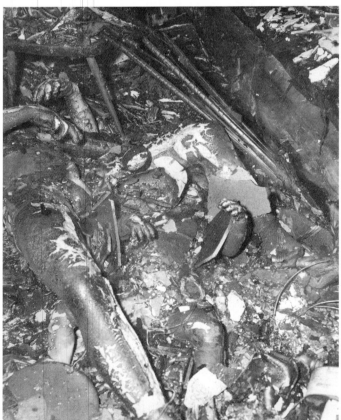

FIGURE XIII-4a–b. Remains of an adult (a) and adult and child (b) in houses destroyed by fire.

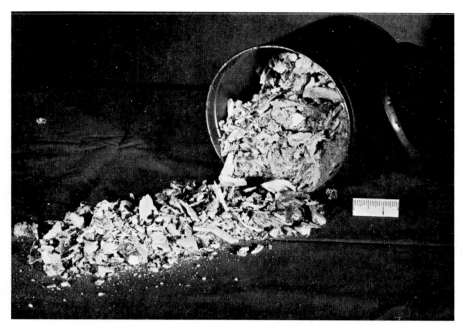

FIGURE XIII-5a. Half-gallon tin can containing human remains following cremation.

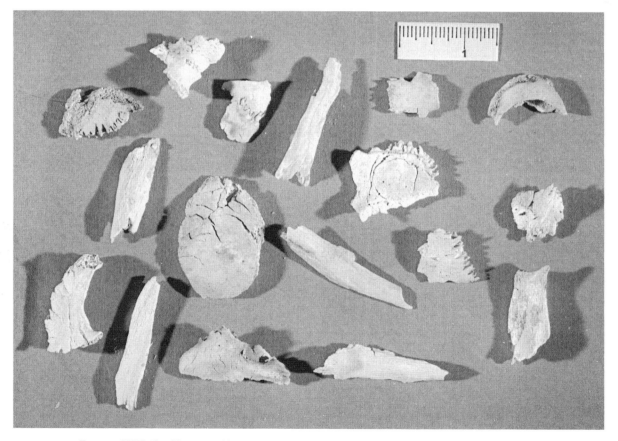

FIGURE XIII-5b. Closeup of bones fragments from the cremains shown in Figure XIII-5a.

utes. This rule for charring of pine is based on a laboratory test which reported exposure of heat from one side vary from 0.4 inch (1 cm) per hour at 750° F (390° C) to 10 inches (25.4 cm) per hour at temperatures approaching 2000° F (1090° C). According to the National Fire Protection Agency (NFPA), the depth of char is not reliable for determining the duration of a fire, however it is significant when evaluating fire spread. The NFPA indicates that by measuring the relative depth and extent of charring, one can determine what portions of material or construction were exposed the longest to a heat source. When applied to death investigation, these criteria may help explain variations in fire damage on bodies.[4]

According to Richards,[5] it takes a considerable time for a body to burn at 1200° F before the bones are exposed. The rib cage and facial skeleton are exposed in about 20 minutes. The arms and legs are severely charred early, but the shin bones take longer. Burning of all flesh from the thigh and shin bones usually occurs after 35 minutes. With this chart in mind, it may be possible to reconstruct where the fire has burned the longest, i.e., where the fire started. Such inspection may suggest acceleration of the fire by the use of an accelerant, such as a flammable liquid.

The use of a flammable liquid, such as kerosene or gasoline, for disposal of a body by fire, often results in patchy charring of disproportionate severity. While some areas are charred deeply, other areas are burned significantly less and protected areas below the body are spared entirely. If the face is charred and the teeth are destroyed, while the chest and abdomen are significantly less burned, the use of an accelerant, as for the purpose of obliterating identity, should be suspected. If the adipose tissue is ignited in an obese individual, prolonged local smoldering may cause severe skeletal damage, including amputation.

Chemical analysis of even small remnants of clothes sometime reveals the presence of residual accelerants (Fig. XIII-6). Dry, leather-like burned skin can also be used for such testing. Broken glass found on the body or clothes may point to a fire victim of a free basing accident.

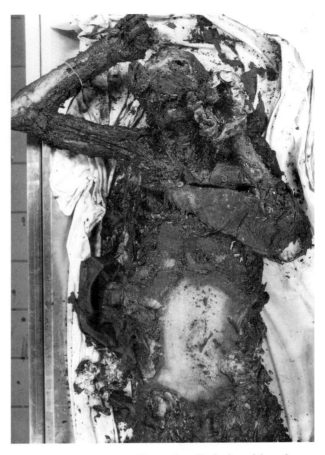

FIGURE XIII-6. Victim of house fire. Body found face down. The abdominal area is spared due to contact with the floor. The right arm and left elbow are also spared for the same reason. There are abundant clothes on the body for chemical analysis. Note that the face is partially burnt to the bone.

Any broken glass at a fire scene should be retained and submitted for analysis. Examination of such specimens may show fingerprints and indicate whether the glass was broken before or after the fire started.

Peculiar, characteristically curved fractures are often seen in bones exposed to high temperatures. The bones of the extremities, as well as the skull, often show this type of fracture. No trauma, other than heat, is known to produce similar skeletal damage (Fig. XIII-7a–b).

Experimentally, these cracks or fractures occur when the bone cools after the fire subsides. Continued exposure to intense heat causes bones to bleach, become brittle, then break into thin sheets of calcific matter, fragmenting the bone

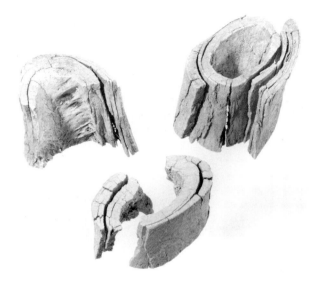

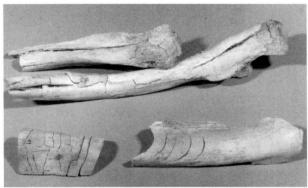

FIGURE XIII-7a–b. (a) Typical fragmentation caused by heat, resembling tree bark. (b) Straight and curved heat fractures of long bones.

and finally transforming it into coarse, whitish-gray powder.

An accelerated fire in the open, as in a field, does not usually result in complete combustion of a body. An example was the attempted disposal of Hitler's body by one of his aides at the end of World War II. In spite of widespread charring as a result of the use of several gallons of gasoline, positive dental identification of the remains was still possible, in fact quite easy.[6] Gasoline, like many other accelerants, burns fast, causing limited body damage unless massive quantities are used. Also, a fire will burn and spread much faster upward than downward and sideways.

Cremation in an outdoor pyre is the orthodox way of corpse disposal among Hindus. The pyre is allowed to burn for three days before the remains are collected for later consignment to the Ganges. Even at this stage, large pieces of bone are still recognizable among the ashes. It has been described that the body of a corpse disposed of in a ceremonial pyre oftentimes will *sit up* due to the effect of immense heat, causing muscle shrinkage. This change of position is similar to that which causes the typical pugilistic or boxer's position commonly seen in fire victims (Fig. XIII-8a–b).

Teeth, like bones, are resistant to fire, presenting excellent means for identification by comparison of pre- and postmortem dental records. Additionally, the lips and facial skin are tightened, the mouth is often shut and the tongue may be protruding due to shrinkage of the cheeks and neck tissues as a result of drying. This seals the oral cavity and provides protection to the teeth from heat and the direct effect of flames.

Death in a fire often occurs a considerable time before the conflagration can be brought under control. The extensive mutilation frequently seen in victims of fire has, therefore, largely occurred after death. Regardless of the severity of surface destruction, the organs of a body recovered from a fire are usually well-preserved for a meaningful autopsy and tissues and body fluids are usually available for comprehensive toxicological analyses (Fig. XIII-9a–b).

The autopsy should be done prior to embalming to exclude contamination of toxicological specimens by alcohol soluble perfumes. Scented crystalline formalin powder is often used by embalmers for preservation of fire damaged remains.

The charred remains of a fifty-two-year-old woman were found on the living room floor of her one-story frame house, gutted by fire. Even though the chest and abdominal walls were incinerated and the organs exposed, at autopsy, the organs were relatively well-preserved (Fig. XIII-10). Carboxyhemoglobin saturation of a blood sample was 25%. It was further established that the victim had suffered from advanced arteriosclerotic heart disease. A blood alcohol determination was not performed in view of the fact that scented salts had been scattered on the body, although a

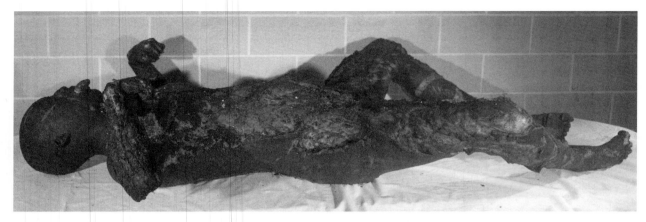

Figure XIII-8a. Charred body in *boxer's position* with bent elbows and knees, clenched fist and protruding tongue due to shrinkage of skin and muscles.

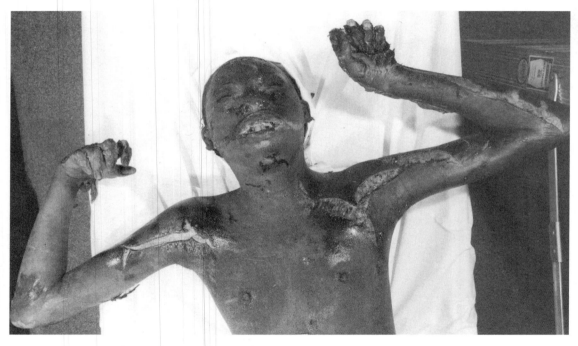

FIGURE XIII-8b. *Pugilistic* or *boxer's attitude* of a burned body. The arms are raised due to shrinkage of muscles as a result of the heat. The skin often splits, as shown in the shoulders and left arm and forearm.

negative result would have indicated a negative alcohol content at the time of death.

The rate of decomposition of a burned body is likely to be delayed, in much the same way as cooked meat keeps longer than fresh. Tissues denatured by heat, i.e., cooked, are less amenable to bacterial growth. Decomposition is accelerated where the body is exposed to elevated temperatures in the absence of burns or with burns limited to some areas. Absence of uniformity in the degree of decomposition in different organs suggests that decomposition was caused by heat rather than the passage of time. Estimation of the time of death of a burned body is usually inaccurate and subject to great variance.

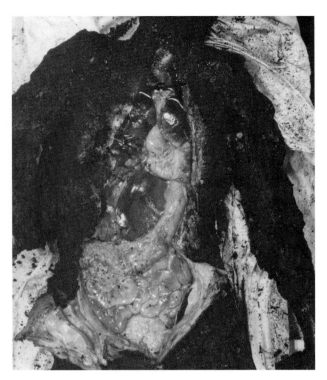

FIGURE XIII-9a. Preservation of the internal organs in spite of charring: Liquid blood from the heart was removed for chemical analyses.

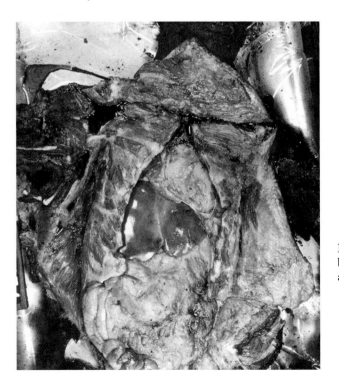

FIGURE XIII-9b. Charred body with organs in an excellent state of preservation.

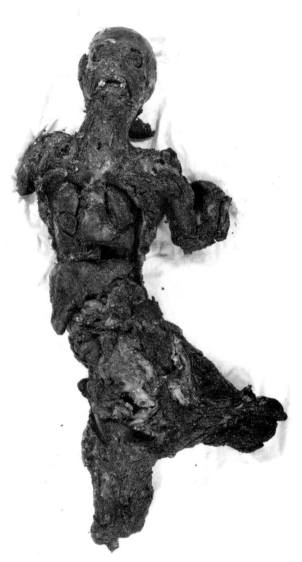

FIGURE XIII-10. Charred remains found among debris of a burned-down house. Note exposure of the chest and abdominal organs as a result of the fire.

Examination of a body found at the site of a conflagration involves primarily the following objectives: (a) identification of the victim, (b) determination of the cause of death.

IDENTIFICATION OF THE VICTIM

Certain principles of identification are particular to a body recovered from the scene of a fire. The weight and length of charred remains are unreliable. Dehydration, i.e., drying of tissues, skeletal fractures and pulverization of the intervertebral discs by heat may significantly alter preexisting dimensions. Body length may be shortened by several inches, and weight loss may exceed 60%. Also, the skin is tightened by shrinkage, changing facial features. An ear, even a hand, may shrink significantly. Head hunters in South America removed the skull, then exposed the skin to intense dry heat by packing it with red-hot sand, shrinking the flesh to the size of a baseball (Fig. XIII-11). Postmortem cataracts as a result of coagulation of proteins in the lens of the eyes have been observed at temperatures as low as 150° F (Fig. XIII-12).

Identifiable peculiarities on the body surface, such as scars, tattoos and moles, are frequently destroyed. However, the presence of a surgical scar may be derived from the autopsy findings, such as a missing appendix, gastrectomy or remote removal of a kidney, unless a laparoscopic approach was used for the procedure.

Since the uterus and prostate are protected by their anatomical locations and fibrous structure determination of the sex of a severely charred body can usually be readily made. The same can be said of the liver, which is not only less flammable by virtue of its location under the rib cage, but especially if cirrhotic, because of its high con-

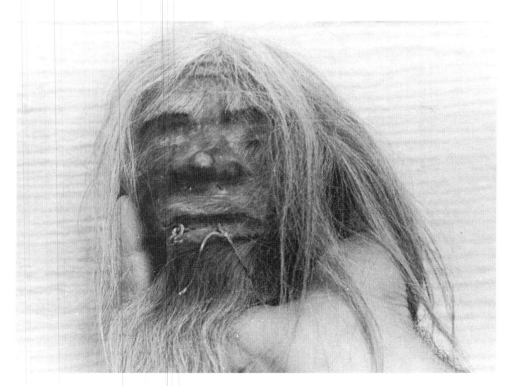

FIGURE XIII-11. Shrunken head held in the palm of my hand.

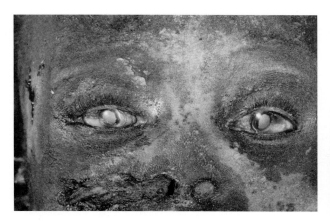

FIGURE XIII-12. Postmortem opacity of the lenses (cataract) of both eyes, caused by heat coagulation of the lens proteins. The deceased was found face up on the kitchen floor, her head in close proximity of the open oven door. The oven was set at 400° F. The room temperature was described as *extremely hot.*

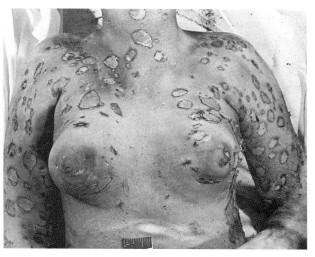

FIGURE XIII-13. Middle-aged woman who died in a house fire. Extensive crater-like second degree burns are seen on the arms and upper chest. Note the shape of the breasts suggesting a much younger individual.

tent of dense, collagenous scar-like tissue. The appearance of female breasts when estimating the age of a fire victim may be misleading. Drying, shrinkage, erection and increased firmness of the breasts occur as a result of the heat, regardless of age (Fig. XIII-13). In a charred body, it may be necessary to incise the breasts to determine the amount of firm, white, glandular tissue. Microscopic examination may be required.

For racial identification, the pathologist should look for patches of intact skin as may be found under the body or under tight articles of clothing, such as a belt, shoes, brassiere or buttoned collar, even in cases of extensive charring. A watch and strap also spare the underlying skin. Unburnt skin about the wrists and ankles suggests the victim may have been bound before the fire. A strap-like, horizontal, undamaged area on the neck may suggest ligature strangulation.

The badly burned body of a twenty-four-year-old black female was found in a field (Fig. XIII-14a–b). Remnants of clothesline were found on the neck. The underlying skin was not burned. Death was determined to be due to ligature strangulation. The burns were caused by a subsequent attempt to dispose of the body or destroy its identity.

Sometimes skin and hair in the armpits are spared. The gums are also frequently preserved. Since the gums are brown or mottled in a large number of blacks, this finding may assist in racial

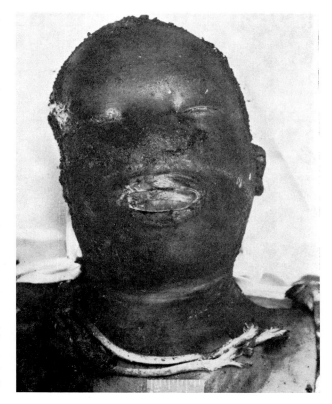

FIGURE XIII-14a. Body of a young woman found charred in a field. The undamaged strap-like area of skin on the neck was caused by the unburned clothesline that was used as a ligature. A pale horizontal band of skin across the left cheek and upper lip suggests the victim had been gagged.

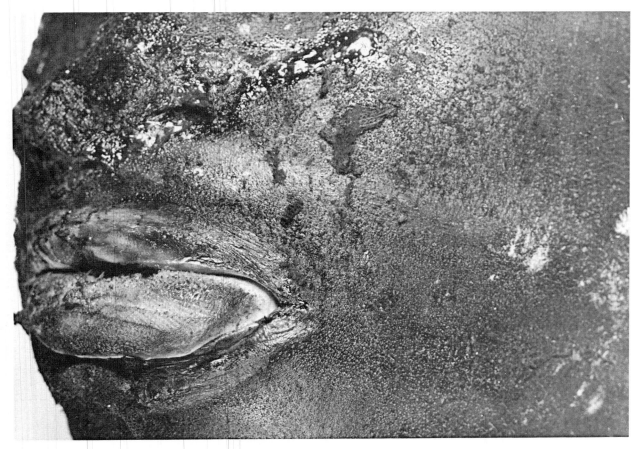

FIGURE XIII-14b. The tongue protrudes from the mouth due to shrinkage of the facial skin due to the heat of the fire. Note the weave pattern of a gag imprinted on the tongue. The gag was burned to ashes after expulsion from the mouth.

identification. Another important observation in blacks is the dark gray deposit of melanin in the arachnoid membrane around the medulla oblongata and, to a lesser extent, in the area of the olfactory nerves at the inferior surface of the frontal lobes. The cervical spine, the base of the skull and the facial skeleton usually remain intact, except in extreme cases.

Hair changes color on exposure to heat, depending on temperature. At about 250° F gray hair turns brassy blonde, and 10 to 15 minutes at 400° F imparts a reddish hue to brown hair. Black hair does not change color.

Complete body x-ray examination may help in locating old fractures, bony abnormalities or foreign bodies that might otherwise escape detection. The finding of metal staples, coronary stents and artificial heart and aortic valves, steel wires, pins, plates, screws and artificial joints indicate a remote surgical procedure. Cardiac pacemakers and defibrillators may have identifying numbers or lettering. X-ray of the teeth may reveal metal pins used for root canal treatment, fillings that were not detected on direct examination and a subgingival metal grid for dental implants (*see* Fig. VI-8). Dental examination is significantly compounded when heat and flames have fragmented tooth enamel and soot and smoke have been deposited on the teeth. Generally, however, teeth and restorations are remarkably resistant to heat, and unless they are struck directly by the flames, preservation is probable in most cases. When heat contractures have tightly locked the jaws detailed visual examination of the teeth, especially the molars is difficult or impossible. The alternative is to disarticulate the mandible and excise the upper jaw. Although mutilating, this procedure is of no consequence, since the remains are not injectable, and viewing of the body in state will not occur.

Frequently, in burned bodies tissue fluids collect between the layers of the skin. In the hands the epidermis comes off like a *glove,* including the fingernails. Either the detached *glove* or the remaining hand, whichever is less damaged, and the palm of the hand may be used to obtain prints. The inner aspect of the *glove* may also be printed, although such prints are the mirror image of the true prints (Fig. XIII-15). The epidermal layer of the feet detaches in like fashion. A similar process occurs as a result of decomposition, following prolonged immersion in water and as a result of dousing with gasoline, especially high octane, as used to fuel aircraft.

Bursting of a blister and removal of the epidermal layer of skin by wiping or rubbing renders a tattoo better recognizable. The pigment of a tattoo is situated in the dermis, which is deeper than the layer of skin that is removed. Wiping areas thought to be tattooed may reveal tattoos or details in a tattoo that were previously unnoticed. A damp paper towel or soft cotton rag is best used for this purpose (Fig. XIII-16).

Regarding the use of DNA for identification of charred remains, ample tissue, including bone is usually available. Even hair may be available in spared areas. However, in bone dust after calcination or bone ashes, DNA is likely to be destroyed. Thus, DNA is useless in cremated remains.

DETERMINATION OF THE CAUSE OF DEATH

To determine the cause of death it must first be established whether the victim was alive at the time of the fire. Even low levels of carboxyhemoglobin (COHb), which results from the inhalation of carbon monoxide (CO), are significant. A few breaths suffice to accumulate a meaningful concentration.

Protesting Buddhist monks and others in the 1960s doused their clothes with kerosene or gasoline, then set fire to themselves. These people had relatively low COHb levels. A similar case of dousing, with which we were personally familiar, had a COHb saturation of 26%. Of course, wind direction and intensity, type of clothing, physical health of the victim, and other factors play a significant role. A *mushroom* of thick, white foam at the nostrils or mouth indicates breathing while the fire was in progress. Foam in the airways is caused, in large part, by pulmonary edema, i.e., accumulation of protein-rich fluid in the lungs as a result of bronchial irritation by smoke, heart failure due to the asphyxiating effect of COHb and direct toxicity of COHb on the heart muscle (Fig. XIII-17).

While the presence of carboxyhemoglobin is proof of life when the fire started, its absence does not imply that death had occurred before the fire. COHb is sometimes absent or present in very low concentrations in victims of flash fires, as in a conflagration in a chemical plant, in warfare or in an explosion, when death may be instantaneous. An individual stoking a furnace may also be the victim of a flash fire. Flame throwers in wartime cause death in a similar fashion. Flames that hit the face can cause death due to inability to breathe. Inhalation of superheated air, such as occurs as a result of exposure to steam, causes edema and swelling of the airways and rapid death due to suffocation. The obstruction is usually at the level of the laryngeal inlet. A blast of hot air causes reflex closure of the airway at the level of the vocal cords, preventing damage below this level. The findings at autopsy are usually characteristic.

Inhalation of moisture-saturated hot air is considerably more damaging than inhalation of dry air of the same temperature. Thus, one or two breaths of moisture saturated air at 130° F may be expected to result in serious airway injury. According to The National Research Council of Canada, 300° F is the maximum survivable breathing temperature. Such temperature can be

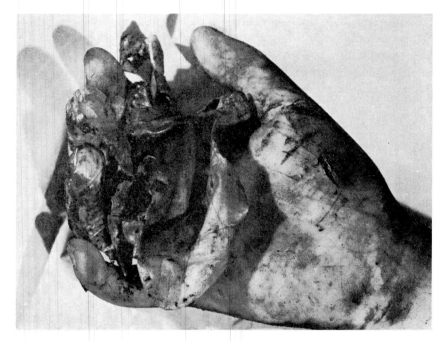

FIGURE XIII-15. The skin of the hand detaches as a *glove*, due to the effect of heat. The *glove* includes the fingernails. Both the *glove* and underlying skin are still suitable for obtaining inked impressions of fingerprints. Care must be taken to preserve this peeled-off skin when handling the body.

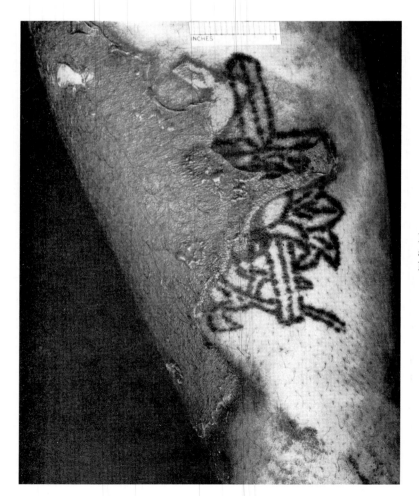

FIGURE XIII-16. Tattoo on forearm made apparent by wiping off the burnt superficial layers of the skin.

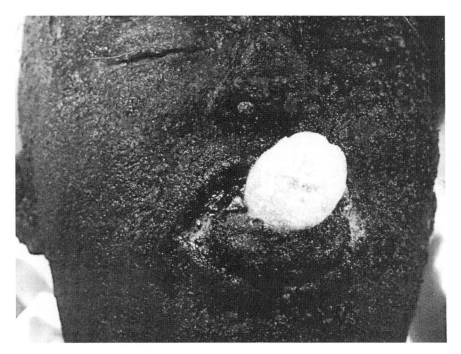

FIGURE XIII-17. Charred black face with ball of white foam at mouth, due to edema of the lungs.

endured for only a short period and not at all if moisture is present.

The vast majority, of all fire-related deaths, result from inhalation of toxic fumes. The severity of injury caused by such inhalation depends on the nature of the fumes, their concentration and duration of exposure. Synthetic furniture, upholsteries, curtains and carpets are now more popular than wood and natural fibers. Plastics are widely used for office equipment, electric, telephone and cable insulation and automobiles. Polyurethane, foam rubber, and many other polymer plastics are potent fuels resembling solidified gasoline. Polyurethane ignites readily in the presence of an open flame and releases twice the heat of wood or cotton. When plastics smolder or burn they introduce a deadly mix of gases to the air. In addition to large amounts of carbon monoxide, burning polymers produce hydrogen cyanide. Fifty-one percent of the victims of the Dupont Plaza Hotel fire in San Juan, Puerto Rico on December 31, 1986, had significantly elevated blood cyanide levels.[7] The

human lethal level of blood cyanide is 5 mg/mL.[8] In evaluating the significance of carboxyhemoglobin and blood cyanide levels it is noteworthy that carboxyhemoglobin decreases and cyanide increases with time during storage of a blood sample. In blood frozen for three months the carboxyhemoglobin saturation decreased up to 20%.

The effects of carboxyhemoglobin and cyanide are additive. Carboxyhemoglobin interferes with the ability of blood to carry oxygen; hydrogen cyanide interferes with the ability of cells to utilize oxygen.

Undoubtedly, even minor concentrations of these gases cause disorientation and confusion, which may be mistaken for alcoholic and or drug intoxication, and may interfere with a fire victim's ability to escape.

Nevertheless, the lethal effect of smoke inhalation is primarily due to carbon monoxide. The November, 1980, fire at the MGM Grand Hotel in Las Vegas serves as a grim reminder of the dangers of fire-related smoke. Most of the 84 deaths and injuries were the result of carbon monoxide intoxication.[9] An intentionally set fire in a private club in New York City in March, 1990 cost the lives of 87 patrons, all as a result of smoke inhalation. According to Icove and DeHaan[3] the aptitude to escape a fire depends upon the ability to see through dense smoke to 15 feet, an environmental carbon monoxide concentration up to 30,000 ppm-min. and a temperature less than 150°C (302°F).

The blood carboxyhemoglobin level rises rapidly. According to Stewart,[10] smoke in a fire can contain carbon monoxide in concentrations of 0.1 to 10% and a few breaths of such smoke, especially in cases of stress, fear, agitation and exertion, would elevate the carboxyhemoglobin saturation to asphyxiating levels. Thus, exposure to a carbon monoxide concentration of 1% (10,000 ppm) for a duration of 2 minutes would cause a blood carboxyhemoglobin saturation of 30% and exposure to 10% carbon monoxide for a period of 30 seconds would result in a blood carboxyhemoglobin saturation of 75%.

Carboxyhemoglobin saturation levels in victims of fire who are found dead at the scene differ, depending on their age and general state of health (Fig. XIII-18). In a healthy middle-aged adult who died in a conflagration a common blood saturation level is 50 to 60%. Lower levels are found in the elderly. In children, carboxyhemoglobin saturation levels are often higher. A high carboxyhemoglobin level in an elderly victim suggests a good state of health and a slow burning or smoldering fire. A smoldering fire is one that causes charring but no flames. In the presence of emphysema, advanced arteriosclerotic heart disease or anemia, death would occur before carboxyhemoglobin can build up to a high concentration. Chain smokers may have a daytime COHb saturation of 8 to 10%. Interpretation of a low carboxyhemoglobin level must therefore be done with care. In a non-smoker a similar blood level may be considered evidence of smoke inhalation.

A non-smoking passenger in an automobile in which another occupant smokes is likely to have an elevated carboxyhemoglobin saturation as a result of breathing the ambient smoky air, so-called second-hand smoke inhalation.

Infants and children build up a fatal carboxyhemoglobin level significantly faster than adults exposed to the same atmosphere. This is because of the higher metabolic rate in early life. It is, therefore, not unusual in cases of conflagration to find that an infant sleeping in the same room with his parents is dead of CO poisoning while the parents may still be salvageable. For the same reason, a dog, cat or bird in the same room is likely to follow the same fate as the child.

Whereas, small amounts of carbon monoxide may bond with hemoglobin in vitro, i.e., in a laboratory, by running the gas over a blood containing Petri dish, no significant amounts of CO will enter the body after death, even in the presence of large open wounds. Thus, a COHb level of over 10% in a burned body even with gaping injuries, indicates that inhalation of smoke, i.e., breathing had occurred.

In addition to the effect of carbon monoxide, smoke inhalation can cause serious damage by direct contact with the respiratory passages and lung tissue.

A young man set fire to a hotel room causing the death of his infant daughter. In order to divert suspicion he placed himself in the bathtub, as if taking a bath. He was found unconscious, but not burned, with a blood carboxyhemoglobin saturation of 43% and severe permanent lung damage.

Delayed onset of respiratory complications following smoke inhalation were first appreciated in the aftermath of the Coconut Grove fire in Boston in 1942. Many of the victims initially appeared to have sustained only minimal burns, however soon their condition deteriorated and many died weeks and months later of respiratory problems.

Widely used chlorine-containing fire retardants generate especially harmful hydrogen chlorine gas when smoldering.

Inhaled smoke is readily seen in the nostrils and mouth as black particles of soot (Fig. XIII-19). Such soot may remain for days in victims who survived. At autopsy, these black particles are mixed with mucous covering the congested lining membrane of the airways (Fig. XIII-20). The soot frequently extends into small airway branches within the lungs. Occasionally, soot is swallowed and small flakes may be recovered

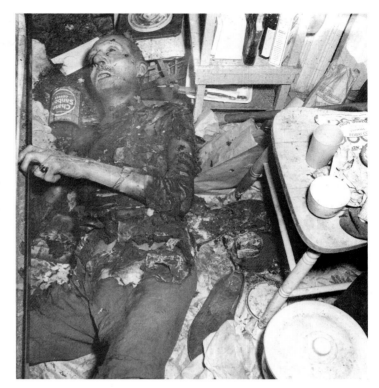

FIGURE XIII-18. Elderly man with history of arteriosclerotic heart disease and emphysema who's shirt caught fire while preparing his dinner. COHb saturation was 22 percent. Burns were limited to the lower chest and abdominal areas.

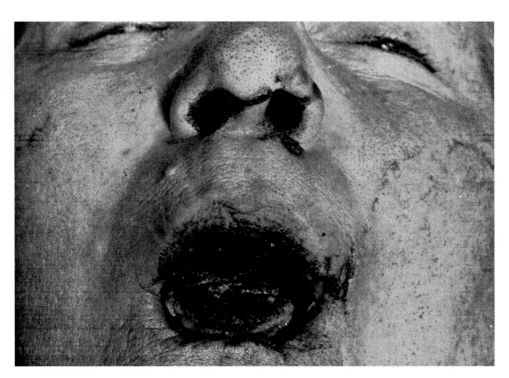

FIGURE XIII-19. Soot in the nostrils and mouth in a body recovered from a smoldering house fire that started in a mattress. This finding indicates breathing while the fire was in progress.

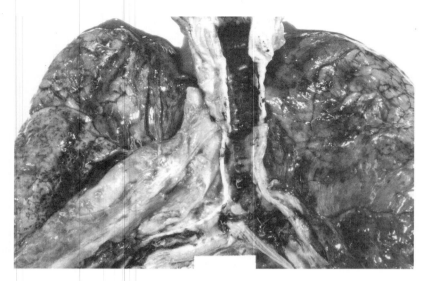

FIGURE XIII-20. Soot deposits in the airways of a fire victim. This indicates that the person was alive when the fire was in progress.

from the esophagus and the lining of the stomach. When a small amount of soot is trapped in mucous it is best documented by using a scalpel to spread a thin film of mucous on a clean white paper towel. To avoid contamination of the airway by soot dropping down from the mouth or throat, it is suggested that the trachea be incised and examined in situ, i.e., before removal from the body. Plugging the upper airway with a ball of absorbent cotton prevents debris from falling into the larynx and trachea below.

Contrary to general belief, blisters in the skin do not necessarily indicate that the victim was alive at the time of the fire (see Figs. XIII-13 and XIII-21). Similarly, the red lining which often surrounds areas of burned skin results from accumulated blood and tissue fluids moved outwards by steam pressure from areas affected by the heat and is not indicative of early onset of inflammation (Fig. XIII-22a–c). Instantly fatal electrocution burns often show this red, peripheral zone, as do burns known to have been sustained after death (Fig. XIII-23). Experimentally produced postmortem burns, in dependent areas of the body with livor mortis, confirm the artifactual nature of this peripheral red zone. Thus, based on this finding, it is not possible to determine, by naked eye or microscopic examination, whether

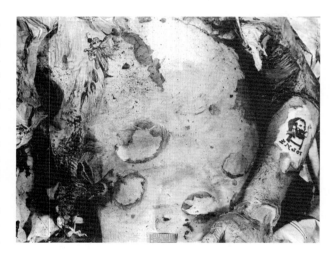

FIGURE XIII-21. Postmortem, second-degree, crater-like burns limited to the epidermis, are often the result of short contact with fast-burning clothes. Note the clarity of the tattoo on the left forearm, where the epidermis was deliberately removed.

a burn occurred before or after death. Also, blisters of a second-degree burn sustained a short time before, or after death, are not distinguishable from skin slippage as seen in the early phases of decomposition. Investigation of the circumstances surrounding a death is required, as is a search for other manifestations of decomposition.

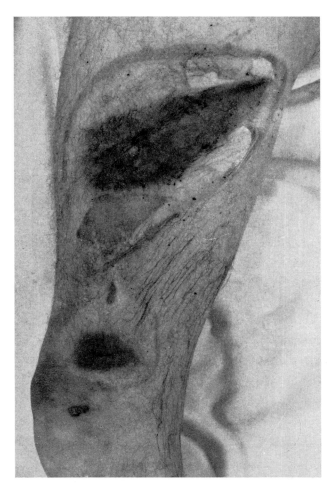

FIGURE XIII-22a–b. Postmortem burns. The peripheral dark zone (red) and marginal blistering surrounding the burned areas is the result of accumulating blood and tissue fluids from areas affected by the heat. This is a frequently observed artifact which must not be mistaken for the onset of inflammation. Arrows mark the red zone on Figure XIII-22 (b). In Figure XIII-22 (a) the zone is obvious.

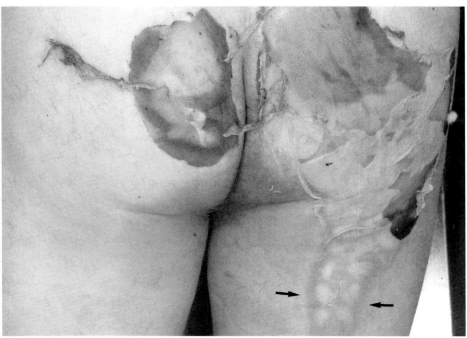

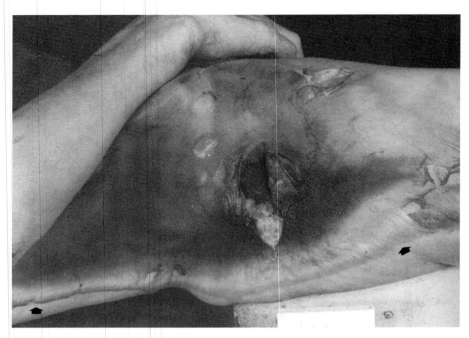

Figure XIII-22c. Right hip and lower chest of a supine fire victim showing charring and a pink discolored longitudinal swelling along the inferior border (between arrows).

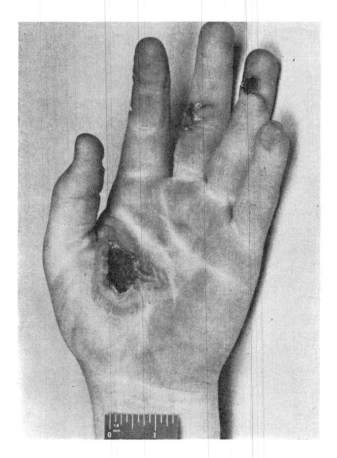

Figure XIII-23. Typical electric burn showing a charred crater with elevated edges and a peripheral pale zone surrounded by a red ring of blood and fluids expelled from the burned center. This is an artifact unrelated to whether the electrocution occurred during life or after death.

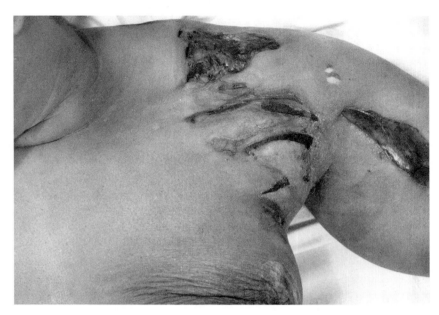

FIGURE XIII-24. Postmortem second-degree burns from contact with radiator ribs following collapse.

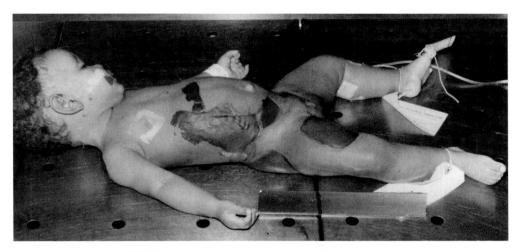

FIGURE XIII-25. Second-degree burns with splash marks on the face.

A fifty-eight-year-old woman was found dead on her bathroom floor, leaning against a hot radiator. Initial investigation suggested foul play. Postmortem examination, however, revealed that death was due to a massive stroke. A patterned injury on the left arm and shoulder was a postmortem second-degree burn, from contact with a steam heat radiator following collapse (Fig. XIII-24).

After bursting, blisters of second-degree burns leave behind a pale pink, moist, raw surface, which turn yellow, then tan and eventually dark brown and become leathery as it dries (Fig. XIII-25). Dousing with gasoline, before or after death, causes skin slippage indistinguishable from second-degree burns due to heat, except for the characteristic odor of the fuel.

Abrasions, especially when dry, leathery and dark brown may resemble a burn. Thus, a linear scratch may simulate a superficial cut by the edge of a heated knife blade and the marginal abrasion of a bullet wound is sometimes mistaken for soot or gunpowder from a contact shot. Micro-

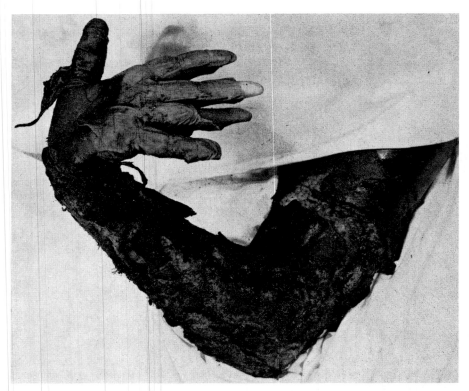

FIGURE XIII-26. Backward pull of the hand due to heat shrinkage of the forearm muscles. Note the difference in burn pattern of the palms and fingers compared to the rest of the extremity due to the fact that a previous clenched fist is now open. The extensor muscles of the forearm in the back are significantly stronger than the flexors in the front.

scopic examination readily establishes the true nature of such injuries.

The presence of fat droplets in blood vessels of the lungs in burn cases must be interpreted with caution, and fat embolism due to blunt trauma or disease such as, sickle cell, should be considered. A small amount of fat in the vessels of the lungs may result from the effect of heat alone and is occasionally observed in individuals who are known to have died before the fire started. The presence of such fat droplets appears to result from a physicochemical alteration of fats normally present in the blood.

Fractures of the extremities in bodies recovered from a fire result from shrinkage of skeletal muscles by the heat. This shrinkage exerts undue pull on tendons and bones. The body assumes a position often referred to as pugilistic, i.e., resembling the position of a boxer, with arms raised and elbows, hips and knees bent. Interestingly,

this position develops during the cooling process, following the fire, which accounts for occasional preservation of hair in the armpits or skin in protected areas that might otherwise be burned (Fig. XIII-26). Rigidity of a body recovered from a fire is caused as a result of denaturation due to heat of muscle proteins and should not be mistaken for rigor mortis.

Fractures of the skull caused by heat are occasionally seen in bodies recovered from fire. Such *cracks* are usually located on either side of the skull above the temples (Fig. XIII-27). Infrequently, they may be bilateral. Characteristically, they consist of several lines radiating from a common center (star burst) (Fig. XIII-28). Outward bursting of the bone flaps and extrusion of brain tissue through the defect may occur as a result of steam pressure building up within the skull (Fig. XIII-29). Cracks of the skull are rarely limited to the external table. Where the appearance of such

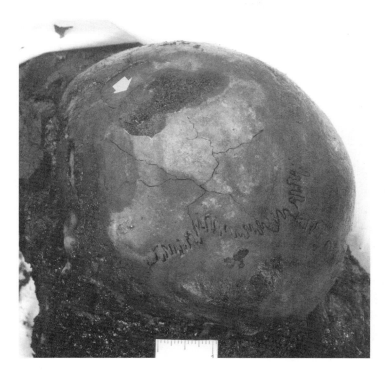

FIGURE XIII-27. *Star burst* shaped fracture in the left parietal area. Note that the fracture lines run up to the suture but do not cross it. Calcination of the frontoparietal area with exposure of the diploe (arrow).

FIGURE XIII-28. Heat fractures of the skull. The fracture in the occipital bone runs up towards the suture, close to a fracture in the parietal bone. Neither fracture crosses the suture. Some bone fragments are bent outward due to internal steam pressure.

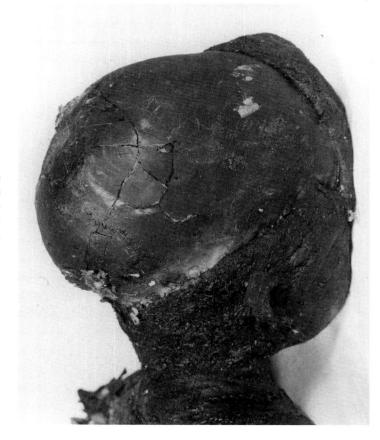

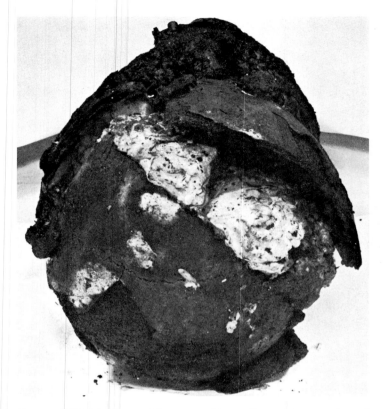

FIGURE XIII-29. Outward bursting of bone flaps and protrusion of cooked brain tissue in a body recovered from a fire. The open skull resembles a partially open oyster.

fractures is atypical, distinction from a fracture sustained during life may be difficult. Contact of flames with the exterior surface of the skull, following charring and ashing of the scalp, sometimes causes localized defects as a result of calcination of the external table and exposure of the spongious layer of the bone (see Fig. XIII-27). Eventually, the entire calvarium may be ashed. Unhealed recently fractured bone is likely to burn more effectively, especially at the edges of separation.

In common house or vehicular fires, heat fractures of the base of the skull usually do not occur, although on rare occasions roofs of the eye sockets may be caved in as a result of steam pressure.

It may be difficult to distinguish between a skull fracture due to heat from one caused by physical trauma. The edges of a heat fracture are usually more irregular and ragged. However, the straight edges of a fracture caused by crushing are likely to become roughened and irregular if the skull was subsequently exposed to flames.

Curiously, heat fractures do not generally involve the sutures of the skull, especially in young individuals with open sutures. When heat fractures cross suture lines, they rarely open and gape by steam pressure alone.

Blood and marrow are frequently expressed from the skull bones by the heat and accumulate between the bone and the dura mater, forming a clot-like mass suggestive of a traumatic epidural hematoma sustained during life (Fig. XIII-30a–b). The skull is commonly badly damaged where an epidural hematoma is found, but fractures are usually absent. The brain may be shrunken, firm and yellow to light brown, due to cooking and dehydration (Fig. XIII-31a–b). The dura is leathery, without evidence of injury. The presence of blood *under* the dura, subdural hemorrhage, in a victim of conflagration always indi-

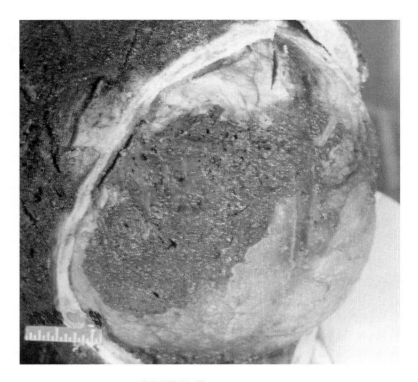

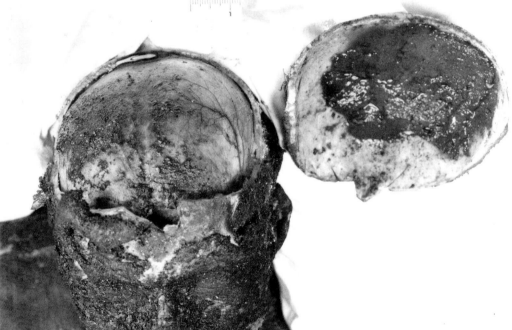

FIGURE XIII-30a–b. Examples of epidural hematomas caused by heat. The calvarium has been removed. The dura mater is intact. The clot is due to blood and marrow expressed by the heat from the bones of the skull. Steam pressure moved the released blood and marrow to one place, forming a single clot. Epidural heat hematomas are unlikely in the elderly due to more complete adherence of the dura to the skull.

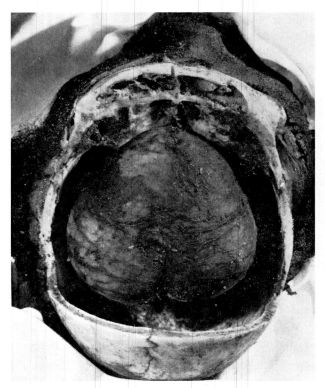
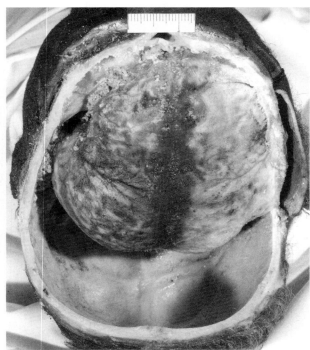

FIGURE XIII-31a–b. Heat shrinkage of the brain within the skull of fire victims. The brains are enclosed in the intact dura mater.

cates an injury sustained during life and is unrelated to the effect of heat or flames. Any subdural blood should be retained for laboratory analysis. A positive alcohol level in the clot indicates consumption of alcoholic beverages prior to injury. Several hours, even days may elapse between the injury and death. During this time, alcohol in the peripheral blood may have been eliminated. The presence of alcohol has been observed in a subdural hematoma in a patient who had sustained fatal head injuries four days earlier.[11] Drug analysis of the epidural clot is equally significant.

Heat that builds up in the chest of a body recovered from a fire is sometimes associated with blood pressed into alveoli, airway, mouth and nostrils. The same occurs with blood and bone marrow expressed from the skull, forming an epidural clot and from livorous areas forming a peripheral red zone, suggestive of an earlier injury, during life. The presence of alveolar blood may also simulate earlier thoracic injury.

Blood caked to the inner linings of the chest cavities, (the parietal pleura), usually signifies trauma unrelated to the fire. Its presence requires exploration of the chest walls for bruises and skeletal fractures.

Splitting of skin occurs as a result of shrinkage. The abdominal cavity may be exposed. It is important to distinguish such postmortem splits from antemortem cuts and slashes (Fig. XIII-32a–e). Splits due to heat involving the abdominal wall invariably run parallel to the muscle fibers. Any split *across* a muscle is the result of physical trauma, and is not heat or fire related.

The anus is occasionally dilated as a result of shrinkage of the perianal tissues and sometimes the rectal wall protrudes through the opening, like in a prolapse. This could be mistaken for evidence of sodomy. Prolapse of the anal lining frequently occurs due to intra-abdominal buildup of gases as a result of putrefaction.

Careless smoking on a sofa or in bed, often following consumption of alcoholic beverages, or

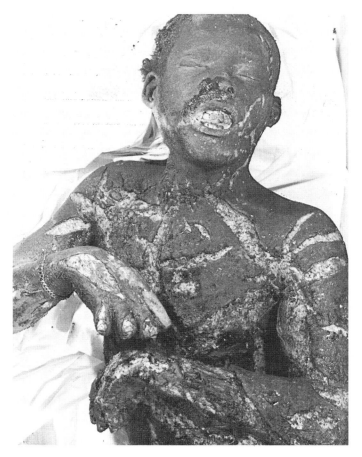

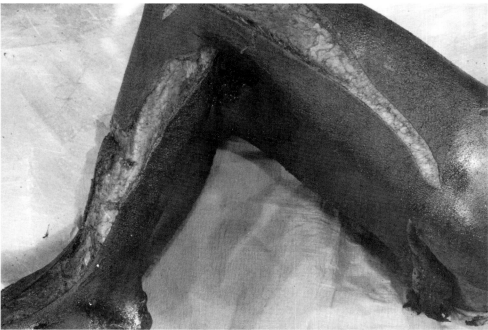

FIGURE XIII-32a–b. Splitting of the skin as the result of heat. Only the skin is involved. The underlying tissues are intact. (b) The skin is split by heat, with sharp edges similar to a cut. Note that surrounding skin appears, but is not, unburnt.

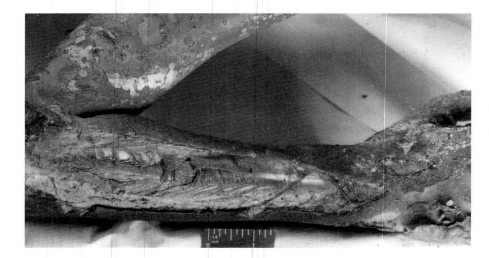

FIGURE XIII-32c. Occasionally, the split will go as deep as the muscle.

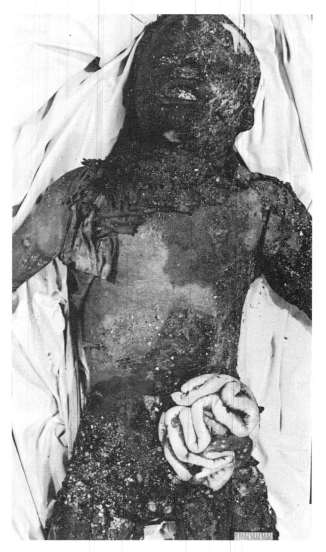

FIGURE XIII-32d. Charred body of a young boy with a split of the abdominal wall resembling a cut. The split is vertical between muscles (rather than *through* muscle substance) and is a result of increased intraabdominal pressure caused by the heat.

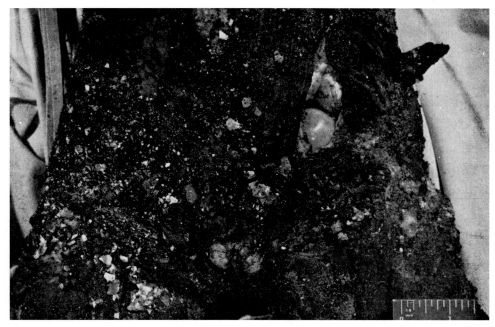

FIGURE XIII-32e. Loops of uninjured bowel protruding through the gap were replaced into the abdominal cavity. There was no evidence of bleeding.

children playing with matches, are probably the most common causes of accidental house fires. The following will review the events associated with this type of conflagration.

According to Henahan,[12] fire develops progressively when a cigarette or burning match falls onto a mattress or other upholstered furniture. The sheet or cover is readily scorched and smolders. Charring occurs, but no flame. At this point the fire is confined and easily extinguishable. A small flame develops. Smoke and toxic gases rise from the burning mattress, accumulating under the ceiling. Heat radiating from the flame raises the temperature in the room. Hot air is lighter than cold air. Soon dense smoke under the ceiling is hot enough to act as a giant space heater, intensifying the heat in the room. At this point, the fire is still confined to a small area of the mattress. A person awakening at this time can still get out, on his knees without much breathing, to avoid inhaling the toxic fumes under the ceiling. Knowing that heat and fire gases rise, an experienced firefighter, without his breathing apparatus, crouches, crawls or even throws himself flat on the floor to keep below the smoke as he exits from the smoke-filled environment.

In the Boston subway fire in 1974, people who crawled out were able to drag with them those who collapsed while running or walking.

As the temperature of the room rises beyond 300° F, volatile gases are released from wood, fabrics, paint, paper and especially plastics. A few minutes later, the room has become a tinderbox waiting for a spark or a tongue of flame from the original small fire to set off an explosion. This is the deadly phenomenon of *flashover*. Almost instantaneously, all flammable objects in the room ignite and the fire is transformed into an inferno from which there is no escape. Following the flashover, the room temperature gradually drops as all combustible materials are consumed.

Non-combustible solids, such as steel, gypsum board and cement fail in their performance at high temperatures. At temperatures in excess of 1700° F, steel beams will bend, causing buildings to collapse.

A tanker truck, carrying 12,000 gallons of heating oil, crashed between Boston and New York, fueling a huge blaze which buckled a highway and overpass. The overpass sagged several feet as a result of heat-damaged steel support beams. We had a similar incident in Detroit.

Although, there has been much dispute regarding the cause of the collapse of the World Trade Center, it is likely that fire fed by burning jet fuel, i.e., approximately 1800° F (1000° C), played a significant role in the building's collapse. Structural steel begins to soften around 800° F (425° C) and loses half its strength at 1200° F (650° C).[13,14]

Injury Due to Scalding

Scalding is the most common type of thermal injury in children.

The severity of injury depends primarily on the temperature and duration of contact. Increase of skin temperature rapidly reduces the time needed to produce a burn. According to Moritz and Henriquez[15] full thickness burns occur in 30 seconds at 130° F (54.4° C) and in one second at 158° F (70° C).

Sensitivity of the skin is a significant factor in burn-injury causation. The mucous membranes of the mouth and throat are considerably more resistant to hot liquids than is skin. We can, therefore, eat and drink foods too hot to touch with our hands. Generally, the skin of a child is more sensitive than that of an adult; children under 5 years, the elderly and persons who are mentally or physically disabled are most at risk. Certain areas of the body are more sensitive than others. For example, the palmar surface of the hands is markedly more resistant to heat than the face, the abdomen or the genitalia.

Household hot water is generally set at 130° to 140° F and may reach 160° F. Most electric water heaters currently in operation in the U.S. have been preset by the factory at 150° F and gas water heaters have been preset to 140° F. At such temperatures severe burns are likely to occur in adults after 2 to 5 seconds of exposure. Almost all scald burns caused by inadvertent turning on of the hot water tap could be avoided if the setting on hot water heaters were not to exceed 120° F.[16,17] In industry, steam from a boiler will cause severe burns. Scalding may occur through clothing. In fact, clothes worsen the damage by prolonging contact with the hot liquid and reducing the cooling effect of evaporation. Pouring a cup of hot coffee on one's lap is likely to cause more damage than pouring the coffee on bare skin. The extent of damage by scalding is in no way comparable to that caused by fire. Singeing of hair does not occur as a result of scalding. This enables distinction of a second-degree scald from a similar burn caused by fire.

It is frequently mandatory to differentiate between accidental scalding due to spilling or splashing, and scalding as a result of deliberate pouring or throwing of hot liquids. Immersion of a child in hot water by an abusive parent or sibling is sometimes the cause of scalding injury. It is important under such circumstances that the distribution of the scalds be evaluated in light of the manner in which the injury was supposedly sustained. This will indicate the compatibility of a scalding pattern with a given history. Thus, a child immersed in hot water will hold the thighs against his or her abdomen and chest while the buttocks and perineum are immersed. Under no circumstances, can such injury be accidental, since if the child had fallen into the water and tried to escape the extremities would have been scalded as well. A straight, horizontal burn pattern across the body or an extremity is always suggestive of forceful immersion (Fig. XIII-33a–b). Presence of an irritant or corrosive chemical in the scalding liquid is likely to increase the severity of the injury.

Injuries caused by chemicals may be corrosive and cause sloughing skin damage suggestive of scalding. Litmus paper and chemical analysis may be required to provide the answer. Dry heat without fire will also cause similar injuries.

Inhalation of hot vapor may cause death without external manifestations of injury. It follows a short asymptomatic period, gradually developing into a progressively worsening shortness of breath and asphyxia resulting from obstruction of the airway by edematous swelling of its lining. Steam contains 4,000 times the heat capacity of air. If inhaled, steam readily injures the lower airway branches within the lungs.

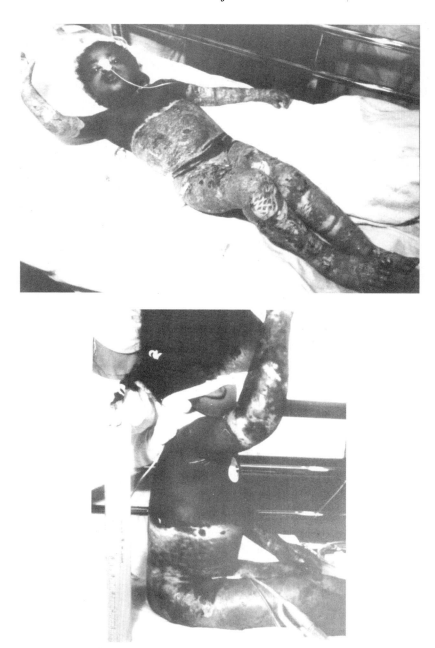

FIGURE XIII-33a–b. Child deliberately immersed in hot water with typical scalding pattern.

Medicolegal Considerations of Bomb Explosions

The postmortem examination of a victim of explosion involves two main objectives: (a) identification, (b) reconstruction of the events.

Procedures for identification of explosion victims are usually the same as those used for identification in general, but differ whenever there is wide dispersion of body parts by the blast. Destruction of the face places particular emphasis on other means of identification. The jaws and

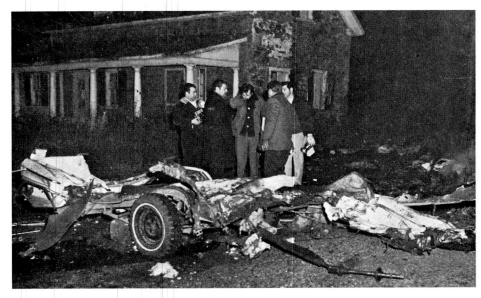

FIGURE XIII-34a. Explosion scene, showing the extent of destruction of the automobile. Fragments were found 162 ft. away from the center of the explosion.

fingers may be scattered and must be retrieved for identification by dental comparison or fingerprints. A single tooth or a fragment of an artificial denture are often all that is needed to confirm identification by dental comparison. When tentative identification of a victim is available, a single fingerprint suffices to confirm identification. Otherwise, all ten fingerprints are required.

With respect to reconstruction of the event, location and extent of the injuries are of foremost significance.

In a case involving an explosion in an automobile,[18] examination of the two victims established who was the driver and who was the right front seat passenger. It was further determined that the bomb was located on the floorboard between the passenger's feet and that he was bending forward and holding the bomb when the blast occurred (Fig. XIII-34a–d). On-the-scene examination of the automobile by explosion specialists confirmed the conclusions of the medical examiner and added that the explosive charge was definitely not in the glove compartment or attached to the undercarriage of the vehicle, either of which would have indicated involvement of another party.

The combined results of independent investigations of the medical examiner and the police left no doubt that the explosion occurred accidentally when the bomb was being transported by the occupants of the vehicle. Test explosions conducted by the FBI indicated that twelve sticks of 40% dynamite placed on the right floorboard of an automobile are required to reproduce damage equivalent to that of the automobile in question.

Death due to explosion may be associated with devastating injuries, as seen in the passenger of the vehicle. Extensive injuries may also be caused by falling debris or cave-in and burial under rubble. However, in some instances, death may occur without any manifestations of trauma. Such deaths result from massive internal bleeding predominantly in the lungs, due to the shock wave following the blast. This is a concussive injury, and death may be practically instantaneous.

Large confluent hemorrhages were observed in the lungs of the vehicle's driver. The same injury was reported as the prevalent cause of death in individuals who were situated within the blast perimeter of exploding bombs in the London blitz of World War II.[19] Perforation of an ear drum with a sudden sharp pain and one-sided loss of hearing, sometimes associated with a trickle of blood from the respective ear hole, is sometimes observed in survivors of an explosion, due to the same phenomenon. Explosions associated with a flash fire or an electric arc sometimes cause extensive singeing of the face. Spared, crow feet-like creases at the outer angles of the

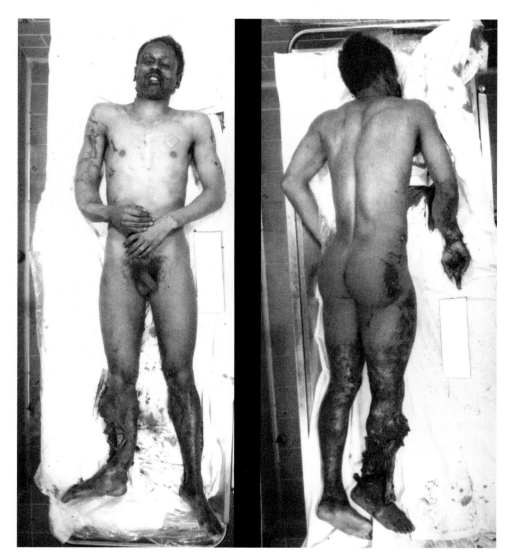

FIGURE XIII-34b. Front and back view of the driver of the automobile, showing the injuries predominately on the right side. The right forearm and the right leg are fractured. The back and buttocks are intact. The intact area above the horizontal demarcating line of injury across the posterior mid thighs is caused by shielding of the back and buttocks due to sitting. Obviously, the right hand was holding the steering wheel, exposing the forearm to the blast. The degloving injury on the lateral aspect of the right leg and significantly less damage to the outer surface of the left leg indicate that the blast was from right to left.

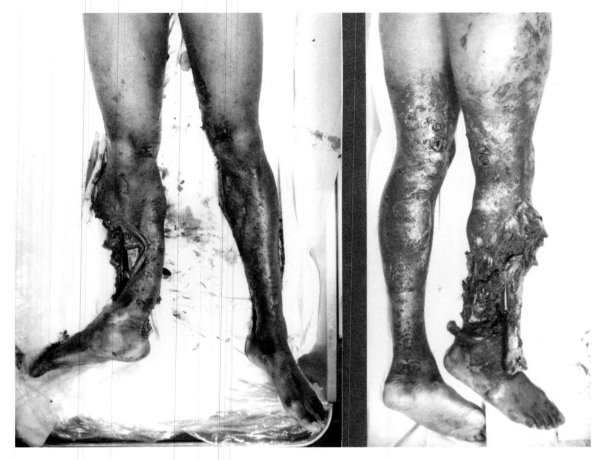

FIGURE XIII-34c. A closer view of the driver's lower extremities shows the avulsion of the lateral surface of the right leg. The medial aspect of the left leg is singed to the shin-line, and in the rear singeing is limited by a vertical plane through the middle of the calf.

eyes, due to squinting, indicate that the victim was alive at the time of the blast.

A large variety of bombs is used, many of which are homemade. It is important after an explosion that attempts be made to determine what materials were used in the construction of the bomb, since this may provide leads to the identity of the perpetrator. Complete body x-ray of the victims is imperative before the clothing is removed. Fragments of the bomb may be trapped among the clothes and within body tissues. In the case of the automobile explosion previously mentioned, x-ray films of the passenger revealed a number of metallic objects in the skull and trunk. Subsequently, at autopsy, a 1.5 volt mercury battery was recovered from within the skull, and other objects, including a small portion of a spring, several rivets and two thin 1/2 inch long, metallic wires, were removed from the chest and abdomen. Some of the fragments used for the firing system of the bomb were identified as originating from a key-wound clock movement characteristic of a specific manufacturer.

Clothing, even if shredded, or any remnants of clothing articles should be retained for chemical analyses, since this too may reveal the presence of traces from the explosive that was used. Victims who are close to the epicenter of an explosion may be found partly or completely nude. Their clothes, especially loose articles, may be blown off by the blast and recovered in shreds a considerable distance away. Tight articles, such as a belt, a buttoned collar, or lace-up boots, are likely to remain on the body.

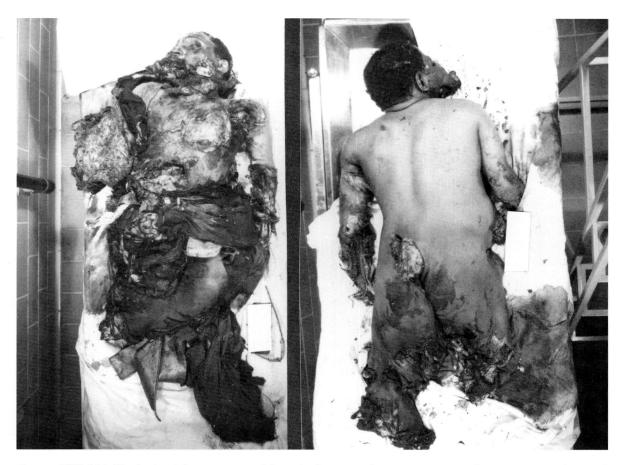

FIGURE XIII-34d. The body of the passenger of the right front seat shows extensive mutilating injuries with partial amputation of the extremities and partial exposure of the abdominal cavity and lower chest. A narrow strip of intact skin was preserved under the belt. The pattern and distribution of the injuries permitted the conclusion that the bomb was situated between the feet of the victim and that he was probably bending forward, holding the bomb. The facial skeleton was fragmented and features were unrecognizable. The battery of the timing device in the bomb was found inside the head.

While explosives are notorious for the blasting and fragmentation they cause, incendiary bombs primarily cause burns. Napalm belongs to this category. Napalm consists of a combination of oil and gasoline in jellied form. It generates temperature close to 1800° F. Phosphorus and magnesium are frequent additives to incendiary bombs and grenades. Under such circumstances temperatures may exceed 3500° F. Systemic poisoning by the added chemicals is sometimes observed.

The *Molotov cocktail* is another variety of incendiary bomb. It is designed to be hand thrown and has been frequently used by terrorists and in guerrilla warfare. The use of such devices has a considerable psychological and devastating effect. A crude, but effective and often used version of this bomb consists of a bottle filled with gasoline and a rag to serve as a wick. The wick is lit, and the "*cocktail*" is thrown at the target. As a point of reference, one pint of gasoline is equivalent to the energy generated by the explosion of two sticks of dynamite. Addition of various acids and other chemicals enhances the destructive effect of these bombs.

REFERENCES

1. Aikawa, N., Aoki, K., and Yamazaki, M.: Recent advances in the management of severely burned patients. *Nippon Geka Gakkai Zasshi, 100* (7): 424–429, July 1999.
2. Svensson, A., and Wendel, O.: *Crime detection.* Amsterdam, Elsevier, 1955.
3. Icove, D.J., and DeHaan, J.D.: *Forensic fire scene reconstruction,* 1st edition. Upper Saddle River, NJ: Pearson Prentice Hall, 2004.
4. National Fire Protection Agency publication 921. Fire and Explosion Investigations. 2001.
5. Richards, N.F.: Fire investigation–Destruction of corpses. *Med Sci Law, 17:* 79, 1977.
6. Bezymenski, L.: *The death of Adolph Hitler.* New York, HarBrace World, 1968.
7. Levin, B.C., Rechani, P.R., Gurman, J.L., Landron, F., Clark, H.M., Yoklavich, M.F., Rodriquez, J.R., Droz, L., deCabrera, F., and Kaye, S.: Analysis of Carboxyhemoglobin and Cyanide in blood from victims of the Dupont Plaza Hotel Fire in Puerto Rico. *J Forensic Sci, 35:* 151, 1990.
8. Toxicological Profile for Cyanide. Agency for Toxic Substances and Disease Registry, U.S. Public Health Service, Washington, D.C. January, 1988, p. 41.
9. Crapo, R.O.: Smoke–Inhalation injuries. *JAMA, 246:* 15, 1694–1696, 1987.
10. Stewart, R.D., Stewart, R.S., Stamm, W., and Seelen, R.P.: Rapid estimation of carboxyhemoglobin level in fire fighters. *JAMA, 235:* 390–392, 1976.
11. Cassin, B., and Spitz, W.U.: Concentration of alcohol in delayed subdural hematoma. *J. Forensic Sci., 28* (4): 1013–1015, 1983.
12. Henahan, J.F.: Fire. *Science, 80,* 1, 2: 29–38, 1980.
13. Eagar, T.W., and Musso, C.: Why Did the World Trade Center collapse? Science, engineering, and speculation. *JOM, 53* (12): 8–11, 2001.
14. Dunn, V.: Why the World Trade Center buildings collapsed, A fire chief's assessment. Http://vincent-dunn.com 2004.
15. Mortiz, A.R., and Henriques, F.C.: Studies of thermal injury: The relative importance of time and surface temperature in the causation of cutaneous burns. *Am J Pathol, 23:* 695, 1947.
16. Feldman, K.W., Schaller, R.T., Feldman, J.A., and McMillon, M.: Tap water scald burns in children. *Pediatrics, 62* (1): 1–7, 1978.
17. Katcher, M.L.: Scald burns from hot tap water. *JAMA, 246:* 1219–1222, 1981.
18. Spitz, W.U., Sopher, I.M., and DiMaio, V.J.M.: Medicolegal investigation of a bomb explosion in an automobile. *J Forensic Sci, 15:* 537, 1970.
19. Zuckerman, S.: Experimental study of blast injuries to the lung. *Lancet, 2:* 219, 1940.

Chapter XIV

ASPHYXIA

WERNER U. SPITZ

ASPHYXIA IS A BROAD TERM encompassing a variety of conditions that result in interference with the uptake or utilization of oxygen (O_2). Oxygen is essential to sustain life. A reduced concentration of oxygen in the blood which reaches the brain causes rapid loss of consciousness. The brain constitutes approximately 2% of body weight, but utilizes 20% of the total available oxygen. Because it is the most sensitive to oxygen deprivation, the brain is the organ most affected in all types of asphyxial death.

In all forms of asphyxia, the heartbeat usually continues for several minutes after respiratory arrest. Clinical records suggest that cardiac function may persist for as long as 10 minutes and sometimes longer. Microscopic manifestations of cerebral anoxia begin to occur after as early as 30 minutes of oxygen deprivation. Continued cardiac activity after respiratory arrest is of critical importance in effecting resuscitation.

It has been suggested that consciousness may persist for up to 10 seconds in cases of abrupt cardiopulmonary arrest, because of oxygen already present in brain tissue. However, experience appears to negate this hypothesis with the thought that oxygen is not the sole determining factor in extending awareness, but that simultaneous active and sound blood pressure is also required.

When Owen Hart fell 180 feet when entering the ring during a televised wrestling performance in Missouri on October 15, 2000, in front of thousands of spectators, it was evident that he never manifested any signs of life after he hit the floor. EMS, stationed at ringside, immediately went to his aid to no avail.

At autopsy, the aorta was severed at the arch and blood flow to the brain was interrupted on impact. A compound comminuted fracture of his left elbow, with a large gaping laceration, showed no blood in or around the wound. There were no other injuries.

In another example, a 50-year-old, unrestrained woman, rear seat passenger in a car which was broadsided by another motor vehicle, fell out through the rear door of the car onto the road as the car came to a halt. She showed no signs of life immediately following the crash. When EMS arrived she was pronounced dead at the scene. At autopsy the only injury was a severed aorta and a left chest cavity full of blood.

There are numerous other examples of victims of motor vehicle crashes who are unresponsive on impact, with severe external injuries which show no evidence of hemorrhage and a severed aorta at autopsy.

For practical purposes, asphyxia falls into one of the following categories:

1. *Compression of the neck,* with or without blockage of the airway, as in:
   a. Hanging
   b. Strangulation
2. *Obstruction of the airway,* as in:
   a. Smothering
   b. Aspiration of foreign material
   c. Swelling of the lining membranes of the throat, as in some allergic and inflammatory reactions, inhalation of superheated air or following a blow to the neck
   d. Postural asphyxia, also known as positional asphyxia or traumatic asphyxia
3. *Compression of the chest* interfering with respiratory movements
4. *Exclusion of oxygen* due to depletion and replacement by another gas or as a result of chemical interference with its uptake and utilization
   a. Carbon dioxide poisoning
   b. Carbon monoxide poisoning
   c. Cyanide poisoning

In spite of similarities of anatomical findings in different types of neck trauma, a basic understanding of tissue responses often permits identification of the mechanism of injury.

COMPRESSION OF THE NECK

Hanging

Death by hanging usually results from arrest of the arterial blood flow to the brain or obstruction of the venous return, or both.

Hanging can be accomplished with the body in any position (Figs. XIV-1a–b to XIV-3a–c). The body can be suspended, with the feet on the ground, sitting, leaning, even lying down. In cases of *semi-suspension,* arterial blood flow to the head persists while the venous return is interrupted. Veins are more compressible than arteries. The face is therefore purple, dusky, cyanotic, swollen, sometimes with bulging eyes, due to edema and congestion of periorbital tissues, and numerous subconjunctival and facial petechiae as well as hemorrhages into skin pores and pimples, all confined to areas above the noose (Fig. XIV-4a). None of these changes occur below the noose. If the body was cut down and the noose removed soon following the hanging, cyanosis will gradually disappear and blood that was trapped above the noose will drain from the head to the neck and shoulders blending with livor mortis in dependent areas of the body. Under such circumstances, an autopsy scheduled for the next day may well encounter a body without cyanosis. However, petechiae, if originally present, will remain.

In a *semi-suspended* body or if the noose was left in place for several hours, especially in warm weather, the blue-purple color of cyanosis will become *fixed,* i.e., irreversible, as a result of hemolysis and diffusion of blood pigment into the skin. In contrast, in cases of *total suspension* where the feet are off the ground, the face is pale and subconjunctival and cutaneous petechiae, facial swelling, and cyanosis are absent.

For the purpose of clarity, asphyxial petechiae are delicate, pinpoint to pinhead size. Larger petechiae are infrequent and when they occur, result from confluence. Petechiae are caused by the rise in venous pressure above the noose, resulting in rupture of capillaries and leakage of a

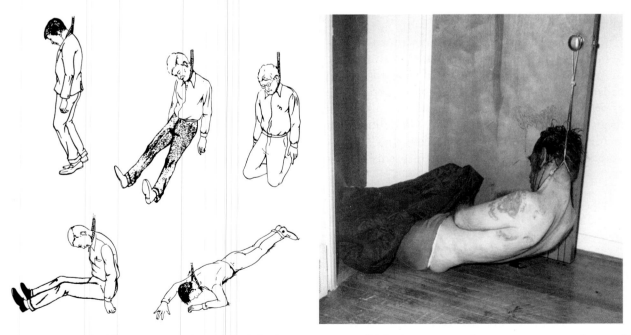

FIGURE XIV-1a–b. (a) Hanging can be accomplished in any position. (b) In this position, the noose runs upward toward the nape of the neck. Had the victim been face down, the noose would have been horizontal as would occur in many homicides.

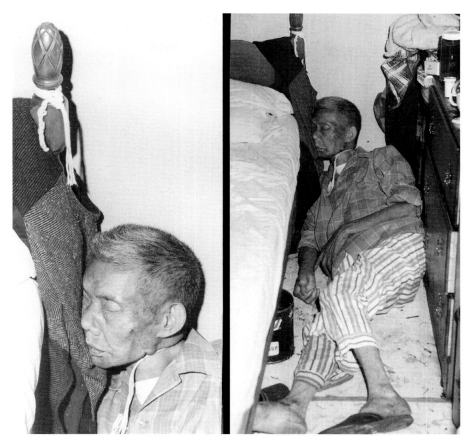

FIGURE XIV-2. Fifty-two-year-old man who lived alone and had been despondent. A neighbor found him hanging from the bedpost in the position shown. The neighbor cut the rope and called the police. Closeup shows the rope imprint on the left jaw and cheek.

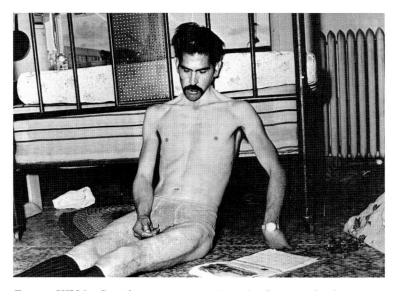

FIGURE XIV-3a. Suicide in a sitting position. A religious calendar is near the body.

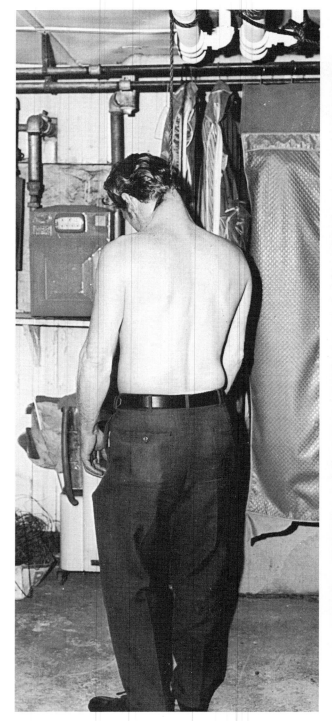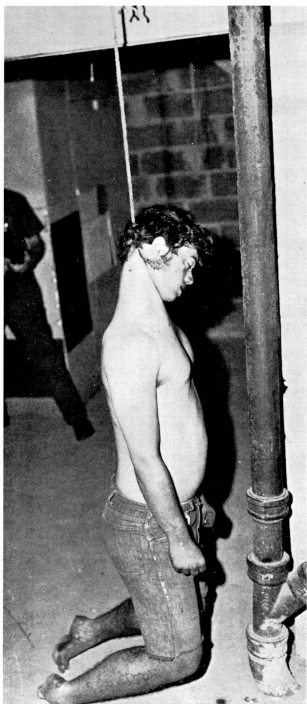

FIGURE XIV-3b–c. (b) Suicide in a standing position. Knees are slightly bent and the head is tilted forward. (c) College student in the basement of his residence, semi-kneeling, suspended from a beam in the ceiling. The body had been hanging for over 24 hours when found. Note discoloration of forearms and legs. The neck is markedly stretched.

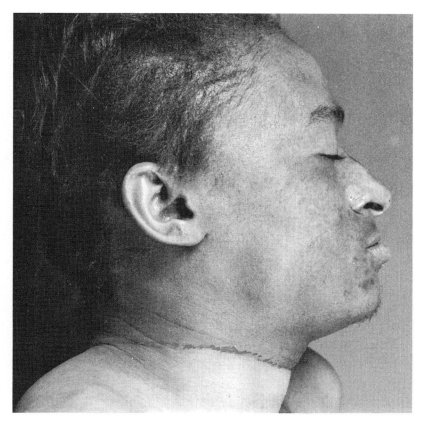

FIGURE XIV-4a. Obstruction of veins, by a horizontal ligature. The victim was lying with his head and neck just above the floor, the noose was tied to a door knob. The body was found one day after the suicide.

droplet of blood into the tissue. Petechial hemorrhages are typically found in the conjunctivae, the skin of the eyelids, the forehead and the upper cheeks (Fig. XIV-4b–c). Petechiae in the lining of the mouth and throat, and in the muscles of the temples are infrequent. Petechiae in these locations are meaningful only in the presence of petechiae in the face and eyes. Over 50% of suicidal hangings show petechial hemorrhages.[1]

Some consider conjunctival petechiae as diagnostic of suffocation, however, petechiae occasionally occur in cases of natural death with marked facial livor, particularly in plethoric and obese individuals and in people who died of acute right heart failure with markedly elevated venous pressure. Such petechiae are usually larger, often much larger, than the asphyxial type. Facial and conjunctival petechiae and tissue

swelling may also occur as a result of gravity settling of intravascular blood in an individual found dead lying across the bed with his head hanging over the mattress.

The density of petechiae in the skin and conjunctivae can serve as indicator for the duration of the process. Thus, in cases of subtle, slow, protracted asphyxia the number of petechiae is far greater compared to that found in cases were pressure on the neck was more aggressive, uninterrupted and of short duration.

Pinpoint hemorrhages about the face and eyelids may also be found following cardiopulmonary resuscitation, independent of the mechanism of death. Such hemorrhages are caused by abrupt movement of the blood column and traumatic rupture of small blood vessels as a result of cardiac compressions.[2] The pres-

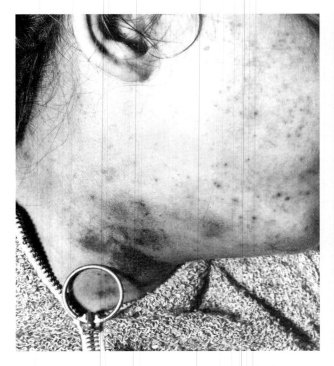

FIGURE XIV-4b. Numerous, scattered petechial hemorrhages and hemorrhages into skin glands on the right side of the face. Four typical fingertip bruises on the neck. The assailant may have been left-handed?

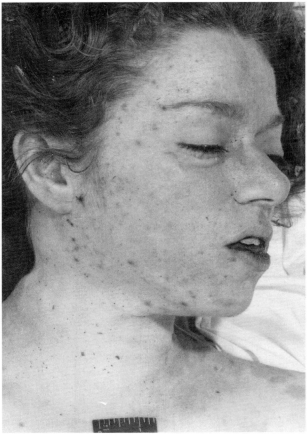

FIGURE XIV-4c. Numerous petechial hemorrhages on the right side of the face, temple and forehead. The face is cyanotic above the noose imprint.

ence of petechiae does not conclusively prove that asphyxia has occurred, only that there was mechanical interference with the blood flow.

A photography technician got his necktie caught in a processing machine. He tried to stop the machine unsuccessfully, then tried to pull on the tie to remove it, eventually tearing it off. He came out of the dark room telling of his ordeal, his face swollen, predominately his ears. His speech was slurred and indistinct due to swelling of his tongue. There were numerous pinpoint petechiae in the conjunctivae and all over his face. The swelling subsided within the hour and the petechiae disappeared by the following day.

Police departments, many years ago, started using clip-on ties for their officers after some were grabbed by their tie during confrontations.

In general, non-asphyxial petechiae are larger, coarser and not limited to areas above the noose. Petechial hemorrhages should not be mistaken for *Tardieu spots* which are spot-like hemorrhages, larger and more irregularly shaped compared to petechiae. Tardieu spots are limited to areas of

livor mortis. They result from blood oozing out of decomposing capillaries.

Two basic types of hanging are recognized:
1. *The knot is situated behind the ears,* usually in the region of the nape of the neck. Blood flow to and from the brain is interrupted by the pressure of the noose on both sides of the neck (Fig. XIV-5). The face is pale, without petechiae or cyanosis.
2. *The knot is situated under the chin.* The lower jaw protects the neck from deep pressure by the noose. Venous outflow from the brain is interrupted, while arterial blood flow to the brain continues. Petechiae are abundant and cyanosis is prominent. When the knot is situated to the side, i.e., in front of one ear and not

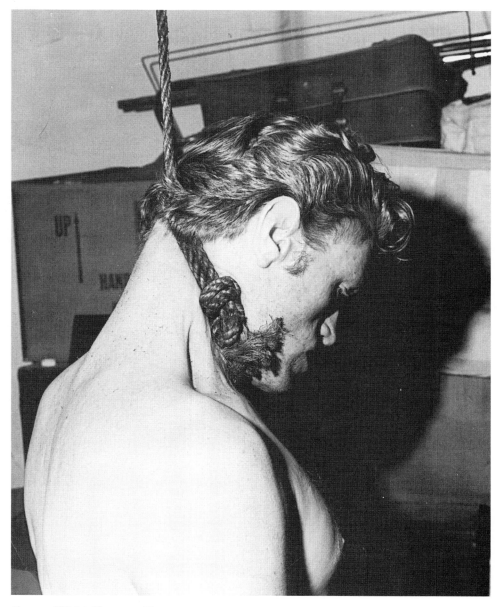

FIGURE XIV-5. Hanging: The noose runs upward behind the ears toward the ceiling. The victim was standing.

the other, subconjunctival hemorrhages may be one sided (Fig. XIV-6).

Depending on the type of noose, the groove on the neck produced by the pressure of the noose may be deep, the skin shrunken, dry, brown, leather-like. This usually occurs when the noose is narrow and furrows deeply into the tissues. When the noose is broad, such as a belt, there may not be a groove, but only slight inden-

tation of the skin between parallel top and bottom lines of demarcation by the edges of the belt. When a twisted piece of clothing or a soft blanket is used, there may be no mark at all on the skin. In the case of a narrow noose, incision of the groove may reveal scattered or clusters of tiny hemorrhages in the upper layers of the skin. The presence of such hemorrhages indicates active blood flow at the time of hanging. These hemor-

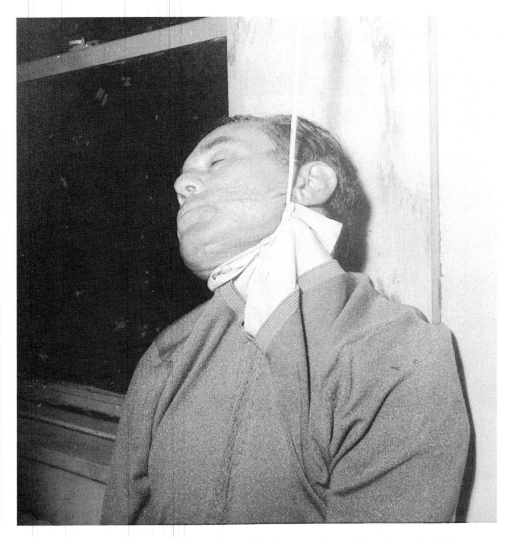

FIGURE XIV-6. The knot is situated in front of the left ear, elevated by the angle of the jaw.

rhages are the result of direct trauma applied by the noose.

In either case, whether the arterial blood flow to the brain or the venous return is interrupted, the brain is ultimately deprived of oxygen, resulting in loss of consciousness. The amount of pressure on the neck that can bring about loss of consciousness is remarkably low.[3] It is said that five or six pounds of pressure per square inch suffice to occlude the carotid arteries and jugular veins. Thirty-two pounds are required to block the airway. In an adult, the head weighs an average of 10 pounds. Thus, blood flow to the brain can be interrupted by pressure of the head alone, with

any type of noose. Loss of consciousness is followed by increased pressure on the neck from the added weight of the limp suspended body. This, in turn, completely shuts off the blood flow to the brain, and death occurs as oxygen is depleted.

Subtle and insidious loss of consciousness account for a large number of accidental hangings, particularly in children. Such deaths, some involving different types of crib toys, have been reported by the Consumer Product Safety Commission. Examples of gradual loss of consciousness are illustrated by the following cases:

A seventeen-month-old child was playing in his crib with a toy telephone. The mother was in an adjacent room.

When she heard no sound from the child for a *few minutes,* she checked and found him face up, dead, with the telephone cord wrapped around his neck. The receiver was beside the child; the phone had slipped from the mattress and was suspended between the bars. The weight of the phone was sufficient to interfere with cerebral blood flow. There was no evidence of a struggle; the non-fitted sheet was in order, and the child was not heard crying.

Similar situations occur in individuals who are heavily intoxicated by alcohol or drugs, in autoerotic deaths, and in cases of sudden collapse due to natural disease (Fig. XIV-7).

An elderly woman with a blood alcohol concentration of .28% died of hanging when she collapsed as she was trying to unlock the door of her apartment with a key she was carrying on a cord around her neck. The broken off key was found in the lock (Fig. XIV-8a–b).

Judging by the circumstances under which these individuals are found, there is certainly no indication that this is a traumatic, painful way to die. It seems as though the individual had fallen asleep. Review of all relevant facts suggests that most hangings, whether accidents or suicides, cause a gradual, subtle and painless death.

Compression of the airway by the noose in hanging cases is not as common as is generally believed. Supportive evidence for this includes the finding of vomitus in the airway of some hanging victims. Suicidal hanging of persons with a tracheostomy below the level of the noose also illustrates this point (Fig. XIV-9). Such individuals continue to breathe while dying. Obstruction of the airway usually elicits a violent struggle, a dramatic condition known as *air hunger.* Air hunger is by no means subtle, insidious, or painless, but generates tremendous fear of impending doom coupled with violent efforts to *open* the airway.

A finding that is now rarely seen in cases of hanging is fracture of the odontoid process of the second cervical vertebra. When hanging was a widely practiced form of judicial execution, such fractures caused almost instantaneous death by impact of the dislodged bony process on vital nerve centers in the medulla oblongata controlling respiration and heartbeat. The weight of the individual to be hanged was directly proportional to the distance he was made to drop. The knot was positioned so as to cause a sudden backlash

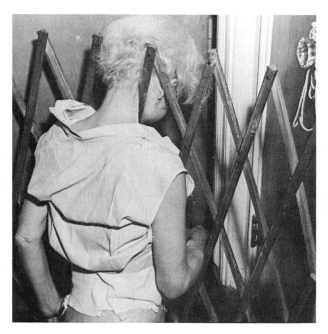

FIGURE XIV-7. Elderly woman who collapsed as a result of a seizure into a folding security gate.

of the head, at the same time as the body was brought to an abrupt halt at the end of the rope. According to Pierrepoint, the former hangman of London, in his testimony before the Royal Commission on Capital Punishment in 1950, the knot must be situated under the left side of the lower jaw to throw the head back and snap the neck at the moment of the drop.[4]

A case of suicidal *execution-style* hanging is illustrated by an elderly man who jumped out of a second floor window and remained suspended at the end of a long rope which he had tied to the headboard of his bed (Fig. XIV-10a). The odontoid process was fractured and the medulla was severely bruised. Similar findings were observed in a young man who jumped out of his third floor bedroom window (Fig. XIV-10b).

Spence, et al.[5] report on skeletal injuries they observed in exhumed remains of six individuals executed by hanging prior to 1962 in Canadian prisons. Fracture and/or dislocation of C-2 was observed in all 6 bodies. However, involvement of the odontoid process occurred in two. The remaining injuries included fractures of C-1, C-3, C-5, basilar skull fractures and hyoid fractures.

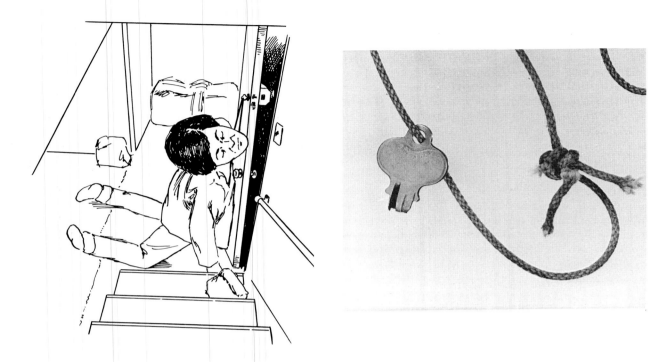

FIGURE XIV-8a–b. (a) Heavily intoxicated woman suspended on a cord on which she carried her house key around her neck. (b) The key was broken off in the lock.

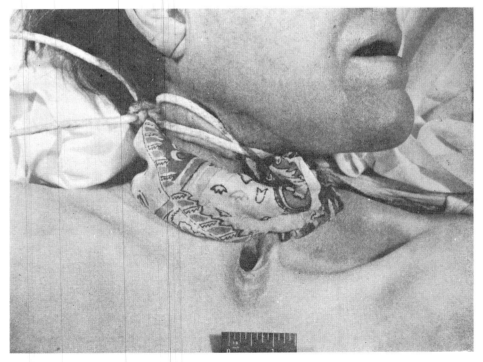

FIGURE XIV-9. Suicidal hanging. The individual was despondent following removal of a cancerous larynx. A tracheostomy is noted below the noose.

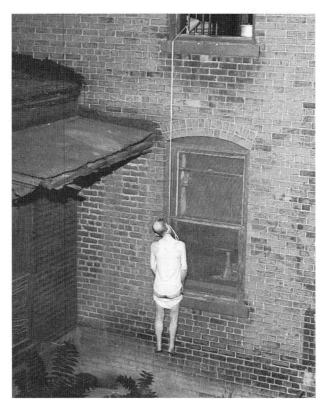 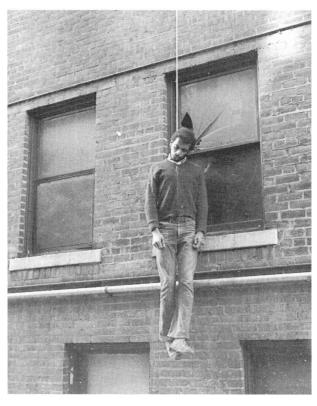

FIGURE XIV-10a–b. Suicidal hangings with autopsy findings similar to those seen in executions. In Figure XIV-10 a, the sudden stop at the end of the rope is best illustrated by the location of the underwear.

The variations are attributed to, minor differences in hanging practices and possible individual anatomic peculiarities.

Due to the relative ease with which hanging can be accomplished, almost any type of noose will suffice. For example, a blanket or bed sheet, left whole, need not be knotted around the neck to cause interference with blood flow to the brain.

In jails, prisoners sometimes commit suicide by hanging using a U-shaped noose fashioned from their shirt, trousers, sheet, or blanket. The ends of the loop are tied to a horizontal bar and the prisoner places his head into the noose positioning it under his chin (Fig. XIV-11). The loop presses against the sides of the neck, as it wraps upward in front or behind the ears. Of course, the same can be achieved by the use of a rope.

In a highly publicized case in Signal Hill, California, Ronald Settles, a college football star, was arrested because of a traffic violation and an altercation ensued with arresting

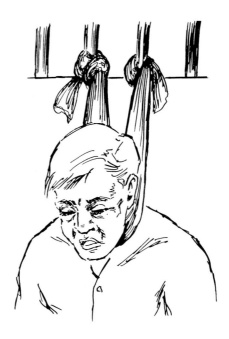

FIGURE XIV-11. Suicidal jail hanging using a U-shaped noose.

officers. The altercation continued during the booking procedure and Settles sustained several bruises to different areas of his body. Several hours later, his lifeless body with his neck resting inside a U-shaped noose, fashioned from his shirt and tied to a bar, was found in his cell. His feet were on the ground and his knees were bent. In a suit filed by Settles' family, it was alleged that death could not have occurred by this method of hanging and that he was strangled, then suspended to simulate suicide.

Children occasionally asphyxiate in their cribs by various means[6] (Fig. XIV-12a-e) and sometimes are found suspended by a curtain pull when their crib is placed close to a window. Entrapment by a power window in a car, where the child inadvertently moves the window by stepping on the control located in the armrest, is a possible scenario and a case of a 26-month-old child whose head was similarly trapped by a power-controlled rear window accidently operated by the driver's remote switch was reported by Simmons.[7]

In another type of case a fifteen-month-old child died of hanging when he slipped between the mattress and the side of his crib remaining suspended by the neck, while his feet dangled above the floor.

Such accidents result from the use of defective, usually old, cribs in which the lower side rail has come loose, permitting it to be pushed outward. We have observed several such cases. In one instance, a wire coat hanger had been used to repair the crib.[6]

Hanging usually leaves distinctive, readily recognizable evidence, even if the individual has been cut down and the scene altered to suggest a different mode of death. A groove or furrow on the neck often suggests the type of loop that was used. The weave of a rope is often imprinted on the skin, permitting a match of patterns (Figs. XIV-13a-b and XIV-14a-b). In victims of strangulation the weave pattern of a ligature or decorative embroidery on the collar of a shirt that was used to strangle may leave a distinctive abrasion on the skin. Good photography and a magnifying lens may aid in identifying a weave pattern. Strangulation with a wire coat hanger may be

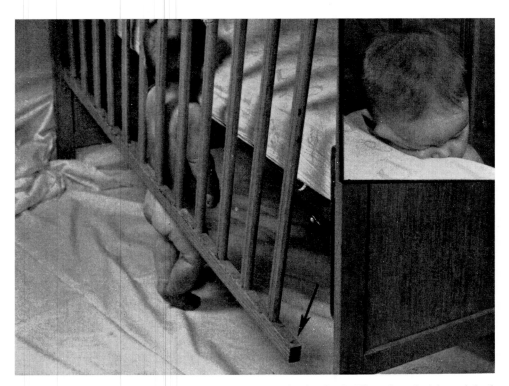

FIGURE XIV-12a. Infant trapped between mattress and side of crib. The side rail of the crib had been repaired, but came loose (arrow), allowing the child to slip into the gap, causing compression of the head and neck.

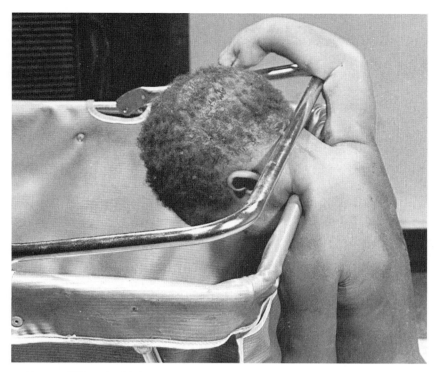

FIGURE XIV-12b. Child's neck trapped under the handle of a portable crib.

FIGURE XIV-12c. Child's head and neck trapped in the crib's headboard.

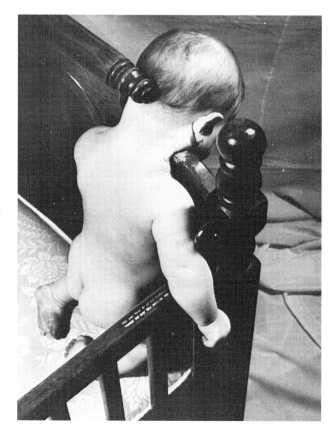

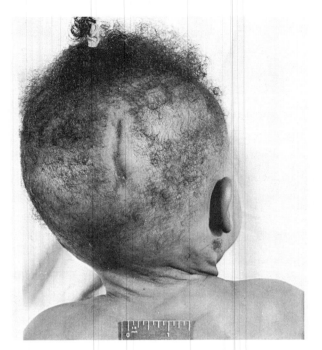
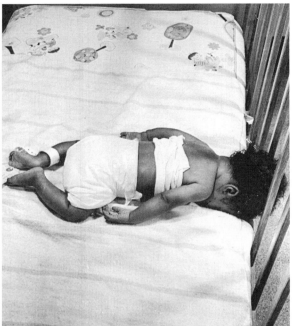

FIGURE XIV-12d–e. A vertical indentation, without underlying bruise (d), suggests that the child's head may have been immobilized between the slats of the side of the crib (e), causing obstruction of the airway.

identified by a thin wavy mark due to the firmness of this type of noose.

In a typical suicidal hanging, the loop passes around the neck and climbs upward toward the knot. A typically indented or abraded area of skin often marks the site of the knot. Pulling and stretching of the skin by the noose sometimes causes a superficial stretchmark-like pattern above or below the ligature (Fig. XIV-15). Grooves on neck skin of hanging victims should be carefully examined. As with abrasions in general, when fresh, such abrasions may be much less conspicuous than after drying.

Hanging may occur without visible marks. A loop of soft fabric, such as a towel or scarf, may cause no noticeable injury. Blankets or sheets used for hanging are often left whole or ripped into strips and sometimes braided to make a noose. If left whole, there may be little or no damage to the skin because of the width and smoothness of the fabric. The knot, if there was one, may well produce a patterned abrasion due to its firmness and rigidity (Fig. XIV-16).

In addition to the mark produced by the noose, bizarre abrasions and bruises are occasionally seen on the neck of a hanging victim. Constriction of the neck by the noose may cause pinching of the skin and vertical folds which rub against the noose and become abraded (Fig. XIV-17). When a noose is wound around the neck more than once, the skin between the loops may be pinched horizontally, causing a thin, sometimes textured, reddish-brown line of dried skin (Fig. XIV-18a–b). Blisters containing serum may result from friction or squeezing of a tight noose (Fig. XIV-19). Similar blisters are sometimes seen in cases of strangulation or on wrists bound too tightly. A thin, non-elastic cord used for hanging may cut into the skin. Obviously, the same is true if a garrote, such as a thin wire or fishing line, were used for strangling. Bleeding is usually minimal or absent from this type of injury, possibly because of blood clotting caused by heat produced by friction.

Horizontal skin folds and creases on the neck of obese persons or infants may resemble a noose

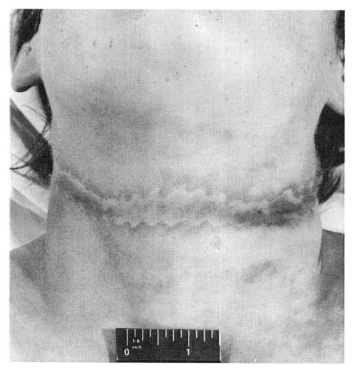

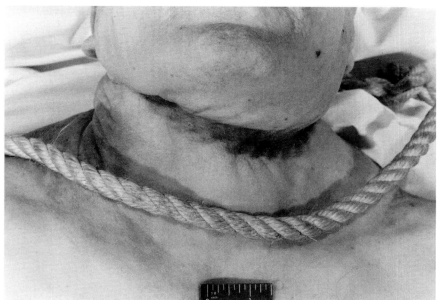

FIGURE XIV-13a–b. Imprints of twisted ropes.

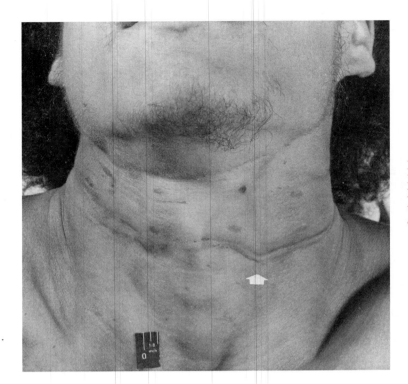

FIGURE XIV-14a. Suicidal hanging with belt. Note symmetrically distributed imprints of eyelets. The thickness of the belt is illustrated by the double line at the bottom and the stiffness of the belt is illustrated by the angle (arrow).

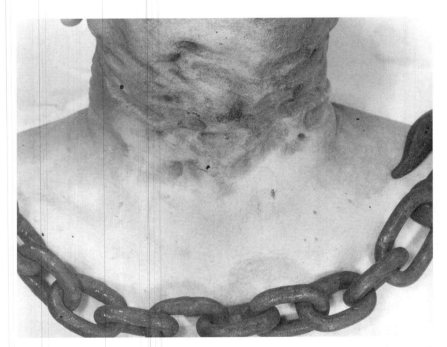

FIGURE XIV-14b. Tow chain used for hanging, wound around the neck several times showing the imprints of the links.

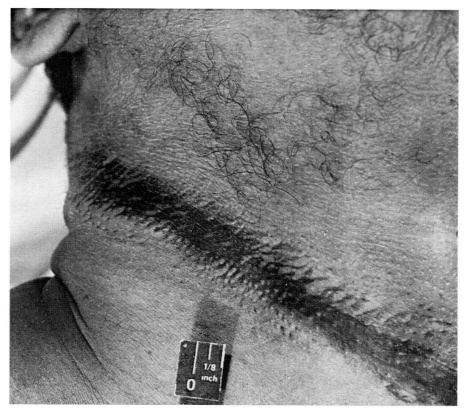

FIGURE XIV-15. Pulling of the skin due to hanging sometimes causes a stretchmark-like pattern above and below the ligature.

FIGURE XIV-16. Elderly woman who hanged herself using a soft blanket attached to a door hinge. The imprint of the knot is well demonstrated on the chin. A faint mark below the jaw made by the noose became visible after drying.

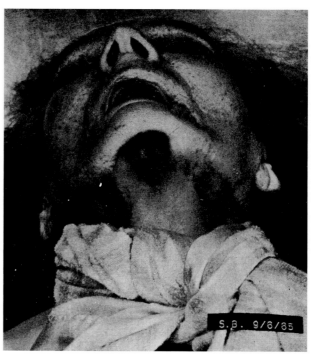
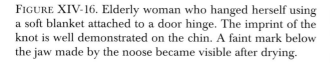

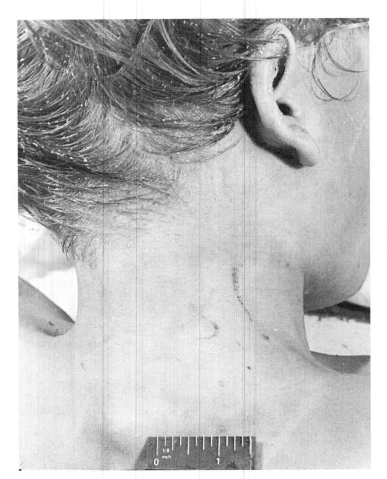

FIGURE XIV-17. Vertical abrasions due to pinching of skin by the noose.

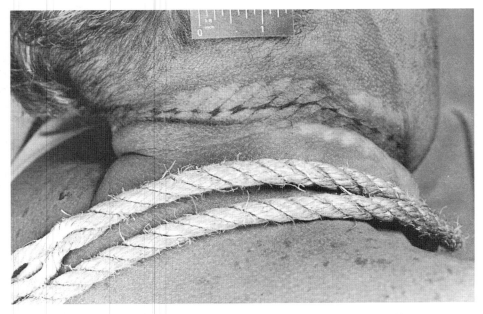

FIGURE XIV-18a. Pinching of the skin between two ligatures of a double noose.

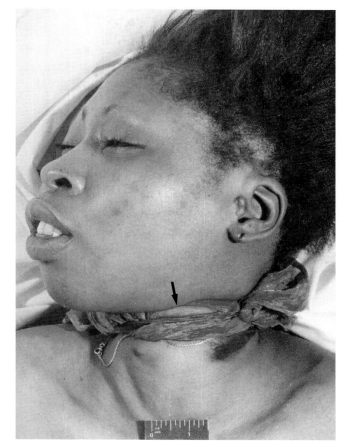

FIGURE XIV-18b. Pinching of the skin between two ligatures of a double noose (arrow).

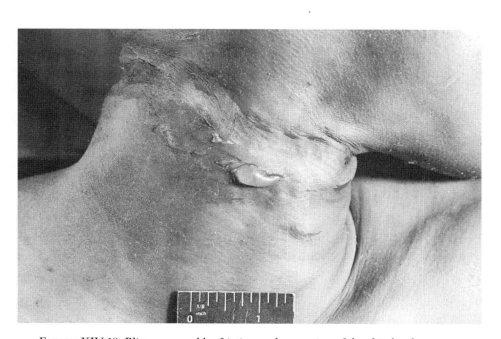

FIGURE XIV-19. Blisters caused by friction and squeezing of the skin by the noose.

mark, particularly after refrigeration of the body has caused congealing of the subcutaneous fat. Allowing the body to warm to room temperature, followed by gentle massage and stretching of the area, readily reveal the artifactual nature of this type of groove. An artifactual groove is rapidly obliterated with the onset of decomposition, whereas a genuine hanging groove remains recognizable as long as bloating, discoloration and skin slippage are not far advanced. Drying and the absence of blood which results from compression in a groove caused by hanging often slow the onset of decomposition by reducing access of bacteria.

Disproportionately extensive bruises of the face are sometimes seen in partially suspended victims of hanging after minor trauma. Such trauma may be sustained just prior to hanging, or when a suspended, limp body swings against a wall or falls to the floor when being cut down (Figs. XIV-20 and XIV-21). Since bacteria thrive on blood, decomposition sets in early in the congested face of a partially suspended body. Visual identification of such remains is sometimes difficult.

Injuries to the strap muscles of the neck are rare in hanging, and fracture of the thyroid cartilage or hyoid bone are the exception rather than the rule. The noose usually passes midway between the hyoid bone and the thyroid cartilage. Thus, in some instances, when such fractures occur they may be due to pressure exerted by the noose on the thyrohyoid membrane and ligaments, most often in the elderly with calcification of the cartilage and greater fragility of bony structures. Submucosal hemorrhage of the lower portion of the epiglottis in suicidal hanging may also be caused by direct pressure of the noose, and bruising of the taste buds and the deep musculature at the base of the tongue may result from crushing of this area against the hard palate by the upward thrust of the ligature.[8]

A small horizontal tear in the lining of the common carotid artery with underlying hemorrhage is also common as a direct result of trauma by the noose. Some attribute these tears to *traction* associated with hanging. If *traction* were the cause, one would expect to find more such parallel tears, not necessarily limited to the level of the ligature. Horizontal intimal traction tears, scattered along the carotid arteries at different levels are sometimes found in hanging associated with a *long drop* and in *feet first free falls* from height. In the latter, they are often associated with one or several transverse tears of the first segment of the aorta. The tear of the aorta results from sudden stoppage of the falling body, while the heart continues to travel.

We have performed an autopsy of a young man who fell feet first from a height of several stories. At autopsy his intact heart was found in the lower abdomen. The heart apex pierced the diaphragm like an arrowhead.

Frictional intimal tears of the carotid arteries surrounded by subintimal dissection and hemorrhage is important supplementary evidence that the victim was alive at the time of hanging. This is in sharp contrast to a homicide followed by suspension of the body to suggest suicide. Hemorrhage does not occur in a dead body and subintimal dissection is unlikely in the absence of blood pressure. Opening the carotid arteries to the level of the mandible may be necessary to demonstrate these intimal tears. This procedure will interfere with injection of embalming fluids, unless the carotids are secured with a string, to enable the embalmer to locate these vessels. Otherwise the carotids, due to their elasticity, retract and disappear into the tissues.

The tongue frequently protrudes from the mouth of a hanging victim. The mechanism of this phenomenon is upward pressure on the neck organs by the noose, causing elevation of the tongue. The tongue is pushed against the palate, then out of the mouth, no different to what happens as a result of gas formation in decomposition or retraction of the soft tissues of the neck by the heat of a fire. The protruding part of the tongue is often dark brown or even black due to drying, caused by exposure to air (Figs. XIV-22a–b, see also III–16).

Blood or bloody mucus may be discharged from the mouth and nose and hemorrhage into the middle ears, associated with rupture of the eardrum, occasionally cause some blood to trickle under a suspended body. Such hemorrhage results from rupture of engorged blood vessels

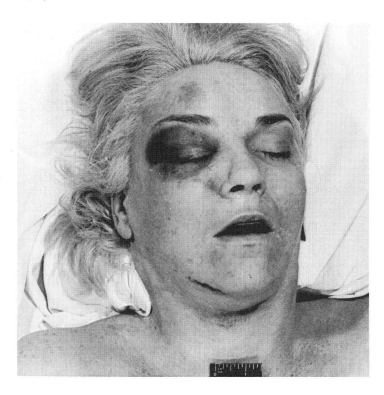

FIGURE XIV-20. Suicidal hanging. Bruise on the right side of the forehead was caused by striking the wall during suspension. There was no evidence of injury to the eyelids when the body was found. Hemorrhage into the eyelids developed later due to seepage.

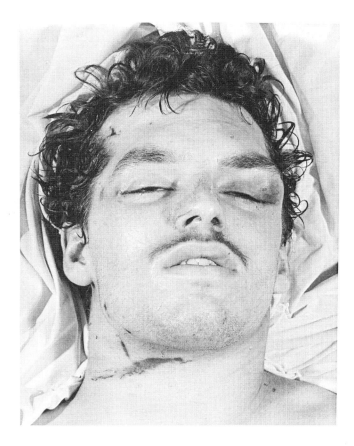

FIGURE XIV-21. Suicidal hanging in jail. The hemorrhage into the left upper eyelid occurred as a result of slipping and striking the floor when the body was being cut down. The scratches of the right side of the face and forehead are caused by the noose.

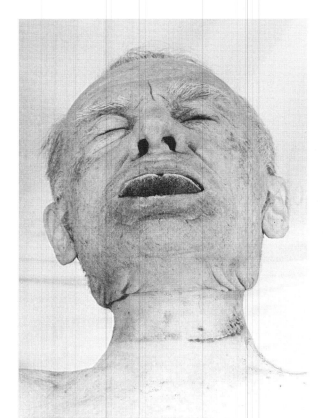

FIGURE XIV-22a–b. Upward pressure on the neck by the noose causes elevation and protrusion of the tongue from the mouth. The exposed part of the tongue becomes dark brown, even black, as a result of drying. The discoloration of the face is due to the fact that both victims were partially suspended to allow blood to enter the head but not exit. (b) Note the pulling and stretching below the noose in the front of the neck.

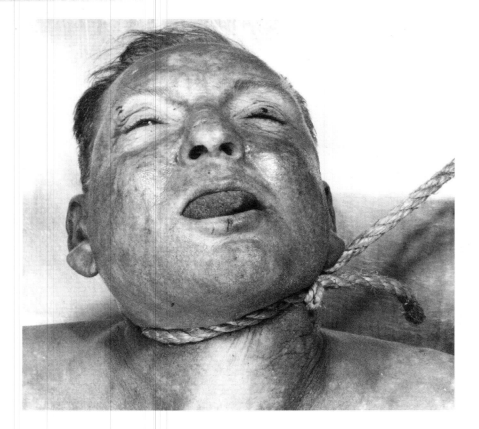

above the noose and should not be mistaken for evidence of foul play. Fluidity of the blood due to absence of postmortem clotting, which is a constant feature in all types of asphyxial death, may contribute to such bleeding. Where putrefaction has set in, dark red-brown and foul-smelling fluids that resemble blood may run down the body. Such fluids originate from decomposing tissues and their presence does not constitute evidence of injury.

Livor mortis in a hanging victim suspended in an upright position settles into the lower half of the body, including the hands and forearms (Fig. XIV-23). If the body is cut down within a few hours after death and placed in a supine position, livor in the extremities fades and new areas of livor mortis appear on the back and buttocks. This may be of importance if, for publicity or insurance reasons, a hanging suicide was cut down and placed in bed to suggest death from natural causes. Swelling of dependent areas in a victim of hanging due to livor mortis and settling of tissue fluids may simulate ankle edema, as in congestive heart failure. In a male victim, such swelling may simulate penile erection due to congestion of the corpus cavernosum, falsely suggestive of an autoerotic death. Although, such penile swelling sometimes occurs in autoerotic deaths, it is not indicative of same. The degree of swelling depends on the length of time the body had been hanging. Some theorize that central nervous system stimulation as a result of oxygen deprivation may be the causative mechanism.

Another postmortem manifestation is the presence of seminal fluid in the victim's undershorts, on his thigh or the floor beneath the body. This discharge from the urethra is caused by rigor mortis of the muscle layer in the wall of the seminal vesicles and is entirely unrelated to any type of sexual activity. This discharge of seminal fluid is especially common in cases of asphyxial death, which lends support to the theory of central nervous system stimulation (*see* Fig. XXVI-7).

Scattered pinpoint hemorrhages are often observed in dependent areas of a hanging victim (see Fig. III- 6). These petechiae result from vascular engorgement and gravity pressure of the settling blood.

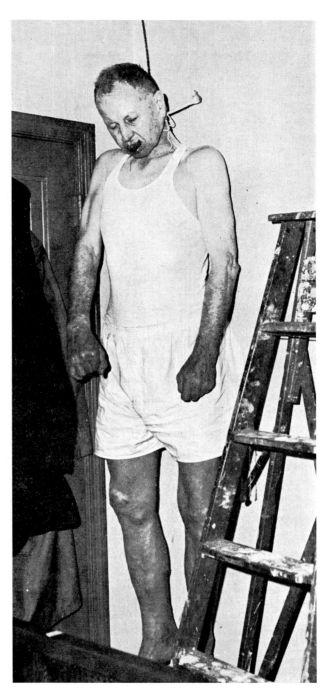

FIGURE XIV-23. Suicide. The body had been hanging in excess of 12 hours. Livor mortis of the forearms and the lower extremities is settled and fixed (compare the color with that of the upper arms and chest). The same phenomenon is noted in Figure XIV-3(c).

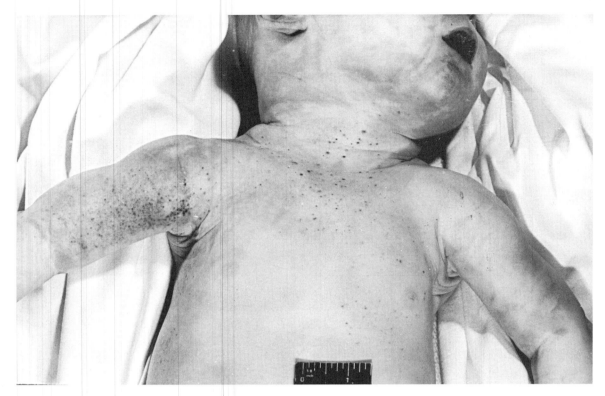

FIGURE XIV-24. Tardieu spots due to early onset of decomposition in an infant who died of natural causes. The body was left face down in the crib overnight. Tardieu spots are always limited to areas involved with livor mortis. Note the sharp horizontal demarcation of livor of the right arm.

Obviously, pinpoint hemorrhages may also result from the usual process of decomposition, where disintegration of capillaries, as occurs with Tardieu spots, allows for permeation of blood pigment into the skin (Fig. XIV-24).

A sixty-eight-year-old woman used a strip of soft thin blanket to hang herself on a door hinge. She was found by her daughter, who cut her down, removed the blanket and placed her in bed. She then called the police and insisted she had found her mother in that position. The daughter stated further that her mother had suffered from a heart condition and had been under the care of a physician. Her doctor refused to sign the death certificate, not having seen the patient recently.

Postmortem examination suggested hanging due to pronounced livor in the lower half of the body, while the back and chest were pale. Abundant pinpoint hemorrhages were noted in the conjunctivae, face and legs. There was no impression of the loop on the skin of the neck, as the ligature was soft and wide, but the knot caused a typical abrasion under the chin (see Fig. XIV-16). Upon questioning, the daughter admitted to changing the scene because she was concerned with losing insurance benefits.

Certain types of knots and nooses may suggest involvement of another party in what is initially thought to be a suicide. To enable subsequent examination of a noose, the knot should be preserved. When removing the ligature from the body, an attempt should be made to slip the noose over the head or cut in an area removed from the knot. The cut ends should then be secured, preferably with string or wire. It is sometimes necessary to secure the knot itself to prevent unraveling (Fig. XIV-25). Some serial killers have been identified by their repeated use of the same type of noose and knot.

Strangulation

Strangulation may be homicidal, suicidal or accidental. Homicidal strangulation may be manual or by ligature. Manual self-strangulation is not feasible. Pressure on the neck is a deliber-

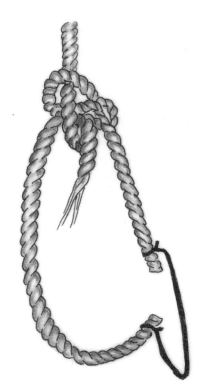

FIGURE XIV-25. The noose should be preserved. This is best done by cutting the noose away from the knot and securing the ends with a string or wire. The knot may be preserved in the same way.

ate action. When an individual loses consciousness, pressure can no longer be applied. Manual strangulation is therefore always homicidal. A sexual motive to the crime must be considered, especially if the victim is female, regardless of age. Detailed examination of the external and internal genital organs, including acid phosphatase determination on vaginal washings and microscopic search for spermatozoa, should be performed. Fingernail scrapings or cuttings and plucked pubic and head hair from the deceased should also be retained for possible later examination by the police crime laboratory. Prior to plucking the hair, it is advisable to comb the pubic area. Any loose hairs and fibers that are obtained may be compared with such recovered from a suspect. The body surface should be carefully canvassed for the presence of any suspicious evidence, with particular emphasis on bite marks and semen stains. Close-up photographs

and swabs for blood typing and DNA should be taken of suspected areas.

The hallmarks of manual strangulation are fingertip bruises and fingernail marks on the neck, although their absence does not preclude strangulation. In many cases of manual strangulation there is extensive external injury to the neck, while in others there are few or no external manifestations of trauma (Fig. XIV-26). Fingertip bruises are approximately dime-size, circular or oval, often fuzzy at the edges, faint and washed-out in appearance. They are produced by grabbing and pressure of fingertips against the skin. Underlying tissues, including the strap muscles, are also frequently bruised. Fingertip bruises are often seen on wrists and forearms in cases of physical altercations. The characteristic fingernail mark is a thin linear or crescent-shaped abrasion on the skin. Inference regarding the way in which the assailant's hands held the victim's neck, i.e., from the front or the rear, based on the direction of the curved abrasions should be avoided. Too many variants, such as the shape of the nails,[9] their length, and inherent qualities of the skin, render such attempt tenuous. In rare instances, fingernails may cause cuts (Fig. XIV-27). Fingernail marks sometimes appear as small superficial gouges or parallel linear scratches. In either case, underlying hemorrhage is usually limited to the upper layers of the skin. A wet body may show no fingernail marks until the skin has dried.

A young black female was found submerged in a bathtub. Initial examination of the body at the scene showed only two small whitish areas resembling scars on the side of the neck. At autopsy, five hours after the body was removed from the tub, unequivocal fingernail marks were noted on all sides of the neck. Drying of the body after removal from the water and the color change of the whitish areas during the lapsed time permitted proper interpretation (Fig. XIV-28a–b).

Another common manifestation of injury in a victim of manual strangulation is abrasion of the chin. The victim sharply lowers the chin in an effort to protect the neck, scraping the chin against the hands of the assailant. Hemorrhage in the tissues under the abrasion is usually minimal, except when the injury resulted from a blow.

Absence of fingernail marks on the skin does not imply absence of bruising in the deeper tis-

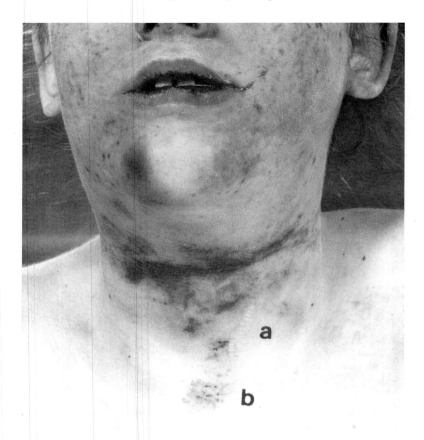

FIGURE XIV-26. Body of an unidentified young girl found beside a highway. The injuries on the neck indicate throttling by twisting the zippered front of the sweater she was wearing. The imprint of the zipper is noted on the left side of the neck (a). The weave pattern of the sweater (b) is seen below the zipper imprint. Note the bruised chin and scattered small hemorrhages on both cheeks.

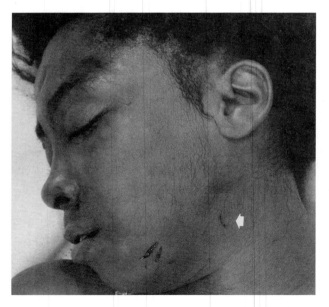

FIGURE XIV-27. Middle-aged woman found in a duffel bag in a public park. A typical fingernail mark is located under the left angle of the jaw (arrow) and a bruise is situated above it. Two superficial cuts on the left side of the chin were caused by long fingernails. There is bruising adjacent to these injuries.

ingful calcification of these structures becomes noticeable between the ages of 30 to 35 and increases with age. The phenomenon of calcification is well established. Therefore, it is not uncommon to find a child or young adult with no fractures of any of these structures, in cases of strangulation.

As in some cases of hanging, pinpoint hemorrhages are often noted in the face of a strangled victim, predominately in the conjunctivae, eyelids and the upper cheeks. The presence of pinpoint hemorrhages or petechiae, as they are often called, is undoubtedly supportive evidence of death by strangulation. Over 70% of strangulation victims have such hemorrhages, however, as a sole finding petechiae must not be considered conclusive evidence.

According to DiMaio[11] who examined 48 cases of ligature strangulation, petechiae were present in 31, absent in 5 and could not be determined in 12 cases, due to decomposition or mutilation of the body by fire. According to this evaluation it is evident that 14% of the ligature strangulation cases had no petechiae, contrary to the general concept in the forensic community, whereby petechiae are always present in this type of death.

Occasionally, these pinpoint hemorrhages are so dense on the eyelids and upper cheeks that they cast a brownish hue on the skin, resembling makeup. Slight downward pull of the upper eyelids stretches and straightens the skin, separating the spots and distinguishing pinpoint hemorrhages from artifact.

Scattered small hemorrhages are sometimes seen at autopsy in the reflected scalp, especially if congested. These hemorrhages are due to tearing of blood vessels caused by separating the scalp from the galea and the vault of the skull. They have no diagnostic meaning and no significance with regards to the cause of death (Fig. XIV-29).

Suicidal ligature strangulation is uncommon. The possibility of second party involvement must always be carefully considered. Distinction between homicidal and suicidal strangulation by ligature is often impossible on the basis of the anatomical findings alone, although fractures of

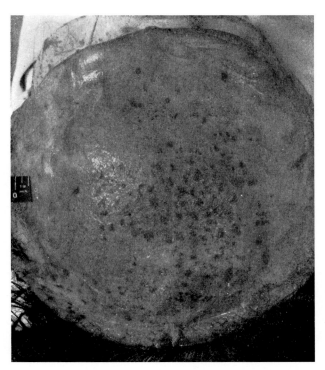

FIGURE XIV-29. Reflected scalp at autopsy showing multiple small hemorrhages produced by tearing of tiny blood vessels that pass between the scalp and the vault of the skull. These hemorrhages bear no relationship to the cause of death.

the larynx in suicidal strangulations are distinctly unusual. The type of noose and knot as well as the number of *turns* around the neck and the circumstances under which the body is found, may suggest the manner of death. A history of mental depression, allusions to suicide or past suicide attempts, provide presumptive evidence in a particular case (Figs. XIV-30 to XIV-32).

A young woman arrested for drunk driving spent the night in jail and was found the next morning with a strip torn from her wool blanket, tied but not knotted around her neck. The remainder of the blanket pulled up to cover the neck. She appeared to be asleep. She was dead and a complaint was filed against the jail authorities alleging that she should have been watched.

Case reports have been published from time to time regarding this issue.[12]

Homicidal strangulation by ligature and subsequent hanging of the victim to simulate suicide is rare. However, because some such cases have been published, crime investigators are aware of

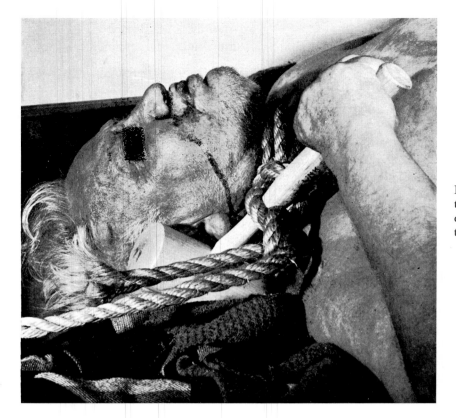

FIGURE XIV-30. Suicidal strangulation: An elderly carpenter found dead in his shop. The noose was tightened by the handle of the mallet.

FIGURE XIV-31. Elderly man who strangled himself with a telephone cord. Note the tourniquet-like knot, which could have been released by pulling one end. (Courtesy of Dr. Dominick DiMaio, New York City.)

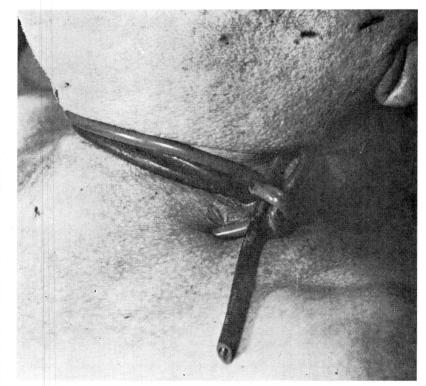

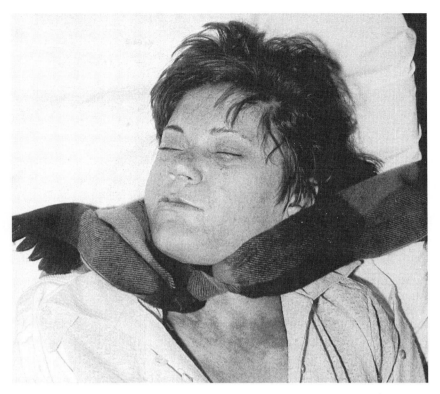

FIGURE XIV-32. Suicidal strangulation with an unknotted wool scarf. Some fabrics would slip open and not sustain the pressure.

this type of homicide. Certain features permit the distinction between hanging and strangulation (Figs. XIV-33a–b to XIV-35) (Table XIV-1).

Defense wounds on the body of a strangulation victim are frequent, although fingernail marks on the victim's neck may be self-inflicted in an attempt to loosen the grip. During an asthmatic attack or following a drug reaction or intoxication, an individual may clutch his or her own neck as if attempting to *open* the airway. Common are the victim's fingernail marks or fingertip bruises on his or her neck when a neck hold is applied from the rear for the purpose of strangulation or slashing the neck.

Also in suicidal hanging, occasionally the victim may be found with nail marks and bruises on the neck and fingers wedged under the noose, as if attempting to remove the constriction. This is a reflex action to preserve life which should not be interpreted as evidence of a conscious effort and deliberation. At all times the position of the victim at the scene must be evaluated in the light of

the injuries found at the postmortem examination. For example, hanging from a door knob while the body is lying down, as shown in Figures XIV-1b and XIV-4a, would cause a horizontal noose mark which may simulate homicide unless the position of the body and other circumstantial evidence are known.

Deep bruises sustained in a struggle or attempted self-defense may not be apparent if death followed rapidly. It is therefore recommended that incisions be made in strategic locations known to be frequently injured, in order to detect such damage. Reflection and undermining of the skin provides wide areas for inspection under the skin, while keeping the integrity of the body intact as much as possible. Wrists, arms, shoulders and the entire back and hips are areas which are often traumatized. The probative value of such incisions clearly outweighs their interference with the cosmetics of the body.

Ligature strangulation sometimes involves the use of the victim's own shirt or blouse by twisting

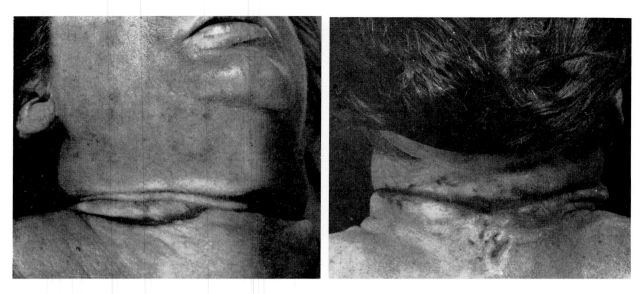

FIGURE XIV-33a–b. Middle-aged woman who was strangled with a non-spiral telephone cord. The photographs of the front and back of the neck show the horizontal imprint of the ligature. The picture on the right shows superficial fingernail scratches in the nape of the neck and upper back. The noose ends run downward and overlap. The assailant subdued the victim from the rear.

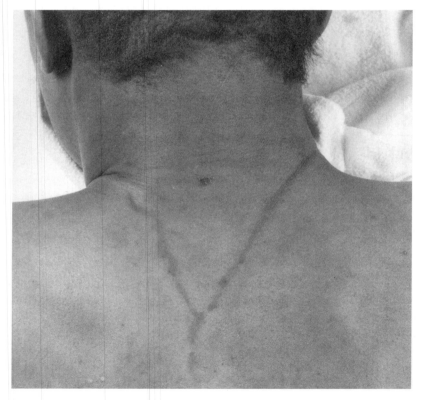

FIGURE XIV-34. Individual placed in prone position with wrists and ankles bound together in *hogtie* fashion. An additional ligature encircled the neck and was tied to the extremities. When the legs drop, pressure on the neck ligature gradually causes strangulation.

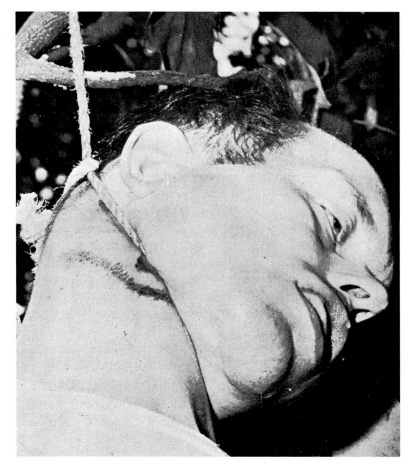

FIGURE XIV-35. Thirty-two-year-old man found hanging from a tree 12 feet above the ground in the backyard of his home. He had climbed up the tree with a ladder. Note the horizontal abrasion made by the rope before it slipped to the upward position shown on the picture.

the open collar around the neck. Typically, the assailant grabs the collar area of the garment and twists to one side or the other. A V-shaped abrasion pointing downward or a zigzag-shaped, abraded pattern results on the victim's neck (Figs. XIV-36 to XIV-40). The victim responds by lowering the head, as if to protect the neck area. The knuckles of the fist rub against the victim's chin, causing an abrasion, which may be one inch or more in length and as much as 1/2 inch in width. Sometimes the victim attempts to pull down and remove the constriction, inflicting fingertip bruises and nail marks above the noose. Successful downward pull of the constriction creates a double pattern, one above the other, confirming the mechanism of injury, the sequence of the altercation and the cause of death.

In the publicized Preppy Murder trial in New York in 1987, the defense argued that the death of Jennifer Levin was caused when Robert Chambers applied a choke hold from behind, tightened the crock of his arm around her neck and flipped her over his head, as she was sitting on his chest, facing his feet. The defense further contended that bruises and abrasions on the front of her neck were caused by creases of Chamber's sleeve and death was instantaneous, unpredictable and accidental, as a result of carotid sinus stimulation.

Had the defense's theory been correct, the pattern of injury of Ms. Levin's neck would have been one of parallel, vertical bruises and abrasions, rather than a double imprint of crossover and V-shaped marks depicting the outline of her own embroidery-edged blouse and fingernail scratches on both sides of her neck, suggesting attempted self-defense (Fig. XIV-36). The unequivocal pattern of injuries on Ms. Levin's neck, indicated that she was strangled by twisting of her own blouse, while *facing* her assailant. This double crossover imprint was caused when Ms. Levin managed to pull the ligature down. This also accounted for her fingernail marks on both sides of her neck. This evidence and the fact that a constriction of the neck would have had to be maintained for some time to cause brain death by oxygen deprivation, led to the realization that the death was neither

TABLE XIV-1

STRANGULATION BY LIGATURE VS. HANGING

Strangulation	*Hanging*
• Mark on neck is horizontal. • Mark on neck is usually below level of thyroid cartilage. • Hyoid bone and/or thyroid cartilage are often fractured. Cricoid cartilage is fractured occasionally.	• Mark on neck passes upward toward knot; may be horizontal, as in strangulation, if victim is lying down. • Mark on neck is usually above thyroid cartilage. • Hyoid bone and thyroid cartilage are usually intact, except in hanging with long drop or in elderly individuals.

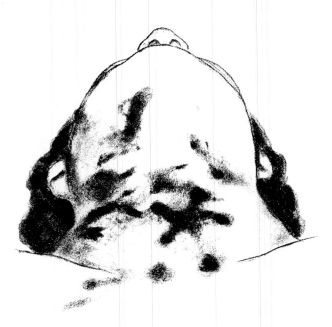

FIGURE XIV-36. Young girl, who was raped and strangled with her own T-shirt. Note zigzag-shaped abrasion on the neck; the circular abrasions are from fingertips. The abraded chin was caused by the twisting fist.

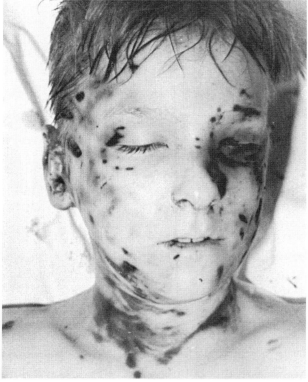

FIGURE XIV-37. Young boy who was mauled by a German Shepherd. In addition to numerous claw and teeth marks, a V-shaped abrasion on the neck was caused when the dog pulled and twisted the boy's shirt collar, causing neck injuries similar to those in Figures XVI-36 and XVI-38.

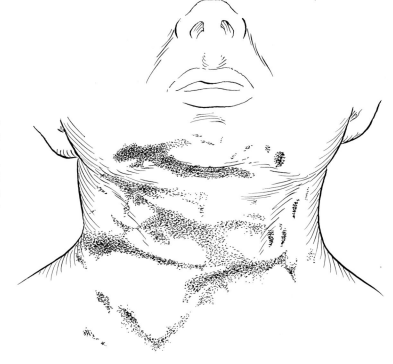

FIGURE XIV-38. Young woman strangled in New York Central Park *(Preppy Murder).* The double imprint of cross-over abrasions and X-shaped marks depict the outline of the decorative neck-edge of her blouse. Fingernail scratches on both sides of her neck were made by the victim in an attempt to remove the ligature.

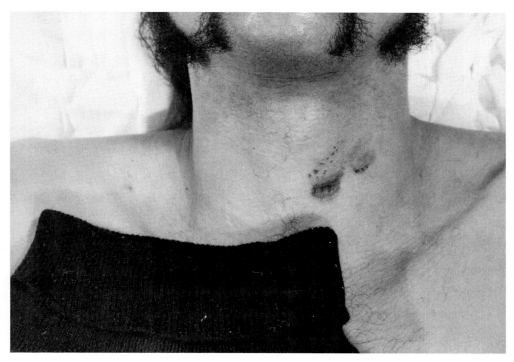

FIGURE XIV-39. Strangulation. The abrasions on the left side of the neck show the weave pattern of the turtleneck sweater. The little dots correspond to knots in the fabric.

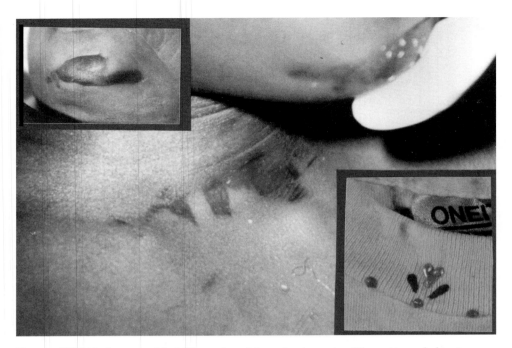

FIGURE XIV-40. Six-year-old child was found in a city dumpster. The patterned abrasions on the neck show the ribbing of the shirt collar (right lower insert). The apparent lack of consistency with the pattern is due to pulling and stretching of the skin and fabric. The ribbing is mostly sideways due to twisting of the shirt. The insert in the left upper corner shows typical abrasion of the chin by the assailant's knuckles.

unintentional nor unexpected. Chamber's was released from prison on Valentines Day, 2003.

Neck Holds

Neck holds as used in Judo and by law enforcement and correctional personnel to subdue combative individuals who resist arrest can cause death. Similar situations sometimes arise in psychiatric institutions during attempts to subdue patients exhibiting violent behavior. Two types of holds are recognized:
• Choke hold or bar arm control
• Carotid sleeper hold

The use of *choke hold* or *bar arm control* is being discouraged, because of its potential for injury of the airway. In this form of restraint a forearm is placed across the front of the neck, while the other hand pulls the forearm back, causing compression of the airway (Fig. XIV-41a–b). This elicits *air hunger*. The victim of a choke hold becomes agitated, fearful for his life and combative due to his inability to breathe. Choke holds can cause serious damage and death within seconds. Laryngeal fractures, internal hemorrhage and swelling of the airway lining due to edema may cause delayed complications, hours, even days later. Death is usually the result of asphyxiation and petechial hemorrhages may be found in the eyes and on the face. The face and front of the neck and shoulders are usually cyanotic, blue-gray and dusky.

Injury of the skin as a result of choke hold is usually absent, except if a police baton or large metal flashlight was used across the neck. Either of these pressed tightly against the skin, may leave two, linear, parallel, horizontal bruises, where the distance between the lines corresponds to the width of the implement. In the case of a flashlight, the knurled pattern of the grip

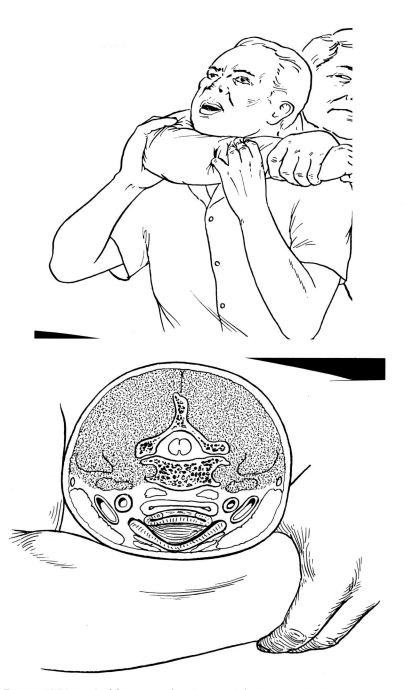

FIGURE XIV-41a–b. (a) Bar arm (or choke hold); force applied to the front of the neck causes compression of the airway. (b) Cross-section of the neck showing compression of the airway, while the vascular channels at the sides of the neck remain un-affected. Published with permission of Dr. Donald T. Reay and Raven Press, *Am J Forensic Med Path, 3:* 3, 1982.

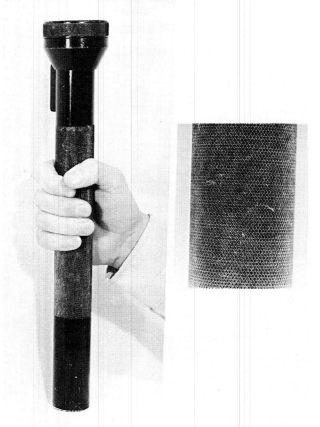

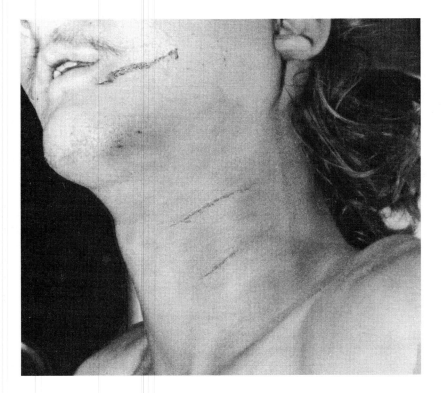

FIGURE XIV-42a–b. (a) Flashlight showing knurling of grip occasionally imprinted on the skin. (b) Two, thin, parallel, linear, horizontal bruises on the side of the neck caused by pressure of flashlight used in an attempt to restrain a combative individual.

may be imprinted on the skin (Fig. XIV-42a–b). Varying photographic exposures, of the same frame, preferably using infrared sensitive film, may reveal a pattern which otherwise remains unseen and unrecognized. Incision of the area or reflection of the skin, as part of the usual Y-shaped autopsy incision, may reveal subcutaneous and muscular hemorrhage.

In contrast to choke hold, a *carotid sleeper hold* does not constrict the airway and breathing continues. The crock of the arm is placed over the front of the neck, while the arm and forearm apply pressure to the sides. The free hand is then used to pull the wrist of the constricting forearm to increase compression. Significantly less force is required to subdue a combative individual with this type of hold (Fig. XIV-43a–b). Both external and internal evidence of injury is usually minimal or absent. The carotid sleeper hold compresses the carotid arteries, reduces blood flow to the brain and causes rapid loss of consciousness. The usual assumption is that consciousness is lost in 10 to 20 seconds following the application of a carotid sleeper hold, but Judo experts say the duration is 3 to 4 seconds and some autoerotic cases, where individuals recorded their events on video, seem to support this time frame. Loss of consciousness begins with seeing black spots, and loss of peripheral vision. The feeling is one of reduced alertness, similar to falling asleep. In general, the greater the need for oxygen by an excited, agitated individual the shorter the time until the victim goes limp. According to Reay and Eisele,[13] blood flow to the head is reduced by an average of 85% in approximately 6 seconds. Release of a carotid hold restores blood flow to the head and complete recovery in a few seconds. A carotid hold, which is not released immediately upon incapacitation, may cause permanent injury and death. Despite the apparent harmlessness of the carotid sleeper hold occasional deaths do occur as a result of application of this form of restraint. Movement during a struggle may turn a sleeper hold into a choke hold with serious, sometimes fatal, consequences.

Any attempt to subdue a combative individual must consider the depressant action of alcohol and drugs. During an altercation, indeed in any situation involving stress and agitation, a sudden surge of blood alcohol, cocaine, etc., may overwhelm the central nervous system. Thus, an individual may be overcome by a dose of a narcotic which under ordinary circumstances may not be fatal.

OBSTRUCTION OF THE AIRWAY

Smothering

Blockage of the nose and mouth causes death by asphyxia due to inability to breathe. This may occur in a variety of ways, such as by gagging, holding a pillow or hand over the face of the victim. Gags, sometimes used to muffle screaming, can cause death. Thus, a gag applied to the mouth, may be sucked or pushed into the throat causing complete blockage of the airway. Whenever possible gags should not be removed until the obstruction can be evaluated. Plastic bags used as gags and tape placed over the mouth and nose may harbor fingerprints. Removal of such gags must be done carefully to preserve evidence.

Smothering is homicidal in the majority of cases. Accidental smothering is rare, as in the case of an infant who is entangled under pillows and blankets. Entrapment in an avalanche or under a collapsed building is another form of asphyxial death.

Plastic bags placed over the head can cause death by obstruction of the airway or re-breathing of bag contents, i.e., carbon dioxide. Depending on the circumstances, such deaths can be

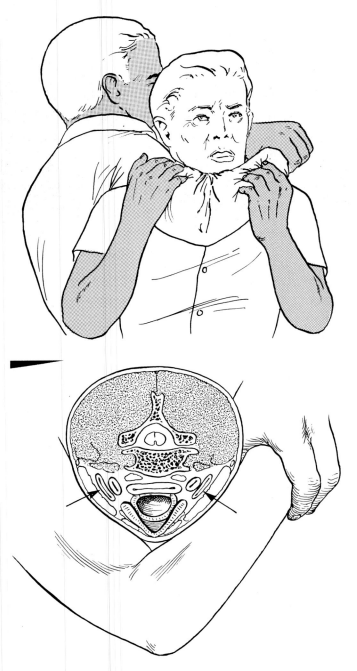

FIGURE XIV-43a–b. (a) Carotid sleeper hold. The arm and forearm apply pressure to the sides of the neck. The airway is in the crock of the arm. (b) Cross-section of the neck showing compression of vascular channels at the sides of the neck, while the airway remains open. Published with permission of Dr. Donald T. Reay and Raven Press, *Am J Forensic Med Path, 3:* 3, 1982.

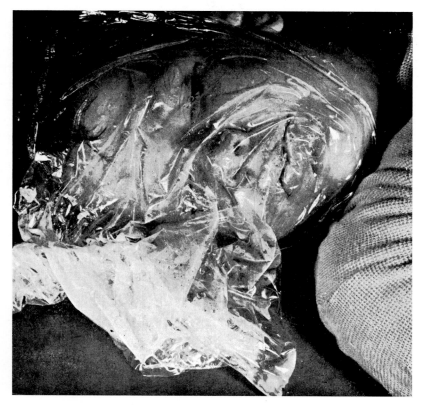

FIGURE XIV-44. Eleven-year-old boy found in a wooded area with a plastic bag over his face following glue-sniffing. Plastic bags and empty tubes of airplane glue were scattered in the area. The bag contained a large amount of water vapor. Subsequent police investigation disclosed that the area had been regularly used by glue sniffers.

accidental, suicidal or homicidal. During the 1960s, accidental smothering increased dramatically with the rise in popularity of *glue sniffing*. The solvent in glue, usually xylene, induces drowsiness and confusion, which result in rebreathing of the contents of the bag and death by oxygen deprivation. Portions of the lungs, liver and a blood sample should be retained at autopsy for chemical analysis to demonstrate the presence of the solvent. Solvent in the lungs indicates that the material was inhaled. A positive finding in the liver or blood confirms systemic absorption. Water vapor which accumulates in a plastic bag applied to the face may cause adherence of the plastic to the skin, sealing off the airway (Fig. XIV-44). The same occurs in small children allowed to play with plastic bags.

Deaths associated with sniffing of aerosols without the use of plastic bags were also common in the 1960s. These individuals used paper bags or made a tent of their clothing, into which they sprayed the aerosol. These deaths were attributed to an overwhelming anaphylactic reaction with arrhythmia of the heartbeat, as was shown experimentally by Taylor and Harris.[14] In recent years, glue and aerosol sniffing have diminished to the point where such deaths have become quite rare.

Burking, named after William Burke (1792–1829) refers to murder by suffocation by sitting on the victim, while covering their mouth and nose. The bodies were then sold for anatomical dissection to medical schools all over Great Britain. Publicity due to the large number of victims resulted in a public outcry and led to the passage in 1832 of a law to regulate the supply of cadavers to Universities.

Autopsy findings in cases of homicidal smothering are non-specific. Mild, acute emphysema and edema of the lungs, scattered areas of atelectasis, petechiae and congestion constitute some of the findings. Bruises and abrasions in the cheeks and chin are significant by their presence as indicators of trauma. Another important area to examine is the inside of the mouth. Hemorrhages and tears of the lining of the oral cavity, including the frenula of the upper and lower lips, as a result of forceful pressure against the teeth may be the only findings indicative of facial trauma. (However, pressure sores on the lower lip and chin from an endotracheal tube or on the nose from a nasogastric tube, may resemble traumatic injury. Care must be taken to properly identify these findings where the tubes have been removed.)

In the past, cases of sudden infant death, so-called *crib death,* were attributed to smothering. This was primarily due to failure of finding an obvious cause of death while observing at autopsy some of the usual changes of asphyxia. In recent years, smothering has been abandoned as the cause of sudden infant death, although the true explanation of this condition is still debated.

Aspiration of Foreign Material

Aspiration of a foreign body may be fatal by occluding or severely narrowing the airway. In an adult, aspiration of vomitus occurs mostly in unconscious or semiconscious individuals, with or without contributory factors such as drugs or alcohol. A healthy, but grossly intoxicated individual who begins a meal, suddenly turns blue, coughs violently, then collapses and dies should be suspected of having asphyxiated on aspirated food. The suddenness and rapidity of the death suggest an acute heart attack, thus the name *café coronary.* The term is poorly chosen because a *café coronary* bears no relationship to a heart attack. Symptoms of a *café coronary* include inability to talk, due to the fact that the airway is blocked, attempted forceful coughing, clutching of the

throat or chest as a sign of distress and collapse. At autopsy, a large piece of poorly chewed food (bolus) may be found obstructing the entrance of the larynx (Fig. XIV-45). A lithmus test of the bolus to determine its acidity will ascertain whether it originated from the mouth or consisted of vomitus, i.e., originated from the stomach. Aspiration of vomitus occasionally occurs in traumatic cases, particularly if associated with a reduced state of consciousness. Displacement of one's denture into the airway is not necessarily associated with alcoholic intoxication.

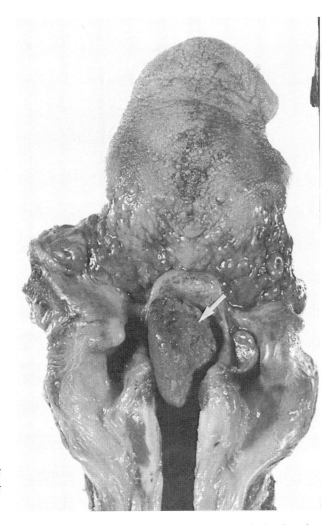

FIGURE XIV-45. Piece of undigested hot dog lodged under the epiglottis in a case of sudden death of an intoxicated individual.

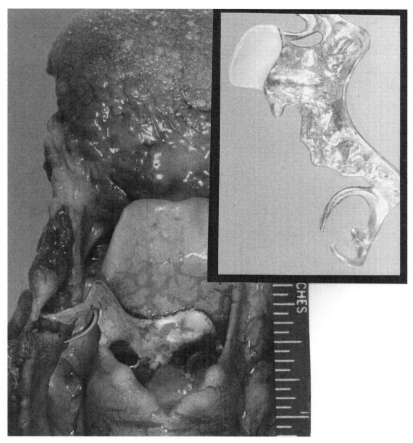

FIGURE XIV-46. Inhaled denture. The case is described in the text.

A forty-year-old woman inhaled her partial denture during a coughing spell (Fig. XIV-46). She lapsed into unconsciousness in front of her husband, who thought she had fallen asleep. At autopsy her blood alcohol level was negative, and she was not under the influence of medication.

Aspiration of food or regurgitation and aspiration of gastric contents often results from suppression of the gag reflex by tranquilizing drugs. It occurs frequently in psychiatric patients.

Infants and children occasionally aspirate a variety of objects, such as nuts, marbles, coins and rattles. Less frequently occurring hazards are certain imported pacifiers with a small diameter plastic guard and a rigid handle.[15] Children sometimes inhale a pea, bean or kernel of corn. If small enough, such pea or bean does not obstruct the air passage completely; however, its presence produces a progressively worsening cough as the adjacent lining membrane of the airway swells from irritation and the pea or bean begins to germinate in the moist and warm environment (Fig. XIV-47).

Swelling of the Lining Membranes of the Larynx

Insect bites, notably those of bees, wasps and hornets, and drug reactions, such as those that sometimes follow administration of penicillin, can cause swelling of the lining membranes of the larynx and death within a few minutes due to anaphylactic shock or asphyxiation. In one case we examined, a hornet-like insect stung the neck of a five-year-old girl. Within minutes, the child developed extreme difficulty breathing and was dead on arrival at the hospital. The autopsy showed near-occlusion of the larynx due to edema. In another case, a forty-two-year-old man attempted to remove a wasp nest on a tree by sawing off the limb. He was stung many times on the face, arms and legs. Within a short time he

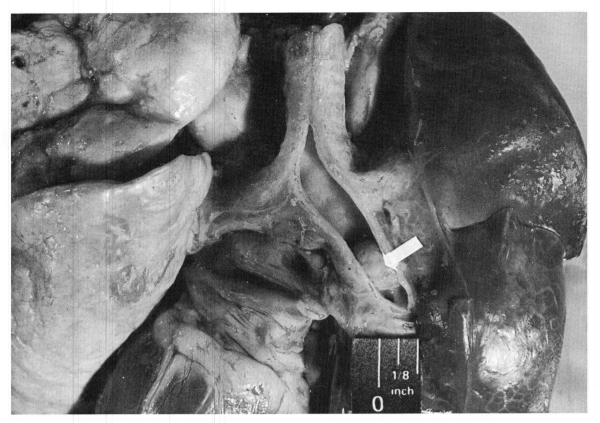

Figure XIV-47. Toddler inhaled pea (arrow) which obstructed the main bronchus causing collapse of the lung. The lung is dark, shrunken, airless, and sunk in water.

developed severe respiratory distress. He reached the hospital in time for a tracheostomy to save his life.

Inflammation of the throat as sometimes seen in diphtheria, infectious mononucleosis and epiglottitis in children may cause swelling of the airway to the point of obstruction. A blow to the front or side of the neck, such as a Karate chop may cause severe swelling of the lining of the airway as a result of edema and hemorrhage. Frac-

ture of the cartilages of the larynx or trachea is not an essential finding. Rupture of the trachea has been reported without a blow to the neck, in straining during labor, during a bout of intense coughing to dislodge a foreign body or even as a result of a sudden backlash of the head rarely seen in automobile collisions.

Swelling of the lining membrane of the airway, hemorrhage and mucosal lacerations are rare complications of endotracheal intubation.

DEATH DUE TO CAROTID SINUS REFLEX

The carotid sinus, situated at the bifurcation of the common carotid artery on both sides of the neck, consists of nerve tissue, stimulation of which regulates blood pressure and pulse rate. Strong pressure on the neck, in the area of carotid sinus, can elicit a drop of the blood pres-

sure by as much as 20 mm Hg. in a normal individual.

In older people, with advanced arteriosclerosis involving the carotid arteries and in rare instances of marked hypersensitivity of this structure, excitation of the carotid sinus, as by a fall or blow on the side of the neck may cause fainting, even cardiac arrest. In extreme cases of hypersensitivity of the carotid sinus the individual is unable to tolerate a necktie or a tight collar.

Criminal defense attorneys sometimes argue that the death of the victim was unpredictable, without malice or foresight on the part of their client, consequently accidental, in cases of obvious manual strangulation. The following must be considered in determining whether a death may have been caused by carotid sinus stimulation:

1. Deaths as a result of carotid sinus stimulation are infrequent.
2. The victim is likely to be elderly with advanced arteriosclerosis involving the carotid arteries.
3. The victim was known to be susceptible to carotid sinus stimulation with previously documented manifestations of dizziness, headache, weakness and fainting associated with pressure on either side of the neck.
4. The presence of injuries, especially fingernail marks (whether the victim's or the assailant's), on the skin of the neck, usually rules out death by carotid sinus stimulation.
5. Injuries in the soft tissues under the skin should be limited to the areas of the carotid sinus.

6. Absence of petechial hemorrhages in the conjunctivae and the facial skin.

Interestingly, no death due to *carotid sinus stimulation* as a result of attempted self-strangulation has as yet been reported.

Since Brouardel (1896) the term *carotid sinus reflex* has permeated the forensic literature and served as argument in the defense of strangulation. However, it remains a mystery of how a claim of death due to carotid sinus reflex may be applicable to cases of obvious strangulation. *Carotid sinus stimulation was a defense claim in the Preppy Murder trial in New York City (1987).*

Many, in fact probably most cases of strangulation in women are sex related and we have often heard the defense claim in cases of obvious manual strangulation, that the death was unexpected during amorous foreplay, without intent to cause harm.

No doubt sudden cardiac arrest elicited by carotid sinus stimulation is a serious and valuable defense tool. However, such claim appears persuasive only at face value. A closer view of the autopsy findings and the infrequency of occurrence of carotid sinus stimulation, as a cause of serious consequences, suggest the contrary.

POSITIONAL ASPHYXIA

Positional asphyxia is a term used to describe situations where the position of an individual interfered with his or her ability to breathe. Various types of positional asphyxia can be recited, such as an individual trapped in the cave-in of a building, or crushed by a stampeding crowd, an individual pinned under an automobile, or one who was *held down* by someone's body weight or other heavy object.[16] The witch trials in Massachusetts in the early 1600s used positional asphyxia as a means of execution.[17,18]

Different examples of positional asphyxia include: Infants who die in unsafe sleeping environments or playpens (Fig. XIV-48); the intoxicated woman who tried to unlock her door and remained suspended on the cord around her neck, holding the key (see Fig. XIV-8a–b); the woman who fell onto a folding security gate (see

Fig. XIV-7); an adult, debilitated by age and disease, in a hospital bed who slips under or between the bed rails, or becomes suspended in a restraining vest; an intoxicated individual who collapses head down into an empty bucket or the burglar who got stuck in a chimney (Fig. XIV-49). Also, children who die of asphyxia when an adult rolls over on top of them during sleep, fall into this category.

The following case reports are additional examples:

A 320 pound, thirty-four-year-old man, driving his automobile was involved in a collision. The car landed upside down in a ditch. The body was wedged head down, between the front seat and the steering wheel, the full weight of the body bearing down on the neck. The chin was pushed against the chest. The chest was otherwise unencumbered. The individual was pronounced dead at the scene. No significant injuries or pathological changes suggestive of dis-

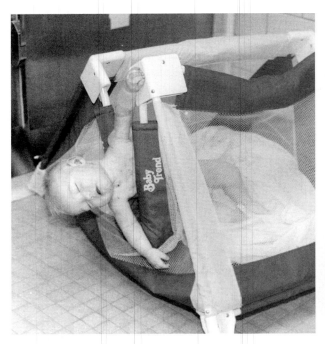

FIGURE XIV-48. Eight-month-old child asphyxiated when the sides of the portable play pen collapsed due to failure of the covered locking mechanism, trapping his chest between the side rails.

ease were found at autopsy and toxicological analyses were negative.

A woman in her forties with a blood alcohol concentration of .30% collapsed face down, her neck over the wooden arm of a chair. Her urinary bladder contained close to 500 mL of urine, with an alcohol concentration of .38%, both suggestive of a prolonged period of unconsciousness preceding her demise. Her death was attributed to gradual postural-asphyxia by partial occlusion of the airway. At autopsy, there was marked edema of the lungs. The brain was congested, edematous and dusky.

A load of construction lumber slid off a tractor trailer onto the roof of an automobile. The roof of the car caved in. Two people in their forties were found dead, sitting upright in the front seats, heads down, their chins wedged tightly against their chests. No injuries were found at the autopsies (Fig. XIV-50a,b,c).

Positional asphyxia would include a middle-aged individual in his cell in jail, with a blood alcohol concentration of .20%, sitting upright on the toilet, his head sharply flexed occluding his tracheostomy. A similar case and other unusual examples were published by Bell and Wetli.[19]

The list of possibilities for death by positional asphyxia is endless (Fig. XIV-51).

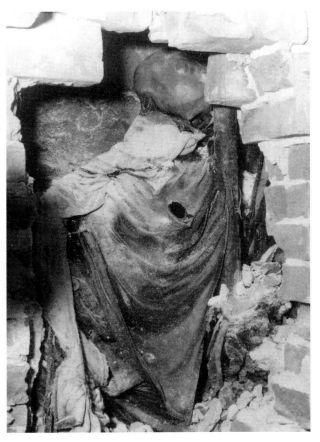

FIGURE XIV-49. Burglar who fell into a chimney and was trapped. The dimensions of the chimney as compared to those of the skeletal remains suggest inability to breathe.

Anatomically, some of these events may be associated with severe injuries of the thoracic wall, including fractures of ribs and vertebrae and tears of the lungs with pneumothorax, subcutaneous emphysema and hemorrhages within the intercostal muscles, as occur from attempted breathing against an obstructed airway. However, the majority of cases are subtle, in fact, often with no traumatic manifestations at all. Two situations, which occur with some frequency are discussed below:

Deaths Caused by Institutional Restraints

Bed rails are used extensively in hospitals and nursing homes. They are intended to prevent falls out of bed and also to serve as a handhold for weak, debilitated patients. Occasionally, a

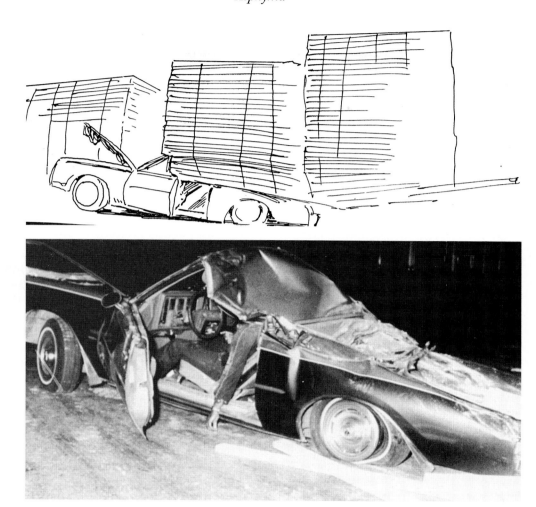

FIGURE XIV-50a–b. Tractor trailer, loaded with lumber, rolled over, crushing the roof of a car driving along side. The two occupants of the automobile died due to positional asphyxia.

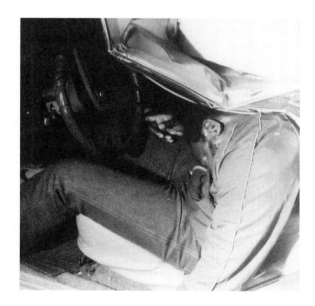

FIGURE XIV-50c. Close-up showing position of driver.

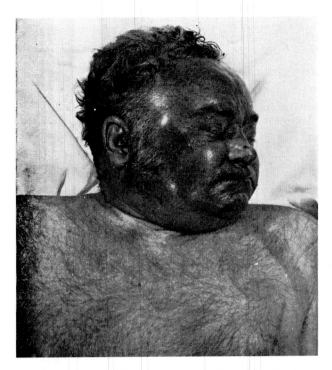

FIGURE XIV-51. Marked congestion and a multitude of pinpoint hemorrhages in the face of a tractor trailer driver who was hauling rolled steel. Following a sudden stop, the metal rolled forward, crushing the driver. Compression of the chest, when severe, will include compression of the heart, mostly the right side, impeding venous return. Therefore, areas above the compression are often so markedly dark discolored.

patient may be trapped between or under the rails or between the mattress and the rails, causing airway or vascular compression (Fig. XIV-52a–e). Parker and Miles[20] report 74 bed rail-related deaths of which the majority were entrapments between the mattress and a rail. These authors point out that bed rail-related deaths are underrecognized.

Indeed, it has been our experience that occasionally in a case where the patient was found wedged between or under bed rails and the death was obviously bed rail-related, it was reported as a death due to natural causes. This may be due to the fact that hospital-based physicians often certify deaths without seeing the patient and only on information received from personnel. Personnel on the other hand may not be aware of the significance of the patient's position relative to the cause of death. Therefore, the medical records should indicate in detail the position and appearance of the body when found. Anytime there are markings, faint or otherwise, on the neck or chest, positional asphyxia should be suspected, although, there may be no evidence of injury on the skin or internally. Cases of suspected positional asphyxia should be reported to the medical examiner for investigation. Close examination of the skin may show that a subtle mark or what appears to be a faint linear scratch is none other than a normal crease. Examination during autopsy is significant in that it provides documentation.

Deaths due to entanglement in vest, jacket or posey restraints are another form of positional asphyxia. Such deaths have resulted from respiratory compromise or pressure on the neck obstructing the airway. Whenever possible the use of such means of restraint in institutions, especially those caring for elderly, often debilitated and demented individuals, is being discouraged.

It must be recognized that a seizure or other form of disease may have placed the patient in the precarious position in which the body was found. Also, the patient's position may be the result of the final collapse, i.e., unrelated to any contributory element provided by the rails.

When investigating an institutional death where asphyxia by bed rails may be a consideration, it must be remembered that one-sided pressure on the neck is insufficient to reduce cerebral blood flow, unless the other side is compromised by arteriosclerosis or other type of stenosis. The circle of Willis, at the base of the brain, allows for transfer of blood from one side to the entire brain.

Death During Prone Restraint

Deaths during restraint occur from time to time in the course of police arrests and in jails, rarely in mental institutions. Whenever such incidents occur, they become subject of media attention and public scrutiny. Such situations usually involve young or middle-aged individuals, many times overweight, psychotic or under the influence of drugs.

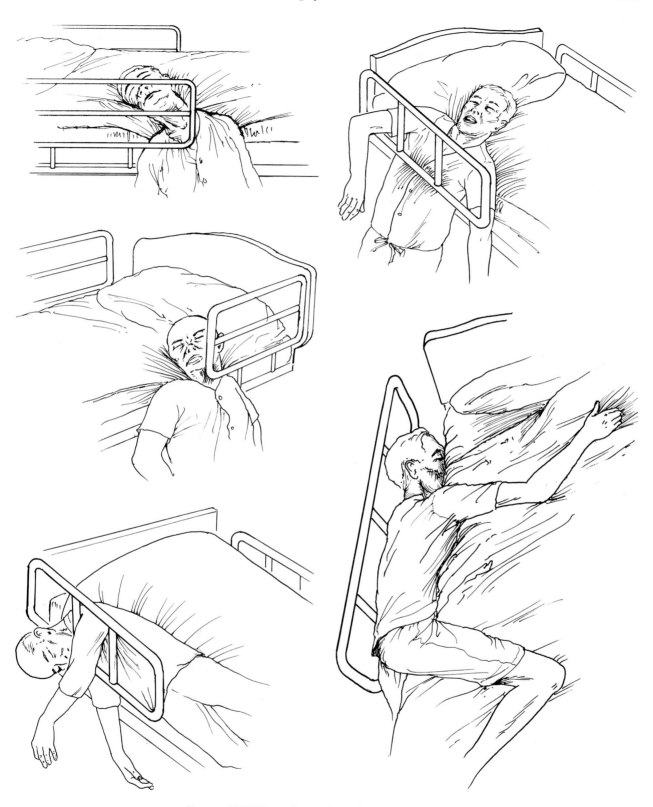

FIGURE XIV-52a–e. Examples of bed rail entrapment.

The *hogtie restraint position,* also known as *hobble or prone restraint,* is a type of restraint, often used by police, where the victim is face down on the ground, i.e., prone, handcuffed behind his back, ankles tied and the wrist and ankle bindings are then tied together. It is a method used to subdue agitated, struggling, aggressive individuals.

In psychiatric facilities, combative patients, while not *hogtied,* may be immobilized in prone position by being held down to the floor or onto a cushioned mattress.

During the restraint the individual may be held down by kneeling or leaning on him, pushing or sitting on his back, using the restrainers body weight to subdue.[21] An overweight individual, with a body mass index (BMI) in excess of 30 (Table XIV-2), is especially susceptible for respiratory arrest when held this way due to protuberance of the anterior abdominal wall, which upon compression causes upward displacement of the abdominal organs and interference with movements of the diaphragm.[22] Of course, severe compression of the chest from back to front or vice versa would include not only the lungs, but also the heart, situated between the chest plate and the spine.

Hence, any of the following findings may be observed in these cases: cyanosis of the face and neck, petechiae in the eyes and face, hemorrhage into one or both middle ears, edema above the level of compression and sometimes hemorrhage within intercostal muscles, predominately along the ribs. Less frequently interstitial emphysema with aligned tiny subpleural bubbles, subcutaneous emphysema and pneumothorax may also occur. Compression of the heart primarily affects the right side, i.e., the venous side, consequently there is venous congestion above the level of compression. This results in reduced arterial blood flow to the brain, brain swelling, sometimes to the point of herniation, and cardiac arrhythmia.

Neuman et al.[23] conducted experiments to determine whether the *hogtie restraint position* was the cause of significant respiratory dysfunction. They concluded that this method of restraint by itself did not cause clinically relevant impairment of ventilation, i.e., did not result in respiratory compromise to the point of asphyxia and that other factors were responsible for the sudden

TABLE XIV-2

BODY MASS INDEX

1. Multiply body weight in pounds by 703
2. Multiply height in inches by itself
3. Divide pounds (1) by height (2)

Under 19	Underweight
19–25	Healthy weight
26–30	Overweight
31–39	Very overweight
40 and above	Extremely overweight

(Morbid obesity is usually considered as being 100 pounds over ideal body weight)

deaths of individuals who were so restrained. The Neuman studies were performed on healthy male volunteers, between the ages of 18 and 40 with a BMI less than 30, who were hogtied after they had exercised on a bicycle, were not subjected to any type of pressure while restrained and were not under the influence of any drug or alcohol. In fact, the Neuman group, at the conclusion of their study acknowledged that they had not attempted to duplicate the conditions under which restraint position deaths had occurred. Their studies, as have others in the past,[24] were geared to the detection of physiologic respiratory impairment under their particular testing regimen. Deaths on gurney mattresses, cushioned car seats or in the restraint position on the ground and on the floor of police cars, where the contoured surface may have increased abdominal compression had not been addressed in their experiments. Additionally, in the real world, individuals in prone restraint tend to become increasingly agitated and panic because they cannot breathe normally.

Most of the restrained subjects who have died while hogtied in police custody, of whom we are aware, were overweight with a BMI usually far in excess of 30, most were under the influence of cocaine, amphetamines, phencyclidine or opiates, sometimes other drugs and occasionally alcohol. Other times, they were psychotic and some had evidence of coronary artery disease or cardiomegaly due to hypertension, or chronic lung disease.[25] The unifying factor in these individuals was that all were subdued by manual pressure of one or more people holding them down, pinning them to the ground, by *loading,* i.e., exerting pressure on their backs, shoulders or arms and some were pepper sprayed as the restraints were being applied.

While pepper spray (oleoresin capsicum) does not in and of itself cause asphyxia, it contributes to respiratory difficulty by irritating the airway lining which has particular significance in individuals with an existing respiratory condition. Pepper spray has been incriminated in spasm of the airways, and causing edema and swelling and reducing patency of the peripheral bronchioles. It further increases the oxygen demand, while oxygen delivery is decreased due to postural compromise of ventilation and respiration.[26]

Another significant observation was that all subjects went into cardiorespiratory arrest during the restraint or were found to be unresponsive when the restraint was completed. None of the individuals recovered after intensive CPR.

Contrary to the belief of some, it is our opinion that pinning down the shoulders or forcefully pressing down the arms is equivalent to *loading* the back. A struggling, agitated individual breathes faster, has a faster heart beat, elevated blood pressure, and heightened metabolism. Such an individual requires more air and more oxygen. Immobilization of the chest, even if only partially reducing the ability to maintain vital functions, culminates in cardiac arrhythmia.

The International Association of Chiefs of Police (IACP) vehemently opposes the use of prone restraint, stating that many deaths had occurred of individuals who, while in police custody, had been restrained in this position.[27,28] Regardless of the exact medical interpretation of the cause of death in individuals so restrained, it is a fact that placing an individual in prone restraint, with wrists and ankles manacled together, so-called *hogtie position*, invariably gives the impression of brutality and large civil damage awards have been paid to persons who have filed lawsuits against arresting officers and their employers.

Two key cases are significant in regards to the controversy which still exists relative to the question of positional asphyxia caused by prone restraint.

In the federal district court case of *Ann Price* v. *County of San Diego*, 1998, the judge ruled that the *"hogtie restraint in and of itself does not constitute excessive force."* This decision was widely viewed as blanket approval for the use of hogtie restraint. The court's decision was based in large measure on the study by Neuman, et al.[23] which was derived from laboratory data obtained by the use of volunteers in experiments which were not representative of what happens in reality to individuals who had died of positional asphyxia while in police custody.

The case of *Cruz* v. *City of Laramie*, filed in 2001 involved a call to police regarding an individual who was naked, yelling about swarming insects, swatting and kicking. Police subdued Thomas Cruz using the hogtie restraint method during which he died. Many of the issues of positional asphyxia were brought forth during this trial. Although, the Court's decision in this case is binding only in the Tenth Circuit, it should serve as a precaution to police departments across the country.

The Tenth Circuit Court of Appeals ruled that the Fourth Amendment protection against excessive force includes protection from hogtie restraint, thus officers may be held liable under Section 1983 for excessive force when employing this technique on individuals whose *diminished capacity* was apparent. *Diminished capacity,* as defined by the Court would include intoxication by drugs or alcohol or any discernible mental or other condition which may place the individual's well being at risk.

A ritualized form of ligature strangulation (incaprettamento), similar to hogtying has been associated with the Italian Mafia and involves binding the wrists and ankles, then tying them together with the body in prone position with an additional ligature encircling the neck attached to the extremities. When the legs drop, pressure on the neck by the ligature gradually reduces cerebral blood flow. Pollanen reported a similar case in East Timor.[28]

EXCLUSION OF OXYGEN

Exclusion of oxygen may occur as a result of depletion and replacement of oxygen by another gas or by chemical interference with the uptake and utilization of oxygen.

Carbon Dioxide Poisoning

Carbon dioxide (CO_2) may cause asphyxia by replacing oxygen. CO_2 is heavier than air, and settles when it accumulates in the absence of turbulence. Manholes, wells, silos and occasionally cellars may contain an excessive amount of CO_2.

A worker who is found lifeless at the bottom of a manhole is likely to have died as a result of asphyxia caused by CO_2 intoxication. A co-worker who goes to the rescue is subject to the same fate, unless he uses supplemental oxygen. A gas mask is useless. In a non-ventilated manhole, consciousness is lost in seconds and death follows rapidly. Maintenance personnel are equipped with pumps which supply air to the crew working underground.

Carbon dioxide may also cause asphyxia when it accumulates in a small closed space, as a result of oxygen depletion from consumption due to re-breathing. A classic example is a glue sniffer, found dead with a plastic bag containing an open tube of airplane glue over his head. With the onset of unconsciousness from inhalation of the volatile hydrocarbon in the glue, the sniffer cannot respond to rising CO_2 or decreasing O_2 levels, and death ensues.

Other examples were the tragic asphyxial deaths in the l950s of children, who hid in discarded refrigerators or washing machines, while playing. These appliances could only be opened from the outside. Since then, laws in most states require that the doors of such appliances be removed or secured before they are discarded (Fig. XIV-53). Nevertheless, despite extensive publicity, the Consumer Product Safety Commission (CPSC) has reported 76 such suffocation deaths in children in the period 1980 to 1988. Most of the victims were aged 4 to 7 years. In all cases, the doors of the appliances could not be opened from the inside. Dr. Dominick DiMaio of New York City, reports a case of suicide in an elderly woman who placed herself in her kitchen refrigerator (Fig. XIV-54).

We have investigated a case where a 5-year-old-child was reported missing only to be found dead inside a suitcase in the basement of his res-idence, where he and other children had been playing hide and seek the previous day (Fig. XIV-55).

The autopsy in cases of carbon dioxide poisoning shows dark fluid blood, the organs are congested, the brain edematous and dusky, no other pertinent changes are evident. The post-mortem diagnosis, i.e., the cause of death, is usually based on circumstantial evidence and findings at the scene. Blood analysis for CO_2 content has no diagnostic significance, since CO_2 rapidly accumulates after death. Of critical importance, is the collection and analysis for CO_2 and O_2 content of air samples from the scene.

Methane Poisoning

Methane (CH_4) is another gas which kills by exclusion of oxygen. Methane is the principal component of natural gas, where its concentration ranges from 50 to 97%. Contrary to the belief of some, natural gas contains no carbon monoxide. Methane is odorless, colorless and tasteless. Methane burns with a hot blue flame (*see* Fig. III-15). The familiar odor associated with natural gas derives from a substance, methyl mercaptan, which is purposely added to methane to enable its detection. Methane forms naturally by decay of organic matter, such as decomposition of a dead body, plants and organic waste. As such, it is the main constituent of fire-damp, the gas found in coal mines and marsh gas, which bubbles up from some lakes and swamps.

Carbon Monoxide Poisoning

Carbon monoxide (CO) causes asphyxia by blocking the respiratory pigment of red blood corpuscles (hemoglobin) from carrying oxygen to the tissues and from returning carbon dioxide to the lungs. Hemoglobin has an affinity for carbon monoxide 250 to 300 times greater than for oxygen. The intensity of this reaction between CO and hemoglobin may be exemplified by the poisoning and death of an individual situated in proximity of an automobile exhaust pipe, even outdoors.

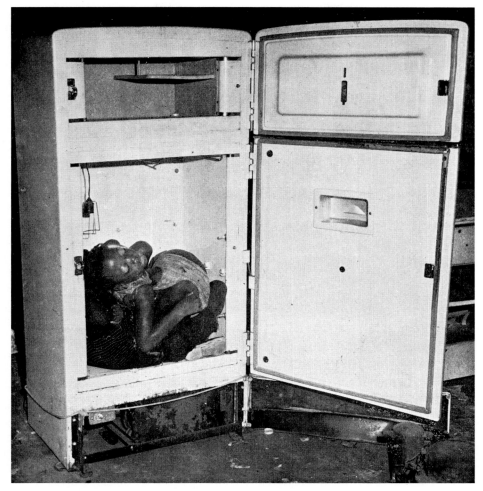

FIGURE XIV-53. Three children were discovered in a discarded refrigerator in an unused garage two days after having been reported missing by their parents. They had been playing hide-and-seek.

A young man injured in a car accident was placed on a stretcher 8 to 10 feet behind an ambulance, as the crew administered first aid to another victim. On arrival at the hospital, the first individual was pronounced dead. At autopsy his blood carbon monoxide concentration was 42%. Injuries sustained in the crash were minor.

We have seen a case where the driver of a vehicle was ejected from his car and landed unconscious on the ground in close proximity of the exhaust pipe, while the vehicle's engine was still running. At autopsy, his blood carbon monoxide concentration was 48%. DiMaio reports three separate cases of suicide from carbon monoxide poisoning which occurred out-

doors in individuals who had placed themselves near the exhaust pipe of their automobile.

Carbon monoxide is an odorless, colorless, non-irritating gas, often referred to as the *Silent Killer*. Since it is slightly lighter than air, the greatest concentration of CO in a closed environment hovers at a level of 4 to 5 feet above the ground. Firemen at the scene of a fire often crawl to avoid inhaling the gas. CO results from incomplete combustion of carbon-containing substance; consequently it is abundant where soot is produced. A yellow flame generates carbon monoxide, while a blue flame burns more completely, with less or no by-products. The presence of carbon

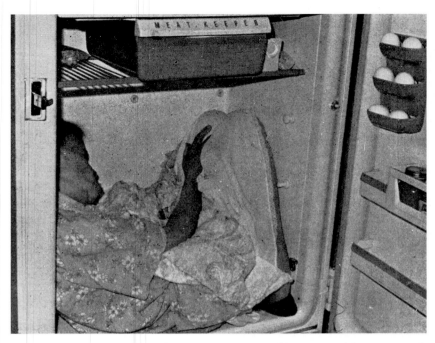

FIGURE XIV-54. Suicide in kitchen refrigerator. (Courtesy of Dr. Dominick DiMaio, New York City.)

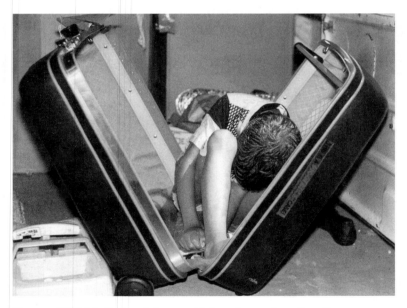

FIGURE XIV-55. Body of 5-year-old found one day after disappearance inside a suitcase. See story in text.

monoxide in fire smoke, engine exhaust, coal gas and tobacco smoke makes it a constant hazard. The amount of carbon monoxide in tobacco smoke varies considerably. For example, cigarette smoke yields approximately 1% by volume, pipe smoke 2% and cigar smoke 6%. Heavy cigarette smokers may have a daytime carbon monoxide blood level up to 8 or 10%. The exhaust from a carbureted automobile engine generates some 4% by volume of carbon monoxide, in contrast with 0.1% CO emitted by various classes of diesel motors. Although catalytic converters and the use of unleaded gasoline have drastically reduced carbon monoxide emission, with over 100 million motor vehicles in the United States, the internal combustion engine is still considered the greatest single source of carbon monoxide.

While postmortem diagnosis of carbon monoxide poisoning is not difficult, blood levels and their significance vary. In a healthy middle-aged individual a blood CO saturation greater than 50% is considered fatal, although significantly higher levels have also been observed. In the presence of illnesses in which tissue oxygenation is compromised, fatal CO concentrations may be significantly lower. Anemia, chronic obstructive pulmonary disease (COPD), particularly emphysema, and arteriosclerotic heart disease are examples of common conditions in which fatal blood carbon monoxide levels may be appreciably lower than in healthy individuals. A blood carbon monoxide level of 15 or 20% from exposure to a smoldering fire in someone with advanced coronary artery disease, may represent *"the straw that broke the camel's back."* Excitation and exertion, as during attempts to extinguish a fire, increases carbon monoxide intake due to faster breathing, while the oxygen carrying capacity of the blood decreases. A blood CO saturation of 20% is equivalent to a loss of 1/5th of the total blood volume.

Another factor to be considered is removal of the victim from the contaminated area. While breathing fresh air, half of the total COHb is eliminated in approximately five hours. Administration of 100% O_2 by way of a tightly fitting mask decreases this half life to approximately 80 minutes. Hyperbaric oxygen with 100% O_2 at 3 ATA reduces COHb half life to 23 minutes.[30] Nevertheless, the poisoned victim may die despite the clearance of CO because of irreversible brain damage sustained while blood CO saturation was high. Some survive in coma for weeks or months before succumbing to infection. On the other hand, we are familiar with a young man who attempted suicide by inhaling automobile exhaust fumes in a closed garage, was found unconscious, taken to a nearby hospital where a COHb saturation of 73% was determined, was breathed with hyperbaric O_2 and recovered without detectable residual damage.

In investigating self-limited house fires or defective burners that generate CO, the possibility that the blood CO concentration in the victim may have fallen as the source abated, is important in interpreting evidence. Also, fire nurtures on oxygen. Thus, asphyxia due to oxygen depletion in a fire contributes significantly to death by carbon monoxide toxicity.

Alcohol, barbiturates, sedatives and numerous other drugs are additional factors that potentiate the toxic effect of acute carbon monoxide poisoning. For instance, a CO saturation of 35 or 40% from which a healthy individual would probably recover after temporary disability, may be fatal in the presence of a blood alcohol concentration of .20%. Numerous automobile accidents are due to the combined effect of alcohol and CO on the driver. The source of CO is usually traced to a deteriorated muffler and a rusted-out floor pan of the vehicle.[31]

The driver of an automobile was found dead in his parked car. The windows were rolled up. The blood CO saturation was 40%, and the blood alcohol level was 0.11%. Investigation revealed that this driver had been stopped by police several hours earlier at the same location for driving on a flat rear tire. He was told to change the tire before driving on. Carbon monoxide seeped into the trunk, then the passenger compartment through the opening of a missing taillight. Directly beneath the opening was the broken and shortened tail pipe.

A forty-four-year-old driver of an automobile was found dead in his car, which was parked in front of his rural home. The engine was running, since it was a cold winter night. The cause of death was 60% carbon monoxide blood saturation. The blood alcohol level was 0.12%. The source of the CO was a defective exhaust system. The tail pipe was

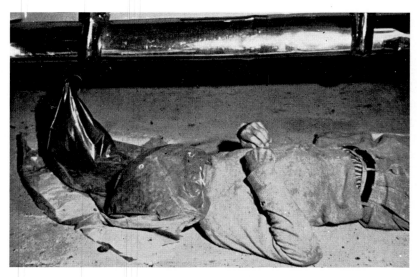

FIGURE XIV-56. Suicide by inhalation of automobile exhaust fumes from a plastic laundry bag connected to the tail pipe.

suspended too close to the undercarriage of the vehicle, and fumes could not escape adequately due to deflection by the bumper and the rear trunk area. The adjacent rear fender was rusted through, allowing fumes to seep into the passenger compartment.

Sitting in a closed car stuck in the mud or snow, with the engine running is hazardous, as exhaust fumes may leak into the interior of the vehicle and overcome the occupants. The mud or snow can block the tail pipe causing the exhaust fumes to seep into the vehicle.

Inhalation of automobile exhaust fumes is a frequent mode of suicide. A garden or vacuum cleaner hose is sometimes used to connect the tailpipe with the vehicle's interior, but other methods have been used (Fig. XIV-56). A level of carbon monoxide sufficient to cause severe brain damage or death accumulates in five to ten minutes in a single-car garage, with the door shut and the engine of the automobile running.

Many times the engine has stalled due to depletion of oxygen in the garage or the vehicle has run out of fuel. The key may or may not still be in the ignition. Often, the occupant, confused or semiconscious, removes the key as he recognizes his predicament, then passes out, continues to inhale fumes, only to be found lifeless at a later time.

Investigation of the scene in cases of carbon monoxide poisoning is imperative to determine the manner of death. A closed garage door is usually suggestive of intent, while scattered tools, black grease on the hands of the deceased or an open hood may be considered presumptive evidence of an accident (Fig. XIV-57). We have observed a number of deaths where people backed their car into the garage to warm up the engine and opened the garage door to release exhaust fumes. The fumes engulfed the rear of the vehicle and seeped into the passenger compartment.

Carbon monoxide notoriously seeps through openings around doors or cracks in walls. It may also rise through a ceiling crack into an attic, or from a tight, confined space, through plasterboard or drywall, into an adjacent area. In this way carbon monoxide may spread through an entire house. An individual who commits suicide in the garage of his house by inhalation of automobile exhaust fumes may cause the death by carbon monoxide poisoning of people in upstairs bedrooms. Similar tragedies have occurred as a result of a faulty furnace in the basement.

There has been some question regarding the passage of carboxyhemoglobin (COHb) through the placenta. Research in regards to the effect of smoking during pregnancy has conclusively shown such transfer. Following exposure to CO fetal COHb concentrations are 10 to 15% higher

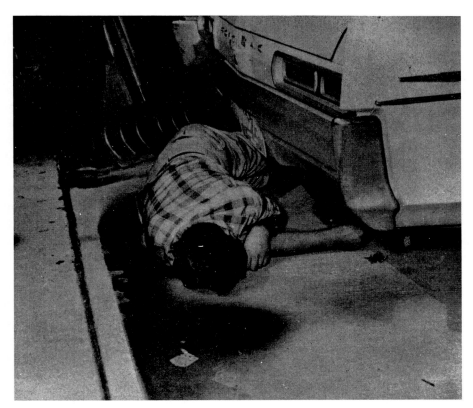

FIGURE XIV-57. Forty-three-year-old man found dead, partly under the rear of his automobile in the family garage. The car's ignition was still on, but the engine was not running due to an empty gas tank. The garage door was closed, as shown by the soot pattern on the floor. The carboxyhemoglobin (COHb) level was 80%. No autopsy was performed. The family claimed he had had a heart attack and collapsed. The high COHb suggested that his heart was healthy or he would have succumbed to a significantly lower level. Furthermore, the position of the deceased, partly under the vehicle, corroborated the hypothesis of suicide.

than maternal levels. A time lag is noted in the uptake of CO by the fetus relative to the mother, but fetal elimination of CO is nearly twice as long. The fetus is more susceptible than the mother to the hypoxic effect of CO. Thus, a single acute maternal exposure to carbon monoxide insufficient to produce clinical manifestations in the mother may cause severe brain injury or death of the fetus.

Pathologic changes attributable to CO poisoning include bright cherry-red discoloration of the blood, skeletal musculature and livor mortis. Fingernail beds involved in lividity in cases of CO poisoning are bright red or pink, one might say they look as though the person were *alive*. One's own fingernails may serve for comparison. The fingernails are a particularly good place to observe this bright color, especially in blacks, in whom the pink discoloration of the skin may not be readily apparent. Cherry-red discoloration of blood and tissues becomes noticeable if the blood CO saturation exceeds 30%. With lower concentrations the color may go unnoticed. Since blood CO concentrations of less than 30% may adversely affect an individual's capability of driving a motor vehicle, by causing confusion, disorientation and reduced judgement, it is essential that blood be analyzed for CO in all occupants of motor vehicles who are killed in crashes.

Cyanide poisoning and exposure of the dead body to a cold and moist environment may cause redness indistinguishable from that due to CO.

Fluidity of the blood due to absence of postmortem clotting is a feature shared by carbon monoxide poisoning with other types of asphyxia. Blisters containing clear serous fluid are frequently seen in the skin in cases of carbon monoxide or barbiturate poisoning where death follows deep coma. Such blisters may be mistaken for second-degree burns, because their rupture leaves a red, raw surface which after drying changes to a brown, leather-like consistency. Blisters are more common over the larger joints of the extremities; the knees and wrists are most commonly involved. Indistinguishable blisters around the ankles and skin slippage over the legs may be caused by proximity of these areas to the heater ducts of the vehicle. We have observed numerous occasions where suicidal individuals have turned up their vehicle's heating system, presumably in the belief of speeding up the suicide process, sustaining second-degree burns on exposed skin, including the face. Occasionally, depending on the position of the body in the vehicle, an entire side of a forearm or thigh may be blistered as a result of burning.

Symmetrical necrosis in the globus pallidus is sometimes observed in individuals who survived an acute episode of CO poisoning. The globus pallidus is particularly vulnerable to oxygen deprivation due to its unique blood supply. The necrotic areas later change to pea- or lentil-size brown cysts, which are usually bilateral. Identical lesions have been observed in cases of prolonged coma from whatever cause, but especially following barbiturate poisoning and in cases of marked arteriosclerosis of the vessels of the corpus striatum. Multiple punctate hemorrhages in the white matter of the brain and in the heart muscle, as well as focal myocardial necroses and fatty vacuolation, are other occasional findings. Heart failure developing two to three days after recovery from an attempted suicide by inhalation of automobile exhaust fumes, is likely the result of the cardiotoxic effect of CO.

The cherry-red discoloration of CO poisoning changes to dark green, then to brown, with the onset of decomposition. While the presence of carboxyhemoglobin can sometimes be shown despite embalming, extensive hemolysis can render carboxyhemoglobin undetectable. Decomposition of the body does not produce carbon monoxide, nor is a significant amount of carbon monoxide absorbed by tissues as a result of exposure to a CO contaminated atmosphere. Carbon monoxide must be inhaled to be toxic.

A mixture of carbon monoxide with two and a half times its volume of air is highly explosive in the presence of a flame. The pilot light of a gas water heater, installed in violation of the code, in the attached garage of a house, ignited the CO generated when a car was backed into the garage and left running. The ensuing explosion demolished the two-story building.

Cyanide Poisoning

Cyanide (hydrogen cyanide–HCN; potassium cyanide–KCN) asphyxiates by blocking the utilization of oxygen by the tissues through poisoning of respiratory enzymes. Cyanide inhibits the action of cytochrome oxidase, carbonic anhydrase and probably other enzyme systems. Cyanide paralyzes vital functions, and death occurs within minutes. A laboratory worker who sniffed an open bottle of potassium cyanide instantly collapsed to the floor, but regained consciousness within 2 or 3 seconds. In about half the cases the body is bright cherry-red, because oxygen remains in the red cells as oxyhemoglobin. Since cyanide is lethal in very low quantities, the total amount of cyanide in the body may be insufficient for a generalized cherry-red discoloration. In such cases lividity closely resembles that seen in deaths due to other causes.[32] Hydrogen cyanide smells like bitter almonds, and this odor exudes from the body. It is particularly noticeable when the body is examined in a warm autopsy room. The interior of the body may emanate a significant amount of cyanide vapor which may intoxicate autopsy personnel. Chemical proof of the presence of cyanide clinches the diagnosis. Not all persons are able to detect the odor of bitter almonds; this ability is inherited as a sex-linked recessive trait.

Potassium or sodium cyanide taken orally causes extensive corrosion of the stomach. Vomiting or postmortem reflux of stomach contents may corrode the esophagus and mouth as well as the throat and cheeks. Corrosion may tear the gastric wall as a result of vomiting. The gastric mucosa reacts intensely alkaline after ingestion of cyanides.

SEX-ASSOCIATED ASPHYXIAS

Various means of accidental asphyxia associated with sexual perversion are encountered. A large proportion of these deaths are discovered under bizarre circumstances, which sometimes defy the imagination by their complexity and hence arouse suspicion of foul play. The scene is often the victim's own home: his bedroom, bathroom or the basement are usual locations. The door is commonly locked from the inside. Sometimes a motel or a secluded wooded area is chosen. In our experience, sex-associated asphyxias involve males exclusively, from boys to old age, although Henry in 1971 described one such case in a nineteen-year-old female.[33]

The victim may be found hanged, strangled, or with a plastic bag over his head. Binding the extremities, tying the wrists or handcuffing are frequent and may be suggestive of bondage. Contrary to expectation, the genitalia are not necessarily exposed. Frequently the body is clothed. There is often no indication of masturbation. Sometimes the body is clothed in female attire, particularly underwear. Within the victim's view may be pornographic pictures, mail-order catalogs opened to women's wear, etc. Occasionally the victim is apparently happily married and has a number of children. The psychiatric background for these undertakings is complex and not totally understood. It is believed that reduced oxygenation of the brain stimulates and heightens the sexual response (Figs. XIV-58 through XIV-61).

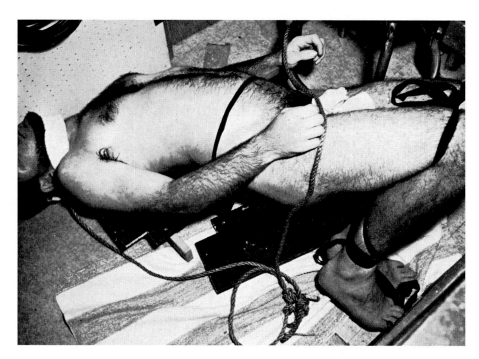

FIGURE XIV-58. Thirty-two-year-old, married, with two children, found in the basement of his home. The ankles and knees were tied. A cloth was wrapped around his genitals and secured by a rubber band. The padded rope around the neck passed over a water pipe in the ceiling and back down, ending in an eye-hook fastened in a vise. Nude pictures were pasted on the wall at the scene.

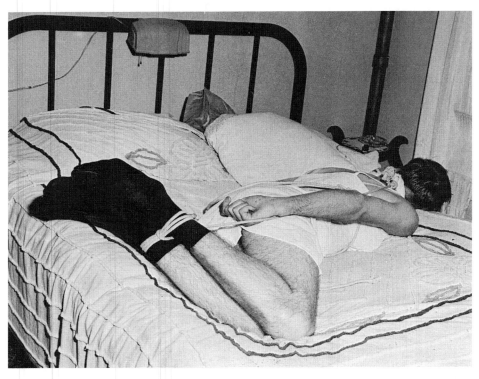

FIGURE XIV-59. Thirty-eight-year-old man dressed in brassiere and slip, tied in a way which allowed him to increase pressure on the neck by moving his legs.

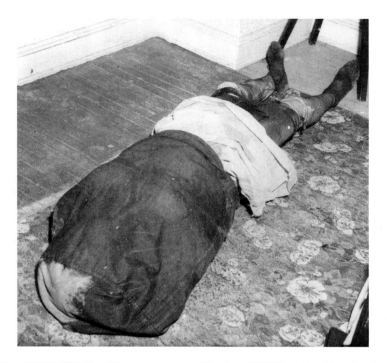

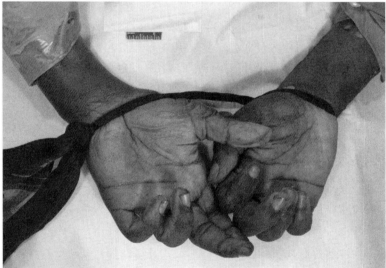

FIGURE XIV-60a–b. Nineteen-year-old male student, found dead wearing a brassiere, girdle, shirt and plastic raincoat, wrapped in a blanket, covered by a laundry bag, with a duffel bag pulled over the upper half of the body. A book was wedged between the girdle and the genitals. The hands were secured in the back by a necktie, which was first knotted into a loop, then the wrists twisted in order to tighten, as shown in (b). This case was first believed to be a homicide until it was ascertained that it was indeed possible for the victim to have tied his own wrists after placing the multiple layers of clothing on himself.

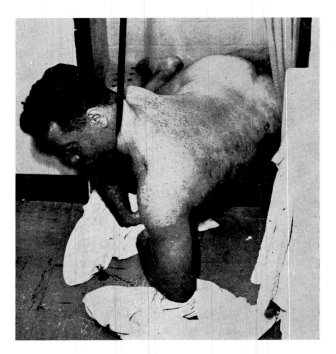

FIGURE XIV-61. This thirty-nine-year-old hung himself accidentally with a belt tied to the shower curtain rod. Towels were used to pad the elbows. The blood on the floor is due to congestion above the noose, and bleeding from the nose and mouth associated with the hanging.

The presence of moist semen or dry semen stains on or near the body of a male victim of asphyxia is believed to be associated with stimulation of certain nerve centers in the brain by the asphyxial process. Contraction of the musculature of the seminal vesicles by rigor mortis, can also cause extrusion of seminal fluid (see Fig. XXVI-7). The latter may occur regardless of the cause of death. Swelling of the penis in a hanging victim is also artifactual, resulting from postmortem settling of blood and fluids into the lower half of the body.

REFERENCES

1. Schroder, R., and Saternus, K.S.: Stauungszeichen im Kipfbereich und Veranderungen am Gehirn beim suicidalen Erhangungstod. *Z Rechtsmed., 89:* 247–265, 1983.
2. Hood, I., Ryan, D., and Spitz, W.U.: Resuscitation and petechiae. *Am J Forensic Med Path, 9* (1): 35–37, 1988.
3. Brouardel, P.: La pendaison, la strangulation, la suffocation, la submersion. Paris, Bailliere, 1897.
4. Teeters, N.K.: *Hang by the neck.* Springfield: Thomas, 1967, p. 156.
5. Spence, M.W., Shkrum, M.J., Ariss, A., and Regan, J.: Craniocervical injuries in judicial hangings: An anthropologic analysis of six cases. *Am J Forensic Med Path, 20* (4): 309–322, 1999.
6. Smialek, J.E., Smialek, P.Z., and Spitz, W.U.: Accidental bed deaths in infants due to unsafe sleeping situations. *Clin Pediatr, 16* (11): 1031–1036, 1977.
7. Simmons, G.T.: Death by power car window: An unrecognized hazard. *Am J Forensic Med Path, 13* (2): 112, 1992.
8. Sperry, K.: An unusual, deep lingual hemorrhage as a consequence of ligature strangulation. *J Forensic Sci, 33* (3): 806–811, 1988.
9. Shapiro, H.A., Gluckman, J., and Gordon, I.: The significance of fingernail abrasions of the skin. *J Forensic Med, 9:* 17, 1962.
10. Holmes, P.: *The trials of Dr. Coppolino.* New York: NAL, 1968.
11. DiMaio, V.J.M.: Homicidal asphyxia. *Am J Forensic Med Path, 21* (1): 1–4, 2000.
12. Di Nunno, N., Costantinides, F., Conticchio, G., et al. Self-strangulation: An uncommon but not unprecedented suicide method. *Am J Forensic Med Path, 23* (3): 260–263, 2002.

13. Reay, D.T., and Eisele, J. W.: Death from law enforcement neck holds. *Am J Forensic Med Path, 3* (3): 253–258, 1982.

14. Taylor, G.J., and Harris, W.S.: Cardiac toxicity of aerosol propellants. *JAMA, 214:* 81, 1970.

15. Mihalakis, I.: Asphyxia from pacifier. *Md State Med J, 20:* 53, 1971.

16. Spitz, D.J., and Spitz, W.U.: Killer pop machines. *J. Forensic Sci, 35* (2): 490–492, 1990.

17. *Witch-hunting in seventeenth century New England: A documentary history, 1638–1693.* David D. Hall, editor, second edition, Boston: Northeastern University Press, 1999.

18. Starkey, M.L.: *The devil in Massachusetts: A modern enquiry into the Salem Witch Trials.* New York: Doubleday Dell, 1989, pp. 204–207.

19. Bell, M.D., Rao, V.J., Wetli, C.V., and Rodriguez, R.N.: Positional asphyxiation in adults: A series of 30 cases from the Dade and Broward County Florida Medical Examiner offices from 1982 to 1990. *Am J Forensic Med Path, 13* (2): 101–107, 1992.

20. Parker, K., and Miles, S.H.: Deaths caused by bedrails. *J Am Geriatr Soc, 45* (7): 797–802, 1997.

21. O'Halloran, R.L., and Frank, J.G.: Asphyxial death during prone restraint revisited: A report of 21 cases. *Am J Forensic Med Path, 21* (1): 39–52, 2000.

22. Letter to the Editor and Reply. *Am J Forensic Med Path, 21* (4): 420–422, 2000.

23. Reay, D.T.: Death in custody. *Clinics in Laboratory Medicine, 28* (1) March, 1998.

24. Chan, T.C., Vilke, G.M., Neuman, T., et al: Does the hobble restraint position result in respiratory compromise? *Academic Emergency Medicine,* May, 1997.

25. Reay, D.T., Howard, J.D., Fligner, C.L., and Ward, R.J.: Effects of positional restraint on oxygen saturation and heart rate following exercise. *Am J Forensic Med Path, 9* (1): 16–18, 1988.

26. Chan, T.C., Vilke, G.M., and Neuman, T.: Reexamination of custody restraint position and positional asphyxia. *Am J Forensic Med Path, 19* (3): 201–205, 1998.

27. Laposata, E.A.: Positional asphyxia during law enforcement transport. *Am J Forensic Med Path, 14* (1): 86–87, 1993.

28. International Association of Chiefs of Police/National Law Enforcement Policy Center. The prone restraint–Still a bad idea. *Policy Review, 10* (1), Spring, 1998.

29. International Association of Chiefs of Police/National Law Enforcement Policy Center. Added concern about four-point restraints. *Policy Review, 13* (3), Fall/Winter, 2001.

30. Pollanen, M.S.: A variant of incaprettamento (ritual ligature strangulation) in East Timor. *Am J Forensic Med Path, 24* (1): 51–54, 2003.

31. Van Hoesen, K.B., Camporesi, E.M., Moon, R.E., Hage, M.L., and Piantadosi, C.A.: Should hyperbaric oxygen be used to treat the pregnant patient for acute carbon monoxide poisoning? *JAMA, 261* (7): 1039–1043, 1989.

32. Sopher, I.M., and Masemore, W.C.: The investigation of vehicular carbon monoxide fatalities. *Traffic Dig Rev, 18* (11): 1–11, 1970.

33. Musshoff, F., Schmidt, P., Daldrup, T., and Madea, B.: Cyanide fatalities: Case studies of four suicides and one homicide. *Am J Forensic Med Path, 23* (4): 315–320, 2002.

34. Henry, R.C.: "Sex" hangings in the female. *Medico-Legal Bulletin,* No. 214. Richmond, Virginia, Office of the Chief Medical Examiner, February, 1971.

Chapter XV

INVESTIGATION OF BODIES IN WATER

DANIEL J. SPITZ

OVER THE YEARS there has been continued confusion regarding the terminology used to describe deaths attributed to submersion. *Dorland's Medical Dictionary* defines drowning as *suffocation and death resulting from filling of the lungs with water or other substance so that gas exchange becomes impossible.*[1] In reality the lungs do not necessarily fill with water and rather than gas exchange being impossible the changes associated with gas exchange are better described in more general terms as being altered or mismatched. Adding to the confusion is the different terminology used by hospital physicians and forensic pathologists when it comes to describing a drowning death. As medical examiners it is important to come to some agreement regarding the terms used to describe these deaths. It is best to be consistent and use simple terminology that is easily understood by all parties associated with the investigation.

Drowning is best defined as death secondary to hypoxemia as a result of asphyxia while immersed in a liquid, usually water. A drowned individual should show no signs of life at the time of removal from the water, however, the term drowning should also be used when death occurs up to 24 hours following submersion. Near-drowning refers to a submersion episode that warrants medical attention and is associated with high morbidity and mortality in both children and adults. It is generally agreed that the term near-drowning is best used to describe a death that occurs greater than 24 hours following submersion. Secondary drowning is the terminology often used by clinicians to describe a delayed death secondary to complications of water submersion, however, this is a term that is often misunderstood. When dealing with fatal complications of submersion, it is recommended that these deaths be classified either as near-drowning, complications of near-drowning, or when possible confirm the pathologic state responsible for the death and use it for the cause of death with near-drowning as a contributory factor. For example, a delayed death from anoxic/ischemic encephalopathy following a near-drowning episode could be called complications of near-drowning or anoxic/ischemic encephalopathy due to near-drowning.

Each year in the United States an estimated 6000–8000 deaths are attributed to drowning, and internationally the annual number of drowning deaths is believed to be 140,000 to 150,000.[2] The true incidence of near-drowning is unknown, but has been reported to be as low as 15,000 or as high as 70,000 cases per year in the United States.[3] The near-drowning victim may recover without sequelae, suffer variable degrees of morbidity or die from one or more of the many associated complications. Overall, drowning is the third leading cause of accidental death in all age groups and the second most common cause of death in individuals under 44 years of age.[2] In children, one month to 14 years, drowning is the second most common cause of death behind motor vehicle accidents.[3] Nearly half of all drownings and near-drownings occur in children less than 5 years old, with the highest rate among toddlers.[3] In California, Arizona and Florida, drowning is the leading cause of death among children up to four years of age.[4] Drowning may occur in any age group, but typically displays a bimodal distribution which includes children under the age of 4 and adolescents and young adults between 10–20 years of age.[2,3] There is a strong male predominance in the latter age group and overall drowning is more common in males than females.

846

Investigation

Investigation of a body recovered from water can be challenging. Autopsy findings alone may be misleading and can cause the inexperienced pathologist to render a diagnosis of drowning when inappropriate. To assume that the cause of death of a body recovered from water is drowning is an unfortunate mistake that can be avoided if a proper investigation is conducted. The diagnosis of drowning requires a full investigation on the part of the police and the pathologist. The investigation should include a detailed account of the circumstances surrounding the death, knowledge of the victim's activities prior to submersion, knowledge of the deceased's social and medical history and a full autopsy including microscopic examination and toxicology.[5] Several questions need to be addressed each time the pathologist conducts an investigation dealing with a body recovered from water. It is most important to determine if the person was alive upon entry into the water. If the investigation supports a diagnosis of drowning, most pathologists feel that the case is closed. However, medical examiners are obligated to go further to attempt to answer two additional questions.

1. Why was the victim in a situation that put him/her at risk for drowning?
2. Why was the victim not able to survive in the water or get out of the water unharmed?

To help answer these questions, Davis described the drowning equation that classifies the risk factors for drowning as human and environmental factors (human factors + environmental factors = drowning).[6]

Human factors include a variety of conditions, the most common of which are related to a victim's mental health, medical conditions, drug or alcohol use and swimming ability. Environmental factors include water current, temperature and depth, dangerous marine life, electrical hazards and equipment failures. In most cases, a complete autopsy examination together with a thorough police investigation will determine how one or more of these factors contributed to the drowning. In some cases, bodies recovered from water are unknown and in these situations identity of the individual is the first step to understanding how and why the person died.

Children under the age of one most commonly drown in bathtubs.[7] The most frequent scenario is that a child was left unattended for a short period of time, typically described as *just a few seconds,* while the parent or caregiver was distracted. Although the majority of these cases are accidental, it is essential that the body be carefully examined for evidence of recent or old injuries, including burns related to hot water immersion. The medical examiner should review the circumstances surrounding the death, police investigation, witness statements, and all other pertinent information and compare this information with autopsy findings for consistency.

Each year young children drown in various types of industrial five-gallon buckets. An unsteady toddler may grab the edge of the bucket for support while standing, falls forward causing his/her upper body to be trapped inside the bucket. Although these deaths are usually accidental, care must be taken to rule out foul play.

In the preschool age group, 60–90% of drownings occur in backyard or community pools.[3,8] In most of these situations, the child was left unattended and drowned upon entry into the water. Even with many communities stressing pool safety, many residential pools have no physical barrier between the pool and the home. It has been found that a secure barrier surrounding the pool is an effective preventive measure, however, no physical barrier can replace the need for constant adult supervision of all children.[9]

Several types of pool alarms have been manufactured to sound an alert when someone falls into a pool. The majority of the alarms function by emitting a loud noise when activated by movement in the water. The sensitivity of some of these alarms has been questioned and thus they are by no means foolproof.

Drowning of adolescents and young adults often occurs in larger bodies of water such as lakes, rivers, or oceans. In this age group, it is important to consider head or cervical spine trauma (Fig. XV-1) and neurogenic shock as a cause of drowning. This is typically associated with diving into water that is shallow or where there are hid-

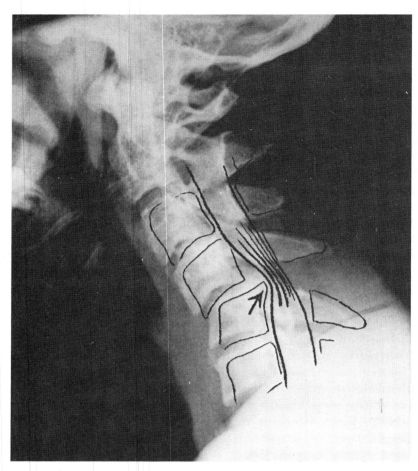

FIGURE XV-1. Fracture and dislocation of the cervical spine causing compression of the spinal cord. This is the type of injury associated with diving into a shallow swimming pool or onto a hidden submerged object.

den underwater rocks or other hazards. Posterior neck dissection with attention directed to the cervical vertebrae and cervical spinal cord is essential if this type of injury is suspected. See Chapter XXV for technique on dissection of the posterior neck. Common findings in such cases include hemorrhage in the deep muscles of the posterior neck and hemorrhage in the ligaments or membranes surrounding the cervical vertebrae. The cervical vertebrae should be evaluated for dislocations or fractures from both the anterior and posterior approach. An impact site may be found on the forehead or top of the head, although in some cases no face or scalp injuries are detected. These are the types of injuries that commonly result in paralysis, if the victim survives.

Pool drains are an additional hazard that may be associated with drowning. Older pools are typically equipped with a single drain that can generate enough suction to hold even a strong swimmer under water if the drain cover is not in place. We have several cases on file where individuals had their intestine sucked through their anus after sitting on an uncovered pool drain. The typical scenario involves an arm or leg inserted into such a drain in an attempt to recover lost jewelry or other objects. This renders the person at risk for severe suction injuries and subsequent drowning. Florida law, as of October 2000, mandates that newly built pools have two drains for the purpose of preventing such injuries.

Shallow Water Blackout

So-called, *shallow water blackout* is usually seen in children or adolescents and is often preceded by a characteristic sequence of events which includes prolonged underwater breath holding or more commonly prolonged underwater swimming. The mechanism of fainting or blackout is initiated by hyperventilation before entering the water. By hyperventilating the swimmer may be able to hold their breath for a longer period of time, however, physiologic changes occur which put the person at risk for *blackout* and subsequent drowning. Under normal conditions, breath holding causes the blood level of carbon dioxide to increase while the oxygen in the body decreases. A high level of carbon dioxide signals the brain to initiate breathing. Carbon dioxide is expelled during exhalation, thus excessive hyperventilation (four or more deep, rapid breaths) serves to decrease the level of carbon dioxide in the blood to a point where the body runs out of oxygen before stimulating the brain to breathe. The lowered oxygen level can result in sudden unconsciousness while underwater and death from drowning.[3,10,11]

Natural Disease and Drowning

In some cases, death in water is due to natural causes, such as heart disease or stroke. Where natural disease is unequivocally responsible for the death, the fact that the death occurred in water is irrelevant. In situations where it can be shown that the person was alive upon submersion and that drowning was a significant factor in the death, the cause of death is best classified as drowning with the decedent's natural disease being a contributory condition. For example, a man with a history of hypertension and a 640-gram heart collapses in the water and is declared dead shortly thereafter. With autopsy findings consistent with drowning, the death is best classified as accidental drowning with the victim's natural disease being the contributory factor. In some cases it is difficult to separate what role the natural disease and the water submersion played in the death. Degenerative brain disease,

advanced arthritis, syncope or vertigo (dizziness) may not be immediately life-threatening conditions, however, they may certainly be contributory factors associated with accidental bathtub drowning in the elderly.

A 62-year-old previously healthy man was standing in knee deep water at the beach when he was observed to grab his chest and collapse. He was pulled from the water less than one minute after he collapsed. The man was pronounced dead upon the arrival of Miami Fire/Rescue. At autopsy it was found that the pericardial sac contained 320 cc of blood which originated from a ruptured acute myocardial infarction. The lungs were congested and edematous and frothy fluid was throughout the tracheobronchial tree. Two cubic centimeters of clear fluid were aspirated from the sphenoid sinus. Due to the fact that a ruptured myocardial infarct is uniformly fatal regardless of the water component, the manner of death was classified as natural.

Seizure disorders represent a serious risk factor associated with drowning. Epilepsy has been associated with a four to fivefold increased risk of drowning and near drowning, especially among patients with poorly controlled seizures and in those who have had a recent change in anti-seizure medication.[3] The majority of these drownings occur while bathing, however, these individuals have an increased risk of drowning in any body of water. Drowning in the shower may result following a seizure if the body obstructs the drain and water accumulates to the point where the victim's nose and mouth become submerged.[12] In these cases, postmortem toxicology may be enlightening. Results often demonstrate that the drowned individual had subtherapeutic blood levels of anticonvulsant medication at the time of death, however, a therapeutic level of medication does not eliminate the risk of seizure. It appears that seizures more commonly occur around or in water and although the exact mechanism is unknown possible explanations include photogenic stimulation from the water surface, hyperventilation during swimming or water-immersion epilepsy.[12] Because seizures are often unwitnessed, bathtub drowning in an epileptic is not usually straightforward and requires a thorough investigation. It is important to have a clear understanding of the victim's medical history with regard to onset and frequency of seizures and medication schedule. Viewing of the scene or scene photographs, if

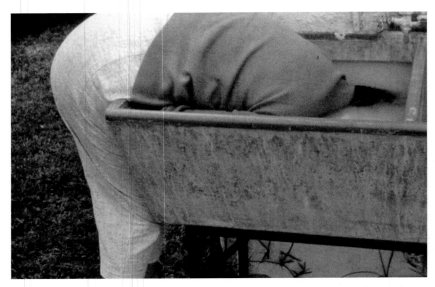

Figure XV-2. Middle-aged woman with a history of epilepsy found slumped over with her head submerged in a large outdoor sink. (Courtesy of Dr. Joseph H. Davis.)

available, may yield important clues. Although in many epileptics the neuropathology examination is normal, in some cases a detailed brain examination demonstrates abnormalities that can account for the seizure disorder.[13]

A middle-aged woman was found slumped over in a large outdoor sink in which she was doing laundry. Investigation determined that the woman had a long history of epilepsy and had frequent grand-mal seizures. Autopsy findings were consistent with a drowning death and no lesions were noted in the brain. The cause of death was classified as drowning associated with idiopathic seizure disorder (Fig. XV-2).

A young woman with a history of epilepsy and gingival hyperplasia related to Dilantin therapy was found in a roadside ditch after an unwitnessed collapse. Her face was submerged in approximately 8 inches of water, but the rest of her body was dry. Autopsy findings included a remote injury involving the left parietal lobe of the brain and pulmonary edema. A small amount of sand and muddy water, identical to that in the ditch, was found in the trachea and in the major bronchi. Toxicology results demonstrated a blood alcohol level of 0.12%. No antiseizure medication was in the woman's body. Based on the scene investigation and the autopsy results, is seems logical to conclude that the deceased suffered an epileptic seizure, fell into the ditch and died as a result of drowning.

Drugs and Alcohol Associated with Drowning

Drugs and alcohol are common factors related to drowning, however, it can be difficult to deter-

mine whether the death was secondary to the toxic effect of the drug or the result of submersion. In all bodies recovered from water, a comprehensive blood screen is necessary to determine what drugs were in the victim's body at the time of death. Although seen infrequently today, narcotic addicts may be found dead partly or completely submerged in a bathtub. In many cases witnesses have stated that the individual was placed in the water in an attempt at revival after collapsing because of an adverse drug reaction. In these cases it can be difficult to determine if drowning played a role in the death since the autopsy findings in drug intoxications and drowning are often similar. In some situations, scene photographs may help determine if the victim's head was below or above the water level (Fig. XV-3). In adults, several studies have shown that in 30–50% of drownings, alcohol was a contributory factor.[14–17]

A middle-aged, previously healthy woman who lived on a houseboat was found floating adjacent to the shoreline. The woman was known to be able to swim and the police investigation yielded no suspicion of foul play. Autopsy findings included pulmonary edema with froth around the nose and mouth and 4 cc of fluid in the sphenoid sinus. No significant trauma was noted on the body. Toxicological analysis yielded a blood alcohol of 0.28%. The cause of death was listed as drowning with acute alcohol intoxication as a contributory cause.

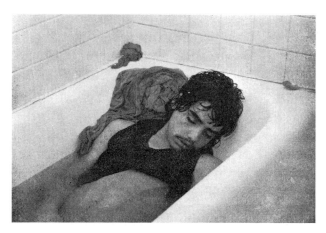

FIGURE XV-3. Narcotic addict placed in a water-filled bathtub in a resuscitation attempt following an adverse reaction to the drug. A stocking tourniquet and a spoon cooker are on the sides of the tub near the victim's head. Toxicologic testing isolated high concentrations of opiates. Scene photographs were helpful to determine that the cause of death was opiate intoxication and that drowning played no role in the death.

Like drinking and driving, there is overwhelming evidence that alcohol is a major risk factor in boating fatalities. Many of these are the result of drowning after the victim falls overboard either while the boat is moving or at rest. The increased popularity of personal watercrafts (i.e., jet skis, wave runners and jet boats) has resulted in a sharp rise in the number of associated injuries and deaths. In 1991, the number of deaths in Florida resulting from personal watercraft accidents was two while in 1995 the number increased six-fold to twelve. Although the majority of deaths resulted from blunt head, chest, or abdominal injuries, a subset of these victims die as a result of non-fatal blunt injuries combined with drowning or near-drowning.[18]

Dangerous Marine Life

Many species of marine animals may come in contact with an unsuspecting swimmer or diver. Of all the marine life encountered only few species deserve consideration because of their ability to cause serious injury or death. In some of these cases, death is actually secondary to drowning, while in others death occurs at some

time after exiting the water secondary to the effect of a toxin that interrupts vital bodily functions. Jellyfish are commonly encountered, but rarely cause more than an annoying sting. Sea wasps are the most dangerous jellyfish and can be lethal within minutes following a sting. As the tentacles attach to the skin, the venom that is released into the body may have a toxic effect on the heart and respiratory center of the brain resulting in shock, tachycardia and respiratory failure. Although rare in the United States, a recent report describes a case of a 4-year-old boy swimming in the Gulf of Mexico who died less than one hour after contact with a sea wasp jellyfish.[19] More frequently, death has been associated with Portuguese man-o'-war *(Physalia physalis),* common along the Atlantic coast of the United States.[20] Suspicion of contact with a jellyfish should prompt scraping of the erythematous and blistered skin to determine what type of nematocyst and possibly what type of jellyfish was involved (Fig. XV-4).

Sea snakes are rarely encountered, but are more deadly. They inhabit the tropical Pacific and Indian Oceans and are not encountered in the United States. Fortunately, these animals do not bite humans unless provoked. Sea snake venom is a curare-like toxin that may cause muscular paralysis followed by ascending paralysis which typically develops over several hours. In severe cases death may result from respiratory muscle paralysis.

Sharks have acquired a bad reputation in regards to swimmers and divers. Sharks do have a predatory nature by instinct, but are not typically attracted to humans and thus pose little risk to swimmers. Each year less than 100 shark attacks are reported worldwide with the majority occurring in the waters off the Florida coast. Injuries from shark attacks are often severe because of tissue loss and profuse bleeding, however most shark-related injuries are not fatal. Sharks feed at dusk and dawn which is when most shark attacks occur. Most shark attacks involving humans are said to occur because in shallow, murky water a shark may mistake a swimmer for a distressed fish. Furthermore, sharks are attracted to shiny, metallic objects

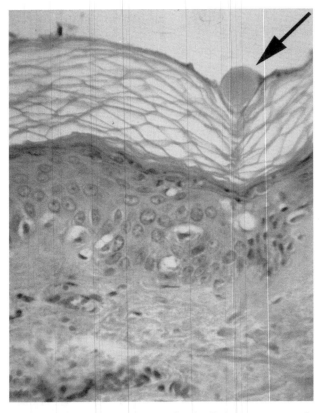

FIGURE XV-4. Photomicrograph of a Portuguese man-o'-war nematocyst (arrow) attached to the surface of the skin. (Courtesy of Dr. Joseph H. Davis.)

which may cause further confusion and prompt an attack. Although rare and less devastating than shark bites are injuries from moray eels and large barracudas.[21]

Non-Accidental Drowning

Although the overwhelming majority of drownings are accidental an estimated 10% are suicides. This should be considered in cases of drowning that involve depressed individuals, those with suicidal ideations and especially those who have attempted suicide in the past. A situation that should raise suspicion of suicide is an adult who drowns in the backyard swimming pool and whose medical history and autopsy reveal no significant natural disease. We have seen several individuals who committed suicide by slowly driving their vehicle into a canal or lake. In many of these cases, the scene investigation raised suspicion that this may in fact be a suicide. In one case, recreation of the event demonstrated that the driver would have had to deliberately negotiate the vehicle into the lake by making several turns prior to entering the water. It was found after discussion with the victim's family that the deceased had attempted suicide in the past and that he had discussed suicide in the days prior to his death. To avoid missing a suicidal drowning, suspicion is warranted in all cases where the drowning cannot be readily explained. A victim's psychiatric history and information regarding a victim's history of suicide attempts should always be obtained.

Homicidal drownings are rare and typically involve the elderly or young children as a component of child abuse.[7,17] In these situations the victims are unable to defend themselves and thus, trauma on the body may be minimal or absent. With children and the elderly, the presence of remote or healing injuries may be the only evidence of previous abuse. Skeletal x-ray films are helpful in observing old fractures. Although the drowning of a young child in a bathtub is usually accidental, this situation must raise suspicion of possible foul play and a detailed interview of the caregiver should be part of the investigation. An estimated 5–6% of drownings are believed to be due to child abuse or neglect.[17]

However, not all child killings are necessarily associated with abuse or neglect. A recent case in Texas (Andrea Yates) and another in South Carolina (Susan Smith), some years earlier, received national media coverage. In the Texas case, the mother drowned her five children, ages 6 months to 7 years, in a bathtub. In the South Carolina case, Susan Smith drove with two children, ages 14 months and 3 years, in the vehicle into a lake. In 1989, Lawrence De Lisle drove his car into the Detroit River with his entire family. Four children drowned, his wife escaped and he was charged and convicted. Cases such as these three are not infrequent.

Disposal of a homicide victim to simulate drowning occurs with enough frequency that each case involving a body recovered from water should be approached with this in mind. This possibility makes distinction between changes due to drowning and those resulting from post-mortem submersion of prime importance. Upon removal of a body from water, abrasions and contusions may not be visible while the body is wet. If the autopsy is performed immediately, and if there is suspicion of foul play, it is recommended that the body be reexamined the following day, after it is thoroughly dried.

The body of a young female was recovered from a shallow lake. The circumstances surrounding the case were suspicious of homicide, however, at the time the body was removed from the water only faint contusions were evident. The body was put in a cooler overnight and allowed to dry. Upon inspection the following morning, extensive abrasions and contusions were easily seen on the neck and chin (Fig. XV-5a–b).

Postmortem Changes in Water

A body in fresh or brackish water will typically sink unless trapped air in the clothing keeps it afloat. In salt water, a body is more likely to remain on the surface or, depending on fat content, float at variable levels beneath the surface. For this reason, bodies in the ocean are often recovered by the use of aircraft. A body that sinks will resurface when gas is formed as part of the decomposition process and even a body weighted down will eventually rise as more and more putrefactive gases are produced. Decomposing bodies have been found floating while weighted down with over one hundred pounds. Two such cases involved homicides where the victims were murdered, put in a suitcase and dumped in a lake. It is important to note that although weight attached to a body will typically not keep it submerged, the longer a body is under water the more it is vulnerable to postmortem animal activity.

The time needed until a body resurfaces usually depends on the temperature of the water. In warm water it may take two or three days while in cold water a body may not resurface for weeks or months. In very cold deep waters, decomposition occurs very slowly and in these conditions a body may never resurface. Bodies recovered from the Russian nuclear submarine, Kursk were

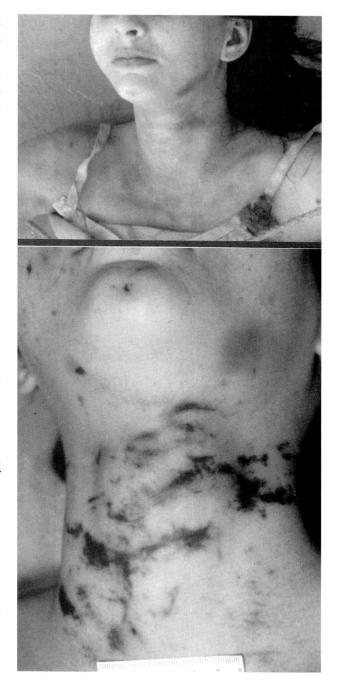

FIGURE XV-5a–b. (a) Young woman's neck upon removal from the water showing faint contusions. (b) The body after overnight in cooler showing extensive injuries. (Courtesy of Dr. Joseph H. Davis.)

identifiable by sight 14 months after an explosion sunk the ship to the floor of the Barents Sea during naval exercises.

In general, putrefaction of a body in water proceeds at a slower rate than putrefaction of a body on land. A body that appears minimally decomposed will often show accelerated putrefaction upon removal from the water. Davis indicates that even refrigeration will not halt the rapid decomposition that ensues after the body is removed from the water.[5] For this reason, a prompt autopsy and collection of toxicology specimens should be performed without delay in these cases.

The rule of thumb for putrefaction of a body is one week in air equals two weeks in water equals eight weeks in the ground. Putrefaction is slower in seawater compared to fresh water because high salinity retards bacterial growth. In stagnant water where bacteria are abundant, putrefaction occurs rapidly.

A human brain placed in a saturated salt (NaCl) solution (26%) at room temperature remained unchanged after 30 years. The waters off the Florida coast have a salt content of about 3%.

A body in water will typically not show mummification, however, drifting in shallow water may expose parts of the body to air while other parts remain submerged. In this situation, mummification of exposed areas may be observed (Fig. XV-6). Fungi may grow on a submerged or moist body (Fig. XV-7). Adipocere is a condition in which the tissues of the body are degraded to a thick, gray, soap-like, greasy substance (Fig. XV-8, see also III-31a–b). Older adipocere may be hard and brittle. Warm temperatures in addition to lack of oxygen and bacterial growth are ideal conditions for the formation of adipocere. Adipocere is usually associated with bodies that have been submerged for several months, however, it may form in as little six weeks in warm water. In a protected cold water environment such as in a car, adipocere may form a protective coating over the body that serves to preserve the bones and internal organs for many years.[22] Over the years, many bodies have been recovered from cars submerged in Miami canals. It is often known how long the cars have been submerged, and thus some conclusions may be drawn regarding duration and extent of decomposition in relatively warm water.

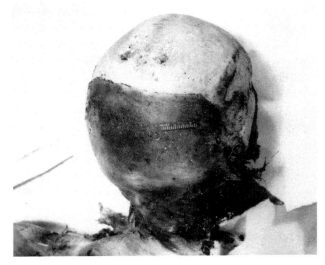

FIGURE XV-6. Body found in July drifting in the waters of the Chesapeake Bay a short distance offshore. The back of the body, which was exposed to air, was mummified, while the submerged front of the body was largely skeletonized. The victim had been reported missing eight months earlier. The back of the head showed a horizontal waterline below which the skull was exposed. Skeletonization was due to the combined effects of postmortem feeding by marine life and putrefaction.

A body recovered from a Miami canal had been missing for just over two years. The body consisted entirely of adipocere which contained disarticulated bones kept together by the deceased's clothing. No organs remained in the chest or abdominal cavities. The adipocere was readily removed from the bones with the use of a brush. The deceased is presumed to have drowned after driving his car into the canal following a Miami Dolphins football game.

Another case involved the remains of a middle-aged man recovered from a Miami canal. The deceased was determined to be a man reported missing over 21 years earlier. He had gone out for a night of drinking with friends and never returned home. The skeleton was completely disarticulated and bones were recovered from the front and back seats of the car. The bones had a brown and partially red discoloration that was most likely related to the thick black mud and sludge which covered the skeleton. Surprisingly, approximately 300 grams of brain parenchyma were recovered from within the skull. At the request of the family DNA testing was performed to confirm his identity. Nuclear DNA on both bone and teeth was unsuccessful, however, mitochondrial DNA from the same specimens provided the necessary sequence for comparison.

A body in water often sustains damage from contact with rocks, underwater objects, boats and

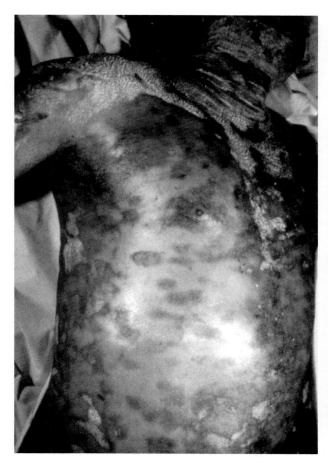

FIGURE XV-7. Dark fungal colonies growing on the body surface.

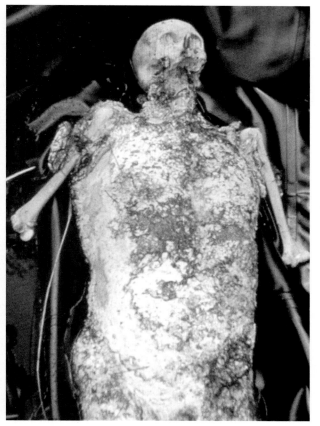

FIGURE XV-8. Adipocere formation of a body found floating in the ocean. It was later determined that this was the body of a man who had died of natural causes and buried at sea 13 months earlier. (Courtesy of Dr. Joseph H. Davis.)

marine life. Submerged bodies usually float face down with the arms and legs hanging. The back of the hands and forearms, forehead, knees and feet are especially vulnerable to scraping along the bottom as the body is moved by the current (Fig. XV-9a–b). Boat propeller injuries may be inflicted before or after death. In most cases the distinction is straightforward based on the appearance of the wounds, while in other cases the circumstances surrounding the incident add the crucial information. Boat propellers typically cause deep, parallel, chop-type wounds that involve soft tissues and often bone (Figs. XV-10a–b and XV-11a–b). Such injuries should be carefully examined paying attention to the depths of the wound for any trace evidence left behind. As in hit-and-run car collisions, trace evidence transfer may occur with boat propellers

and a chip of paint may be all that is necessary to determine which boat was responsible.

A 14-year-old female was snorkeling in Biscayne Bay while on a family outing. Family members saw her in distress and noticed that she was bleeding profusely leading them to believe that she had been attacked by a shark. Examination of the body demonstrated multiple boat propeller injuries involving the right thigh, right arm, chest and head. It was determined that the deceased was the victim of a hit-and-run incident, however, no boat could be linked to the scene. At autopsy small specks of white paint were recovered from several of the wounds and compared using pyrolysis gas chromatography to paint samples taken from the propeller of a suspect boat. A positive match was made.

Often it is possible to reconstruct the activity or position of the victim at the time the injuries were sustained.

The body of a middle-aged woman was found a few hundred feet from the shoreline on the ocean floor. Examina-

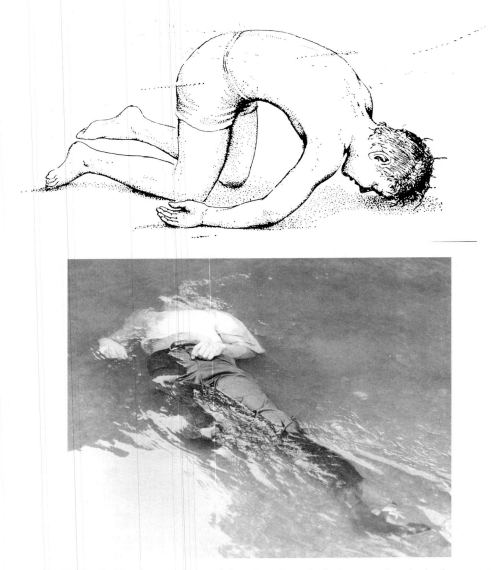

Figure XV-9a–b. Floating in water and dragging along the bottom renders the body suscepti-ble to injuries which typically involve the head, back of the hands, knees and top of the feet. (b) Occasionally, bodies are turned as a result of wave action and will be found face up when washed ashore.

tion of the body revealed typical parallel boat propeller cuts on her head, chest and the underside of one arm. Alignment of the injuries indicated that she was swimming backstroke-style on the surface and that she had obviously not been div-ing, as alleged.

A floating body may come in contact with gasoline or oil that coats the surface of the water. In these situations the skin will be reddened and readily sloughs off, resembling skin slippage or a second-degree burn. Postmortem fish and crab

activity will often manifest as injuries involving the eyelids, lips, tip of the nose and earlobes (Fig. XV-12a). These injuries are initially superficial, but larger skin defects will occur with continued animal activity and decomposition (Fig. XV-12b). In some cases postmortem fish activity may result in extensive loss of skin and deep soft tis-sues (Fig. XV-13).

With time, algae may grow on the skin and clothing imparting a green or green-black discol-

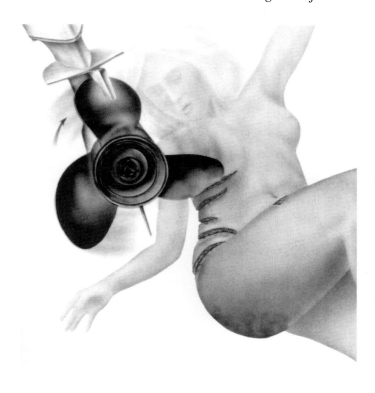

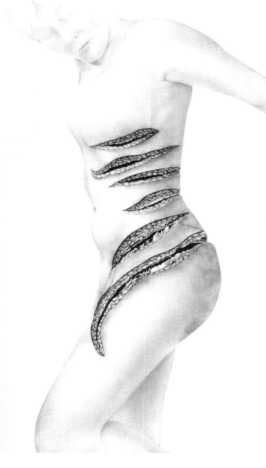

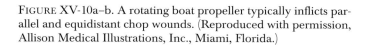

FIGURE XV-10a–b. A rotating boat propeller typically inflicts parallel and equidistant chop wounds. (Reproduced with permission, Allison Medical Illustrations, Inc., Miami, Florida.)

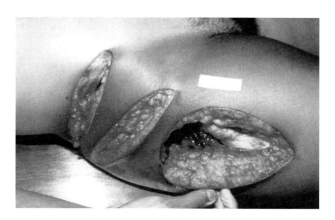

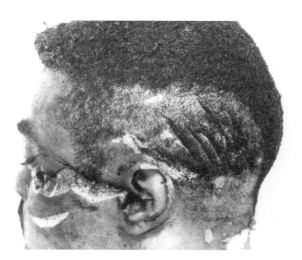

FIGURE XV-11a–b. (a) Characteristic propeller chop wounds on the thigh sustained while snorkeling (b) and similar injuries on the face.

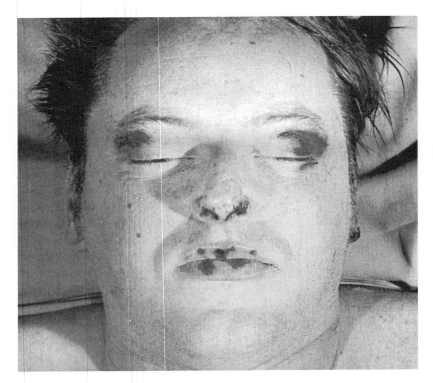

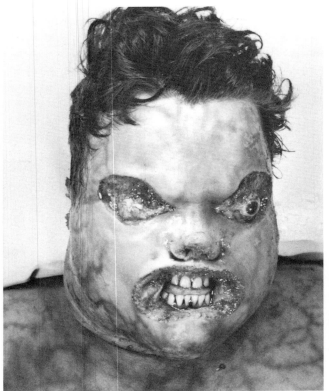

FIGURE XV-12a–b. (a) Early phase of postmortem activity by fish, crabs or crayfish. Such injuries usually involve the eyelids, lips, nose and earlobes. (b) Continued postmortem fish activity results in larger skin defects.

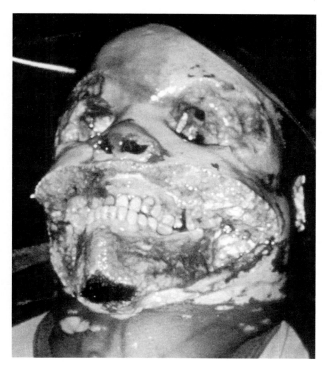

FIGURE XV-13. Extensive loss of facial soft tissue due to postmortem fish feeding.

oration to these areas (Fig. XV-14 a-b). Algae are not usually seen on bodies recovered from tropical waters because decomposition will precede algae growth. Growth of algae on the face may make recognition of a body difficult. It may be possible to remove the algae to help with visual identification, however, as the algae are wiped away so is the underlying epidermis. In temperate climates, where the onset of decomposition is not as rapid as in tropical regions, algae growth on the body is accelerated and decomposition is further delayed due to antimicrobial properties of algae.

Under certain conditions, bodies in water can travel great distances. Giertsen and Morild reported situations in which two bodies drifted more than 300 miles in the open ocean.[23] In open waters, determination of direction and speed of the current can be used to approximate the distance traveled and thus help locate the body. In the Detroit River, it is often possible to predict with fair accuracy when and where the body of someone who drowned upstream is likely to surface. In general a raft or float will drift a

distance of 100 feet in 60 seconds at a current speed of 1.0 knot (1.15 mph).[24]

It is important to distinguish antemortem from postmortem *injuries,* however, in some cases this determination is difficult or even impossible. Antemortem and postmortem lacerations often look similar because antemortem lacerations typically appear bloodless due to leaching of blood from an open wound. As described previously, some postmortem *injuries* have characteristic features that should be recognized. Prolonged submersion in water may alter the appearance of gunshot and stab wounds, however, recognition of these injuries is usually possible. Any suspicion of a gunshot or stab wound should prompt x-ray of the body. Damage to the internal organs or blood in the body cavities is associated with penetrating trauma and would not be seen with postmortem artifacts.

The decomposed body of a homeless man was found floating adjacent to a houseboat that was docked approximately one mile from the underpass where he was living. The two lacerations on the deceased's scalp were caused by rescue workers while attempting to recover the body from the water. Without knowing that the lacerations were inflicted after death, it would have been difficult to make this distinction. A thorough police investigation discovered that the man was an alcoholic and that the slope of the embankment where he had been living would have made a fall into the water likely.

Bodies recovered from water are often partially or completely nude. The victim's clothes may be found floating nearby or may never be recovered. Certainly the lack of clothing on a female's body in water should raise suspicion of foul play, however, it is important to note that nude bodies in water may have in fact been clothed at the time of entry into the water. Why the body is nude is often an intriguing question. Several situations exist to explain this phenomenon. The churning of the surf or pounding of the waves while the body is against the shore is a likely possibility. Sometimes the struggle to stay afloat may account for partial disrobing.

Autopsy Findings Associated with Drowning

Drowning is often called a diagnosis of exclusion, and although this is partly correct, it should

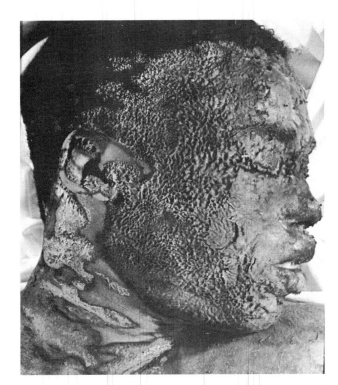

FIGURE XV-14a. Algae growth on the body may resemble mud.

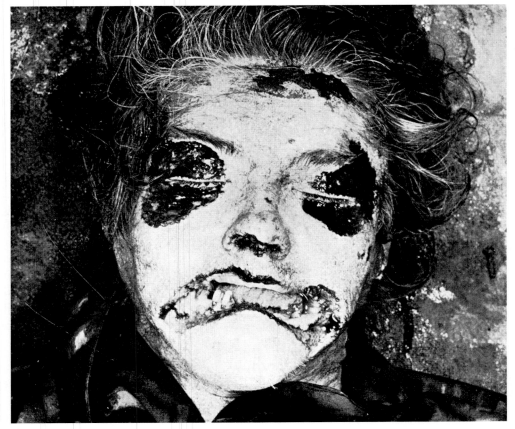

FIGURE XV-14b. Growth of algae on exposed areas of the face previously damaged by marine life.

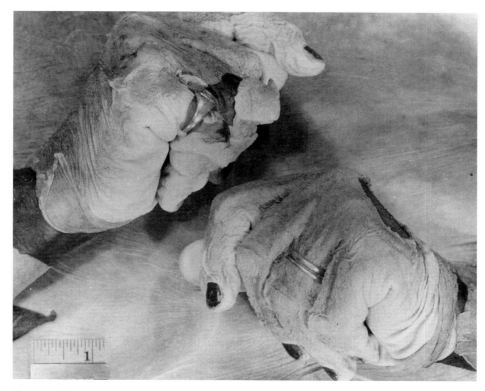

FIGURE XV-15. Detachment of the epidermis from the deeper skin layers of the hands after eight hours immersion in warm water.

be understood that victims of drowning typically demonstrate characteristic autopsy findings. Although certain autopsy findings are clearly associated with drowning, there are no autopsy findings that are pathognomonic. Each drowning is a unique and individual event and autopsy findings are most useful when correlated with the circumstances uncovered by a detailed police investigation.

Autopsy findings associated with drowning can be seen both externally and internally. Body surface findings are associated with a body in water whether or not the cause of death is drowning. External findings may include the presence of mud and aquatic debris within the mouth or in the nares and wrinkling of the skin on the hands and feet (Figs. XV-15 to XV-17a). Typically skin wrinkling is seen if the body has been in the water for one or more hours, however, in warm water wrinkling can begin in less than 20 minutes. With continued immersion and depending on the temperature of the water, the epidermis

peels off like a *glove* including the toenails and fingernails (Fig. XV-17b). In many cases ink can be applied to the fingertips to obtain fingerprints for the purpose of identification. In cold water, several days may pass before the epidermis separates from the underlying tissues, whereas in warm water, such as a bathtub, this may occur after several hours (Fig. XV-18). Skin separation (epidermal sloughing) that occurs with prolonged submersion is similar to that seen in early decomposition and second-degree burns. Few conjunctival petechiae are not uncommon in someone who drowns, and although multiple conjunctival petechiae have been seen in cases of drowning, this is a rare. Drowning and near-drowning victims often receive cardiopulmonary resuscitation (CPR) and as a result may have both conjunctival or periorbital petechiae. In general, the petechiae associated with CPR are coarse and not numerous. Scleral hemorrhages and hemorrhage in the anterior neck muscles which are often seen in cases of strangulation do not occur

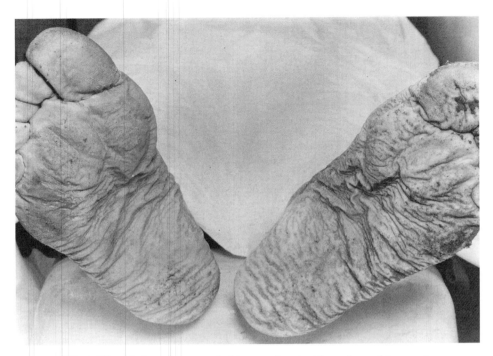

FIGURE XV-16. Wrinkled *washerwoman's* skin associated with prolonged immersion.

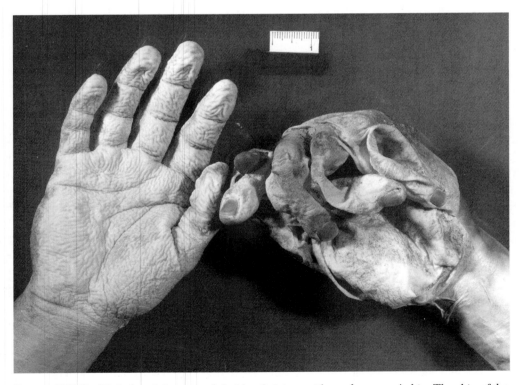

FIGURE XV-17a. Right hand shown on left side of picture with *washerwoman's* skin. The skin of the left hand is starting to slip off due to improper handling of the body.

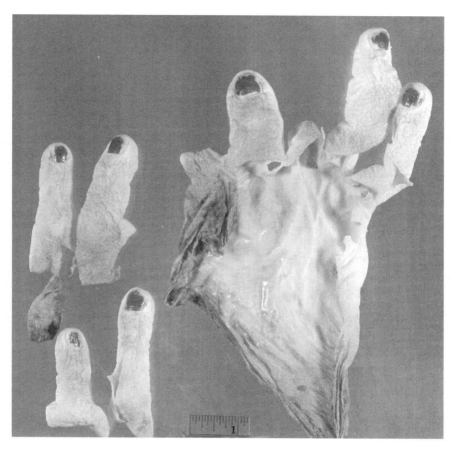

FIGURE XV-17b. Glove-like separated epidermis can float in the water independently of the body.

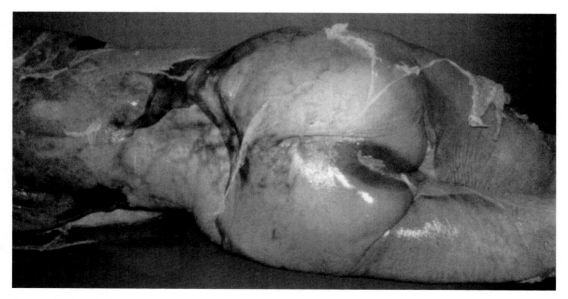

FIGURE XV-18. Diffuse skin slippage in an elderly woman who drowned in the bathtub and remained submerged for 14 hours.

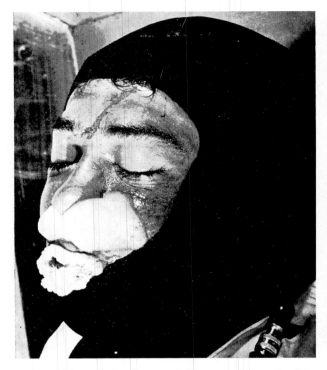
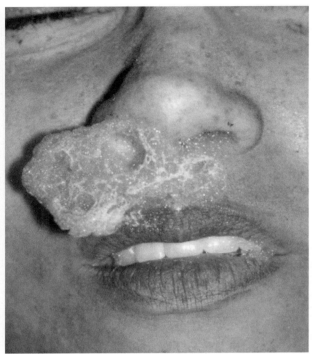

FIGURE XV-19a–b. Froth around the nose and mouth of drowning victims. The froth may be white or blood-tinged, usually thick and resembling shaving cream.

in drowning and should always raise suspicion of foul play.

An external examination finding that supports death by drowning is the presence of white or bloody foam around the nose and mouth (Fig. XV-19a-b). The amount of exuding foam is much increased during chest compression as in CPR. The foam is produced in the lungs due to the presence of protein (albumin) mixed with water and air. The hypoxic environment may lead to rupture of alveolar capillaries and the alveolar hemorrhage will cause the foam to be blood-tinged. Since bloody or non-bloody foam is occasionally associated with other causes of death including drug overdoses (most commonly heroin), the circumstances surrounding the death play an important role when interpreting this finding.

The significance of blood-stained foam in the airways and around the nose and mouth of a body recovered from water became apparent in 1969 during a court hearing in Wilkes-Barre, Pennsylvania regarding the death of Mary Jo Kopechne. At this hearing, arguments were heard regarding whether or not Miss Kopechne's body should be exhumed for autopsy to determine the cause of her death. The judge refused to order an exhumation based on the testimony that a large amount of pinkish foam was seen around her nose and mouth after she was recovered from the water. This finding led to the conclusion that Ms. Kopechne had to have been alive at the time she went into the water. Based on this finding and the fact that no bodily injuries were observed by the medical examiner who responded to the scene, it was determined that Miss Kopechne did in fact drown when the car driven by Senator Ted Kennedy went off a bridge at Chappaquiddick Island, near the Massachusetts coast.

The analogy given to the court by the expert who testified on behalf of the Kopechne family was that water and egg white (protein) in a bottle will not froth, unless shaken. Breathing was equated to shaking, i.e., definite evidence that Ms. Kopechne breathed in the water and drowned.

Although bloody, white or clear foam around the nose and mouth is common in individuals who drown, it is not sufficient to assume someone drowned based solely on this finding.

The autopsy on a body retrieved from water typically yields the most supportive findings for the diagnosis of drowning. The lungs are often voluminous and may overlie the pericardial sac anteriorly (aqueous emphysema). Lung weights may exceed 1000 grams each. The pulmonary

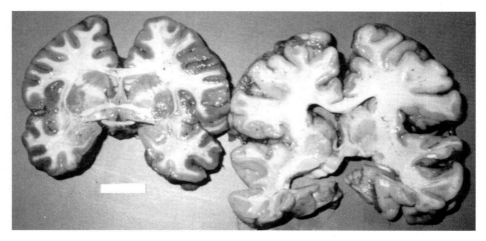

FIGURE XV-20. In cases of saltwater drowning, the cerebral cortex often has a red-brown discoloration which is attributed to hemoconcentration.

parenchyma is usually dark red-blue, congested and markedly edematous. Frothy fluid is often noted upon cutting the main bronchi and a copious amount of watery and frothy fluid is easily expressed from the cut surface of the lung tissue. It should be noted that similar appearing lungs may be seen in some natural deaths and deaths preceded by cardiopulmonary resuscitation (CPR). In a study by Copeland, it was found that 80–90% of fresh and saltwater drowning victims have significantly increased lung weights secondary to pulmonary edema.[22] Washed-out appearing subpleural hemorrhages characterized by variably sized purple areas at the periphery of the lungs may be present. Sand, mud, seaweed, broken shells and other aquatic debris may be seen in the trachea and main bronchi with extension into segmental bronchi. Although this foreign material may passively enter the mouth, pharynx and tracheobronchial tree, identification of such material in the deep airways is suggestive of some active respiratory effort while in the water. The stomach may contain water which suggests antemortem swallowing, however, water and aquatic debris may passively enter the stomach of a submerged body, especially in rough waters. Aspiration of gastric contents occurs commonly during the unconscious gasping phase of drowning and should not be interpreted as an antemortem event.

The brain often shows varying degrees of edema, typically more pronounced in children. In saltwater drownings, the osmotic shifts and hemoconcentration that occur may cause the cerebral cortex to have a red-brown discoloration (Fig. XV-20).

The fully clothed fresh body of a young woman was found on a deserted beach just below the waterline. The waves were washing over the body and had swept abundant sand over the clothing and into the pockets. At autopsy a contact gunshot wound was noted in the center of the forehead. The airway, including the segmental bronchi, contained sand and seaweed, forming a solid cast. A small quantity of sand was present in the stomach and the first part of the small intestine. As death was believed to have occurred rapidly, most of the sand and seaweed must have been washed into the body after death.

Aspiration of the sphenoid sinus to document the presence of fluid is an easy procedure that should be performed on all suspected drowning victims. Although no current studies have determined the sensitivity or specificity of this procedure, the presence of measurable amounts of clear or blood-tinged fluid within the sphenoid sinus is another autopsy finding to support a diagnosis of drowning. In some cases of drowning, the sphenoid sinus contains no fluid. The sphenoid sinus is best approached by breaking the anterior portion of the sphenoid body with any blunt autopsy instrument. The contents of the sphenoid should then be aspirated under direct visualization using a needle and syringe. See Chapter XXV for sinus aspiration technique. In someone who dies in the churning ocean surf, sand grains and fragments of seaweed may be seen in the middle ears and in the fluid recovered from the sinus. In adults the volume of the sphenoid sinus may reach seven cubic centimeters, however, the sinus size is quite variable and depends primarily on the size of the individual. This type of aspiration cannot be performed in infants or children because the sphenoid sinus is only developed after six or seven years of age.

Hemorrhage in the middle ear and mastoid air cells has also been observed with some frequency in drowning victims.[26,27] In 1963, this was demonstrated by Niles who found such hemorrhages in 23 out of 24 cases of drowning.[27] Middle ear hemorrhage is typically seen as a bluish discoloration in the base of the skull at the posterolateral regions of the middle cranial fossae. The middle ear cavity, including the tympanic membrane, can be directly visualized after removing the temporal bone adjacent to the internal acoustic meatus. The hemorrhages are believed to arise from delicate mucosal capillaries that rupture in association with increased pressure within the middle ear. Depending on the degree of pressure increase, the tympanic membrane may be ruptured. Such findings are common in SCUBA diving deaths which more commonly occur in deep water. The tympanic membrane is often artifactually damaged when the bone is dissected, thus it is recommended that the tympanic membrane be initially visualized using an otoscope followed by removal of the overlying bone for direct visualization.

Microscopic findings in the lungs of drowning victims are non-specific, but may consist of variable degrees of pulmonary edema, intra-alveolar hemorrhage, focal alveolar distention (aqueous emphysema) and increased pulmonary macrophages. Mud and aquatic debris may occasionally be seen in the bronchioles and alveolar ducts (Fig. XV-21).

Diatoms are single cell, microscopic organisms that may be alive or in fossil form (Fig. XV-22a–b). There are thousands of different species of diatoms, each having its own characteristic

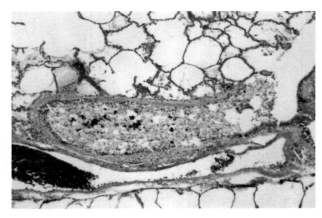

FIGURE XV-21. Microscopic section of the lung showing mud and foreign debris in a small airway. (Courtesy of Dr. Joseph H. Davis.)

exoskeleton composed mainly of silicon. Diatoms are widespread throughout the environment. They inhabit virtually every natural body of water and are easily carried through the air from one location to another.

The diatom test is based on the idea that during the drowning process water is inhaled and diatoms enter the circulation and get carried through the blood to the internal organs. Diatoms are resistant to acid, and thus they can be extracted from various organs using an acid preparation which digests the tissue, but leaves the silica-based extracellular shell of the diatom intact. Although diatoms may be found in many tissues, including lung and liver, those in favor of the diatom test suggest using marrow extracted from intact long bones.[28] (The idea of using bone marrow for testing[29] originated in Europe in the early 1960s and stems from the belief that the only way for diatoms to enter the bone marrow is by way of the circulating blood. This however, ignores the possibility of previous contamination. Once diatoms are in the system, they will remain in the tissues. Further, dating the time of such contamination is not possible.)

Over the years the significance of diatoms has been a source of great debate among forensic pathologists with many European doctors accepting the use of diatoms and pathologists in the United States largely disregarding diatom data. Recent studies supporting the use of diatoms as

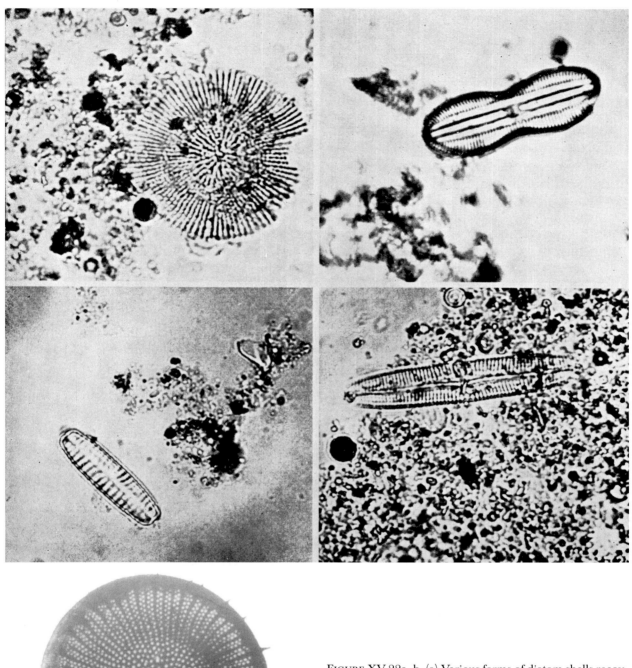

FIGURE XV-22a–b. (a) Various forms of diatom shells recovered from the ashes of incinerated air filters. The material in the background is mostly carbon. The diatom in the upper left picture is 42 microns in diameter. (b) Scanning electron micrograph of a diatom.

an adjunct to the diagnosis of drowning fail to address the fact that diatoms are commonly found in the tissues of non-drowned individuals.[28,30] The presence of diatoms in non-drowned persons gives the diatom test a low sensitivity in the diagnosis of drowning. Furthermore, the absence of diatoms is not a reliable means to rule out the possibility of drowning. There is some data suggesting that the quantity of diatoms in the tissue may be significant, however, further work in this area is necessary before any conclusions can be made.[31]

At this time, the ubiquitous nature of diatoms makes their routine use in the diagnosis of drowning misleading and unreliable.

The use of autopsy findings to differentiate fresh and saltwater drowning is rarely of significance and in reality it is extremely difficult or impossible to make such distinction. Copeland found that there is no significant difference in lung weights between fresh and saltwater drowning victims.[22] Increased fluidity of the blood has been noted in fresh water drowning, however, this is subjective and in reality of little or no value. Although no current study exists, it seems logical that a test of the salinity of the sphenoid sinus fluid could help distinguish fresh and saltwater drowning.

It is estimated from both animal and clinical research studies that in approximately 10-15 percent of drownings there is no inhalation of water.[2,8,17,32–34] Some speculate that the presumed reason for this so called *dry-drowning* is laryngospasm which precludes aspiration of water. Spastic closure of the airway is not detectable at autopsy because of relaxation of the tissues in the early postmortem period. In these cases the victim's lungs are not voluminous and do not demonstrate the characteristic frothy pulmonary edema that is seen in most drowning victims. In 1999, Modell et al. questioned the diagnosis of drowning without aspiration (dry-drowning) and proposed that the cause of death in many of these individuals may be related to sudden cardiac death that occurs while in the water. The authors warned that a diagnosis of drowning at autopsy without the characteristic pulmonary edema associated with water aspiration is risky and may

not be appropriate.[35] The possibility of sudden cardiac death from conditions not associated with an anatomic lesion must be considered in these cases.[36]

Drowning Tests

Experiments on drowning victims date back to the early 1900s. These early studies attempted to determine the sequence of events that occur in drowning victims as well as the pathophysiology associated with fresh and saltwater drowning. Many studies also attempted to discover a so-called *drowning test* that could routinely and reliably diagnose drowning.

In the early and mid 1900s it was believed that postmortem serum or ocular fluid electrolyte values could be helpful to diagnose drowning and assist in differentiating drowning in fresh and saltwater. Based on these beliefs, most studies concentrated on using serum or ocular fluid electrolytes to associate a particular abnormality with drowning.

In 1921, Gettler proposed that serum chloride concentration from the right and left sides of the heart was useful in the diagnosis of drowning.[36] In 1944, Moritz pointed out that differences in the chloride concentration could be secondary to the postmortem interval alone.[37] In 1953, Durlacher et al. suggested that measuring plasma specific gravity from the right and left sides of the heart was a more specific test associated with drowning.[38] These studies have subsequently been shown to be unreliable and of no significant diagnostic value.

In 1974, Adjutantis postulated that the rate of diffusion of magnesium ions into ocular fluid from saltwater is proportional to the time elapsed since death. It was thus demonstrated that the ocular fluid magnesium concentration could be used to determine the length of time a body was submerged in saltwater.[39] Unfortunately, it has been shown that due to various postmortem changes, the relationship of magnesium levels to submersion time is subject to great variation and is therefore unreliable.[40] In a more recent electrolyte study by Farmer et al. it was concluded that confirmation or exclusion of drowning is not possible on the basis of postmortem vitreous fluid electrolytes because of post-immersion diffusion across the permeable membrane of the eyeball.[41]

The end result of all the electrolyte studies is that at the present time a *drowning test* does not exist. Determination of serum or vitreous electrolytes in drowning victims is generally not warranted, because results are variable and cannot be interpreted with any degree of accuracy.

Pathophysiology Associated with Fresh and Saltwater Drowning

A review of the sequence of events described in both animals and witnessed human drownings is best described as follows: As the body is submerged, breath holding occurs and lasts until carbon dioxide in the blood and tissues accumulates sufficiently to stimulate the respiratory centers in the brain. Exhalation of the remaining air in the lungs occurs immediately followed by uncontrolled inhalation of water.[42]

Of course, breath holding is bypassed in an unconscious victim. In such a case the drowning process begins at the instant of submersion.

The behavior of animals and humans during the drowning process is somewhat variable, however, in general the events associated with drowning can be divided into several stages. It typically begins with a struggle to stay above water. As the victim's head becomes submerged the actual drowning process begins. Breath holding occurs and typically lasts between one and two minutes until the accumulation of carbon dioxide stimulates involuntary respiratory effort. Inhalation of large volumes of water results as the respiratory center in the brain stimulates involuntary breathing. Swallowing of water, coughing and vomiting is followed by convulsions and spasmodic inspiratory effort. Progressive loss of consciousness over a period of two to three minutes, is followed by cardiopulmonary arrest and subsequent death. In most situations, death results within five minutes following submersion.

Death by drowning is a complex event which includes a spectrum of pathophysiologic phenomena that are still the subject of debate. Animal studies dating back to 1931 support that there are clear physiologic and biochemical differences between fresh and saltwater drowning.[43,44] Most of the early drowning studies were conducted on animals and demonstrated that drowning in fresh or brackish (0.5% NaCl) water caused hemodilution due to increased intravascular volume. The osmotic gradient between the inhaled hypotonic fresh water and the hypertonic plasma allowed large amounts of water to cross from the alveoli into the vasculature. Ultimately profound electrolyte abnormalities, including hyponatremia and hypokalemia were believed to induce fatal cardiac dysrhythmias, most commonly ventricular fibrillation.[28,32,42] In saltwater (3-5% NaCl) environments, the hypertonicity of the water was found to result in an osmotic gradient that caused hemoconcentration as water shifted from the intravascular space into the alveoli. This resulted in massive aspiration-induced pulmonary edema, physiologic shunting with subsequent hypoxemia.[2,3,8,33]

The mechanism of death in saltwater drowning has remained relatively unchallenged, however, the pathophysiology associated with freshwater drowning is less well-established. It is still believed that freshwater drowning results in some degree of hemodilution, however, recent studies primarily done on near-drowning victims have shown that although mild hyponatremia, hypokalemia and decreased chloride levels occur, the levels are typically insufficient to cause fatal arrhythmia.[45] Also, the quantity of water inhaled is less than previously suggested and most current investigators are of the opinion that the amount of water inhaled is not enough to overload a healthy heart.[2,3,8,17,35]

Although significant electrolyte abnormalities are seen in animal models of freshwater drowning, the levels are not as prominent in clinical practice. The degree of electrolyte changes has been shown to be related to the amount of water aspirated during the drowning process.[2] Modell and Moya observed that in dogs significant hyponatremia and ventricular fibrillation were typically seen after aspiration of 20 cc of water/pound of body weight, whereas using the same dog model, it was found that aspiration of

10 cc of water/pound of body weight had little effect on sodium concentration.[46]

Modell and Davis demonstrated that approximately 85% of human drowning victims aspirate 10 cc of fluid or less per pound of body weight.[45] In a study on near-drowning victims, it was found that even a small amount of fluid (1 to 3 cc of water/kg body weight) can lead to severe abnormalities in gas exchange resulting in hypoxia.[2] Based on these data it was concluded that most freshwater drowning victims do not have severe electrolyte abnormalities and that ventricular fibrillation is not the terminal event in the majority of these cases. Ultimately, although current studies acknowledge the pathophysiologic differences between fresh and saltwater drowning, it is now the belief of most experts that the mechanism of death associated with fresh and saltwater submersion is similar, with irreversible cerebral hypoxia being the common endpoint.

Although the mechanism of death in fresh and saltwater drowning is similar, the pathophysiology associated with drowning in freshwater is more complicated than originally believed. In addition to hemodilution, pulmonary surfactant within the alveoli is diluted and damaged. This results in atelectasis secondary to increased surface tension within the alveoli which causes the alveoli to collapse.[2,33] The end result is ventilation-perfusion mismatch and hypoxemia. Also, clinically with people who survive the initial drowning in freshwater, i.e., in cases of near-drowning, blood-stained urine is occasionally found on the second or third day following the drowning episode, probably the result of hemolysis.

Another factor to consider is that neurogenic pulmonary edema can occur with any insult to the brain including hypoxia. This can further complicate pulmonary edema that already exists from water aspiration. Although in most cases pulmonary edema is probably caused by both mechanisms, in freshwater drowning and when minimal water is inhaled, neurogenic pulmonary edema may be the primary factor.[47]

Previously it was believed that submersion in fresh water carried a higher mortality, however, a recent study by Conn, et al. showed no significant difference in survival between fresh and salt-water submersion.[48] Also, there is no significant difference in the time necessary for death to occur following submersion in fresh or saltwater.

In regards to near-drowning, the most severe complications that ultimately result in death are anoxic/ischemic brain injury, aspiration pneumonia, adult respiratory distress syndrome (ARDS) and less commonly disseminated intravascular coagulation (DIC) and renal failure.

Injury and Death in Cold Water

In 1912, the Titanic sank in the frigid waters of the North Atlantic and 1,503 fatalities resulted. Seven-hundred and four people in life rafts survived, but all those afloat with the help of life jackets were dead upon arrival of rescue boats that reached the scene after one hour and 50 minutes. It is clear that these fatalities were not the result of drowning. The cause of death was hypothermia related to cold water immersion.

The normal internal body temperature is 98.6° F (37° C) which is generally referred to as the core temperature. Body temperature is greater toward the center of the body and lower at the periphery. Skin temperature fluctuates much more than core temperature and typically ranges between 87.5° F (31° C) and 91.4° F (33° C). On average, humans maintain a skin temperature of 91.4° F (33° C). A core temperature can be obtained using a thermometer inserted deep into the rectum or, in a dead body, a liver temperature may be taken by making a small incision into the abdomen and inserting the thermometer into the liver tissue.

A body in cold water loses heat more rapidly than a body in air. This occurs through several mechanisms including via respirations, through the skin via conduction and convection and by urination and sweating.[49] Comparison of rectal temperatures while naked subjects were in 40° F (4° C) air temperature versus 40° F (4° C) water temperature demonstrated that in one hour the subjects in air showed no decrease in rectal temperature, whereas the subjects in the water demonstrated an 11° F (6° C) decrease in rectal temperature.[50] A dead body in water will lose heat more rapidly than a dead body on land. The rate at which the temperature decreases, is primarily dependent on the temperature of the water. Because of the high thermal conductivity of water, 20–25 times greater than air, the body heat is lost approximately three times faster in water than in air at the same temperature.[50]

When the human body is immersed in cold water a predictable sequence of events occurs. During the initial period of immersion, pain ensues followed by intense shivering. Subjects immersed in 43° F (6° C) water experience severe pain over the entire body due to intense vasoconstriction of the peripheral blood vessels. The pain is transient and disappears as the skin temperature begins to approximate the water temperature.[51] The temperature of the deeper tissues falls in a linear fashion, but always lags behind skin temperature. Initial physiologic responses to cold water immersion include increased respiratory rate, heart rate and blood pressure. As the body continues to cool, confusion and disorientation occur as the core temperature approaches 93° F (33.9° C) and semiconsciousness is typically seen around 86 to 90° F (30 to 32° C).[52] Studies conducted during World War II showed that death usually occurs when the core body temperature reaches 86° F (30° C).[52,53]

Expected Human Responses to Immersion in Cold Water

Mild hypothermia [core temperature between 91.4–95° F (33–35° C)]
- Shivering
- Decreased muscle strength
- Increased heart rate, respiratory rate and blood pressure
- Respiratory rate may increase to the point of hyperventilation
- Variable central nervous system impairment which typically includes loss of initiative, reduced coordination and disorientation

Moderate hypothermia [core temperature between 86–91.4° F (30–33° C)]
- Respiratory rate decreases
- Heart rate slows
- Blood pressure decreases with subsequent vasoconstriction to help prevent cardiac collapse

- Oxygen demand and consumption by the tissues is reduced
- Decreased consciousness which rapidly progresses to unconsciousness

Severe hypothermia [core temperature below 86° F (30° C)]
- Cardiac arrest with the onset of ventricular fibrillation which progresses to asystole
- Clinically the patient appears dead

According to the United States Coast Guard, survival in freezing water is unlikely for longer than 30 minutes for an individual of average body build. In 43° F (6° C) water, incapacitation is likely to occur within 30 minutes and death in less than one hour, and immersion in 59° F (15° C) water results in profound hypothermia in less than six hours.[52,54] In general, survival in cold water is dependent on the temperature of the water and duration of exposure.

Although rare, sudden death may result upon immediate immersion in very cold water and is believed to be secondary to the initial cold shock. It is well-documented and understood that immersion in freezing water causes rapid increase in heart rate and blood pressure and a dramatic increase in serum catecholamines which can precipitate ventricular fibrillation. In some cases, victims of cold water immersion experience powerful uncontrolled gasping that can lead to aspiration of a large amount of water. In addition, breath holding in cold water is decreased, causing the process of drowning to occur more rapidly.[55]

In 1999, Tipton et al. found that drowning is much more likely in cold water even in victims who do not have generalized hypothermia. The study demonstrated that local muscle cooling decreases muscle strength and impairs swimming performance before the onset of generalized hypothermia. If immersed in choppy water, even a life-jacketed victim may drown if he/she is unable to avoid aspiration of water secondary to wave splash. The data generated from this study may explain why some people drown before the onset of significant hypothermia, while wearing a life jacket.[56]

It should be recognized that there are several factors associated with increased risk of death secondary to cold water immersion other than

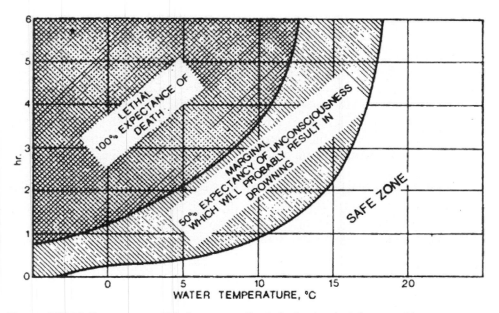

FIGURE XV-23. Expectation of life for a normally clothed individual during cold water immersion is dependent on the temperature of the water and the time immersed (from Barnett, 1962).[49]

the water temperature and the length of exposure (Fig. XV-23).[51,57] A study by Keatinge demonstrated that activity in cold water, such as swimming, significantly increases the rate at which the body cools. Subjects in 41°F (5°C) water cooled at a 47% greater rate with sustained activity when compared to those who remained still. Although activity increases heat loss in cold water, at water temperatures above 75°F (24°C), exercise will maintain and often raise body temperature. In this situation activity is preferred to remaining still.[58] Large body size extends survival time in cold water while smaller body size is associated with decreased survival time.

Another factor to consider is the amount of body fat. Studies have demonstrated that fat serves as thermal insulation that will slow the rate at which core temperature declines and allow for prolonged survival in cold water. For this reason, children and the elderly are at increased risk for hypothermia. Clothing helps to maintain body temperature and may lengthen survival time, however, bulky, heavy clothing can increase the likelihood of drowning.

A recent study by Franks et al. looked at the effects of moderate alcohol consumption and the risk of drowning. It was found that after three minutes in 59°F (15°C) water, following moderate alcohol intake, the respiratory rate was slightly reduced whereas the tidal volume, heart rate, rectal temperature and skin temperature were not significantly different from the control population. Conclusions drawn from this controlled study were that moderate alcohol consumption does not significantly change the risk of drowning upon immersion in cold water.[59] Despite the conclusions of this study, alcohol is known to affect the body in several ways that can increase the risk of hypothermia and death. Acute alcohol intoxication is associated with decreased mental alertness, poor judgment and irresponsible actions, all of which increase the risk of exposure. The chronic alcoholic may have altered metabolic processes due to liver damage and poor thermoregulation from injury to the hypothalamus. Several other drugs including barbiturates, lithium and certain antihypertensive medications are associated with hypothermia and may increase the likelihood of death upon immersion in cold water. Although all of these conditions should be considered in estimating survival time, the most important factor is that there is great physiologic and psychological variability between individuals immersed in cold water.

Over the past two decades there have been several reports of successful resuscitation following prolonged periods in the cold or following cold water submersion. The victims in many of these cases suffered no significant neurologic injury. It is important to understand that although a hypothermic victim may be asystolic upon removal from cold water, death should not be pronounced until such patient is thoroughly warmed and still is unable to be resuscitated. It is not uncommon for resuscitative efforts to cause a non-beating heart to revert to ventricular fibrillation and occasionally back to a normal rhythm. Recovery following prolonged submersion in cold water is occasionally seen in children, but is extremely rare in adults. Children are believed to have a greater likelihood of survival in the cold because they cool more rapidly owing to less adipose tissue and a greater surface area to body mass ratio. This apparent discrepancy is answered by the fact that if the body cools rapidly, the metabolic rate and oxygen demand of the brain and heart are reduced, which may serve to protect these organs from the lack of oxygen and possibly enable resuscitation without significant neurologic injury.

Although probably less important, another factor that may help explain how someone may survive prolonged submersion in cold water is the dive reflex. This reflex is associated with three simultaneous physiologic responses including, decreased heart rate, peripheral vasoconstriction and increased blood pressure. The dive reflex serves to protect the vital organs from anoxia by shunting blood from the periphery to the lungs, heart and brain. The reflex has been shown to be more prominent in infants and children which may help explain why the rare cases of survival after prolonged cold water submersion are much more common in the young.

In the winter of 2001, a one-year-old Canadian child wearing only a shirt and diaper wandered out of her home into freezing cold temperatures recorded to be 1° F (−17° C) with a wind chill factor of −20° F (−28° C). She was found after several hours lying face down in the snow and was noted to be cold, stiff and lifeless when she was found by her mother. Upon arrival of paramedics her core temperature was noted to be 63° F (17° C). She was warmed and aggressively resuscitated and after five hours her temperature had returned to 98.6° F. After 24 hours the child was awake and responding appropriately and six months after the incident she appears to have made a full recovery.

In 1993, a six-year-old boy weighing 22 kg fell into a river near Innsbruck, Austria. The water temperature was 36.5° F (2.5° C). The child was in the water for 65 minutes and when rescued was in asystole and had a rectal temperature of 62° F (16.4° C). He was rewarmed using cardiopulmonary bypass and when the rectal temperature reached 91° F (32.9° C), sinus rhythm returned. The boy recovered over several months and after five months his neurologic function had improved to the point where he returned to kindergarten.[60]

Injury and Death Associated with SCUBA Diving

Self-contained underwater breathing apparatus (SCUBA) diving dates back to the mid-1900s and began following development of the equipment which allowed prolonged underwater survival. The equipment associated with SCUBA diving includes the typical gear needed for snorkeling (mask, fins and snorkel) in addition to a regulator, buoyancy compensator device (BCD), air tank, pressure and depth gauges and a weight belt.

SCUBA divers in the United States are advised to complete an approved SCUBA diving course, which is primarily under the direction of the Professional Association of Diving Instructors (PADI) or the National Association of Underwater Instructors (NAUI). Currently there are over three million certified divers in the United States.[61] Although proof of a diving certificate is usually needed to rent equipment or have air tanks filled, it is still easy for a non-certified diver to obtain the necessary gear to dive. DAN (Divers Alert Network) is a non-profit organization that provides safety and health-related support services to divers around the world. DAN conducts numerous dive-related research projects and may be an important resource in the investigation of a SCUBA related death. Each year DAN publishes an annual report detailing diving injuries and fatalities.[62]

In 1999, there were 109 recreational diving fatalities in the United States, 78 of which are detailed in the 2001 DAN publication. In the last 10 years, the number of SCUBA-related fatalities in the United States was around 100 deaths per year.[62]

The majority of diving-related deaths are the result of a significant error in judgment by the diver or violation of generally accepted safe diving guidelines. In some situations the fatal decision or poor judgment is attributed to the effects of alcohol or drugs. This being said, no investigation involving a SCUBA-related death is complete without a thorough investigation on the part of the police and the medical examiner. All SCUBA death investigations should include information detailing the victim's medical, social and psychiatric history, dive experience including a profile of the last dive, description of the terminal event and resuscitative efforts, examination of the SCUBA equipment, water conditions and a complete autopsy with toxicology. The SCUBA equipment must be examined by an impartial certified diving expert who is prepared to generate a report detailing the findings.

Investigation of the SCUBA equipment should begin with photographs of the victim with the gear still in place and an inventory and description of all equipment used by the diver. The final tank pressure should be recorded and the tank should be inspected for corrosion of the internal lining. The gas within the tank should be sampled and tested for toxic substances particularly carbon monoxide. The regulator and buoyancy compensator should be checked for leaks or other defects. Today many divers use sophisticated dive computers to record vital information regarding their dives. The computer should be tested to assure proper function. In most situations, valuable information including number of dives, maximum depth of each dive, dive duration and decompression time can be obtained from the computer. If the weight belt is recovered the amount of weight should be recorded. It is all too common that divers drown because of insufficient air. This may occur under a variety of situations ranging from a faulty pressure gauge, poor judgment or situations such as cave diving or entanglement. Determination that the air tank is empty may be the most important piece of

documentation in a SCUBA-related fatality. Most police dive teams have expert divers that can be helpful in the evaluation of SCUBA equipment and dive computers. Local dive shops may also be useful in this regard.

A common mistake made by pathologists is to disregard natural disease found in persons who die while SCUBA diving. Cardiovascular disease in the form of hypertension and/or coronary artery atherosclerosis is the most common medical condition associated with a diving fatality. What role the heart disease played in a diver's demise is often difficult to determine unless the pathologist is aware of the circumstances surrounding the death.

The death that stems from a diving-related event may occur while in the water or after the diver exits the water. In situations where the person is believed to have died while in the water, drowning is often the terminal event. The autopsy findings in a drowning victim should now be understood, but as noted previously the real question in a drowning death is what caused the person to drown. The investigator dealing with a diving-related death should have a basic understanding of the physiology associated with diving.

SCUBA technology allows a diver to use compressed air to breathe while under water. Boyle's law holds that the relationship between pressure and volume is inverse, and thus as the pressure increases, the volume decreases and vice versa. Using this law a flexible container filled with air at sea level, where the pressure is one atmosphere, will have its volume halved at 33 feet; where the pressure is two atmospheres, reduced to one-third; at three atmospheres (66 feet); and decreased to one-quarter the original volume at four atmospheres (99 feet). It should be clear that the largest volume changes occur in shallow water. Applying this law to diving means that air inhaled in deep water will expand to a larger volume as the diver ascends. The regulator is designed to deliver compressed air to divers as they inhale so that the pressure is equal to the surrounding or ambient pressure. Continuous breathing of the compressed air allows for automatic pressure equalization in the lungs. However, if a diver inhales compressed air and then ascends without exhaling the lungs will become overexpanded. As the lungs expand, air may escape through ruptured alveoli, into the pulmonary vasculature, putting the diver at risk of extra-alveolar air syndrome. The major SCUBA-related injuries are the result of either extra-alveolar air syndrome or decompression sickness. These conditions both result from the obstructive effect of gas bubbles in blood vessels. When bubbles form by dissolution from a supersaturated state, the clinical condition that results is known as decompression sickness. When gas escapes from the lung and enters the systemic circulation, arterial gas embolism results.

Extra-alveolar air syndrome is a general term used to describe a situation in which air escapes from the alveoli to enter the pleural space, the pulmonary veins, the connective tissue of the pulmonary hili, mediastinum or more distant tissues. One or more of the following conditions may result: (1) pneumothorax, (2) systemic arterial gas embolism (air embolism), (3) pulmonary interstitial emphysema (acute pulmonary emphysema), (4) mediastinal and subcutaneous emphysema. Arterial gas embolism occurs when air bubbles enter the pulmonary veins, left atrium or left ventricle and are pumped to the tissues, brain, heart, or other organs. Small volumes of gas can occlude small blood vessels and cause acute infarction in the affected organs, with the most serious sequelae resulting from embolism of the vertebral or coronary arteries.

Knowledge that the death occurred while diving is enough to prompt suspicion of possible air embolism. Before beginning the autopsy, one should take postmortem x-rays of the head, neck, chest and abdomen, which are occasionally helpful in documenting extra-alveolar air in the pleural cavities, heart chambers, or large blood vessels.[63,64] Autopsy findings associated with this condition may include air within the cardiac chambers or air bubbles in the cerebral or coronary blood vessels. Unfortunately, air in the cerebral or coronary vessels is difficult to interpret, due to the fact that it can represent a postmortem artifact. Because arterial gas emboli usually occur while a diver is ascending and upright, the emboli commonly travel to the brain. The arter-

ies of the circle of Willis should be inspected for gas bubbles prior to removing the brain or cutting the large vessels in the neck. Unfortunately, even using this approach, finding gas bubbles in the cerebral arteries is not necessarily indicative of a cerebral air embolism due to the high likelihood of air contamination in these vessels. Some authors have advocated tying the large blood vessels in the neck prior to opening the skull, however, this technique has not been shown to significantly reduce air contamination in the cerebral arteries. Once the brain is removed, evaluation of the cerebral vessels is nearly useless, because removal of the brain invariably causes some degree of artifactual air ingress.

The arteries over the surface of the heart should be inspected in-situ for gas bubbles and photographed before cutting the innominate or subclavian veins. The presence of few small gas bubbles in the coronary circulation is not necessarily significant since artifactual air contamination may occur upon entering the chest cavity. For this reason, the diagnosis of an arterial gas embolism should not be solely based on this finding. Occasionally, in true cases of arterial gas embolism, the left atrium or left ventricle may contain large amounts of air and in this situation embolized air bubbles may also be seen throughout the coronary circulation. To minimize contamination, gas bubbles within the coronary arteries are best visualized by cutting a window in the chest plate over the heart and inspecting the coronary arteries before the heart is removed. Documentation of air within the cardiac chambers is best accomplished by opening the heart chambers under water and looking for the release of air bubbles. The technique to demonstrate air emboli is described in Chapter XXV.

True air emboli may be difficult to demonstrate and interpret following cardiopulmonary resuscitation and are impossible to distinguish from the gas bubbles formed with decomposition. A witnessed collapse following diving is with rare exception followed by resuscitative efforts and if the death is unwitnessed the body is often not found until decomposition has begun. In some cases of cerebral air embolism, petechial hemorrhages may be seen in the white matter of the brain.

Fortunately, even without autopsy confirmation of cerebral or coronary artery air emboli, the diagnosis of an air embolism can still be reliably made based on characteristic circumstantial evidence. In general, circumstances that support a diagnosis of air embolism include the rapid onset of unconsciousness which typically occurs within 10 minutes following a rapid, uncontrolled ascent to the surface. The symptoms may develop as the diver ascends or shortly after reaching the surface. Although rare, arterial gas emboli have been reported in SCUBA divers following breath holding and ascent in as little as three or four feet of water.[61]

Rupture of alveoli may cause a pneumothorax which occurs as air escapes from the damaged lung tissue and enters the pleural cavity. A small pneumothorax may not cause symptoms, but a large or tension pneumothorax may cause rapid death if not treated immediately. A pneumothorax may be easier than an air embolism to document *(see Chapter XXV)* and because these two entities often coexist, the presence of a pneumothorax in a SCUBA-related death should raise suspicion of air embolism. Pneumopericardium, mediastinal emphysema and subcutaneous emphysema are other related conditions that occur if extra-alveolar air dissects into the pericardial sac, mediastinum, or into the soft tissues under the skin. Subcutaneous emphysema is often palpable over the chest and neck and gives the skin a crackling texture. Subcutaneous emphysema can dissect downward to involve the abdominal wall and cause distension of the scrotum. Pulmonary interstitial emphysema (acute pulmonary emphysema) may also occur as alveoli rupture. The lungs should always be inspected *in situ* for evidence of bullae on the pleural surfaces, air bubbles between the pulmonary fissures and focal parenchymal hemorrhages.

Several autopsy findings that can provide evidence of barotrauma in SCUBA-diving deaths. These include examination of the middle ears for rupture of one or both tympanic membranes and inspection of the face, conjunctivae and sclerae for petechiae, which suggests barotrauma, a condition divers call *mask squeeze.* Although not life-threatening, these conditions provide evidence of barotrauma and may help shed light on the mechanism of death when a pneumothorax or air embolism cannot be documented.

Decompression sickness or caisson disease, commonly called the bends, is a condition typically associated with long and/or deep dives. SCUBA divers typically use compressed air, which is composed primarily of oxygen (21%) and nitrogen (79%). In some situations divers may use air mixed with helium or pure oxygen. Both nitrogen and helium are physiologically inert gases, not used by the body, that progressively dissolve when breathed at high partial pressures making it possible for the gases to enter various tissues of the body. Henry's law states that the amount of gas that is dissolved in a liquid at a given temperature is directly proportional to the partial pressure of that gas. This law serves the basis for decompression sickness.[65] With increased depth, the partial pressure of both nitrogen and oxygen increase. The amount of gas that the body tissues absorb is largely dependent on the length of time the body is submerged in deep water. The longer a diver is underwater, the more nitrogen is absorbed by the blood and other tissues. With ascent, the pressure surrounding the body decreases and the excess nitrogen can no longer stay dissolved. This phenomenon is similar to opening a bottle of soda. As the bottle is opened the pressure is decreased and the dissolved gas comes out of solution making the soda effervesce *(fizz).* If a diver is in deep water for an extended period of time, the ascent must be interrupted with timed stops at specific depths to effect a controlled decompression. This procedure permits gas to escape safely from the alveoli rather than into the tissues. The time necessary to decompress during such a controlled ascent is determined from published dive tables. Most dive computers will record the maximum depth and the length of each dive, and will calculate the required decompression time. If one's body cannot eliminate the nitrogen through the alveoli as fast as it comes out of solution, the excess nitrogen will form bubbles in the tissues. The essential feature of decompression sickness is the supersaturation of tissue with dissolved gas and subsequent formation of gas bubbles as the pressure decreases during ascent. As the gas comes out of solution organ dysfunction results from blockage of arteries, veins and lymphatics or by compression of the tissue. In addition to marked individual variability, the amount of gas that diffuses into the tissues is based on many additional factors such as solubility of the specific gas, pressure gradient, perfusion of the tissue, time of exposure, and cell membrane thickness. Fatigue, dehydration, hypothermia and alcohol consumption may all contribute to the development of decompression sickness. The physiology associated with absorption of gas by various tissues was studied by J.S. Haldane, an English physiologist in 1908 and his theory remains the basis for dive tables still in use today.[66]

A caisson is a watertight chamber used in the construction of bridges, tunnels, or other such structures that require an underwater foundation. Caissons allow for construction crews to work at great depths in a watertight environment while underwater. Caissons are open at the bottom where crews dig, allowing the caisson to sink deeper into the ground. When the digging is complete, the caisson is usually filled with concrete and used as part of the finished structure. Prior to entering a caisson, workers must first enter an airtight chamber called an air lock. The air pressure in the air lock is gradually increased until it equals the pressure of the caisson. As workers leave the caisson, they must pass through the air lock where the pressure is gradually reduced. If workers go through a change of pressure too quickly, they may develop what has become known as decompression sickness or caisson disease.[67]

Customarily, decompression sickness is classified as Type I or Type II.[65,66] Most cases fall into Type I, which is less dangerous. The symptoms associated with Type I decompression sickness include fatigue, mild joint pain, skin rash, muscle pain and swelling. Type II disease includes any of the symptoms seen in Type I in addition to neurologic symptoms. Type II neurologic symptoms include muscle weakness which may progress to paresthesias with tingling or numbness, paraly-

sis, hearing or vision impairment, gastrointestinal or bladder dysfunction, memory loss and in severe cases, death.[65,66] Death from decompression sickness is rare, but may occur secondary to respiratory failure as a consequence of brain stem or spinal cord infarction. In most cases early treatment is associated with partial or complete resolution of symptoms while delay in treatment makes therapy much less effective. Neurologic injury may present early in the course of disease, whereas damage to bone in the form of dysbaric osteonecrosis may present years later.[65] In divers with a patent foramen ovale, air bubbles in the venous system may enter the arterial circulation and embolize to the heart or brain. Regardless of the duration of the dive, decompression sickness does not occur with shallow dives of less than 33 feet. Most cases of decompression sickness are associated with long dives in water over 80 feet deep.[61] Symptoms associated with decompression sickness usually evolve after several hours, but may occur as early as 5 minutes or up to 24–36 hours after ascent.[66] Early symptoms of decompression sickness include muscle cramps and joint pain which over the next few hours may progress to neurologic symptoms and occasionally death. Repeated dives over a short period of time are a significant risk factor for decompression sickness, because with each dive residual nitrogen remains in the body. This makes symptoms of decompression sickness more likely with each subsequent dive.[65] In some situations, a SCUBA diver may have risk factors for both decompression sickness and arterial gas emboli. In these cases, the victim's symptoms and the rapidity with which the symptoms appeared are important clues to the distinction between the two entities. In general, divers with cerebral artery gas embolism present with rapid onset of neurologic symptoms including paralysis, unconsciousness or sudden death, whereas in victims of decompression sickness there is typically a delay of several hours before neurologic symptoms develop.

When detectable, autopsy findings of decompression sickness consist of foci of ischemic necrosis, which in fatal cases often involve the brain or spinal cord. These findings may not be grossly or microscopically detectable unless the victim dies after some delay. The lungs are edematous and may be focally hemorrhagic with areas of atelectasis and emphysema. Gas bubbles in superficial meningeal veins or venous sinuses are not specific for decompression sickness since air usually enters leptomeningeal vessels when the skull is opened.

Another factor to consider is that nitrogen at high partial pressure has an intoxicating effect similar to alcohol. Although individuals have varying levels of susceptibility, the effect of breathing compressed air containing nitrogen may become apparent as a diver descends below 100 feet. At extreme depths, usually below 200 feet, the effect of *nitrogen narcosis* may initially result in a feeling of euphoria which rapidly progresses to disorientation, hallucinations, unconsciousness and death. Resolution of symptoms occurs rapidly if the diver ascends. Alcohol, fatigue and hypothermia may exacerbate this condition.[65] Nitrogen has a high affinity for lipids and is five times more soluble in fat than blood. At high pressure, nitrogen seeps into the nonaqueous structures of the brain and alters communication between cells. The use of compressed gas free of nitrogen prevent nitrogen narcosis. A gas mixture called nitrox has lower levels of nitrogen and higher levels of oxygen than air. Nitrox is typically used by experienced divers to reduce decompression time during decompression stops.

Helium is not associated with narcosis and, for this reason, a gas called heliox, which is a mixture of helium and oxygen, is often used for deep dives. Unfortunately, helium is expensive, difficult to store and does not decrease the risk of decompression sickness.

Oxygen toxicity occurs at high partial pressures associated with deep dives, usually below 200 feet. Breathing compressed air at this depth can cause seizures. Using nitrox with a high oxygen concentration in deep water may cause oxygen toxicity at less depth than is normally associated with this condition. In contrast to deaths from nitrogen narcosis, which occurs mostly among sport divers who exceed recreational limits, the extreme depths associated with oxygen toxicity make this condition rare in the recreational SCUBA diver.

Carbon monoxide toxicity is a rare complication of SCUBA diving caused by contamination of air tanks. Carbon monoxide contamination may occur when SCUBA tanks are filled by faulty oil-contaminated air compressors. Even a small amount of carbon monoxide contamination may be detrimental because the effect of the gas proportionately increases as the pressure on the body rises. Traces of contaminants that would be harmless at the surface can be toxic under water. Symptoms of carbon monoxide intoxication include dizziness, nausea, headaches, and sudden onset of drowsiness followed by unconsciousness and death. Although rare, the possibility of carbon monoxide intoxication does exist, and when suspected, the air tanks should be tested for contamination. At autopsy, cherry-pink discoloration of the skin or body cavities should raise suspicion of carbon monoxide toxicity and prompt a test for carboxyhemoglobin.

The snorkeler or skin diver typically stays on or near the surface of the water and for practical purposes the risks associated with snorkeling are similar to those described with swimming. Over the years, several deaths have been seen in individuals who engaged in *breath-hold* diving. Some of these deaths are related to the previously described *shallow water blackout* and the others are the result of decompression sickness. Decompression sickness in this situation was originally described in the South Pacific pearl divers of the Tuamotu Archipelago, who would make repeated deep dives for up to six hours a day. Pulmonary barotrauma or arterial gas emboli do not occur unless compressed air is inhaled prior to ascent,[68] thus these conditions do not occur in snorkelers.

By far the overwhelming majority of SCUBA-related deaths are accidental. Only with the right amount of suspicion and a detailed investigation will the unusual diving suicides or homicides be uncovered.

Summary

A death investigation involving a body in water can be challenging and should always be approached with an open mind. The police and the medical examiner need to work in conjunction to assure a full and thorough investigation.

Although there are no diagnostic autopsy findings or laboratory tests, a complete autopsy can yield clues supportive of a drowning death. It is important that postmortem changes and artifacts of water submersion be recognized to avoid steering the investigation in the wrong direction. Ultimately, the diagnosis of drowning should be based on multiple factors, including the autopsy findings and a thorough investigation of the circumstances surrounding the death. In SCUBA-related fatalities, the death investigation should also include a complete evaluation of the diving equipment. Following this approach will not only serve to help make a confident diagnosis of drowning, but will help determine why the drowning occurred.*

REFERENCES

1. *Dorland's Illustrated Medical Dictionary,* 28th Edition. Philadelphia, PA: W.B. Saunders Co., 1994.
2. Sachdeva, R.C.: Near-drowning. *Crit Care Clin, 15* (2): 281–296, 1999.
3. Weinstein, M.D., and Krieger, B.P.: Near-drowning: Epidemiology, pathophysiology and initial treatment. *J Emerg Med, 14* (4): 461–467, 1996.
4. Fields, A.I.: Near drowning in the pediatric population. *Progress in Pediatric Critical Care, 8* (1): 113–129, 1992.
5. Davis, J.H.: Bodies in the water: An investigative approach. *Am J Forensic Med Path, 7* (4): 291–297, 1986.
6. Davis, J.H. The autopsy in diving fatalities. In *Hyperbaric and Undersea Medicine, 1* (35), Medical Seminars Inc., 1981.
7. Bross, M.H., and Clark, J.L. Near-drowning. *Am Fam Physician, 51* (6): 1545–1551, 1995.
8. Levin, D.L., Morriss, F.C., Toro, L.O., et al.: Drowning and near-drowning. *Pediatr Clin North Am, 40* (2): 321–335, 1993.
9. Thompson, D.C., and Rivara, F.P.: Pool fencing for preventing drowning in children. *Cochrane Database of Systemic Review,* Issue 1, 2001.
10. Davis, J.H.: Fatal underwater breath holding in trained swimmers. *J. Forensic Sci., 6:* 301–306, 1961.
11. Craig, A.B.: Underwater swimming and loss of consciousness. *JAMA, 176* (4): 255–258, 1961.
12. Ryan, C.A., and Dowling, G.: Drowning deaths in people with epilepsy. *Can Med Assoc J, 148* (5): 781–784, 1993.
13. Saxena, A, and Ang, L.C.: Epilepsy and bathtub drowning: Important neurologic observations. *Am J of Forensic Med Path, 14* (2): 125–129, 1993.
14. Wintemute, G.J.: Childhood drowning and near-drowning in the United States. *Am J Dis Child, 144:* 663–669, 1990.
15. Wintemute, G.J., Kraus, J.F., Teret, S.P., et al.: Drowning in childhood and adolescence: A population-based study. *Am J Public Health, 77:* 830–832, 1987.
16. Dietz, P.E., and Baker, S.P.: Drowning: Epidemiology and prevention. *Am J Public Health, 64:* 303–312, 1974.
17. Olshaker, J.S.: Near-drowning. *Emerg Med Clin North Am, 10* (2): 339–349, 1992.
18. Shatz, D.V., Kirton, O.C., McKenney, M.G., et al.: Personal watercraft crash injuries: An emerging problem. *J of Trauma, Infection and Critical Care, 44* (1): 198–201, 1998.
19. Bengston, K., Nichols, M.M., Schnadig, V., and Ellis, M.D.: Sudden death in a child following jellyfish envenomation by Chiropsalmus quadrumanus. *JAMA, 266* (10): 1404–1406, 1991.
20. Stein, M.R., Marraccine, J.V., Rothschild, N.E., and Burnett, J.W.: Fatal Portuguese man-o'-war (Physalia physalis) envenomation. *Ann Emerg Med, 18* (3): 312–315, 1989.
21. Harrison, L.J.: Dangerous marine life. *J of the Florida Medical Association, 79* (9): 633–641, 1992.
22. Haglund, W.D.: Disappearance of soft tissue and the disarticulation of human remains from aqueous environments. *J Forensic Sci, 38* (4): 806–815, 1993.
23. Giertsen, J.C., and Morild, I.: Seafaring bodies. *Am J Forensic Med Pathol, 10* (1): 25–27, 1989.
24. Teather, R.G.: *The underwater investigator.* Concept Systems Inc., Fort Collins, CO, 1983.
25. Copeland, A.R.: An assessment of lung weights in drowning cases: The Metro Dade County experience from 1978–1982. *Am J Forensic Med Pathol, 6 (4):* 301–304, 1985.
26. Mueller, W.F.: Pathology of temporal bone hemorrhage in drowning. *J Forensic Sci, 14:* 327–336, 1969.
27. Niles, N.R.: Hemorrhage in the middle ear and mastoid in drowning. *Am J Clin Path, 40:* 281–283, 1963.
28. Kamada, S., Seo, Y., and Takahama, K.: A sandwich enzyme immunoassay for pulmonary surfactant protein D and measurement of its blood levels in drowning victims. *Forensic Sci Int, 109:* 51–63, 2000.

* *Acknowledgments:* The author is grateful to Naoya Wada for his computer skills and photographic expertise and Dr. Joseph H. Davis for his advice, encouragement and photographic contribution.

29. Tamáska, L.: Über den Diatomeennachweis im Knochenmark der Wasserleichen. *Dtsch Z gerichtl Med. 51:* 398–403, 1961.

30. Spitz, W.U., and Schneider, V.: The significance of diatoms in the diagnosis of death by drowning. *J Forensic Sci, 9* (1): 11–18, 1964.

31. Pollanen, M.S.: The diagnostic value of the diatom test for drowning II. Validity: Analysis of diatoms in bone marrow and drowning medium. *J Forensic Sci, 42* (2): 286–290, 1997.

32. Spitz, W.U., and Blanke, R.V.: Mechanism of death in fresh-water drowning. *Archives of Pathology, 71:* 661–668, 1961.

33. Modell, J.H.: Drowning. *N Engl J Med, 328* (4): 253–256, 1993.

34. Giammona, S.T., and Modell, J.H.: Drowning by total immersion. *Amer J Dis Child, 114:* 612–616, 1967.

35. Modell, J.H., Bellefleur, M., and Davis, J.H.: Drowning without aspiration: Is this an appropriate diagnosis. *J Forensic Sci, 44* (6): 1119–1123, 1999.

36. Gettler, A.O.: A method for the determination of death by drowning. *JAMA, 77:* 1650, 1921.

37. Moritz, A.R.: Chemical methods for the determination of death by drowning. *Physiol Rev, 24:* 70–88, 1944.

38. Durlacher, S.H., Freimuth, H.C., and Swann, H.E.: Blood changes in man following death due to drowning. *Archives of Pathology, 56:* 454–461, 1953.

39. Adjutantis, G., and Coutselinis, A.: Changes in magnesium concentration of the vitreous humour of exenterated human eyeballs immersed in sea water. *J Forensic Sci, 4:* 63–65, 1974.

40. Sturner, W.Q., Balko, A., and Sullivan, J.: Magnesium and other electrolytes in bovine eyeballs immersed in sea water and other fluids. *J Forensic Sci, 8:* 139-150, 1976.

41. Farmer, J.G., Benomran, F., Watson, A.A., and Harland, W.A.: Magnesium, potassium, sodium and calcium in post-mortem vitreous humour from humans. *Forensic Sci Int, 27:* 1–13, 1995.

42. Spitz, W.U.: Drowning. *Hosp Med,* 8–18, July 1969.

43. Cot, C.: Les asphyxies accidentecelles (submersion, electrocution, intoxication oxycarbonique) etude clinigue, therapeutiques et preventive. *Edition Medicales N. Maloine,* Paris 1931.

44. Swann, H.G., Brucer, M., Moore, C., et al.: Fresh and seawater drowning: A study of the terminal cardiac and biomedical events. *Texas Rep Biol Med, 5:* 423–437, 1947.

45. Modell, J.H., and Davis, J.H.: Electrolyte changes in human drowning victims. *Anesthesiology, 30* (4): 414–420, April 1969.

46. Modell, J.H., and Moya, F.: Effects of volume of aspirated fluid during chlorinated fresh water drowning. *Anesthesiology, 27:* 662, 1969.

47. Rumbak, M.J.: The etiology of pulmonary edema in fresh water near-drowning. *Am J Emerg Med, 14:* 176–179, 1969.

48. Conn, A.W., Miyasaka, K., Katayama, M., et al.: A canine study of cold water drowning in fresh versus salt water. *Crit Care Med, 23* (12): 2029–2037, 1995.

49. Beckman, E.L.: Thermal protective suits for underwater swimmers. *Military Medicine, 132:* 195–209, 1967.

50. Molnar, G.W.: Survival of hypothermia by men immersed in the ocean. *JAMA, 131:* 1046–1050, 1946.

51. Behnke, A.R., and Yaglou, C.P.: Responses of human subjects to immersion in ice water and to slow and fast rewarming. *Naval Medical Research Institute.* Project X-189, No. 11, 1950.

52. Golden, F.S.C.: Accidental hypothermia. *J Royal Nav Med Service, 58:* 196–206, 1972.

53. Haywood, J.S., Eckerson, J.D., and Collis, M.L.: Thermal balance and survival time prediction of man in cold water. *Can J Physiol Pharmacol, 53:* 21–32, 1975.

54. United States Navy Diving Manual Rev 2, Washington, D.C., Naval Sea Systems Command Superintendent of Documents, GPO, 1989.

55. Laursen, G.A., Pozos, R.S., and Hempel, F.G.: *Human Performance in the Cold.* Undersea Medical Society, Bethesda, Maryland, 1982.

56. Tipton, M., Eglin, C., Gennser, M., and Golden, F.: Immersion deaths and deterioration in swimming performance in cold water. *Lancet, 354* (9179): 626–629, 1999.

57. Barnett, P.N.: Field tests of two antiexposure assemblies. Artic Aerospace Lab. AAL-TDR; 61-656, 1962.

58. Keatinge, W.R.: *Survival in cold water.* Oxford: Blackwell Scientific Publications, 1969.

59. Franks, C.M., Golden, F.S., Hampton, I.F., and Tipton, M.J.: The effect of blood alcohol on the initial responses to cold water immersion in humans. *European J of Applied Physiology and Occupational Physiology, 75* (3): 279–281, 1997.

60. Bolte, R.G., Black, P.G., Bowers, R.S., et al.: The use of extracorporeal rewarming in a child submerged for 66 minutes. *JAMA, 260:* 377–379, 1988.

61. Dovenbarger, J.: Recreational scuba injuries. *J of the Florida Medical Association, 79* (9): 616–624, 1992.

62. Divers Alert Network. Report on decompression illness, diving fatalities and project dive exploration. 2001 edition.

63. Williamson, J.A., King, G.K., Callanan, V.I., Lanskey, R.M., and Rich, K.W.. Fatal arterial gas embolism: Detection by chest radiography and imaging before autopsy. *Medical Journal of Australia, 153:* 97–100, 1990.

64. Roobottom, C.A., Hunter, J.D., and Bryson, P.J.: The diagnosis of fatal gas embolism: Detection by plain film radiology. *Clin Radiol, 49:* 805–807, 1994.

65. Melamed, Y., Shupak, A., and Bitterman, H.: Medical problems associated with underwater diving. *N Engl J Med, 326* (1): 30–34, 1992.

66. Loewenherz, J.W.: Pathophysiology and treatment of decompression sickness and gas embolism. *J of the Florida Medical Association, 79* (9): 620–629, 1992.

67. Saul, W.E.: "Caisson," World Book Online Americas Edition, http://aolsvc.worldbook.aol.com/wbol/wbPage/na/ar/co/087120, October 14, 2001.

68. Bayne, C.G.: Breath-hold diving. In *Hyperbaric and Undersea Medicine, 1*(4), Medical Seminars Inc., 1981.

Chapter XVI

ELECTRICAL AND LIGHTNING INJURIES

EDMUND R. DONOGHUE AND BARRY D. LIFSCHULTZ

ELECTRICAL INJURY

ELECTRICAL INJURY, also referred to as electrocution, abides by *rules of the extremes:* it may be trivial or fatal, readily observable or inconspicuous, even absent.

Electricity or electric power is produced by generators activated by coal, natural gas, oil, falling water, or nuclear energy. Burning of waste products, wind and solar power have also been used to manufacture electricity. A complex network of lines carries electric power across the country, into homes, businesses and for use in industry. Transformers within this system regulate the amount of power according to need. Thus, voltage is increased for transmission over long distances, since power is lost in the lines, or reduced for local distribution.

Long distance high-voltage lines convey 100 kV or more, across the United States (one kilovolt equals 1000 volts). This voltage is stepped down at substations and by transformers to less than 10,000 volts, usually about 7650 volts for cities and towns, followed by further step down to 120–240 volts for residential and office use and 480 volts for industrial use. High-voltage electrocutions in the United States usually involve 7620–7680 volts, since this is the usual voltage in transmission and distribution lines in populous areas. When electricity is sent from a distribution line to a residence or business final step down by a field transformer, often located on a utility pole or in a vault under a city street, will reduce the power to 120–240 volts.

Whereas, high voltage is defined as greater than 600 volts and sometimes greater than 1000 volts, measured from line to ground, low voltage is defined as no higher than 1000 volts and usually does not exceed 600 volts. To avoid confusion, let it be said that despite the apparent inconsistency in defining high and low voltage, currents between 600 and 1000 volts are extremely infrequent and present no practical applicability. Low voltage in the United States is virtually always alternating current (AC) regulated at 60 Hz, i.e., 60 oscillations per second.

Electrocutions involving direct current (DC), such as obtained from batteries, are practically never encountered.

An elderly individual who received an abrupt sharp pain in his right hand and arm while working on his car battery collapsed at the scene and was DOA at a nearby hospital. Autopsy showed a small electrical burn on the right index finger and advanced but not occlusive coronary artery disease. It could be argued that the electrical jolt caused vasospasm and ventricular fibrillation in a predisposed individual.

Household electricity in the United States is 120 volts AC and 220–240 volt circuits are used for household clothes dryers, ranges, hot tubs and some power tools.

Nevertheless, despite the common usage of electricity, electrocutions are relatively rare, causing about 1,000 fatalities in this country each year. Additionally, about another 150 lightning deaths occur annually. High-voltage electrocutions are usually associated with extensive burns and present little difficulty for forensic pathologists. Low-voltage alternating current electrocutions from household current may occur with little or no visible evidence of injury. Lightning bolts with enormous amounts of electricity usually cause minimal or no injuries at all due to their extremely short duration. Thus, death from household electrocution and lightning may cause serious diagnostic problems.

Three elements are required for an electrocution to occur: (a) a charged electrical source, (b) a current pathway through the victim, (c) a ground.

A ground has the same electrical potential as the earth or zero. Examples of good grounds include metal water pipes and faucets, metal electrical conduits, the metal parts of electrical outlets and fixtures, radiators, metal drains, and grounded appliances. For electrocution to occur, all three elements must come together simultaneously. A person, well-insulated from ground, may contact a charged conductor without experiencing any difficulty, just as birds can perch on non-insulated high tension lines with no adverse effect.

The current pathway for electrocution must pass through vital organs susceptible to disruption by the flow of electricity. When an electric current flows through the brain or spinal cord, death due to asphyxiation may occur as a result of interference with the central nervous system's control of respiration. However, asphyxiation may also result from direct paralysis of chest muscles. When current flows through the heart, fatal ventricular fibrillation and cardiac arrest may occur. Low-voltage alternating current (120v., 60 Hz) traveling through the chest for a split second is particularly likely to cause ventricular fibrillation. Fatal heart rhythm disturbances may result from alternating currents as low as 0.1 amperes. With increased availability of defibrillators more lives may be saved by rapid defibrillation.

According to Carr,[1] the generally accepted rules of thumb for limb contact electrical shocks are:
- 1–5   mA   level of perception
- 10   mA   pain is felt
- 100   mA   severe muscular contractions *
- 100–300 mA   fatal electrocution can occur

* Some electrical engineers suggest that this amount of current is high. Accordingly, muscle spasms causing inability to *let go* of an electrically charged device occurs with currents exceeding 5-7 mA in women and 7-9 mA for men, depending on body mass. According to Zitzewitz[2] damage caused by electric shock depends on current flowing through the body, where 1 mA can be felt, 5 mA is painful, above 15 mA muscle control is lost and 70 mA can be fatal.

Inmates in European prisons (220 volt) sometimes construct *immersion heaters* to heat water for

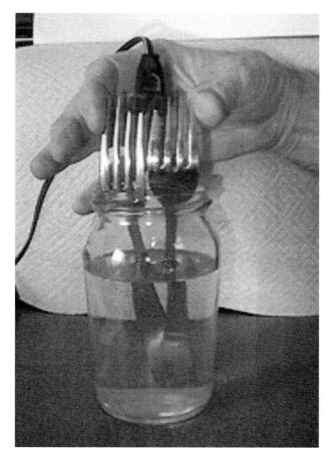

FIGURE XVI-1. Reconstruction of a *home-made immersion heater* responsible for accidental electrocution.

hot drinks. A glass jar is filled with water. Two forks are immersed in the container, prong-end up. An electric cord, such as comes with an electric razor or radio is connected to one prong on each fork (Fig. XVI-1). Touching the fork may cause fatal electrocution.[3]

With regards to electrocution as a means of capital punishment, it should be noted that eleven states still utilize the electric chair to execute prisoners. Most states use a voltage of 2000–2200 AC at 7–12 amperes.

Skin has a strong insulating effect against electrocution. Dry skin may provide resistance to electric current at values in excess of 100,000 Ohms.[4] Thus, to cause injury current must overcome the shielding effect provided by the external surface of the body in addition to that contributed by insulated clothes, shoes, gloves, etc. which are so important for those who work with electricity at their places of employment.

Blood offers less resistance to the flow of electricity than other tissues; thus, large amounts of current may flow through blood vessels. The heat produced by this current flow may break up red and white blood cells, activate platelets and damage the lining of blood vessels along the path of the current. As little as 5 mA may be painful and cause tetanic muscle contractions, freezing the victim to the source of electricity, increasing the duration of electrical contact. If the electrical event is survived, clotting may occur in blood vessels along the path of current flow. We have observed thrombosis of the right brachial artery of an electrician who had touched a live wire with his right hand several weeks earlier. In high-voltage electrocutions, skeletal fractures may occur due to forceful contraction of muscles.[5,6]

Circuit breakers or fuses are designed to protect against overloads and short circuits. They protect the equipment, not people. Thus, a circuit breaker will shut off the circuit when the current reaches dangerously high levels. Overloads occur when too many appliances are plugged into a single circuit. Short circuits occur when a bare hot wire touches a second bare wire or any metal that is grounded. Current then bypasses the normal circuit and flows directly to ground without doing work. In both overloads and short circuits, the intense heat that develops in the wires due to high current flow may cause a fire if left unchecked by a fuse or circuit breaker. Such overload protectors protect wiring only, in contrast to GFIs (ground fault interrupters) and GFCIs (see below) which are designed to protect against electrocution.

Fuse or circuit breaker panels are grounded, that is, a wire connects the service panel to a copper rod that is driven into the earth or is connected to a water supply pipe that leads to the ground. Grounded wiring systems are those in which all metal outlets and switch boxes, cable armor, and exposed metal parts of the wiring system are connected back to the grounding terminals in the service panel. Grounded household electrical systems are protected against fires and electrical shock by providing a low resistance pathway for aberrant current to flow to the earth. Since the pathway is of low resistance, current flows will be large and should trip fuses or circuit breakers, thereby shutting off the circuit.

Household wiring is color-coded. In 120-volt circuits, the *neutral* wire is white and the *hot* wire is usually black. The white neutral wires of the various circuits throughout the house are also connected to the grounded service panel. By using grounded outlets and grounded electrical cords, the benefit of grounding can be extended to tools and household appliances. To ground a tool or household appliance, a green wire is secured to its metal case and connected to the long round prong on a three-prong plug. If the insulation within the tool or appliance becomes defective and the metal casing becomes electrified, the current will pass harmlessly down the ground wire and should trip the fuse or circuit breakers.[7] In electrocution cases, involving a grounded tool or appliance, two defects must be present in the device; a defect in the insulation that allows the tool or appliance to become charged and a defect in the ground circuit.

Certain appliances should not be grounded. Metal-cased appliances with exposed heating elements, such as a toaster or an electric space heater, should not be grounded, because contact with the heating element and the grounded metal casing could cause electrocution.

If an electrical tool or appliance leaks current, the grounding wire will carry off most of the current. However, small leaks, insufficient to blow a fuse or trip a circuit breaker, may be sufficient to shock or electrocute under proper conditions. A ground fault circuit interrupter (GFCI, sometimes referred to as, GFI) monitors both the hot and neutral sides of a circuit. If the two sides differ by as little as .005 amperes, a magnetic switch in the GFCI disconnects the circuit in 1/40 of a second. Most building codes now require that ground-fault interrupters protect all 15 and 20-amp outdoor receptacles and all bathroom circuits. Many codes also include kitchen, basement and garage outlets. These devices are designed to prevent electrocution, but to do so must be properly installed and functioning correctly. We have seen electrocutions occur even in the presence of GFCIs.

Another method of safeguarding tools against the danger of electrocution is double insulation. In doubly insulated tools, all electrical conductors are insulated and the casing of the tool is non-conductive plastic. Such tools require neither a 3-prong plug nor a 3-wire extension cord.

Certain problems arise with grounding. A grounded electrical appliance is an ideal *ground* for electrocution when another charged conductor is contacted. Additionally, an improperly wired outlet, extension cord or plug, in which the ground wire becomes connected to the hot side of the circuit, will create a charged electrical casing that may become the *charged conductor* in an electrocution.

Electrocution should be suspected whenever an individual falls while near a charged source, especially if arching backwards at the time of the fall. Victims of electrocution may remain conscious and speak or move for several seconds, even unplug the offending appliance, after a fatal electrical shock.[8]

Two men were working on a 600-volt transformer at the top of a utility pole when one leaned forward and his chest touched a live wire. He was able to push himself back from the wire. When his co-worker asked him, "Are you all right?" He answered, "Yes, I think I will be all right, except I've got a burn." Thereupon he collapsed, and by the time he was carried to the ground and resuscitation commenced, it was too late.

In another instance, an individual was working behind a large electrical panel. Another man elsewhere in the room heard him curse and state, "I've electrocuted myself." He came walking out from behind the panel and reached the middle of the room, some ten or fifteen feet away, before he collapsed. Even though immediate resuscitative efforts were started, it was apparent that he had sustained ventricular fibrillation, and in the absence of a defibrillator, his heart rhythm could not be restored.

Low-voltage electrocution should be suspected whenever a potentially grounded person exposed to a potential electrical source collapses suddenly, especially if the person cries out or utters an expletive prior to collapsing.

The autopsy of a victim of electrocution usually yields no specific results. Pulmonary and cerebral edema as determined by increased weights of these organs may be caused by ventricular fibrillation or asphyxiation, whichever the mechanism of death may be. Wright[9] described visceral petechiae in individuals who had died of asphyxiation. All clothing worn by the victim must be retrieved and examined.

A multidisciplinary study at the Dade County, Florida Medical Examiner's Office over a period of 22 years suggests that the 50% higher rate of electrocution deaths in that county was the result of underreporting of electrocution deaths in the rest of the United States, presumably due in large part to inadequate scene investigation.[9]

Low-voltage electrocution cannot be determined without thorough examination and evaluation of the scene: What was the potential for an electrocution (wet concrete, wet carpet or grounded appliances)? Was there an operational overload or ground fault protector? Were outlets properly wired? The outlets should be checked for proper wiring utilizing an outlet checker. All portable electrical equipment, extension cords, outlet strips, adapters and connectors should be retrieved from the scene and submitted for examination. Best is to consult with a qualified electrical engineer and often the Fire Marshall will be of assistance.

Next, the equipment must be examined for defects. In a short circuit the current from the hot wire bypasses the normal circuit and flows directly to the ground. A ground system usually blocks shock dangers by carrying current, which has leaked out of the system to ground through a special system of wires. However, if the ground system is malfunctioning, the current from a shorted wire may find a pathway through the victim to ground. Because testing may alter the equipment, each step of the examination should be documented and preferably, photographed. X-ray studies of cords and plugs may also be useful for demonstrating defects.[10]

In low-voltage electrocutions involving a defective device, commonly, a charged wire inside of the appliance becomes exposed and short-circuits to the outer metal case. Typically, a defective ground is also present.

A barefoot man using an electric saw on a wet concrete floor was found dead with electrical burns. The appliance and all associated extension cords were obtained for examination. The outlet was properly wired. No GFCI was in use. The victim had bypassed the third or grounding prong of the saw's plug when he inserted it into a two-pronged

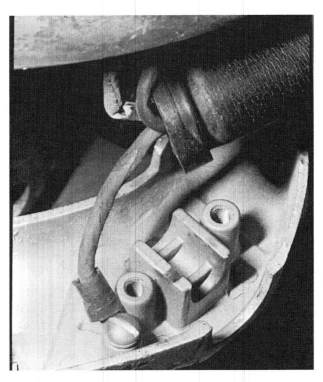

FIGURE XVI-2a. Crimped white neutral wire with insulation defect had been trapped between the halves of a saw handle following reassembly. A screw to the tool's metal casing attaches the grounding wire. Bypassing the plug's ground prong defeated this protective device.

FIGURE XVI-2b. Charred electrical marks are present on the opposing half of the saw handle, where the charged wire had been trapped. Deep groove, beads of melted metal, and carbon charring in the area of contact are caused by electrical arcing.

extension cord. This procedure defeated the tool's protective ground system and destroyed the plug's polarity. The saw was dismantled for examination. The insulation of the white neutral wire showed a defect where it had become entrapped in the handle's screw mountings. This short probably occurred when the tool had been reassembled after cleaning.

There was direct electrical contact between the power cord and the metal handle of the saw. Current could easily flow to ground through the victim when the cord was charged (Fig. XVI-2a–b).

A maintenance man screamed and collapsed while using an upright vacuum cleaner. The outlet was properly wired. No GFCI was in use. The three-pronged grounded plug of the device had been replaced with a non-polarized two-prong plug. In a non-polarized plug either prong can be inserted into the hot side of the outlet. Inspection of the plug revealed that the black hot wire was secured to one terminal while the white neutral wire was twisted together with the green ground wire and secured to the other terminal. The replacement plug defeated the ground and polarity safety features of the vacuum cleaner. This connection caused the metal components of the vacuum cleaner to be electrically charged anytime the *neutral* prong was inserted into the hot

side of the outlet. Current could then easily flow from the charged metal casing through a grounded individual who made contact with it (Fig. XVI-3).

Many electrocutions occur at home. About half of the electrocutions at home occur while bathing. Often an electrical appliance like a hair dryer drops into the bathtub. Many people are unaware that dropping an electrical appliance, which is turned off, into the water can cause electrocution. Though the current flow inside the device has stopped, the terminal of the attached electric cord is still charged. The bathroom outlets of modern homes and recently purchased hair dryers are equipped with protective GFCIs. However, many older dwellings and older hair dryers are not protected.[6]

Young children and infants are especially vulnerable to items like extension cords that they may put in their mouth (Fig. XVI-4). Additionally, damaged or bare wires may be accidentally

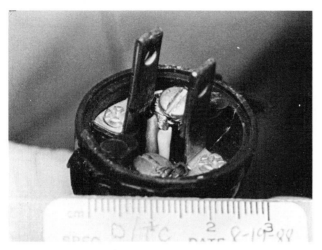

FIGURE XVI-3. Improperly wired vacuum cleaner replacement plug. White neutral wire and ground wire were twisted together beneath screw terminal of an unpolarized plug. This alteration charged the vacuum cleaner's metal casing whenever the *neutral* prong was mated with the hot side of the receptacle.

contacted during play. Older children are more likely to be at risk of electrocution during climbing activities that may bring them into the vicinity of high-voltage lines.[11] In an unusual case an infant was electrocuted by improper use of a medical device in the neonatal intensive care unit of a hospital.

A 12-day-old infant in a hospital intensive care unit for hypoglycemia was taken out of his crib and placed in an incubator for transport to the ultrasound laboratory. When the power cord to his apnea monitor was disconnected from the back of the unit, the monitor automatically switched to battery power. After the infant returned from the laboratory, the three chest electrodes of the apnea monitor were erroneously connected to the three receptacle slots of the energized power cord. The infant became rigid and appeared to have a seizure. An odor of burning was also noted. At autopsy, an electrical burn was noted on the chest in the area where the electrodes had been connected.

Electrocutions are more common in the warm months of the year.[9] In the United States, these deaths occur most frequently in July and August, which are particularly hot and humid in many areas. Electrocutions may be more common during warm weather because skin is likely to be moist with sweat and offers less resistance to the flow of electric current. Also, in warm weather, people wear less clothing and may be barefoot, additional factors that make them more vulnerable to electrocution.

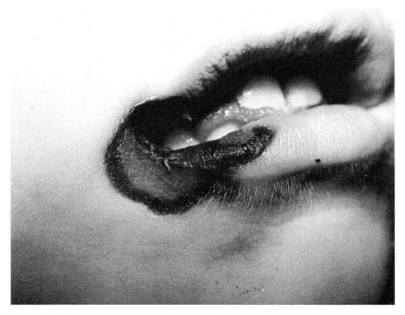

FIGURE XVI-4. Circumscribed electrical burn that occurred when this child bit an electrical cord while standing barefoot on a wet basement floor.

A barefoot young woman had been operating an electric lawn mower on a hot summer day. She was found lifeless on the lawn with the cord of the mower across her shoulders. Examination of the cord showed partly missing friction tape used to cover a defect in the insulation, where the mower blade had previously struck the cord. A small electric burn was discovered when the nape of the neck area was shaved and cleaned of all hair.

High-voltage electrocutions are more common than low-voltage cases. Virtually, all high voltage victims have visible electrical burns on their bodies (Fig. XVI-5a–d). High-voltage electrocutions mostly involve accidents in the workplace and contact with downed power lines, as in a storm. High-voltage lines are not insulated and present a considerable hazard to workers using booms, hoists, tall metal ladders, etc. One-third to one-half of low-voltage electrocutions have no electrical burns. If one requires the presence of burns to make the diagnosis of low-voltage electrocution, one-third to one-half of the cases are likely to be misdiagnosed (Fig. XVI-6a–b).

The production of electrical burns depends on voltage, amount of current flow and the area, and duration of contact. An electrical burn occurs only if the temperature of the skin is raised enough for a sufficiently long period to produce damage. If the voltage is low, the current flow small, the area of contact large, and the time of exposure short, it is unlikely that an electrical burn will be produced. When present an electrical burn may have a characteristic crater-like appearance with central charring, or may resemble an abrasion or second-degree or third degree burn (Fig. XVI-7a–c).

Examination of an electrical burn does not permit determination of the direction of current flow, i.e., it is not possible to determine whether entrance or exit of the electric current caused a burn.

Electric burns frequently represent high temperature burns, and this produces characteristic findings of severe thermal denaturation of collagen, causing it to stain blue with hematoxylin. The epidermis is often elevated with micro-blisters within the squamous epithelium, as well as in the external horny layer. The blisters result from the *cooking effect* on the tissue and represent channels through which steam exited. Large vacuoles

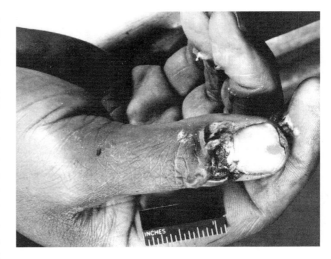

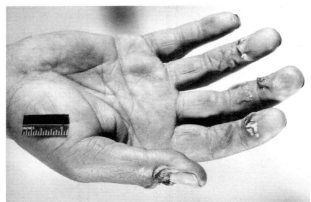

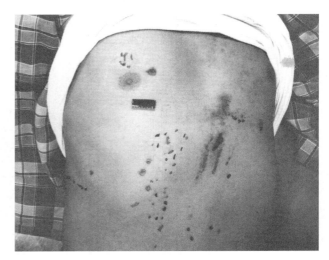

FIGURE XVI-5a–c. Man who climbed up an electrical utility pole to spy on his wife. He touched a high tension wire with his hand while sustaining spark burns to his chest and abdomen.

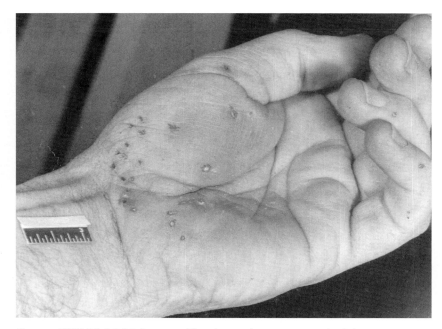

FIGURE XVI-5d. Multiple crater-like electric burns sustained while converting a transformer from 4000 to 13000 volts.

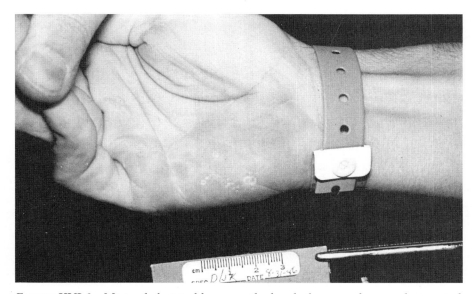

FIGURE XVI-6a. Minimal electrical burns on the hand of a man who was electrocuted when he briefly contacted the charged metal microphone of a defectively wired, low-voltage public address system.

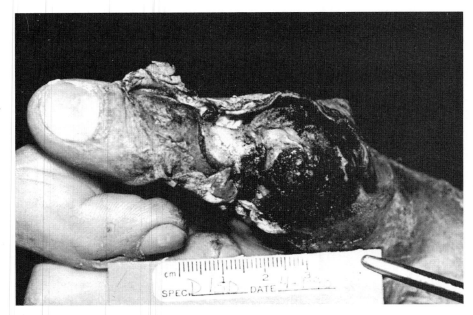

FIGURE XVI-6b. Charred electrical burn on the hand of a man who contacted a high-voltage line.

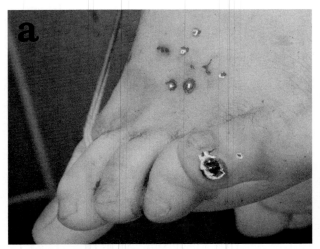

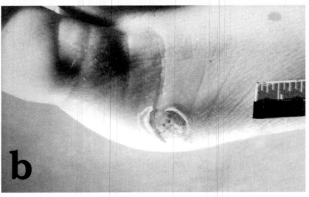

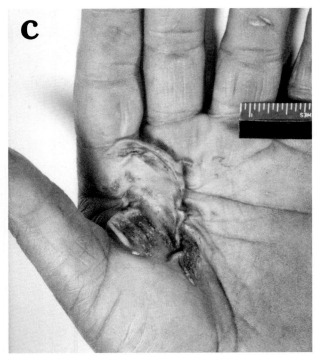

FIGURE XVI-7a–c. (a) Young man who made contact with a downed power line. Note spark burns on top of foot and crater-shaped entrance burn on the little toe. (b) Crater-shaped exit burn. (c) Crater-shaped entrance burn sustained by touching a defective electric drill.

produced by heat may also appear within epidermal cells. Further, nuclei of epidermal cells at the site of an electrical burn frequently show stretching and narrowing of the contour to produce a palisade-type appearance. This change is often referred to as *streaming of the nuclei* (Fig. XVI-8a–b). Small injuries on the hands and feet should be sampled in search of microscopic changes suggestive of electrical burns. The autopsy findings in electrocutions are otherwise not specific.

Histochemical color tests using reagents that react with copper (to produce a purplish color) or iron (to produce a blue color) may be helpful in identifying a particular electrical conductor. More specifically, the outline of a particular conductor is sometimes readily recognizable at the site of an electrical burn. Thus, the thread at the base of a light bulb may be found *branded* into the skin, leaving no doubt regarding the mechanism of electrocution (Fig. XVI-9).

Also, close examination of a potential electrical conductor at the scene may show the presence of shreds of epidermis from the area of *contact* welded to the metal.

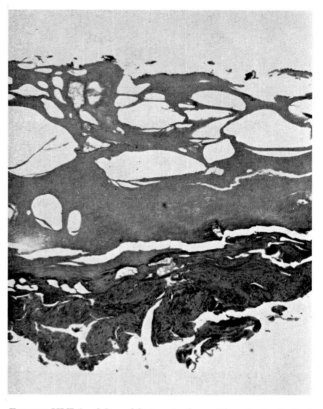

FIGURE XVI-8a. Micro-blisters in the epidermis, typical of electrical burns.

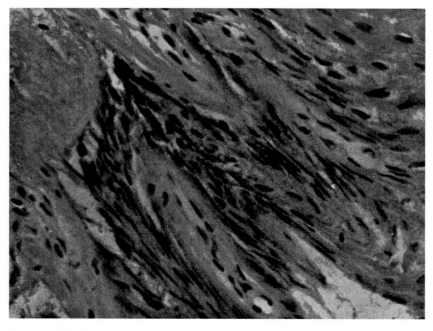

FIGURE XVI-8b. Streaming of nuclei of epidermis characteristic of electrical burns.

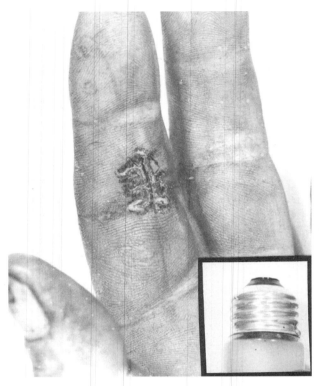

FIGURE XVI-9. Individual electrocuted while replacing a light bulb. Threaded end is *branded* into the skin of the finger.

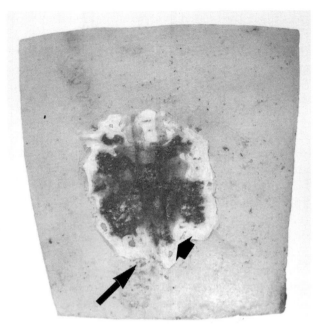

FIGURE XVI-10. The thickness of the wire is seen running through the center of the charred area (wide arrow). The pale peripheral *halo* is the result of displacement of the underlying marrow and blood by the heat generated by the passage of the current (narrow arrow).

A large fragment of epidermis from the scalp was found attached to a high-tension wire passing above a rooftop. A young man who tried to free a kite entangled in these wires, was electrocuted and fell to the street below. The question was whether the death was the result of the fall. The skin on the wire confirmed the electrocution when the lifeless body was found at the scene. Subsequent autopsy showed a burn in the top of the skull shown in actual size in Figure XVI-10.

In a questionable case, a suspected piece of tissue on the wire, unless charred, may be subjected to DNA analysis.

Having described the gross and microscopic manifestations of an electric burn, it must be emphasized that electric burns, like thermal burns which occurred during life are indistinguishable from those which occurred postmortem. This includes the red halo often seen surrounding the pale peripheral zone encircling the charred crater or blistered center of an electric burn. This red zone results from the outward movement of intravascular blood by the heat generated by the burn. The determination of ante vs postmortem electrocution would have to be based on circumstantial scene evidence or witnesses, but not the autopsy (Fig. XVI-11a–c).

Electricity may leap a gap and arc through air causing sparks. An electric arc resembles bright, fast traveling sparks making a rhythmic crackling sound. High-voltage electricity is especially prone to arcing. In general, the higher the voltage the more likely arcing will occur. Lightning is perhaps the most dramatic example of an electric arc. Air is a poor conductor of electricity, and the voltage needed to arc, even a short distance, is large. Arcs cannot be initiated through normal air at a voltage of less than three hundred fifty, unless there is hot ionized gas or debris in the air.[12] When electricity arcs, temperatures of up to 5000 degrees Centigrade may be reached. The heat produced by an electric arc may cause characteristic small pitted burns on the victim's body and clothing. Arc marks may also be seen on other objects which are part of the circuit (Fig. XVI-12a–c).

High-voltage electrical injury may cause multiple discrete lesions due to arcing from the con-

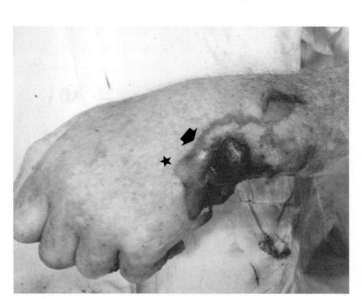

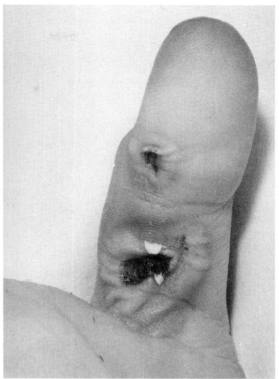

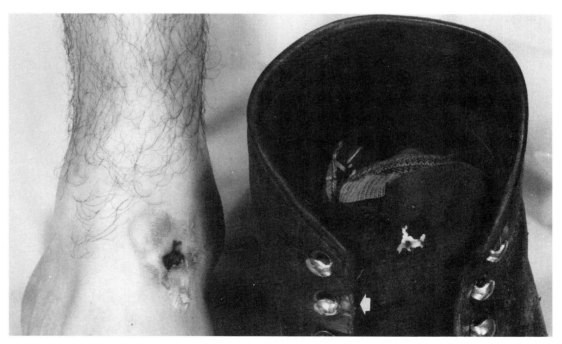

FIGURE XVI-11a–c. (a) High-voltage electric burn with charring on the wrist. Note the pale peripheral zone and the adjacent strip of congested skin (arrow) which is where the blood from the pale area accumulated. The red rim is interrupted by a blister (star). This phenomenon must not be mistaken for *vital reaction,* it can be readily duplicated within a postmortem burn in an area of livor mortis. (b) Electrocution burns showing central charring with surrounding pale *halo.* The pale areas are blistered. (c) Struck by lightning next to second right eyelet (white arrow). The burn hole in the tongue overlapped the injury of the foot showing central charring with a peripheral pale *halo* bordered by dark, congested border zone.

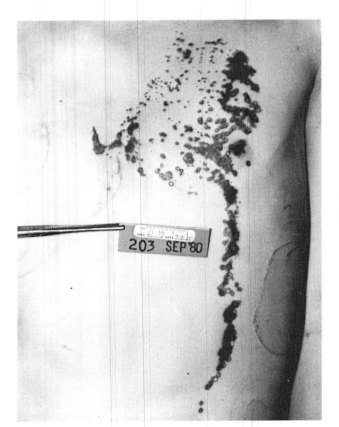

FIGURE XVI-12a. Electric arc mark on skin of victim of high voltage electrocution. *Dancing* of electrical current over the skin caused scattered, circular, crater-like burns.

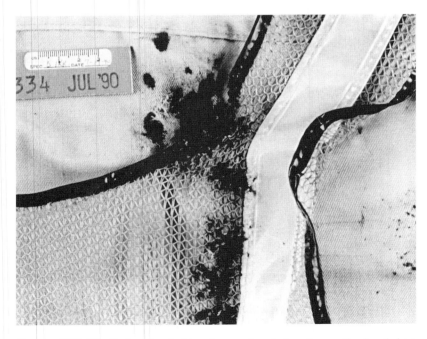

FIGURE XVI-12b. Defects in clothing due to electrical arcing on the fused shirt and safety vest of the same victim.

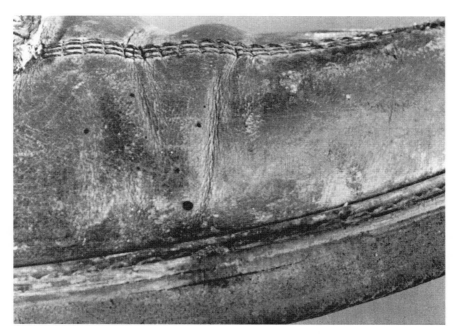

FIGURE XVI-12c. Charred arc marks on the shoe of a man who was electrocuted when the crane against which he was leaning made contact with a high-voltage line.

ductor to the body of the victim, though no direct contact is made. In such cases, the arc seems to *dance* over the body surface, producing multiple seared or punched-out lesions. Secondary burning due to ignition of clothing can also occur.

Electrocutions can occur as a result of contact with the third rail of rapid-transit tracks (Fig. XVI-13). The third rail usually is charged with more than 600 volts direct current. Alcohol is present in over half the individuals electrocuted on rapid transit tracks. Several cases of fatal electrocution have occurred as a result of urinating on the third rail.

A 14-year-old male, on medication for epilepsy was standing on a rapid transit platform with three friends. He informed them that he had to urinate. He then jumped off the platform and ran down to the tracks to find a darker area. Moments later his friends saw him lying on the tracks. A passerby reported hearing "muffled pops like a gunshot." The friends carried him down an embankment and summoned a police car. The victim was transported to the emergency room where he was noted to have cardiac asystole. The victim's underwear shorts were wet at the time of autopsy. Multiple pitted burn defects due to arcing electrical current were present on the posterior elbows and forearm and the anterior knees and legs. Microscopic changes consistent with electrocution were noted in the involved skin.

INJURY BY LIGHTNING

A natural high-voltage electrical discharge of direct current (DC) in the atmosphere is called lightning, or lightning flash. Usually, lightning strikes occur during thunderstorms, however, strikes may occur when it is not raining. The motion of water and dust particles during thunderstorms causes the buildup of a large negative charge on the undersurface of clouds. Lightning, an electrical arc from negatively charged cloud to the underlying positively charged earth occurs when charge differentials become excessive.[13]

A lightning strike begins as a relatively slow moving *leader stroke* traveling from the cloud to earth. A *pilot stroke* rising from the ground meets the leader stroke. Once the connection is established, a rapidly moving and powerful *return*

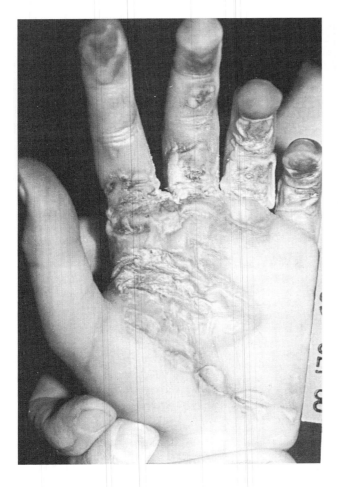

FIGURE XVI-13. Severe electrical burns resulting from contact with the third rail of a rapid transit track.

stroke occurs, as the differences in charge are resolved. Because the leader stroke moves more slowly, lightning is usually perceived as an arc traveling from the cloud to earth, though it actually moves in both directions.[14]

Lightning injuries differ significantly from other high-voltage electrical injuries. Although the electrical potential of lightning may be 10 to 100 million volts, a current of 10,000 to 100,000 amperes, and temperatures of 15,000 to 50,000 degrees Fahrenheit, the duration of the strike is extremely short, less than one ten-thousandth of a second. Because the victim's exposure is so brief, no burns at all or only very small burns, no larger than a pinhead, or minor singeing of hair may be all that is seen (Figs. XVI-14 and XVI-15a–c). Due to a phenomenon known as flashover, a majority of lightning energy may actually travel over the surface of the victim's body and decrease the amount of injury compared with passage of a similar current through the body.[15]

Lightning victims may be injured by direct strike, side flash or splash, ground strike, or contact. In a direct strike the current strikes the victim directly. Metal objects worn or carried by the victim may attract a direct strike. In a side flash or splash current jumps from an adjacent object to the victim and a transient fern-like marking may be seen on the skin. In a ground strike, current is conducted through the ground to the victim, entering one leg and exiting through the other. In a contact strike, the victim is in contact with an electrical conductor struck by lightning.

Lightning strikes are by no means always fatal. It has been estimated that less than half of the individuals struck by lightning are killed. The vast majority of victims survive with little or no

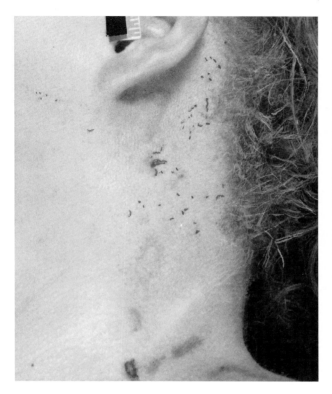

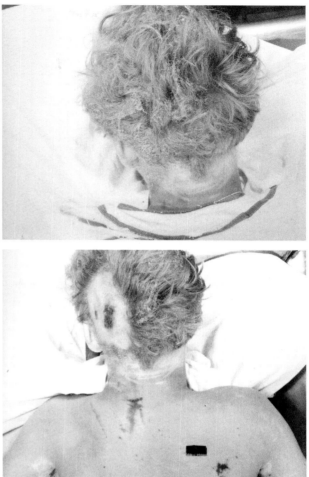

FIGURE XVI-14. Singeing of hair and non-descript superficial burn marks resembling scratches.

sequelae. Prompt cardiopulmonary resuscitation and prolonged artificial respiration sometimes can revive a person who has apparently been *killed* by lightning. It has been suggested that resuscitative efforts should be continued until onset of livor mortis.

Strikes that pass through airplanes are not unusual and generally cause little or no damage. The witnessed lightning strike to *Apollo 12* on November 14, 1969, as it passed through the clouds above Cape Kennedy, interfered with the spacecraft's electrical system but had no serious harmful effect. Over the years, there have been numerous reports of lightning-related commercial aircraft accidents by ignition and explosion of fuel compartments, temporary blinding of pilots, or interference with electrical systems.[16]

A distinctive fern-like discoloration of the skin, which follows the distribution of cutaneous blood vessels, may be present on the body of individuals struck by a lightning side flash or splash.[17,18] This pattern may remain on the body

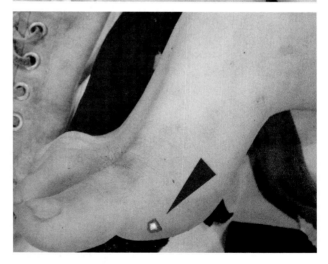

FIGURE XVI-15a–c. (a) Singeing of hair in a victim of lightning. (b) Subsequent shaving of scalp revealed the lightning strike in the scalp running down the neck causing abrasion-like injuries. (c) Pinhead size exit wound on the foot.

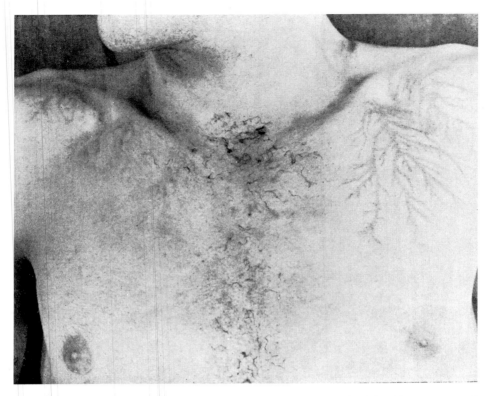

FIGURE XVI-16. Fern-like red pattern due to lightning injury on shoulder. Note singeing of hair on chest.

or disappear with time (Fig. XVI-16). While the mechanism by which this pattern occurs is unknown, it is likely that hemolysis due to intense heat generated by the current along the blood flow may be the cause. A similar pattern may also be observed in other high-voltage electrocutions. The explosive effect of the lightning strike may cause rupture of the eardrums and blood to run from the ear canals, suggesting a head injury.

An individual sustained a lightening strike on the top of his head. The site was marked by singed hair and a focal superficial burn in the left posterior scalp. Subsequent autopsy showed multiple foci of subarachnoid hemorrhage over the left side of the brain. There was no evidence of dura or brain injury and the skull was intact (Fig. XVI-17).

The blast effect due to extreme changes in air pressure caused by a lightning discharge, occasionally throws the victim several feet, resulting in blunt injuries, and may rip his or her clothing, including shoes (Figs. XVI-18 and XVI-19a–b). We have seen partially disrobed victims of light-ening strikes with shredded clothes and shoes thrown off the body. Torn clothes may arouse suspicion that an assault has occurred.[19] Secondary burns from ignition of clothing are sometimes seen.

Most lightning deaths occur outdoors during thunderstorms. Trees attract lightning, as do metal fences, gates, tall light poles and power lines. But, hardtop automobiles provide good shelter, if the windows are rolled up. Tires, however provide inadequate insulation. Open areas such as golf courses and football fields are common sites for lightning strikes. Lightning need not strike directly. It can be transmitted through the ground to persons nearby. During a thunderstorm in Arizona, 38 cows were struck and killed by a single lightning discharge.

When lightning strikes utility lines, it is possible to be killed indoors while talking on a telephone or touching an electrical appliance. Computers, television sets and power tools are notorious in facilitating electrical accidents. A

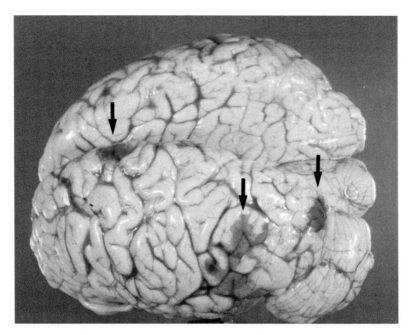

FIGURE XVI-17. Subarachnoid hemorrhage underlying a lightning strike in the scalp.

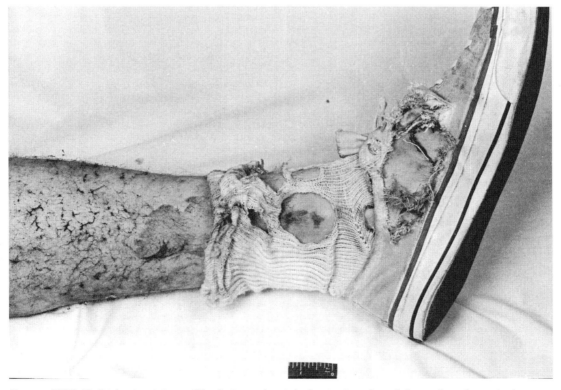

FIGURE XVI-18. Lightning injures: The hair on the right leg is singed, and the sock and tennis shoe are burned.

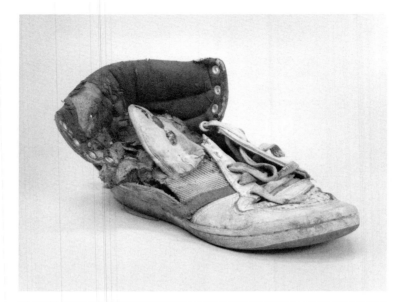

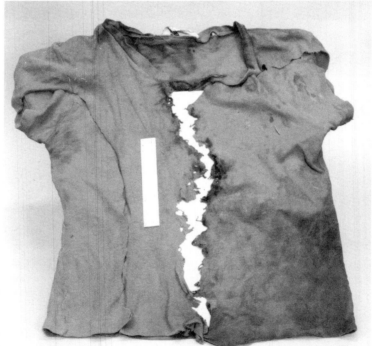

FIGURE XVI-19a–b. Young man struck by lightning in the head area. His exploded sneaker showed evidence of burning. The lightning blast traveled down his shirt tearing a distinctive path.

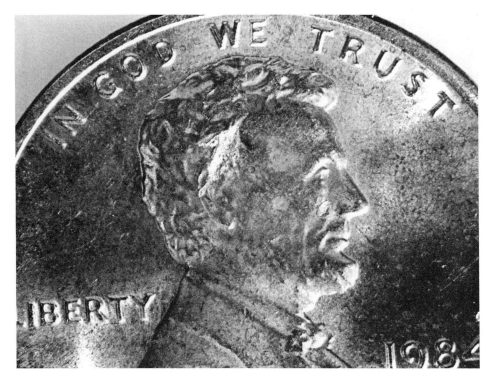

FIGURE XVI-20. Coin in pocket of lightning victim showing electrical arc marks above right ear. (Photo courtesy of Yuksel Konakci, M.D.)

shower or bath during an electric storm may be fatal if lightning strikes the copper water pipes. The same is true of indoor swimming pools unless properly constructed and grounded.

Rubber soles on shoes and boots provide no protection against lightning strikes due to their enormously high voltage and amperage.[20] Metal objects on the body, such as an earring or belt buckle or a coin, or key in the pocket of a lightning victim, may be partially melted or reveal electrical arc marks (Fig. XVI-20). The underlying skin often shows a deep burn, even if the metal object is undamaged. Electronic devices carried by the victim may be rendered inoperable due to short circuit, even ignition and fire. Iron or steel objects, such as a key, or steel-cased cigarette lighter, may be magnetized. The use of a compass readily shows this phenomenon. Coins, links of a necklace, or a zipper may be fused and a watch may be stopped.[21]

TASER STUN GUNS

WERNER U. SPITZ

The use of taser guns as a substitue for lethal force by law enforcement has increased in recent years with approximately 7,000 police departments currently employing this device. The X26 Taser model delivers 50,000 volts of electricity (0.0021 amps) through a pulsating discharge causing painful and severe muscle contractions and temporary incapacitation. These stun guns are advertised as being safe and indeed many individuals have been shocked without known adverse effect. However, it is significant that all testing done to determine the safety of these weapons has been carried out by the Taser manufacturers or on their behalf.

According to the *New York Times* (Alex Berenson, January 21, 2005) more than 100,000 police officers nationwide carry the weapon and the manufacturer, Taser International, began selling a version of the X26 to civilians in the fall of 2004. The same article indicates that some cardiologists and biomedical engineers believe that these stun guns may interfere with the heart's rhythm. The number of reported deaths following taser application has risen significantly with the increase in the use of these devices. More than 100 people are said to have died in the past five years, after being shocked with taser guns (Kevin Johnson, *USA Today*, May 12, 2005).

In our experience, deaths have followed taser use. In some of these cases autopsy showed cardiomegaly, i.e., enlargement of the heart, due to hypertensive disease or coronary artery disease. In others, there were multiple shockings to the chest or back in the heart area. The effect of electricity in the body is cumulative with successive applications. Thus, repeated shocking may entail serious complications, including ventricular fibrillation (VF) and seizures. It would seem that more research is needed before the safety of these weapons can be ensured.

REFERENCES

1. Carr, J.J.: Safety for electronic hobbyists. *Popular Electronics,* October, 1997, as found in Britannica.com.
2. Zitzewitz, P.W., and Neff, R.F.: *Merrill physics, principles and problems.* New York: Glencoe McGraw-Hill, 1995.
3. Grellner, W., Fischer, O., and Wilske, J.: *Ungewöhnlicher Stromtod In Der Haftanstalt.* Report at the 81st meeting of the German Association of Legal Medicine, Rostock, September, 2002.
4. Bruner, J.M.R.: Hazards of electrical apparatus. *Anesthesiology, 28:* 396–425, 1967.
5. Cooper MA. Electrical and lightning injuries. *Emerg Med Clin North Am, 2:* 489–501, 1984.
6. Budnick, L.D.: Bathtub-related electrocutions in the United States, 1979 to 1982. *JAMA, 252:* 918–920, 1984.
7. Electricity: Home wiring basics, installation, and repairs. *Reader's Digest New Complete Do-It-Yourself Manual.* Pleasantville, NY: Reader's Digest Association, 1991, 235–270.
8. Spitz, W.: Befunde bei vorubergehender Wiederbelebung nach Elektrounfall. *Munch Med Wochenschr, 106:* 495, 1964.
9. Wright, R.K.: Death or injury caused by electrocution. *Clin Lab Med, 3:* 343–353, 1983.
10. Wright, R.K., and Davis, J.H.: The investigation of electrical deaths: A report of 220 fatalities. *J Forensic Sci, 25:* 514–521, 1980.
11. Thompson, J.C., and Ashwal, S.: Electrical injuries in children. *Am J Dis Child, 137:* 231–235, 1983.
12. Bernstein, T.: Electrical injury: Electrical engineer's perspective and an historical review. *Ann N Y Acad Sci, 720:* 1–10, 1994.
13. Kobernick, M.: Electrical injuries: Pathophysiology and emergency management. *Ann Emerg Med, 11:* 633–638, 1982.
14. Lifschultz, B.D., and Donoghue, E.R.: Deaths caused by lightning. *J Forensic Sci, 38:* 353–358, 1993.
15. Cooper, M.A., and Andrews, C.J.: Lightning injuries. In Auerbach, P.S., ed. *Wilderness medicine: Management of wilderness and environmental emergencies,* 3rd ed. St. Louis, MO: Mosby-Year Book, 1995, 261–289.
16. Cherington, M., and Mathys, K.: Deaths and injuries as a result of lightning strikes to aircraft. *Aviat Space Environ Med, 66:* 687–689, 1995.
17. Resnik, B.I., and Wetli, C.V.: Lichtenberg figures. *Am J Forensic Med Pathol, 17:* 99–102, 1996.
18. Lichtenberg, R., Dries, D., Ward, K., Marshall, W., and Scanlon, P.: Cardiovascular effects of lightning strikes. *J Am Coll Cardiol, 21:* 531–536, 1993.
19. Massello, W., III.: Lightning deaths. *Medico-Legal Bull, 37:* 1, 1988.
20. Ojala, F.C., Professor Eastern Michigan University, Geography and Geology, personal communication, 2001.
21. Wetli, C.V.: Keraunopathology. *Am J Forensic Med Pathol, 17* (2): 89–98, 1996.

Chapter XVII

ROAD TRAFFIC VICTIM

Werner U. Spitz

CORRELATION OF POSTMORTEM FINDINGS WITH ROADSIDE EVIDENCE

THE PURPOSE OF THIS CHAPTER is to assist those concerned with investigating traffic deaths to corroborate autopsy findings with roadside evidence.

At the urging of the National Highway Traffic Safety Administration (NHTSA), the diagnostic readout box (DRB) was developed. The DRB, which is the equivalent of the flight data recorder (black box) in aircraft, has proven invaluable for helping to determine what happened in the seconds preceding a crash. The DRB is capable of recording faults in the engine, the antilock brake system and other safety devices. Data from such recorders would show, for example, the speed at which the car was traveling at the time of impact, that the driver was applying the brakes or accelerating, whether he or she was wearing a seatbelt, the instant at which the air bag deployed and numerous other occurrences. Cases have been reported where it was claimed that the air bag deployed early, such as due to hitting a pothole. However, data in the DRB showed that the air bag deployed upon frontal impact, as designed.[1] This technology has opened the door to a new source of information for the reconstruction of motor vehicular crashes.

Evaluating injuries sustained in a motor vehicular crash requires the ability to recognize and distinguish between blunt and sharp force trauma. These are the two most common types of injury that occur in all types of motor vehicular crashes.

Police accident investigators are trained to furnish thorough reports, including witness statements. However, eyewitness accounts of a motor vehicle crash, in fact any traumatic event involving severe injury or death, are often unreliable and sometimes conflicting. While such state-

ments must be considered, they cannot indiscriminately be taken as factual. Eyewitness accounts are frequently tainted by emotions, sorrow and feelings of guilt, resulting in distorted, exaggerated and misleading information. Therefore, correlation of autopsy findings with vehicular and roadside evidence is necessary. To achieve this goal it is advantageous for the investigating officer to attend the autopsy and perhaps for the pathologist to accompany the officer to personally observe the scene and the vehicle or vehicles involved in the crash, even after the fact, after the vehicles have been removed. Only consideration of the injuries in light of roadside evidence will provide the background for proper evaluation of autopsy findings and assist in subsequent testimony.

As in the majority of traumatic medicolegal cases, most of the injuries sustained in a motor vehicular crash are found on the body surface. Such injuries may consist of an identifiable pattern which indicates the causative mechanism. Examples are, the circular abrasion on a driver's chest or face from impact on the steering column or the steering wheel, a bruise in the shape of the car's headlight on a pedestrian's thigh (Fig. XVII-1a–c and XVII-2a–b) or overstretching injuries in the skin, imprint of the thread of a bolt in a strategic location (Fig. XVII-3a–b), or pedestrian whiplash fracture/separation of the neck, usually at the base of the skull in conjunction with bumper injuries, indicative of a rear impact.

Recognition and careful analysis of wound characteristics, location and distribution frequently permit reconstruction of a case with a degree of accuracy not commonly appreciated. On the other hand, overinterpretation of post-

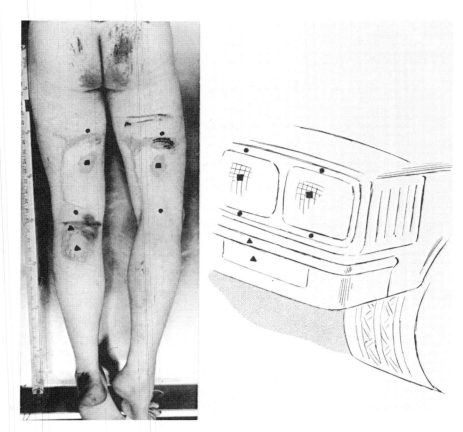

Figure XVII-1a. Pedestrian struck from behind by automobile with double horizontal headlights. Level of injuries suggests that the victim was standing when struck and vehicle was braking. The dimensions, curvature of the frame and lens of the headlight apparent on the body, correspond with the shape of the headlight of the vehicle.

mortem findings is equally undesirable. It is usually impossible to attribute a specific causative mechanism to each and every wound on a victim's body.

For complete injury documentation, incisions should be made in areas of the body known to be frequently traumatized in certain types of situations, even in the absence of external evidence of damage. For example, longitudinal incisions for examination of the calves in an individual who was struck by a car will furnish information regarding the presence of a bumper impact and deep exploration of the hips in a pedestrian will often document a subcutaneous pocket filled with blood and crushed fat. These and other incisions assist in *mapping out* hidden injuries, providing documentation of *all* areas of significant impact.

Due to the multitude of different types of surfaces with which a motor vehicular crash victim comes in contact, such an individual often presents with a larger number and diversity of injuries than victims of other types of trauma. This adds to the complexity of the interpretation, but at the same time enhances the challenge.

The Pedestrian

Vehicular crashes involving pedestrians can often be reconstructed with considerable accuracy. Pedestrian injuries may be sustained in one of two ways: (1) the pedestrian was struck by the front of the motor vehicle; (2) the pedestrian was sideswiped by the vehicle. Questions that will be raised are:

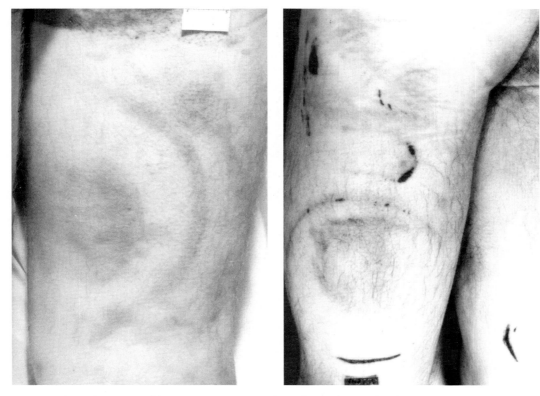

FIGURE XVII-1b–c. Typical bruise pattern of round headlight, showing outline and curved lens.

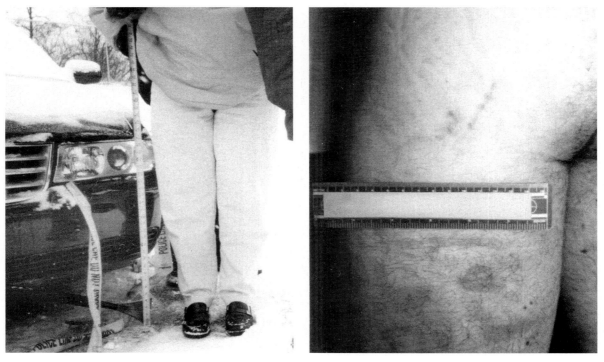

FIGURE XVII-2a–b. (a) Re-enactment by model, standing next to vehicle which struck a pedestrian, demonstrating level of impact as seen on Figure XVII-2b.

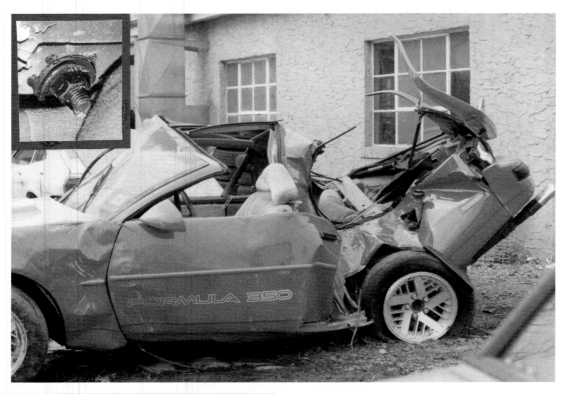

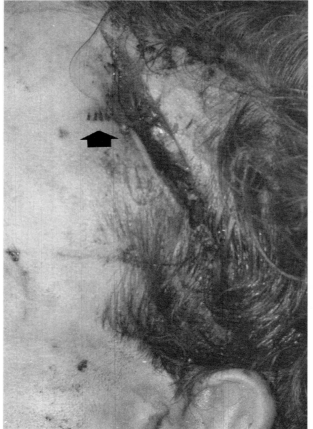

FIGURE XVII-3a–b. (a) A hatchback car struck a tree on the driver's side in front of the rear wheel causing the vehicle to rotate sharply to the right, ejecting the driver through his window. He landed on the ground, next to the front wheel with minor injuries. When found he claimed he was not the driver. A second occupant was found hanging head first, out of the driver's door window. His left hip was bruised, from impact against the console, a laceration of his forehead showed a large underlying bruise and skull fracture. (b) A small inconspicuous pattern (arrow) below the laceration was caused by impact on an exposed bolt, which held the hatch (insert - Figure XVII-3a). Only the passenger could have sustained these injuries.

- Was the pedestrian walking, standing, or lying on the road?
- What was the direction of travel of the vehicle?
- Were the brakes being applied at the moment of impact?
- Did the driver see the pedestrian prior to the collision?
- Was evidence from the vehicle found on the body?
- What was the approximate speed of the striking vehicle at the time of the impact?

The victim's clothes may aid in determining what happened in a given crash. The postmortem examination therefore, should begin with a careful examination of the victim's outer garments (Fig. XVII-4). In the case of a hit-and-run vehicle, the clothing requires particular attention. Even before the body is undressed meticulous examination of the clothing may reveal important trace evidence. Small fragments of lacquer, glass, or other parts from the vehicle may be inadvertently discarded, unless specific measures are undertaken to avoid such loss. For this reason, if feasible, it would be advantageous if the body were transported from the scene to the location of the autopsy, wrapped in a clean white sheet, then undressed on the sheet, which is removed, folded and secured prior to the start of any incisions. Carelessness in handling this part of the postmortem examination may result in loss of valuable, in fact, irreplaceable links in the investigation. Presence of grease or tire marks on the clothing may further help reconstruct the crash.

Inspection of the vehicle, whenever possible by the pathologist, adds still another dimension to the investigation. This often provides understanding of mechanisms of injury and phenomena that otherwise remain vague.

The following case exemplifies how an accurate reconstruction can be accomplished by correlating autopsy data with inspection of the vehicle.

A pedestrian struck by a jeep was dead at the scene. The driver contended that he had not seen the victim before the crash.

The pattern and distribution of the injuries supported the driver's contention, indicating that the pedestrian had not

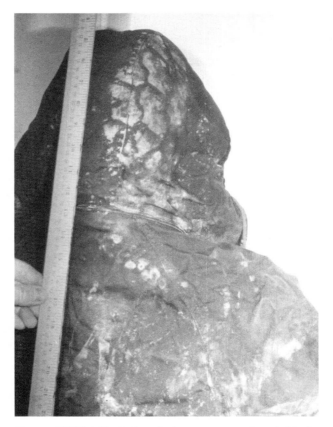

FIGURE XVII-4. Typical truck tire pattern on a hooded jacket confirms that the child wearing this garment had been run over. Witnesses had given conflicting statements and several indicated that the injuries were the result of a fall. The garments had not been examined at the autopsy two years earlier. The garments were miraculously found at the police evidence storage room and were examined prior to trial.

been in front of the vehicle, but rather was struck by the side of the car. The victim was struck on his left side; the patterned injuries of the left side of the face resulted from striking the right corner of the vehicle's roof. A dent in the corner of the roof disclosed several pinhead-size fragments, microscopically identified as fat tissue and skin. Since there were no brush marks on the front of the vehicle, it was assumed that the corner of the roof had been the site where the victim first came in contact with the automobile. A tire mark on the left thigh, initially thought to have resulted from being run over, was due to sideswiping by the spare wheel affixed to the right rear side of the vehicle (Fig. XVII-5a). The spare wheel had been bent outwards by the impact and there was minimal hemorrhage under the skin, which showed the distinct pattern of the tire, indicating the glancing nature of the impact (Fig. XVII-5b). A circular abrasion of the left forearm explained the broken-off right door handle of the Jeep.

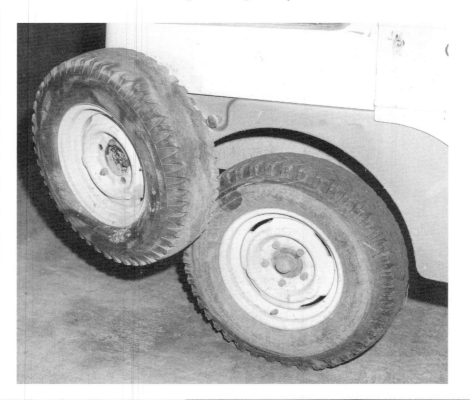

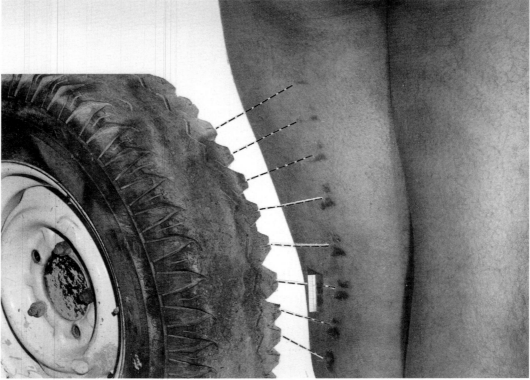

FIGURE XVII-5a–b. (a) Jeep involved in a collision with a pedestrian. The spare tire was displaced outward. (b) The tread pattern of the spare tire imprinted on the left thigh of the victim matches the tire, showing a *rubber stamp* effect.

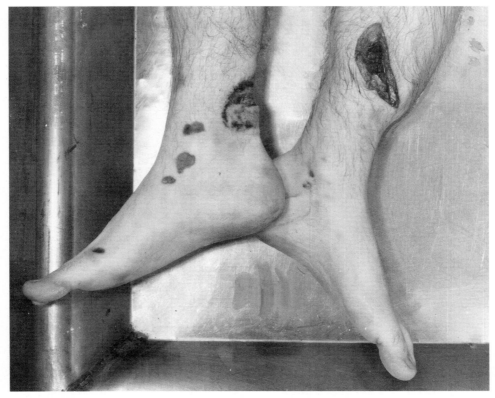

FIGURE XVII-6. Bumper injuries. Pedestrian struck from behind by an automobile. The driver was braking, as shown by the low level of the injuries. The laceration on the left leg is due to an open fracture. The different levels of the injuries suggest that the victim was walking. The abrasions on the inner side of the right foot and left ankle are due to the forward thrust of the feet within the boots.

The deceased had a blood alcohol concentration of 0.17%. No barbiturates were detected. The autopsy also disclosed evidence of old brain surgery, which corroborated the subsequently obtained history of posttraumatic epilepsy. Several capsules of anticonvulsant medication were found in the pockets of the deceased.

Any part of a car may strike a pedestrian, but most pedestrian crashes involve the bumper and front of the vehicle. In a typical situation, the adult pedestrian sustains *bumper injuries* on the legs (Fig. XVII-6). These injuries may be severe, with fractures and extensive soft tissue damage, or they may be minimal or even absent on external examination of the body. In addition to the age of the pedestrian, the severity of these injuries depends upon the speed of the car, the shape of the bumper and the amount of clothing over the area that was struck. In the winter, when heavy garments are worn, injuries caused by

impact of car bumpers may be inconspicuous, since much of the force is absorbed by clothing. A car sliding on snow or ice is likely to strike a pedestrian at a significantly lower speed, causing less extensive injuries, than a vehicle traveling on a dry road.

Incision and reflection of the skin of each calf, followed by exploration of the calf muscles, should be performed in every pedestrian fatality. This procedure reveals the site, thus, the direction of the impact or possibly no impact at all. To afford maximum exposure it is recommended that the incision of the skin be vertical and extend from above the popliteal fossa the entire length of each calf (Fig. XVII-7a–b). A single midline, vertical incision followed by undermining can be easily stitched together and sealed, causing little interference with subsequent embalming. The muscles are best separated from

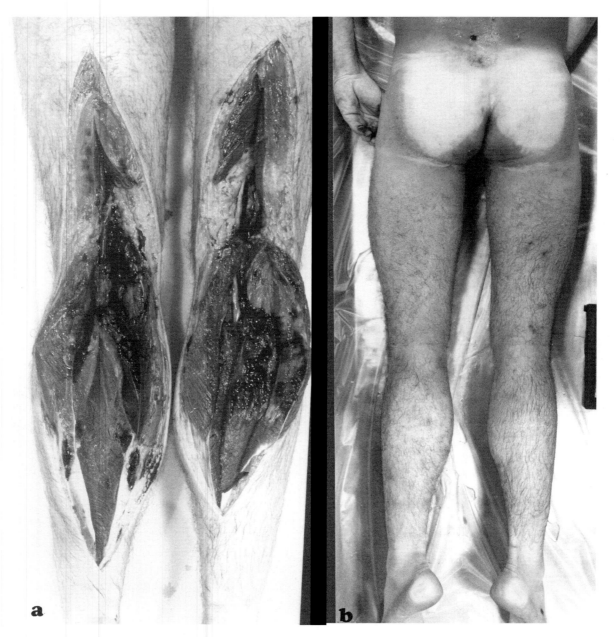

FIGURE XVII-7a–b. (a) Incision at autopsy of the back of the legs shows extensive bruises and tears of the calf muscles due to bumper impact. (b) The calves prior to incision show no external injuries.

the bones, elevated over the thigh then cut across, i.e., horizontally, from the Achilles tendon to above the knee.

Absence of bumper injuries suggests that the *pedestrian struck* the side of the automobile, as may happen if he or she inadvertently emerged from between two parked vehicles into the path of a passing car. This car may have evidence of

wiping along the side in contact with the pedestrian. A startled pedestrian, especially one who is intoxicated, may strike his or her head on the ground or a parked vehicle as a result of an unmitigated backward fall. Impact by a protruding side mirror or other projecting part may cause damage to a motor vehicle and serious injury to a pedestrian, including a depressed skull fracture and death. A vehicle is sometimes identified by the damage it received. The level of the injury on the pedestrian is of special significance in attempting to determine the type of vehicle. For example, the mirror on a large sports utility vehicle (SUV) will cause pedestrian damage higher than that by a compact car (more than 50 inches versus less than 40 inches). Bumper injuries may portray the pattern or contour of the bumper, such as the horizontal rubber strips or trim on some models (Fig. XVII-8a–c). Patterned bruises or abrasions may be explicit, easy to recognize, or subtle, requiring attention to detail (Fig. XVII-8d). A rectangular abrasion or bruise is suggestive. The sharp outline of an injury is unlikely to be coincidental.

The leg bones are frequently fractured as a result of bumper impact. The bone fragments may be displaced, and the skin is often bruised and torn, causing an open, also known as compound fracture. Fractured lower leg or thigh bones frequently overlap, which is an important consideration when determining the level of the impact. Incision and deep exploration or x-ray examination of the fracture site is necessary to determine the level of the fracture above the heel (Fig. XVII-9). However, it must be emphasized that the fracture does not always represent the level of the impact. No fracture at all may occur if the particular extremity is not weight bearing at the time of impact and fracture may occur above or below the level of the impact if the extremity was weight bearing. Thus, it is suggested that a diligent effort be made to determine the presence of skin and subcutaneous bruising, especially a possible bumper pattern, before concluding whether the victim was walking or standing, or the brakes were being applied. In the case of an impact by a bumper with a narrow, protruding, horizontal lip the tibia often fractures in the shape of a wedge where the apex of the triangular fragment represents the level of the blow and points in the direction in which the automobile was traveling (Fig. XVII-10a–b).

The occurrence of bumper fractures depends on the speed of the vehicle, the weight of the vehicle and the shape of the bumper. A weight-bearing leg is likely to fracture at a lower speed and with a lighter weight vehicle. Bumper fractures occur at considerably lower speeds in elderly individuals with osteoporosis and skeletal fragility.

The height of injuries above the soles of the feet should be measured. It should be emphasized however, that since fractures do not always occur at the actual site of the impact, examination of the skin is of equal, if not greater significance when evaluating the level of contact with the vehicle. The height of the heels and thickness of the soles of the victim's shoes play an important role in such determinations. The levels of injury vary with the height of the bumper. Photographs of the injuries with a yardstick placed alongside the legs are advantageous for later reference and testimony. The average bumper level above the ground is approximately 15–17 inches. However, the protuberant part of the bumper may be 18 to 19 inches above the ground.

The front end of an automobile is likely to *dip* when the brakes are applied, sometimes inflicting bumper injuries as low as the ankles and rarely the heels. Worn shock absorbers may contribute significantly to low bumper injuries. Also, popular fads which involve raising or lowering of automobile or truck bodies may play a role.

Bumper injuries with or without fracture may be one-sided. In a side impact the leg which is struck by the bumper may strike and bruise and sometimes fracture the other leg. Such injury should not be construed as evidence of bumper impact (Fig. XVII-11). When this happens, the leg which is struck by the vehicle, usually at the level of the knee, is bruised on both sides. The outer surface is bruised by vehicle contact, the inner surface is bruised as a result of striking the opposite knee.

Bumper injuries at different levels on both legs suggest that the victim was walking or running when struck. The leg with the higher-placed injury usually represents the weight-bearing extremity. This leg acts as an axis upon which the body turns, resulting in a glancing blow by the radiator grill, headlight, or front fender. This injury may be located on either hip, thigh, or buttock, depending on the direction in which the vehicle was traveling in relation to the victim.

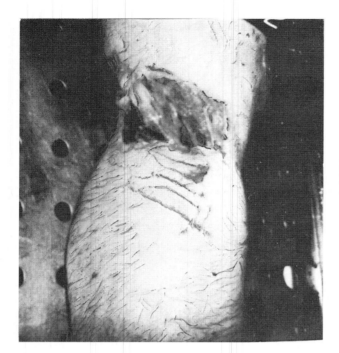

FIGURE XVII-8a. Bumper injury behind the left knee. The horizontal linear, parallel bruises and abrasions correspond to the rubber bumper strips.

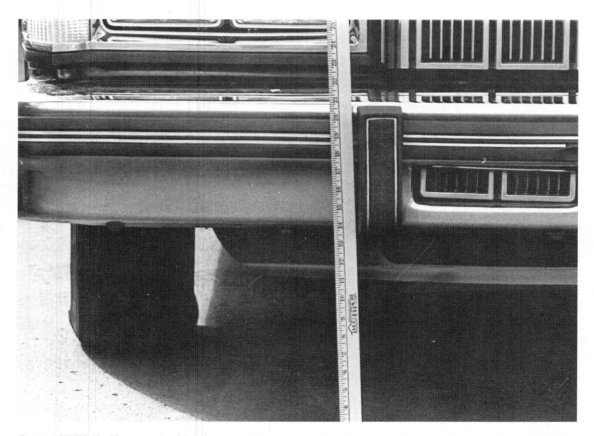

FIGURE XVII-8b. Horizontal rubber bumper strips on vehicle, which caused injuries shown in Figure XVII-8a.

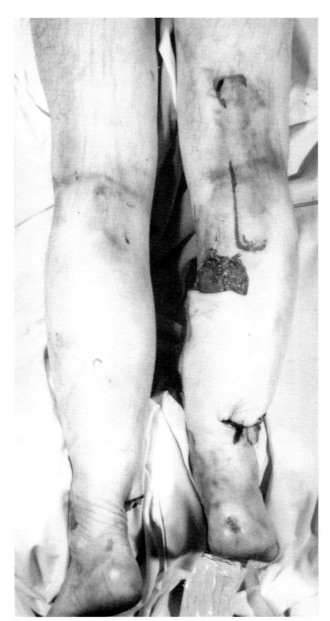

FIGURE XVII-8c. Injuries showing bumper guard on right leg. The extent of the injuries, including the fractures of the right leg, suggest the leg was weight bearing. Also note, that the fractures are much lower than the actual impact.

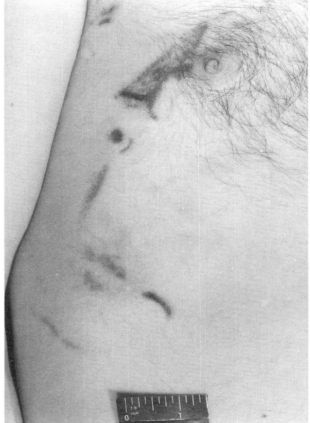

FIGURE XVII-8d. Abrasions on chest from license plate.

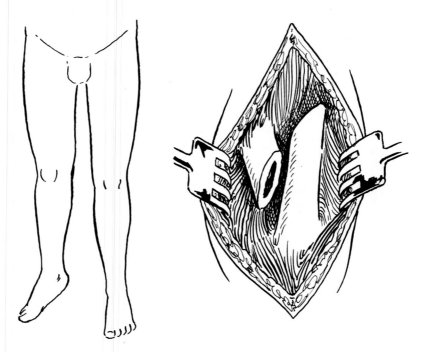

FIGURE XVII-9. Overlapping of fractured femur. Note, the right lower extremity is shortened and rotated outward.

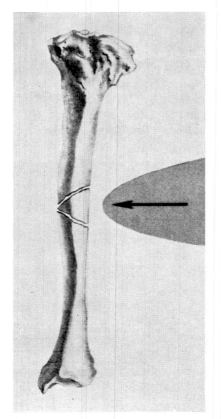

FIGURE XVII-10a. Wedge-shaped fracture of tibia in a pedestrian with bumper injuries. The apex of the triangular fragment of bone often, points in the direction of travel of the vehicle.

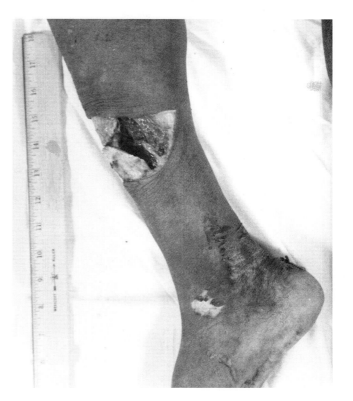

FIGURE XVII-10b. Open triangular fracture of the tibia in a pedestrian struck from behind.

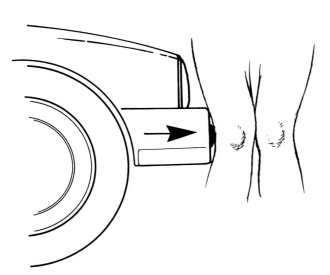

FIGURE XVII-11. A one-sided bumper impact may cause injury to the opposite leg.

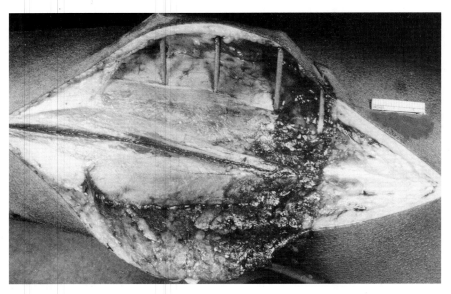

FIGURE XVII-12. Pedestrian struck by an automobile. A small abrasion on the right hip, 32 inches above the sole of the foot was due to a glancing blow by the front of the hood. Incision revealed a large *pocket* containing blood and torn adipose tissue. The pocket is limited by intact muscle fascia. The edges of the injury were elevated to show the extent of undermining.

The back of a hand may occasionally receive the blow. A glancing impact may sometimes be masked by the absence of external evidence of injury or the finding of an insignificant abrasion or a superficial bruise. Palpation of the area often suggests the presence of liquid under the skin, and incision reveals a large *pocket,* containing blood and crushed fat, between the skin and the muscle fascia (Fig. XVII-12). The fascia is usually intact, although the deeper muscles may be torn and bruised. In an obese victim the *pocket* may be enormous and present a source of major bleeding and fat embolism.

An elderly, considerably overweight pedestrian who was hit by a car died in shock as a result of blood loss. At autopsy she had four quarts of blood and crushed fat in a *pocket* under the skin of her right hip.

Glancing blows cause large *pockets* with extensive hemorrhage due to shearing forces. Perpendicular impacts also cause *pockets* with bleeding and crushed fat equivalent in size to the impacting force. Thus, bumper injuries are often associated with subcutaneous pockets of blood and liquified fat.

In some instances the *pocket* is torn open, with extensive undermining of the edges, providing an effective *hideout* for fragments of lacquer, glass or other trace evidence from the vehicle. Any one of these items may be of importance for identification of a vehicle in a hit-and-run situation. Specialized examination of a chip of lacquer sometimes reveals layers of colors and different primers. Spectrographic and chemical analyses of such a fragment may provide conclusive evidence of involvement of a specific vehicle model.

Impact by the radiator guard or front fender often results in extensive fractures of the pelvis. Fractures of the pubic rami, opposite the hip or buttock which were struck, are noted frequently. The ilium, particularly the sacroiliac joint, on the opposite side as the impact is rarely spared. The pattern of pelvic fractures resembles the bursting of a wooden hoop when opposite sides are compressed.

In elderly individuals, the head of the femur may be pushed through the socket of the joint, into the interior of the pelvis.

A rear impact of a pedestrian is often associated with fracture of the spine. The cervical spine may be fractured and often dislocated at the base of the skull, at the level of the atlanto-occipital joints when the head is forcefully thrust backward, in whiplash fashion. With this mechanism of injury, the atlanto-occipital joints are rarely fractured. Instead, they are separated with the ligaments and joint capsule often pulling off fragments of cartilage and bone from the joint edges. (See Chapter XXV which discusses the technique for dissection of the atlanto-occipital area.) When the medulla is severed or crushed, such injuries are fatal on impact, i.e., prior to striking the ground.

Hemorrhage from a wound sustained by impact on the ground results from continued heart action, despite brain death. Effective heartbeat may persist for several minutes. Bumper injuries of the legs and whiplash damage of the neck are sometimes the only significant injuries in a pedestrian who was struck by an automobile. Depending on the type of vehicle, the thoracic and lumbar areas may be crushed and severed by impact on the hood. We have seen at least two cases where a pedestrian's body was transected above the pelvis by the square and relatively sharp front edge of the hood of a large, boxy automobile traveling at high speed.

Overstretching causes stretchmark-like superficial tears in the skin. The injuries are so superficial that hemorrhage does not occur. A pedestrian, who was struck from behind by an automobile traveling at 25 to 30 mph, may sustain such injuries in his groins or lower abdomen. If the impact was *off center,* overstretching tears are likely to be one-sided (Fig. XVII-13a–d). Deep lacerations of the groins and shattering of the pelvis occur if the vehicle was traveling at a speed in excess of 45 to 50 mph (Fig. XVII-14a–c). Sometimes pelvic organs and shattered bone may be found hanging from such wounds. Stretchmark-like tears in one or both groins may occur if the victim's upper thighs were run over. The crushing weight and spinning of the vehicle's wheel causes pulling and stretching of the skin (Fig. XVII-15). The presence of tire marks on the skin or clothing confirms that the body was run over (Fig. XVII-16a–c). I have seen one case where a motorcyclist, who rolled his cycle, severed his head at C-6 with distinct overstretching tears in the skin at the edges of severance. Overstretching tears may sometimes be seen on the front of the neck in cases of severe whiplash.

Such injuries occur in pedestrians who were struck from behind by speeding cars and in drivers in head-on collisions.

A relationship may be expected between the speed of a vehicle and the nature of the injuries (Fig. XVII-17a-c). As a matter of fact, it can be said that, the faster the speed of the vehicle, the more severe the injuries.

In addition to injuries sustained by impact of the bumper, an adult victim is usually struck below the center of gravity. The center of gravity of a standing adult is located below the waistline at the brim of the pelvis. At usual city speeds, the pedestrian is propelled upward, sliding onto the hood of the automobile, frequently sustaining abrasions of the elbows and shoulders (Fig. XVII-18a–b). Symmetrical abrasion of both elbows and shoulders suggest a central rear impact. The head may be severely injured by impact on the A-pillar, which holds the windshield and supports the roof of the car, or by sliding off the hood and striking the ground. Either of these injuries may be fatal.

At relatively low impact speeds, the pedestrian may be carried by the vehicle for a considerable distance before dropping to the ground when the vehicle slows or stops. Usually a pedestrian accident transpires in less than two or three seconds.

On occasion, the victim may strike the ground with another part of his or her body. Fractures of the sacroiliac joints occur occasionally, predominately in elderly people, as the result of falls onto the buttocks. This is the same type of injury sustained by an individual who starts to sit down, when the chair is pulled out from under him. With age the space between the articular surfaces of the sacroiliac joints increases. Manipulation at autopsy permits significant movement in the joints and may lead to an erroneous impression of fracture, unless the soft tissues are removed and the joints are exposed.

When the automobile travels at greater speed, the pedestrian may be thrown considerably higher and land on the roof or trunk, or on the road behind the vehicle, subject to being run over by another car.[2] Blood and tissue, such as skin, fat, or hair, may sometimes be found on the rear bumper of the primary car.

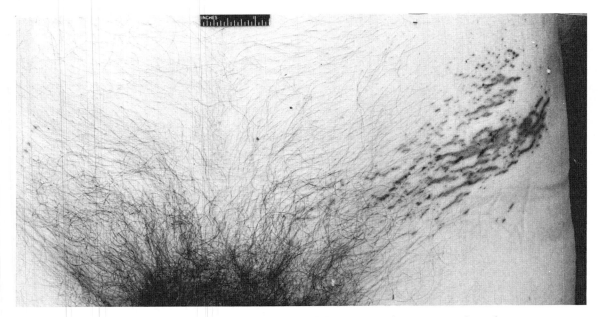

FIGURE XVII-13a. Typical overstretching in the left groin area due to impact from the rear.

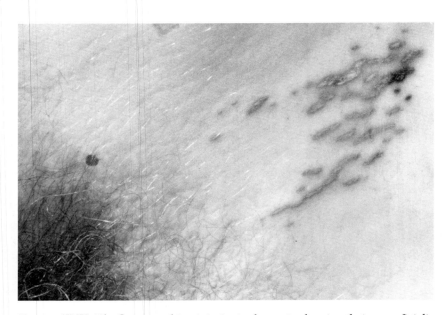

FIGURE XVII-13b. Overstretching injuries in the groin showing their superficiality. Only the epidermis is involved. The pattern is typical.

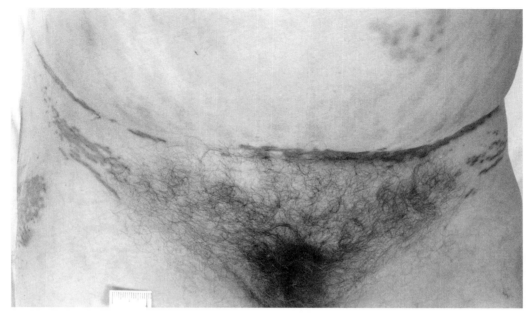

FIGURE XVII-13c. Overweight pedestrian struck in the rear showing bilateral overstretching marks in the groins and abrasion caused by the elastic band of the underwear.

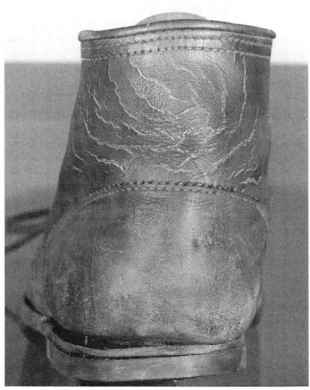

FIGURE XVII-13d. Leather is skin and when overstretched shows the same pattern as depicted above.

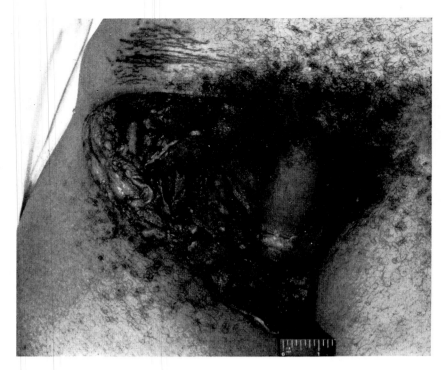

FIGURE XVII-14a. Full thickness laceration of the groin in a pedestrian who was struck from behind by an automobile traveling at highway speed.

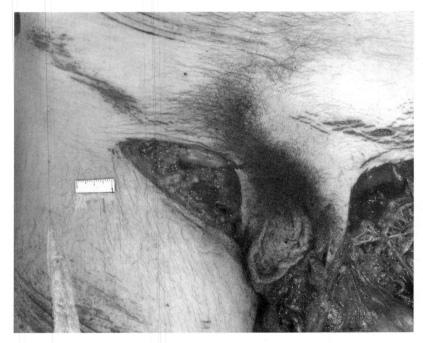

FIGURE XVII-14b. Highway speed impact. Bilateral lacerations of similar severity suggest a central rear impact. On the left, one injury is transdermal with destruction of deep tissues. Note the above overstretching injuries of different depths.

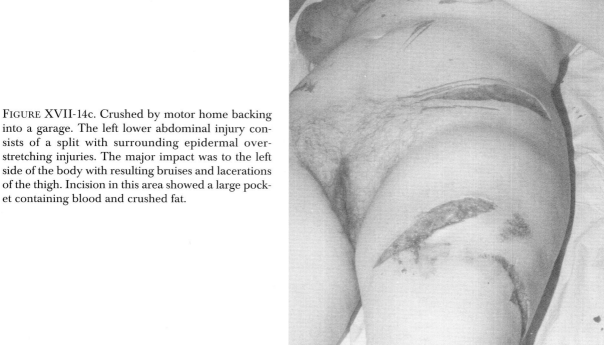

FIGURE XVII-14c. Crushed by motor home backing into a garage. The left lower abdominal injury consists of a split with surrounding epidermal over-stretching injuries. The major impact was to the left side of the body with resulting bruises and lacerations of the thigh. Incision in this area showed a large pocket containing blood and crushed fat.

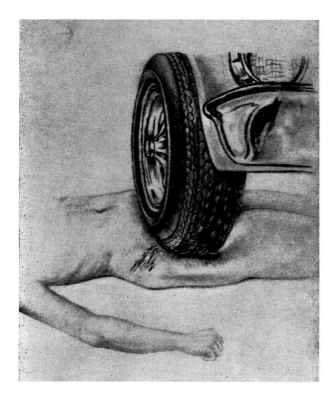

FIGURE XVII-15. Diagram showing mechanism of stretch-mark-like tears in the groin of a pedestrian struck and run over by an automobile. Overstretching of the skin is caused by the weight of the vehicle and the pull of the tire.

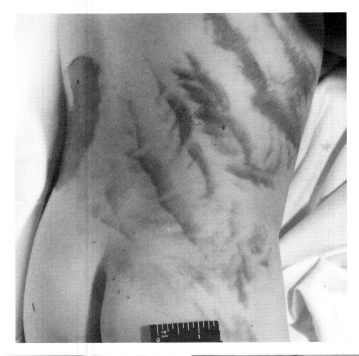

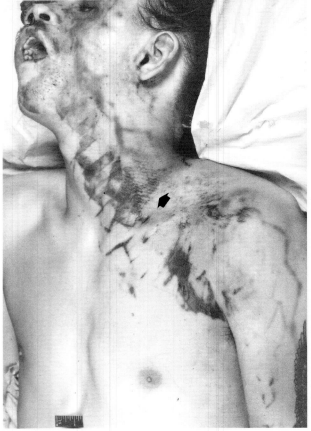

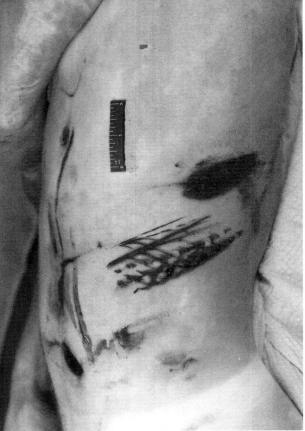

FIGURE XVII-16a–c. Different patterns of tire marks on the skin. All of the patterns could be matched with the vehicles involved. (b) is a truck. Note the overstretching marks on the left side of the neck (arrow). (c) is a motorcycle.

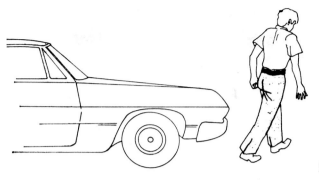

FIGURE XVII-17a. An adult pedestrian struck below the center of gravity sustains bumper injuries on his legs and an impact on the hip by the front of the hood.

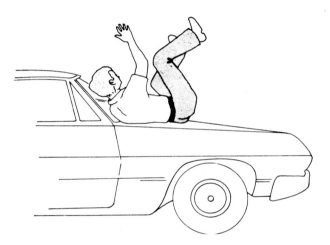

FIGURE XVII-17b. At city speeds, the adult pedestrian is propelled upward after impact by the front of the vehicle and slides onto the hood. When the vehicle slows or comes to a halt, the victim rolls to the ground.

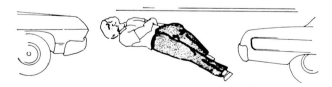

FIGURE XVII-17c. At highway speeds, the victim is thrown higher and may land on the roof or trunk of the automobile or strike the rear bumper, from where blood or skin may be recovered. The victim may land on the road behind the car, and be run over by other vehicles.

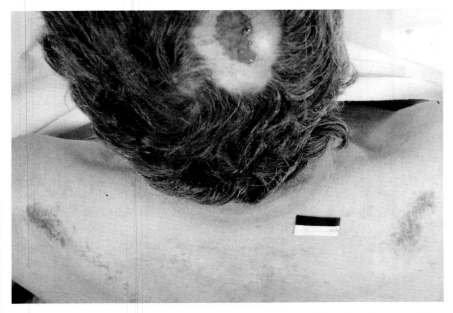

FIGURE XVII-18a. Pedestrian who was struck by an automobile. The abrasions of the shoulders were sustained by sliding on the hood. The elbows may be similarly injured. Symmetry of injuries suggests a central rear impact. The abrasion of the scalp is from impact on the windshield.

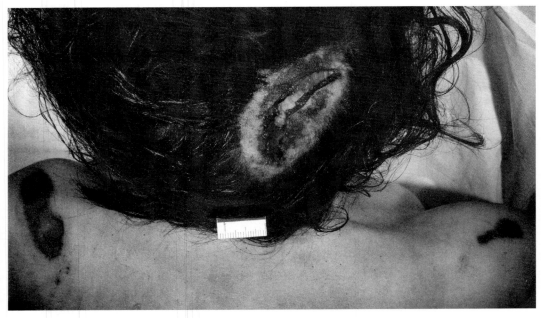

FIGURE XVII-18b. Similar injury as seen in Figure XVII-18a. The laceration suggests a faster moving vehicle.

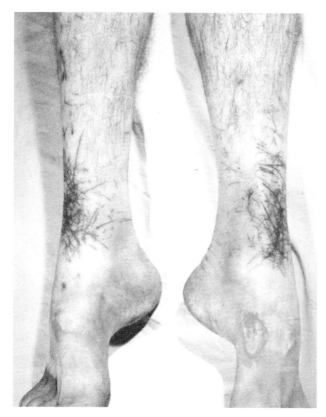

FIGURE XVII-19. Typical brush burns from walking through brush.

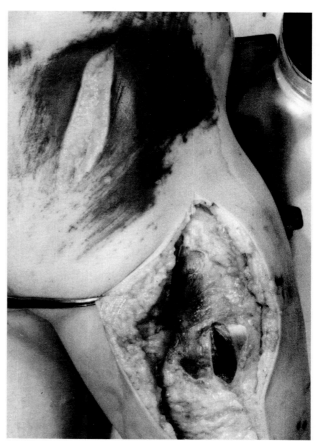

FIGURE XVII-20. Pedestrian who was struck by an automobile. Characteristic brush burns on the flank and buttock due to scraping on the road surface. There are no hemorrhages under the brush burns. The injury of the thigh is the site of impact. Incision shows hemorrhage.

The circumstances of a pedestrian accident are different in the case of an adult who was struck by a fast-moving van, truck, or bus, all of which have a high and flush front end. The victim, when struck, is thrown forward or sideways rather than upward, or, if the vehicle travels at high speed, he may be carried by centrifugal force on the radiator grill before falling to the ground, and perhaps run over, when the vehicle slows down or comes to a halt.

When a small child is struck by an automobile, the mechanism of injury is similar to that of an adult who is struck by a van, truck, or bus. In children the primary impact is likely to be located above the center of gravity, frequently involving the head area.

Both adults and children are often run over when struck by a reversing bus or truck. This occurs when the point of impact is high, above the center of gravity.

For an effective reconstruction of a motor vehicle crash, injuries sustained by dragging or scraping on the ground must be identified and distinguished from those sustained as a result of a direct impact by or on the vehicle.

The term, *brush burn* is taken from the type of scratches sustained from walking through brush (Fig. XVII-19). With regards to traffic, injuries sustained by dragging or scraping are referred to as *brush burns*. They are usually superficial, even if spread over large areas and without significant hemorrhage in the skin and subcutaneous tissues (Fig. XVII-20). The word *burn* in *brush burn* refers to the fact that the upper layer of the skin is scraped off, resulting in a painful injury oozing serum, and causing significant fluid loss, similar to

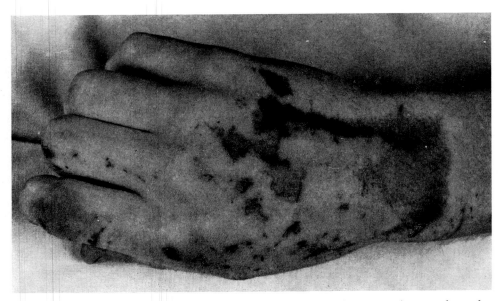

Figure XVII-21a. Brush burns on the back of the right hand and wrist, predominantly on the protuberant areas.

a second-degree thermal burn. A brush burn consists of numerous thin, straight, superficial scratches, each produced by a rolling and scraping grain of sand or dust. Unusual brush burn patterns occur depending on the road surface. For example, non-skid concrete with grooves cut into the surface or a road surface scored with parallel lines in preparation for resurfacing, may be mistaken for an imprint from a striking vehicle or its undercarriage. Scene inspection may resolve the issue.

Depending on the force of the impact on the ground, deep tissues may be extensively torn and bones may be fractured. Protuberant areas of the body, such as in the face and over joints, ribs, and, to a lesser extent, over tendons, are predominantly injured. Recessed surfaces are spared (Fig. XVII-21a–c).

Deep skeletal injuries occur when dragging extends over a long stretch of road. We have observed an entire hemipelvis *planed away* when a man, hanging out the passenger side of his vehicle, tried to stop a car jacking.

Very severe, often characteristic injuries result when an automobile runs over a body. The grinding action of the spinning wheel causes tearing and separation of the skin from the subcutaneous tissues and musculature (Fig. XVII-22).

The musculature may be bruised but remains intact if the wheel is spinning. Bruising of the skin may be slight or absent. However, if the brakes are applied, the wheels of the vehicle lock and vast lacerations result from the shearing and pulling action of this tangential type of force. Amputation of an extremity or decapitation, may occur (Fig. XVII-23). A body may be dragged and spun as a result of being run over. Thus, tire marks or grease from the undercarriage of the vehicle may sometimes be seen on the surface of the body in contact with the vehicle, while the opposite side of the body shows brush burns from contact with the road. Contrary to expectation, running over a body with the brakes applied more often causes disarticulation rather than fracture. Thus, comminuted fractures of both legs are more likely the result of bumper impact than running over by the locked wheel of an automobile. Fractures in children run over by motor vehicles may be absent due to the considerable pliability of their soft, partly cartilaginous skeleton. In a case involving a three-year-old child, who was run over by a pickup truck, there were no fractured ribs or vertebrae, but all thoracic organs and the liver were crushed into a semi-liquid pulp (Fig. XVII-24).

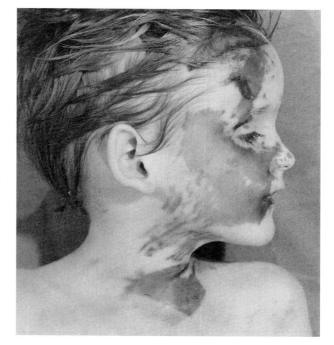

FIGURE XVII-21b. Pedestrian struck by automobile. Brush burns on the right side of the face due to scraping on the road. Lacerations on the right side of the forehead. The eye area is spared.

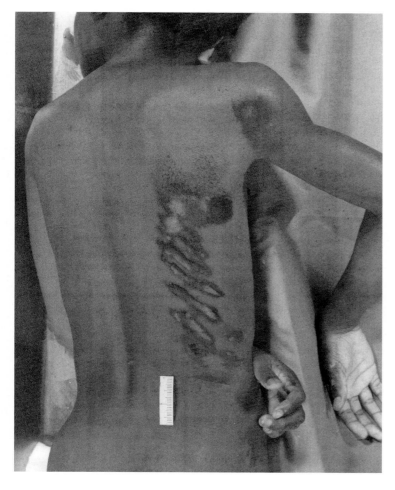

FIGURE XVII-21c. Scraping on road causes the outline of the ribs. The deeper abrasions are pale.

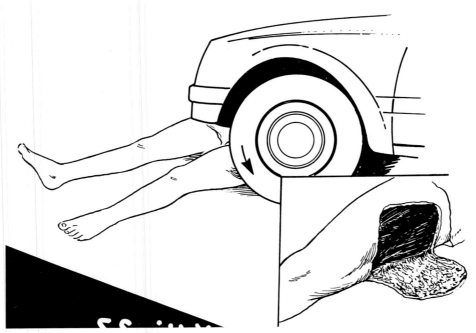

FIGURE XVII-22. Separation of the skin is due to the pull of the tire as it spins.

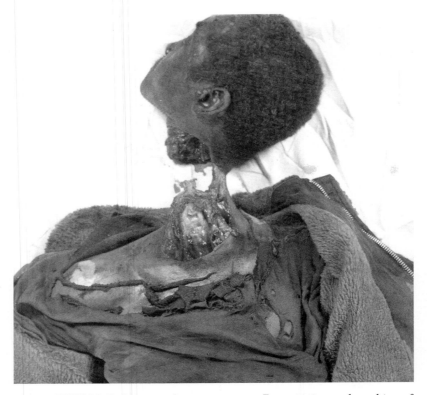

FIGURE XVII-23. Pedestrian who was run over. Decapitation and crushing of the vertebral column by the wheel of the vehicle.

Avulsion of an ear almost always occurs if a tire passes over the head of the victim. The ear is literally *pulled off* by the moving wheel. The tear is behind the ear if the vehicle rolls from back to front in relation to the victim, and it is located in front of the ear if the vehicle travels in the opposite direction (Fig. XVII-25). Tissue bridges are often noted in these tears.

Tire marks often remain as trace evidence on the body of the victim or his clothes (Fig. XVII-26). Tire marks are especially helpful in establishing the identity of the vehicle involved in the crash. No two tires are alike. Small imperfections in the pattern of the tread are specific for each tire (Fig. XVII-27). A useful procedure for comparing the pattern on the body with that of a suspected tire is to copy the imprint from the skin or clothing onto a sheet of transparent paper. Such a tracing permits easy side-by-side comparison with the tire print and can be retained on file for documentation. The importance of photography before autopsy cannot be overemphasized. Some spreading of the impression on the skin due to flattening of the body by the weight of the vehicle has to be considered. The side of the body in contact with the road usually shows typical brush burns or the patterned imprint of gravel (Fig. XVII-28).

A treadless tire obviously leaves no tire marks. There are other situations where a victim had been run over, but no tire marks could be identified on the body or clothing (Fig. XVII-29a–c). An opinion as to whether *running over* had occurred must be based on all findings, including the scene and autopsy.

The Driver and the Passenger

While injuries of pedestrians usually conform to a set pattern, those found in drivers and passengers are considerably less uniform. When a motor vehicle comes to a sudden stop as a result of a collision, unrestrained occupants of the vehicle continue to move in the direction of travel and at the same speed. An automobile is a spacious environment in which an unrestrained occupant may be thrown in any direction, sustaining different types of injury of varying severity.

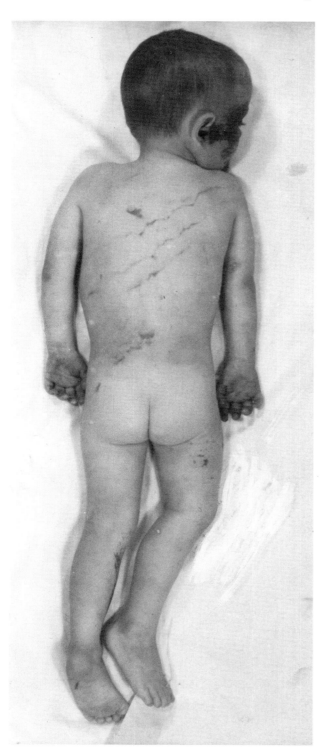

FIGURE XVII-24. Child run over by a truck with tire marks across the back. The right side of the face was against the pavement, hence the abrasion. The contour of the body is intact.

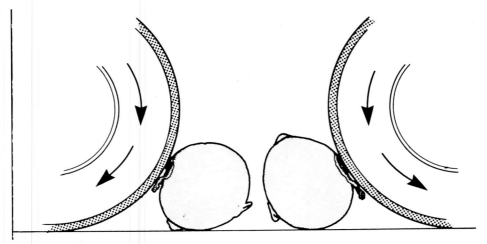

FIGURE XVII-25. Avulsion of the ear depends on the position of the head or the direction of the moving vehicle.

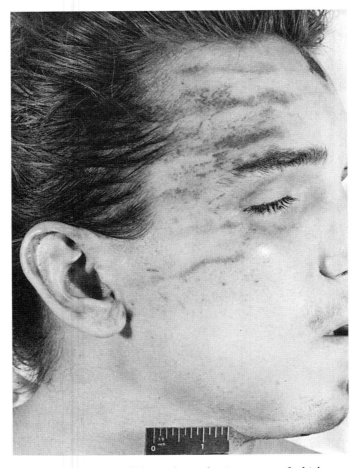

FIGURE XVII-26. Parallel equidistant bruises, some of which suggest a zig-zag, and equal spacing between the lines, represent the pattern of a tire tread.

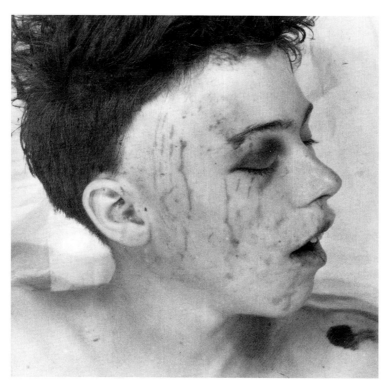

FIGURE XVII-27. Pedestrian run over by a car, showing tire marks. The skull was fractured.

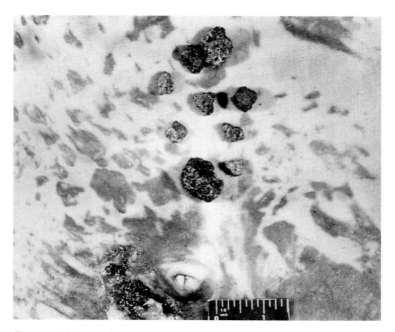

FIGURE XVII-28. Stamp-like abrasions from gravel. The body did not slide and the gravel did not move.

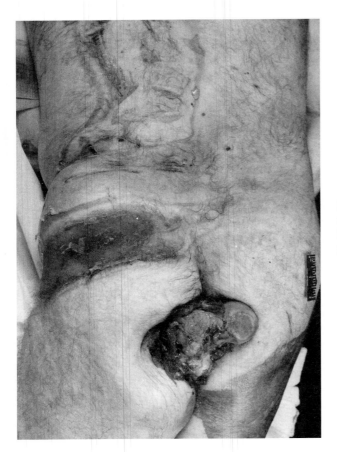

FIGURE XVII-29a. Ejected driver whose vehicle came to rest on his body causing charring and second-degree burns by the exhaust system and laceration of the perineum with protrusion of the bowel.

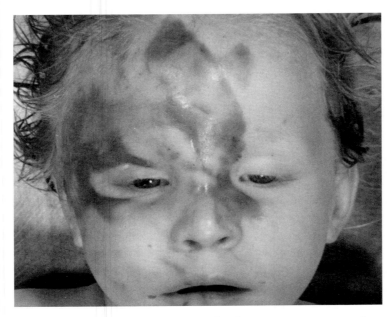

FIGURE XVII-29b. Child playing in the driveway was run over face down by vehicle backing out of a garage. The pale areas on the forehead and around the eyes are recessed, therefore undamaged.

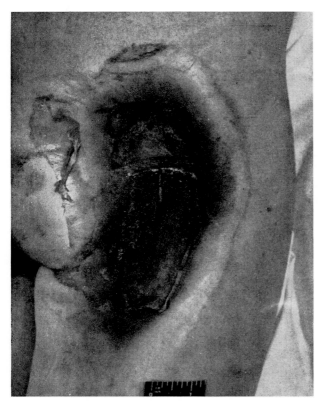

FIGURE XVII-29c. Muffler burn. The dark outer ring (red) and the adjacent pale zone are due to blood moved by the heat from the area of charring and do not represent evidence of active circulation. The heart was severed in the initial impact.

A consensus viewpoint among automotive safety engineers is that with diminishing size of American cars, so goes their safety. On the other hand, any interior surface of a vehicle which is close to the occupant during a crash is likely to cause less injury than one farther away. Thus, the relative velocity between the vehicle interior and the occupant tends to be less the closer and better padded the *shell*. Automakers may reflect this design in the future by manufacturing larger vehicles with better cushioned, smaller interiors. Even at the present time, occupants of larger cars, say a 2004 Cadillac Seville or Lincoln Town Car weighing over 4000 pounds, stand a significantly better chance in a collision than those in a down-sized vehicle, such as a 2004 Ford Focus or Dodge Neon weighing approximately 2700 pounds. In a head-on collision of two such cars, each traveling 40 mph, unrestrained occupants of the small car would be thrown against the rigid interior of their vehicle with twice as much force as would the occupants of the larger vehicle. Over 50% of highway deaths occur in head-on crashes.

A rule of thumb for estimating the speed of an automobile prior to crashing into a stationary barrier, such as a wall, is based on the severity of intrusion. It is usually considered that one inch of deformity is equivalent to one mile per hour. Accidents are categorized as:

- Low severity   0–8 inches of deformity
- Moderate severity   9–16 inches of deformity
- High severity   17 or more inches of deformity

In a side impact, intrusion of 12–15 inches indicates high crash forces.

In rear-end collisions, the occupants of the *bullet* car are less likely to be severely injured than the occupants of the *target* vehicle. The engine in the front affords significant protection, and the cushioning effect of the rear of the target vehicle allows for gradual deceleration of the bullet car.

In a documented case, two cars of similar weight were involved in a rear-end collision. The *bullet* car was traveling at a speed exceeding 70 mph. Except for a few scrapes and bruises, the driver of this vehicle was uninjured. The target vehicle was entering a construction zone and slowing when struck in the rear. The driver of the *target* vehicle was dead at the scene.

While there may be limitations, valuable information pertinent to the reconstruction of an automobile crash may be obtained from injury analysis of vehicle occupants.

A Chrysler sedan was traveling downhill on a city street, which intersects and dead-ends with a major highway. The vehicle ran off the right side of the street, re-entered the roadway, crossed the midline, went up an embankment and hit a tree. The automobile then rolled over on its right side and came to rest near a telephone pole, 75 feet before reaching the intersection. The latter part of the incident was observed by two policemen in a patrol car traveling in the opposite direction. Immediate investigation by the officers found the sole occupant, a young woman, thrown onto the right front door of the vehicle. Her face was covered with blood. Swelling and contusion of the right hand were noticed. She was pronounced dead at the scene.

Postmortem examination showed multiple fresh typical blunt force injuries of the forehead, the left ear, scalp, right hand and left forearm. The base of the skull was extensive-

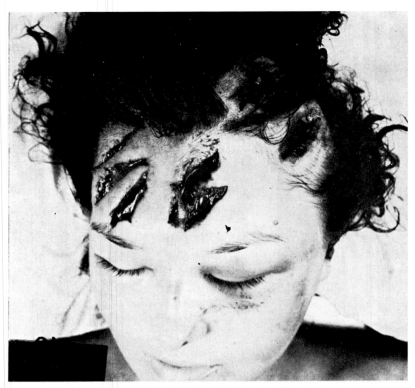

FIGURE XVII-30. Multiple injuries of the forehead and scalp due to bludgeoning with a metal pipe. The pattern under the left eye was caused by the thread at the end of the pipe.

ly fractured. No other pertinent findings were noted, except for aspiration and swallowing of blood.

In view of the lack of a plausible anatomical and chronological explanation of the injuries by this apparent accident, the automobile was re-examined. The vehicle showed comparatively little damage, consisting of dents of the left and right sides and fenders. No glass was broken. Clotted blood was noted on and behind the driver's seat, and blood splatters, indicating both forward and backward directions in reference to the upright position of the car, were found on the ceiling.

It was concluded that the woman had been beaten to death in the car and then the car was dispatched down a hill in an effort to conceal the murder. Additionally, a stone was found wedged under the gas pedal, to accelerate the motor. The husband was convicted of bludgeoning his wife, probably with a piece of metal pipe, then attempting to simulate an accident (Fig. XVII-30).

Patterned injuries from the steering wheel or steering column (Fig. XVII-31a–b), from knobs on the dashboard or the doors or other protruding objects of definite shapes within the vehicle may be of assistance in determining the direction of thrust and possibly establish how the occupants were seated.

Identification of the driver is essential. An important finding may be the imprinted pattern of the gas or brake pedal on the sole of the driver's right shoe; the left shoe may show the pattern of the clutch in a vehicle with standard transmission. Similarly, the presence of shoe sole patterns on the accelerator or brake pedals may be observed on rare occasions. The driver's shoes must therefore be recovered and examined. The driver's feet are frequently wedged under the front seat when the car comes to a sudden halt as a result of a collision. Laceration and fracture of the ankle are often observed in such situations (Fig. XVII-32). Unfortunately, the shoes of car occupants are often considered irrelevant and discarded or left in the vehicle.

When an unrestrained driver's head strikes the windshield, strands of hair may be trapped in the broken glass (Fig. XVII-33). Such hair, and

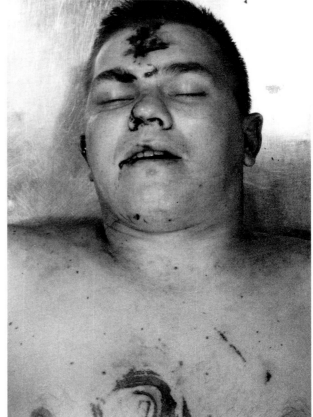

FIGURE XVII-31a. Unbelted driver who struck the steering column. The head jackknifed causing the forehead to strike the top of the steering wheel.

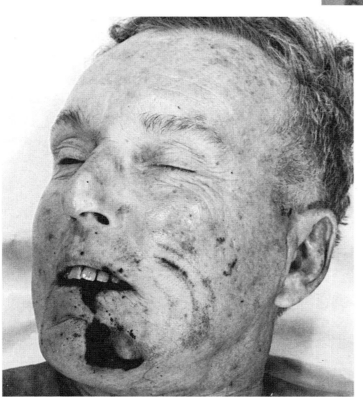

FIGURE XVII-31b. Steering column injury on face.

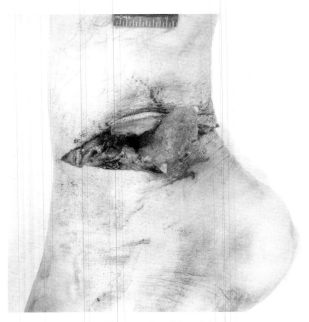

FIGURE XVII-32. Fractured ankle of front-seat occupant. The seat moved forward during the collision wedging the foot.

sometimes blood, may assist in identifying the driver. It is important that the inner surface of the windshield be examined for the presence of hair and blood. Often the windshield is dislodged from the frame, draped over the steering wheel or thrown on the road. Hair and/or blood may also be found on the A-pillars (which are the lateral roof supports between the windshield and the front door), window channels, doors, steering wheel, or dashboard. Any such evidence must be collected and compared with known samples taken from the vehicle occupants. Identification of such evidence and its location within the vehicle will provide information regarding the pattern of movement of vehicle occupants following the crash.

A toddler in the rear seat on the passenger side was thrown forward and broke the plastic covering of the driver side B-pillar, when the vehicle abruptly veered right following a minor crash involving the right front fender. Hairs with roots from the child's head were found trapped inside cracks in the B-pillar cover, negating the plaintiff's theory

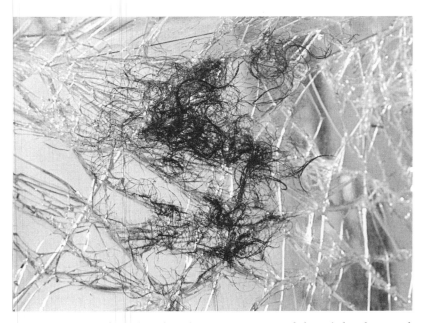

FIGURE XVII-33. Strands of hair from an unrestrained driver's head trapped among fragments of glass in windshield.

that the hair had been deposited when the child was brushed against the B-pillar as the body was removed from the vehicle. The finding of trapped hair affirmed the defense theory that the child had not been restrained. The child died of head injuries.

Blood deteriorates rapidly as a result of decomposition, especially in a warm environment, and should be preserved and refrigerated or analyzed promptly. Mold may further obscure the characteristic appearance of blood stains. However, uncontaminated dry blood is suitable for DNA testing for years.

Trauma associated with an impact on the chest by the steering wheel or column is often severe, despite absent or minimal, external evidence of injury. Frontal impacts may cause transverse fracture of the sternum, usually in the area of the manubrium, and rib fractures, along the sides of the chest. Other locations of rib fractures vary, depending on the angle of impact. Occasionally, the lower portion of the steering wheel crushes the upper abdominal area, causing frontal tears of the liver. Central liver tears also occur frequently. Such tears may rupture the liver capsule and bleed into the abdominal cavity several days after injury. Multiple fractures of the rib cage, as well as tears and bruises of the heart and lungs are common. Sometimes the heart is shredded due to crushing between the chest plate and spine. In young adults, the ribs and chest plate may be intact. In the absence of naked eye evidence of heart muscle injury, microscopic examination may reveal bruises and torn muscle fibers which may have triggered rhythm abnormalities of the heartbeat and death. Among less common injuries are central tears of the lung, i.e., without communication with the pleural surface. Fatalities following compression of the chest without apparent injury to the chest wall have been abundantly documented. On the other hand, extensive bruises of the anterior chest wall may also cause death of an elderly individual, even without fractures of the rib cage or other evidence of trauma.

Laceration of the aorta at the level of the aortic ligament is frequent. The aorta is fixed and unyielding in this area. Tears of the aorta are not limited to steering wheel impact. The jarring effect on the chest organs as a result of an intersection-type collision, i.e., a side impact, may shear the ascending segment of the aorta. In some instances, horizontal and V-shaped superficial tears of the aortic intima are due to the same mechanism (Fig. XVII-34). Sometimes, such superficial tears expand and deepen as a result of the blood pressure within the aorta, causing delayed dissection and perforation of the aorta and sudden death, sometimes hours after the crash.

The female driver of a motor vehicle involved in a collision sustained superficial abrasions and bruises. Two male passengers debated between themselves at the scene who would be transported to the hospital first, since the ambulance could only transport two victims. The male occupant who stayed behind to wait for the second ambulance arrived at the hospital approximately 20 minutes after the first dispatch. He was talking en route and appeared uninjured. Suddenly, as the ambulance arrived at the hospital, he became unconscious and was pronounced DOA.

At autopsy, the aorta was severed at the arch (ligamentum arteriosum). Superficial horizontal intimal tears were noted above and below the level of severance. There was massive bleeding into the left chest cavity. No other injuries were present.

Extensive injuries may be sustained, especially in unrestrained drivers, as a result of striking the steering wheel (see Fig. XVII-31b). Such trauma may help to identify who was driving the vehicle. Facial lacerations and fractures of the facial skeleton, especially the nose and maxilla, by impact on the steering wheel occur.

Although today's steering columns are collapsible, in high speed, head-on collisions, the entire steering assembly may be moved inward, sometimes with the engine, causing severe chest injuries whether restraints were worn or not.

Occasionally, an automobile strikes a semi-tractor-trailer or other large truck, usually in the rear and most often as a result of intoxication of the driver. The front of the car passes under the larger vehicle, and the steel lower corner of its carriage shears off the roof, causing decapitation of the occupants. We have observed several cases where the driver's entire facial skin without bone was actually *shaved-off* and found at the scene, separated from the body (Fig. XVII-35a–b).

Injuries to the neck, so-called whiplash injuries, are still common despite prophylactic headrests mandatory on all models of automobiles. Although adjustable, the majority of head-

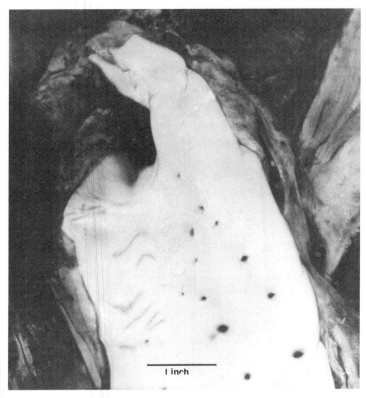

FIGURE XVII-34. Superficial tears of the aortic lining in a driver with steering wheel injury.

rests provide little or no protection in crash situations. We believe the majority of people do not know that headrests should be adjusted and do not adjust them to protect their neck. If the distance between the head and the headrest is excessive, a whiplash-type neck injury may occur before the backward thrust of the head is mitigated or stopped by the headrest.

While fractures and dislocations have been described as occurring particularly in the levels of the fifth and sixth cervical vertebrae, there appears to be some question regarding the severity of other neck injuries associated with the whiplash mechanism. Routine exploration at autopsy of the cervical spine in motor vehicle fatalities has shown a significant incidence of injury of the atlanto-occipital joints, which include laceration of tendons and joint capsules, intra-articular hemorrhages and tears with separation of the cartilaginous lining of the articular surfaces. Such injuries, while of apparent minor

importance, are certainly indicative of trauma to this vital area. Laceration, crushing, bruising, or other obvious injury of the medulla is uncommon. In fatal cases in which no other evidence of significant injury can be found, consideration should be given to possible concussion of the medulla as the cause of death. Microscopic examination of the medulla may reveal hemorrhages not visible to the naked eye.

Whiplash injuries of the neck are not limited to front or rear-end collisions. The cervical spine is just as vulnerable to side impacts. Skeletal and soft tissue damage sustained in intersection-type crashes are usually indistinguishable from injuries which occur in frontal or rear-end collisions. Removal of the atlas through a posterior midline incision permits demonstration of skeletal and soft tissue injuries to this part of the body as well as inspection of the underside of the base of the skull. This procedure does not affect subsequent laminectomy for examination of the

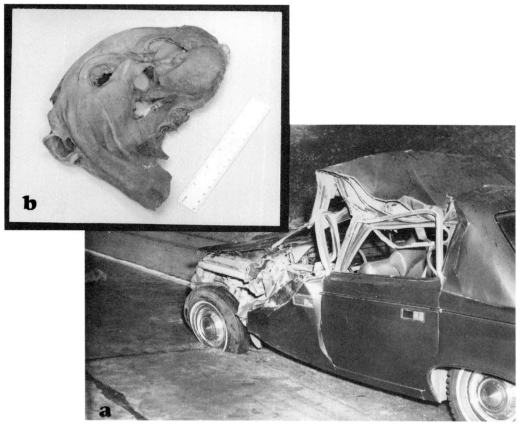

FIGURE XVII-35a–b. (a) Car which rear-ended an unlit parked semi shaving off the face of the driver. (b) The mummified face was found a year later in a ditch at the site of the crash.

spinal cord and does not cause mutilation which may interfere with later viewing of the remains. Leakage of embalming fluids through this incision has not, in our experience, been subject of complaints by relatives and funeral directors.

Seat Belts

The importance of seat belts in the prevention of crash injuries cannot be overemphasized. According to States,[3] three principles essential to protect motor vehicle occupants are: (1) an intact occupant compartment, (2) energy absorption external to the occupant compartment, and (3) occupant restraint within the compartment. The latter is to prevent ejection and the *second impact*. The first impact is that of the car with whatever it strikes, such as another car, a tree or

other fixed object. The second impact occurs when the occupant strikes the interior of the car. When an automobile is traveling at 30 mph collides head-on with a large tree or bridge abutment, the car begins to crumble and slow down. Within one-tenth of a second after the impact the car has stopped. But the unrestrained occupant, obeying the laws of motion, continues to move forward at the same speed the car was traveling. Within one-fiftieth of a second, the occupant slams into the windshield, dashboard, or steering wheel with a force, which even at the low speed of 30 mph, exceeds 100 times the force of gravity. An occupant wearing a seat belt slows down with the vehicle, rather than being stopped short by some hard structure inside the car.

A back-seat passenger in an automobile was catapulted forward in a head-on collision and died as a result of striking her forehead against the exposed ball joint of the rearview mirror which penetrated the skull. There were no other significant injuries.

Seat belts are designed to restrain the body in two ways: (1) the lap portion of the belt anchors the body below the waistline; (2) the shoulder strap keeps the head and upper torso from striking the windshield and steering wheel. However, because the head and neck are unrestrained, cervical spinal injuries may occur to restrained front seat occupants due to the inertial forces of the mass of the head acting on the neck. Similarly, in a side impact, as in collision of two vehicles in an intersection or a side impact of a car against a tree, restraint of an occupant of the *target* car is likely to provide little protection. The head of this individual is thrust toward the impacting force and fatal injuries are common. We have observed a number of cases where a restrained occupant of the *target* car, sustained fatal head injuries by impact on the *bullet* car. The same occurs in a rollover accident where the restrained occupant of the vehicle sustains fatal head injuries from striking the ground or is crushed under the vehicle, sometimes with minor injuries, but evidence suggestive of asphyxiation.

The first time seat belts were offered in an American car, the *Tucker,* was 1947. Today, the use of seat belts is mandated across the United States, except for New Hampshire. Also, all 50 states and the District of Columbia have child restraint laws which require children to travel in approved child restraint devices.

Submarining or *slipping* of the body from under the restraint system is infrequent, but occurs occasionally in rear-end collisions.

The singer, Harry Chapin was killed when a truck rear-ended the 1975 Volkswagen Rabbit he was driving. As a result of the impact, Mr. Chapin's restrained body *slipped* from under the lap belt he was wearing *(submarined)*, slammed against the back rest of his seat, causing the seat bracket to break. This allowed his body (6'3" - 210 lbs.) to slide rearward, striking his head above the rear window and bouncing his back on the back of the driver's seat. The impact in mid-back, fractured and dislocated a thoracic vertebra while the impact of the head pushed the vertebral column downward, toward the feet. Forward movement of the spine caused the sharp lower front edge of the displaced vertebra to cut into the aorta, resulting in fatal internal bleeding (Fig. XVII-36).

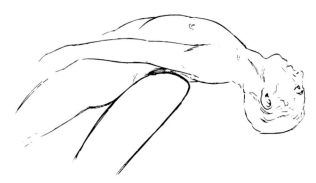

FIGURE XVII-36. Occupant submarined under lap belt, slammed against the back rest, causing the seat bracket to break. The body slid rear-ward, striking his head above the rear window and bouncing his back on the back of the driver's seat. This caused vertebral dislocation. The dislocated vertebra cut into the aorta causing massive internal hemorrhage.

A similar injury occurred to a middle-aged forklift operator, moving crates. The operator stood in the open rear of the forklift, facing forward. On backing up the man's back struck a protruding 3/4 inch sheet of plywood, used as a shelf. He was dead at the scene and autopsy showed a fractured thoracic vertebra displaced forward cutting into the aorta (Fig. XVII-37).

Another crash involved a speeding truck which rear-ended a stopped passenger car, causing a 4-year-old boy, seated in the back seat, to slip out from under his restraint and *submarine* rearward. The truck penetrated the smaller vehicle striking the child in the forehead, causing his death.

Injuries are sometimes caused by the use of seat belts. Seat belts are rugged and abrasive. Such injuries range from superficial bruises and abrasions to severe fractures, internal damage, even rare decapitation (Fig. XVII-38a–d).

When they occur, bruises and abrasions are situated along the path of the seat belt, i.e., the side of the neck, the front of the shoulder, the hip and sometimes the chest and abdomen. Parallel lines from the edges of the seat belt, the weave pattern or stitching along the edges, may be imprinted on the skin. The location of these injuries will often aid in determining whether the victim was the driver and also, his movements in the vehicle in response to the impact (Fig. XIV-39a–b). Sometimes clothes will display evidence of direct seat belt contact, such as rubbing, however care must be taken in interpreting these markings:

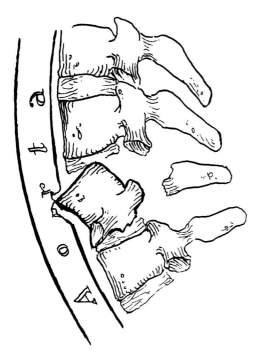

Scale ··· approx ½

FIGURE XVII-37. Fracture and dislocation of a thoracic vertebra lacerating the aorta. The identical mechanism of injury occurred in Figure XVII-36.

A driver of a sports car crashed the right side of his vehicle into a tree. In reconstructing the accident, questions arose regarding whether he was restrained and what his movements were following the crash.

The mechanics of the crash indicated that the body had moved to the right striking the top of the B-pillar from where the victim's hair was recovered. There were parallel, horizontal, linear markings on his dark blue cotton windbreaker jacket in the area of the left shoulder blade, the center back and the right posterior waist area. The markings were at first thought to have come from the weave pattern of the seat belt. However, further examination revealed that they were transfers from the windbreaker liner as the driver's body twisted rearward and to the right striking and deforming the right passenger seat and center console. The presence of the markings confirmed that the driver was not wearing a seat belt and his movements in the vehicle were as a result of impact.

Fractures of the clavicle or ribs, lacerations of the liver, spleen and small intestines, as well as the aorta caused by seatbelts have been

described. We have observed two cases of decapitation, with minimal other injuries and dismemberment, involving loss of an arm. When these types of injury occur, they usually result from improper positioning of the belt. The edge of the belt cuts through the skin and severs the joint. The bone is not damaged.

Another injury which may be related to improper use of restraints is the Chance fracture in which a lumbar vertebra is split horizontally from the spinous process forward. It occurs predominately in frontal collisions due to acute forward flexion of the upper half of the body over the lap belt. Chance fracture was more common before the three-point seat belt system was introduced. Now, this injury is rare.

Hangman's fracture which is the bilateral fracture of the pedicles of second cervical vertebra was frequently seen when judicial hanging was practiced. A few cases, related to automobile crashes, have been reported in recent years and there appears to be some debate about, whether the fracture results from the absence of a headrest, striking the head on the roof of the car or the steering wheel, or whether the injury is attributable to improper seat belt use.[4]

As to pregnancy, a recent study concludes that most women wear automobile restraints during pregnancy, but despite excellent compliance, the restraints are often worn improperly.[5]

When responding to the scene of a traffic crash, extrication of an injured or deceased occupant from a vehicle often requires removal of a seat belt. Whether a seat belt was worn may become crucial evidence in subsequent litigation. Therefore, it is important that witnesses at the scene and EMS personnel be questioned without delay regarding whether the occupants were restrained. If so, who unbuckled the victims? Such information should be noted in investigative and other official reports.

On occasion it may be necessary to cut a seat belt when removing a victim. Since seat belt webbing may fray with time, it is recommended that the belt be cut diagonally or in a zigzag pattern, to exclude that the belt may have been torn in the crash as a result of webbing failure. Examination of the webbing may also be significant in

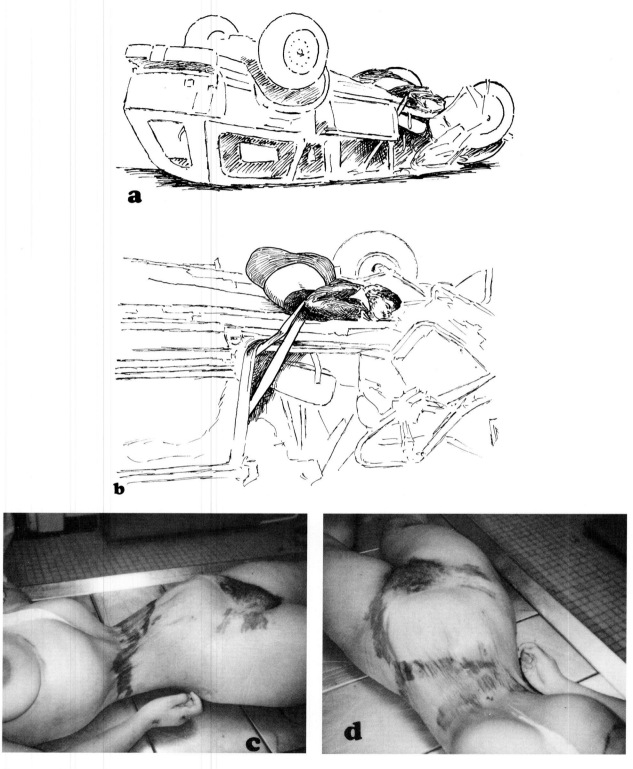

FIGURE XVII-38a–d. Unrestrained young driver who rolled her SUV which came to a rest upside down (a). She was eject-ed through the driver's door and became entangled in the seat belt (b). The body shows the abrasions, produced by the seat belt, and overstretching injuries in both groins (c–d), from the pull over the pubic bone of the anterior abdominal wall.

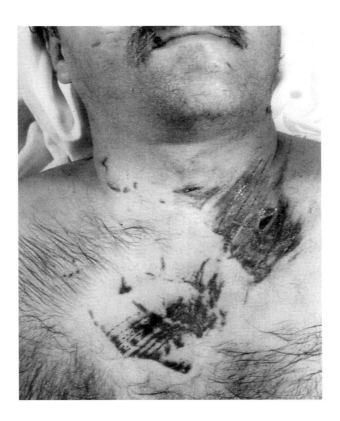

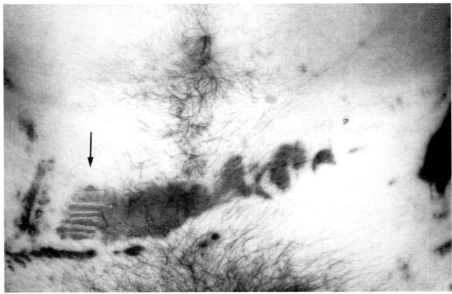

FIGURE XVII-39a–b. (a) Weave pattern of seat belt running from left to right, typical for the driver. (b) Lap belt imprint showing weave pattern (arrow).

determining seat belt effectiveness. Such inspection often reveals an area of friction wear at the *D-ring* level. This ring is situated above the door, slightly behind the occupant and secures the upper end of the shoulder harness. When suddenly stressed, the seat belt strap may be abraded by the *D-ring*. Location of such damage indicates the amount of slack in the harness. Damage at the far end of the strap is likely to result from too much slack and would suggest an ineffective belt. The size of the occupant, position and adjustment of the restraint must be considered when evaluating the functioning of a seat belt.

Air Bags

Air bags deploy in response to compression of front bumper sensors, usually at speeds above 8 to 14 mph. Steering wheel and dashboard mounted air bags are not designed to deploy on side impacts.

Air bags are designed to protect average adults in 35 mph frontal crashes. While protecting the chest from impact on the steering wheel, air bags also mitigate the violent whiplash motion of the head in a frontal crash, by providing a more gradual deceleration of the head and neck (Fig. XVII-40). Injuries of the neck are significantly reduced and the face is protected from contact with hard or lacerating surfaces. Federal law mandates that all passenger cars manufactured after September 1, 1997 be equipped with both driver and passenger side air bags, as well as manual lap and shoulder belts.

The combined use of seat belts and air bags provides greater protection. Air bags deploy rapidly, faster than the blink of an eye (up to 200 mph/322 kph). No sooner has it inflated, it deflates, the entire process lasts one to two seconds. The exploding force of the inflating air bag can injure an occupant who is seated too close, unrestrained, or improperly restrained. The *risk zone* for driver air bags is the first 2–3 inches (5–8 cm) of inflation. Most agree that 10 inches (25 cm) of clearance are required to allow the air bag to safely inflate and even then, severe injuries and fatalities have been reported.[6]

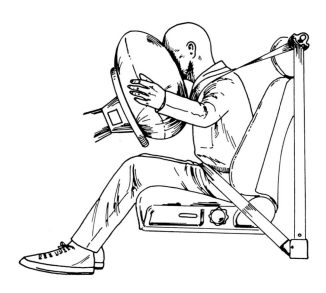

FIGURE XVII-40. Air bags provide significant protection when used in conjunction with seat belts.

Among the injuries associated with air bag deployment, fractures of the arms and forearms (predominately on the right side) are of particular interest.[7-9] Such injuries point to the driver, especially if the occupant of the right front seat shows no such injury. Facial bruises and abrasions are occasionally seen as a result of air bag deployment and abrasion of the chin due to the air bag's slap is no exception.[10-11] Laceration of the brain stem and cervical dislocations have been associated with air bag-related trauma and hemothorax with and without rib fractures are among the injuries caused by air bags.

Creams, hair gels, makeup and lipstick from the front seat occupants may be deposited on the bag and serve to identify the seating position. The weave pattern, seams, stitches and the deflating holes of the bags may be imprinted on the skin and produce confusing bruises and abrasions, sometimes suggestive of ligatures, fingernail marks or some other type of deliberate injury (Fig. XVII-41). The clothes or jewelry worn by the occupant may leave their own markings and depending on the type of clothes may simulate assault. Occasionally, an earring may be ripped out causing extensive damage to the area (Fig. XVII-42).

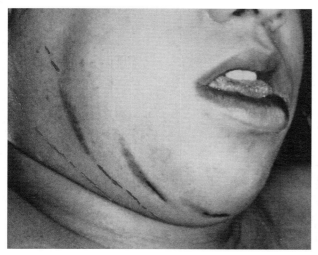

FIGURE XVII-41. Parallel abrasions, some of which show the weave pattern of the air bag.

Children and small stature adults are especially susceptible for facial and neck injuries. Therefore, children less than 13 years of age should be seated in the back seat. Pregnant women are at risk for fetal injury.

Glass

Federal standards for windshields are multi-pronged and aimed at preventing ejection of occupants, withstanding the force of an air bag and supporting the roof in rollover situations. Federal regulations currently allow three types of glass for use in motor vehicles: laminated, tempered and glass-plastic.[12]

Laminated

Disfiguring and even life-threatening injuries of the face and neck have decreased dramatically since the introduction of laminated windshields in 1966. All cars, vans and trucks use laminated windshields usually consisting of two sheets of glass with an inner middle layer of tough flexible plastic (polyvinyl butyral (PVB) and layers of adhesive material. Laminated glass is allowed in all vehicle windows but is typically used only in windshields. A multitude of thickness combinations are being manufactured,

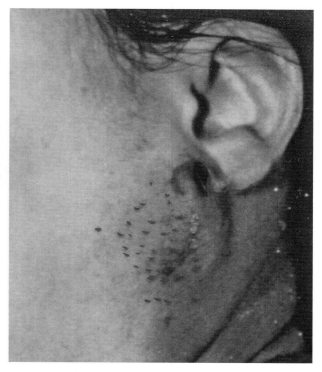

FIGURE XVII-42. Earring ripped out of the earlobe with evidence of abrasion on the cheek. A blow by the air bag slapped the earring against the skin.

depending on vehicle specifications, in order to provide desirable levels of optical, structural, acoustical and safety performance.

A low bond strength between the layer of plastic and the glass provides for greater energy absorption on impact and considerable bulging of the windshield before tearing of the plastic allows penetration (Fig. XVII-43a–c). The perforation velocity of these windshields is given at about 30 mph and has not changed significantly over the last 15 years. Most automobile collisions occur below this speed.

Although, the windshield still breaks like ordinary plate glass, the glass shards adhere to the inner plastic which keeps them in place instead of flying into the vehicle's compartment (Fig. XVII-44). A laminated windshield acts as an energy absorbing *safety net* which keeps the occupants inside the vehicle during a crash. However, in high-speed collisions, penetration and perforation of the windshield by the head still occurs. This may cause deep, often parallel, horizontal

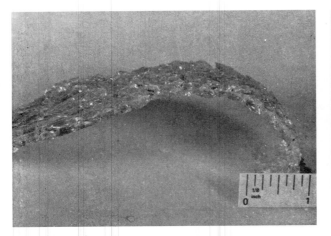

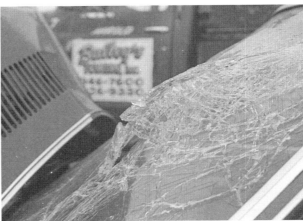

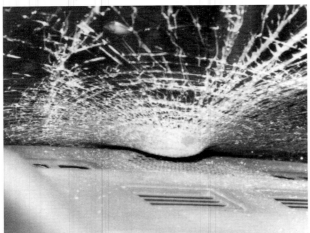

FIGURE XVII-43a-c. (a–b) Section of broken windshield illustrates the amount of *give* upon impact, prior to rupture. A layer of plastic is sandwiched between two sheets of glass. (c) Inward broken windshield after striking a pedestrian. The shape of the penetration suggests an elbow.

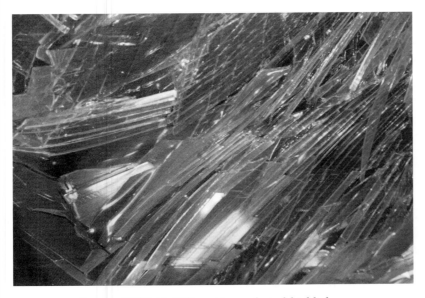

FIGURE XVII-44. Different type of windshield glass.

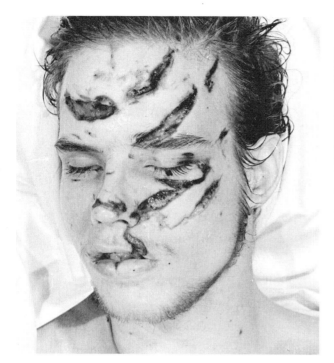

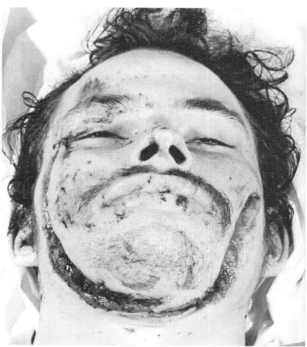

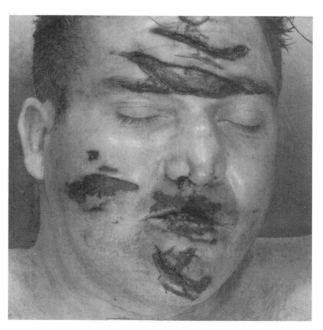

FIGURE XVII-45a–c. (a–c) Perforation of the head through a windshield causing deep, parallel, diagonal cuts of the face. (b) Driver's head extended through the windshield causing severe cuts below the chin. The head which perforates a windshield bobs up and down until the vehicle comes to a stop.

or diagonal cuts of the face and neck, due to bobbing of the head in the hole (Fig. XVII-45a–c).

More often, crashes occur at city speed (below 35 mph), where windshield injuries of unrestrained front-seat occupants are caused by sliding on the sharp edges of the fragmented inner pane of glass. Such injuries consist of parallel, vertical, brush burn-like, superficial cuts involving the protuberant areas of the head, such as, the central portion of the forehead and the tip of the nose (Fig. XVII-46a–e). In automobiles equipped with a rearward-inclined windshield,

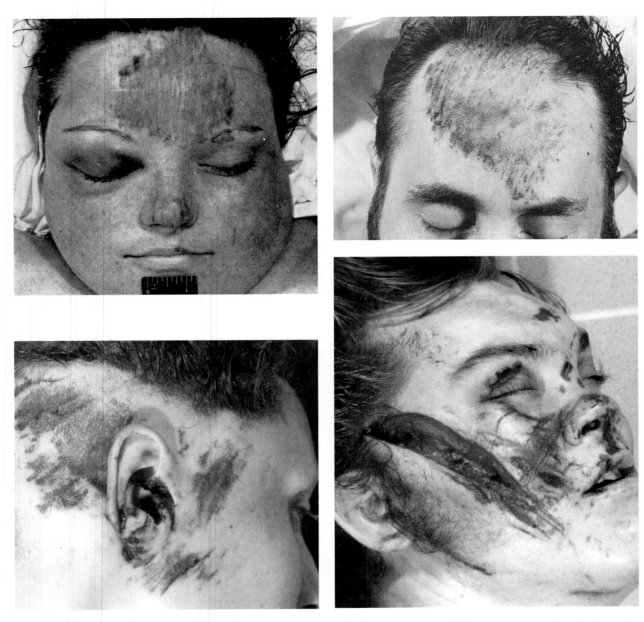

FIGURE XVII-46a–d. (a–b) Unrestrained driver who struck a parked car at low speed. The vertical superficial cuts on the forehead and nose are caused by sliding on the shattered windshield glass. (c) Oblique cuts of the side of the head from broken windshield glass. (d) Deep disfiguring and superficial cuts by windshield glass.

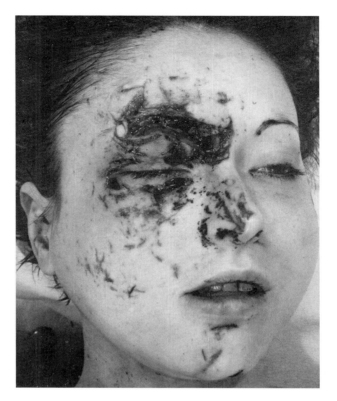

FIGURE XVII-46e. Impact against the windshield causing deep and superficial irregular cuts.

the head may slide down the glass and impact the dashboard. The presence of sharp slivers of glass on the skin or in wounds, however superficial, indicates that they originated from the windshield. Tempered glass does not break into slivers or shards.

Significant brain injury from laminated windshield impact is unlikely and will at most cause a short period of unconsciousness, i.e., concussion. Studies of actual collisions indicate that head deceleration on the windshield is usually nonconsequential, except for the laceration potential of the glass. While manufacturers offer laminated side windows on a select number of luxury vehicles, most are available only in Europe and this has been done to prevent smash and grab theft.

Windshields tend to break in a *spider web* pattern, where the central area represents the point of impact (Figs. XVII-47 and XVII-48).

Tempered

Tempered glass which years ago was used for windshields in the United States is now being used on American cars for the side and rear windows exclusively. This is a heat-treated plate glass which retains a high resistance to bending. When this glass breaks, it shatters into 1/4 inch cubes with sharp edges (Fig. XVII-49). These are usually ejected from the frame, and are found in large numbers at the site of a crash. An occupant of the vehicle who is struck by such flying pieces of glass sustains a typical pattern of right-angled, superficial cuts, commonly referred to as *dicing* because of the rectangular shape of individual injuries (Fig. XVII-50a–f). The presence and location of a *dicing pattern* may help reconstruct an accident.

A driver in a left-sided intersection-type collision would sustain a *dicing pattern* on the left side of his face and arm. In a right-sided intersection-type collision, the right front-seat passenger would sustain the same type of injury on the right side. A passenger seated next to the driver in a car involved in a right-sided collision may shield the driver from flying fragments of glass from a broken door window. In the absence of a front-seat passenger, the driver may sustain facial cuts

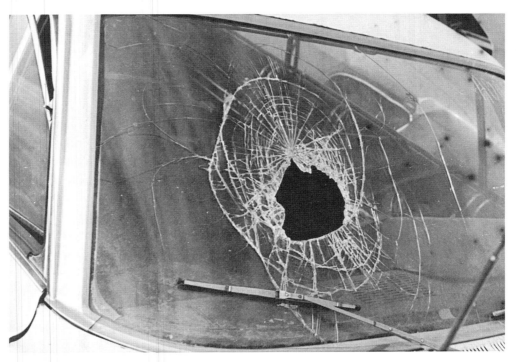

FIGURE XVII-47. Typical *spider web* fracture of the windshield caused by impact of the driver's head. The head did not go through the hole.

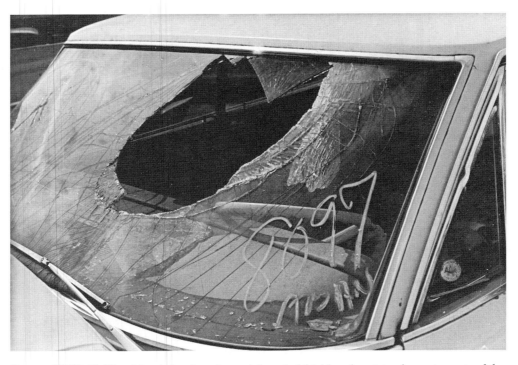

FIGURE XVII-48. The driver's head perforated the windshield and sustained massive cuts of the face and neck.

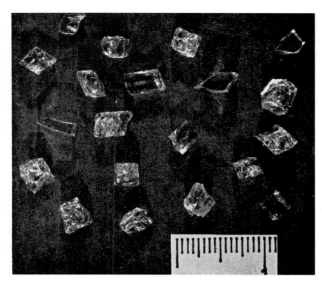

FIGURE XVII-49. Angulated fragments, mostly cubes, of tempered glass used for the side and rear windows of automobiles.

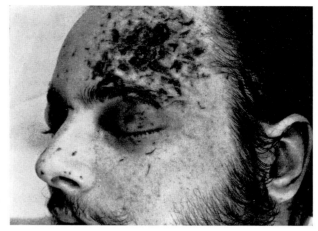

FIGURE XVII-50a. Driver of automobile who skidded into a pole. The driver's side of the automobile sustained the impact. The injuries of the forehead were caused by chunks of tempered glass. Note the rectangular shape of some of the wounds.

from *flying* glass, but such injuries are unlikely to have the typical dense *dicing pattern*. The broken glass cubes travel like shotgun pellets; the greater the distance the wider the spread of the cubes.

Two unrestrained, heavily intoxicated men were driving over a railroad crossing when the right side of their vehicle was struck by a train. Both were killed and thrown under the dashboard. From their positions, it was not possible to ascertain who had been the driver. At postmortem examination, the back of the right hand of one of the men showed a *typical pattern of dicing cuts,* favoring him as the right front-seat passenger who raised his hand in a defensive motion when he saw the approaching train (Fig. XVII-50g).

Impact of the face or head against tempered glass causes crushing of the skin and splits which extend from the site of impact. Additionally, rectangles may be identified within a maze of epidermal tears resembling overstretching (Fig. XVII-51a). When the face strikes, facial bones including the nose may be fractured (Fig. XVII-51b).

Glass-Plastic

Studies by automobile manufacturers, show that 60% of driver and passenger ejections occur through windows other than the windshield. A *glass-plastic* consisting of laminated or tempered glass with a clear plastic laminate on the inner side, i.e., facing the occupants has been devised. The benefits of the inner layer of plastic are obvious in that it:
- protects against flying glass
- helps in holding the glass together
- helps in preventing ejection while retaining structural support features afforded by the vehicle's glazing

Dashboard

Dashboard injuries to the knees of unrestrained front-seat occupants are significant insofar as their presence suggests a head-on collision, especially if the injuries are of similar severity on both sides. Bruises, abrasions and lacerations of the knees are often seen in such cases. Fractures of the lower ends of the femurs with separation of the condyles are less frequent. When they occur, such fractures are due to the fact that in the sitting position, the wedge-shaped kneecap is forced between the condyles upon frontal impact, prying the condyles apart, exposing the marrow cavity of the lower end of the femur and causing massive, fat and bone marrow embolism (Figs. XVII-52 and XVII-53). The impact velocity and

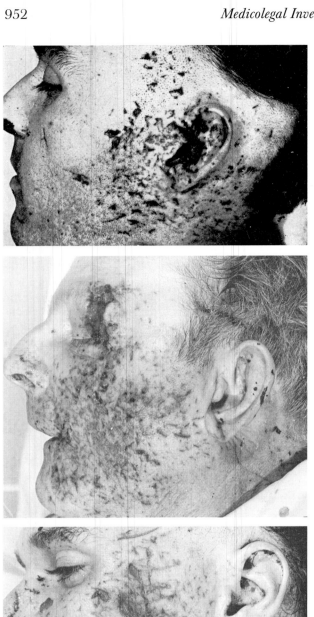

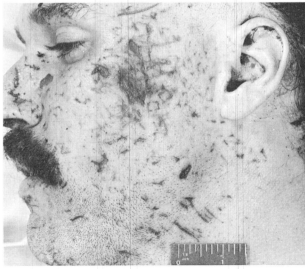

FIGURE XVII-50b–d. Characteristic *dicing* pattern on the left side of the face caused by flying fragments of tempered glass from the left door window. Such injury in a left-sided intersection-type collision will identify the driver.

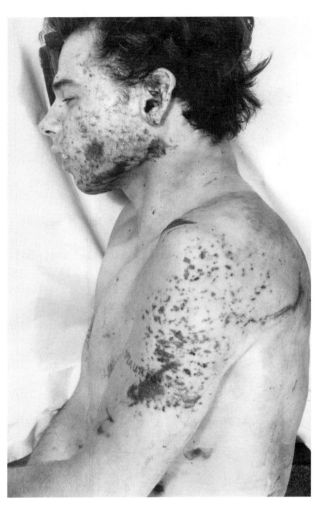

FIGURE XVII-50e. Dicing pattern on the left side of the face and left arm.

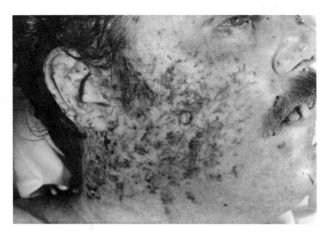

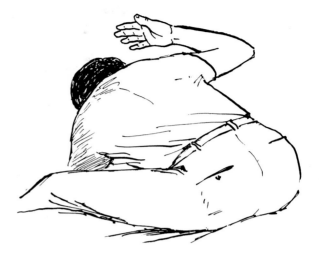

FIGURE XVII-50f. Dense dicing pattern on the right side (one piece of glass is embedded in the skin). This pattern on the right side in a right-sided collision identifies the passenger. Had there been no passenger in the front seat, the driver would not have sustained a pattern of this density.

FIGURE XVII-50g. The presence of a *dicing* pattern on the skin often allows identification of the seating positions of the vehicle's occupants.

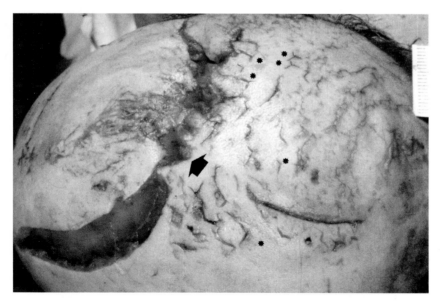

FIGURE XVII-51a. Site of impact *(fat arrow)* shows extending splits on scalp. The remaining injuries are superficial, nondescript and occasionally there are scattered imprints of cubes and angles *(asterisks).*

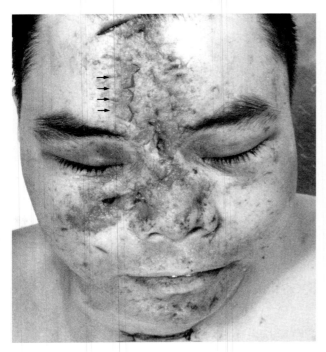

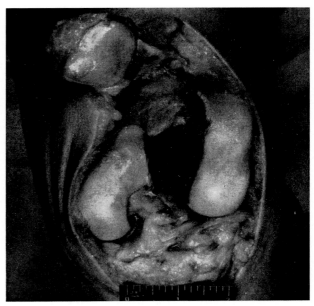

FIGURE XVII-52. Incised knee of driver with dashboard injury. The condyles of the femur are pried apart as result of impact on the kneecap (reflected in the photograph).

FIGURE XVII-51b. Central facial impact on tempered glass. The nose is fractured. The central forehead and the right cheek and nose are crushed and there are four dice vertically aligned above the medial right eyebrow (arrows).

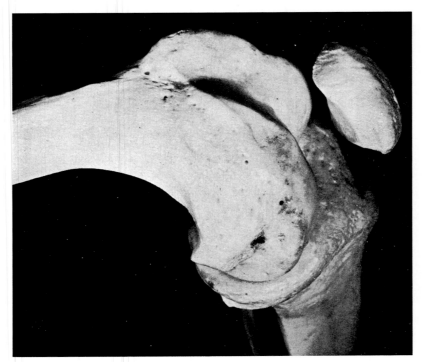

FIGURE XVII-53. Knee joint showing mechanism of fracture in dashboard impact. The wedge-shaped kneecap separates the femoral condyles. Bilateral injuries of similar severity suggest a frontal collision.

the shape and rigidity of the area that was struck are significant factors in the interpretation of these injuries. Evidence of external injury to the knees may be minimal and sometimes lacking.

Another type of dashboard injury is dislocation, with or without fracture, of the head of the femur. The head of the femur is literally pushed through its socket into the pelvis by the impact of the knee. Depending on the angle of impact, the shaft of the femur may also be fractured. Again, external manifestations of trauma at the knee or elsewhere may be absent or minimal.

Ejection

Litigation involving motor vehicular deaths often raises the question of whether the fatal injury occurred:
- Inside the vehicle?
- Outside the vehicle, as a result of *partial* ejection?
- Outside the vehicle, as a result of *complete* ejection.

Injuries sustained inside the vehicle are the most common. Certain types of injuries and injury locations are often referable to impact on a particular surface, such as the windshield, steering wheel, A or B-pillar or dashboard. Impact on a protruding part inside the car, such as a door or window handle may cause a particular injury pattern (Fig. XVII-54a–b).

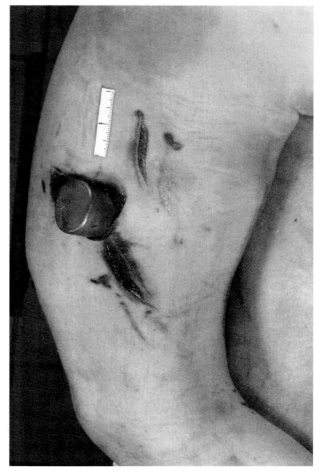

FIGURE XVII-54a. Passenger of automobile in a left intersection-type collision. The handle of the gearshift is embedded in the thigh, as the passenger moved to the left.

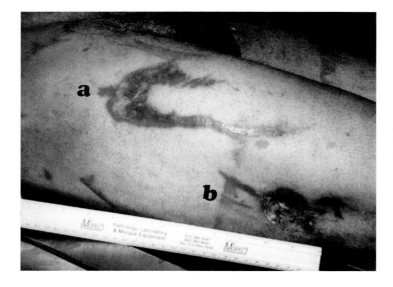

FIGURE XVII-54b. Imprint of armrest (a) and injury by window crank (b) on passenger's thigh in a right-sided collision.

The body of an occupant, even if restrained, moves towards the impacting force. In an intersection-type collision, occupants of a passenger car are injured on the side of the impact. The head and neck may be ejected through the door window, while the torso strikes the door. In the case of a collision with a truck or van, a typical dent may be made by the head on the grill of the higher vehicle (Fig. XVII-55a–d). In the same way, a vehicle that skids sideways into a tree or pole is likely to cause an occupant, seated on the same side, to sustain head injuries as a result of partial ejection.

In *rollover* situations, it is sometimes difficult to determine whether injuries were sustained inside or outside the vehicle. The head of the occupant may be crushed between the car and the ground. An occupant may be found inside the vehicle, after sustaining the fatal injury outside the vehicle while partially ejected. Blood may be expected on the outside of the car and brush burn abrasions are likely from scraping on the ground. It is noteworthy, that on snow or ice, brush burns may be reduced or lacking.

Ejection of an occupant from a vehicle can occur though a door, window, windshield or sunroof. Distinction must be made between forceful ejection during the initial phase, after the collision, or the body falling out following a deadly impact inside the vehicle, when the vehicle comes to a halt. The question of whether ejection occurred through an open door or window can sometimes be answered by the finding of patterned injuries on the body. Horizontal striped bruises may be caused by impact against a window frame; the width of such bruises corresponds to the width of the frame. Ejection through the windshield is likely to cause cuts, unless the windshield has popped out and ejection occurred through an open space. The entire crash sequence transpires in fractions of seconds.

Ideally, the scene and vehicle(s) should be viewed by the pathologist, who reconstructs the accident. Scene photographs and detailed accident reports are of considerable assistance if viewing of the scene and vehicle(s) are not feasible.

Often an occupant of a car, especially the driver or front-seat passenger, is ejected by centrifu-

gal force while the car is spinning after a crash. Ejection occurs along a parabola-like curve. The ejected occupant often strikes the ground head first, sustaining fatal injuries. A single injury in the area of contact with the ground may be all that is noted at the postmortem examination of the body. This injury usually consists of a large area of abrasion, with some evidence of brush burn pattern and a central star-shaped or linear split of the skin with underlying non-depressed fracture of the skull. Extensive hemorrhage may be associated with this type of injury, since heart activity continues for a short time, despite instantaneous death.

Despite recent advances in automobile design, with particular emphasis on safety measures, the number of traffic crash fatalities in the United States rose from 37,241 in 1995 to 38,309 in 2002.[13]

Also, in particular with reference to *rollovers,* deaths involving SUVs have increased 178% since 1991, according to the NHTSA. Most of these deaths were due to head and neck injuries. More than 7000 deaths and serious injuries occur each year in *rollovers* in which the roofs collapse. It should be noted that only the number of *rollover* crash fatalities involving cars has significantly decreased during this period.

Motorcyclist

In 2002, 3,244 motorcycle riders died from injuries sustained in crashes. Injuries of motorcyclists are usually more extensive and severe than those sustained by occupants of automobiles, and for obvious reasons: motorcyclists are unprotected for all practical purposes. The protection afforded by leather clothes is minimal in a major collision. Whereas, *brush burns* on the body surface may be reduced by such clothing, internal injuries and skeletal fractures remain unaffected.

With regards to helmets, all helmets offer reasonable protection. Helmets reduce the risk of serious head injury, but no helmet guarantees complete safety or protects the wearer from all possible impacts. Helmet protection is mostly provided by the liner which consists of expanded polystyrene (EPS) also known as, Styrofoam.

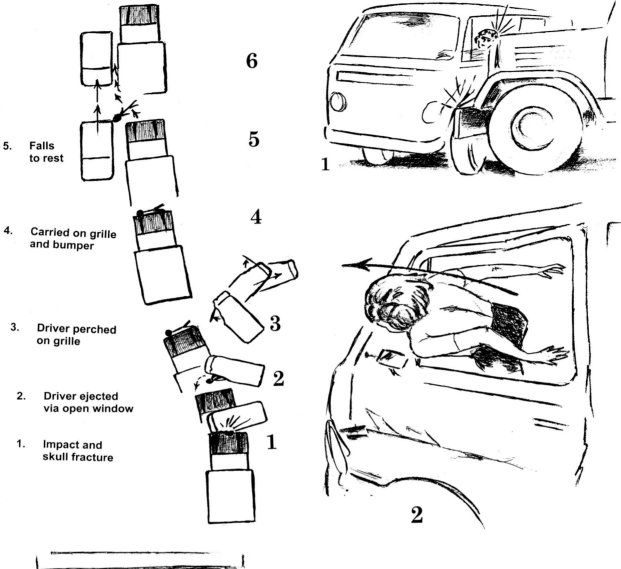

5. Falls to rest

4. Carried on grille and bumper

3. Driver perched on grille

2. Driver ejected via open window

1. Impact and skull fracture

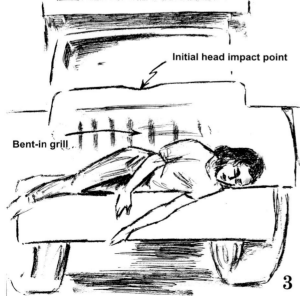

Initial head impact point

Bent-in grill

FIGURE XVII-55a–d. Re-enactment of intersection-type collision involving a tractor trailer and minivan. The minivan driver is injured when her head comes through the open window (1). The minivan driver is ejected through her window (2), strikes the front of the truck denting the hood, and simultaneously bending the grill (3), both vehicles are still moving, such that the driver of the minivan is carried on the bumper and the grill (4) until point 5 at which she falls to the ground and rolls as the truck slows and continues for a short distance.

The EPS is made of thousands of tiny air cells which compress and explode when submitted to pressure, similar to bubble wrap.

This construction of the helmet padding acts as a one-time cushion between the head and an obstacle, to the extent that a relatively thin padding is able to absorb a portion of the impact energy and reduce a 10 mph impact to zero. In order to afford maximal protection the helmet must fit tightly and snugly. Failure to meet this requirement does not give the wearer the protection that is needed. Placement of an intermediate object such as, a towel, scarf, or hat, between the head and the padding of the helmet significantly reduces the helmet's performance. The helmet molds itself to the shape of the owner's head and for this reason one should not use a helmet that belonged to someone else. By using someone else's helmet the interior of the helmet will not conform to the shape of the new user's head.

Frontal protection is probably the weakest area in current helmet design. The frontal opening is significantly too large and the visor constitutes a hazard rather than providing protection. Furthermore, most helmets have only an inadequate comfort padding inside the chin bar. Nevertheless, helmets are one of the most effective countermeasures for protecting cyclists. It is generally agreed that 75% of cycle-related deaths are the result of head trauma.

Fractures of the skull follow the usual rules of thumb:

- Impact of the face causes fractures of the facial skeleton.
- Impact of the forehead causes a sagittal fracture of the base of the skull.
- Impact of the chin is likely to cause mandibular fractures. Such fractures may mitigate and absorb the blow. In more severe impacts of the chin, transmission of the blow through the temporomandibular joints to the base of the skull may result in massive fracture of the pyramids and the sella turcica, *hinge fracture*. The injury of the chin may be limited to the skin, i.e., minimal as compared to the extent of internal damage.
- A side impact of the head causes a similar fracture of the base of the skull, as seen in blows to the chin area. Careful evaluation to determine the actual point of impact is required.

Inspection of the helmet often indicates the location of the impact and is of prime importance. Rupture or tear of a helmet is likely to be associated with skull fracture at the point of impact. Such fracture is often depressed with severe damage to underlying tissues. We have observed that some helmets are more likely to rupture than others under similar circumstances.

Sudden deceleration often causes *whiplash* injury of the neck. Instantaneous death may be due to injury of the medulla associated with fractures and/or dislocations of the atlanto-occipital areas. No autopsy of a motorcyclist is complete without a detailed exploration of this part of the body.

Patterned injuries on the body surface are often caused by the cycle falling on the driver, imprinting parts of the vehicle on the body. Chain marks, etc., and muffler burns are seen with some frequency in motorcyclists.

In intersection-type collisions where the motorcyclist strikes the side of an automobile, the cyclist moves forward, striking the gas tank (Fig. XVII-56), while the pelvis lifts from the seat and the head strikes the side of the vehicle close to the roof (Fig. XVII-57). In collisions where the cycle strikes the front or rear bumper of a car, the rider is likely to be thrown forward and upward over the top of the automobile. Occasionally, the chest sustains the impact on the side of the car, while the head strikes the roof.

Lacerations of the liver, spleen, or kidney sometimes result from sudden violent turning of the handlebars as a result of a collision. Such injuries may not be recognizable externally and therefore present a considerable clinical hazard. Similar injuries occur with some frequency in riders of bicycles.[14]

A passenger of a motorcycle is often thrown off before the vehicle comes to a stop. A sudden frontal collision often causes the passenger to be thrown forward over the driver.

Motorcycle crashes, like many automobile collisions, are often related to consumption of alcohol. Crashes involving motorcycles are likely to occur with significantly lower blood alcohol levels than do automobile collisions. There can be no doubt that the usually accepted prima facie level of 0.08% blood alcohol concentration is

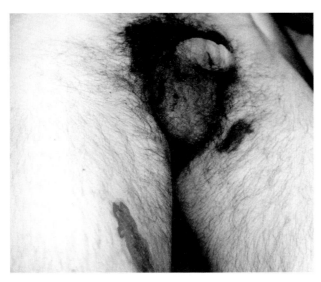

FIGURE XVII-56. Abrasions on the medial surfaces of the thighs of a motorcycle driver from impact on the gas tank in a frontal collision as shown in Figure XIV-57.

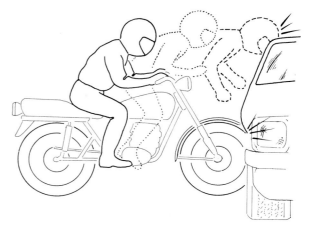

FIGURE XVII-57. Motorcyclist striking the side of a car in an intersection-type collision. The cyclist moves forward, the pelvis lifts from the seat and the head strikes the side of the vehicle. The medial thighs rub against the gas tank.

excessive when applied to motorcyclists. The ability to maintain balance is impaired at low blood alcohol concentrations.

The Car Fire Victim

Fuel-fed fires in automobiles were recently brought into the spotlight when the gas tanks, on a number of police Crown Victoria Interceptors, ruptured and exploded during high speed rear-end crashes. Ford is now studying the possibility of using fuel tank bladders in some of these vehicles. The bladder is a reinforced tank similar to those used in race cars. They are made with puncture proof materials which prevent leakage that could spark a fire.[15]

Fire deaths due to motor vehicle crashes in the United States are estimated at 650–750 annually. Only 2% of vehicle fires are caused by collision. The majority of vehicle fire deaths occur in crashes which are survivable.[5] Fire in car crashes is most often associated with rollover damage and to a lesser extent with rear impacts. Both of these types of crashes are associated with metal deformity which often causes the doors to jam. This interferes with occupants getting out of the vehicles and rescue operations. Car fires are four times more common, in rear-end collisions compared to head-on crashes. A car fire may be electrical in origin. Even when fuel-fed, a car fire is rarely explosive. More often, such fires smolder for sometime before erupting into flames. This generates toxic gases such as, carbon monoxide and cyanide and a very hot environment from burning synthetic and flammable materials which make up the vehicle's interior.

A seventy-three-year-old man driving a 1984 Cadillac Cimarron at a speed exceeding 70 mph struck a Mazda RX-7 from behind, propelling the RX-7 into the side of a Chevrolet pickup. The RX-7 was witnessed to be traveling through a construction zone at a speed of approximately 20 mph and the driver was reported to have been applying the brakes at the moment of impact.

The occupants of the Chevy pickup found the woman driving the RX-7 sitting peacefully in the driver's seat, wearing a lap belt and shoulder harness. Her head was down to one side, her chin touching her chest. She appeared to be lifeless. Two men who attempted to remove her from the vehicle could not open the door. They saw no evidence of fire at the time. Flames erupted after a short while, and when the body was removed it was charred. Blood carboxyhemoglobin was negative, indicating that the victim was dead when the fire started.

Automobile collision-induced fires are statistically infrequent. However, in the case of a rollover, gasoline from the tank may leak out. Gasoline vapor may ignite from the heat of the catalytic converter causing an explosion. The catalytic converter operates at about 1,600

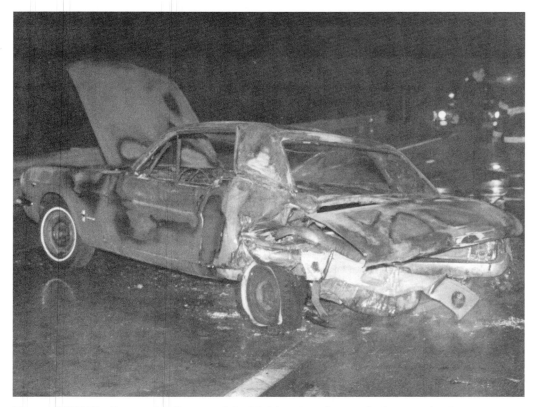

FIGURE XVII-58a. Rear-end collision with fuel-fed fire. As is frequently the case, the doors jam trapping the occupants and hindering rescue.

degrees Fahrenheit under normal conditions and in poorly maintained vehicles may reach 4,000 degrees Fahrenheit. One gallon of gasoline has the explosive potential of 30 sticks of dynamite.

Reconstruction of a fiery crash involving a motor vehicle usually leaves many unanswered questions. Burned out cars are difficult and tedious to investigate (Fig. XVII-58a–b).

Eye witness accounts are notoriously unreliable and in some instances, misleading. It is not unusual for witnesses to relate hearing screams and even seeing occupants of a burning car trying to escape where it is evident from the nature of the injuries that death was instantaneous on impact. I have had such eye witness accounts related to me in cases where the victims were extensively mutilated, even or decapitated.

Therefore, a significant burden is placed on the postmortem examination of bodies retrieved from car fire scenes.

The immediate questions which arise following a fiery motor vehicle crash are:
• Was the victim alive at the time of the fire?
• Did he or she die as a result of injuries sustained in the impact?
• Did inhalation of smoke and/or exposure to flames contribute to incapacity and death?
• Why did the victim remain in the vehicle?
• Was the victim incapacitated by the crash and unable to extricate himself?
• Was he or she pinned in the car?

Bodies retrieved from a car fire are usually severely charred. The following should be emphasized:

Despite charring of the body surface, the organs are usually in a good state of preservation, permitting a complete autopsy. Body fluids are usually available for toxicological analyses. The autopsy should include the throat and neck organs, as well as the cervical spine, with partic-

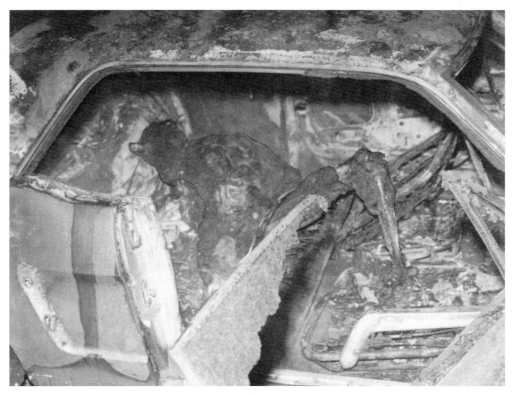

FIGURE XVII-58b. The driver's body is charred by the flames, however, a meaningful autopsy and collection of specimens for toxicological analyses are probably still feasible.

ular attention to the atlanto-occipital joints. Pathologists often forego examining the upper cervical vertebrae in victims of automobile collisions. Damage of the medulla oblongata, located in this area of the spine, could account for instantaneous death. The trachea should be vertically incised and inspected in situ, i.e., prior to removal from the body, to avoid contamination with particles of soot from the mouth and throat. To secure against contamination during the autopsy it is helpful to plug the airway at the time of inspection by inserting a bunched piece of gauze or cotton ball through the incision. The presence of soot in the lower airway indicates inhalation, but in the absence of carboxyhemoglobin, such inhalation becomes questionable, and the presence of soot could be artifactual.

Blood should be retained for toxicological analyses, specifically carbon monoxide, cyanide, alcohol and drugs. It is recommended that urine also be retained for alcohol analysis and drug screen.

A negative carboxyhemoglobin usually suggests death prior to the fire. Rarely in flash fires, deaths may occur in the presence of low levels of carboxyhemoglobin. Otherwise, low levels of carboxyhemoglobin indicate respiratory arrest after a few breaths. Respiration and heartbeat may continue for some time, even in the presence of fatal injuries. Brain death on impact would not necessitate simultaneous cardiopulmonary arrest.

Whereas, a fuel-fed fire generates relatively little smoke and only low amounts of carbon monoxide, interior plastics, upholstery and padding of an automobile produce dense smoke and a heavy concentration of carbon monoxide. These items are slow burning and resist ignition in compliance with federal safety standards.

Hirsch,[16] in a frequently quoted article, reports the absence of significant blood carbon monoxide levels and soot in the air passages of victims of a fiery multi-vehicular car crash. Hirsch postulates that the absence of conspicuous elevations of carboxyhemoglobin may have been the result of the victims' death in the first seconds after the crash, while the fire had sufficient oxygen available to burn efficiently and produce little carbon monoxide. Such fire may also have initiated *instantly lethal reflexes* by subjecting the victims to an intense flash of heat.

Whereas, such inhalation of an *intense flash of heat* is conceivable, under certain circumstances, the presence at autopsy of burns and severe swelling of the upper portion of the airway might be expected under such circumstances. In the absence of these manifestations, the likelihood of *flame* or *heat inhalation* is remote.

The investigator must be aware that an elevated carboxyhemoglobin level may originate from inhalation of exhaust fumes from a defective muffler, rather than as a result of inhalation of products of combustion. In fact, carboxyhemoglobin may have caused the crash, instead of indicating that the inhalation of smoke resulted from a fuel-fed fire after a collision.

It should also be noted that an 8 to 10% carboxyhemoglobin concentration may be found in heavy smokers, especially in the closed compartment of an automobile.

A toxicological check for medication may be significant. For example, the presence or absence of antiepileptic medication is significant, if it is believed that epilepsy played a role in the crash.

Accident or Suicide?

The use of the automobile as an instrument of self-destruction is well known. Morton[17] reported that life insurance companies had noted a disproportionately high number of fatal automobile collisions occurring in the first year of double indemnity policies. Certainly, there are many more suicides on the road than can be determined. In the absence of concrete evidence of suicide, medical examiners tend to certify motor vehicular deaths indiscriminately as accidents. Estimates of underreporting of vehicular suicide range from 25 to 50%.[18] Edland[19] indicates that one-sixth of traffic fatalities in his study resulted from purposely caused collisions. In most cases, it is difficult, if not impossible, to decide whether a decedent consciously and willfully caused his own death.

I have personally investigated a number of car crashes where individuals were observed to drive deliberately into a fixed object such as a large tree or bridge abutment. In one case on an expressway, the driver of a compact car was observed to drive his vehicle in front of a tractor trailer, then abruptly applied the brakes to be rear-ended. He miraculously survived the impact uninjured and committed suicide one month later by another method.

It is noteworthy that a vehicle, extensively damaged in a crash, may show a misleading speedometer reading caused by the gauge stuck at a speed well in excess of that traveled.

Supportive evidence of suicide are a driver with a history of depression, the imprint of the gas pedal pattern on the sole of his shoe, and the absence of skid marks leading to the site of collision. Skid marks which are inconspicuous in the rain may be readily noticeable when the road is dry. Also, possible skid marks should be viewed from various directions and angles above the road to afford optimal visibility in different lighting conditions before a decision is made that skid marks are absent.

On the other hand, how can it be excluded that the driver fell asleep at the wheel or ignored existing road conditions? Alcohol and drug intoxication must be considered. Alcohol is known to be associated with at least half of all traffic deaths, but alcohol may also have been consumed to muster courage necessary for suicide.

The driving record of the victim may indicate previous violations and suggest a problem driver rather than suicidal intent. More attention should be paid the psychiatric makeup of the victim. Suicidal individuals as a group appear to be immature, unstable persons with recent records of failure in interpersonal relationships.

Individuals contemplating suicide sometimes demonstrate unusual behavior for the purpose of drawing attention to themselves.

A twenty-four-year-old woman with a history of depression parked her car on the side of a bridge which connects two major cities separated by a river. The lights of the car were turned on and the horn was jammed to sound steadily. The young woman jumped over the railing and drowned.

In a crash situation, should the question arise whether the car's headlights had been on, examination of the lamps may show whether the tungsten filaments were stretched by heat. Also, the glass of the lamp melts before the tungsten of the filament, thus, if the filament was hot when the glass was shattered microscopic beads of glass may be found adherent to the filament.

The possibility of carbon monoxide intoxication due to a faulty muffler should not be overlooked. Carbon monoxide causes drowsiness at low concentrations. Blood from *all* occupants of a car should be retained to determine the presence and concentration of carboxyhemoglobin.

Sudden Natural Death at the Wheel

Automobile accidents occur occasionally as a result of sudden death of the driver. In the early 1960s, Peterson and Petty,[20] in a classical review of this subject, determined that death in 19% of all drivers involved in collisions was due to natural causes and that in the vast majority of cases this was due to an acute heart attack. West et al.[21] concurred with these observations and attributed sudden natural death to 15% of road accidents in which drivers die. Interestingly, accidents involving these drivers are usually of relatively minor severity, an observation also made by Baker and Spitz.[22] According to their study, natural death of a sober driver does not entail a measurable risk of death or severe injury to his passengers or other persons. Despite impending death the sober driver is usually able to reduce speed and avoid a major collision. The reverse is true if the driver operates his vehicle while under the influence of alcohol.

Of course, it is hard to draw conclusions regarding a specific case from what is known to occur statistically.

Individuals with preexisting known or unknown heart disease may be particularly susceptible to chest impact. With age, tissues, especially the heart and aorta, become less elastic and more brittle, the rib cage becomes porotic and preexisting cardiovascular disease is more frequent, which makes the cardiovascular system more vulnerable to impact forces, including air bags.

In certifying the death of a driver, a clear distinction must be drawn between the cause of death and the cause of the crash. Whereas, a natural disease process may have caused a crash, the death may have resulted from injuries.

Some life insurance policies deny accidental death benefits when natural disease contributed to the crash.

Perception and Reaction Time

Reaction is the response to visual or auditory perception. According to Baker[23] four types of reaction times are recognized:

1. Instinctive and automatic, requires no thinking and has the shortest response, about 1/10 of a second.
2. Slowing when a traffic signal turns yellow is based on habit. This reaction usually requires 1/2 second to recognize and apply the brakes.
3. When a choice needs to be made as for example, when a pedestrian is in the roadway and a driver must decide whether to turn or slow down. This process can take 1/2 second to 2 seconds.
4. The longest reaction time occurs, for example, when a driver comes up behind a weaving vehicle, suspects the driver to be drunk and must decide whether to pass the car and if so, on what side.

Reaction time is affected by age, where the young and the elderly react slower; strength of stimulus, such as a pedestrian wearing dark clothes on an unlit road at night as opposed to the bright illumination of a segment of road or a traffic sign; physical condition, where sickness, fatigue, or intoxication by alcohol or drugs prolong reaction time and where training and driving experience reduce reaction time.

Whereas, an exact perception/reaction time is unpredictable in each and every case, the average is usually considered as 1.5 seconds with a range of 1/10 second to 2 seconds and longer.

It should be mentioned that anticipation of an event can cut reaction time by at least 50%. For

TABLE XVII-1

BLOOD ALCOHOL CONCENTRATION

Individual Weight	Number of Drinks in One Hour				
	One	*Two*	*Three*	*Four*	*Five*
90–109 lbs.	0.05	0.09	0.13	0.16	0.20
110–129 lbs.	0.05	0.08	0.11	0.14	0.17
130–149 lbs.	0.04	0.07	0.09	0.12	0.15
150–169 lbs.	0.04	0.06	0.08	0.11	0.13
170–189 lbs.	0.04	0.06	0.08	0.10	0.12
190–209 lbs.	0.03	0.05	0.07	0.09	0.11
210–229 lbs.	0.03	0.05	0.07	0.08	0.10
230 lbs. & over	0.03	0.05	0.06	0.08	0.09

One drink is defined as a 12-oz. beer, a 4-oz. glass of wine, or a 1-1/4-oz. shot of 80-proof liquor.

example, it has been shown that a 1.5 second average reaction time is reduced to 1/3, i.e., 0.5 seconds, in a tennis player who sees the ball coming or a hockey player who sees the puck, but the spectators do not, because of the players' anticipation.

Alcohol and Fatal Crashes

Driver impairment due to alcohol consumption has been widely recognized as the single most significant factor contributing to motor vehicle crashes. Data collected in 1988, indicated that 49.6% of all traffic deaths were associated with drinking. Despite national efforts to reduce the carnage on United States roads, alcohol related fatalities in 2002 deceased by only 8.6%, which equates to a total of 17,419 fatalities.[24] In fact, statistics released by the Department of Transportation indicate that road deaths involving alcohol remained at about the same level over the last 8 years.

Consequently, the federal government passed legislation requiring states to adopt lower blood alcohol levels (0.08%) as prima facie evidence of drunk driving or face losing federal support for highway construction. Michigan put in effect this legislation in 2003. The American Medical Association (AMA) has long advocated reducing the level to 0.05%.

It has been shown that the higher the alcohol level of the driver, the more severe the injuries sustained in a crash.

Although, the effects of alcohol vary markedly, the average 160-lb. person who consumed three drinks of (1-1/4 ounces each) 80-proof liquor, or three 12-oz. bottles of regular beer or three 4-oz. glasses of wine in one hour runs the risk of exceeding a blood alcohol concentration of 0.08%. Table XVII-1 shows the percentages of blood alcohol for various body weights after one hour of consumption.

In our experience, driving ability can be impaired in susceptible individuals, when the blood is free of alcohol, in the hangover phase. Young, inexperienced alcohol drinkers are particularly affected by the aftereffects of alcohol on judgment, perception, reaction time and the ability to drive safely.

About 10% of adult Americans who drink have been consistently reported to be alcoholics or problem drinkers. Studies of drinking practices and consumption patterns have shown that moderate drinkers only rarely exceed blood alcohol concentrations of 0.10% and usually have 0.06 to 0.08%, while significantly higher values are seen in problem drinkers and alcoholics where values of 0.15 to 0.30% are common. Even a single blood alcohol concentration of 0.25 to 0.30% deserves consideration that the individual may be alcoholic.

When questioning an intoxicated person regarding the amount of alcohol he or she has consumed, a tendency to underestimate such quantities is generally evident. It is difficult to determine whether the response is to mitigate their responsibility in a given incident or if it is more likely that the ability to remember genuinely diminishes the higher the blood alcohol concentration.

Alcohol potentiates the effect of marijuana and vice versa. The combined use of alcohol and marijuana causes impairment of driving skills, exceeding the effect of each of these drugs alone; psychomotor skills and information processing are particularly affected. Cocaine, methamphetamine, heroin and many prescription drugs, when taken with alcohol, cause manifestations incompatible with driving or operating machinery. However, drugs play only a small role in automobile crashes.[25]

REFERENCES

1. Little-known 'black-box' technology on cars helps diagnose accidents. The Dallas Morning News OnLine, May 11, 2000.

2. Spitz, W.U.: Reconstruction of accidents: Integration of pathologic and roadside evidence. In Brinkhouse, K.M. (Ed.): *Accident pathology.* Washington, D.C.: Govt. Print. Office, 1971, pp. 26–35.

3. States, J.D.: Problem delineation: Automobile restraint systems. *Bull NY Acad Med, 64:* 684, 1988.

4. Yarbrough, B.E., and Hendey, G.W.: Hangman's fracture resulting from improper seat belt use. *Southern Medical Journal, 83* (7), June 1990.

5. Taylor, P.L.: Automobile Fire Safety. Savannah Fire and Emergency Services, February 19, 2004.

6. Denton, J.S., and Segovia, A.: Check sample, forensic pathology no.: FP99-7 (FP-248). American Society of Clinical Pathologists. *Forensic Pathology, 41* (7), 1999.

7. Huelke, D.F., Moore, J.L., Compton, T.W., Samuels, J., and Levine, R.S.: Upper Extremity Injuries Related to Air Bag Deployments. SAE Technical Paper Series 940716, March, 1994.

8. Saul, R.A., Backaitis, S.H., Beebe, M.S., and Ore, L.S.: Hybrid III Dummy Instrumentation and Assessment of Arm Injuries During Air Bag Deployment. Society of Automotive Engineers, Inc., 1996.

9. Zuby, D.S., Ferguson, S.A., and Cammisa, M.X.: Analysis of Driver Fatalities in Frontal Crashes of Airbag-Equipped Vehicles in 1990-98 NASS/CDS. SAE Technical Paper Series 2001-01-0156, March, 2001.

10. Kress, T.A., Porta, D.J., Duma, S.M., Snider, J.N., and Nino, N.M.: A Discussion of the Air Bag System and Review of Induced Injuries. SAE Technical Paper Series 960658, February, 1996.

11. Otte, D.: Review of the Air Bag Effectiveness in Real Life Accidents Demands - for Positioning and Optimal Deployment of Air Bag Systems. SAE Technical Paper Series 952701, 1995.

12. Federal Motor Vehicle Safety Standard 205. Title 49, Volume 5, Parts 400 to 999. Cite: 49CFR571.205. U.S. Government Printing Office. Revised as of October 1, 1997.

13. Fatality Analysis Reporting System (FARS) Web-Based Encyclopedia, National Center for Statistics and Analysis. National Highway Traffic Safety Administration, 2004.

14. Spitz, D.J.: Unrecognized fatal liver injury caused by a bicycle handlebar. *Am J Emerg Med, 17:* 3, 244, May 1999.

15. Cops consider bladders for Crown Victoria fuel. *The Detroit Free Press,* July 20, 2002.

16. Hirsch, C.S., Bost, R.O., Gerber, S.R., Cowan, M.E., Adelson, L., and Sunshine, I.: Carboxyhemoglobin concentrations in flash fire victims: Report of six simultaneous fire fatalities without elevated carboxyhemoglobin. *Amer J Clin Path, 68:* 317, 1977.

17. Morton, J.: The suicide driver. *Traffic Safety, 68:* 37, 1968.

18. Jobes, D.A., Berman, A.L., and Josselson, A.R.: Improving the validity and reliability of medical-legal certifications of suicide. *Suicide and Life-Threatening Behavior, 17:* 310, 1987.

19. Edland, J.F.: Vehicular suicide. In Brinkhouse, K.M. (Ed.): *Accident pathology.* Washington, D.C.: U.S. Govt. Print. Office, 1971, pp. 42–45.

20. Peterson, B.J., and Petty, C.S.: Sudden natural death at the wheel. *J Forensic Sci, 7:* 274, 1962.

21. West, I., Nielsen, G.L., Gilmore, A.E., and Ryan, J.R.: Natural death at the wheel. *JAMA, 205:* 266, 1968.

22. Baker, S.P., and Spitz, W.U.: An evaluation of the hazard created by natural death at the wheel. *N Engl J Med, 283:* 405, 1970.

23. Baker, J.S.: *Traffic accident investigation manual.* Evanston, IL: The Traffic Institute, Northwestern University, 1976.

24. USDOT Releases 2002 Highway Fatality Statistics. U.S. Department of Transportation, Office of Public Affairs, Washington, D.C., July 17, 2003.

25. Marzuk, P.M., and Mann, J.J.: Cocaine danger on the road. Quoted in *Accident Reconstruction Journal, 2:* 4, 1990.

Chapter XVIII

MEDICOLEGAL INVESTIGATION OF
MASS DISASTERS

GLENN N. WAGNER AND RICHARD C. FROEDE

THE PATHOLOGIST, either forensic or hospital based, will likely be called upon to assist in the investigation of mass disaster incidents during the course of their career. The causes of these tragedies are both natural and man-made and occur with sufficient frequency to require a disaster plan in most healthcare delivery systems. Disasters often result in extensive damage of property and loss of life. Response to these events is predicated on the laws, statutes or regulations of that particular jurisdiction and the resources available. The magnitude of the event governs the response, the severity of which could exceed the capability of local resources. Contaminated remains of victims from biological, chemical or radiation exposures may require specialized handling and safety procedures and add to the resource requirements. A mass disaster or multiple casualty incident usually involves eight or more victims.

Natural disasters usually include earthquakes, tornadoes, floods, volcanic eruptions, typhoons, hurricanes, forest and brush fires and avalanches. The most common natural disasters with multiple casualties are floods, largely because of population densities in flood plains. In contrast, man-made catastrophes are those caused or contributed to by human factors, including transportation accidents (aircraft, ship, train, bus, or other vehicle), structural failures of bridges and roadways, structural fires, industrial accidents, acts of terrorism, mass suicides/homicides and war.

The nature of the multiple casualty incident directs its focus. Natural disasters shift the investigation towards recovery, identification and disposition of the victims, whereas, man-made disasters shift the investigation towards obtaining documentation of the injuries, pre-existing disease conditions, the analysis of the injury mechanisms and human factors contributing to or causing the incident.

The development of a disaster operational plan is essential to any such investigation. The plan must delineate policies and procedures necessary for victim and casualty identification, adequate documentation and processing of the victims and investigating the catastrophe. Such a plan must consider facilities, required services, specified personnel, administrative assistance, logistical resources, ancillary services, law enforcement and emergency response teams. This involves communications, cooperation, coordination, consensus, mobilization and standardization of training, responsibilities, supplies and equipment.

The most frequent disaster situation that a jurisdiction may encounter outside of a flood or tornado is an aircraft crash. Although natural disasters can occur anywhere and a variety of transportation accidents occur frequently, aircraft accidents, especially commercial transport mishaps, remain the most visible because of the number of planes flying, functional airports and the large number of people transported. It may be expected that this situation will worsen in the future because of the shortage of runways and the expected increase in air traffic (ed).

We have elected to pattern the mass disaster medicolegal investigation after this type of incident. However, with little change, the pattern is appropriate for a wide variety of catastrophes.

In each case, the pathologist acting as the medical examiner or coroner or as his deputy will have custody of the remains. Although it is the duty of the pathologist to identify the victims, provide proper documentation, and try to interpret and correlate the patterns of injury, a wide variety of investigative agencies will be in charge of the overall investigation. These may be municipal, county, state or federal agencies, depending on the nature of the catastrophe. For example, the National Transportation Safety Board (NTSB) has jurisdiction over transportation accidents, whereas the Federal Bureau of Investigation (FBI) assumes jurisdiction over acts of terrorism involving American citizens in this country and overseas.[1] There are well over 60 federal law enforcement agencies, each with defined jurisdiction. In most cases however, local authorities will be the first responders and often determine the success of the investigation.

AIRCRAFT CRASH INVESTIGATION

Transport accidents remain the major cause of accidental death each year in the United States. There are an estimated two thousand aviation fatalities a year, with some 45 crashes having as many as 150–200 people onboard. The larger aircraft, with the capacity for more passengers, make such investigations a study in mass disaster planning, procedures and logistics. Such was the case on March 27, 1977 in Tenerife, Canary Islands, when two 747 jumbo jets collided on the runway, killing some 580 individuals.[2] Such was also the case in 1985, when a contract airliner crashed in Gander, Newfoundland, killing 256 people, including 248 servicemen returning from the Sinai. Recent overwater crashes of commercial airliners, for example TWA 800, Swiss Air, Alaska Air, exemplify the challenges of transport mishap investigations.

Aircraft accidents have recurring themes and epidemiological patterns which are relatively specific to aircraft type, flight actions and omissions and the environment. Aircraft accident investigations are oriented towards the engineering and flight operations based on the premise that the cause is discoverable.

Following an incident, the scene evaluation will encompass a variety of investigative authorities and agencies (Fig. XVIII-1). Each investigative group should be responsible for specific areas and make detailed records of their actions. The medical investigation will involve a multidisciplinary investigative team. Central to these efforts are the recovery, identification and documentation of the fatalities. The pathologist, as the custodian of these remains, is the unifying focus for all of these specialty teams and their efforts.

It is interesting that despite generations of aircraft and constantly improving avionics, some 80% of aircraft accidents are still attributed to pilot error where physiological factors such as hypoxia, fatigue, vestibular and visual illusions, accelerative forces, fear and natural disease are often contributory, if not causal factors in the crash. Because of such factors, aircraft accident investigations have incorporated a human factors team approach that emphasizes the flight environment, crash biodynamics, and crash injury analysis in an attempt to reconstruct the conditions and circumstances of the crash. This reliance on aviation pathology seems to have been instituted following the 1954 Comet disasters off Italy where pathological studies of recovered victims pointed to in-flight breakup from metal fatigue and aircraft deficiencies. Systematic analysis of aircraft accidents has been attempted since the 1930s and has led to the development of concepts of crash survivability and crashworthiness. Such analyses are often possible despite greater speeds and larger aircraft because the majority of aircraft crashes occur during takeoff and landing, at relatively low speeds and with shallow angles of ground impact. Nonetheless, the results of collision can be catastrophic such as mishaps at Tenerife (1977), the Singapore 747 crash in Taiwan (2000) or the Paris Concorde mishap (2000) at their respective airports. In these cases, survival is often complicated by fire and toxic fumes following the crash.

The medical examiner or coroner engaged in the work-up of a plane crash has the following major functions: identification of the victims, documentation of their injuries and disease

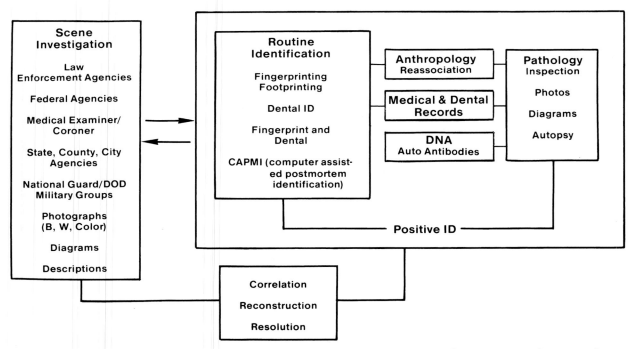

FIGURE XVIII-1. Following an incident, the scene evaluation will encompass a variety of investigative authorities and agencies. Each investigative group should be responsible for specific areas and make detailed records of their actions. The medical investigation will involve a multidisciplinary investigative team. Central to these efforts are the recovery, identification and documentation of the fatalities. The pathologist, as the custodian of these remains, is the unifying focus for all of these specialty teams and their efforts.

processes, and correlating these findings with aircraft and crash-site evidence, communication with families and return of property and release of information to the news media. This involves autopsies and toxicological analyses of the flight crew and examination of the aircraft. The role played by disease and drug or alcohol intoxication in causing the crash must be categorically addressed. Complete autopsies, including microscopy and neuropathological examination are recommended. X-ray examination may be necessary to determine the presence of metal fragments, such as bullets, shrapnel or bomb parts. As to toxicological testing, blood and urine are most suitable. If body fluids are unobtainable, tissue specimens should be retained and refrigerated or better yet, frozen without delay, until they can be forwarded to the laboratory. The presence of COHb in blood or tissue fluids indicates smoke in the plane before the crash and the fact that passengers and crew were alive at the time of the fire. In the event of fire onboard the plane,

the absence of COHb strongly supports death in the air prior to the crash. Of course COHb will also be negative if the plane erupted in flames on ground impact. As a general proposition, it is rare that blood in sufficient quantity for toxicological analysis will be found in victims of a plane crash from a high altitude.

For passengers, the need for autopsies is not as stringent as that for the crew in control of the plane. Passengers are usually presumed to have died as a result of physical injuries incurred in the crash, unless the circumstances of the crash suggest otherwise. Nevertheless, x-ray examination of bodies and body parts in suspected cases of terrorism may be advantageous for obvious reasons indicated above and determination of the COHb saturation is significant for the same reason. Occasional autopsies may have to be performed on certain passengers as part of the identification process to verify the existence of past surgical procedures and preexisting conditions known from medical records and historical data. Lastly, all phases of the process need to be accomplished expeditiously. It is essential that the remains be returned to their next of kin without undue delay. Thus, if a temporary morgue is established for this endeavor, proximity to the crash site is of the essence. Transportation of bodies and body parts for examination to some distant morgue facility takes time and hampers communication.

Since most crashes occur on landing or take-off, chances are that an airport is nearby. A hanger or similar large building is most advantageous to allow for direct interaction between the various speciality groups needed for rapid completion of this task (ed). Expertise and materials in the above areas may be obtained upon request from the National Disaster Medical System, 5600 Fishers Lane, 4-81, Rockville, Maryland 20857, 1-800-USA-NDMS (D-Mort Teams).

These requirements underscore the need for a multidisciplinary approach to mass disasters in general and to aircraft accident investigation in particular.

INVESTIGATING TEAMS

In the United States, the National Transportation Safety Board (NTSB), headquartered in Washington, D.C., has jurisdiction over all civil aircraft accidents and is *probable cause* oriented.[3] The NTSB investigates on-site all civil airline and air-taxi crashes, all mid-air collisions and most fatal general aviation accidents. The Federal Aviation Administration (FAA) investigates general aviation accidents in which the gross weight of the aircraft is 12,500 pounds or less. In military aircraft crashes (Fig. XVIII-2), where no civil aircraft is involved, the respective military service appoints a Mishap Investigation Board to investigate the accident.[4] Unless the crash occurs on land, where there is Federal Exclusive jurisdiction, local authorities are involved in the investigation and have jurisdiction over the bodies of the victims. These cases would normally be medical examiner or coroner cases in most jurisdictions because the deaths are of a violent nature.

Because of the human factors concept, the medical aspect of the investigation is primarily concerned with the medical and behavioral factors in the causal sequence of events and the relationships between crash dynamics and other factors causing injury or death. The accident investigation board usually has a medical member trained in aerospace medicine, either a military flight surgeon[5] or FAA Aviation Medical Examiner, depending on the type of crash, as well as other professionals as needed, including psychologists, physiologists and life support specialists. The pathologist provides the identification of the victims and the documentation and correlation of injuries and disease. In most investigations, recovery and identification of the victims is the most time-consuming and labor-intensive aspect of the investigation (Fig. XVIII-3). Disfigurement and mutilation of the remains and delay in obtaining information frequently hamper the identification process.

Some of the delay caused by difficulties in obtaining information may be alleviated by installation of unrestricted phone lines at the temporary morgue to enable workers engaged in the identification process to communicate directly with hospitals, physicians, dentists, etc. worldwide on an as needed basis. The airlines are usually cooperative in providing this service. It is perhaps not surprising how helpful people and institutions are at times of such emergency (ed.)

JURISDICTION

Planning is the first procedure to consider when preparing for a mass disaster.[6] It is important to know the geography of the potential disaster area and the agencies, laws, statutes, or reg-

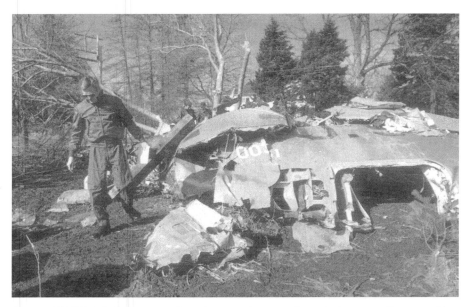

FIGURE XVIII-2. Military aircraft mishap involving an Army helicopter. Absence of fire despite significant deformation. The military has significantly reduced injuries from post-crash fires through crashworthy fuel systems. This effort was a direct consequence of losses sustained in Vietnam.

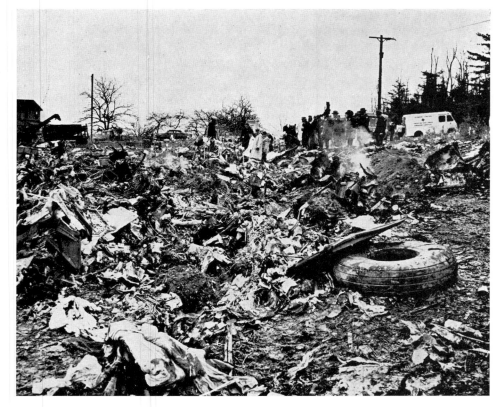

FIGURE XVIII-3. Scene at which a Boeing 707 crashed after it was struck by lightning. There were eighty-one people killed. Parts of the aircraft were spread over a circle one-half mile in diameter.

ulations in the involved area. Most disasters will come under control of law enforcement, emergency management, or disaster control agencies. Medical personnel will care for injured casualties and emergency management agencies will implement the disaster plan.

The key to resolving jurisdictional problems is knowing the geographic locations of the deaths and the applicable statutes. Incidents such as aircraft crashes or natural disasters often involve multiple jurisdictions. A plan must consider the possibility of disasters of this type and the need to coordinate actions among two or more jurisdictions. In the United States, the jurisdiction of local, state, federal, and military agencies varies considerably.

IDENTIFICATION

The identification process is divided into two major categories, positive and presumptive. Positive identification is a legal identification of a unique person based on comparison of pre and postmortem information, including dental examination, fingerprints, palmprints, footprints, or DNA profiling. Under certain circumstances, positive identification can be made on radiographic evidence, such as the configuration of frontal sinuses, vertebral bodies, pelvis, orthopedic or dental appliances, or trabecular bone patterns where adequate antemortem data exist for comparison.[7] All other means of identification are considered presumptive, including visual, anthropometrics, personal data (race, sex, age, blood type, parity, hair color and style, eye color, skin blemishes, tattoos, scars, medical history), personal effects including wallets, clothing and jewelry, flight manifest or other data. In these cases, this presumptive information usually identifies the victim as a member of a sub-group of the population rather than as a unique individual. In the absence of positive identification, presumptive identification can be legally certified if several points of comparison are used and there are no disparities that cannot be explained. Identification by exclusion is possible only after all victims have been accounted for. As might be expected, such an identification process involves several disciplines, including dentists, pathologists, fingerprint technicians, anthropologists, serologists and possibly radiologists and criminalists (Fig. XVIII-4).

An important logistical consideration is the inventory of personal effects, including jewelry, clothing, wallets, money, photographs, etc. This inventory provides two major functions: a source for presumptive identification and material reaffirmation of victim presence for the family or estate. It is equally important that this material not be removed from the bodies until the remains have been photographed and the identification process begun.

The identification process is done in an assembly-line fashion in which the remains are processed through pre-arranged work stations, including overall body photography, inventory of associated remains and personal effects, finger and footprinting, dental examination (radiographs and charting), full-body radiographs and autopsy when indicated. In the event of viewable remains it has been found advantageous to dedicate one station to a closed circuit television system, with the camera situated in the morgue area and the screen in another suitable location. A black-and-white screen is preferable, in that it is less personal and less offensive than color. Not only does this procedure substantially expedite the identification process, but relatives allowed to view their kin in this way derive considerable emotional benefit from the experience (Fig. XVIII-5).

Depending on the number of victims, the process of identification can be handled by wall charts depicting the progression and various data, or better, by computer. Whereas wall charts become soiled and often display inaccuracies because of the number of people who have access to such displays, it is possible to assure that a computer be handled by a single reliable operator. A number of software systems exist that are designed to compare the developed postmortem

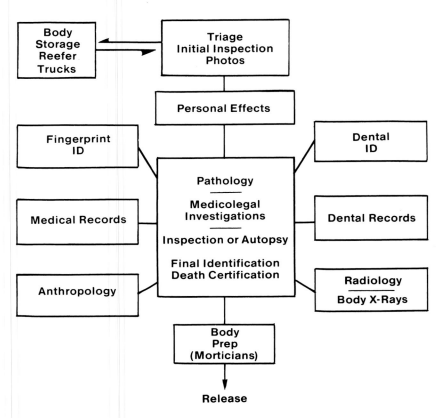

FIGURE XVIII-4. An algorithm approach to the medicolegal investigation of a mass disaster.

data with acquired antemortem data as it becomes available. This use of computers has become particularly important in dental identifications where a large amount of information can be rapidly sorted and compared and possible matches identified.

Computers played a vital role in the identification process of 156 victims of the Northwest 255 crash at Metropolitan Airport outside of Detroit in August, 1987. The dental team utilized computers and a specially developed program never used before. Tracking of the identification was started on a wall chart that soon became unmanageable. On the second morning after the crash, a PC with an ordinary database-filing program was brought to the temporary morgue. The computer operator created fields for necessary information and the passenger data was loaded on the computer, printouts were provided to the various teams 3–4 times daily, to keep workers informed as to which victims had been identified

and by what means—dental, fingerprints, etc. This allowed concentration of resources on those victims who were still unidentified. A similar effort in the ArrowAir crash in Gander, Newfoundland in December 1985 with processing of the 256 recovered remains at Dover Air Force Base enabled the multidisciplinary, multiagency investigation effort to identify all 256 people.[8]

Display of distinctive personal property allows for tentative identification in some cases and also for on-site return of valuables to the next of kin. Handling and storage of large quantities of personal property, until claimed by relatives, sometimes months, even years later, can present a significant problem.

Another useful tool is the fax machine that may be used to gather various types of antemortem data, including photographs, dental charts and fingerprints. When available e-mail can be used in the same way. Documentation of all steps is critical. Photographs provide a visual

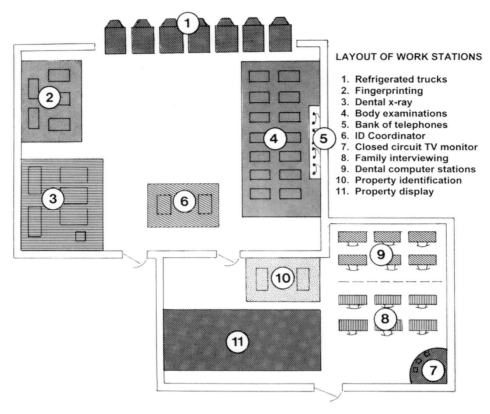

LAYOUT OF WORK STATIONS

1. Refrigerated trucks
2. Fingerprinting
3. Dental x-ray
4. Body examinations
5. Bank of telephones
6. ID Coordinator
7. Closed circuit TV monitor
8. Family interviewing
9. Dental computer stations
10. Property identification
11. Property display

Figure XVIII-5. Layout of work stations used in NW 255 crash at a temporary morgue situated at an airport hangar.

means of documenting identification and autopsy findings.

The identification process begins with inspection of the crash site before the fatalities have been removed. Unlike crime scenes, crash sites rarely maintain their integrity for long; security is essential and is an early consideration in any disaster plan (Fig. XVIII-6a). Once the scene is secured and emergency medical and fire suppression teams have completed their roles, the medicolegal investigators working with law enforcement personnel should grid the scene and inventory and photographically document all findings within each grid before removal. This is particularly important for remains, personal effects and aircraft wreckage. Gridding has proved to be advantageous because items and connected parts in proximity of each other prior to the crash will tend to remain that way on the ground. Police tape is best used for gridding (Fig.

XVIII-6b). In most cases, a pre-arranged alphanumeric system is used for the grid and a sequential numbering system for all of its contents. Numbered stakes may be placed at the site of each find to provide for easy and rapid reference at the scene (Fig. XVIII-6c). Experience has shown that the use of ordinary toe tags for labeling of human remains at a disaster scene is inadequate because rain, humidity and secretions from the remains destroy these tags, making them illegible. An alternative, inexpensive, and durable toe tag made of thick aluminum foil is now available. Pertinent identifying information may be inscribed onto the surface with an ordinary ballpoint pen. The tag will retain its integrity indefinitely. A thin wire may be used to tie the tag to the body bag or a red *biohazard* bag or a small thick gauge plastic bag, depending on the size of the specimen. It is advisable that both the body, or body part, and the body bag or other

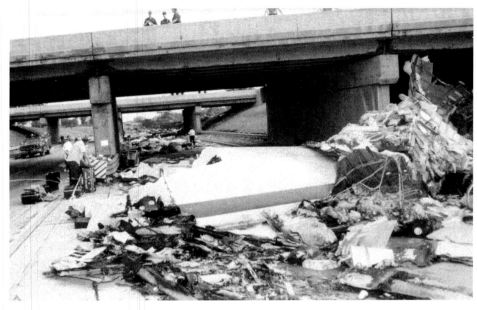

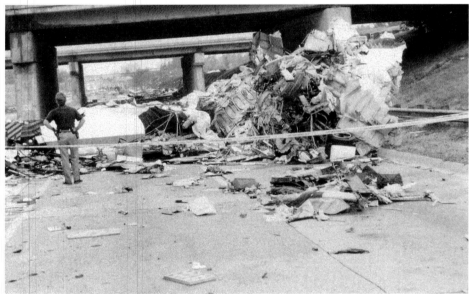

FIGURE XVIII-6a–b. These pictures show the extent of destruction of a plane which crashed on takeoff from a height of 150 feet. Care must be taken where removal of bodies trapped in the wreckage requires cutting with torches, as oxygen tanks may be mingled among the twisted metal.

container be tagged. Safety considerations dictate that as few people as possible be involved in the process until the scene is secured and cleared of hazards including flammables, ordinance, explosive materials and wreckage. It usually is advisable to establish several perimeters around the crash site with access limited to identified necessary personnel. A bright colored vest and picture ID are helpful for recognition of authorized workers.

Recovery and storage of fatalities from the crash site often requires additional resources such

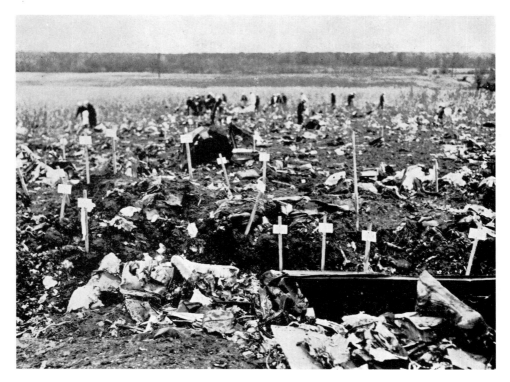

FIGURE XVIII-6c. Only after tagging and placement of numbered stakes may tissues and belongings be removed to the mortuary.

as refrigerated trucks, perimeter security and adequate working space. A temporary morgue may be necessary, depending on the number of victims. This facility should be selected for its proximity to the crash site and the availability of running water, adequate lighting, communications, bathrooms, and food services as well as administrative and security requirements.

In crashes where there is extensive fragmentation and ground disruption, excavation may be necessary to recover buried remains and wreckage. This may involve shovels, rakes and possibly heavy equipment, such as a backhoe or front-end loader, and the services of the public works department. The excavated material is systematically examined by sifting through wire screens, then labeled according to grid and numerical sequence, photographed and inventoried (Fig. XVIII-7).

After a two-day search of the surface, following the Pan Am crash (Boeing 707) in Maryland in December of 1963, 4,247 pounds of tissue were recovered, an estimated 1/3 of the total weight of the 81 people onboard. The crash site was excavated utilizing a front-end loader. The excavation area was 15 feet wide, 16 feet deep and over 120 feet long. A total of 7,998 pounds of tissue were recovered, approximately 3/4 of the estimated weight of all people in the plane (Fig. XVIII-8).

In the crash of ValuJet 592, in 1996 the aggregate weight of recovered fragments was 4,073 pounds of tissue, an estimated 26% of total passenger weight. No whole bodies were recovered. Instead, over 4,000 fragments of human remains were scattered within the swampy environment of the Florida Everglades.[9]

In most cases where there are multiple fatalities, refrigerated trucks will be needed to secure and preserve the remains. These are usually leased from a local source. An adequate number is necessary to allow separation of identified incomplete remains from the unidentified. The crash of NW 255, indicated above, required six refrigerated trucks for the six-day duration of the operation. Frequent temperature checks in the trucks will insure adequate functioning of the cooling units and prevent freezer burns of the remains.

The intensive recovery and identification process underscores the importance of society's

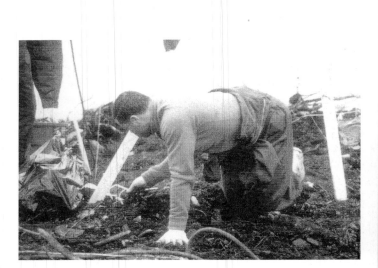

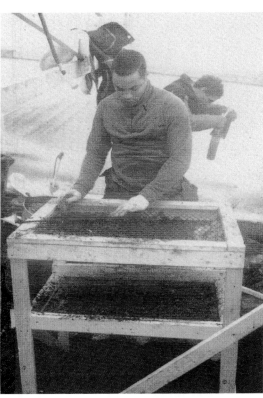

FIGURE XVIII-7a–b. (a) Scene of recovery efforts. (b) Search for small fragments on ground and use of makeshift sieve.

aversion to mass graves. After the sinking of the Russian submarine *Kursk* in the Barents Sea on August 12, 2000, the Russian government intended to declare the ship a natural mass grave site and leave the sailors onboard on the ocean floor. Outrage of the victims' families and the Russian public reversed this declaration and led to the decision to recover the remains at a suitable time and provide individual burial for each one of the crew.

In the case of extensive fragmentation of the bodies, a portion of a denture or a finger may confirm the presence of a particular individual on the plane and allow issuing of a death certificate (Fig. XVIII-9a–c). An unidentified individual means a hampered investigation and delay in settling the victim's estate. Such persons fall under the Uniform Absent Persons Act which requires petitioning the court for receivership of the estate until the person is identified or legally declared dead. Resolution of such cases may have a waiting period up to seven years.

At present, most positive identifications and frequently many presumptive identifications are made on the basis of dental examination. The forensic odontologist plays a critical role in this process. Dental radiographs, including panorexes and bitewings, underscore the need for good antemortem and postmortem dental records. A number of dental identification systems have been developed in which key personal facts are encoded and implanted in a tooth. Lack of agreement on which tooth and what system as well as constitutional issues appear to prevent further development of this technology.

Despite such difficulties, over 80% of the passengers of NW 255 which crashed near Detroit in 1987 were identified by dental records as compared to 12% who were similarly identified in a crash in Maryland in 1963.[10]

Between 1993 and 1995, 86 people died in 14 suicidal terrorist bombings in Israel. Identification was made by visual recognition, supported by other physical data in 40.8%, 36.6% by fin-

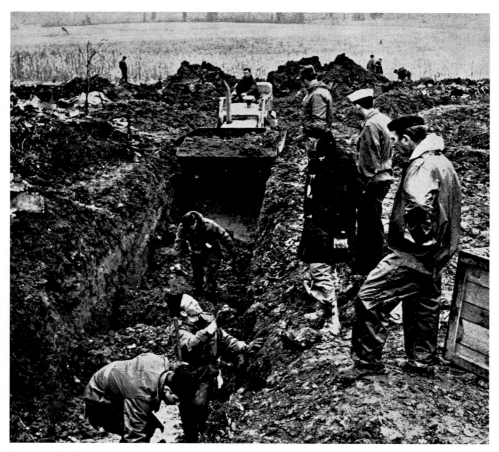

FIGURE XVIII-8. Excavation of crash site in Maryland yielded almost double the amount of tissue recovered on the surface.

gerprints, 11.2% by dental comparisons, 9.8% by medical matches and 1.4% by DNA profiling.[11]

Fingerprints often provide the means for positive identification. However, antemortem fingerprint records may not be available, even when there is a high probability of their existence based on known military service or other employment that require security clearance. It has been estimated that less than 25% of the American population has fingerprints on file. If postmortem fingerprints are obtained, the only fingerprints available for comparison may be from latent prints developed from the personal effects of the victim at the crash site or his or her home; this assumes that a presumptive identification has been made on some basis. Further, only a single fingerprint is needed to confirm identification by comparison with an existing fin-

gerprint record, but all ten prints are required if no tentative identification is available.

There is surprising variability in presumptive antemortem identification data, particularly height, weight, eye and hair color, blood type, evidence of previous childbirth, and known surgical procedures such as cholecystectomies, gastrectomies, appendectomies, hysterectomies, herniorrhaphies and circumcisions. Laparoscopic surgical procedures have made surgical scars in the skin difficult or impossible to recognize. Medical histories including old fractures, prosthetic devices, heart disease and skeletal or joint pathology may have to be correlated with autopsy findings and additional medical data. Pacemakers and new prosthetic devices have serial numbers which can be tracked through the manufacturer. Frequently, useful data include descrip-

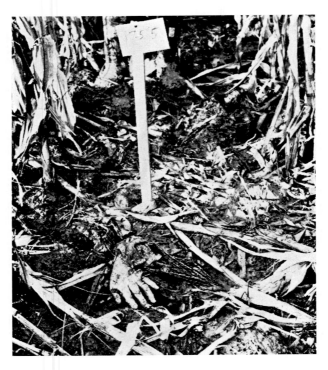

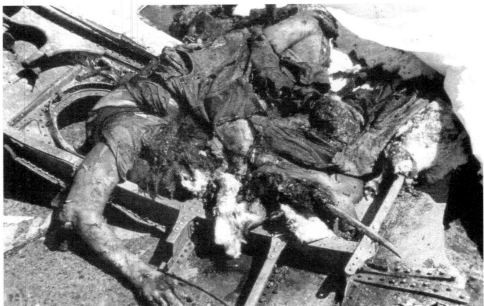

FIGURE XVIII-9a–b. (a) Stake erected at the site where a body fragment (left hand) was found. (b) Mutilated and decapitated unrecognizable body among aircraft debris.

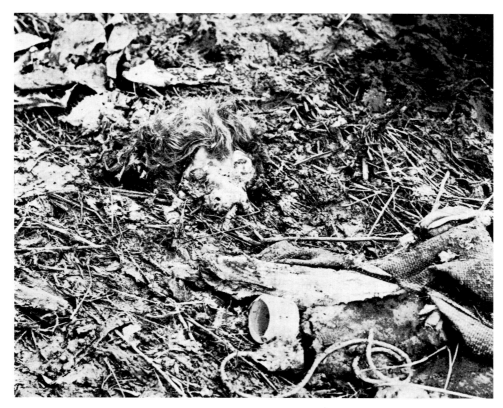

FIGURE XVIII-9c. Scalp and portion of a face found in the wreckage of a plane crash.

tions of tattoos, jewelry and photographs of the individual showing facial and scalp characteristics, ear shapes (Fig. XVIII-10) and dental diastemata. Antemortem photographs of the victim obtained from families and personal effects on the bodies or in baggage often provide the means necessary to make an identification. These characteristics often lead to presumptive identification, particularly when reconstructive procedures are required. The refractive indices of eyeglasses and dental prostheses may prove valuable in comparing pre and postmortem data. Dental prostheses sometimes have the victim's name or social security number imprinted.

Forensic anthropologists are often able to provide substantial information in such investigations despite extensive injuries and commingling of body parts. Combining these capabilities with those provided by serologists and criminalists/microscopists (hair analysis) may permit adequate sorting of the remains. Blood and sex typing is now possible on formalin-fixed, paraf-

fin-embedded tissues using monoclonal antibodies for the major blood groups and the Y chromosome and looking for antibody staining of endothelial surfaces. DNA profiling of remains both nuclear and mitochondrial has significantly improved the likelihood of identifying most if not all victims providing there is antemortem material to be compared with postmortem data. Some states, Michigan is one example, require hospitals to obtain a drop of blood from each newborn on a PKU card which is kept on file indefinitely and obviously available for comparison (ed.). Microscopic studies on scene evidence may identify a causal factor in a crash, such as a bird strike revealing feather fragments or nucleated red blood cells.

Time constraints were a detriment for use of DNA profiling until recently. New procedures enable positive identification and matching of tissues, including tissues subjected to high temperatures, to the point of calcination, in less than 3 hours.[12]

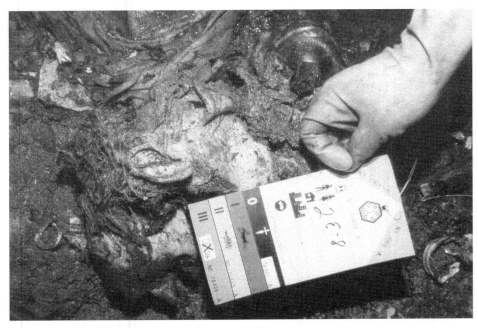

FIGURE XVIII-10. Unidentifiable remains of a white woman. The ear may serve for comparison if premortem photographs are available. If identification by ear comparison is not possible, it certainly can be used for exclusion.

In order to make these results functional, a system must be developed for retrieving medical, dental, radiographic, law enforcement, military, federal, and family records creating a registry of data. These comparative databases help epidemiologists and disaster planners identify issues that are unique to a particular disaster or are common in most multiple casualty incidents. Evidentiary material obtained from families may include items such as hair, shaving fragments, blood or tissue samples, and photographs. With the appropriate technology and analysis of all evidentiary items, the information process may begin. An appropriate computer system greatly facilitates this process.

A system for adequately educating and training all personnel prior to an incident is fundamental in the planning process. It is wise to continuously improve and update training programs. Unfortunately, training and experience are minimal in most jurisdictions and published disaster plans are often disregarded during an actual multiple fatality incident. A program of repetitive orientation and familiarization should include all levels of disaster personnel from executive to site staff. Scheduled and spontaneous *full dress* rehearsals are helpful to achieve coordination when a disaster occurs.

The disposition of identified remains will be determined by the next-of-kin, disposition of non-associable parts and unidentified remains must be made by the local jurisdiction. In this juncture it must be understood, as indicated earlier in this chapter, that *identified* may mean a portion of a finger with an identifiable print or an identifiable portion of a denture. Theoretically a single tooth may be identifiable. The remaining tissues of this victim may not present identifiable characteristics which end up being buried in one or several caskets of unidentifiable remains. In the crash of NW 255 in Detroit, everyone onboard this plane and 3 people on the ground were identified, consequently 156 death certificates were issued, yet, there were 11 full caskets of remains buried as unidentifiable tissues.

METHODS OF IDENTIFICATION

Portable full body and dental x-ray units and a medical x-ray film processor or other source for developing film can be used to identify victims in a multiple fatality disaster. Even if the medical examiner's or coroner's office has a fixed unit, it is advisable to locate a source for portable units. A C-arm fluoroscope is not essential, but in incidents where live ammunition and explosive devices might be embedded within bodies, it can be a lifesaver. Portable screens or lead sandwiched between half-inch sheets of plywood are necessary for proper shielding and radiation safety. These shields are easily moved or nailed into position. Radiographs often provide the first confirmatory estimation of recovered remains based on gender, age, size, medical condition, etc. that can be confirmed or expanded by further study. Likewise, photography plays an important role in the investigation by providing documentation on the individual case as well as the overall process. A portable ladder is useful for identification photography.

During triage employ a system of numbering the cases to maintain proper records, including documentation of personal effects, clothing, and photographs. Accession numbers are also given to separate body parts or fragments. These body parts or fragments may be specifically matched with remains after initial, presumptive, or even confirmatory identifications are made.

The identification process is a multidisciplinary exercise involving pathologists, fingerprint experts, dentists, anthropologists, radiologists, laboratory personnel experienced in blood and DNA typing, criminalists, and morticians. Bodies from disasters are often mutilated, fragmented, crushed, decomposed, macerated, biologically or chemically contaminated, burned, or charred. Multiple methods are used for identification:

Fingerprinting, footprinting, and palmprinting: Although personnel are trained to obtain prints, only experts in fingerprint identification, usually from the identification division of the FBI or local crime laboratories, are qualified to analyze, classify, compare and certify these prints. The most difficult identification problem will be comparing fingerprint records with latent prints from physical evidence and personal effects. Although many people in the United States have been fingerprinted, approximately 30% of the records submitted to the FBI cannot be classified and retrieved for comparison.

Dental identification is best performed by a forensic odontologist. The procedure may also be carried out by general practice dentists and anthropologists who have been trained to perform these duties.

Anthropological studies, including anthropometric measurements, are performed by forensic or physical anthropologists. Experienced forensic pathologists may be capable of skeletal examination and data collection, but they may need assistance in interpreting these findings.

Radiological studies provide useful and often pivotal clues to identification of the remains, probable mechanisms of injury and estimates of applied forces.[13] X-rays may identify the pilot at the controls at the time of the crash (Fig. XVIII-11a–b). Radiographs are particularly important in inflight breakups because they may identify blast injuries or other evidence supporting the presence of an explosive device. It is interesting to note that bodies usually are not disintegrated by a crash even from an altitude of 30,000 feet. When disintegration occurs, it is usually due to the twisting and turning of the aircraft and the subsequent impact or an explosion in mid-air (Figs. XVIII-12 and XVIII-13). Of course, passengers seated in proximity of the explosion will be most affected. Radiographs also identify displaced dentition and other foreign materials, including bullets, surgical staples, and pre-existing skeletal conditions. Body diagrams depicting soft tissue and skeletal findings supported by photographs, radiographs and the autopsy report correlate with other aspects of the investigation. X-ray studies are useful for commingled or charred remains, old and new fractures, congenital or acquired skeletal defects and detection of foreign objects such as metallic fragments of bullets. Radiologists and anthropologists have used superimposition techniques for identification purposes.

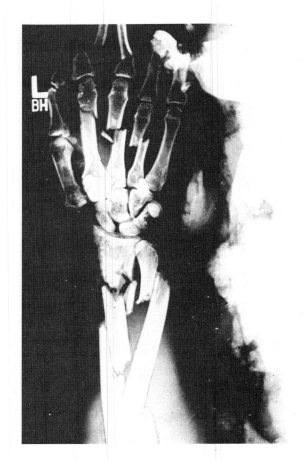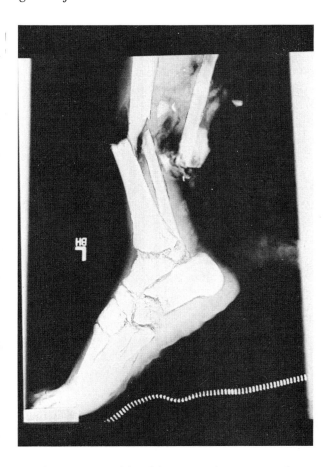

FIGURE XVIII-11 a–b. (a) Multiple, largely transverse fractures of the forearm and hand from a crash victim are characteristic of those seen when the pilot is at the controls at the time of impact. Such a finding may eliminate the likelihood of pilot in-flight incapacitation. (b) Transverse boot-top patterned fractures of the lower leg from a crash victim indicating direction of applied force as well as relative magnitude. Such injuries are seen primarily in two situations: (1) feet on the rudder pedals (a pilot) or (2) buckling of the floor boards.

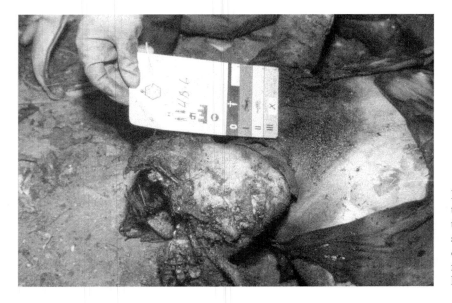

FIGURE XVIII-12. Vast laceration of the top of the head with fragmentation of the skull and complete extrusion of the brain. Such injuries are common in aircraft crashes and result from striking the head on the overhead structures.

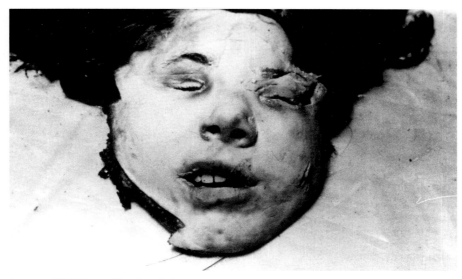

FIGURE XVIII-13. The facial skin of a Native American female was sheared off and found trapped among plane wreckage. Identification was possible by draping and molding the tissue around paper toweling in order to reshape the face.

Criminalistic studies are used for determining cell types, blood groups, hemoglobin types, and for DNA identification procedures. Hair and fiber comparisons, bloodstain evaluation, and other examinations of physical evidence are best handled by criminalists in federal, state, or local crime laboratories.

Examination of the victims' clothing may provide clues just as in a criminal investigation. Such examination may require the services of a crime laboratory, particularly where microscopy and trace residue analyses are indicated. There is always the possibility that an aircraft crash is not accidental, but rather a suicide and/or homicide. With in-flight breakups such as PAN AM flight 107 over Lockerbie, Scotland in December of 1988, these examinations may be crucial to any attempted reconstruction and evaluation of the cause of the crash.[14,15] Since aircraft crashes are criminal investigations, identification, recovery, documentation and reconstruction become critical aspects of the investigation and identification of the perpetrators.

COUNSELING OF FRIENDS AND PERSONNEL (POSTTRAUMATIC STRESS)

Mass disasters cause not only injuries, deaths, and damage to property and to the environment, but also significant psychological impact on survivors, rescuers, and service providers, similar to the effects of war or other violence. Hyams[16] (1996) has reviewed numerous psychiatric syndromes identified and evaluated during the past century including shell shock, acute combat stress reaction, chronic fatigue syndrome, and posttraumatic stress disorder. These syndromes have similar symptoms including fatigue, headache, shortness of breath, forgetfulness, impaired concentration, and sleep disorders. Appropriate support, including the availability of counseling, should be provided not only to personnel involved in recovery operations, investigation, identification and treatment of victims, and postmortem examinations, but also to surviving family members and friends. A number of canine handlers in search and recovery efforts have reported clinical depression in their dogs with repeated *failure* to find living victims.

DOCUMENTATION

Photography plays a critical role and is the most economical commodity in the documentation process. Photographs of the remains as recovered and received as well as those obtained during the identification process and autopsy provide a visual basis for accident reconstruction, particularly that based on patterns of injuries. In most investigations, photographs are obtained with a 35-mm camera and any ordinary color film. Video documentation is increasing in frequency with both positive and negative aspects. The video often captures unintended comments.

Special photographic studies such as color infrared or ultraviolet exposures are possible with a minimum of additional material and cost. Such studies are useful in scene documentation, particularly of aerial views (Fig. XVIII-14). The Armed Forces Institute of Pathology accident investigation teams regularly use color infrared slide film for aerial scene documentation to better define ground gouges, fuel spills, and fire damage as well as locate *missing* aircraft structures and recently damaged flora such as tree strikes. The only additions required to the standard 35-mm setup is a yellow filter (#12) and, color infrared film. Unlike thermal infrared studies, photographs enhance physical changes in the environment by shifting the observed visual spectra and, in so doing, frequently enhance *patterned injuries* of the soil and foliage.

Video studies often identify aspects of the scene or examination that might otherwise be missed. Such video coverage may prove invaluable where the probable cause of the crash remains elusive despite extensive investigation. Analysis of aircraft crashes is based on developing facts and defining the assumptions that are used in formulating the accident investigation and testing reconstructions against the evidence. For example, an initial scene observation at the crash site of Avianca Airlines flight 52, a Boeing 707 attempting to land at LaGuardia International Airport in New York, was the absence of the smell of jet fuel on the bodies or luggage which suggested the aircraft had no fuel at the time of impact. Further investigation revealed that the aircraft had run out of fuel that resulted in the mishap.

Digitized photographs allow for further forensic imaging to enhance patterns of injury, instrumentality, or other pertinent data. This capability has allowed for appropriate images to be integrated into reports within the content rather than as enclosures or appendices. These images also lend themselves to telemedicine/teleconferencing opportunities potentially expanding available resources.

SEARCH AND RECOVERY OF VICTIMS

In contrast to typical search and recovery operations, SAR efforts follow general guidelines on public safety and public health and are reflected in the multidisciplinary, multijurisdictional aircraft mishap investigations surrounding TWA 800, Swiss Air, Egypt Air and most recently Air Alaska. Recovery efforts in adverse environments such as ocean depths involve specialized equipment and training such as supplied by the US Navy and contractors with unmanned submersibles, dredging capabilities and other sophisticated detection systems. The complex excavation and search recovery efforts following the bombing of the Federal Building in Oklahoma City or similar efforts in earthquake areas worldwide,[17] including the enormous devastation and loss of life in the Gujarat region of India, reflect the complexity and magnitude of a multidisciplinary and multi-factorial disaster plan and its implementation. In the latter in excess of 30,000 people were killed. Identification issues in such cases are often significant and usually involve heavy dependence on positive identification techniques versus presumptive. These are labor and time intensive efforts. Positive techniques include fingerprints, footprints,

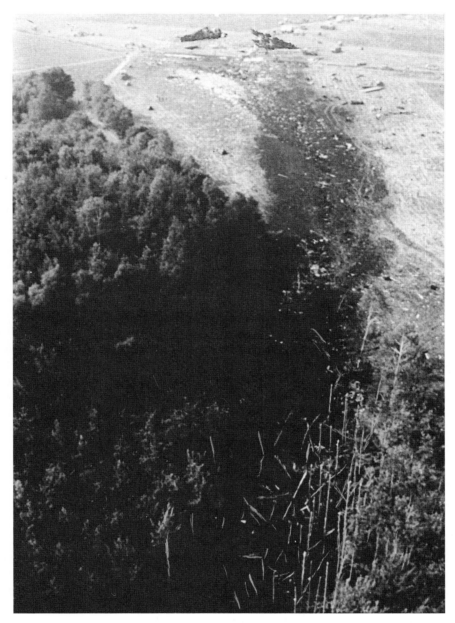

FIGURE XVIII-14. Aerial photography in aircraft crash investigation. In the background is the runway from which the airliner departed. The crash site shows a linear progression of aircraft breakup and the relative attitude of the aircraft.

palmprints, dental comparisons, radiographic superimposition, and DNA profiling. In a similar fashion recovery of wreckage or other physical evidence is critical in search and recovery efforts and is focused on recovery and validation of real and demonstrative evidence that will corroborate or contradict the prevailing opinion(s) on the cause of the multiple casualty incident. These efforts are well-developed in commercial transportation mishaps and FEMA-directed disaster management. Useful references are DeHart's[18] *Fundamentals of Aerospace Medicine* (1985) and Kenneth Beers and Sylves & Waugh's[19] (1996) *Disaster Management in the U.S. and Canada.* An older but extremely useful reference on wilderness SAR is TJ Setnicka's[20] *Wilderness Search and*

Rescue, Appalachian Mountain Club, Boston MA, 1980.

COLLECTION AND PRESERVATION OF EVIDENCE

Evidence often exists in multiple forms and is usually categorized into real or demonstrative depending on its value for identifying or defining the corpus delicti or modus operandi. Evidence may be physical or hearsay, circumstantial or testamentary but is evaluated by principles of relevance and materiality for admissibility. Physical evidence, especially trace evidence is dependent on the exchange principle of Locard's which states that you take and deposit evidence wherever you go and whatever you do. Chemistry, microscopy, spectroscopy and photography play critical roles in the documentation and characterization of that principle in evidence recognition, collection, preservation, and evaluation. The chain of custody is an important concept to minimize and preferably prevent the disappearance of evidence or problems of intrusion based on casual walk through the scene, moving of objects and handling, or removing of items.

Preservation of evidence is often focused on preserving transient evidence influenced by the postmortem interval, adverse weather, geography, size, or other factors. This evidence varies from insect instars, trace evidence, footprints, volatile gases, bitemarks, and large surfaces requiring photography and casting for preservation. The procedures include identification, chain of custody, and competency of materials based on relevancy and materiality. Excellent texts which discuss the principles, tactics and procedures of crime investigation are available.

Scene investigation must be directed toward preservation of evidence, photographic documentation and cataloguing the scene in an organized and controlled manner. Scenes are often divided into grids sequentially and labeled for later correlation. Failure to follow these procedures will jeopardize later identification attempts and reconstruction.

CORRELATIONS

Many pathologists feel that their contribution to the investigation should be limited to identification and documentation of trauma and preexisting conditions supplemented by toxicological studies. In most cases, this would satisfy statutory requirements necessary to complete death certificates. Additional correlations are often left to other investigators who are expected to take the factual information and give it meaning within the context of the particular aircraft crash. In these cases, what is often lost is the unique relationship between man, machine and the environment. These relationships have a significant impact on the safety aspects of transportation, let alone any tort or criminal issues that may be present. In order to go beyond these basic steps, the pathologist must study the crash site and

wreckage and communicate with other investigators. This dialogue usually opens additional avenues of investigation or at least focuses on the pertinent unanswered questions. From a medicolegal point of view, these issues may represent the causes of death, likely mechanisms of injury, lethality of the injuries, probable survival times, significance of pre-existing diseases or conditions, correlation of toxicological studies relative to disease or performance and possibly psychophysiological factors which may be consequential. The latter are often evaluated by testimonial evidence, lifestyle reconstructions and physiological markers assessed by laboratory testing and simulations. These assessments often require some degree of profiling, including *psychological* autopsies. Although considered controversial by some, such profiling may provide valuable insights into psychophysiological factors of the investigation.

Survivability is evaluated by considering the loss of occupiable space, crash forces to which the victim was exposed (as they relate to deceleration and impact) and the post-crash environment. These parameters often identify why some travelers survive and others do not. These correlations require integration of crash-site evidence, wreckage and autopsies. Crashworthiness is frequently evaluated utilizing the acronym CREEP.

C = CONTAINER
R = RESTRAINTS
E = ENVIRONMENT
E = ENERGY-ABSORPTIVE MATERIALS
P = POST-CRASH FACTORS

This design engineering endeavor examines the man, machine and environmental interfaces. The observed physical and chemical injuries are correlated with aircraft structure, cargo and post-crash environment such as fire, water immersion, altitude and wreckage characteristics. The aircraft and its contents should reflect the forces that were present during the crash sequence. These forces, as previously stated, have magnitude and direction. The questions raised are: What force was necessary to create this condition and from what direction did it come? The goal of crashworthiness is to attenuate the crash forces, as much as possible, to accommodate human tolerances. This is the principle behind seat anchors, energy absorbing cushions, frangible structures, airbags and shoulder-lap belt restraints. It is assumed that certain directional as well as magnitude markers of the crash forces will be evident in the documented injuries of the victims, as well as in the aircraft wreckage and crash-site evidence. The AFIP accident investigation teams use a series of body injury markers to evaluate these force vectors (Table XVIII-1). These markers have been identified over a period of time in a variety of aircraft crashes and appear to hold up under the limited mathematical and engineering modeling that is frequently applied. They provide the medicolegal investigator at least a starting point for this type of analysis. Evaluation of the post-crash environ-

TABLE XVIII-1

AFIP MORPHOLOGICAL MARKERS OF CRASH FORCES

Observation	G Force	Axis
Vertebral fractures	15–30	Gz, Gx
Pulmonary contusions	25–30	Gx, Gy
Rupture of atlanto-occipital membrane	30–35	Gz, Gx
Laceration of aorta	50+	Gx, Gz
Transection of aorta	80+	Gx, Gz
Skull fractures*	50+	Gx, Gz, Gy
Pelvic fractures	100+	Gz, Gx
Fragmentation	350+	Gx, Gz, Gy

* Based on Swearingin chart FAA Rep AM 65–20 July.

TABLE XVIII-2

DECELERATION FORCE TOLERANCE LIMITS

Position		Limit	Duration
Eyeballs-out	(–Gx)	45 G	0.1 sec.
Eyeballs-in	(+Gx)	83 G	0.04 sec.
Eyeballs-down	(+Gz)	20 G	0.1 sec.
Eyeballs-up	(–Gz)	15 G	0.1 sec.
Eyeballs-left	(–Gy)	9 G	0.1 sec.
Eyeballs-right	(+Gy)	9 G	0.1 sec.

ment relative to survivability is dependent on the nature of the observed injuries, their relative lethality and the supporting toxicological and testimonial evidence. Since many aircraft crashes result in fires, autopsy and toxicological studies, indicating some period of survival based on evidence of smoke inhalation, suggest potentially survivable crash forces and support the ongoing safety studies in self-sealing fuel tanks, egress systems, protective clothing and fire-retardant, non-toxic materials.[21]

What are the limits of human tolerance? There probably is not a single answer. Tolerance is a function of force magnitude, pulse duration and direction. Relatively high pulses can be withstood for short periods, fractions of a second. Longer pulsed forces are less tolerated. Published deceleration force tolerance limits seem to have been largely derived from studies at the Crash Survival Investigator's School in Tempe, Arizona (Table XVIII-2).

Injury patterns play an important role in aircraft crash investigation. The absence of control surface injuries such as by the throttle, control stick, or rudder pedals on the pilot(s) may indi-

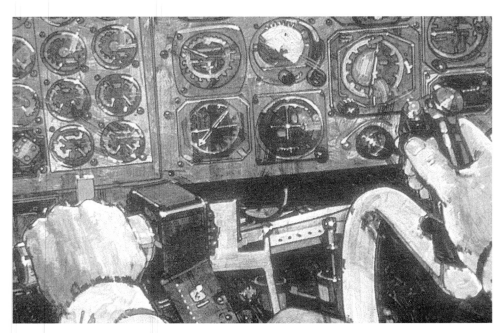

FIGURE XVIII-15. Diagram of pilot controls of airplane.

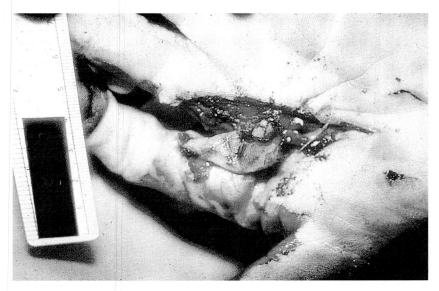

FIGURE XVIII-16. Injury to pilots hand. Pattern of injuries is dependent on configuration of control surfaces, such as yokes, sticks and rubber pedals.

cate in-flight incapacitation (Figs. XVIII-15 and XVIII-16). The absence of restraint injuries may suggest that the individual was moving around and that the emergency was sudden and unexpected. Similar cause-and-effect scenarios may be possible based on other injury patterns. This analysis is the basis for reconstruction of events based on injury patterns. The first goal is to recognize and document the observed injuries. Some may be subtle and not readily appreciated during the autopsy. Body radiographs and photographs, as well as clothing and equipment examinations often support the assumptions on which the analyses should be based. A starting point would be to collate the observed injuries into injury categories:

1. Patterned blunt force injuries such as the control surface injuries of the pilot's hands and feet, restraint belt injuries, and documented impacts with aircraft structures such as consoles, bulkheads, and cargoes.
2. Penetrating injuries from rotor blades, explosions, wire strikes, or gunshot wounds.
3. Thermal injuries including flash or flame burns, evidence of heat and smoke inhalation and electrocution.
4. Drowning
5. Hypothermia/Hyperthermia
7. Decompression/Dysbarism
9. Hypoxia

The general patterns of injury usually considered in light of the above list include: seat restraints, flailing injuries, vertical and lateral deceleration injuries, rollovers, free-falls (115–120 fps) and thermotoxic injuries (Fig. XVIII-17a–b). Egress injury pattern analysis is often possible depending on the available systems in the aircraft. These may involve ejection seats, escape modules, bailouts, and a variety of slides. Despite several different manufacturers, ejection seats have much in common with one another. The acceleration is usually 50–70 fps with an 18–20 G peak in about four feet. Survivability is dependent on the ejection being within the operating ejection envelope that varies from aircraft to aircraft and is based on altitude, attitude, airspeed and sink rate.

Toxicology plays an important role in vehicular crashes. In aircraft accidents, toxicological studies are usually done by the medical examiner/coroner's office and toxicology laboratory such as, the FAA facilities in Oklahoma City or the AFIP in Washington, D.C. The general categories of study include carboxyhemoglobin saturations, cyanide, volatiles and drug screens. Difficulties in interpretation rest with correlating measured concentrations with expected levels of impairment or performance decrements. Therapeutic drug monitoring may be extremely important, since positive findings in vehicular operators may point to self-medication and underlying medical conditions which would disqualify the pilot or crew member from flight operations. Some flight operations may be more hazardous than others. This is true of military flights in general and crop dusters in particular. In the latter, it is prudent to obtain heparinized blood for anticholinesterase measurement. Many times no blood or urine are available for analysis in which case these categories of toxicological study are done on tissue homogenates or samples obtained by gentle squeezing of organs such as the spleen. Postmortem artifacts must be considered. Alcohol levels as high as 200 mg/dl have been reported from advanced postmortem decomposition. In such cases, acetaldehyde, acetone and the higher alcohols (propyl and butyl) are frequently found in small quantities.

Clinical chemistry studies are important in evaluating possible physiological causes of a crash. The mainstays for these evaluations are peripheral blood, urine and vitreous humor. This line of investigation is important in evaluating medical conditions that might be present and contributory. Sturner has studied the stability of clinical chemistries after death (Chapter III, Part 2). Of particular interest are the clinical markers of diabetes, hypoglycemia, dehydration and fatigue. With the exception of sickle cell disease and trait, most hematological studies rapidly degrade following death. Recommended analyses include peripheral blood and vitreous for glucose, and possibly a glycolated hemoglobin, vitreous electrolytes, urea nitrogen and creatinine, urine specific gravity and dipstick analysis and possibly CK isoenzymes, troponin 1 and lactic acid.

Physiological parameters are notoriously difficult to assess. Key factors include hypoxia, dysbarism, spatial disorientation, olfactory illusions, G-induced loss of consciousness, hyperventilation and oxygen toxicity. Most of these are evaluated by analysis of flight operations, simulations and testimonial evidence. Clues as to the event may come from radio transmissions or recorded aberrations of flight. Certain chemical analyses may compliment such assessments and when combined with toxicological results provide valuable insight into the man-machine interface.

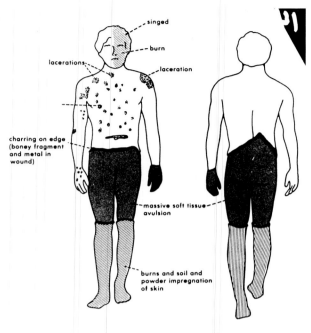

Injury Pattern Distribution

FIGURE XVIII-17a. Injury pattern distribution as a result of a bomb explosion under a victim's seat. Such schematic diagrams provide valuable insight to the investigators in sorting out the victim's injury patterns.

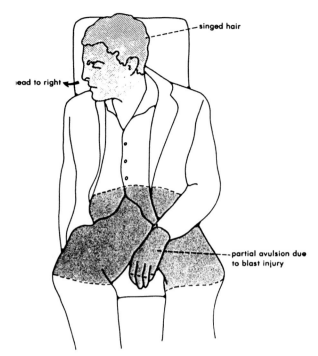

Proposed Body Position Based on Injury Patterns

FIGURE XVIII-17b. Reconstruction diagram indicating a victim's position in the seat based on injuries documented in the schematic total body diagram of body injuries.

Pre-existing diseases and conditions are important aspects of any medicolegal death investigation. In many cases, positive findings are likely incidental, based on developed evidence of the crash investigation. In some cases, they may be contributory to causal factors. In general, there are only three systems which cause sudden and unexpected death: the central nervous system, cardiovascular and respiratory systems. The autopsy examination supported by medical records, histology, clinical chemistry and toxicology should try to exclude with precision the presence of tumor, infection, vascular defects and congenital or acquired anomalies that might predispose to a spontaneous pneumothorax, cardiac arrhythmia, syncope or air embolism. Of these three systems, an extensive cardiovascular pathology evaluation is the most important. Other pre-existing conditions which might not be fatal but may cause in-flight incapacitation include pancreatitis, gastric, or duodenal ulcers, diarrhea, vomiting, cholecystitis, kidney stones and middle ear or eye disease.[22] These tend to be issues involving general aviation rather than commercial or military aircraft where extensive monitoring of aircrews is routine.

BOMBS AND EXPLOSION INJURIES: APPLICATIONS AND PRINCIPLES

The increasing number of bombings are examples of multiple casualty incidents. These unanticipated explosions are usually acts of terrorism such as the bombings at the World Trade Center, the Murrah Federal Building in Oklahoma City (1995) and the Summer Olympic

Games in Atlanta (1996). Relatively common over the past few years are bombings of abortion clinics and numerous fire scenes with an explosion component. Explosions occur in a number of different scenarios such as fires, fuelings, space flights, aircraft mishaps and acts of terrorism both domestic and foreign. The worst explosion mishap in the past century occurred in Halifax, Nova Scotia on December 6, 1917 when a French ammunition ship, Mont Blanc, collided with a Belgian steamer killing 1,654 people. On April 16, 1947, the SS Grandchamp carrying ammonium nitrate exploded in the harbor of Texas City, Texas killing 561 persons and injuring 3,000. Property damage exceeded $57M and workmen's compensation payouts exceeded an additional $8M. The following day, the SS High exploded in the same harbor killing one and injuring 100. The explosion of the Space Shuttle Challenger during takeoff on January 18, 1986 and the complicated recovery and reconstruction of a witnessed event remains prominent in many minds. In April of the same year, the Chernobyl incident occurred in the Ukraine, directly affecting those living within a 60-mile radius.

Explosions are generally characterized as one of three types: mechanical, chemical or nuclear and are either classified as low explosives (gunpowder, smokeless powder) or high explosives (ammonium nitrate, dynamite, plastics) based on their blast pressure velocities. Low explosives are deflagrating explosions with maximum velocities under 3200 fps and include natural gas, cellulose nitrate, black powder and grain dust. High explosives are detonating events with fissile (fracturing) and brissance (shattering) components and velocities exceeding 3200 fps up to 30,000 fps. Examples include dynamite, nitroglycerin, trinitrotoluene, RDX, HMX, PETN, mercury fulmigate, and ammonium nitrate fuel oil (ANFO). Detonation of high explosives requires blasting caps which may be either electrical or non-electrical and often a booster or primer. Low explosives are chemical mixtures whereas, high explosives are compounds. Deflagrating explosions show a progressive slow burn characteristic with normal heat transfer mechanisms and are dependent on external factors, ambient pressure

and temperature conditions. The pressure differential created in such explosions results in a pushing pressure damage readily evident on examination. Detonating explosions have a relatively high or fast burn rate with high energy release and high peak pressures. Shock waves are the usual, resulting in both fracturing and shattering damage. In both types of explosions there are two components, a positive pressure wave radiating outward and a negative wave that is often three times longer in duration than the positive wave. Explosions in soil and water differ from those in air by their lack of compressibility. They produce a clearly defined shock wave similar to that of an earthquake.

The primary wave may be modified by structures or shapes that reflect, focus, or shield. These are considered secondary characteristics. Primary characteristics include blast pressure measured in psig or millibars, fragmentation with velocities often in excess of 2700 fps, and thermal damage. Basic parameters include maximum pressure with hydrocarbon based explosions typically 7–9x ambient pressure (7100–9120 millibars) whereas, a gaseous detonation generates pressures of 14,000–18,240 millibars. One standard atmosphere equals 1013.3 millibars. Gas mixtures range from 1.3–6% for gasoline to 15-28% for ammonia, dusts 40–50 grams/m^3, and metallic powders from 30–120 grams/m^3.

Scene and crime laboratory investigations of explosions track with those of fire and arson investigations with special attention directed toward documentation, segmented or layered scene assessments, and handling of physical evidence to preserve volatiles, residues and other trace evidence varying from tool marks to fingerprints. Suspected residues are collected with methanol or ethanol swabs and preserved in vials. Acetone will break down many explosive components. A variety of instrumentation is used for chemical and physical analysis including gas chromatography, mass spectrometry and raman spectroscopy.[23,24] Radiographic analysis of fragments and intact bombs remain the workhorse for explosive incident analysis. The focus of these investigations is to find and interpret signatures leading to the identification of the perpetrator and data as to modus operandi.[25] Collectively these laboratory analyses become part of a materials repository and a library for future investigations.

Explosions cause: (1) pressure wave, (2) concussion, (3) vacuum, (4) fragmentation, and (5) heat. These translate into primary, secondary and tertiary effects based on six principal results: (1) complete body disruption, (2) explosive injury, (3) masonry injury, (4) flying missiles, (5) burns and (6) blast injuries. The primary effects are related to pressure, secondary to fragmentation, and the tertiary effects are translational. These findings are applied to both biological and physical structures with the view of developing directional vectors that will aid in the reverse design engineering efforts. Markers include the following:

Psig Value	Observation
0.5–1.1	glass breakage
>1.0	knocks people down
1–2.0	corrugated panels collapse
2–3.0	collapse of unreinforced cinder blocks
5–6.0	pushes over telephone poles
>5.0	rupture of tympanic membranes
>10.0	buildings collapse

>35.0	threshold for fatality
>50.0	50% fatality rate
>65.0	99% fatality rate
>300.0	crater formation
>300.0	total body disruption

From these directional vectors and a meticulous search of the scene in layered standardized formats documenting, recovering and collecting physical evidence, the characteristics of the epicenter and blast pattern can be reconstructed. Flame fronts are useful directional vectors particularly in deflagrating explosions where fuel is pushed along the pressure front resulting in a fireball and a patterned burn area. Pressure drops as a cube of distance so that the burn area is always smaller than the pressure front. Energy assessments are acoustical, kinetic, thermal and fissile. T.K. Marshall, chief pathologist for Northern Ireland described in 1976 and 1978 blast injury categories still widely used: (1) complete disruption, (2) explosive injury with mangling of body parts, small discrete bruises, abrasions, puncture wounds and dust tattooing, (3) fragmentation and shrapnel wounds, (4) blast effects on ear drums, lungs and gastrointestinal tract, traumatic emphysema, (5) blunt force injuries from structural collapse, (6) burns and inhalation of toxic substances, and (7) sharp force injuries from metal and glass.

SUMMARY

The occurrence of environmental and other disasters appear to be on the increase. Thus, the scope of the medicolegal death investigation in mass casualty incidents is increasing.

Medical examiner and coroner offices have an important role in managing mass disasters. Each office should develop a plan to recover, process, identify, and examine victims. When possible, confirmatory methods should be used for identification. A multidisciplinary team of forensic pathologists, odontologists, and anthropologists should review and verify each identification before the remains are released. The final judgment as to the adequacy of a particular identification is the responsibility of the senior forensic pathologist.

REFERENCES

1. Clark, M.A., Wagner, G.N., Wright, D.G., Ruehle, C.J., and McDonnell, E.W.: Investigation of incidents of terrorism involving commercial aircraft. *Aviat Space Environ Med, 60,* 7, Section II, A55, July 1989.

2. Wolcott J.H., and Hanson C.A.: Summary of the means to positively identify the American victims in the Canary Islands crash. *Aviat, Space Environ Med, 51* (9): 1034–1035, September 1980.

3. McCormick, M.M.: The National Transportation Safety Board and the investigation of civil aviation and transportation accident. *Am J Forensic Med Pathol, 1:* 239–243, 1980.

4. Shemonsky, N.K. et al.: Jurisdiction on military installations. *Am J Forensic Med Pathol, 14* (1): 39–42, 1993.

5. *U.S. Naval Flight Surgeon's Manual,* 3rd edition, Washington, DC, 1993.

6. Friedman, E.: Coping with calamity-How well does health care disaster planning work? *JAMA, 272* (23): 1875–1879, 1994.

7. Kahana, T., Ravioli, J.A., Urroz, C.L., and Hiss, J.: Radiographic identification of fragmentary human remains from a mass disaster. *Am J Forensic Med Pathol, 18* (1): 40–44, March 1997.

8. Mulligan, M.E., McCarthy, M.J., Wippold, F.J., Lichtenstein, J.E., and Wagner, G.N.: Radiologic evaluation of mass casualty victims: lessons from the Gander, Newfoundland accident. *Radiology, 168:* 229–233, 1988.

9. Mittleman, R.E.: The crash of ValuJet Flight 592: A forensic approach to severe body fragmentation. Miami-Dade County Medical Examiner Department, Miami, Florida 2000.

10. Fisher, R.S., Spitz, W.U., Breitenecker, R., and Adams, J.E.: Techniques of identification applied to 81 extremely fragmented aircraft fatalities. *J Forensic Sci, 10:* 121, 1965.

11. Hiss, J., and Kahana, T.: Suicide bombers in Israel. *Amer J Forensic Med Pathol, 19* (1): 63–66, 1998.

12. Kahana, T., Freund, M., and Hiss, J.: Suicidal terrorist bombings in Israel: Identification of human remains. *J Forensic Sci, 42* (2): 260–264, 1997.

13. Brogdon, B.G. (Ed): *Forensic radiology.* Boca Raton, FL: CRC, 1998.

14. Eckert, W.G.: The Lockerbie Disaster and other aircraft breakups in midair. *Am J Forensic Med Pathol, 11* (2): 93–101, June 1990.

15. Moody, G.H., and Busuttil, A.: Identification in the Lockerbie air disaster. *Am J Forensic Med Pathol, 15* (1): 63–69, March 1994.

16. Hyams, K.C. et al: War syndromes and their evaluation: From the U.S. Civil War to the Persian Gulf War. *Ann Intern Med, 125* (5): 398–405, 1996.

17. Angus, D.C., Pretto, E.A., Abrams, J.I., Ceciliano, N., et al.: Epidemiologic assessment of mortality, building collapse pattern, and medical response after the 1992 earthquake in Turkey. *Pre-hospital and Disaster Medicine, 12* (3): 222–231, 1997

18. DeHart, R.L. (Ed): *Fundamentals of aerospace medicine.* Philadelphia: Lea and Febiger, 1985.

19. Beers, K.: *Sylves & Waugh's: Disaster management in the U.S. and Canada.* 1996.

20. Setnicka, T.J.: *Wilderness search and rescue.* Boston, MA: Appalachian Mountain Club, 1980.

21. Hill, I.R.: Toxicological findings in fatal aircraft accidents in the United Kingdom. *Am J Forensic Med Pathol, 7* (4): 322–326, December 1986.

22. Rayman, R.B.: Sudden incapacitation in flight. *Aerospace Med, 43:* 953–955, 1973.

23. McLuckey, S.A., Glish, G.L., and Carter, J.A.: The analysis of explosives by tandem mass spectrometry. *J Forensic Sci, 30* (3): 773–788, July 1985.

24. Nowicki, J., and Pauling, S.: Identification of sugars in explosive residues by gas chromatography-mass spectrometry. *J Forensic Sci, 33* (5): 1254–1261, September 1988.

25. Stoffel, J.: *Explosives and homemade bombs,* 2nd edition. Springfield, Thomas, 1972.

Chapter XIX

TRAUMA OF THE NERVOUS SYSTEM[1]

Part 1

FORENSIC NEUROPATHOLOGY

VERNON ARMBRUSTMACHER AND CHARLES S. HIRSCH

THE STUDY OF THE BRAIN in the context of forensic medicine, not surprisingly, involves a large and varied exposure to the pathologic effects of neurotrauma. In our experience, we find brain abnormalities that cause or contribute to death or help to clarify the manner of death in approximately 25% of all forensic autopsies. The total range of these conditions covers the gamut of neuropathology and is beyond the scope of this chapter. Approximately 35% of functionally important neuropathologic lesions relate either to *neurotrauma* or to conditions that complicate or must be distinguished from trauma. This chapter will describe the pathology of *neurotrauma* and lesions that occur secondary to trauma. In doing so, we will emphasize the features that may answer questions of special forensic interest, although our precision in answering these questions is often not as great as we would wish.

We have noticed over recent years that a progressively increasing proportion of the persons we examine would have died at the scene or very quickly in the hospital with little or no medical intervention. Such individuals now survive much longer and frequently have had extensive inva-

sive procedures. The benefits of dramatic advances in modern diagnostic and therapeutic techniques have saved many lives, but the forensic neuropathologic examination of those who die is greatly complicated by the superimposition of an array of structural changes resulting from post-injury events. Often these people are maintained on a respirator for various lengths of time after total cessation of brain circulation and function. Sorting the effects of these changes from the primary lesions of the original injury is becoming more complex. One way to conceptualize the distinction between primary and secondary lesions is to think of primary lesions as causes of brain swelling and secondary lesions as results of brain swelling.

Fortunately, on the other hand, the quality of the clinical images obtained from CT and MRI and detailed physiologic data, such as blood flow and intracranial pressure (ICP), fill in many of the gaps between the head injury and the *respirator brain*. It has become more and more important, even critical, to analyze all of this information before arriving at final conclusions in a given case.

EXAMINATION OF THE BRAIN

While the subject of this chapter is the neuropathology of brain trauma, it goes without saying that the examination of the injured brain must be done in the context of all other bodily

injuries, especially the head, the effects of treatment and whatever additional information is known about the circumstances of the injury. The pathology of surface and soft tissue injuries and

---

[1] This chapter was originally authored by Richard Lindenberg, M.D. and many of his excellent photographs have been retained.

most aspects of cranial fractures are considered in other chapters of this text. The techniques for removal of the brain and spinal cord are widely known and, if carefully followed, artifacts can be avoided. A few additional comments are presented here.

Examine and describe the head in layerwise detail noting the presence and absence of injuries, the age of injuries and the effects of surgical intervention. When the scalp is reflected, note the presence or absence of scalpular or subscalpular injury, which may be the only sign of impact. Avoid a deep cranial cut with the oscillating saw. If there is underlying subarachnoid or intracerebral hemorrhage, a deep cut may allow blood to flow into the subdural space before the cranium is removed, thus confusing the presence or absence of a subdural hemorrhage. This may be of critical importance. As the cranium is entered, carefully separate the underlying dura. This will prevent tearing artifact of the brain. Look at the brain carefully before removing. This is a point at which critical information can be permanently lost, such as the presence, location and volume of subdural hemorrhage, the presence of large, basal, acute, subarachnoid hemorrhage, the integrity (or not) of the vertebral arteries. The presence of large, basal subarachnoid hemorrhage in the context of a possibly traumatic death requires the examiner to account for the entire course of the intracranial vertebral arteries and to note the presence or absence of blunt head and/or neck injury. After removing the brain, always strip the dura in order to visualize the base of the skull. When removing the spinal cord using the posterior approach, position the body so as to neutralize the cervical and lumbar lordotic curves. Always remove the spinal cord with the dura. Cut the spinal laminae as far lateral as possible and do not allow the oscillating saw blade to penetrate beyond the laminae. Pulling the cord as it is being removed easily causes stretch artifacts.

If the examination of the brain requires the demonstration of small lesions and their distribution (i.e., multiple sclerosis, multiple contusions, diffuse axonal injury), the brain should be suspended in neutral, buffered formalin for at least two weeks prior to sectioning. Weigh the brain prior to fixation since it may gain or lose weight in the fixative. The normal range of the brain weight is from 1100 g to about 1700 g. The reason for such a wide range is not clear. The amount of blood and water is an important variable.

Coronal sections are the most informative plane in which to visualize the brain because they best display the condition of the base of the brain, an important area when assessing trauma. In general, always examine the brain using a consistent systematic technique so as not to overlook abnormalities. Of course, modify the system when it makes sense, e.g., bullet tracks, cerebellar tonsils, looking for aneurysms, ponto-medullary lacerations, etc. Separate the brain stem at the midbrain. Section the brain at approximately 1 cm intervals. Make some sections at specific levels such as the optic chiasm, mammillary bodies, interpeduncular fossa and 2–4 mm rostral to the aqueduct of Sylvius (middle of the hippocampus). Always display the sections the same way (e.g., right is right and left is left). Make a longitudinal 3–4 mm deep incision in the right side of the brain stem (midbrain to cervical/medullary junction) to mark the right vs. left side. Have a default pattern of always taking sections from the same side (i.e., right) unless otherwise specified. When describing lesions, picture yourself reading your report several years later with no diagrams or photographs. Note color (reflects the age of the lesion), consistency, location and size of abnormalities. Note negatives that are pertinent to the issues being considered. Be concise.

Secondary Effects of Neurotrauma

Except for instances of rapidly lethal injury, almost all cases of fatal neurotrauma manifest some secondary injuries of the brain. These are lesions that are not directly due to the trauma itself, but evolve later as complications of the lesions that are the direct result of trauma. Some secondary injuries develop almost immediately while others appear after a delay of hours, days, or longer. The primary and secondary traumatic lesions must be properly sorted in the forensic analysis of a case in order to accurately assess the

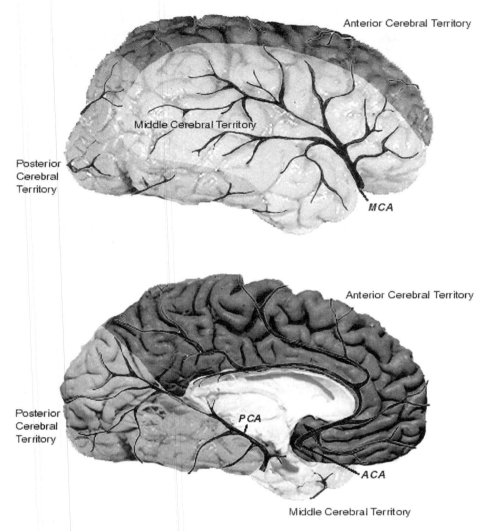

FIGURE XIX-1. *Diagram.* Lateral (upper) and medial (lower) surfaces of the cerebral hemispheres indicating the areas of supply of the anterior (ACA), middle (MCA) and posterior (PCA) cerebral arteries.

extent and mechanism of the trauma. These secondary effects often are responsible for much of the morbidity and even the death of the victim. To a large extent, these changes result from disturbances in cerebral circulation and are manifestations of brain swelling, shifting, herniation, increased intracranial pressure, vascular compression, anoxia/ischemia or even the total non-perfusion of the brain. Grossly, these injuries result in characteristic patterns of brain distortions, disruptions, hemorrhages and necroses. Separating these lesions from primary traumatic injuries requires some familiarity with normal neuroanatomy, the cerebral blood supply and the physiology and pathophysiology of brain circulation.

In our discussion of the pathology of neurotrauma, we first will describe the appearance and the dynamics of these secondary changes.

The Circulation

The anatomy of the cerebral vasculature is reflected in the distribution of many of the lesions that complicate neurotrauma (Figs. XIX-1 to XIX-5).

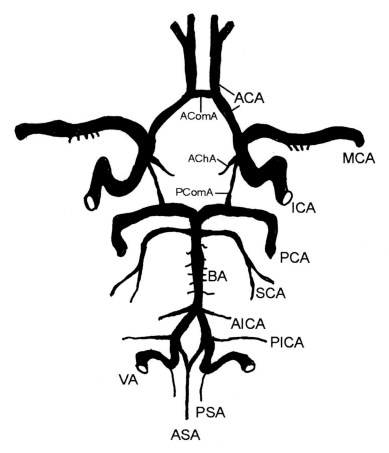

FIGURE XIX-2. *Diagram.* The circle of Willis and some of its branches. AComA = anterior communicating artery; ACA = anterior cerebral artery; MCA = middle cerebral artery; ICA = internal carotid artery; PComA = posterior communicating artery; AChA = anterior choroidal artery; PCA = posterior cerebral artery; SCA = superior cerebellar artery; BA = basilar artery; AICA = anterior inferior cerebellar artery; PICA = posterior inferior cerebellar artery; VA = vertebral artery; PSA = posterior spinal artery; ASA = anterior spinal artery. Groups of numerous small penetrating arteries arise from the cerebral surface of the circle of Willis and its proximal branches.

The paired *internal carotid arteries* forming the *anterior circulation* (Fig. XIX-2) each give rise to the *anterior cerebral arteries* which are joined in the midline by the *anterior communicating artery* and supply the medial 2–4 cm of each cerebral hemisphere from the frontal pole to the parietal/occipital junction. The terminal branches interdigitate with those of the middle and posterior cerebral arteries forming the *watershed* or *border zone* among the three arteries (see Figs. XIX-1 to XIX-4).

The continuation of the internal carotid after the origin of the anterior cerebral artery becomes the *middle cerebral artery,* which supplies the lateral surface of the cerebral hemisphere from the lateral frontal lobe to the lateral occipital lobe and from the paramedian cerebral convexity to the paramedian base of the frontal lobe and the inferior-lateral surface of the temporal lobe. Its terminal branches interdigitate with those of the anterior cerebral and the posterior cerebral arteries forming watershed areas along the paramedi-

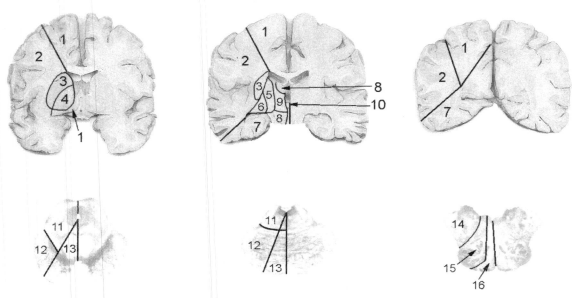

FIGURE XIX-3. Coronal sections of cerebral hemispheres and cross sections of brain stem showing the arterial distribution. 1. anterior cerebral artery; 2. middle cerebral artery; 3. lenticulostriate artery; 4. recurrent artery of Heubner (branch of anterior cerebral artery); 5. thalamogeniculate artery (branch of posterior cerebral artery); 6. anterior choroidal artery (branch of internal carotid artery); 7. posterior cerebral artery; 8. posterior choroidal artery (branch of posterior cerebral artery); 9. thalamoperforating artery (branch of posterior cerebral artery); 10. hypothalamic artery (branch of posterior communicating artery); 11. superior cerebellar artery (see also Figure XIX-4); 12. short circumferential branch of the posterior cerebral artery; 13. paramedian branch of the posterior cerebral artery; 14. posterior-inferior cerebellar artery (see also Figure XIX-4); 15. lateral bulbar branch of vertebral artery; 16. paramedian branch of vertebral artery.

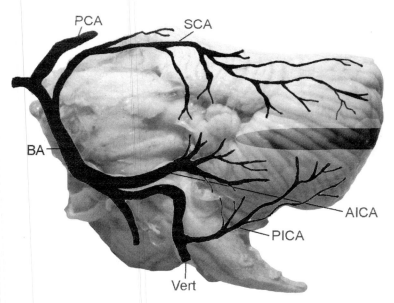

FIGURE XIX-4. Lateral view of cerebellum and brain stem with major arteries. The shaded area represents the border zone between the superior and inferior cerebellar circulation. PCA = posterior cerebral artery; SCA = superior cerebellar artery; AICA = anterior-inferior cerebellar artery; PICA = posterior-inferior cerebellar artery; Vert = vertebral artery; BA = basilar artery.

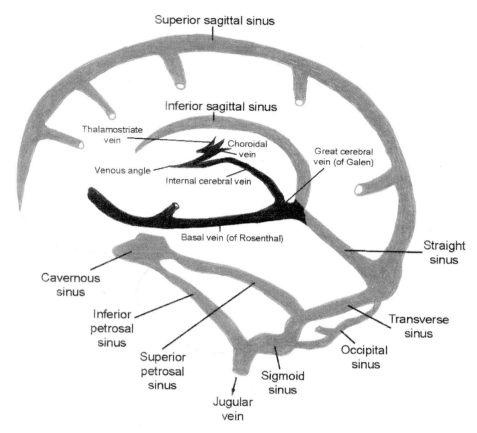

FIGURE XIX-5. *Diagram.* Relationships of the venous circulation of the brain. The light shade represents the dural sinuses and the dark shade represents the major veins.

an convexity surface of each cerebral hemisphere approximately 3 cm from the sagittal midline, the inferior frontal surface approximately 3 cm from the midline and along the inferior lateral surface of the temporal lobe (see Figs. XIX-1 to XIX-4).

The paired *vertebral arteries,* forming the posterior circulation, each give rise to a *posterior-inferior cerebellar artery (PICA)* along the ventral surface of the medulla which supplies the posterior-inferior portion of each cerebellar hemisphere and the lateral medulla. (The spinal cord circulation will be described later). The vertebral arteries join in the midline at the caudal base of the pons to form the single *basilar artery,* which gives rise to a pair of *anterior-inferior cerebellar arteries (AICA).* Each AICA supplies the anterior-inferior portion of the cerebellar hemisphere. The terminal branches of each PICA and AICA interdigitate with those of the superior cerebellar arteries to form a water-

shed area (see Fig. XIX-3). The pair of *superior cerebellar arteries* arises from the basilar artery at the rostral pons and each supplies the superior half of the cerebellar hemisphere. Its terminal branches interdigitate with those of the PICA and AICA to form a watershed zone along the lateral margins of the transverse mid-plane of each hemisphere (see Fig. XIX-3). The basilar artery terminates at the interpeduncular fossa by giving rise to a pair of *posterior cerebral arteries,* which supply the inferior-medial surfaces of the occipital and temporal lobes. The terminal branches of the posterior cerebral arteries interdigitate with those of the anterior and middle cerebral arteries forming the above noted watershed areas. Each posterior cerebral artery gives rise to a *posterior communicating artery* that connects to the internal carotid artery and completes the *circle of Willis* (see Figs. XIX-1 to XIX-4).

The relative size of each of the branches varies considerably among individuals. Wide connections among the four major supplying arteries leads to a more robust cerebral circulation if narrowing or occlusion develops in one or more of the major arteries.

The major cerebral arteries just described spread out over the cortex in the subarachnoid space and penetrate the cortex and white matter extending almost to the ependymal surfaces of the lateral ventricles.

Numerous small *penetrating arteries* (see Figs. XIX-2 and XIX-4) arise from the cerebral surface of the internal carotid, proximal anterior, middle and posterior cerebral and the anterior and posterior communicating arteries. These arteries (see Figs. XIX-3 and XIX-4) penetrate the base of the brain and supply the *diencephalon* and *basal ganglia.* [The *diencephalon* is that part of the brain derived from the prosencephalon that consists of the thalamus, hypothalamus and the subthalamus. *Basal ganglia* is a term with variable meaning among clinicians, neuroradiologists, neuroanatomists and neuropathologists but the most common use (and the way it is used in this chapter) includes the caudate nucleus, putamen, globus pallidus and claustrum.] The terminations of these arteries interdigitate with the penetrating surface branches of the anterior, middle and posterior cerebral arteries where they form an internal watershed area (see Fig. XIX-4).

Numerous similar arteries arise from the inner surface of the vertebral, PICA, AICA, basilar and superior cerebellar arteries to supply the brain stem.

Normally, the perfusion of the brain is maintained by a relationship between the *mean arterial blood pressure (MAP)* and the *intracranial pressure (ICP).* The intracranial pressure is 5–15 mm Hg and the MAP is about 100 mm Hg resulting in a *cerebral perfusion pressure (CPP)* of approximately 90 mm Hg. The factors that create the ICP constitute a closed system. The contents of the rigid calvarium (brain, blood, CSF) are not compressible and, therefore, an increase in any of these components or the addition of an expanding mass will result in an increase in ICP *(The Monro-Kellie doctrine).* The rise in ICP does not occur, however, until certain compensatory compliance mechanisms have been exhausted.

The cerebral circulation has some unique properties. Because of its large energy requirements, the brain captures 20% of the cardiac output and consumes 15% of its oxygen even though the weight of the human brain is only 2% of the body. The total *cerebral blood flow (CBF)* ranges from 750 to 1000 mL/min with approximately 550 mL/min coming from the internal carotid arteries and 200 mL/min from the vertebral arteries. This degree of perfusion is required because neurons depend on a steady supply of glucose and oxygen, which are its sole energy source and are stored in an amount that provides a reserve that lasts only approximately 15 seconds prior to disruption of function.

The energy requirements of the brain drive the CBF through *chemoregulatory* and *autoregulatory* control. Chemoregulatory responses include cerebrovascular dilatation in response to a rising PCO_2, a fall in pH, an increase in metabolic byproducts or a severe drop in PO_2. Cerebrovascular constriction results from a fall in PCO_2, a rise in pH and a decrease in metabolic byproducts. The autoregulatory response consists of vasodilatation in response to a fall in CPP and vasoconstriction in response to a rise in CPP. Autoregulation, then, can maintain a constant CBF in the face of rising or falling CPP but begins to fail below CPP of 60 mm Hg or above 160 mm Hg. If a rising ICP causes the CPP to fall, a compensatory systemic hypertension with bardycardia *(Cushing response)* develops. If a condition of elevated ICP results in a CPP lower than 40 mm Hg, the CBF will begin a dramatic decline.[1] Autoregulatory flow also constantly responds by dilating or contracting according to increased or decreased metabolic needs of active or inactive areas of the brain by physiologic mechanisms that are not completely understood.

Intracranial pressure (ICP) normally is maintained at a level of 5 to 15 mm Hg in adults, up to 5 mm Hg in children and up to 3 mm Hg in the newborn. Pathologic elevation of the ICP due to changes in blood flow, brain swelling and enlarging mass lesions such as hemorrhages are common in fatal head injuries. As the forces of increasing brain volume develop, there is limited compliance allowing the brain to adapt to the change before the ICP begins to increase. When this capacity is exhausted, the ICP rapidly increases similar to when a bicycle tire has been maximally inflated. If the rise in pressure is unchecked, the ICP can exceed the systemic blood pressure resulting in no cerebral blood flow, a situation that produces total cerebral necrosis.

Brain Swelling

The normal circulation of the brain has a number of unique features that influence the outcome of brain swelling, whether generalized or local. The brain is soft with no connective tissue support and has an enormous capacity to swell. The skull is protective, but also limits brain swelling. The fundamental question is whether the cardiovascular system can maintain perfusion of the brain in the face of rising intracranial pressure as the swelling brain is progressively compressed by the rigid skull.

An increase in brain volume complicates many neuropathologic conditions such as metabolic derangements, infections, tumors, infarcts, hemorrhages and trauma. These conditions may be focal or diffuse, acute or chronic and may involve an increase in cerebral blood volume (congestion), an increase in brain water (edema) or both. *Congestive brain swelling* eventually will progress to *cerebral edema*.

The pathologic evidence of the compliance of the intracranial contents to an enlarging brain or an expanding intracranial mass is based on displacement of the blood and cerebrospinal fluid (CSF).

The *cerebrospinal fluid* is an ultrafiltrate of plasma that is produced by the *choroid plexus* at a rate of approximately 20 cc/hr. Normally there is a volume of approximately 140 cc of CSF in the cranium and spinal canal, about 20 cc of which is in the ventricles. It flows into the *subarachnoid space* from the fourth ventricle through the two *lateral foramina of Luschka* and the *midline foramen of Magendie*. The CSF forms a thin layer of watery fluid in the subarachnoid space that covers the surface of the brain and spinal cord and surrounds the subarachnoid blood vessels. The outer membrane of the subarachnoid space is formed by the thin, delicate, transparent *arachnoid membrane* that covers the surface of the brain bridging the cerebral and cerebellar sulci and loosely covering the spinal cord. The inner membrane is the even more delicate *pia mater* that tightly covers the brain extending into the sulci and folia of the cerebrum and cerebellum. It also follows the cortical blood vessels as they penetrate the brain. The subarachnoid space is wide in some areas where the arachnoid membrane bridges larger gaps on the brain surface and these spaces are called *cisterns* (Fig. XIX- 6). The chiasmatic, interpeduncular and pontine cisterns are located at the base of the brain covering the optic chiasm, infundibulum, mammillary bodies and interpeduncular fossa and are called the *basal cisterns*. The *cisterna magna* is located over the dorsal medulla and between the inferior cerebellar hemispheres. The *quadrageminal cistern* overlies the dorsal midbrain. The basal cisterns and quadrageminal plate cisterns are sometimes called the *perimesencephalic cistern* (see Fig. XIX- 6). The presence and configuration of these cisterns are important observations for neuroradiologists and pathologists in assessing the degree of brain swelling. As the brain swells, the CSF is expressed from the ventricles and subarachnoid space due to increased reabsorption into the *dural sinuses* through the *arachnoid granulations*. This results in flattening and widening of the gyri, narrowing of the sulci, effacement of the cisterns and compression of the ventricles. It should be noted that the presence of these changes does not necessarily mean the ICP is elevated. It indicates the brain is swollen and is spreading into the available empty spaces by occupying some of the CSF compartment.

The intracranial pressure is measured in vivo by surgically placing various intracranial pressure measuring devices in the epidural, subdural, subarachnoid, intracerebral or intraventricular spaces. Intraventricular measurements are considered the gold standard but all of the above techniques are used. It is recognized, however, that pressure sensing units in the epidural or sub-

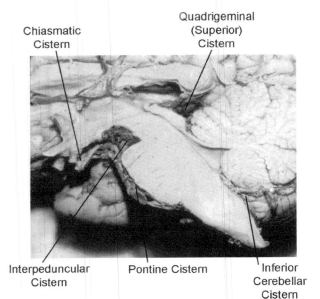

Chiasmatic Cistern

Quadrigeminal (Superior) Cistern

Interpeduncular Cistern   Pontine Cistern   Inferior Cerebellar Cistern

FIGURE XIX-6. *Diagram.* Sagittal view of brain stem, cerebellum and diencephalon designating the cisternal spaces. These are large subarachnoid spaces that result where the arachnoid membrane bridges a large gap over the pia arachnoid. The *chiasmatic cistern* is beneath and anterior to the optic chiasm. The *interpeduncular cistern* is anterior and between the cerebral peduncles of the midbrain. The *quadrigeminal (superior) cistern* is over the tectum of the midbrain and above the cerebellar vermis. The *inferior cerebellar cistern (cisterna magna)* is the space between the inferior cerebellum and the dorsal medulla. The interpeduncular and quadrigeminal (superior) cisterns are sometimes designated *perimesencephalic cisterns.*

dural space become less accurate at pressures above 30 mm Hg.

Using these devices, three clinically important types of ICP fluctuations have been described by Lundberg.[2] The *A wave,* also called a plateau wave, is greater than 50 mm Hg, is sustained for five to 20 minutes and is thought to result when there is cerebrovascular dilatation in a patient who is on the edge of compliance due to an expanding mass. They often develop during sleep when CO_2 retention-related cerebrovascular dilatation can cause the equivalent of a mass effect in a marginally compensated patient. The *B waves* are sharply peaked, less than 50 mm Hg, 0.5 to two-minute ICP elevations that result from phasic fluctuations in vasomotor tone and cerebral blood volume in patients with marginal

brain compliance. The *C waves* are less than 20 mm Hg, 4 to 8 Hz waves that may be part of the normal ICP pulsation due to heartbeat and respiration.

Once the cerebral compliance is exceeded, the intracranial pressure rises dramatically and *intracranial herniation* develops. It can be triggered by a minor or clinically undetected event. The volume of the intracranial mass lesion necessary to cause herniation varies according to the rate of accumulation of the mass and its location. A large, slow-growing neoplasm, such as a meningioma may be an incidental finding with a large mass effect but little or no herniation while the sudden accumulation of a hematoma can be lethal at a fraction of the size. The sudden accumulation of a hematoma of 150 mL is almost invariably fatal.[3,4] On the other hand, a patient with a clinically undetected slow growing tumor may suddenly precipitate lethal brain herniation by minor or clinically undetected trauma or by sudden, small, spontaneous tumor hemorrhage or even due to a small increase in cerebral blood volume as during a Valsalva maneuver.

ICP levels of 15–20 mm Hg are usually well tolerated and do not require therapy. Patients with ICP of 30 mm Hg require treatment. At levels of 37 mm Hg the pressure is severe and ischemia will develop. At 60 mm Hg, especially with cerebral shift, death is imminent. Patients with rising ICP have cerebrovascular instability and may experience episodes of loss of cerebrovascular tone and sudden increase in cerebral blood volume that can trigger brain shift, necrosis and herniation.[5]

To avoid ischemic brain necrosis, patients with increased intracranial pressure must maintain cerebral blood flow (CBF) roughly above 15 mL/100gm/min (normal 50 mL/100gm/min) or a minimum perfusion pressure (CPP) of 40 mm Hg (normal about 90 mm Hg). Fall of CBF or CPP below these levels can occur when the ICP rises above the mean arterial pressure due to expanding intracranial mass, by a fall in systemic arterial pressure or a combination of the two. Since there may be *intracerebral pressure gradients* due to shifting brain against irregular skull surfaces or focal swelling due to contusions and

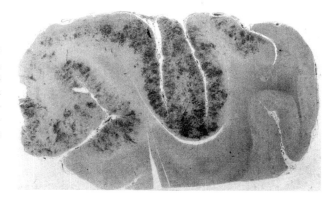

FIGURE XIX-7. Photomicrograph of cerebral cortex. (H&E) Hemorrhagic infarct. The cortex is diffusely hemorrhagic, involving the gyral crowns and sulcal cortex equally. This pattern may occur if thomboembolic occlusion results in ischemic injury to the non-perfused vasculature and fibrinolysis results in reperfusion or if ischemic injury is preceded by a period of venous obstruction, e.g., dural sinus thrombosis or transtentorial herniation.

hemorrhages, the cerebral blood flow may fall below the critical threshold and cause ischemic necrosis in a patchy pattern, not reflecting individual vascular territories.

The ischemic lesions may be hemorrhagic or anemic. When they are cortical and hemorrhagic, they are grossly distinguishable from traumatic lesions (hemorrhagic cortical contusions) by the fact that hemorrhagic infarcts involve the cortex evenly over the crowns of the gyri and into the sulci (Figs. XIX-7 and XIX-9) whereas a contusion tends to involve the crowns of the gyri, sparing the sulcal cortex (Figs. XIX-8 and XIX-10). Microscopic examination is helpful in distinguishing between infarcts and contusions, because infarcts typically spare the subpial layer of the cortex whereas this layer is typically destroyed in contusions. Sometimes, selective sulcal infarcts occur (Fig. XIX-11). If such a patient survives, the pattern of thin sulcal cortex topped by a crown of normal gyral cortex *(ulegyria)* will reflect the event (Fig. XIX-12). Diffuse, sulcal infarction may result when a patient with pre-existing intracranial hypertension suffers a drop in systemic blood pressure.[6,7]

Congestive Brain Swelling

Some with diffuse traumatic head injury develop brain swelling without evidence of increased brain water as seen in brain edema.[8–10] The onset can be rapid and appears to be due to increased cerebral blood volume due to loss of autoregulatory control of blood flow. This allows blood to accumulate in the capillary and venular compartments, probably also impeded from drainage by the relatively inflexible dural sinuses.[8] If the systemic blood pressure rises in the face of the intracerebral vasomotor paralysis, the intracranial pressure may rise to disastrous levels. This situation often is preceded by the development of pathologic pressure waves of the types noted above. Postmortem detection of this condition is difficult because the congestion may dissipate with the terminal fall in blood pressure. The only evidence may be recent necrosis of the uncal or medial temporal cortex due to pressure against the tentorial edge. The presence of widened gyri and narrowed sulci may reflect some degree of brain swelling, but in the absence of pressure injury to the brain surface, there may not have been increased intracranial pressure.[11]

Cerebral Edema

If the condition of acute brain congestion persists, the increased intravascular pressure breaks down the blood-brain barrier and vasogenic edema develops. Cerebral edema is a condition of increased brain volume due to increased brain water content. The most commonly encountered mechanism involves situations that damage the integrity of the blood-brain barrier and allow vascular fluid to leak into the interstitial space. It may be localized, for example, around a tumor or contusion. The edema around such lesions may create a mass effect larger than the initiating lesion itself. Diffuse edema may involve most of the brain, usually resulting from diffuse brain injury or from a global ischemic insult. Also, it

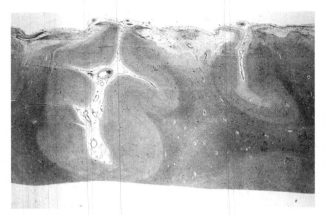

FIGURE XIX-8. Photomicrograph of cerebral cortex. (H&E) Old contusion. Note the triangular cavitary lesion in the crown of each of the three contiguous gyri. The adjacent white matter is pale. Abundant hemosiderin has accumulated at the apex of each contusion. The subpial layer of each gyral crown is not spared as it tends to be in ischemic lesions.

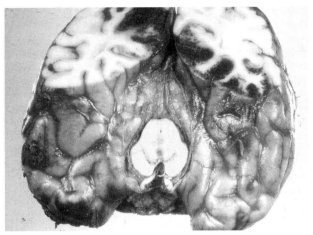

FIGURE XIX-9. Gross photograph of basal cerebrum and cut surface of each occipital lobe after fixation. There are bilateral tentorial grooves of the unci and parahippocampal gyri and bilateral posterior artery distribution acute hemorrhagic infarcts (the left side involves mostly the superior distribution of the calcarine branches). The hemorrhagic necrosis involves the cortex of the gyral crowns and sulci.

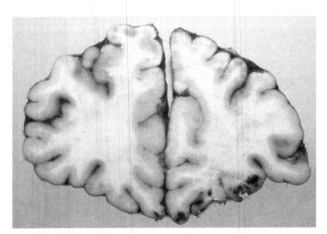

FIGURE XIX-10. Gross photograph of a coronal section of both frontal lobes of a fixed brain. The decedent was a pedestrian struck by a motor vehicle. Note the acute contusion hemorrhages in the gyral crowns of the inferior frontal cortex.

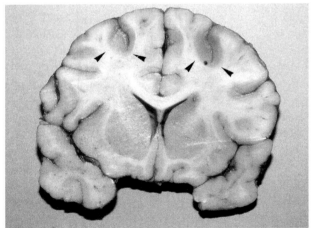

FIGURE XIX-11. Coronal section of cerebrum. 52-year-old woman who was in coma for 4 days following cardiac arrest during a diagnostic cardiac catheterization for occlusive coronary artery disease. There are acute, bilateral cortical infarcts in the border zones (arrowheads) between the anterior and middle cerebral arteries. The necrosis involves the sulcal cortex with relative sparing of the crowns of the gyri. If the patient had survived, the necrotic cortex would have been removed leaving shrunken, yellow-brown sulcal cortex and preserved, prominent cortex over the gyral crown (*ulegyria*–see Figure XIX-12).

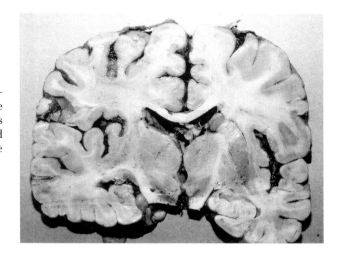

Figure XIX-12. Coronal section of cerebrum. Ulegyria. 79-year-old woman with a history of a remote stroke. Note the atrophy of the sulcal cortex of the left middle frontal gyrus and the preservation of the coronal cortex of the involved gyri resulting in a *mushroom* configuration. This is the late stage of the type of lesion depicted in Figure XIX-11.

may evolve from a pre-existing state of congestive brain swelling. If unchecked, the mass effect of the increased brain volume will result in rising ICP, pathologic pressure waves, diminishing cerebral perfusion, herniation and total cerebral necrosis.

Pathology of Increased Intracranial Pressure

When the increased pressure is longstanding and develops slowly, in instances such as obstructive hydrocephalus or the slow growth of a benign brain tumor, actual erosion and reabsorption of bone occurs. Particularly vulnerable are the dorsum sellae and the clinoid processes of the sphenoid bone, which may be completely reabsorbed. The orbital plates and the sphenoid wings become thin and may disappear. The convolutional markings of the cerebral cortex on the inner table become abnormally prominent *(lacunar skull)*.

The autopsy pathologist can recognize the presence of antemortem increased intracranial pressure by detecting brain damage in certain characteristic patterns. These changes are the result of pressure and distortion on the brain surface or certain vulnerable blood vessels. When a mass lesion begins to evolve, distortion of the adjacent brain structures occurs at the expense of the brain components that can be displaced, first the cerebrospinal fluid and, then, as the pressure mounts, the blood. Since the dura and the skull form several open compartments, a pressure gradient develops across these boundaries and herniation occurs from one compartment to another. This causes distortions and impressions on the brain surface in predictable and recognizable places (Fig. XIX-13).

Any cerebral mass, but especially a lateral mass, will produce a *midline shift* that presses medially against the *falx cerebri* and downward against the edge of the *tentorium cerebelli*. Pressure against the falx results in herniation of the cingulate gyrus beneath the edge of the falx causing a characteristic deformity (Figs. XIX-13 to XIX-16). The compressed and herniated cingulate cortex will become necrotic and hemorrhagic if the compressive force is sufficient to compromise circulation in the callosomarginal artery. The shift also distorts the *corpus callosum* usually by tilting the ipsilateral side downward and the contralateral side upward as it is pushed away from the mass (Figs. XIX-14 to XIX-16). When severe, hemorrhage and necrosis can develop in the midline of the corpus callosum and in the subjacent attachment of the *septum pellucidum* due to compression of the pericallosal artery (Figs. XIX-15 and XIX-16). The ipsilateral *lateral ventricle* is compressed and displaced medially and usually downward while the contralateral lateral ventricle is displaced laterally and usually upward (Figs. XIX-13 to XIX-16). Sometimes, the contralateral lateral ventricle becomes distended because of obstruction at the foramen of Monro due to distortion of the midline structures (Fig. XIX-16). This may necessitate a ventriculostomy drainage proce-

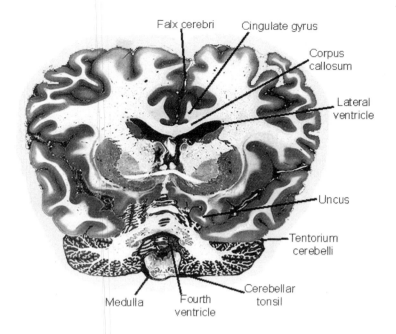

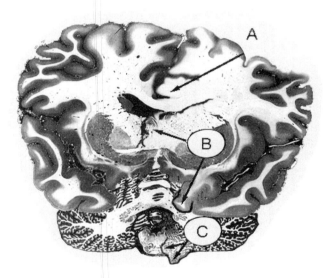

FIGURE XIX-13. *Diagram.* Two mid-coronal sections of the brain. The upper section shows the normal anatomic relationships. The lower section shows anatomic configurations of three types of internal brain herniations. In *A,* a chronic subdural hematoma has forced the ipsilateral cingulate gyrus beneath the falx *(cingulate gyrus herniation).* If severe, the resulting pressure can compress the *pericallosal* and/or the *callosomarginal arteries* (branches of the anterior cerebral arteries) causing ischemic necrosis and/or hemorrhage of the corpus callosum and/or cingulate gyrus respectively. In *B,* a temporal lobe mass has forced the ipsilateral medial temporal lobe through the incisura of the tentorium cerebelli *(transtentorial herniation)* and displaced the third ventricle and the right diencephalon to the left (cerebral midline shift). In *C,* a posterior fossa mass has forced the ipsilateral cerebellar tonsil into the foramen magnum *(tonsillar herniation)* and compressed the medulla.

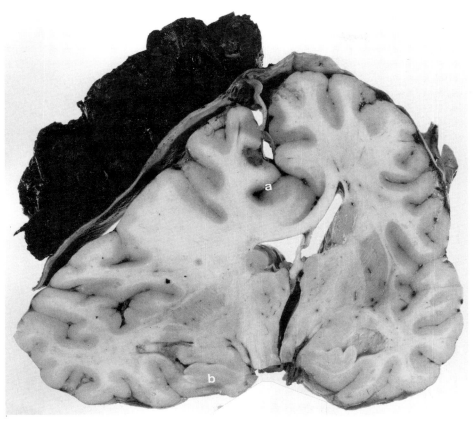

FIGURE XIX-14. Mid-coronal section of cerebrum. Combined mass effect of the large epidural hematoma and swollen left cerebral hemisphere causes a left to right midline shift resulting in left subfalcine cingulate gyrus herniation (a), left transtentorial herniation of the hippocampus (b), tilting of the corpus callosum and distortion with rightward displacement of the lateral and third ventricles. The decedent suffered a fall on the left side of the head and survived two days.

FIGURE XIX-15. Streak-like contusion hemorrhages in the cortex of the left hippocampal gyrus caused at the moment of impact by striking against the tentorial margins (herniation contusions), now located medially from tentorial notching (a) due to displacement to the right and herniation of the hippocampal gyrus. Displacement of the left thalamus (b) to the right, two punctate contusion hemorrhages in the corpus callosum (c), and subfalcial herniation of the cingulate gyrus.

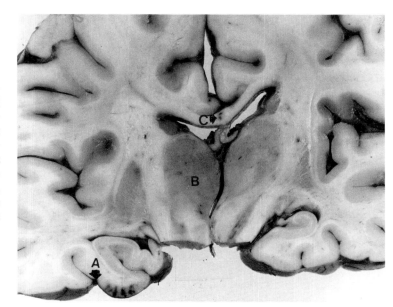

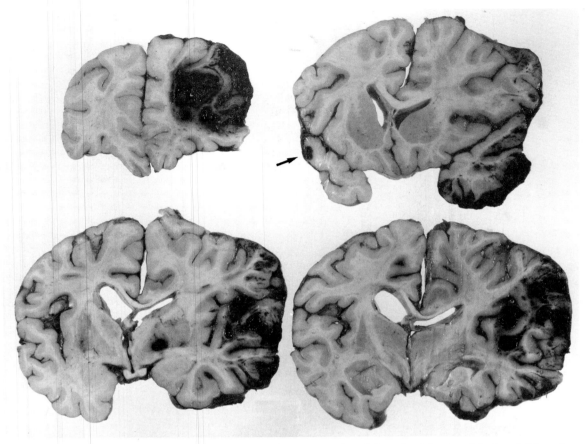

FIGURE XIX-16. Coronal sections of cerebral hemispheres. Decedent fell on the left side of the head. There is a small left lateral temporal contusion (arrow). Severe right lateral cerebral contusions. Right to left midline shift with cingulate gyrus herniation, tilting of the corpus callosum, compression of the right lateral ventricle, enlargement of the left lateral ventricle due to compression of left foramen of Monro and displacement of the interhemispheric fissure and third ventricle. Survived 14 hours.

dure. Neuroradiologists have recognized that a *midline shift* due to a lateral mass with associated enlargement of the contralateral temporal horn of the lateral ventricle indicates increased ICP and is an ominous prognostic sign.[12] The *third ventricle* is compressed and displaced away from the mass and is curved so that the concave surface faces the mass (Figs. XIX-14 to XIX-16). The basal ganglia, diencephalon and rostral midbrain are compressed, elongated and deformed away from the mass (Fig. XIX-17). These distorted structures may develop ipsilateral or contralateral linear and round small hemorrhages. The aqueduct of Sylvius may be compressed. Often the deformity and compression of the *diencephalon* is severe enough to obstruct the blood flow of the pene-

trating arteries and cause diffuse or focal ischemic necrosis. If the patient subsequently is maintained on a respirator for days, these necrotic areas of the brain disintegrate more rapidly than the surrounding brain (Figs. XIX-17 and XIX-18).

The downward component of the effect of a cerebral mass forces the ipsilateral hemisphere caudally through the incisura of the tentorium cerebelli *(transtentorial herniation)*. Such transtentorial herniation first pushes the uncus and then progressively more of the medial temporal lobe (the parahippocampal gyrus) past the tentorial edge, which leaves a deep groove in the cortical surface (Figs. XIX-13, XIX-14 and XIX-19). The tentorial edge may cause hemorrhage and necrosis of the cortical surface and sometimes all of the

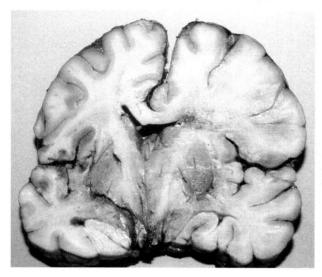

FIGURE XIX-17. Coronal section of cerebrum. Patient with recent subdural hemorrhage and right cerebral swelling. Maintained on a respirator for four days. There is right to left midline shift, cingulate gyrus herniation, tilting of the corpus callosum, compression of the right lateral ventricle, and leftward deformity of the interhemispheric fissure and third ventricle. The diencephalon is markedly elongated due to transtentorial herniation. There is beginning disintegration of the diencephalon and basal ganglia due to compression ischemia.

herniated tissue undergoes hemorrhagic infarction (Fig. XIX-19). The distance from the medial uncal or temporal margin to the tentorial groove and the presence or absence of associated cortical change should be noted.

Transtentorial herniation of the temporal lobe *compresses the midbrain* with resultant flattening of its ipsilateral surface. The ipsilateral *oculomotor nerve,* which arises from the medial surface of the adjacent interpeduncular fossa, passes slightly caudal and then around the posterior cerebral artery and rostral to perforate the dura and enter the cavernous sinus where it is firmly anchored. As the transtentorial herniation proceeds, caudal displacement of the brain stem pulls the fixed oculomotor nerve with it. The compression and stretching of the nerve interferes with the function of the parasympathetic fibers that constrict the pupil resulting in an ipsilateral *fixed, dilated pupil,* the well-known ominous clinical sign that heralds transtentorial herniation.[13] Progression of the herniation may cause total oculomotor paral-

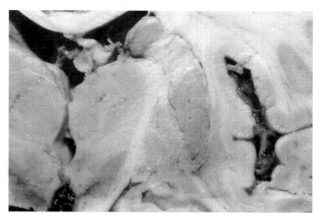

FIGURE XIX-18. Coronal section of cerebrum. The patient was maintained on a respirator for 5 days after suffering a cardiac arrest. The right caudate, anterior limb of the internal capsule and putamen show more advanced disintegration due to compression of the lenticulostriate artery.

ysis. The nerve is stretched, thin and sometimes hemorrhagic over the posterior cerebral artery. If the herniation is relieved, the pupil function returns to normal unless there has been necrosis of the nerve.

In severe cases, the midbrain is compressed and displaced away from the mass and the contralateral cerebral peduncle is pressed against the contralateral tentorial edge. In this situation, the tentorial edge may interrupt the descending corticospinal tract fibers (that will cross the midline in the medulla) and result in hemiparesis ipsilateral to the mass *(Kernohan's notch)* (see Fig. XIX-19). The distortions of the transtentorial herniation may cause compression of the veins draining the inferior surface of the occipital and temporal lobes followed by compression of the ipsilateral, contralateral or bilateral *posterior cerebral arteries* resulting in infarction, usually hemorrhagic, in its territory (see Fig. XIX-9).

The areas of hemorrhagic necrosis that may be seen in the cingulate gyrus, corpus callosum, medial temporal lobe, inferior occipital/temporal cortex and occasionally elsewhere in the cortex at pressure points should not be mistaken for contusions. A typical cortical contusion is a surface lesion that highlights the protruding crowns of the gyri while sparing the sulcal cortex, whereas a hemorrhagic infarct involves the cortical ribbon not sparing the sulci (see Figs. XIX-7 to XIX-10).

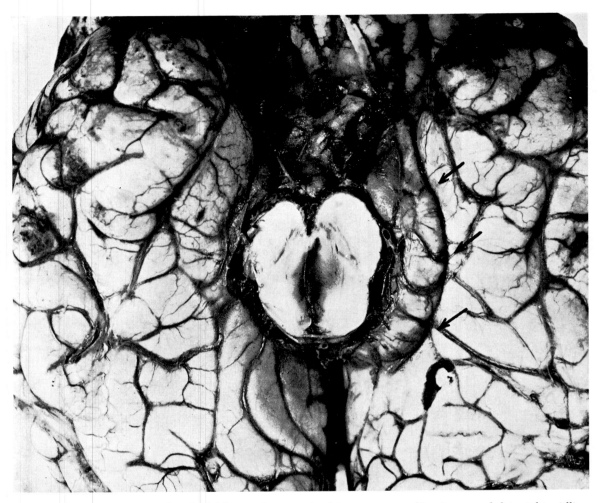

FIGURE XIX-19. Decedent suffered a left hemispheric epidural hematoma resulting in severe left to right midline shift and transtentorial herniation. A deep tentorial groove indents the left hippocampus and parahippocampal gyrus (arrows). The herniated cortex appears congested and necrotic. The midbrain is compressed and shifted to the right. There is secondary necrosis and hemorrhage (Duret) of the midbrain tegmentum. The right cerebral peduncle is compressed and necrotic due to pressure against the right tentorial edge (Kernohan's notch). If the corticospinal fibers, running in the middle one-third of the peduncle, are damaged, the result would be left hemiparesis (ipsilateral to the hematoma). Survival for 26 hours.

When the expanding mass is frontal/parietal and bilateral the pressure forces the cerebrum backward and downward resulting in herniation of the posterior-inferior frontal lobes into the middle cranial fossa resulting in a groove from the ridge of each sphenoid wing that indents the posterior-inferior frontal cortex. Such anterior-superior masses may cause bilateral parahippocampal gyrus herniation which may be more prominent posteriorly. Also in these cases, the diencephalic structures around the posterior third ventricle, including the *mammillary bodies* and *infundibulum,* may be displaced downward to a point below the level of the incisura (Fig. XIX-20). The *pituitary gland* is often infarcted. The diencephalon is narrowed and elongated due to compression, often with linear and round hemorrhages.

If the entire brain is diffusely swollen, depending on the size of the incisura there will be marked *central herniation* of the diencephalon but little medial temporal herniation or midline shift

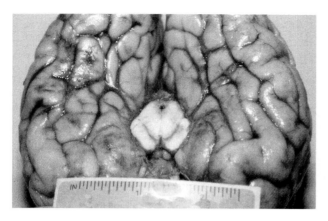

FIGURE XIX-20. Brain swelling with posterior and downward herniation of the mammillary bodies into the interpeduncular fossa.

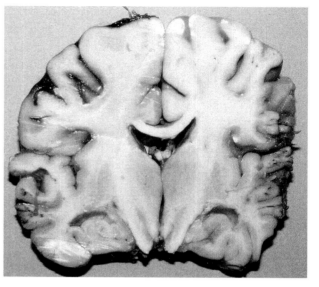

FIGURE XIX-21. Diffuse brain swelling without midline shift. There is central transtentorial herniation without medial temporal herniation. The diencephalon (thalamus, subthalamus) and rostral midbrain are laterally compressed and elongated. The stretching and compression of the diencephalon may result in symmetrical, bilateral focal necrosis and/or hemorrhages. Compression and ischemia of these structures may result in coma, persistent vegetative state or death.

(Fig. XIX-21). As noted above with anterior masses, the mammillary bodies may be forced posterior and inferior into the interpeduncular fossa and the pituitary gland may be infarcted.

A common terminal event in the process of transtentorial herniation is the development of central necrosis and hemorrhage in the tegmentum of the midbrain and the tegmentum and base of the pons, often referred to as *Duret hemorrhages,* although, ischemic necrosis is the initial lesion followed by the hemorrhage (Figs. XIX-19 and XIX-22). Unless a person has been maintained by mechanical ventilation, this process never involves the medulla and the hemorrhage rarely extends to the surface of the brain stem. Duret hemorrhage occurs when there has been lateral compression with dorsal-ventral elongation of the midbrain and pons and caudal displacement of the brain stem. The paramedian penetrating arteries derived from the rostral basilar artery and basilar tip normally have a slightly caudal angle. The caudal displacement of the rostral brain stem next to the relatively less mobile basilar artery leads to attenuation of the central perforating arteries with resulting ischemic necrosis and subsequent hemorrhage.

Herniation of one or both cerebellar tonsils and the medulla through the foramen magnum, leaving a distinctive circular groove in the inferior cerebellar surface, is called *tonsillar herniation* (Figs. XIX-13 and XIX-23 to XIX-25). The tonsils usually show some hemorrhage and necrosis and often there is hemorrhage and necrosis of the dorsal medulla. Similar medullary injury may occur as a primary traumatic lesion due to fracture of the foramen magnum (Fig. XIX-26). Involvement of the medulla in this fashion is associated with apnea. If the herniation is associated with a supratentorial mass, the apnea will occur in an already comatose patient. Tonsillar herniation also is seen when there is a posterior fossa mass, and in these cases there may be associated blockage of the flow of cerebrospinal fluid due to compression the fourth ventricle and aqueduct of Sylvius. Posterior fossa masses also can cause *upward herniation of the superior cerebellar vermis* and midbrain resulting in a circular incisural groove. The upward and downward pressures of a posterior fossa mass may cause compression with resulting infarction in the distribution of the superior, anterior-inferior and/or posterior-inferior cerebellar arteries.

Finally, the brain can herniate through any defect in the skull, whether surgical or traumatic,

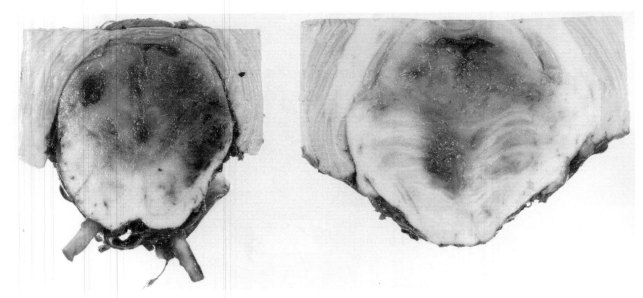

FIGURE XIX-22. Transverse sections of midbrain and pons. Large, secondary (Duret) hemorrhage of the tegmentum of the midbrain (a) and pons (b) and extension into the base of the pons in a patient with acute subdural hematoma. Survived 5 days.

if the dura is also disrupted. When this happens, there is very little resistance to expansion of the swollen brain, and the sharply demarcated, fungating, cerebral mass soon becomes necrotic and hemorrhagic *(fungus cerebri)* (Fig. XIX-27).

Anoxic/Ischemic Encephalopathy

Some facets of the pathology of anoxic/ischemic injury of the brain are relevant to analysis of the brains of persons who have sustained neurotrauma. There are extensive reviews of this large topic.[14] Some general concepts are important to have in mind as one attempts to interpret the unfolding sequence of events following an episode of neurotrauma, or, indeed, whether or not trauma has been inflicted at all. In most instances with survival periods longer than a day, the direct effects of trauma become intermixed with the subsequent secondary effects of swelling, edema, anoxia and ischemia. Accurately sorting these lesions is essential for proper analysis of the cases.

Hypoxia/Anoxia

Anoxia is an absence of oxygen whereas *hypoxia* is a state of inadequate oxygen supply. Often

the terms are used interchangeably. *Ischemia* is inadequate blood perfusion. In some brains it is possible to separate the effects of anoxia from ischemia but usually the effects of ischemia are enhanced by a pre-existing state of anoxia, so the term *anoxic-ischemic* injury is used.

The brain depends entirely on the aerobic metabolism of glucose for its energy. It uses no other energy source and its capacity for anaerobic glycolysis is insufficient to meet its energy requirements. Since the brain stores very little glucose and cannot store oxygen, its high metabolic requirements are met by an average perfusion rate of 55 mL/100g/min. A sudden, complete, anoxic exposure leads to loss of consciousness in 10 seconds, with cessation of electrical activity after 20 seconds. This is similar to events resulting from a total circulatory arrest. However, if the anoxic brain continues to be perfused, it can withstand prolonged periods of complete anoxia without damage. During the period of anoxia with perfusion, cellular activities temporarily switch to anaerobic processes producing lactic acidosis. When the substrate is exhausted, the brain tissue becomes inactive. All electrical activity ceases and the brain reaches a steady state without damage. With the return of oxygen and substrate, the cells resume function.

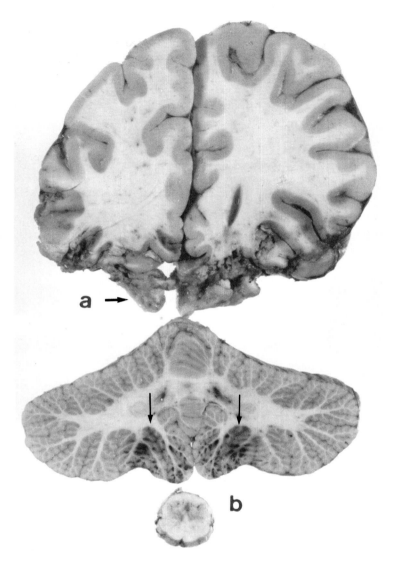

FIGURE XIX-23. Coronal sections of frontal lobes and cerebellum and transverse section of medulla. Gunshot wound of orbital frontal lobes (a). There are herniation contusion hemorrhages of the cerebellar tonsils (arrows) and the medulla (b). Death was instantaneous.

In the case of ischemic anoxia (stagnant anoxia) anaerobic glycolysis proceeds, intracellular acidosis develops, all electrical activity ceases and cell death occurs in a few minutes because of the failure to remove toxic metabolic byproducts. Analysis of those clinical situations characterized by pure anoxia, even if prolonged and severe, shows that when the anoxia is not accompanied by circulatory collapse and ischemia the brain is not damaged. If circulatory collapse does occur, brain damage rapidly develops.[15-19]

Ischemia

The neuropathology of ischemia is a vast topic[14] and our discussion of it is restricted to some comments that are of forensic interest. When the cerebral perfusion rate falls below the

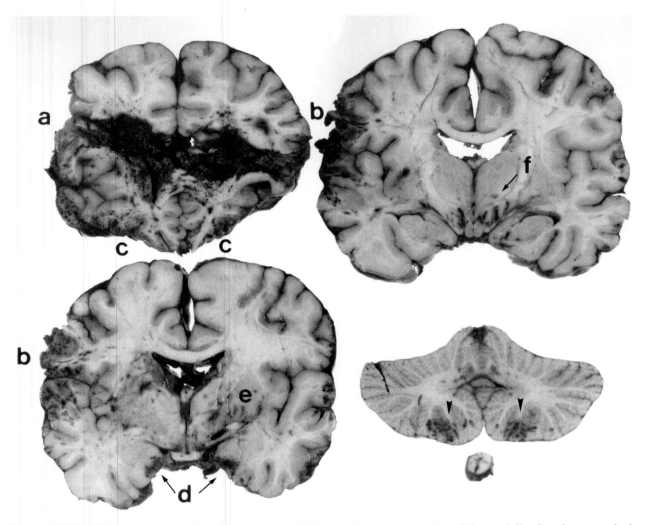

FIGURE XIX-24. Coronal sections of cerebrum and cerebellum and transverse section of the medulla. Gunshot wound of frontal lobes (a) with a large, hemorrhagic, permanent cavity. The left lateral temporal area is the craniotomy site (b). Blast effect with temporary and permanent cavities caused distant contusion hemorrhages of the orbital frontal cortex (c), the surrounding deep nuclear structures (e, f), and herniation hemorrhages of the unci (d), the cerebellar tonsils (arrows) and the medulla. The decedent survived three and one-half hours.

threshold of viability, necrosis occurs rapidly. If the blood flow to the entire brain is affected, the result is *global ischemia*. If a portion of the brain is affected, the result is *focal ischemia*. The importance of anoxic/ischemic damage as an acute consequence of brain injury is well recognized.[20,21] A period of apnea, often followed by a period of depressed respiratory drive follows head injury. The more severe the head injury, the longer the apnea. As noted above, apnea alone is not the determinant of subsequent brain damage. Hypoxia rapidly affects cardiac output, which results in cerebral ischemia. Diffuse head injury also may cause acute brain swelling with a rise in intracranial pressure (ICP) which, if sustained, will progress to vasogenic edema. In such patients with elevated ICP and ventilatory insufficiency, even a slight drop in blood pressure with decreased cerebral perfusion pressure (CPP) may result in cerebral ischemia.

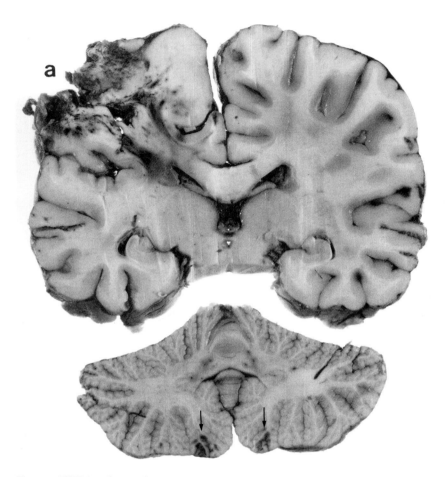

FIGURE XIX-25. Coronal section of cerebrum and cerebellum. Decedent struck on left parietal region with a baseball bat. Large contusion laceration and white matter hemorrhage at the site of impact (a). No contrecoup contusions. Bilateral herniation contusions of the cerebellar tonsils (arrows). One hour survival.

FIGURE XIX-26. Transverse section of cerebellum and medulla. Patient fell from a height. Pronounced dead at the scene. Acute contusion of the dorsal medulla due to fracture across the foramen magnum.

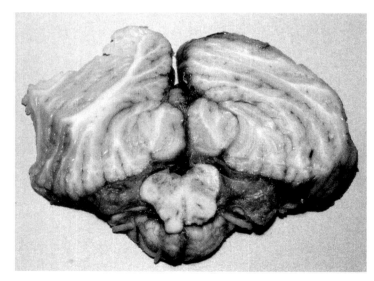

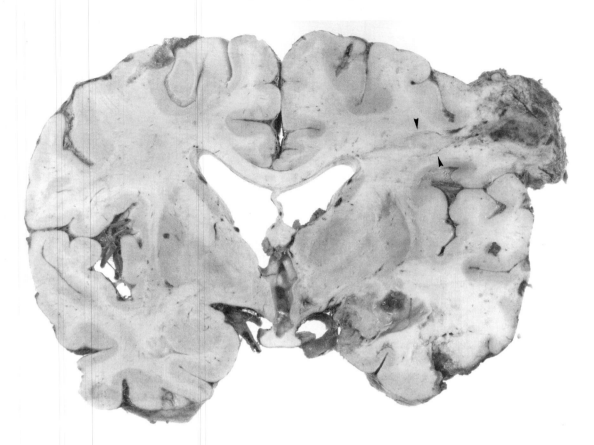

FIGURE XIX-27. Coronal section of cerebrum. Herniation of right lateral frontal lobe through craniotomy opening with infarction of the deep white matter (arrowheads) and swelling of the right temporal lobe. Survived one month.

Respirator Brain

In a given case, the length of time the brain can tolerate severe hypoperfusion depends on a number of variables that may not be known, such as how rapidly hypoperfusion developed, how long it persisted and how quickly a normal blood pressure was restored. If the cerebral circulation stops immediately, consciousness is usually lost in 10 seconds with permanent damage occurring if ischemia lasts for longer than about 5 minutes, although there are rare exceptions if there is hypothermia. A complete interruption of cerebral circulation of more than 4–5 minutes is rarely survived. The heart may be even less tolerant of ischemia than the brain, and cardiac status may be determinative of the cerebral outcome of resuscitation. Hyperthermia and hyperglycemia

(including contemporaneous intravenous infusions containing glucose) increase the morbidity and mortality of global ischemia.[19,22–24]

If the heart is resuscitated after this period and the patient is maintained on a mechanical ventilator, the result may be a totally non-perfused brain that begins to undergo autolysis. The term *respirator brain* has been applied not because the respirator is *cerebrotoxic* but because such advanced structural degeneration cannot develop without mechanical ventilation; i.e., without respiratory support humans stop breathing long before the development of total cerebral necrosis. Such patients have no cerebral perfusion, flat EEG, no cranial nerve reflexes and are comatose. In these circumstances the cardiac function could be maintained for several days (much longer more recently). The situation led to the generally recognized condition of *brain death*. In 1981, the President's commission for the Study of Ethical Problems in Medicine and Biomedical and Behavioral Research introduced the Uniform Determination of Death Act.[25] The guidelines include apnea, absence of neurological function, irreversibility and ancillary tests (most often to determine irreversibility). This involves recognizing a proximate cause of brain injury, ruling out a confounding intoxication and repeating the tests after 6 to 24 hours.[26]

We prefer to avoid the term *brain death,* because it fosters the erroneous impression that there are two kinds of death, with brain death less certain and subordinate to cessation of cardiac action and respiration. The unnecessary uncertainty created by brain death terminology has the potential to cause ethical dilemmas for families confronted with the need to make decisions about *pulling the plug* and organ donations. Instead, we emphasize that death is death and can be determined by neurologic or cardiorespiratory criteria. Hence, we advocate the use of *death by neurologic criteria* rather than *brain death.*

The respirator brain is soft, swollen, discolored gray-brown with a musty odor due to ischemia and autolysis. Often structures of the base of the brain, particularly the diencephalon and rostral midbrain, are extremely friable, even after fixation. The cerebellar tonsils are usually friable and fragments are scattered in the subarachnoid space around the spinal cord. The dural sinuses and the cerebral veins are often distended with thrombus.[27] Indeed, if significant intravenous stasis and coagulation occur during the circulatory arrest, cardiorespiratory resuscitation may create a period of reperfusion with venous obstruction followed by diffuse congestion and hemorrhage until the ICP rises above the blood pressure and perfusion stops. The result is a hemorrhagic brain that resembles venous infarction. Autolysis is not an *in vivo* reaction to injury, but it is more advanced in areas that were ischemic prior to death, such as those that were under more extreme pressure due to mass effect or central herniation. Microscopic studies are useful to document any *in vivo* pathologic changes such as inflammation or acute anoxic neuronal injury, because these changes record events that occurred prior to cardiovascular collapse and total brain necrosis.

Irreversible global anoxic/ischemic injury may not be followed by a permanent, irreversible state of total non-perfusion. If cerebral circulation and perfusion pressure are restored, the result is a total or subtotal brain infarction, and the body reacts as it would to any focus of necrosis with phases of intense acute, subacute and chronic inflammation, phagocytosis, neovascularity, gliosis and cavitation. Furthermore, the inflammatory and repair processes are non-uniform, resulting in changes at different stages in different areas of the brain. Such patients may be maintained on a respirator for a prolonged period of time. In reconstructing the events that led to the cardiorespiratory arrest, it is important to recognize the post-arrest nature of these changes. In some instances, the earliest post-arrest CT scan may provide illuminating information in resolving the question.

When the brain is subjected to a global ischemic insult, the amount of brain damage depends on numerous variables. Factors that increase the damage include a period of pre-existing hypotension (i.e., shock), the completeness of the ischemia, the presence of hyperthermia, long duration of ischemia, the presence of hyperglycemia and the presence of pre-existing cardiovascular disease. The ischemic necrosis will be visible first in the watershed areas of the cerebral arteries, particularly in the tri-vessel watershed area of the posterior occipital lobes (Figs. XIX-1, XIX-3, XIX-4 and XIX-28). In cases of pre-existing elevated intracranial pressure, the most vulnerable area of the brain may be the diencephalon and basal ganglia due to pressure on the penetrating arteries from the base of the brain. This may result in bilateral, symmetrical ischemic necrosis in the globus pallidus, thalamus or subthalamic areas (Figs. XIX- 29 and XIX-30). Also in situations of pre-existing increased intracranial pressure, widespread necrosis of the cerebral sulcal cortex may result from a drop in the cerebral perfusion pressure (see above). If the cardiorespiratory collapse is complete but the circulation is reestablished before a situation of no

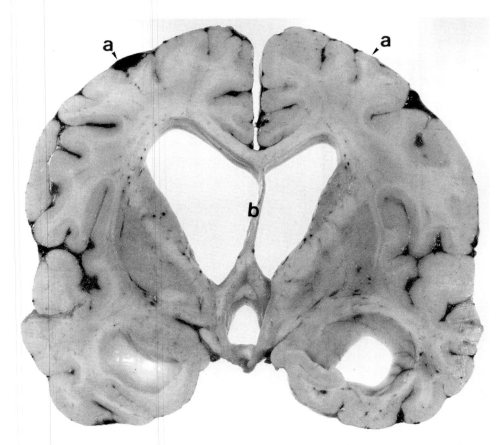

FIGURE XIX-28. Coronal section of cerebral hemisphere. Survived one year. Severe anoxic/ischemic encephalopathy due to post-traumatic cardiac arrest. Cortical atrophy is most severe in the dorsal paramedian border zones between the anterior and middle cerebral arteries (a). The septum is intact (b). The ventricles are secondarily enlarged (ex vacuo).

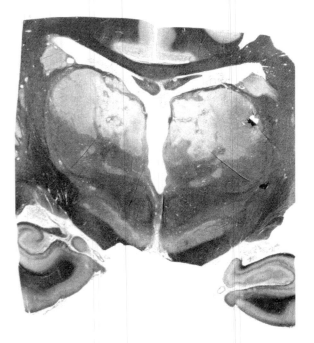

FIGURE XIX-29. Histologic section of both thalami, corpus callosum and fornix with lateral and third ventricles. Child two month's post-traumatic anoxic/ischemic injury. Bilateral, symmetrical, ischemic, thalamic necrosis.

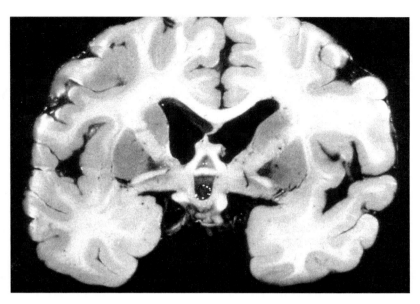

FIGURE XIX-30. Coronal section of mid-cerebrum. Bilateral, symmetrical necrosis of globus pallidus four months after global anoxic/ischemic injury due to cardiorespiratory arrest.

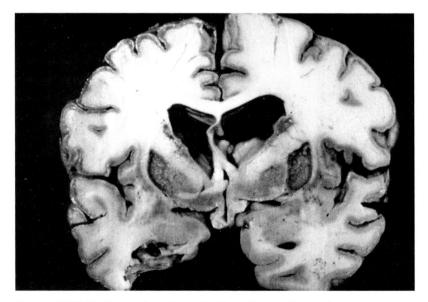

FIGURE XIX-31. Coronal section of mid-cerebrum. Six weeks in coma after cardiac arrest. There is widespread ischemic necrosis of cerebral cortex and deep cerebral gray matter.

reflow develops, there will be widespread or almost total necrosis of the gray matter including cerebral cortex, the deep cerebral nuclei and the gray matter of the cerebellum and much of the brain stem (Figs. XIX- 28 and XIX-31). The white matter may appear structurally intact but it will also undergo dissolution if survival is prolonged.

If there is generalized anoxic/ischemic cerebral damage but the brain stem is intact, the patient is in a state of transition from coma to a state characterized by sleep-awake cycles. The patient can open his eyes to auditory stimuli and can breathe but shows no verbal response or any behavior that indicates awareness. This state has been called *coma vigil,* or, more recently, *persistent vegetative state.*[28]

The various cellular components of the central nervous system have different sensitivities to anoxic/ischemic injury, neurons being more vulnerable than glia. Occasionally, a patient who survives an anoxic/ischemic insult in coma for days or weeks may show little or no grossly visible brain abnormality at the time of autopsy. Microscopic examination, however, will reveal widespread selective neuronal loss with preserved glia and white matter. The early pathologic picture will consist only of neurons with brightly eosinophilic cytoplasm without any other cellular reaction. These *red neurons* indicate cell death. The eosinophilic change is visible within four hours, in some experimental situations, but are more often seen after 10–12 hours in clinical settings. Red neurons may persist (or continue to evolve) for days or weeks after the anoxic/ischemic event. With time the neurons disappear leaving behind the surviving blood vessels and reactive astrocytic gliosis. No inflammatory cells or histiocytes are involved and no cavitation develops. In our experience, one can reliably survey the brain for diffuse anoxic/ischemic changes by microscopic sampling of the rostral medulla, the cerebellum (the block including the dentate nucleus and folia), the thalamic/subthalamic area, the hippocampus and a cerebral border zone.

As noted above, a patient may suffer a global anoxic/ischemic event that causes total or subtotal cerebral necrosis and subsequently have cerebral reperfusion due to cardiac resuscitation. In such cases, the brain swells over several days due to edema in the reperfused, necrotic areas. After 24–36 hours neutrophils infiltrate the necrotic tissue and persist for 5–7 days, a process that is non-uniform and can begin repeatedly in multiple areas, probably reflecting patchy, non-uniform restoration of circulation. After 3–5 days, histiocytes begin to appear and phagocytize the lipid-rich necrotic tissue. After 2–3 weeks, there are sheets of lipid laden histiocytes. After one month, cavitation of the necrotic areas is visible. Some degree of phagocytic activity and increasing cavitation may persist for months or even years. Surrounding the zone of complete necrosis is a zone of partial or selective injury characterized by reactive astrocytosis (a process that begins within 2-3 days and persists indefinitely) and neuronal and white matter loss.

Occasionally the question posed to the medical examiner is whether a decedent who has been in prolonged coma originally suffered diffuse head trauma with diffuse axonal injury or suffered a global ischemic event such as a cardiac arrest due to natural disease. In certain cases, this distinction can be made with some confidence.[29]

NEUROTRAUMA

The forensic analysis of neurotrauma is directed towards reconstructing its traumatic mechanisms, the age and severity of injuries, and the relation of injuries to the patient's symptoms and cause of death. Just as the brain must be evaluated in light of findings in each layer of the head from the scalp to the brain itself, head injuries in general should be evaluated in light of general autopsy findings. For example, an impact on the torso or buttocks may cause injuries of the head and brain. Specific anatomic features of the head and neck as well as the brain and its coverings are factors that contribute to the pattern and distribution of injuries and their secondary consequences. Secondary lesions frequently mediate the lethal outcome of head injuries.

When assessing the clinical course, prognosis and outcome of the victim of neurotrauma, the medical examiner should review the decedent's physical injuries, clinical course, and effect of treatment. An important milestone is the clinician's assessment of the decedent's condition at the onset of treatment. A standard tool for a rapid, consistent and meaningful evaluation at the onset of therapy and throughout the patient's course is the *Glasgow Coma Scale (GCS),*[30] which has been generally accepted and survived the test of time.[31] The scale is designed to provide a quantitative measure of the severity of neurologic damage. The scores quantitate the quality of the victim's response with eye and motor movement and to verbal interactions. A head injury is considered mild with GCS score of 13–15, moderate with 8–12 and severe at <8 (see Table XIX-1).

Definitions

Neurotrauma may result from *blunt forces,* which may be due to impact (contact) or movement (inertia). The most common result is a *closed head injury* with no exposure of the brain to the external environment. The second category of neurotrauma is *penetrating/perforating injury* which results in a wound that communicates from the external environment to the brain. These are due to high (usually gunshot wounds) or low (nail gun, screwdriver, etc.) velocity missiles that have penetration as their salient characteristic. *Chop wounds* are inflicted with edged blunt instruments (hatchet, machete) and have the combined characteristics of blunt and penetrating trauma.

The injuries are either *focal or diffuse.*[32] *Impact (contact) injuries* occur in one of three circumstances: a moving object strikes the resting head, a moving head strikes a stationary object; or a collision between a moving head and a moving object. The resulting injuries are due to local deformity and are *focal. Inertial (motion) injuries* do not require impact and result from the resistence of the brain to forces that accelerate the head from a position of rest or changes its uniform motion *(acceleration/deceleration).* The acceleration/deceleration causes widespread internal movements of the brain that result in stretching, compression and shearing of the nerve fibers and intracranial blood vessels. Inertial injuries are *diffuse.* Examples of injuries that require contact and are focal are scalp lacerations, most skull fractures, epidural hemorrhages and cortical contusions. Inertial injuries are subdural hemorrhage and the constellation of hem-

TABLE XIX-1

THE GLASGOW COMA SCALE

Definition of coma: A patient in coma cannot open his/her eyes, speak or obey simple commands and is graded as GCS <8 (GCS = 8 if he/she utters incomprehensible sounds.) Such patients are classified as having severe head injuries.

EYE OPENING	
Spontaneous	4
To verbal command	3
To pain	2
None	1

BEST MOTOR RESPONSE	
Obeys verbal commands	6
Localizing response to pain	5
Flexor withdrawal to pain	4
Abnormal flexor response(decorticate)	3
Extensor response to pain(decerebrate)	2
None	1

BEST VERBAL RESPONSE	
Oriented, conversing	5
Confused conversation	4
Inappropriate words	3
Incomprehensible words	2
None	1

TOTAL	3–15

orrhages and nerve fiber disruptions that constitute the condition called *diffuse axonal injury (see below).*[33-38] Combined injuries are common, such as when an impact to a movable head causes localized contusions due to impact and diffuse injury due to the resulting acceleration/ deceleration.

Acceleration/deceleration can be *translational (linear), rotational or angular.* A passenger in a high-back automobile seat of a car traveling at 50 mph that is struck from behind by a vehicle traveling 80 mph experiences *translational (linear) acceleration* of the head which is protected from whiplash *(rotational acceleration/deceleration)* by the high seat back. A blow to the side of a movable head incurs an *impact (contact) injury* at the point of contact and a *rotational acceleration/ deceleration injury* as the head is propelled away from the blow, the center of rotation being in the head. A person who suffers an unbroken fall on the back of the head after pivoting on his heels incurs an *angular acceleration/deceleration injury,* the center of angular movement being outside the head, i.e., the heels.

BLUNT FORCE HEAD INJURIES

New information from experimental models of head injury and recent clinicopathologic studies of head-injured patients have advanced our understanding of the pathophysiology of brain injuries. These clinical studies have used new techniques of monitoring the head-injured patient. Serial neuroimaging of the head with CT and/or MRI and monitoring intracranial pressure and cerebral blood flow are some of the techniques that have provided a dynamic picture as the primary and secondary effects of trauma unfold over time. Much new information continues to be produced at the molecular level as well.

Blunt force can be applied to the head in a variety of ways, often in the same episode. The force may be applied slowly over more than 200 msec as in slow, crushing forces that cause extensive skull fractures, while loss of consciousness may not occur at all unless the brain is also lacerated. Blood vessels and neural tissue can withstand more deformity due to strain than the skull. Indeed, each type of tissue has different properties based on its inherent elasticity when exposed to a deforming force. As a result, while bone is stronger than vascular or neural tissue, it is less tolerant of deformity and will fracture. Animal experiments have shown that the tolerance of blood vessels and neural tissue to deformity resulting from blunt force also is partially governed by the duration of impulse.[32,34]

TYPES OF BLUNT FORCE HEAD INJURY

Scalp Injuries

Blunt impact injuries of the head of sufficient energy to cause brain injuries are usually reflected by injuries of the skin or subcutaneous tissues of the face or scalp because there is only a thin layer of subcutaneous soft tissue between the skin and the bone over which it stretches. Although many persons who sustain fatal brain injuries from blunt impacts have no externally visible injury due to the presence of thick hair, a hat, or a broad impact, layerwise dissection usually discloses subscalpular or subgaleal hemorrhages at points of impact. Scalp injuries inflicted by blunt trauma are abrasions, lacerations, or contusions. In addition to the location of the impact, features of the injuries may provide information as to the nature of the impact surface and the mechanism of the injury. Some blunt force injuries of the brain, such as acceleration-deceleration injuries or falls on the lower extremities or buttocks, are not due to impacts of the head or face.

Skull Fractures

The forensic analysis of skull fractures is complex and is discussed elsewhere in the text. In general, the location and pattern of skull fractures provide information relevant to the neuropathology examination in terms of the point of impact, the distribution of cortical contusions, the sequence of multiple impacts, the age of the injury, the nature of the impacting object and the relevance to prognosis and risk of complications such as post-traumatic epilepsy, CSF leaks, or infections.

Blunt Force Neurotrauma

For purposes of conceptual organization and discussion as well as an aid in the analysis of cases of blunt force head injury, we think of brain injuries as focal or diffuse. Focal injuries are most often due to an impact to the movable head. We can see them with the naked eye. They are circumscribed and cause dysfunction related to regional destruction of the brain or a regional mass effect. Examples of focal traumatic brain injury are epidural hematoma and contusions.

Diffuse brain injury, in contrast, results in widespread, global disruption of brain function such as confusion, amnesia, or loss of consciousness. These injuries can be produced without an impact although impacts often complicate these events and augment the forces of acceleration/ deceleration. Subdural hematoma is a diffuse brain injury because it can be produced without an impact and often the removal of the hematoma fails to improve the patient's condition, reflecting the additional diffuse brain injury that accompanies the subdural hemorrhage. Acceleration/ deceleration, especially if there is a rotational component, is the common denominator of the pathophysiology of these injuries, and the pathology is axonal damage due to deforming strains. There may be few, if any, lesions visible to the naked eye.

Many brain injuries are complex, such as seen in a motor vehicle accident, a fall down stairs or a beating, so it is common to see both focal and diffuse brain injuries in the same patient. Furthermore, patients with either diffuse or focal brain injuries (or both) may develop superimposed secondary damage that may also be focal (pressure necrosis, herniation sequelae) or diffuse (global ischemia). Sorting out these patterns in order to reconstruct the pathobiology of the injury is a challenge.

Diffuse Brain Injury

Brain injuries that cause widespread, global brain dysfunction include conditions with widely varying severity and outcome but are classified as a group because they present with a continuous spectrum of dysfunction. The difference depends on variations in the quantity of brain damage rather than the type of injury. In the milder forms of diffuse traumatic brain injury there is no morphologic marker to correlate with the clinical symptoms, although neuropathologic studies are rare. However, clinical studies can demonstrate in a semiquantitative way a continuum of conditions that range from mild to severe that begin to reveal visible neuropathologic changes with increasing severity of trauma. This defines the relationship between concussion and diffuse axonal injury.[33,36,38,39]

Loss of consciousness is a consistent feature of diffuse head injury except in its mildest form when the patient displays symptoms of confusion. Consciousness requires an intact cerebral cortex and diffuse connections with the thalamus and hypothalamus and the rostral brain stem reticular formation. Focal brain stem injuries can cause widespread cortical dysfunction including loss of consciousness.[40] Diffuse white matter brain injury causes loss of consciousness by widespread disruption of cerebral hemispheric connections rostral to the brain stem and reticular formation.

Concussion

Axonal damage, whether transient or permanent, is believed to be the common denominator of diffuse brain injury. In practice, a classification has been developed through clinical studies that divides these patients into two groups—one with relatively mild and one with severe injury. The widely recognized term *concussion* identifies the first group and *diffuse traumatic axonal injury* the second. Concussion is defined as *"a clinical syndrome due to mechanical, usually traumatic, forces characterized by immediate and transient impairment of neural function such as alteration of consciousness, disturbance of vision and equilibrium."*[41] Based on patient morbidity and survival outcome, the Glasgow Coma Scale identifies a severe head injury as coma lasting longer than 6 hours. Accordingly, cerebral concussion is defined as traumatic coma lasting less than 6 hours.

Le Roux,[42] based on clinical and neuropathological studies, presented the following classification of diffuse brain injuries:

- **Mild concussion:** temporary disturbance of neurological function without loss of consciousness.
- **Cerebral concussion:** trauma-induced, transient, reversible neurologic dysfunction that results in loss of consciousness for less than 6 hours.
- **Mild diffuse axonal injury:** head injury with coma that lasts between 6 and 24 hours that is not due to mass lesions or ischemia.
- **Moderate diffuse axonal injury:** head injury with coma that lasts longer than 24 hours without prominent brain stem signs such as decerebrate or decorticate posturing.

- **Severe diffuse axonal injury:** same as moderate diffuse axonal injury but with brain stem signs.

Mild Concussion

Mild concussion is a very common injury.[36,38,43] Usually, a physician does not evaluate the patient. The symptoms are transient and the patient does not become unconscious. There is always some element of confusion, which may not be detected without close questioning. Retrograde amnesia, loss of recall of events prior to the injury, always occurs and persists after recovery. The length of retrograde amnesia is proportional to the severity of the injury. Anterograde amnesia is variable.

Cerebral Concussion

Cerebral concussion is a transient (less than 6 hours) traumatic loss of consciousness. During the loss of consciousness the patient may have transient decerebrate posture, bradycardia, elevated blood pressure, apnea, or flaccidity. Varying amounts of retrograde and antrograde amnesia will follow the return of consciousness. The pathophysiological lesion is believed to be diffuse functional disruption of cerebral cortical and brain stem connections. A rare neuropathological study in a patient who expired from other injuries after a cerebral concussion demonstrated beta amyloid precursor protein immunostaining in the fornix, important for memory, and loss of neurons consistent with ischemia in the CA-3 segment of the hippocampus, also important for memory.[44]

Although concussion is a mild diffuse head injury that results in a transient loss of function, the significance of loss of consciousness is debated. It may be followed by a post-concussion syndrome characterized by persistent headaches, dizziness, fatigue, irritability, personality changes and mild cognitive dysfunction. While the more severe form of concussion is characterized by loss of consciousness for up to 6 hours the incidence of post-concussive syndrome does not seem to correlate with loss of consciousness.[42]

Epidemiologic studies have indicated that head injury, even at an early age, is a risk factor for Alzheimer's disease.[45] Individuals who have the genotype apolipoprotein E subtype e4 (APOE e4) have an increased risk to develop Alzheimer's disease.[46] Furthermore, the frequency of the APOE e4 genotype in patients with beta amyloid deposits following head injury is higher than most non-head injured Alzheimer patients suggesting a genetic susceptibility to the effects of head injury.[47] Also there is evidence that patients with acute traumatic brain injury who have the genotype APOE e4 have increased morbidity and mortality. These patients even start with lower GCS suggesting that the risk factor is active immediately.[48] Concern has been expressed that young athletes should be tested for APOE genotype before being allowed to participate in high-contact sports.[49,50]

Diffuse Axonal Injury

The most severe form of diffuse traumatic brain injury is *diffuse axonal injury (DAI)*. The neuropathologic definition of DAI is based on a combination of detailed clinical neuropathological studies and experimental studies that have reproduced the axonal lesions in animals without impact with dynamic loading and angular acceleration. Lateral rotational acceleration is more effective than sagittal rotation.[37,51] Patients who suffer from DAI are exposed to forces of severe acceleration/deceleration with or without impact. DAI typically is seen in patients injured in motor vehicle accidents but also is seen in victims of assaults.[52,53] DAI has not been seen in association with boxing fatalities where, in the few cases in whom detailed neuropathologic studies have been performed, the usual finding is subdural hematoma and brain swelling.[54,55]

Patients with severe DAI are rendered immediately unconscious and do not have an intracranial mass. They usually do not experience a lucid interval and do not fully recover. When they awaken from coma, their subsequent condition depends on the extent of their diffuse axonal injury. This may range from minimal neurological

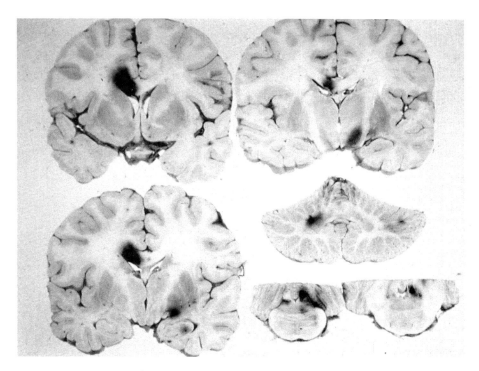

FIGURE XIX-32. Patient with severe, diffuse head injury due to a motor vehicle accident who survived three days. Note the hemorrhages in left cingulate gyrus/corpus callosum, the right basal ganglia, the right subthalamic area, the deep left cerebellar white matter and the right dorsolateral brain stem.

deficits to a persistent vegetative state. Patients in the latter group typically remain in a persistent vegetative or debilitated state until death from post-traumatic complications. Often, during the acute phase, CT or MRI demonstrates small hemorrhages in the subcortical cerebral white matter, the corpus callosum, the fornices, the cerebellar white matter (especially the peduncles), the diencephalon and the tectum of the midbrain or pons. These lesions also are found in the postmortem brain (Figs. XIX-32 and XIX-34 to XIX-36). *Gliding contusions,* slit-like traumatic hemorrhages in the white matter of the superior frontal gyri, may be present (Fig. XIX-33). Lesions in the deep portions of the brain are associated with the more severe injuries. These CT and MRI visualized hemorrhages reflect the distribution of damage to the axons demonstrated on microscopic examination. However, diffuse axonal injury can occur in the absence of any hemorrhage.

Neuropathological criteria for diagnosis have been developed and consist of finding wide-spread axonal injury in the cerebral hemispheres, corpus callosum, fornices, posterior limb of the internal capsule, the rostral brain stem including the superior cerebellar peduncle and the cerebellum including the middle cerebellar peduncle. These axonal lesions may or may not be associated with the above noted hemorrhages.[56,57]

Experimental and clinical studies have resulted in classifying patients according the severity of the injury based on the duration of coma and the presence or absence of brain stem signs.[37,58] The cases are classified as mild, moderate or severe DAI.

MILD DAI: The coma lasts from 6 to 24 hours. Brain stem posturing signs are rarely present. Usually there is no motor deficit and memory deficits are mild. Two-thirds of the patients have an overall good outcome. Deficits are moderate in 15% of cases and severe in 5%. Death, often from other injuries, results in 15%.

MODERATE DAI: Coma lasts longer than 24 hours. Patients occasionally show brain stem pos-

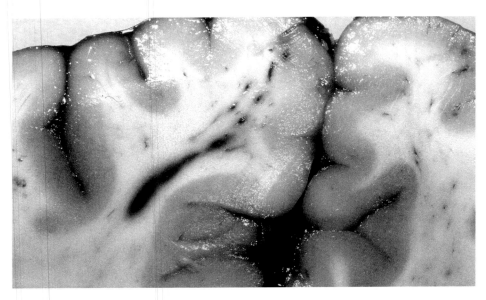

FIGURE XIX-33. Acute *gliding contusion* in the white matter of the left superior frontal gyrus. This type of injury is associated with diffuse brain injury.

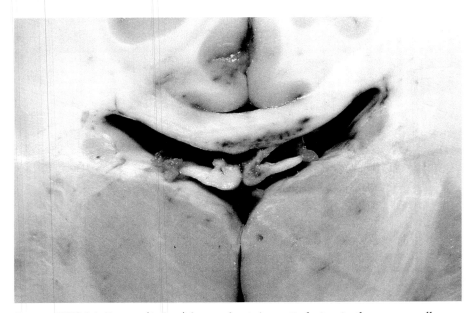

FIGURE XIX-34. Recent (4 days) hemorrhagic/necrotic lesion in the corpus callosum and fornix of a person who suffered a diffuse head injury due to a fall from the 17th floor.

tural reflexes. There are mild motor deficits. Memory loss is moderate. Outcome is good in 40%, moderate in 20%, and severe in 15%. Mortality is 25%.

SEVERE DAI: Coma is longer than 24 hours. Brain stem postural reflexes (decerebrate and decorticate) are always present. Motor and memory deficits are severe. Outcome is good in 15%, moderate in 15%, and severe in 20%. Mortality is 60%. Patients with severe DAI tend to have a neuropathological pattern of diffuse axonal damage with focal lesions in the corpus callosum, the

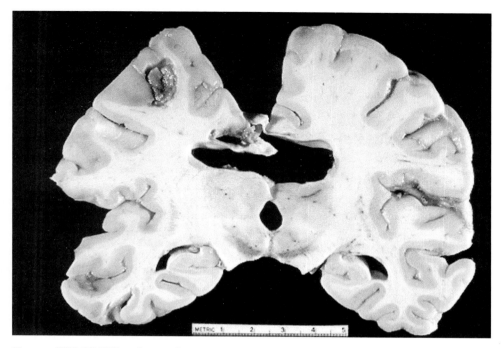

FIGURE XIX-35. Yellow-brown foci of organizing hemorrhage/necrosis in the white matter of the left superior frontal gyrus (gliding contusion) and the corpus callosum in a patient who was in a vegetative state for 4 months following a diffuse head injury.

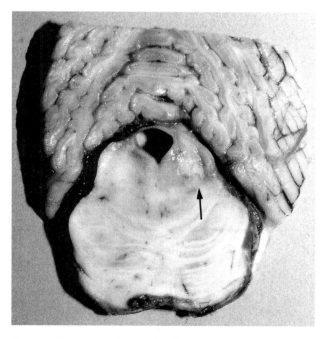

FIGURE XIX-36. A focus of yellow-brown necrosis in the dorsolateral pons in a patient in a vegetative state for 15 months following a diffuse head injury.

posterior limb of the internal capsule and the lateral tectum of the midbrain and pons.

In these cases, a severe outcome is characterized by the *persistent vegetative state (PVS)* as defined by Plum.[28] *Coma* is a state of complete unresponsiveness to external stimuli with eyes closed. When the coma ends for these severely injured patients, they progress into a persistent unresponsive state. The brain stem function returns with sleep-wake cycles, normal respiratory control and eye opening in response to auditory stimuli. However, these patients show no evidence that they understand or can respond to events in their environment. They produce no intelligible verbal or meaningful, specific, motor response of any kind. There appears to be no detectable interaction between the cerebral hemispheres and the brain stem, although the latter is functioning. Patients with PVS can be supported for long periods of time with careful nursing. Eventually they die of complications of their debilitated state.

Pathology of DAI

The lesions of DAI consist of injuries to the axons and blood vessels. First we will characterize the lesions, then their patterns.

The forces of strain that deform and damage the neuronal axons are the essential lesions of DAI. The vulnerability of axons and blood vessels to injury from the forces of strain is different and the difference in vulnerability is related both to the severity and the duration of the force. Therefore, while hemorrhages and DAI are often found in the same injured person, the two types of injury do not always occur together.[32,34]

The most sensitive technique for demonstrating axonal injury is the immunohistochemical reaction for *beta amyloid precursor protein (beta-APP)*. This protein is produced at a slow but steady rate in the cell bodies of neurons and distributed throughout the cytoplasm by fast axoplasmic transport. Normally the beta-APP is not present in great enough concentration in the axon to be visible with the immunohistochemical technique. The normal method of movement along the axon is one of active transport at each point along the way similar to a chain of humans who pass sandbags from one to another to build a dike. If a segment of the axon transport system is damaged, the transported proteins, including beta-APP, accumulate proximal (on the side of the neuron cell body) to the obstruction in great enough quantity and concentration to become visible with the immunohistochemical stain. Also, by activation of immediate early genes, neurons near the injury increase production of beta-APP in response to trauma.

Copious literature describes the molecular pathobiology and ultrastructural sequence of changes in the evolution of the injured axon from the time of injury to the formation of the *retraction ball*.[59,60] This information is important because at each step in our understanding there is a potential site for therapeutic intervention. Also, in the future, each step provides an opportunity to develop techniques of forensic interest to reveal the mechanism and the history of a traumatic lesion.

Immunohistochemical staining for beta-APP begins to demonstrate the axonal injury approximately three hours after the event. The normal neural tissue is negative and the injured segment of the axons become positive allowing for relatively easy recognition (Fig. XIX-37). Clinical and experimental studies have indicated a predictable series of changes that evolve in the injured axons. The early pattern is positive staining of axons with otherwise normal features. During subsequent hours, the axons become swollen and then are disrupted with the proximal end forming a bulbous enlargement, the *retraction ball* or the *axonal body*. At this stage the abnormality is visible with standard H&E or silver stains (Figs. XIX-38 and XIX-39). With the H&E stain, cross sections of the axonal swelling and the retraction ball appear as sharply demarcated, round, finely granular, eosinophilic structures that are several times the diameter of the surrounding normal axons. They may be in groups or individually scattered throughout the neuropil. Sometimes they surround small parenchymal blood vessels. When the injured axons are diffusely scattered, the lesions are usually not grossly visible. When they occur in groups, they may be visible grossly as punctate, gray lesions. When longitudinally viewed, they may appear as bulbous enlargements of a transected axon or segmental swelling in a damaged axon. The silver stains demonstrate argyrophilic images of the same nature (Fig. XIX-39). The H&E and silver stains are more difficult to interpret because all of the axons stain positively and there is considerable normal variation in axon diameter, even in the same field, and the axons are cut in a variety of planes.

Once formed, axonal swellings may persist for days, weeks and even months.[37,58] Secondary events such as subsequent ischemia, herniation or hemorrhages may cause additional secondary axonal damage. *It must be understood that axonal damage* **per se** *is not a specific marker for trauma and interpretation must rely upon the total clinical and pathologic picture.* Any natural disease that results in segmental damage to axons will cause the formation of axonal bodies. Axonal bodies are seen at the margins of infarcts, abscesses, some tumor metastases, multiple sclerosis plaques or non-traumatic intracerebral hemorrhages. Diffuse

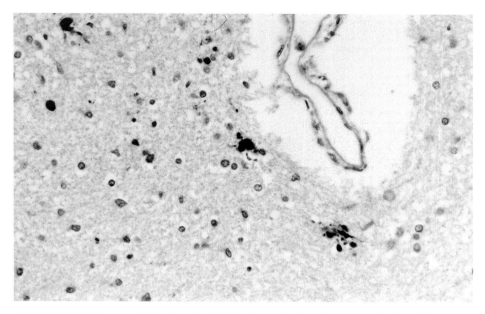

FIGURE XIX-37. Immunohistochemical stain demonstrating the accumulation of beta amyloid precursor protein in the injured axons of the posterior limb of the internal capsule in a patient who died 2 days following a diffuse brain injury in a motor vehicle accident. This pattern of discrete, injured axons (individual or in small groups) in locations known to be typical of diffuse traumatic injury, are characteristic of traumatic DAI rather than ischemic DAI (see Figure XIX-40).

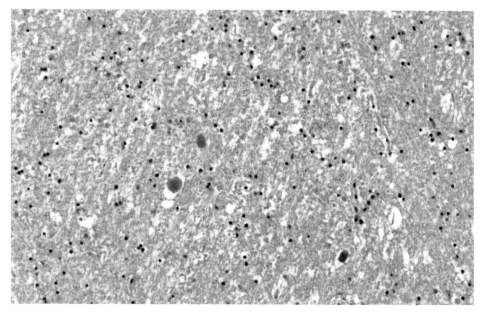

FIGURE XIX-38. H&E stained section from the same block of tissue as *Figure XIX-37*. The axonal bodies stand out as discrete, round, dark staining bodies.

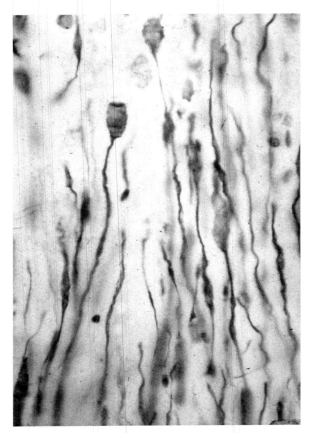

FIGURE XIX-39. A silver stain (Bodian) demonstrates the longitudinal configuration of axonal bodies.

anoxic/ischemic encephalopathy also may result in diffuse or patchy axonal injury (Fig. XIX-40). Some controlled studies of DAI due to trauma have pointed out the difficulty in distinguishing traumatic from non-traumatic DAI. They have emphasized that linear and geographic patterns that are situated in areas commonly involved in vascular compression in patients with these conditions must be considered vascular rather than traumatic. Unfortunately, these are areas that are often involved in traumatic DAI as well. Sometimes one cannot be certain.[37,58,61]

Some axons are transiently damaged and recover. Other injured axons may remain in a swollen, damaged state for long periods either without becoming disrupted or without repairing the axonal injury. Others eventually undergo axotomy. Still other axons will tear immediately with the trauma and the distal axon along with

the proximal stump will undergo the well-defined process of wallerian degeneration. In the latter situation, microglial cells invade the lesion several days after necrosis has occurred and gradually become distended with foamy cytoplasm over the following days and weeks. Reactive astrocytes are visible in about one week. The end stage is a rarefied or microcystic reactive astrocytic lesion with scattered histiocytes containing lipid and/or hemosiderin if there was initial hemorrhage.

The forces that cause DAI can tear the vascular component of the tissue as well as the axons. This will result in hemorrhages, usually small, that tend to localize in the same distribution as the axonal injury. Since they occur at the time of trauma, they are detectable before the axonal injury is visible and therefore may constitute the only evidence of DAI in cases with a brief period of survival. In instances of longer survival the distribution of the axonal injury is more extensive than the hemorrhages. In the absence of characteristic hemorrhages, the axonal injury is the only evidence of DAI, and the lesions may not be visible to the naked eye.

Since, as noted above, pathologic segmental axonal accumulation of beta APP reflects many types of damage, some of which are diffuse, it is appropriate to qualify the term *DAI* as *traumatic DAI* or *diffuse traumatic axonal injury (TAI)* when due to trauma. Furthermore, cases have been described in which traumatic axonal injury is localized, such as only in the cervicomedullary area. This does not fit the definition of traumatic DAI and is designated *localized traumatic axonal injury (TAI).*[60-62] This pattern of injury may be important in some cases of the impact/shaken baby syndrome.

Acute Traumatic Brain Swelling

Brain swelling can complicate mild, moderate or severe diffuse head injury.[38,39] Diffuse brain swelling with delayed catastrophic deterioration following a lucid interval is also a known complication of brain trauma, especially in children and young adults. Initially, the swelling is due to cerebral vasodilatation after compromise of

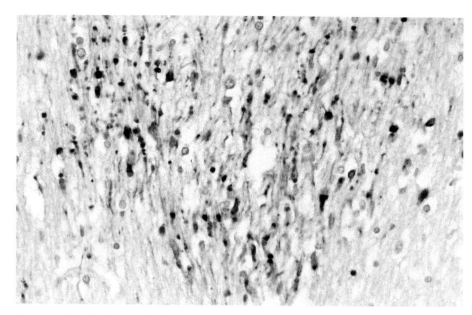

FIGURE XIX-40. Beta APP from a patient with non-traumatic anoxic/ischemic injury complicated by increased intracranial pressure. The injured axons are in the posterior limb of the internal capsule, a location also often injured in diffuse traumatic DAI. The axons were injured due to local vascular compression resulting from increased intracranial pressure and central transtentorial herniation, which produced damage to irregular large groups and linear arrays of groups of positively stained axons (contrast this with Figure XIX-37). Patients with traumatic DAI may also develop ischemic complications. In such cases, sampling multiple areas of the brain and correlating both the staining pattern and the distribution of the lesions may clarify the pathogenesis of the injury.

autoregulatory control of cerebral blood flow. If the congestion persists, it will cause increased vascular permeability and edema and lead to complications of increased intracranial pressure. Similarly a condition known as the *second impact syndrome* has been described.[63] In this situation a person, often an athlete, suffers a concussion. Before recovering from the effects of the concussion the individual suffers a second, often minor, diffuse head injury. This is followed by precipitous onset of coma and respiratory difficulty. The mortality is 50%. While these conditions are complications of diffuse head injury, as far as is known, they do not involve demonstrable diffuse axonal injury. It is postulated that the second impact syndrome involves a first impact that disturbs autoregulatory cerebral vascular control causing a state of abrupt increased cerebral blood volume utilizing the capacity of intracra-

nial compliance. The second blow increases the cerebral congestion, overcomes further compliance and results in malignant brain swelling with elevated intracranial pressure. One recent review questions the role of a second injury in this syndrome.[64]

Diffuse Vascular Injury

Another manifestation of a diffuse brain injury is the presence of widespread perivascular hemorrhages, mostly in the white matter of the frontal and temporal lobes in patients who die immediately or very soon after a head injury. Sometimes hemorrhages also are present around the aqueduct of Sylvius and along the floor of the fourth ventricle and in the base of the rostral pons.[65] These patients often have a small amount of blood in the ventricles.

INTRACRANIAL HEMORRHAGES

Intracranial hemorrhages resulting from blunt force head injury are the most common cause of clinical deterioration and death after a lucid interval and often are associated with skull fracture.[66-68] It is assumed that the bleeding originates from blood vessels disrupted at the time of the injury. The rate of onset of clinical signs and symptoms depends on multiple factors, some of which include the size and number of blood vessels torn, whether they are arteries or veins, whether a period of arterial vasospasm followed the injury and preceded the onset of hemorrhage, whether the external pressure on the injury, such as, brain swelling, could temporarily tamponade the hemorrhage and the effects of a variety of therapeutic interventions.

Clinical studies classify traumatic intracranial hemorrhages as acute, subacute, or chronic. Acute traumatic hemorrhages are the most common and present within the first 24 hours postinjury. Those that present clinically after 24 hours are considered delayed although presumably the bleeding began at the time of injury. Hemorrhages presenting between 2 and 14 days are designated subacute and those presenting after 14 days are considered chronic.[69]

Epidural Hemorrhage

Epidural hemorrhages (EDH) occur into the epidural space, which is a potential space that exists between the inner table of the calvarium and the tightly attached outer periosteal layer of the dura (Fig. XIX-41). They are seen in approximately 1–2% of all treated head injuries and 5–10% of autopsies of fatal head injuries.[70]

Most EDH occur during the second and third decades of life. They are rare before two years,[71] because prior to that age the dura is more firmly attached to the inner table of the skull and thus less likely to provide a space for a hematoma to accumulate if a blood vessel is torn. This firm attachment to the inner table of the skull is reflected by the presence of a microscopic epidural layer of spindle cells, osteoclasts and small islands of osteoid tissue that are pulled from the inner table of the skull as the dura is removed at autopsy. This layer should not be misinterpreted as a subdural neomembrane (see below). EDH is rare after the age of 60.[70] As we age, the dura becomes more firmly attached to the inner table of the skull making it less likely for the torn blood vessel to create a hematoma.

Forces of acceleration and deceleration alone cannot produce an epidural hematoma. An impact to the head must cause enough inward bending deformity of the skull to create a focal detachment of the dura of approximately 1 to 2 cm for space to establish a hematoma.[72] The deformity also must be sufficient to lacerate an adjacent epidural blood vessel that will be the source of the hematoma. This is most often a branch of the middle meningeal artery that is normally partially embedded in the surface of the inner table of the skull. Other vessels include meningeal veins, diploic veins or a dural sinus. A fracture is present in up to 90% of cases of EDH[73] and is a crucial factor in tearing the adjacent blood vessels. However, in approximately 10% of cases skull deformity without a fracture is sufficient to detach the dura and tear the blood vessels. This is seen more often in children under 15 years whose more flexible calvarium with unfused sutures tolerates more deformity without fracture but allows enough deformity to lacerate meningeal blood vessels.

In most cases of EDH, the source of the bleeding is arterial, usually from one or more branches of the middle meningeal artery, and most of these hematomas are in the temporal area of the skull. In the remainder of the cases, the bleeding is of venous origin including the middle meningeal veins, the dural venous sinuses and the diploic veins of the skull that are connections between the dural venous sinuses and the emissary veins of the scalp. When the bleeding is venous in origin the onset of symptoms due to the mass effect of the hematoma is later, so these are more often classified clinically as subacute or chronic. In adults, they often result from impacts on the

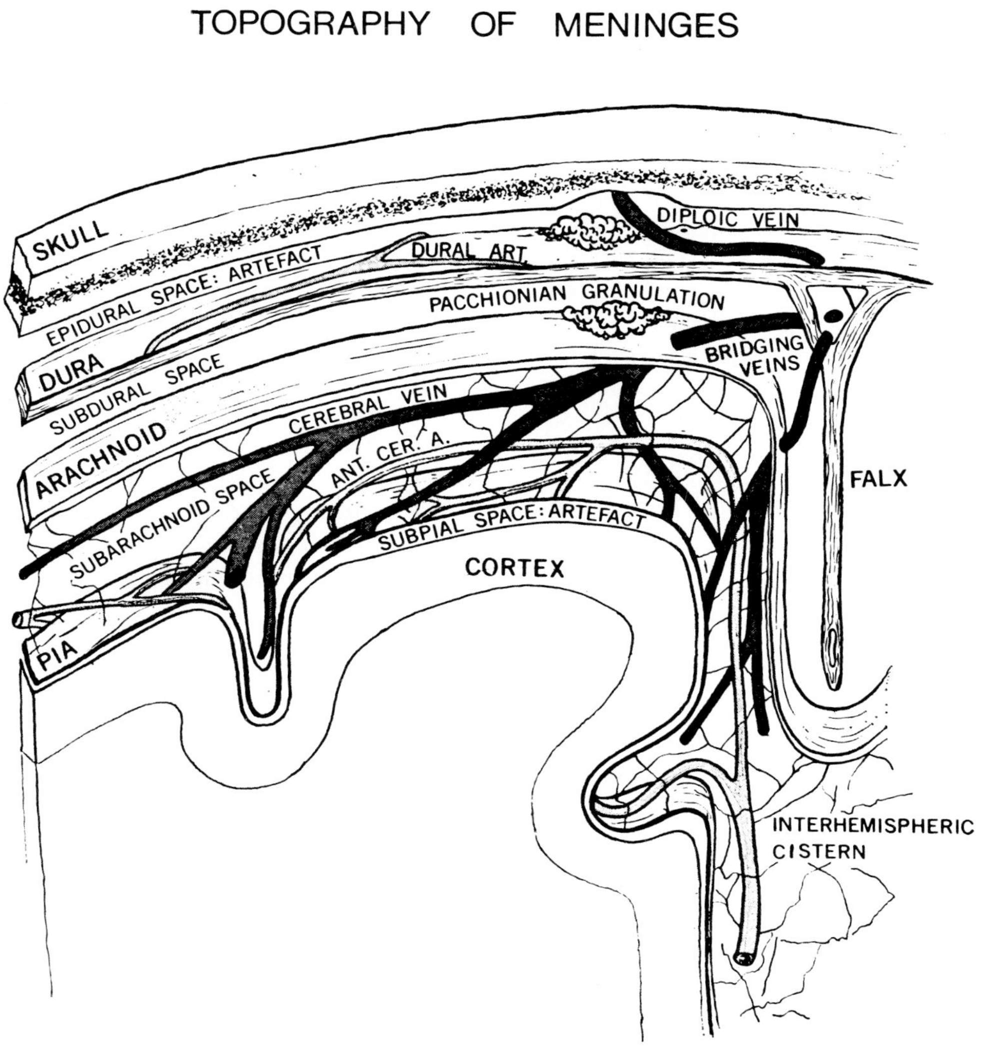

TOPOGRAPHY OF MENINGES

FIGURE XIX-41. Diagrammatic representation of the relationship between the skull, dura, arachnoid and pia and the extracerebral blood vessels.

occiput. There is usually a fracture and the bleeding is frequently from a lacerated dural sinus. EDH is almost always unilateral.

Most EDH occur over the cerebral hemispheres and the remainder are found over the occiput and posterior fossa (Fig. XIX-42). EDH of the posterior fossa are venous in origin. There are no branches of the meningeal artery in that location. Of those that occur over the hemispheres, most are found over the temporal/parietal region (Fig. XIX-14). In a typical situation, a blunt impact to the head creates enough defor-

mity of the skull to cause a fracture, separate the dura from the inner table and lacerate one or more branches of the middle meningeal artery. The combination of arterial hemorrhage and a newly created epidural compartment allows the hematoma to expand and thicken rapidly. After the suture lines, which anchor the dura more firmly, restrict the spread of the hematoma, it thickens and assumes a biconvex lens shape. Thrombosis of the torn blood vessel and the tamponade effect of the attached margins of dura may stop the enlargement of the hematoma.

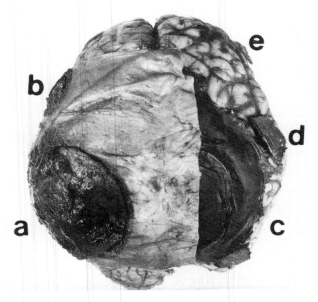

FIGURE XIX-42. Cerebral convexity with most of the left cerebral dura in place. There are sharply circumscribed epidural hematomas over the left lateral parietal (a) and left lateral frontal (b) lobes. On the right cerebral hemisphere there is a recent parietal/occipital subdural hematoma (c) and thin lateral parietal (d) and lateral frontal (e) subarachnoid hemorrhage. The decedent suffered a fall on the left side of the head and survived for 15 hours.

Before this happens, however, the size of the hematoma and the speed with which it accumulates will often produce serious, potentially lethal mass effects. Clinical studies have shown that a volume more than 50 mL, a thickness greater than 1.5 cm and a cerebral shift greater than 1 cm requires immediate treatment.[74-77] Hematomas of more than 150 mL result in markedly increased morbidity and mortality.[3]

The magnitude of the force necessary to produce an epidural hematoma without associated primary brain damage is not as great as the forces typically necessary to produce unconsciousness due to diffuse axonal injury in healthy adults. In clinical studies, the incidence of associated injuries such as subdural hemorrhage, contusions or diffuse axonal injury ranges from 30 to 70%.[77] Untreated, the mortality is high. In recent clinical studies of treated EDH using CT and MRI images as diagnostic tools, the mortality is approximately 10%.[75,76] If the patient is treated within a few hours, the prognosis is good

because often there is little or no associated brain damage. If there is substantial associated intradural injury however, the outcome is more dependent on the consequence of the brain injury than the EDH. The factors negatively affecting the outcome are the timeliness of diagnosis and treatment, the presence and severity of intradural injuries, the presence of coma at the time of surgery, a hematoma larger than 150 mL, the speed with which it manifested itself after the injury and the presence of postoperative ICP greater than 35 mm Hg.[74-77]

Sometimes the trauma does not cause loss of consciousness or any neurologic symptom that would cause the patient to seek medical help until several hours later when the mass effect of the hemorrhage causes rapid deterioration and constitutes a neurologic emergency. In this situation there is a post-traumatic lucid interval followed by loss of consciousness. Another possible scenario is immediate, transient loss of consciousness (a concussion) after the injury followed by an asymptomatic, lucid interval of minutes or hours, in turn followed by loss of consciousness due to the mass effect of the hematoma. If the patient suffers immediate loss of consciousness followed later by the appearance of an epidural hematoma with a mass effect without ever having regained consciousness, the victim most likely sustained additional diffuse brain injury.

When EDH occurs in the newborn, it is usually associated with a skull fracture and there has often been an application of forceps. Epidural hemorrhage constitutes approximately 2% of all neonatal intracranial hemorrhages.[78] The hemorrhage can be large because the neonatal skull can expand and the hematoma may decompress through the fracture into the subgaleal space. The hematoma may constitute a large enough portion of the neonatal blood volume to produce anemia or shock.

In older children EDH is a rare manifestation of head injury, less than 5% of the pediatric head injury population, and there are some differences in the presentation of EDH in children as compared to adults. The greater resistance of the child's skull to fracture when deformed and the greater adherence of the dura to the inner table of the skull make the more common adult middle meningeal artery laceration unusual in children. In children the bleeding is more often venous or sinusoidal and therefore the hematoma is more often subacute or chronic. Often there is no fracture or concussion at the time of impact making the onset of symptoms the first sign of the hematoma. Children have a greater percentage of posterior fossa EDH than adults. The child's posterior fossa EDH typically results from an occipital impact without a fracture and with dural sinus laceration. It can present as a posterior fossa mass of unknown etiology days after the injury, which is not recalled.[79]

In deaths associated with fire, the intense heat causes the dura to thicken and contract and pull away from the inner table of the skull. Sometimes the pressure of the contracting dura on the compressed brain results in rupture of the dura and extrusion of brain tissue into the epidural space. The heat also causes expansion of the contents of the marrow spaces of the skull with consequent numerous *fissure fractures* of the inner and outer tables. This forces bloody fluids from the marrow to flow diffusely into the epidural space, driven by steam pressure, producing the appearance of an EDH (see Fig. XIII-30a–b). In investigating a fire death, it is important that a postmortem artifact be distinguished from a genuine EDH sustained during life. The heat-induced epidural hemorrhage spreads thinly and diffusely over the epidural surface, typically with a bilateral, symmetrical distribution over the vertex and adjacent to the sagittal sinus of the dura mater. The antemortem epidural hemorrhage is localized and unilateral, being restricted by the suture attachments of the dura if they are still intact. The artifact is associated with numerous, diffusely distributed, interconnected, fissure-like fractures whereas the antemortem traumatic EDH is associated with a simple, often linear, localized fracture that overlies the hemorrhage and is related to a meningeal artery.

Subdural Hemorrhage

As noted above, subdural hemorrhages can be produced experimentally without impact by inertial forces alone and are thus classified as a *diffuse* rather than *focal head injury.* In actual practice, it is unusual to see acute subdural hemorrhages in young adults in the absence of an impact injury. A frequent scenario is rotational acceleration/deceleration initiated or arrested by an impact. These injuries often are accompanied by diffuse brain injury reflecting the large amount of force needed to produce a subdural hemorrhage in a healthy adult. Exceptions are the very old and the very young, especially less than one year, both of these groups having special anatomic characteristics that lower their threshold for suffering such hemorrhages. In the elderly, the neck is less strong and there is less resistance to rotational acceleration/deceleration and the subarachnoid space is larger, allowing for increased intracranial tissue deformity. Infants have relatively large heads with almost no resistence to rotational acceleration/deceleration. Their subarachnoid space is larger and their skull is malleable, both features allowing for increased intracranial soft tissue deformity. The summation effect of rapid, sequential, alternating rotational acceleration/deceleration movements, with or without impacts, is also important in some infant head injuries. There are no experimental data regarding such injuries in the elderly or the very young but there are a number of relevant clinical studies.

The subdural space is located between the inner surface of the dura and the outer surface of the leptomeninges (see Fig. XIX-41). In vivo, the two surfaces are in contact and cytoplasmic processes of the arachnoid cells bridge the gap between the layers as they connect to specialized contacts on the surface of the dural cells.[80] The subdural space remains closed even as the brain shrinks due to atrophy, consequently, the subarachnoid space enlarges and fills with cerebral spinal fluid.

Pathogenesis

It is assumed that in order for a subdural hemorrhage (SDH) to occur, somewhere one or more blood vessels that communicate with the subdural space must be disrupted. In this sense, subdural hemorrhages are always due to trauma. There are circumstances when the trauma may be so trivial that the individual does not recall the injury or be of such a nature that he does not associate it with the subdural hemorrhage. Individuals on anticoagulants, with bleeding dyscrasia, uremia[81] or a widened subarachnoid space due to cerebral atrophy are particularly vulnerable to *spontaneous subdural hemorrhage*. Patients who undergo ventricular cerebral spinal fluid (CSF) shunting procedures to relieve elevated intracranial pressure (ICP) are at risk for developing SDH as the surface of the brain rapidly pulls away from the inner table of the skull and places stress on the bridging veins. SDH is an occasional complication of intracerebral hemorrhage due to natural causes such as hypertension or ruptured arteriovenous malformation if the intracerebral hematoma dissects into the subarachnoid space and bursts through the leptomeninges into the subdural space. A similar, also uncommon, event can complicate a subarachnoid hemorrhage due to rupture of a saccular aneurysm. Through a mechanism that is not clearly understood, SDH can complicate hemodialysis or peritoneal dialysis.[82-84] Individuals with epilepsy have an increased risk of SDH as a traumatic complication of seizures.

The majority of acute subdural hemorrhages occur as a result of severe head injury. The most common causes of the trauma are, in order of frequency, motor vehicle accidents, falls, assaults, sporting events and industrial accidents.[85] Men are involved far more often than women and the mean age is about 40 years. The reported frequency of SDH varies considerably according to the nature of the series and ranges from 5 to 22% of treated head injuries. Factors that unfavorably influence the quality of the outcome for patients with SDH are the level of consciousness at the time of treatment (GCS<8), the presence of elevated ICP, evidence of transtentorial herniation and the presence of associated brain injury.[86]

The most common pathophysiologic element in the production of the SDH is sudden acceleration and/or deceleration of the skull relative to the brain. This results in stretching and laceration of the veins that bridge the subdural space as they penetrate the leptomeninges and attach to the relatively fixed dural sinuses (see Fig. XIX-41). The hemorrhage is usually venous in origin but another source is bridging arteries and veins in areas of incomplete dural/arachnoid cleavage particularly over the lateral temporal lobes. Forces that cause cerebral cortical contusions, especially fracture contusions, also may lacerate the arachnoid along with subarachnoid veins or arteries allowing hemorrhage to enter the subdural space. Typically, though, tearing of the bridging blood vessels involves angular or rotational acceleration/deceleration in the sagittal plane and the veins involved are those entering the superior sagittal sinus. Of interest, the frequency of SDH from motor vehicle accidents (MVA) is approximately 25% as compared to 75% in assaults or falls.[87] The energy-absorbing protective mechanisms present in a motor vehicle provide for slower acceleration/deceleration than are present in falls on hard surfaces or blows with hard objects. More frequently, MVA injuries present with immediate loss of consciousness without an intracranial mass and are found to have diffuse axonal injury (DAI), an injury associated with longer duration of the deforming force.

Compared to the epidural space, the subdural space offers little resistance to the flow of blood from the torn blood vessels so the hemorrhage spreads diffusely over the cerebral surface. Most subdural hemorrhages are located over the cerebral hemispheres. Some develop beneath the temporal lobe or between the occipital lobe and the tentorium cerebelli. Interhemispheric subdural hemorrhage, arising from torn veins between the medial cerebral hemisphere and the falx cerebri, is rare in adults.[88] The rate of accumulation of SDH is extremely variable. Clinicians classify the SDH as acute, subacute or chronic if the hematoma becomes manifest within 4 days, from 4 to 21 days or more than 21 days after the injury respectively. Pathologists base the age of the subdural on the pathologic features of the hemorrhage.[85,86]

In contrast to EDH and chronic SDH, the forces that produce an acute SDH in an otherwise healthy adult cause other brain injuries in over 50% of cases. These injuries are often more important than the SDH in determining the clinical outcome. Patients with a *simple* SDH without associated brain injury have an overall mortality of approximately 20%, whereas, for those with other cerebral injuries it is up to 80%.[89] Approximately 50% of patients with SDH have a skull fracture that is not related to the location of the SDH. Two-thirds of the fractures are in the posterior fossa and most of the contusions are frontal and temporal.[85,86] More than one-half of patients with SDH have cerebral cortical contusions and these may be associated with laceration of cerebral cortical blood vessels and tears of the leptomeninges. These often provide multiple sources of both arterial and venous SDH and, at autopsy, present as coagulated blood adherent to the leptomeningeal surface of the brain. Ischemic neuronal injury is often seen in cerebral cortex underlying the SDH. Diffuse cerebral swelling of the underlying cerebral hemisphere may develop shortly after the head injury, during surgical removal of the SDH or in the postoperative period. Post SDH removal, brain swelling is often a disastrous complication with a high mortality rate.[90] The acute phase of brain swelling appears to be related to loss of cerebrovascular autoregulation and, if not controlled, will proceed to cerebral edema. The resulting increased ICP may cause cerebral shift and fatal herniation.

Factors that enhance the patient's outcome are a young age, absence of pupil abnormality, high level of consciousness (GCS >8), a post-injury lucid interval (reflecting absence of diffuse brain injury), absence of parenchymal lesions on CT scan, open basal cisterns on CT scans and early treatment.[91] A 50 mL acute SDH almost always causes symptoms and a 100 mL SDH is often fatal.[92] The best series has a mortality rate of 35%. The average series mortality is 50% and the survivors are frequently disabled.

Pathology

As the hemorrhage enlarges to form a mass lesion, thus becoming a hematoma, its semi-liquid surface presses on the cerebral surface with homogeneous force preserving the gyral convolutional pattern (Fig. XIX-43). This is in contrast to epidural hematomas with smooth dural surfaces (see Fig. XIX-14) or chronic SDH with well-formed inner neomembranes that flatten the gyral crowns and create smooth, concave cerebral deformities. The gross and microscopic organization and resolution of a SDH follows a somewhat predictable but potentially variable course. It must be recognized that many variables affect the pace and the pattern of subdural hemorrhage organization. These include the age of the individual, the size of the hematoma, its bleeding source, recurrent head injury, rebleeding, and the intracranial pressure. The gross and microscopic features also vary in the same SDH.

During the *first 24 hours* the SDH consists of partially liquid and partially soft fragments of red-black, gel-like, clotted blood that do not adhere to the inner dural surface. At this stage, clots that may stick to the inner dural surface are loose and slide along the surface when pressed. The microscopic picture consists of no cellular reaction from the dura, intact erythrocytes, trapped leucocytes, and discontinuous layers of fibrin. In preparing the microscopic section, the clot will not remain attached to the dura.

At *2 to 4 days,* these soft clots stick loosely to the dura and resist pressure to move them along its surface. After fixation, the blood is black-brown instead of red-black. Microscopically, there are usually no neutrophils. Scattered macrophages are present in the clot and occasional spindle cells invade the clot from the dura. The margins of the clotted erythrocytes are becoming indistinct. Rare hemosiderin granules are demonstrable. Irregular layers of fibrin persist on the inner and outer surfaces (Figs. XIX-44 and XIX-45).

At *one week* a thin, outer (dural side), yellow neomembrane is grossly visible around the edges of the clot. The now more orange-brown coagulated blood definitely adheres to the dura. The blood is not yet covered by an inner membrane although the neomembrane may be starting to cover its edges. Microscopically, large, thin-walled capillaries are starting to invade the clot along with the more abundant fibroblasts, giving the appearance of typical granulation tissue. More intracellular hemosiderin accumulates.

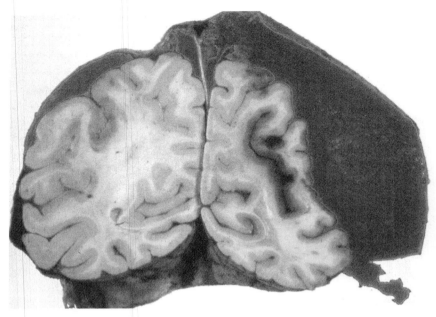

FIGURE XIX-43. Coronal section of cerebrum at the level of the occipital lobes with attached convexity dura with large, acute subdural hematoma. The pressure of the hematoma deforms the cerebral surface but preserves its convolutional configuration.

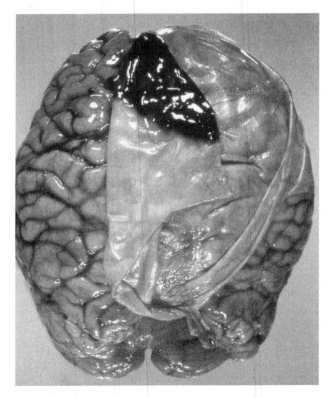

FIGURE XIX-44. Dorsal surface of the unfixed brain. A dark red, soft, coagulated hemorrhage sticks loosely to the inner surface of the left frontal dura as it is reflected over the right hemisphere. Three days after injury.

The erythrocytes are starting to lyse (Figs. XIX-46 and XIX-47).

During the *second and third week,* the outer (dural) neomembrane thickens and becomes more vascular. It proceeds to partially cover the inner surface of the clot which is beginning to liquefy. The clot is orange to yellow brown. Foci of red-black blood are common, reflecting the tendency of the granulation tissue to bleed. Microscopically, the capsule is more vascular and the blood vessels are large with thin walls. Its thickness is variable depending on the sampling site. Macrophages, some with hemosiderin, are numerous. The inner neomembrane is thin and incomplete (Figs. XIX-48 and XIX-49).

At the *fourth week,* the outer (dural) and inner (arachnoidal) membranes are complete and grossly visible. The thickness of the membranes is variable. Unless there was an arachnoidal laceration, there is no adhesion to the arachnoidal surface and the arachnoid does not contribute to the process of organization. Most of the blood is semiliquid and orange brown. Usually, there are islands of membrane-bound blood with intervening, thin, yellow neomembrane reflecting the variable thickness of the original hematoma

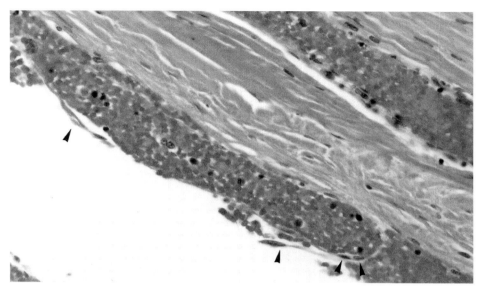

FIGURE XIX-45. H&E stained section of subdural hemorrhage. No inflammation. Early invasion of the hematoma with spindle cells (arrowheads). Three days after injury.

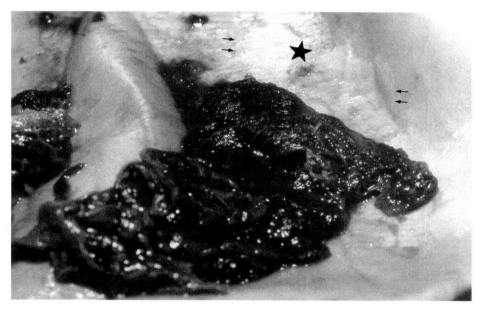

FIGURE XIX-46. Inner surface of the cerebral dura with an adherent subdural hematoma (after fixation). There is a thin, pale, yellow outer neomembrane (star) around the coagulated hematoma (membrane margins–arrows) but the inner (cerebral) surface has no visible membrane. One week after injury.

and the focal occurrence of rebleeding (Fig. XIX-50).

After one month, estimation of the age of the SDH is less precise. During the following months most acute SDH resolve completely as all of the blood is removed and the inner and outer membranes fuse eventually forming a barely perceptible, transparent, colorless or slightly yellow, adherent neomembrane that will remain indefinitely (Figs. XIX-51 and XIX-52). In some cases,

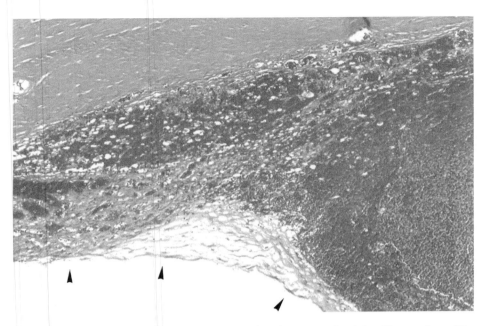

FIGURE XIX-47. H&E stained section from the edge of a one-week subdural hemorrhage. The vascular neomembrane (arrowheads) partially covers the inner surface of the hemorrhage.

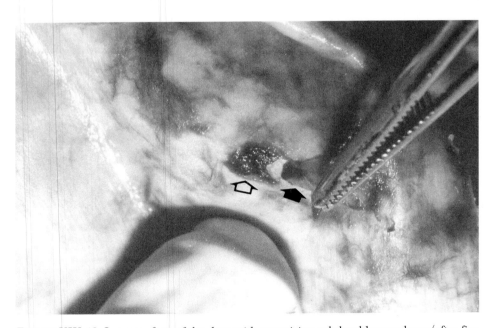

FIGURE XIX-48. Inner surface of the dura with organizing subdural hemorrhage (after fixation). There is a thin, 1–2 mm thick, yellow-brown outer membrane (solid arrow). A barely visible, inner membrane (open arrow) partially covers an island of dark brown coagulated blood. Three weeks after injury.

however, several events can occur to change this process of resolution that will alter the expected appearance of the SDH either entirely or focally. This means the gross or microscopic appearance of one particular area of a SDH may not accurately reflect its history.[93]

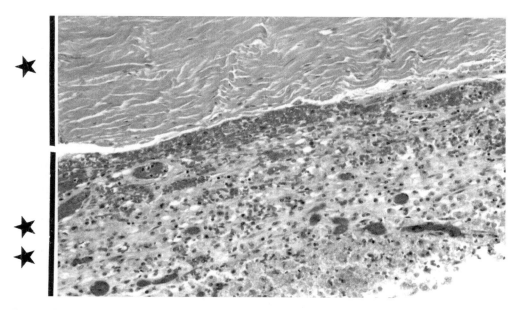

FIGURE XIX-49. H&E stained section from the edge of a three-week subdural hemorrhage (dura–single star). Most of the hemorrhage is replaced by vascular granulation tissue (stars) which contains numerous histiocytes.

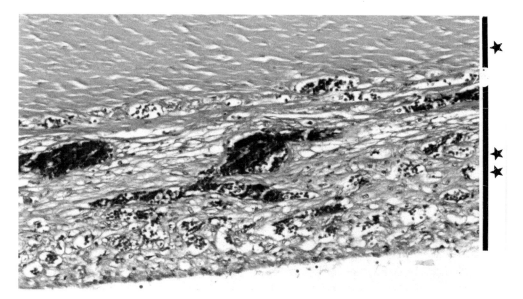

FIGURE XIX-50. H&E stained section of a four-week subdural hematoma (dura–single star). The hemorrhage is replaced by the vascular neomembrane (stars).

If the arachnoid has been lacerated, as it may if there were underlying cortical contusions, mesodermal cells from the subarachnoid space may participate in the formation of the inner neomembrane. This will result in an adhesive scar between the cortex and the dura, a lesion that increases the risk of post-traumatic epilepsy.

Chronic Subdural Hematoma

The clinical definition of chronic SDH is subdural hemorrhage that presents with signs and symptoms more than 21 days after the initiating injury. At this time, the SDH would have an outer and an inner membrane. They occur most

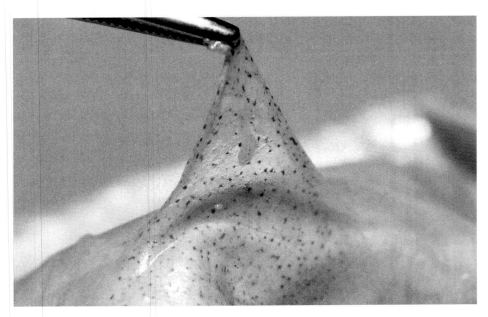

FIGURE XIX-51. Organized, 1–2 mm thick, transparent, subdural neomembrane with punctate deposits that represent aggregates of hemosiderin containing histiocytes. This neomembrane could represent a subdural hemorrhage that occurred months or years previously.

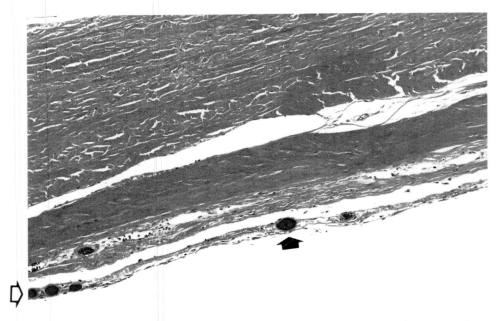

FIGURE XIX-52. H&E stained section of dura. Note the thin neomembrane (open arrow) on the inner dural surface with an occasional dilated blood vessel (solid arrow).

frequently in the elderly. Seventy-five percent are found in patients older than 50 years. In up to 50% of cases, there is no history or recollection of head trauma. Many suffer from chronic alcoholism. Other associated conditions are epilepsy, ventriculo-peritoneal shunts or coagulopathy.[94,95]

The pathogenesis of a chronic SDH is variable. Relatively minor trauma may initiate grad-

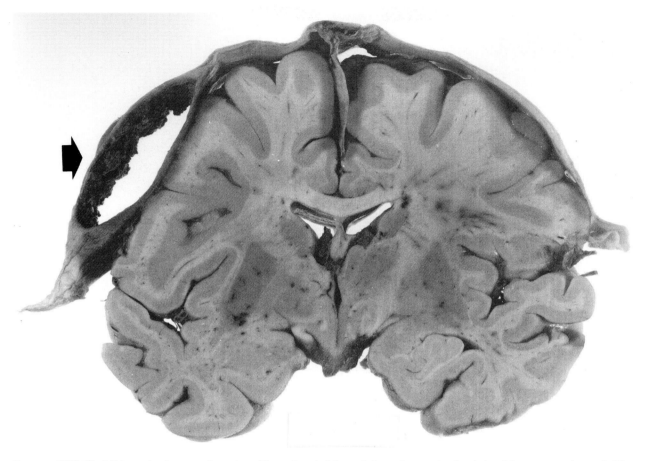

FIGURE XIX-53. Mid-cerebral coronal section. There is a left lateral frontal organized subdural hematoma (arrow). The inner and outer membranes have not fused. The underlying cerebral surface is flattened but the hemisphere is not swollen and there is no left to right midline shift. The ventricles are not displaced and there is no cingulate gyrus or hippocampal herniation.

ual subdural bleeding that enlarges gradually. Neomembranes develop as the bleeding continues so the blood is never completely reabsorbed and the inner and outer membranes never fuse (Fig. XIX-53). If there is cerebral atrophy with a larger than usual subarachnoid space and the enlargement of the hematoma is slow, allowing the brain to accommodate, the membrane-encased hematoma may be remarkably large long after the injury. The symptoms may be vague and the individual may appear demented. Often the chronic SDH is bilateral. Typically, the contents of the chronic subdural hemorrhage are a brown liquid, although foci of recent hemorrhage are often present.

Sometimes an acute SDH may encapsulate as expected but repeated hemorrhages due to relatively minor trauma may occur during the early phase of neomembrane formation when granulation tissue is composed of dilated, thin-walled sinusoidal blood vessels. Repeated hemorrhages prevent the inner and outer membranes from fusing and may result in the same condition noted above. The presence of cerebral atrophy enhances the possibility of this outcome.[96]

Sometimes, a rebleed into an organizing SDH ruptures through the inner membrane creating a second hematoma that develops a second inner membrane. These may go on to a stage of chronic bleeding or multiple rebleeds as described earlier.

Subdural Hygroma

A subdural hygroma is a collection of clear, xanthochromic or bloody fluid in the subdural space following a head injury. The fluid appears to be a mixture of blood, breakdown products of blood and cerebrospinal fluid. The fluid accumulation is often bilateral and an individual may present acutely or weeks after head injury usually with changes in mental status or symptoms of elevated intercranial pressure, such as, headaches, nausea and vomiting.[97]

The exact pathogenesis is not always clear but the generally accepted concept is that head injury causes a tear in the arachnoid membrane. This allows the cerebrospinal fluid to flow into the subdural space but a valve action at the laceration prevents the fluid from re-entering the subarachnoid space.[97] The accumulation increases producing a mass effect. There is no secondary membrane formation and this differentiates it from a chronic subdural hematoma. The accumulation is often bilateral.[98]

If symptomatic, the treatment of choice is drainage through a burr hole or by trephine. The morbidity and mortality are more related to other aspects of the injury and rarely due directly to the hygroma.[97]

Contusions

Contusions are impact related, *focal,* traumatic *injuries* of the brain. The pathologic components of an acute contusion are hemorrhage, necrosis, edema and a variable amount of surrounding ischemia. The contusion occurs when an impact to the head creates an inward deformity of the skull (Fig. XIX-54). The relatively convex surface of the inward-bent inner table of the skull impacts on the round crest of one or more of the adjacent gyri. The force transmits non-uniform deformity to the soft gyrus so that the gyral tissue under the apex of the crest undergoes tensile and shearing strains. The neural and vascular components of this differentially stressed gyrus are disrupted where the deformity is greatest while adjacent areas are partially injured. If the skull

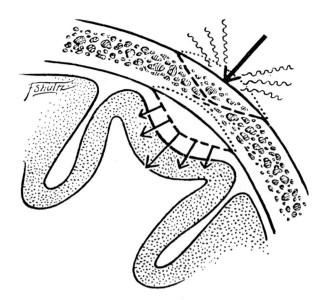

FIGURE XIX-54. Diagram demonstrating the impact deformity caused by blunt forces on the skull. The apex of the gyral crown is most severely deformed while adjacent sites undergo progressively less deformity resulting in shearing stresses within the damaged area.

deformity is sufficient to produce a fracture, the contusion tends to be more severe.[99]

Local tensile models of head injury that apply sudden negative pressure to the dura without the intervening skull produce contusions. Thus, the rebound of the deformed skull may also produce an underlying negative pressure and contribute to the development of a contusion.[100] The compression and tensile mechanisms are not mutually exclusive concepts. Sudden underpressure may also be a factor in producing contrecoup contusions in falls when an accelerated head impacts a hard surface.

The disrupted areas bleed at the time of impact due to tearing of the blood vessels, which are mainly capillaries and veins, but sometimes arteries. Localized swelling due to congestion and edema from damaged microcirculation develops rapidly. Neurons and their processes are injured, unleashing the processes of axonal injury and cell death. In the partially injured zone, blood vessels leak allowing vasogenic edema to develop with resulting ischemia lead-

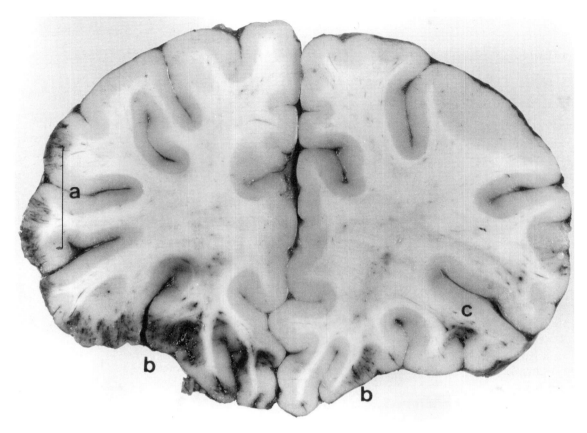

FIGURE XIX-55. Coronal section of frontal lobes. Typical left lateral and bilateral inferior frontal acute cortical contusion hemorrhages. The typical hemorrhages are in the gyral crests (a, b) but there is an occasional hemorrhage in the sulcus (c).

ing to a zone of eosinophilic neurons and injured axons. Disruption of the overlying pia-arachnoid constitutes a cortical laceration. In that case, the cortical and subarachnoid hemorrhage may extend into the subdural space creating or contributing to a subdural hematoma. When subdural blood adheres to the surface of the brain it is a sign of an underlying cortical laceration.

The typical area of contusion necrosis is cone-shaped with the base toward the gyral crest and the apex toward the white matter (Figs. XIX-15, XIX-55 and XIX-56a–b). The superficial molecular layer of the cortex, which is typically spared in infarcts, is destroyed. As the lesion evolves, the classic pattern of coagulation necrosis, inflammation and phagocytosis unfolds. Although the onset of hemorrhage is immediate, it may continue or be intermittent. Axonal injury is

detectable within 3 to 6 hours using the immuno-histochemical reaction for beta amyloid precursor protein and may persist and evolve for days or weeks. Lipid filled histiocytes begin to infiltrate the injury in 2–3 days, are prominent in 7–10 days and persist for weeks or months. The necrotic area begins to cavitate within 2–3 weeks. The cross section of a typical organized contusion is a triangular, cavitary lesion in the crest or a series of contiguous crests of gyral cortex with sparing of the intervening sulcal cortex (Figs. XIX-8, XIX-55 and XIX-56a–b). This is in contrast to hemorrhagic cortical infarcts that involve the crests and the sulcal cortex (Fig. XIX-7) and sometimes the sulcal cortex preferentially. Reactive astrocytes and variable numbers of lipid-filled and hemosiderin-laden histiocytes line the lesions, the latter reflecting the hemorrhagic

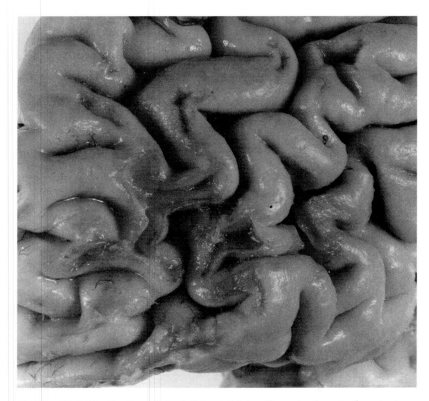

FIGURE XIX-56a. Surface of the left frontal lobe. Organized cortical contusions predominantly involve the gyral crests. These lesions are usually discolored yellow-orange due to hemosiderin deposits.

nature of the original injury (Fig. XIX-56b). In some, the cavity extends into the adjacent white matter reflecting the presence of a contusion hematoma in the acute lesion and these are sometimes extensive. The surrounding white matter is shrunken and gray due to Wallerian degeneration (Fig. XIX-57).

A contusion is a focal lesion and may not be associated with loss of consciousness. Most are minor and cause little, if any morbidity. If the individual did not also suffer a diffuse brain injury, the prognosis is good. Healed cortical contusions are a common incidental finding in the autopsy population of a medical examiner's office as well as in general hospital cases. They are the most common of all structural traumatic brain injuries.[85] It should be noted that fatal head injuries may occur in the absence of contusions.

The severity of the contusion is related to the amount of energy the cortex absorbed from the skull deformity. When the cortical contusions are confluent they may give rise to a large hematoma that requires neurosurgical treatment. Such contusions are particularly common in persons who are alcoholics, have hypertensive vascular disease, take anticoagulants or have a natural hemorrhagic diathesis. Contusion hematomas are most common in the frontal and temporal lobes. A hematoma that extends from the lateral surface of the temporal lobe to the diencephalon raises the possibility of a natural rather than a traumatic cause. A careful examination for signs of trauma must be combined with assessment of clinical and autopsy evidence of hypertension and a search for a possible ruptured saccular aneurysm or other vascular malformation. Sometimes serial head CT scans may reveal the origin of the hemorrhage either on the surface or in the basal ganglia before it spread to both areas. Individuals who are coagulopathic may develop large hemorrhages from small contusions. If confluent, cortical contusion hemorrhages involve an entire

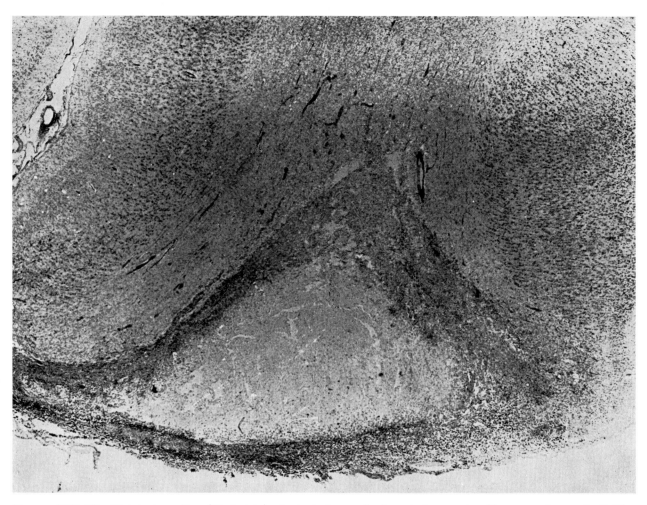

FIGURE XIX-56b. Histologic section (Nissl stain) of a typical organized cortical contusion (three months survival). The lesion is triangular, located in the gyral crest and the subpial layer of the cortex is destroyed. In contrast, ischemic lesions involve the gyral crest and sulcal cortex, preserve the subpial cortical layer and have a pattern of linear necrosis.

lobe, usually the frontal or temporal lobe, the term, *burst lobe* is used. The burst lobe is always associated with and frequently contributes to a subdural hematoma. The burst lobe may also develop following surgical removal of an acute subdural hematoma which decompresses existing small traumatic contusion hemorrhages. The expansion of these hemorrhages plus acute edema causes a fungating mass that herniates through the craniotomy defect *(fungus cerebri)*.

Contusions are found most commonly over the frontal and temporal lobes. They are less common over the parietal lobes and even less so over the occipital poles. They are occasionally present on the medial surfaces of the parietal and occipital lobes due to impact against the relatively rigid falx cerebri or tentorium cerebelli. The irregular surfaces of the floor of the anterior and middle fossae contribute to the increased tendency for contusions to develop in these areas as the brain is propelled by the force of the impact. Sometimes, confluent contusions are found in a *tetrapolar* location, i.e., the tips of the frontal and temporal lobes. Confluent contusions are also frequent over the orbital cortex of the frontal lobes and the inferior and lateral surfaces of each temporal lobe. In this case, a mass effect is produced, often resulting in elevated ICP with falling level of consciousness. Neurosurgeons have come to recognize that contusions can

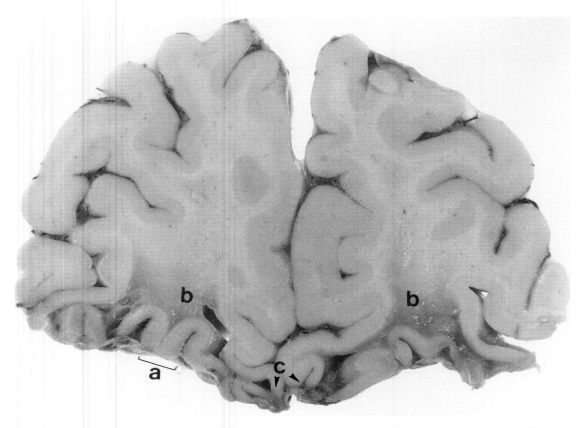

FIGURE XIX-57. Coronal section of frontal lobes. Old cortical contusions of the orbital frontal cortex. There is relative destruction of the gyral crests and sparing of the sulcal cortex (a). Focal, subcortical cavitation reflects resolution of areas of contusion necrosis and contusion hematomas. Shrunken, gray areas of the white matter reflect Wallerian degeneration of damaged axons (b). The olfactory bulbs and tracts are destroyed (c).

abruptly swell about one week post-injury when the hemorrhage begins the resolve but when vasogenic edema can develop rapidly. Of particular concern are contusions of the medial temporal lobe that can rapidly cause transtentorial herniation and pressure on the brain stem with little elevation of ICP.[101]

Impacts that produce fractures often produce enough deformity of the skull to contuse the surface of the brain. These *fracture contusions* may follow the length of the fracture. Since fractures may radiate away from the point of impact, contusions that underlie a fracture do not necessarily reflect the point of impact. Fracture contusions also do not reflect the moving or non-moving status of the head at the time of impact. A depressed, comminuted skull fracture and its underlying contusions form at the site of impact

whether it resulted from a fall or a blow. A linear fracture and its underlying contusions may or may not reflect the site of the impact and may result from a blow or a fall.

When the impact deforms the calvarium sufficient to force the surface of the non compressible brain against the rigid margin of a compartment within the calvarium at the time of the impact, those surfaces may suffer a contusion hemorrhage and are called *herniation contusions* (see Figs. XIX-15, XIX-23 to XIX-25). Examples are herniation contusion hemorrhages of the *medial temporal lobe* against the tentorial edge, the *cingulate gyrus* against the falx or the *cerebellar tonsils* against the margin of the foramen magnum. It is often important in the forensic analysis of a case to distinguish herniation contusions from the cortical injury from herniations due to increased

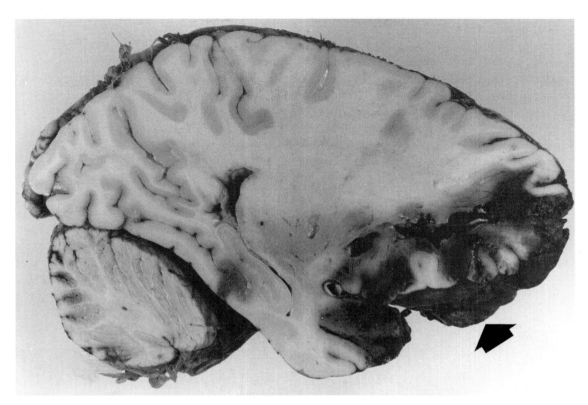

FIGURE XIX-58. Right parasagittal brain section. Decedent fell on the back of the head. No coup contusion. Severe anterior temporal and inferior and anterior frontal contusions (arrow). Survival time was nine hours.

ICP developing as a delayed effect of trauma. *Herniation contusions* often are associated with sudden death, whereas, *herniation necrosis* implies a period of survival. In contrast to herniation necrosis, herniation contusions usually are not associated with mass lesions, brain edema, dramatic brain shifts or evidence of increased ICP.

An impact of a moving, accelerating head against a hard surface causes contusions of the cerebrocortical surface opposite the point of impact. These *contrecoup contusions* occur mostly in the tetrapolar and inferior frontotemporal distribution (Figs. XIX-16, XIX-58 and XIX-59). The contrecoup pattern occurs most commonly with accelerating impacts of the back or the side of the head but rarely to the front. If a blow to the resting, movable head that does not produce fractures, causes cerebrocortical contusions, they will be situated beneath the point of impact. These are *coup contusions* and are much less common than contrecoup contusions (Figs. XIX-25 and XIX-60). A blow to the movable head almost never produces contrecoup contusions and if it does, they are smaller than the coup contusions. An impact of an accelerating head against a hard surface almost never produces coup contusions and if it does, they are smaller than the contrecoup contusions. Falls from a height great enough to exceed the acceleration phase do not produce contrecoup contusions. Frontal impacts of the accelerating head on a hard surface rarely produce any contusions. Crushing of the head between a low velocity force and a firm surface may shatter the skull and lacerate the brain but produces few contusions.

A fall that produces contrecoup contusions must create an acceleration phase so that the skull falls more rapidly than the brain. This forces the lagging brain against the inner surface of the skull opposite the side of the impact displacing the CSF to the side of the impact. The angular acceleration of an unbroken fall on the

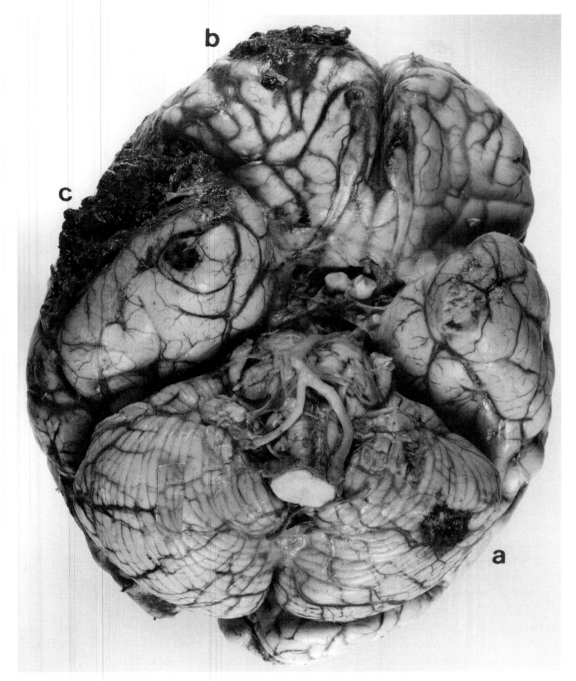

FIGURE XIX-59. Base of the brain. Decedent fell on the left occipital area. There is a small coup contusion of the left posterior-lateral cerebellum (a) and large contrecoup contusions of the right frontal pole and the lateral frontal/temporal surface (b, c).

occiput creates a force greater than 1 g at the time of impact. The occipital side of the skull is protected by a thicker layer of CSF that can be displaced on impact and by a smooth inner table of the occipital skull. The frontal and temporal areas of the brain have several disadvantages. There is no buffering layer of CSF to cushion the impact between the surface of the brain and the

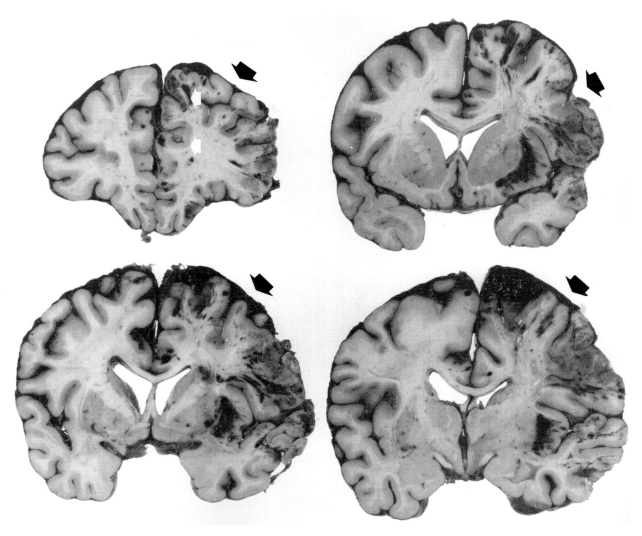

FIGURE XIX-60. Coronal sections of cerebral hemispheres. Severe, broad blow to the right frontal/temporal area with a board (black arrows). No contrecoup contusions. Some right medial frontal contusions (white arrows). Found dead.

inner table of the skull. The relative absence of CSF increases the friction between the brain and skull as the brain slides over the skull surface. The surface of the skull on the floor of the anterior and middle fossae is rough. The occipital impact compresses the frontotemporal cortex against the rough surfaces of the anterior calvarium creating positive forces. Finally, the abrupt acceleration of the frontotemporal surfaces of the brain away from the surface of the inner table of the skull after impact may produce an area of negative pressure which by itself can cause con-

tusions. The two mechanisms may both apply in an alternating manner.[102]

Slit-shaped traumatic hemorrhages, often bilateral, in the subcortical white matter of the dorsal frontal lobes have been designated *gliding contusions*.[103] They are paramedian, usually in the white matter of the superior frontal gyrus, and may extend into the overlying cortex. Gliding contusions do not appear to be focal, contact lesions but rather are commonly associated with other lesions characteristic of diffuse axonal injury (see Fig. XIX-33).

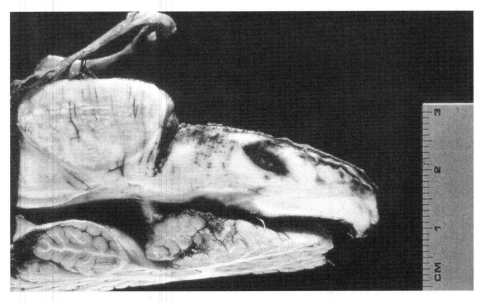

FIGURE XIX-61. Sagittal section of pons, medulla and roof of the fourth ventricle. There is a partial, ventral, hemorrhagic laceration of the pontomedullary junction.

Lacerations

It is common to see subdural blood that adheres to the leptomeningeal surface of the brain overlying areas of subarachnoid blood and cortical contusions. This is indicative of an area of *cortical and leptomeningeal laceration* with bleeding into the subdural space. Often the area is adjacent to a skull fracture. Healing of these lesions may result in fibrous adhesions between the dura and brain, a lesion associated with a higher risk of post-traumatic epilepsy.

Hemorrhage and *laceration of the corpus callosum* is frequently part of a more widespread injury as seen in diffuse axonal injury. Rarely, it may be an isolated traumatic lesion, associated with an impact on the vertex or high occipital skull (see Fig. XIX-15). Also it is seen in cases of pericallosal artery infarction during transfalcine herniation resulting from a supracallosal midline shift, especially in individuals who are coagulopathic.[104,105]

Pontomedullary lacerations (Fig. XIX-61) occur either as an isolated injury or in association with other traumatic brain lesions.[106] The laceration is always ventral but may extend to a complete, traumatic separation between the pons and medulla, an injury which is immediately lethal.

When incomplete and involving the medullary pyramids and a portion of the tegmentum, the clinical result may be a *locked in syndrome,*[106] that is, total paralysis except for voluntary eye movements without loss of consciousness.

When pontomedullary laceration occurs in the absence of other brain stem injuries, there is frequently an associated ring fracture around the foramen magnum and/or fractures or dislocations of C 1 and C 2. This pattern of injury is due to severe hyperextension. If other traumatic injuries of the brain stem are seen in association with pontomedullary laceration, there are usually extensive fractures of the base of the skull and the calvarium, and the mechanism of injury is more complex than pure hyperextension.[107]

Intracerebral Hemorrhage

A single, large, intracerebral hematoma, not related to a cortical contusion, rarely if ever occurs as a direct result of blunt force head injury. Small, multiple, intra-axial hemorrhages due to trauma are common. They usually are a result of diffuse axonal injury and develop in predictable locations. Multiple white matter hematomas may be contiguous to cortical contusions and are contusion hematomas. If the individual is coagulopathic, these hemorrhages may be large.

Single hematomas in an adult located in the basal ganglia or diencephalon, the base of the pons or the white matter of the cerebellum are usually found with some stigmata of hypertension and are non-traumatic in origin. Such hematomas arise from rupture of small penetrating arteries with degenerative intramural changes with[108] or without[109] Charcot-Bouchard miliary aneurysms. The hemorrhages may extend into the ventricles, the subarachnoid space or, occasionally, the subdural space. Ingestion of cocaine is a risk factor for hemorrhage in these same areas because the drug induces surges of elevated blood pressure.[110] Any medication that can cause elevation of blood pressure can potentially be at risk for these hemorrhages.

A large hematoma, not related to a contusion and in a location other than the above is usually secondary to one of several natural causes. These include large or small (cryptic) vascular malformations, aneurysms, emboli (bland or septic), neoplasms, abscesses or coagulopathic states. An extensive search for these causes is warranted because when such a hematoma is present in the context of blunt force head injury, a question arises as to whether the lesion is the cause or the result of trauma. With comprehensive gross and microscopic examination of the margins of the hematoma and review of all clinical information, most such cases can be resolved.

If traumatic intracerebral hemorrhage presents clinically hours or days after the blunt force head injury, it is a *delayed traumatic intracerebral hemorrhage (DTICH)*. They may be single or multiple and often are related to contusions. DTICH is defined as a hemorrhage following trauma that becomes manifest after an admission CT scan that was interpreted as normal.[111] There are a variety of potential causes. Vasospasm may temporarily block the hemorrhage. Increased ICP may temporarily tamponade the damaged vessels. Treatment of the increased ICP will relieve the pressure and may allow the bleeding to begin. Coagulopathic individuals are more prone to develop DTICH. MRI scans obtained from post-traumatic patients who had normal CT scans and

who subsequently developed hemorrhages showed parenchymal lesions.[112] It is thought these lesions represent areas of damage, including vascular injury, that subsequently result in rupture and hemorrhage.[113]

Subarachnoid Hemorrhage

Traumatic brain injury, whether caused by impact or pure acceleration/deceleration forces, is the most common cause of subarachnoid hemorrhage (SAH). Traumatic SAH is usually thin and does not cause complications due to mass effect. It is an indicator of a traumatic brain injury and in some cases of fatal diffuse brain injury. SAH may be the only visible manifestation of head injury. Indeed, one study concluded that the presence of traumatic SAH is an independent factor related to a significant increased risk of elevated intracranial pressure and death.[21] SAH often overlies a contusion which may also be the source of bleeding. However, contusions do not always cause SAH and SAH may be present in the absence of contusions.

Blood provokes an inflammatory response when it flows into the subarachnoid space. It is first dominated by neutrophils and, after several days, macrophages begin to remove the erythrocytes. In some circumstances, this may be mistaken for meningitis. The end stage of SAH removal consists of hemosiderin pigment filled macrophages in the subarachnoid and Virchow-Robin spaces. The presence of blood in the subarachnoid space, including the arachnoid granulations may interfere with CSF absorption and cause acute hydrocephalus.[114] Previous subarachnoid hemorrhage, especially if it is repeated, is considered a potential cause of *normal pressure hydrocephalus,* a form of communicating hydrocephalus which may present as disturbance of gait and dementia.[115] The gate disturbance results when the enlarging angle of the lateral ventricles distorts the corticospinal axons to the lower extremities as they pass from their origins in the dorsomedial motor cortex to the posterior limb of the internal capsule. Shunting may relieve the symptoms of dementia and the spastic gait.[116]

The most common cause of *massive subarachnoid hemorrhage* is rupture of a *saccular aneurysm* at one of the proximal bifurcations of the cerebral arteries at or near the circle of Willis. An estimated 25 to 50% of saccular aneurysms rupture.[117] Approximately 90% develop in the anterior circulation. Rupture of the aneurysm causes abrupt onset of symptoms that includes headache, nausea, vomiting, mental status changes and focal neurologic signs depending on the location and spread of the hemorrhage. Forensic pathologists regularly encounter a subset of patients who suffer sudden death due to saccular aneurysm rupture. These individuals are found dead or are observed to collapse and die at the scene, bypassing any form of medical treatment. This is one of the few causes of CNS-related sudden death and is due to hypothalamic dysfunction with cardiac arrhythmias resulting from excessive sympathetic stimulation.[118,119]

Saccular aneurysms are considered acquired lesions, rarely seen before age 20 years, that result from a combination of degenerative changes at the arterial bifurcation and hemodynamic stress. Some risk factors for their formation are heavy smoking, heavy alcohol consumption, polycystic kidney disease, some forms of collagen deficiency, aortic coarctation and, rarely, genetic factors. The possibility that hypertension may cause saccular aneurysms to develop has been considered but clinical study has shown no relationship.[120] The relationship between rupture of the aneurysm and trauma is not established. A recent clinical study found that 8% of patients with post-traumatic subarachnoid hemorrhage had ruptured saccular aneurysms.[121] These patients were notable in that their hemorrhage was thick along the base of the brain and had spread into the Sylvian fissures, thus provoking a four-vessel angiogram which revealed the aneurysms. There is a convincing association between rupture of saccular aneurysms and ingestion of cocaine probably related to the surge in the blood pressure that results from its use.[122]

When one encounters large basilar SAH at the time of autopsy, it important to visualize the state of the vertebral and internal carotid arteries as they enter the intracranial compartment because lacerations or saccular aneurysms may be present at these points. Most ruptured aneurysms result in thick SAH that covers the base of the brain from the optic chiasm to the caudal medulla. If the aneurysm is in the anterior circulation, rostral to the basilar tip and the posterior cerebral arteries, the hemorrhage extends into the interhemispheric and Sylvian fissures and over each perisylvian cerebral hemisphere (Fig. XIX-62).

Other natural causes of massive SAH are ruptured arteriovenous malformations and dissection of intracerebral hemorrhage into the subarachnoid space.

Thick, basilar, subarachnoid hemorrhage may occasionally result from *blunt force head or neck injury*. The most common source of the hemorrhage is *vertebral artery injury* near its attachment to the dura as it enters the subarachnoid space. The most common forensic history is a physical altercation involving a blow to the side of the upper neck or jaw that quickly results in death. It is usually associated with acute hemorrhage in the neck muscles that cover the dorsal-lateral cervical/occipital area. The vertebral artery may be torn along its intracranial course, or at its attachment to the dura which, at that point, is fused with the arachnoid. More commonly, however, the wall of the extradural vertebral artery is damaged as it courses beneath the posterior arch of the atlas. A traumatic intramural hemorrhage then dissects rostrally into the subarachnoid space where the vertebral artery penetrates the dura.

To determine the site of the vascular injury, the first step is to recognize its possibility. Suspicion should arise in a traumatic death situation when removal of the calvarium reveals the presence of large SAH over the base of the brain in a distribution that resembles a ruptured saccular aneurysm. The brain should be removed without disrupting the arachnoid and only after confirming the intracranial integrity of both vertebral and internal carotid arteries. The extent and thickness of the SAH should be noted and the blood removed. If no aneurysm is found and no damage to the intracranial vertebral arteries is present the next step is a posterior neck dissection to demonstrate the terminal extracranial seg-

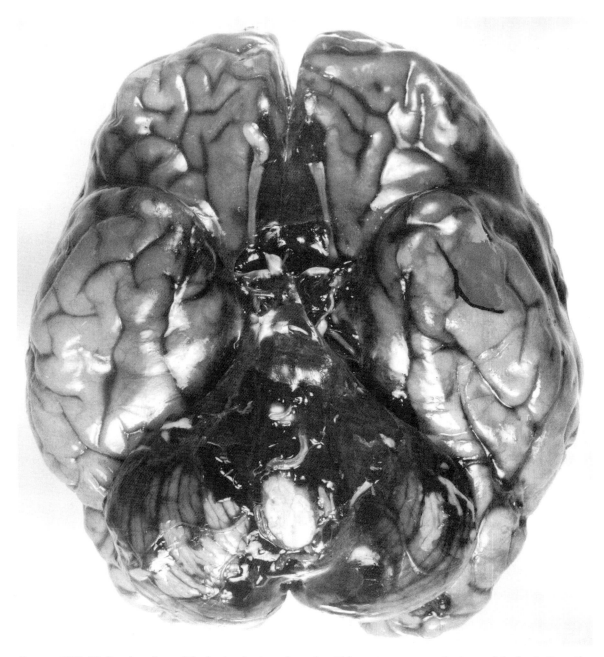

FIGURE XIX-62. Basal surface of the brain. Acute, subarachnoid hematoma covers the base of the brain from the infundibulum to the medulla. The decedent died instantly after a blow (fist) to the face. Traumatic disruption of the vertebral artery near its intradural origin or a ruptured dissecting hemorrhage from an injured extradural vertebral artery segment at C-1 is a high probability. If the subarachnoid hemorrhage results from rupture of a saccular aneurysm of the anterior circulation, the hemorrhage usually spreads into the Sylvian fissures and the perisylvian surface of the cerebral hemispheres.

ments of the vertebral arteries. Some acute soft tissue injury of the upper posterior-lateral neck will be present. The key area to visualize is the segment of the vertebral artery between the foramen transversarium of C-1 and its attachment to the atlanto-occipital membrane. A portion of this segment lies beneath the posterior arch of the atlas which may be fractured at this point. If so, the fracture should be photographically documented. Removal of the arch will expose the vertebral artery to examine for signs of injury. If this segment of the artery is lacerated, the hemorrhage will flow into the epidural space and soft tissues of the neck and will not cause subarachnoid hemorrhage. If, however, the twisting and distortion of the impacted neck is sufficient to partially tear the wall of the vertebral artery near its dural attachment, the hemorrhage may dissect along the arterial wall and rupture into the subarachnoid space. The blood enters the subarachnoid rather than the subdural space because the arachnoid membrane is fused with the dura at the point of vertebral artery penetration.[123-126]

If no vertebral artery injury is present, the most likely source of the hemorrhage is one or more of the small arterial or venous branches over the ventral base of the brain stem.

Birth Trauma

Injuries to the infant during childbirth result from mechanical forces during the process of delivery. Some risk factors for head injuries due to birth trauma include prolonged labor, abrupt labor, uncontrolled delivery of the head, macrosomia, prematurity, abnormal presentation, forceps delivery or vacuum extraction. Also, injury can occur in an uncomplicated birth. In recent years, the combination of improved prenatal care, improved anesthesia, more frequent resort to cesarean section and less frequent use of forceps has significantly lowered the incidence of injuries from these sources. Neonatal birth injuries may involve one or more of the layers between the skin and the brain. A unique potential complication of the hemorrhages that may complicate the birth process is that the relatively large size of the head compared to the small neonatal blood volume provides the opportunity for a given hemorrhage to produce anemia, shock or exsanguination.

Subgaleal blood vessels such as emissary veins may tear during difficult deliveries and form *subgaleal hematomas*. Because the soft tissue is elastic and there are no lateral barriers to tamponade the bleeding, it is possible for the infant to suffer serious, even fatal loss of blood into the hematoma.

During labor, especially of a primiparous mother, molding of the infant's head may cause shearing distortion between the skull and the external periosteum. This not only loosens the periosteum, but also may tear subperiosteal blood vessels leading to a *cephalohematoma*. The hemorrhage is confined by the fibrous attachment of the periosteum at the sutures. Cephalohematomas develop most commonly in the parietal area and there is often an underlying linear fracture. Cephalohematomas, unless associated with other, more serious injuries, are inconsequential and usually resorb completely without complications.[127]

The typical birth-related *skull fractures* are minor with little clinical consequence. *Severe, depressed, comminuted fractures,* often associated with dural or brain injury, were usually caused by the application of mid or high forceps in severely complicated deliveries, a situation rarely encountered in recent years. The most common *fracture* seen today is not a fracture but a dent in the pliant skull, most often the parietal area, due to slowly applied pressure from the prominences of the maternal pelvis. They have been called *ping pong fractures* reminiscent of a dent that can occur in a ping pong ball. They are rarely associated with serious brain injury and rarely require treatment. *Linear fractures,* also most common in the parietal area, may be associated with a cephalohematoma. They are rarely associated with any additional dural or brain injury.

The above birth injuries may be unexpectedly encountered during an autopsy of an infant who may have died of the sudden infant death syndrome (SIDS). They must be recognized as innocuous birth injuries and not as a manifestation of child abuse.

Under some circumstances, fractures in infants may evolve into *growing fractures* when they occur during the period of rapid brain growth. Most occur during the first year and rarely after the third year. Such fractures may be linear or diastatic and are associated with a dural tear. The growing, swollen, pulsating brain pushes the fracture margins apart causing a widening fracture defect with scalloped, loculated bone margins (Fig. XIX-63). A bulging leptomeningeal out-pouching or cyst may interpose between the fracture margins which progressively widen. The brain and leptomeninges adhere to the fracture edges and there is often focal underlying brain damage. Eventually, the lesion may become an epileptogenic focus.[128,129]

Epidural hemorrhage is unusual and has been related to forceps deliveries. They may be large enough to cause hemodynamic instability, anemia and shock. As in adults, they are often, but not always associated with skull fractures.

Clinically deleterious *subdural hemorrhage* in the neonate is almost always a complication of excessive molding of the infant's head during a difficult delivery. With horizontal compression and vertical elongation, the hemorrhage emanates from torn bridging veins. Elongation of the head stresses the tentorium cerebelli, the straight sinus or the vein of Galen and may result in a posterior fossa SDH. In both situations, the distortion of the head may also cause *intradural hemorrhage* or *dural lacerations*. The exact incidence of neonatal SDH is not known but in forensic practice, it is common to see a subdural neomembrane in infant autopsies.

The same forces that mold the head may cause *subarachnoid hemorrhage* which is relatively common and rarely harmful. It is common to see erythrocytes in the CSF of neonates. SAH may be a risk factor to develop communicating hydrocephalus in the future.

Traumatic, neonatal *intracerebral hematoma* is rare and has been seen with forceps delivery.

Neurotrauma in Infants

An *infant* is a child who is less than 12 months old. The physical properties of an infant's body differ from an adult in a number of ways that influence the pattern of head injuries resulting from trauma. Some are well understood and clearly defined while others are more vague and subjects of controversy. These are issues of considerable social concern because head injuries

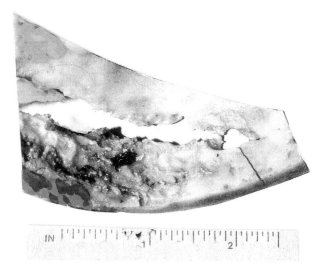

FIGURE XIX-63. The inner surface of the parietal skull of a 45-year-old woman. The skull defect was associated with an underlying dural defect so the surface of the sclerotic leptomeninges adhered to the subscalpular connective tissue. There was an underlying acute intracerebral hematoma. Notice the gap between the edges of the skull defect and the scalloped surface of the edges and the margins of the inner table.

are the most common cause of death and disability among children and many of these injuries are non-accidental. It is not possible to ascertain the exact incidence of non-accidental head injury but estimates are in the range of 25% of medically treated childhood head injuries. From the forensic point of view the challenge of distinguishing between accidental and non-accidental head injury is often difficult.[130]

Crucial to determining the accidental vs. non-accidental nature of the injury is assessing whether or not the description of events that caused the injury is compatible with the physical findings. To this end, clinical studies of known accidental injuries have been conducted to elucidate some quantitative references to compare with a given hypothetical situation. From these studies, some generalizations have been drawn.

It is apparent that the infant's body responds differently in some respects from an adult and these differences change rapidly after the first year. First of all, the state of virtual total dependency during the pre-ambulatory period means the infant can suffer serious trauma only though the actions of another by accident, neglect, or intent. Compared to the adult, the infant's head is relatively large and heavy, the neck is weak and elastic, the skull is pliable, the white matter is soft and unmyelinated and the subarachnoid space is larger. These factors lower the threshold for traumatic brain injury and change its pattern in infants as compared to adults.

When infants suffer blunt force injuries that would cause contusions in a more mature individual, they instead develop white matter *contusion tears,* usually not hemorrhagic, at the cortical/white matter junction in the frontal and temporal lobes. The lack of myelin and softness of the infant white matter adjacent to the more dense gray matter creates an interface that is vulnerable to shearing injury. At the same time, the bone surfaces of the anterior and middle fossae are relatively smooth, reducing the risk of surface contusion hemorrhage injury to the cortex.[131]

Non-Accidental Head Injury in Children

The first term applied to inflicted injuries in children was the *battered child syndrome* which recognized multiple injuries of multiple ages in the traumatized child. The *shaken baby syndrome* was defined as a constellation of injuries resulting from the *whiplash* movement of the infant's head when violently shaken. Broad attention was drawn to the fact that violent shaking, with or without evidence of impact, could cause severe neurologic injury or death in infants.[132] The absence of obvious, visible traumatic injuries may obscure the etiology of the incident. Children who survive but are brain damaged may not be brought to medical treatment and the neurologic deficit may not become apparent until later developmental milestones are not met. Such children sometimes acquire the diagnostic designation of *cerebral palsy.* Some children are brought to the emergency room with an admitting complaint of a seizure and are treated without recognition of the trauma. The children frequently have a history of an acute illness with coughing, vomiting and irritability. In fact, the acutely ill, irritable, crying infant is at risk for such injury

when the angry, frustrated caregiver loses control and resorts to physical abuse.

Injuries from shaking are most common in the youngest infants with the incidence rapidly decreasing during the second, third and fourth year of life. This is because the unique anatomic features of the infant as noted above rapidly evolve toward that of the adult thus raising the threshold for the amount of force necessary to produce the injuries. One case fatality has been reported of an adult prisoner who was violently shaken during interrogation.[133] The repetitive nature of the act, both with repetitive bouts of shaking and with multiple shakes within an episode, is paramount in the production of the injury. The energy produced by a single shake is insufficient to produce the injuries typically seen, but each whiplash adds some quantum of damage to blood vessels and axons which do not recover between shakes. The damage summates as in any repetitive injury situation until the shaking stops or the injuries develop.

Head injuries resulting from rotational acceleration/deceleration consist of subdural hemorrhage, usually small and midline; subarachnoid hemorrhage, also small and usually paramedian; periopticointrascleral hemorrhages; and retinal hemorrhages. The children also may have subperiosteal new bone formation of long bones and *bucket handle* fractures of long bone epiphyses where they are gripped or pivot when shaken. More recent case reports demonstrate a high incidence of impact injuries of the head in children with this injury pattern which led to the term *shaken/impact syndrome.* The impact during shaking increases the severity of the injury. While the absence of evidence of contact does not rule out an impact with certainty, it is not necessary to conclude that an impact must have occurred when there is no evidence of a bruise in the scalp and the caregiver gives a history of shaking without impact.

The latter observation has led to a hypothesis that shaking alone cannot produce enough energy to cause the severe, often lethal brain injuries presented by these victims and that these injuries require an impact to occur.[134] The presumption is that death must result from diffuse axonal injury

(DAI), since it is not due to the small subdural hemorrhage, the scant subarachnoid hemorrhage or the retinal hemorrhages. Indeed, the experimental models used for shaking do not come close to matching energy required to create the experimental injuries of DAI produced by a single lateral rotational acceleration in adult primates. A counterpoint to the discussion is that the special anatomic features of the infant noted above allow greater movement of the brain within the skull and actually lower the threshold for such injuries in the infant, a fact suggested by the rapid decrease in incidence of the syndrome after the first year of life. Other factors of relevance could be that abusive shaking, in contrast to the two dimensional experimental model, is a repetitive, three-dimensional injury with clusters of acceleration/deceleration injuries that have a summation effect.

We are left with a clinical/pathologic fact that a disturbing number of infants continue to present with small subdural hemorrhage, small subarachnoid hemorrhage, periopticoscleral hemorrhages, and retinal hemorrhage and they die. In every published series, a number of the victims have no sign of head impact after thorough, competent examination. A few of the caregivers have admitted to shaking only and, as noted above, the incidence of this scenario diminishes rapidly after the first year of life.

Several recent observations offer a different hypothesis. First, was a report of a clinical/radiological/pathological study of non-accidentally head-injured children who met the criteria for the shaken impact syndrome and had a high incidence of apnea prior to admission.[135] The most consistent findings in the group were apnea, intracranial hemorrhages (SDH, SAH, retinal hemorrhages) and diffuse brain swelling of the type associated with hypoxia and hypotension as reported by the NIH Traumatic Coma Data Bank in their cases of severely head-injured children.[136] Some of the children had cervical cord injury. The authors concluded that trauma-induced apnea causes diffuse cerebral anoxic/ischemic injury that is the most important factor in the infant's outcome and it was more important than whether the injury was due to shaking alone versus shaking with impact and more important than the SDH, SAH, diffuse axonal injury, parenchymal shear or brain contusion.

More recently, two detailed neuropathological studies (both from the same series of patients) of fatal inflicted head injury in children was carried out including the use of beta amyloid precursor protein (beta APP) immunohistochemical technique for demonstrating axonal injury.[137,138] They noted significant differences between infants less than nine months and those older than one year. In the younger group, the most common finding was apnea at the time of presentation, and global anoxic/ischemic injury was the most common histologic finding. DAI was seen only in two cases, both of whom had severe head injuries with multiple skull fractures. Injury of the brain stem and cervical cord nerve roots and cervical epidural hemorrhage were found in a significant number of cases. These authors also concluded that the most common mechanism of death in infants with inflicted head injury and subdural, subarachnoid and retinal hemorrhages with or without evidence of impact is apnea resulting from stretching injury of the cervicomedullary region during craniocervical hyperextension and flexion.

This hypothesis explains many of the findings associated with the shaking/impact syndrome. Much depends on the authors' interpretation of the beta APP immunostains and their criteria for distinguishing staining due to ischemic injury from that due to primary traumatic axonal injury, a difficult diagnostic issue.[60,61] Hopefully these criteria will be confirmed with additional studies. Also it is apparent that we are without meaningful experimental data. There is no shaking head injury model in general and there is no model that reproduces the conditions of infancy. We will have to continue, for the foreseeable future, to rely on clinical studies to clarify, as much as possible, some of these issues. These studies need to be focused and detailed. They must recognize that infants and children at different ages are different biophysical entities and should not be combined with each other in clinical studies. Detailed neuropathologic information is needed, particularly about the medulla, spinal cord and the nerve roots (especially the upper cervical level). More must be learned about the early sequence of events. For example, the acute effect of trauma-induced apnea would produce loss of consciousness within seconds, an observation that has been made by some perpetrators.[135] If the trauma produces the syndrome of acute, malignant brain swelling followed by increased ICP and brain stem suppression and apnea, one would expect a short lucid interval.[8] If the collapse is due to DAI, more detailed studies may demonstrate axonal damage. In any case, the severity of the trauma that produces these injuries and death is substantial. Many children survive shaking/impact injury but with varying degrees of brain damage. We know very little of the neuropathologic changes in these victims.

PENETRATING BRAIN INJURIES

Whereas, blunt force head trauma results in closed brain injuries, sharp force head trauma causes penetrating (or perforating) wounds that leave a communication between the brain tissue and the external environment. In practice, the vast majority of penetrating/perforating head injuries are gunshot wounds. Other sources are nail guns, crossbows, knives, screwdrivers and a host of other sharp objects that one can propel, thrust, or fall upon.

Gunshot Wounds

Approximately one million gunshot wounds were inflicted in the United States in 1993 and about 17,000 homicides were committed with guns.[139] About 6,000 individuals die of gunshot wounds of the head each year.[140] The overall mortality of a gunshot wound of the head is very high and most victims die at the scene or on arrival at the emergency medical facility.

The biophysics and forensic pathology of gunshot wounds is described in detail elsewhere in this text. This includes the appearance of the entrance and exit wounds, the relationship between the energy of the missile and its mass and velocity and the presence of a permanent and a temporary cavity. The destructive capacity of the bullet is related linearly to its mass but to the square of its velocity. The amount of damage a bullet causes in a wound is related to the amount of energy it gives up in the body. That is its energy at the point of entrance minus its energy at the point of exit or, in the case of a penetrating wound, its total energy at the point of entrance. Amount of yaw (degree of axis deviation from the line of flight) and deformability of the bullet are factors in the amount of energy given up by the bullet in the head. Straight flying, small caliber, non-deforming, perforating, jacketed bullets give only the energy related to the loss of velocity during passage. Some features of the effects of gunshot wounds on the brain are addressed in this section.

The brain, in contrast to other tissues, is confined by the rigid skull. This creates a more damaging environment when exposed to the effects of the temporary cavity caused by the bullet. The radiating forces around the expanding track compress the brain tissue against the unyielding skull and dural reflections potentially creating multiple injuries (Figs. XIX-23 and XIX-24). These include fractures of the orbital plates and calvarium and contusion hemorrhages of the inferior frontal and temporal cortex against the base of the skull, the cingulate gyrus against the falx, the unci against the tentorial edge, the basal ganglia, diencephalon and rostral brain stem with central herniation through the incisura and the cerebellar tonsils and dorsal medulla through the foramen magnum.[141,142] The sudden, marked elevation of intracranial pressure is responsible for a period of apnea and, frequently, immediate death.[143] The permanent cavity returns to a non-distended state almost immediately and appears as a blood-filled track with hemorrhagic margins that is larger than the caliber of the bullet depending on the amount of its deformity, yaw and tumbling. Surrounding this is a variable zone of pink or gray discoloration due to injury from

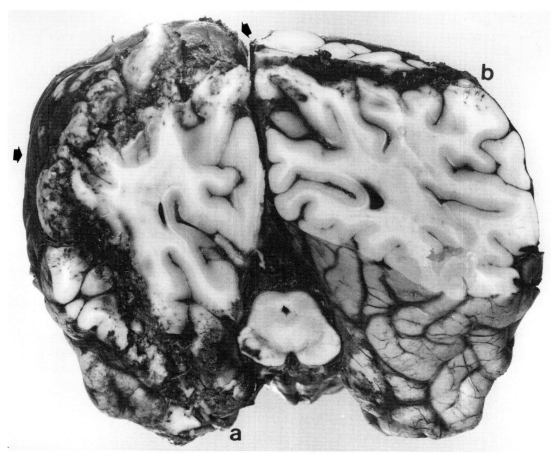

FIGURE XIX-64. Gunshot wound of the brain. Double ricochet. The bullet entered the left anterior temporal lobe (a) and lodged in the right parietal lobe (b) after deflecting off the inner table at two separate points (arrows). There are contusion hemorrhages of the left cerebral peduncle and the right posterior-inferior-lateral temporal lobe.

the temporary cavity which may have been 30 times the diameter of the permanent cavity, largely dependent on the velocity of the bullet.

At the entrance wound, the passage of the bullet through the skull produces internal beveling and secondary missiles in the form of bone fragments which do additional brain damage and create additional tracks. These fragments remain in the area of the entrance wound, a feature which helps to determine the direction of the bullet.

Bullets from smaller caliber handguns with low muzzle velocity may not have sufficient energy to perforate the head. The bullet may ricochet back from the inner table of the skull or glide along the inner table surface producing additional tracks (Fig. XIX-64). Thus, a line drawn from

the entrance wound to the final resting point of the bullet in such a case will not accurately reflect the direction of fire.

A bullet may impact but not perforate the skull. Depending on the amount of imparted energy, the extent of skull deformation and the location of the impact, the result to the victim may range from inconsequential to lethal. The impact may produce a transient cerebral concussion. The deformity may produce fracture and/or cortical contusion (and thus local injury and symptoms) or an impact over the brain stem or upper cervical cord may produce a fatal concussion. A high velocity perforating bullet that passes through the head or neck without contacting the skull or vertebrae may cause sudden death by the concussive effect of the temporary cavity. This may or may not cause contusions.

Penetrating, Sharp Force (Non-Gunshot) Injuries

A great variety of implements and surfaces cause penetrating (and occasional perforating) brain injuries. These are low velocity injuries with much of the energy dissipated in the process of perforating the skull. The brain injury consists of a track approximately the size of the penetrating object. No temporal cavity forms. The outcome of the injury hinges on which structures of the brain are injured (Fig. XIX-65).

Objects penetrate more easily through the thinner areas of the skull such as the eye socket or the squamous portion of the temporal bone. Major complications result from damage to intracranial blood vessels, destruction of vital brain centers and infections. Blood vessels, whether dural sinuses, veins or arteries, may be pierced and cause fatal acute hemorrhages. The bleeding may be acute or delayed with onset of symptoms ranging from immediate to subtle. Often the patient arrives with a dramatic presentation such as a screwdriver protruding from the head. In other situations the victim may be unaware of a penetrating brain injury by a small object (needle, nail, thorn) and may not seek medical attention or the injury may not be detected on examination. In such a situation, eventual *infection* or *delayed hemorrhage* is a risk. Sometimes the penetrating object may damage the wall of an artery. This may result in *arterial thrombosis* at the site of injury, a complication that occurs within hours or days. The injury also may weaken the wall of the artery and cause a *traumatic aneurysm* that may rupture days, weeks or years later.

All penetrating wounds of the brain pose the *risk of infection* which may develop rapidly or slowly. The infection may present as *subdural empyema, meningitis, cerebritis, brain abscess* or all of the above in various combinations. Penetrating wounds also pose a significantly higher risk of *post-traumatic epilepsy* than closed head injuries.

SPINAL CORD INJURY

Spinal cord injury is an enormous and growing medical, societal and legal problem in the United States. The prevalence of patients with serious spinal cord injuries is growing dramatically not only because of a rising incidence but because of increased survival. The approximate number of such patients was 30,000 in 1974[144] 175,000 in 1980[145] and 250,000 in 1992.[146]

Approximately 50% of spinal cord injuries result from vehicular accidents (including motorcycles and bicycles). More than half of these are single vehicle collisions. Fifteen to 20% involve falls. Elderly people with pre-existing spinal degenerative disease are heavily represented in this group. Sports and recreational activities constitute about 15 to 20% and two-thirds of these events are related to diving. The frequency of football spinal injuries is falling with recent attention given to the problem. Finally, violent assaults including beating, stabbing and gunshot wounds (mostly with handguns) represent 15 to 20%. The handgun injuries are the most rapidly growing group. Most victims of spinal injury are male.[147]

The medical examiner encounters cases of acute, subacute or remote spinal cord injuries on a regular basis, each case presenting a number of forensic issues. Assessing each case involves correlating the pathologic anatomy with as much clinical information as is available. The spinal cord must be removed in its entirety within the dura. There are a number of accepted techniques for postmortem removal of the spinal cord. The posterior approach allows for removal with less tension on the cord, especially at the cervical level which is often critical. The body should be positioned to neutralize the lordotic curvature of the lumbar and cervical spine. A midline longi-

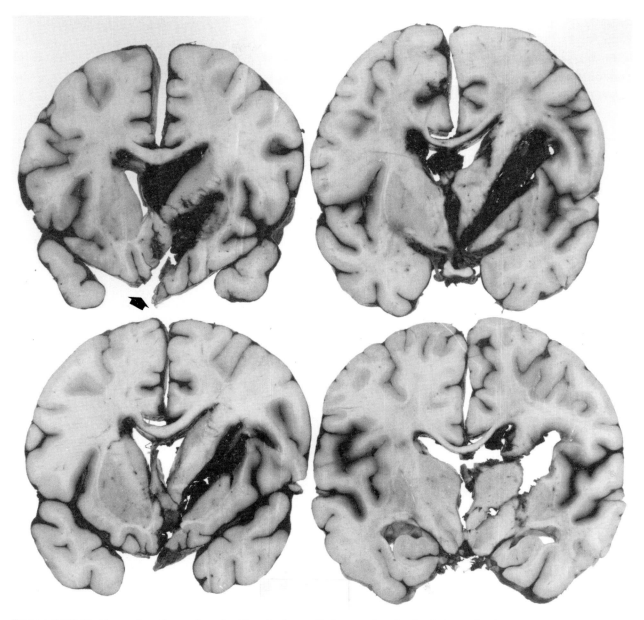

FIGURE XIX-65. Coronal sections of cerebral hemispheres. Stab wound with a knife (arrow). The track is filled with blood and is directed rightward, upward and backward from inferior-medial right frontal lobe to right superior-lateral basal ganglia. There is blood in the ventricle. The distal portion of the wound track is enlarged due to movement of the knife. The decedent survived for two and one-half hours.

tudinal skin incision from the occiput to the sacrum followed by lateral reflection of the paraspinal musculature to expose the vertebral spines and laminae is carried out. Using an oscillating saw, cut both laminae of each vertebral body as far lateral as possible to avoid cutting the dura or the spinal cord. Each vertebral lamina should be cut separately avoiding a single longitudinal saw cut that tends to extend too deep. Next, starting at the lumbosacral level, carefully lift the strip of vertebral spines and laminae, cutting the soft tissue as necessary. This exposes the spinal cord within the dura. Transect the dura and cauda equina at the sacral level and, with forceps, gently lift the cut edge, gripping the dura while cutting the lateral attachments of the dura as far lateral as possible. This will require minimal tension.

Sometimes it is necessary to remove the spinal cord in continuity with the brain. In this case, the midline skin incision is extended to the vertex of the skull to the level of the coronal scalp incision. The scalp is reflected laterally and a coronal skull incision from the lateral edge of the foramen magnum around the cranium to the opposite edge of the foramen magnum is made with an oscillating saw. Removal of the incised cranium will allow removal of the brain and spinal cord in continuity.

Spinal Cord Anatomy

In contrast to the calvarium, the spinal dura is not adherent to the vertebral canal. The epidural space contains fat and blood vessels including an extensive venous plexus. The dura contains a pouch for each nerve root including the dorsal root ganglion and the junction of the dorsal and ventral roots. The *dentate ligament* periodically anchors each lateral dural surface to the spinal cord. The dura and the leptomeninges loosely cover the surface of the spinal cord. The lumbar spinal cord is located opposite T-12 and the conus medullaris is opposite L-1.

The circulatory anatomy of the spinal cord determines the pathologic anatomy of many of its traumatic conditions (Figs. XIX-66 and XIX-67). Approximately 75% of the cross sectional area of the spinal cord is supplied by the *anterior spinal artery* which traverses the length of the cord in the midline *ventral fissure.* Its rostral origin is over the ventral surface of the medulla with the merger of a pair of small arterial branches of each vertebral artery just caudal to the origin of the basilar artery. This pair of arteries supplies the rostral one-third of the cervical cord. Several *segmental branches* from the vertebral artery provide segmental input into the anterior spinal artery to supply the caudal two-thirds of the cervical and the rostral one-fourth of the thoracic cord. A large radicular artery *(the artery of Adamkiewicz)* arising from the aorta at approxi-

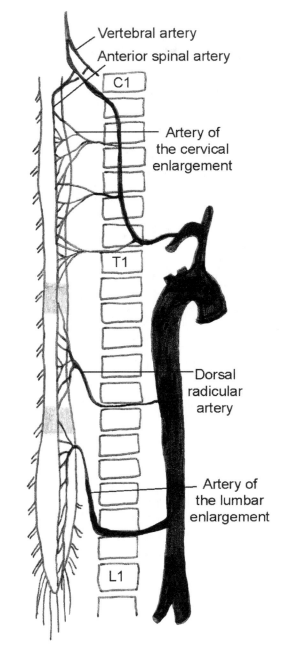

FIGURE XIX-66. *Diagram.* Blood supply of the spinal cord (see text).

mately T-12 inputs the anterior spinal artery to supply the caudal one-fourth of the thoracic and the lumbosacral cord. A smaller, more variable radicular branch arises from the thoracic aorta and supplies the segment between these two ter-

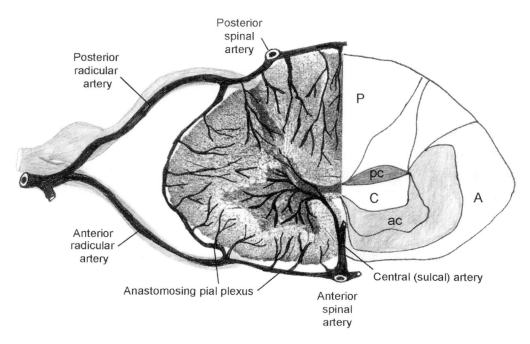

FIGURE XIX-67. *Diagram.* Cross section of spinal cord illustrating the segmental arterial blood supply on the left and the territories of the arteries on the right. P = posterior spinal artery; A = anastomosing pial plexus of the anterior spinal artery; C = Central (sulcal) artery; PC = overlapping territories of the posterior spinal and the central (sulcal) arteries; AC = overlapping territories of the central (sulcal) and anterior spinal arteries.

ritories (the middle one-half of the thoracic cord). This segment has the least robust supply and, in situations of systemic hypotension, may undergo watershed ischemia. Multiple sulcal branches arise from the anterior spinal artery and supply the ventral-medial white matter and most of the gray matter except for the dorsal portion of the dorsal horns. A pair of dorsal-lateral arteries form an irregular network over the dorsal cord. These give rise to penetrating branches that supply the dorsal white matter, dorsal portion of the dorsal horns and superficial lateral and inferior lateral white matter.

Focal damage to the spinal cord reflects its internal functional architecture. Loss of lower motor neurons at the level of injury results in flaccid paralysis at that level. Transverse injury across the cord reflects the loss of function of the interrupted longitudinally running tracts. The dorsal white matter columns are sensory, carrying ascending (caudal-rostral), ipsilateral information from the body to the contralateral brain that is specific for proprioception (body position) and

light touch. The medial bundle of the dorsal column *(fasciculus gracilis)* carries this sensory information from the lower extremity and trunk with the most medial fibers being the most distal (caudal). The lateral bundle of the dorsal column *(fasciculus cuneatus)* caries the same type of sensory information from the arm and shoulder. It originates at the caudal cervical level and ends at the caudal medulla. A large bundle of fibers in each dorsal-lateral column *(corticospinal tracts)* carry descending (motor) fibers from the contralateral brain to the ipsilateral lower motor neuron to initiate voluntary movement. An ascending tract in each ventral-lateral column *(the lateral spinothalamic tracts)* carries ascending information sensing pain and temperature from the contralateral body to the ipsilateral brain. There are many other ascending and descending fiber bundles but these are the most sharply demarcated, easiest to recognize anatomically and easiest to test clinically.

When axons in these tracts are transected, a characteristic process of degeneration occurs which is called *Wallerian degeneration.* The seg-

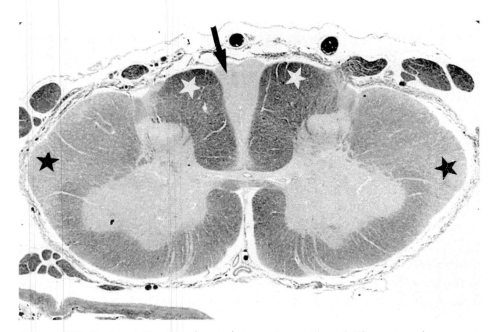

FIGURE XIX-68. Luxol Fast Blue (myelin) stain of cervical cord. The section shows a pattern of ascending Wallerian degeneration indicating the cord injury is below this section. The discrete unmyelinated dorsal-medial area (arrow) represents bilateral degeneration of fasciculus gracilis, carrying ascending (sensory) information for proprioception and touch from the ipsilateral lower extremities and trunk. The tracts immediately lateral to fasciculus gracilis (white stars), carrying the same type of sensory information from the shoulders and upper extremities, are fasciculus cuneatus and are intact. Since fasciculus cuneatus originates at the caudal cervical level and they appear to be completely spared, the lesion is caudal to the cervical cord. There is less distinct bilateral degeneration in the lateral columns (black stars) in the areas of the lateral spinothalamic tracts (pain and temperature) from the contralateral sides of the body, also indicating the section is above the lesion. Since the ascending degeneration is bilateral, the lesion is probably a complete transection. The dorsal part of the lateral columns, carrying the descending (corticospinal) tracts are intact, also indicating the section is above the lesion.

ment of the axon and its myelin sheath that is distal to the injury gradually breaks down into small segments and is slowly removed by a process of phagocytosis. The segment proximal to the injury dies back for a short distance but it and its cell body are preserved unless the transection is extremely close to the cell body. This means, for example, myelin or axon stains of cross sections of the cervical spinal cord after a traumatic transection of the mid-thoracic cord will show degeneration of fasciculus gracilis, preservation of fasciculus cuneatus, degeneration of the lateral spinothalamic tracts and preservation of the corticospinal tracts. A section from the distal thoracic cord will show preservation of the fasciculus gracilis and lateral spinothalamic tract and degeneration of the corticospinal tracts (Figs. XIX-68 and XIX-69). Wallerian degeneration becomes visible as tract specific vacuolar degeneration of the white matter after approximately two weeks. Demyelination, gliosis and axonal loss are complete after 2–3 months and the pattern persists indefinitely.

Circulatory Injuries of the Spinal Cord

Focal Ischemic Injury

Focal ischemic injury of the spinal cord due to occlusion of spinal arteries is unusual. Athero-

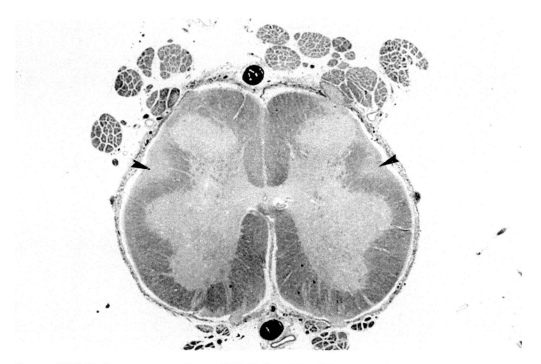

FIGURE XIX-69. Same patient as Figure XIX-68. Luxol Fast Blue stain of lumbar spinal cord. Section shows a pattern of descending degeneration. There are discrete, bilateral, unmyelinated foci in the dorsolateral lateral columns (arrowheads) representing degeneration of the corticospinal tracts. The ascending tracts are spared. Both of these findings indicate the section is below the lesion, which, given the pattern in Figure XIX-68 and its bilaterality at this level, is probably a complete transection.

sclerosis and thromboemboli have been demonstrated. The pattern of ischemic necrosis is most commonly consistent with *anterior spinal artery occlusion* with necrosis of the ventral two-thirds of the gray matter and variable amounts of the ventral-medial white matter. Dissecting aneurysms of the aorta may compress one or more of the segmental arteries that provide input into the anterior spinal artery. Occlusion or compromise of the *artery of Adamkiewicz* may complicate abdominal aortic aneurysm surgery. This may result in paraplegia, loss of bowel and bladder control and a lower thoracic sensory level due to infarction in the distribution of the anterior spinal artery in the lower thoracic/lumbar cord. A few cases of *fibrocartilage fragment embolization from intervertebral disc tissue* of intrinsic spinal arteries have been reported.[148] The infarctions are multifocal and the pathophysiology of the condition is not understood, although most of the patients have had acute rupture of intervertebral discs.

Spinal Cord in Circulatory Collapse

The effect of acute global ischemia on the spinal cord due to cardiorespiratory failure is varied and unpredictable. Most often in cases of global anoxic/ischemic encephalopathy with total brain necrosis *(respirator brain)* the spinal cord is not involved. Usually, there is a fairly sharp demarcation between soft, ischemic brain and normal spinal cord somewhere at the level of the lower medulla and upper cervical cord. At the other extreme, the entire spinal cord is swollen, tensely filling the dura with changes of ischemia and necrosis. Analogous to what has occurred in the cranium, the ischemia-induced swelling has led to a situation of increased intradural pressure, no perfusion, necrosis and degeneration. Sometimes the necrosis involves the distribution of the anterior spinal artery. Sometimes there is selective gray matter necrosis possibly reflecting the greater metabolic requirement of the neurons and excitotoxicity with the release of glutamate and intracellular influx of calcium. Sometimes the selective gray matter necrosis is found in watershed areas between the upper thoracic or lower thoracic levels.

Spinal Cord Trauma

Injuries to the spinal cord are *penetrating* or *blunt force (non-penetrating)*. The level of the injury and the completeness of the transection determine the chances of survival and the extent of the post-injury morbidity. *Penetrating injuries,* such as from knives or gunshot wounds, produce damage by cutting or lacerating the spinal cord and its blood vessels at low or high velocity. The injury may cause complete or partial transections that result in recognized syndromes. A high velocity missile wound, such as from a gunshot wound, may cause a blunt force injury without actually penetrating the spinal canal due to transmitted energy.

Blunt force trauma causes deformity of the spinal canal which may be transient or permanent. The result is compression injury to the cord due to hyperextension, hyperflexion, rotation, translational and compression forces, frequently in various combinations. The segments of the spine most exposed to these types of movements are the mid-cervical and the distal thoracic spine and these areas are the most common sites of such injuries. The upper cervical spine has a relatively wide spinal canal and somewhat fixed occipital/atlanto/axial segment, both features being partially protective for excessive movement. The thoracic spine is relatively rigid because of the rib cage. The protective rigidity is lost at T11-12. The blunt force deformity may result in dislocation and subluxation with or without fracture. The cord damage may be minor and transient or may result in complete transection. Blunt force injuries may also cause laceration of the cord and its covering when fractured vertebral fragments are driven into the spinal canal.

Pathology

Penetrating injuries result from the direct effect of the penetrating, disruptive object. They there-fore involve disruption of the vertebra, ligaments, meninges and the spinal cord parenchyma resulting in complete or partial transections. The acute effects are hemorrhage and swelling. Over the subsequent days and weeks the subdural and subarachnoid hemorrhage evolves as it would elsewhere. The disrupted tissue margins become red-brown (days), granular (days and weeks) then yellow-brown (weeks) as blood breaks down, granulation tissue develops, inflammatory cells appear and disappear and lipid-filled histiocytes accumulate. Microscopic events follow the usual sequence of organizing necrosis and healing. Axonal swellings develop proximal to the cell bodies and Wallerian degeneration evolves in the distal tracts. The disrupted nerve roots with sprouting axons and Schwann cells and meningeal connective tissue proliferate to create a traumatic neuroma which may invade the spinal cord. After months, there is a contracted, complex scar composed of dural/arachnoid/spinal cord adhesions, traumatic neuroma and gray-brown, hemosiderin-stained gliosis with no recognizable neural tissue at the level of the lesion if it was complete. If the penetrating object entered the spinal canal but damaged the cord by displacement rather than disruption, the result is a crushing or compression injury that is less likely to produce dural adhesion or traumatic neuroma.

Non-penetrating trauma causes crush injury of the spinal cord which, if the displacement is severe enough, may result in a complete transverse disruption. If the injury is very high (C1-2) and caused sudden death, there may be very subtle, if any, gross or microscopic findings. A few minutes or hours later small, acute hemorrhages may be visible and the damaged area may be soft. Swelling develops over the first hours and days. Internal hemorrhage in the gray matter may develop and damage motor neurons at the level of hemorrhage. Such hemorrhages taper in the rostral and caudal direction and, when they reabsorb, will leave a spindle-shaped hemosiderin stained glial lined cavity, a *syrinx*. The central gray matter hematoma in addition to acute swelling may produce damage due to compression against the rigid dura and spinal canal.

Spinal Shock

Severe spinal injuries are immediately accompanied by spinal shock which is a diffuse axonal injury analogous to cerebral concussion. The higher the level of cord injury and the more severe the trauma, the more likely spinal shock will occur and the longer it will last. Spinal shock consists of an immediate, transient, diffuse loss of motor and sensory activity and loss of sympathetic autonomic function. The loss of motor and sensory function due to spinal shock usually does not last for more than one hour but the autonomic effects of bradycardia, systemic hypotension and vasodilation, which may lead to hypothermia, may persist for weeks or months. Eventually, over days and weeks, if the corticospinal tracts were transected, flaccid paralysis changes to spasticity and hyperactive deep tendon reflexes.[149]

SYNDROMES

Complete, acute transection of the spinal cord results in immediate complete loss of sensation, autonomic sympathetic activity, muscle tone and voluntary movement below the affected level.[149,150] Some of these changes are due to spinal shock The loss of muscle tone evolves to a state of spasticity and hyperreflexia at a level below the lesion.

The clinical hallmark of the *cervical central cord syndrome* is a cervical cord injury resulting in greater weakness in the upper extremities than the legs with variable sensory loss.[151] Many patients are elderly and suffer a hyperextension injury that results in anterior-posterior cord compression. The pathology is believed to be a central hematoma that damages the upper extremity motor neurons in the anterior horns and produces lateral pressure on the medial corticospinal tract which compromises the medial upper extremity fibers more than the lateral leg fibers. However, anatomic studies have shown the arm and leg fibers of the corticospinal tract are intermixed[152] and recent MRI/pathology correlation studies have shown the absence of a central hematoma, intact ventral horns and degenerative changes in the myelin, especially the larger fibers of the corticospinal tract. Possibly, as observed in primates, the corticospinal fibers are more important for hand function than for walking[153] explaining the clinical prominence of the upper extremity deficits.

The *anterior cord syndrome* is associated with acute compression of the ventral cord such as from acute central rupture of an intervertebral disc or vertebral fracture with fragments in the spinal canal. The anterior and lateral columns and gray matter are damaged resulting in bilateral paralysis below the lesion and preservation of touch and proprioception (posterior columns are preserved). This injury could also result from compression and occlusion of the anterior spinal artery.

When the lateral half of the spinal cord is damaged, the result is contralateral loss of pain and temperature (the lateral spinothalamic tract), ipsilateral loss of touch and proprioception (fasciculus gracilis and fasciculus cuneatus) and ipsilateral paralysis (corticospinal tract) and is called the *Brown-Séquard syndrome*. This can result from many causes, including lateral vertebral fractures, lateral herniated nucleus pulposus or penetrating injuries.

As noted above, the caudal thoracic spine is relatively susceptible to the injurious movements of blunt force spinal injury. Most of the lumbar spinal cord segments are adjacent to vertebral body T12. The sacral segments are at L1 and the spinal cord ends at the L1-2 disc. Injuries at this level are the most common cause of traumatic paraplegia usually producing the *conus medullaris syndrome* which consists of paralysis of the lower extremities, anal sphincter and bladder with variable sensory loss.

In the evaluation of a fatality related to spinal cord injury in terms of the cause of death, there are two groups of problems that are the direct result of the neurologic injury that should be recognized.

Autonomic dysfunction can produce serious symptoms related to circulation and temperature regulation. Complete or subtotal lesions of the cervical or upper thoracic cord may produce the effect of a *sympathectomy* manifesting with bradycardia (unopposed vagal action), hypotension (loss of vasoconstriction) and hypothermia (heat loss due to vasodilation). These effects must be sorted out from other possible injuries such as shock due to blood loss or infection. These individuals may not be able to generate fever, thus masking the presence of infection. They often remain at least partially poikilothermic and are vulnerable to high or low environmental temperatures. Later, in the chronic phase, the patient may develop *autonomic dysreflexia,* a form of autonomic spasticity in which an overactive reflex triggered, for example, by a distended bladder or bowel (fecal impaction) produces an autonomic crisis with hypertension, bradycardia, hyperthermia and profuse sweating of the head and arms. The hypertension may be life-threatening.

The second complication concerns the *neurologic control of respiration.* The following levels are relevant to neural control of various aspects of respiration. Lesions of C1-2 may interrupt fibers from the brain stem that transmit impulses of respiratory drive. Lesions at C3-4 result in paralysis of the diaphragm and intercostal muscles. Such individuals are found in a state of complete respiratory arrest at the scene and may be resuscitated but often remain in coma because of global ischemic brain injury. Lesions at C5-T2 cause loss of intercostal muscle control but the diaphragmatic function remains. Lesions between T2-T12 have varying degrees of intercostal muscle weakness.

Fat Emboli Syndrome

In most acute trauma patients who suffer long bone fractures, crushing soft tissue injury or deep burns, fat globules are released and find their way into locally disrupted veins, often aided by increased tissue pressure due to swelling.[154] Fat is carried to the lungs where it can be demonstrat-

ed in capillaries as an incidental finding at least 90% of the time. Such patients are, at most, mildly symptomatic. Occasionally the fat globules enter the arterial system through pulmonary arteriovenous shunts, a patent foramen ovale or by overwhelming the filtering capacity of the lungs.[155] In this situation, about 10% of cases, the patient may be symptomatic due to the *fat emboli syndrome (FES).* In patients with such injuries plus a severe head injury the incidence of FES is about 30%.[156,157] Non-trauma-related conditions may also cause the syndrome. These include hemorrhagic pancreatitis and sickle cell crisis.

The onset of symptoms of FES occurs between 12 and 72 hours after the injury in a typically stable patient. Respiratory distress is followed by mental status changes characterized by delirium, lethargy, confusion and seizures.[157] Petechiae may appear in the skin and conjunctivae. The fat globules may be visible in the retinal arteries and in the urine. If fatal, the cause of death is pulmonary failure with diffuse intravascular coagulopathy and multi-organ failure. The mortality rate has been variously reported between 13 and 87% because of the variable severity of the accompanying injuries.[154]

The arterial fat globules block the cerebral microvasculature causing diffuse ischemic injury that is accentuated by the pulmonary insufficiency. The brain may appear grossly normal during the first 1–2 days. Subsequently, numerous petechiae appear, mostly in the white matter throughout the brain (Fig. XIX-70). After one week, the petechial lesions evolve to multiple foci of necrosis in the white matter and deep layers of the cortex especially in the frontal lobes and the pons. Frozen sections for neutral fat, before or after fixation in formaldehyde, demonstrate most of the fat is in the cortex. The fat is present in both normal and ischemic/hemorrhagic brain tissue. The elaborate capillary network in the gray matter allows for collateral flow, thus avoiding micro-infarction. The small, penetrating blood vessels of the white matter are arranged in parallel with little collateral anastomosis. Occlusion of these vessels by fat globules is more likely to result in ischemic damage. The petechiae in the white matter represent hemorrhagic infarcts

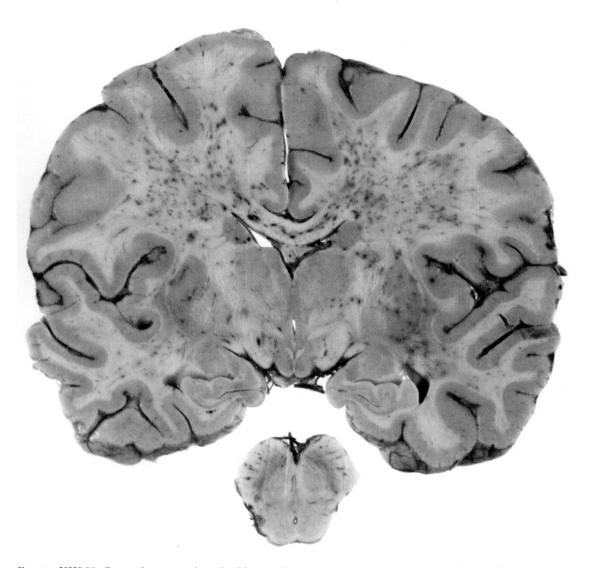

FIGURE XIX-70. Coronal section of cerebral hemispheres and transverse section of midbrain. Diffuse petechiae of the white matter due to fat emboli syndrome. Survived 4 days.

in the distribution of the small, occluded, penetrating arterioles.[156]

Patients who survive FES may show multifocal ischemic infarcts of the white matter and deep cortical layers, gliosis and atrophy of the white matter with ex vacuo ventricular enlargement.[158]

Post-Traumatic Seizures

Post-traumatic seizures are one of the most common complications of head injury. An important distinction is made between *early* (within one week) and *late* (after one week) post-traumatic seizures. The forensic pathologist is frequently confronted with the issue of whether a seizure disorder may or may not be related to a previous head injury. The following is a summary of some clinical literature that addresses some aspects of this question.

Early Post-Traumatic Seizures

Seizures during the acute phase of a serious head injury are a dangerous event which may complicate as many as 25% of cases with an intracranial hemorrhage. During a seizure there is an increase in cerebral metabolic rate which causes a dramatic increase in cerebral blood flow followed by elevation of intracranial pressure. The latter effect may cause significant increase in morbidity and mortality. Prophylactic treatment of acute head injury patients with anticonvulsants significantly lowers the incidence of early post-traumatic seizures but seems to have no effect on the incidence of late post-traumatic seizures.[159] Children have a higher incidence of early post-traumatic seizures than adults.[160] Risk factors for early post-traumatic seizures are prolonged coma, skull fractures, hematomas, contusions and focal neurologic signs.

Late Post-Traumatic Seizures

Adults have a higher risk for late post-traumatic seizures than children.[161] Approximately 5.5% of all patients with a diagnosis of epilepsy have a history of a head injury. The overall incidence of at least one late post-traumatic seizure in all patients medically treated for head injury is about 2%.[161] It increases to 5% for all patients treated in civilian hospitals for head injury[162] and to 35–53% in those hospitalized for combat missile injuries.[163] Almost one-fourth of late post-trau-

matic seizure patients do not have more than one seizure[164] and one-half do not have more than three.[162]

There are well-known risk factors for the development of late post-traumatic seizures. These include, in decreasing degrees of risk, penetrating missile wounds, early post-traumatic seizure, intracerebral hematoma, subdural hematoma, Glasgow coma scale of 10 or less, depressed skull fracture, cortical contusion and epidural hematoma. More than one-third of patients with one or more of these complications have a risk of at least one late post-traumatic seizure.[162]

The risk of developing post-traumatic seizures decreases with time. Approximately 50% of post-traumatic seizure patients have the first seizure within the first year,[162,163] however the increased risk persists for many years.[163,164] [2]

Editorial Postscriptum:
According to the Detroit Free Press of January 10, 2004, the CDC reported that the number of people who die from blows to the head during fights is probably higher than most realize. Each year, 50,000 people die in the United States due to brain trauma. Seven out of every 100,000 people were hospitalized for head trauma due to assault.

REFERENCES

1. Firlik, A.D., and Marion, D.W.: In *Head injury*, Fourth Edition. Editors: Cooper, P.R., and Golfinos, J.G. 2000, p. 223.
2. Lundberg, N.: Continuous recording and control of ventricular fluid pressure in neurosurgical practice. *Acta Psychiat Neurol Scand, 36:* 1–193, 1960.
3. Rivas, J.J., Lobato, R.D., et al.: Extradural hematoma: Analysis of factors influencing the course of 161 patients. *Neurosurgery, 23:* 44–51, 1984.
4. Servadei, F., Piazza, G., et al.: Extradural hematomas: An analysis of the changing characteristics of patients admitted from 1980 to 1986: Diagnostic and therapeutic implications in 158 cases. *Brain Inj, 2:* 87–100, 1988.
5. Miller, J.D., Becker, D.P., et al.: Significance of intracranial hypertension in severe head injury. *J Neurosurg, 47:* 503–516, 1977.
6. Lindenberg, R.: Compression of brain arteries as a pathogenic factor for tissue necrosis and their areas of predilection. *J Neuropathol Exp Neurol, 14:* 233–243, 1955.
7. Janzer, R.C., and Friede, R.L.: Perisulcal infarcts: Lesions caused by hypotension during increased intracranial pressure. *Ann Neurol, 6:* 339–404, 1979.
8. Bruce D.A., Alavi, A., et al.: Diffuse cerebral swelling following head injuries in children: The syndrome of "malignant brain edema." *J Neurosurg, 54:* 170–178, 1981.

---

[2] The authors wish to recognize and thank Dr. Judy Melinek for her contribution in creating the images for Figures 1–6, 13, 66, and 67.

9. Marmarou, A., Masset, A.L., and Ward, J.D.: Contribution of CSF and vascular factors to elevation of ICP in severely head injured patients. *J Neurosurg, 66:* 883–890, 1987.

10. Obrist, W.D., Langfitt, T.W., Jaggi, J.L., et al.: Cerebral blood flow and metabolism in comatose patients with acute head injury. *Nature Med, 1:* 135–137, 1984.

11. Graham, D.I., Lawrence, A.E., et al.: Brain damage in non-missile head injury secondary to high intracranial pressure. *Neuropathol Appl Neurobiol, 13:* 209–217, 1987.

12. Sadhu, V.K., Sampson, J., et al.: Correlation between computed tomography and intracranial pressure monitoring in acute head trauma patients. *Radiology, 133:* 507–509, 1979.

13. The Brain Trauma Foundation. The American Association of Neurological Surgery. The Joint Section on Neurotrauma and Critical Care. Pupillary diameter and light reflex. *J Neurotrauma, 17:* 583–590, 2000.

14. Auer, R.N., and Beneviste, H.: Hypoxia and related conditions. In *Greenfield's neuropathology,* Sixth edition. Editors: Graham, D.I., and Lantos, P.L., pp. 263–314, Vol I. Arnold Press, 1997.

15. Gurdjian, E.S., Stone, W.E., and Webster, J.E.: Cerebral metabolism in hypoxia. *Arch Neurol Psychiat (Chic), 5:* 472–477, 1944.

16. Johannsson, H., and Siesjo, B.K.: Blood flow of the rat brain in profound hypoxia. *Acta Physiol Scand, 90:* 281–282, 1974.

17. Jason, G.W., Pajurkova, E.M., et al.: High-altitude mountaineering and brain function: Neuro-psychological testing of members of a Mount Everest expedition. *Aviat Space Environ Med, 60:* 170–173, 1989.

18. Sadove, M.S., Yon, M.K., et al.: Severe prolonged cerebral hypoxic episode with complete recovery. *JAMA, 175:* 1102–1104, 1961.

19. Brierely, J.B., Adams, J.H., et al.: Neocortical death after cardiac arrest: A clinical, neurophysiological, and neuropathological report of two cases. *Lancet, 2:* 560–565, 1971.

20. Rose, J., Balronen, S., and Jennett, B.: Avoidable factors contributing to death after head injury. *Br Med J, 21:* 615–518, 1977.

21. Eisenberg, H.M., Gary, H.E., and Aldrich, E.F.: Initial CT findings in 753 patients with severe head injury: A report from the NIH Traumatic Coma Data Bank. *J Neurosurg, 73:* 688–698, 1990.

22. Plum, F.: Vulnerability of the brain and heart after cardiac arrest. *New Engl J Med, 324:* 1978–1980, 1991.

23. Graham, D.I.: The pathology of brain ischaemia and possibilities for therapeutic intervention. *Br J Anaesth, 57:* 3–17, 1985.

24. Plum, F., and Posner, J.B.: *The diagnosis of stupor and coma,* 3rd Ed. Philadelphia: F.A. Davis, 1980.

25. Guidelines for the determination of death. *JAMA, 12:* 2184–2186, 1981.

26. Hanley, D.F.: Brain death update: An update on the North American viewpoint. *Anaesth Intens Care, 23:* 24–25, 1995.

27. Towbin, A.: The respirator brain death syndrome. *Human Pathology, 4:* 583–594, 1973.

28. Jennett, B., and Plum, F.: The persistent vegetative state after brain damage: A syndrome in search of a name. *Lancet, 1:* 734–737, 1972.

29. Adams, J.H., Jennett, B., et al.: The neuropathology of the vegetative state after head injury. *J Clin Pathol, 52:* 804–806, 1999.

30. Teasdale, G., and Jennett, B.: Assessment of coma and impaired consciousness: A practical scale. *Lancet, 1:* 81–83, 1974.

31. Teasdale, G., Murray, C.T., Parker, L., et al.: Adding up the Glasgow Coma Scale score. *Acta Neurochir, 28:* 13–16, 1979.

32. Graham, D.I., Adams, J.H., et al.: The nature, distribution and causes of traumatic brain injury. *Brain Pathology, 5:* 397–406, 1995.

33. Gennarelli, T.A.: Animate models of human head injury. *J Neurotrauma, 11:* 357–368, 1994.

34. Gennarelli, T.A., and Thibault, L.E.: Biomechanics of acute subdural hematoma. *J Trauma, 22:* 680–686, 1982.

35. Gennarelli, T.A.: Head injury in man and experimental animals—Clinical aspects. *Acta Neurochir, 32:* 1–13, 1983.

36. Gennarelli, T.A., and Thibault, L.E.: Biologic modes of head injury. In Becker, D.P., and Povlishock, J.T. (eds), Central Nervous System Trauma Status Report. National Institute of Neurological and Communicative Disorders and Stroke. Bethesda, MD, National Institute of Health, 391–404, 1985.

37. Gennarelli, T.A., Thibault, L.E., et al.: Diffuse axonal injury and traumatic coma in the primate. *Ann Neurol, 12:* 564–574, 1982.

38. Ommaya, A.K., and Gennarelli, T.A.: Cerebral concussion and traumatic unconsciousness: Correlation of experimental and clinical observations on blunt head injuries. *Brain, 97:* 633–654, 1974.

39. Ruff, R.M., and Jurica, P.: In search of a unified definition for mild brain injury. *Brain Injury, 13:* 943–952, 1999.

40. Kandel, E.R., Schwartz, J.H., and Jessell, T.M. (eds.): *Principles of neural science,* Fourth Edition. New York: McGraw-Hill, 2000.

41. *Stedman's Medical Dictionary,* 26th Edition. Baltimore: Williams & Wilkins, 1995.

42. Le Roux, P.D., Choudri, H., and Andrews, B.T.: Cerebral concussion and diffuse brain injury. In *Head injury,* eds. Cooper, P.R., and Golfinos, J.G., Fourth Edition. New York: McGraw-Hill, 2000, pp. 174–200.

43. Kelly, J.P., Nichols, J.S., et al.: Concussion in sports: Guidelines for the prevention of catastrophic outcome. *JAMA, 226:* 2867–2869, 1991.

44. Blumberg, P.C., Scott, G., et al.: Staining of amyloid precursor protein to study axonal damage in mild head injury. *Lancet, 344:* 1055–1056, 1994.

45. Plassman, B.L., Havlik, R.J., et al.: Documented head injury in early adulthood and risk of Alzheimer's dis-

ease and other dementias. *Neurol, 55:* 1158–1166, 2000.

46. Strittmatter, W.J., Saunders, A.M., et al.: Apolipoprotein E: High-avidity binding to beta-amyloid and increased frequency of type 4 allele in late-onset familial Alzheimer disease. *Proc Natl Acad Sci USA, 90:* 1977–1981, 1993.

47. Mayeux, R., Ottman, R., et al.: Synergistic effects of traumatic head injury and apolipoprotein-epsilon 4 in patients with Alzheimer's disease. *Neurology, 45:* 555–557, 1995.

48. Teasdale, G.M., Nicoll, J.A., et al.: *Lancet, 350:* 1069–1071, 1997.

49. Caulfield, T.A.: The law, adolescents, and the APOE e4 genotype: A view from Canada. *Genet Test, 3* (1): 107–113, 1999.

50. Samatovicz, R.A.: Genetics and brain injury: Apolipoprotein E e4. *J Head Trauma Rehabil, 15* (3): 869–874, 2000.

51. Gennarelli, T., Thibault, L., et al.: Pathophysiologic responses to rotational and translational acceleration of the head. 16th Stapp Car Crash Conference. New York, Society of Auto Engineers, 296–308, 1972.

52. Imajo, T., Challener, R.C., et al: Diffuse axonal injury by assault. *Am J Forensic Med Pathol, 8:* 217–219, 1987.

53. Graham, D.I., Clark, J.C., et al.: Diffuse axonal injury caused by assault. *J Clin Pathol, 45:* 840–841, 1992.

54. Geddes, J.F., Vowles, G.H., et al.: Neuronal cytoskeletal changes are an early consequence of repetitive head injury. *Acta Neuropath, 98:* 171–178, 1999.

55. Jordon, B.D.: Chronic brain injury associated with boxing. *Sem in Neurol, 20:* 179–185, 2000.

56. Adams, J.H., Doyle, D., et al.: Diffuse axonal injury: definition, diagnosis and grading. *Histopathology, 15:* 49–59, 1989.

57. Adams, J.H., Graham, D.I., et al.: Diffuse axonal injury in non-missile head injury. *J Neurol Neurosurg Psychiatry, 54:* 481–483, 1991.

58. Gennarelli, T., Spielman, G., et al.: The influence of the type of intracranial lesion on the outcome from severe head injury: A multicenter study using a new classification system. *J Neurosurg, 56:* 26–32, 1982.

59. Graham, D.I., and Gennarelli, T.: Trauma. In *Greenfield's neuropathology,* ed. Graham, D.I., and Lantos, P.L., sixth edition. 197–262, 1997.

60. Geddes, J.F., Whitwell, H.L.,et al.: Traumatic axonal injury: Practical issues for diagnosis in medicolegal cases. (Review) *Neuropathol Appl Neurobiol, 26:* 105–116, 2000.

61. Geddes, J.F., Vowles, G.H., et al.: The diagnosis of diffuse axonal injury: Implications for forensic practice. *Neuropathol Appl Neurobiol, 23:* 339–347, 1997.

62. Pilz, P., Strohecker, J., et al.: Survival after traumatic ponto-medullary tear. *J Neurol Neurosurg Psychiatry, 45:* 422–427, 1982.

63. Cantu, R.C.: Second-impact syndrome. *Clin Sports Medicine, 17* (1): 37–44,1998.

64. McCrory, P.R., and Berkovic, S.F.: Second impact syndrome. *Neurology, 50* (3): 677–683, 1998.

65. Tomlinson, B.E.: Brainstem lesions after head injury. *J Clin Pathol, 4:* 154–165, 1970.

66. Klauber, M.R., Marshall, L.F., et al.: Determinants of head injury mortality: Importance of the low risk patient. *Neurosurgery, 23:* 31–36, 1989.

67. Marshall, L.F., Toole, B.M., et al.: The National Traumatic Data Bank II. Patients who talk and deteriorate: Implications for treatment. *J Neurosurg, 59:* 285–288, 1983.

68. Rockswold, G. L., Leonard, P. R., et al.: Analysis of management in 33 closed head injury patients who "talked and deteriorated." *Neurosurgery, 21:* 51–55, 1987.

69. Graham, D.I., and Gennarelli, T.A.: Pathology of brain damage after head injury. In *Head injury,* 4th Ed, Editors, Cooper, P.R., and Golfinos, J.G. New York: McGraw-Hill, 2000, pp. 133–154.

70. Jamieson, K.G., and Yelland, J.D.N.: Extradural hematoma: Report of 167 cases. *J Neurosurg, 29:* 13–23, 1968.

71. Campbell, J.B., and Cohen, J.: Epidural hemorrhage and the skull of children. *Surg Gynecol Obstret, 92:* 257–280, 1951.

72. Ford, L.E., and McLaurin, R.L.: Mechanisms of extradural hematomas. *J Neurosurg, 20:* 760–769, 1963.

73. McLaurin, R.L., and Ford, L.E.: Extradural hematoma: Statistical survey of 47 cases. *J Neurosurg, 21:* 364–371, 1964.

74. Chen, T.Y., Wong, C.W., et al.: The expectant treatment of "asymptomatic" supratentorial epidural hematomas. *Neurosurgery, 32:* 176–179, 1993.

75. Cucciniello, B., Martellotta, N., et al: Conservative management of extradural hematomas. *Acta Neurochir, 120:* 47–52, 1993.

76. Lobato, R.D., Rivas, J.J., et al.: Acute epidural hematoma: An analysis of factors influencing the outcome of patients undergoing surgery in coma. *J Neurosurg, 68:* 48–57, 1988.

77. Servadei, F.: Prognostic factors in severely head injured patients with epidural hematomas. *Acta Neurochir, 139:* 273–278, 1997.

78. Takagi, T., Nagai, R., et al: Extradural hemorrhage in the newborn as a result of birth trauma. *Childs Brain, 4:* 306–318, 1978.

79. Peter, J., and Domingo, Z.: Subacute traumatic extradural hematomas of the posterior fossa: A clinicopathological entity of the 5 to 10-year-old child. *Childs Nerv Syst, 6:* 135–138, 1990.

80. Haines, D.E., Harkey, H.L., et al.: The subdural space: A new look at an outdated concept. *Neurosurgery, 32:* 111–120, 1993.

81. Fraser, C.L., and Arieff, A.I.: Nervous system complications in uremia. *Ann Intern Med, 109:* 143–153, 1988.

82. Kopitnik, T.A., de Andrade, R., et al.: Pressure changes within a chronic subdural hematoma during hemodialysis. *Surg Neurol, 32:* 289–293, 1989.

83. Leonard, A., and Shapiro, F.L.: Subdural hematoma in regularly hemodialyzed patients. *Ann Intern Med, 82:* 650–658, 1975.

84. Wheeler, R.P.: Subdural hematoma in a patient on continuous ambulatory peritoneal dialysis. *Am J Med Sci, 294:* 448–450, 1987.

85. El Gindi, S., Salama, M., et al.: A review of 2000 patients with craniocerebral injuries with regard to intracranial haematomas and other vascular complications. *Acta Neurochir, 48:* 237–244, 1979.

86. Stone, J.L., Rifai, M.H.S., et al.: Subdural hematomas. I. Acute subdural hematomas: Progress in definition, clinical pathology and therapy. *Surg Neurol, 19:* 216–231, 1983.

87. Gennarelli, T.A., Thibault, L.E., et al.: Biomechanics of acute subdural hematoma. *J Trauma, 22:* 680–686, 1982.

88. Houtteville, J.P., Toumi, K., et al.: Interhemispheric subdural hematomas: Seven cases and review of the literature. *Br J Neurosurg, 2:* 357–368, 1988.

89. Jamieson, K.G., and Yelland, J.D.N.: Surgically treated traumatic subdural hematomas. *J Neurosurg, 37:* 137–149, 1972.

90. Hoff, J., and Richards, T.: Factors affecting survival from acute subdural hematoma. *Surgery, 75:* 253–258.

91. Servadei, F.: Prognostic factors in severely head injured adult patients with acute subdural haematoma. *Acta Neurochir, 139:* 279–285, 1997.

92. Kraus, J.F.: A comparison of recent studies on the extent of the head and spinal cord injury problem in the United States. *J Neurosurg, 53:* S35-43, 1980.

93. Hardman, J.M.: The pathology of traumatic brain injuries. *Adv Neurol,* 15–50, 1979.

94. Fogelholm, R., and Waltimo, O.: Epidemiology of chronic subdural haematoma. *Acta Neurochir, 32:* 247–250, 1975.

95. Marshall, L.F., Toole, B.M., et al.: The national traumatic coma data bank. 2: Patients who talk and deteriorate: Implications for treatment. *J Neurosurg, 59:* 285–288, 1983.

96. Markwalder, T.M.: Chronic subdural hematomas: A review. *J Neurosurg, 54:* 637–645, 1981.

97. Hoff, J., Bates, E., et al.: Traumatic subdural hygroma. *J Trauma, 13:* 870–876, 1973.

98. Da Costa, D.G., and Adson, A.W.: Subdural hygroma. *Arch Surg, 43:* 559–567, 1941.

99. Adams, J.H., Doyle, D., et al.: The contusion index: A reappraisal in human and experimental non-missile head injury. *Neuropathol Appl Neurobiol, 11:* 299–308, 1985.

100. Meaney, D.F., Ross, D.T., et al.: Modification of the cortical impact model to produce axonal injury in the rat cortex. *J Neurotrauma, 11:* 599–612, 1994.

101. McLaurin, R.L., and Helmer, F.: The syndrome of temporal lobe contusion. *J Neurosurg, 23:* 296–304, 1965.

102. Dawson, S.L., Hirsch, C.S., et al.: The contrecoup phenomenon: Reappraisal of a classic problem. *Hum Pathol, 11:* 155–166, 1980.

103. Lindenberg, R., and Freytag, E.: A mechanism of cerebral contusions: A pathologic-anatomic study. *Arch Pathol, 69:* 440–469, 1960.

104. Komatsu, S., Sato, T., et al.: Traumatic lesions of the corpus callosum. *Neurosurgery, 5:* 32–35, 1979.

105. Lindenberg, R., Fisher, R., et al.: Lesions of the corpus callosum following blunt mechanical trauma to the head. *Am J Pathol, 31:* 297–317, 1955.

106. Britt, R.H., Herrick, M.K., et al.: Traumatic lesions of the pontomedullary junction. *Neurosurgery, 6:* 623–631, 1980.

107. Simpson, D.A., Blumbergs, P.C., et al.: Pontomedullary tears and other gross brainstem injuries after vehicular accidents. *J Trauma, 29:* 1519–1525, 1989.

108. Wakai, S., Nagai, M., et al.: Histological verification of microaneurysm as a cause of cerebral haemorrhage in surgical specimens. *J Neurol Neurosurg Psychiat, 52:* 595–599, 1989.

109. Challa, V.R., Moody, D.M., et al.: The Charcot-Bouchard aneurysm controversy: Impact of a new histologic technique. *J Neuropathol Exp Neurol, 51:* 264–271, 1992.

110. Levine, S.R., Brust, J.C.M., et al: Cerebrovascular complications of the use of the "crack" form of alkaloidal cocaine. *N Engl J Med, 323:* 699–704, 1990.

111. Gentleman, D., Nath, F., et al.: Diagnosis and management of delayed traumatic intracerebral hematoma. *Br J Neurosurg, 3:* 367–372, 1989.

112. Tanaka, T., Sakai, T., et al.: MR imaging as a predictor of delayed post-traumatic cerebral hemorrhage. *J Neurosurg, 69:* 203–209, 1988.

113. Gudeman, S.K., Kishore, P.R.S., et al.: The genesis and significance of delayed traumatic intracerebral hematoma. *Neurosurgery, 5:* 309–313, 1979.

114. Brinker, T.S., Seifert, V., et al.: Acute changes in the dynamics of the cerebrospinal fluid system during experimental subarachnoid hemorrhage. *Neurosurgery, 27:* 369–372, 1990.

115. Pickard, J.D.: Adult communicating hydrocephalus. *Br J Hosp Med, 27:* 35–44, 1982.

116. Raftopoulos, C., Deleval, J., et al.: Cognitive recovery in idiopathic normal pressure hydrocephalus: A prospective study. *Neurosurgery, 35:* 397–405, 1994.

117. Brill, J.: Massive aneurysms at the base of the brain. *Brain, 92:* 535–570, 1969.

118. Estanol, B.V., Marin, O.S.M., et al.: Cardiac arrhythmias and sudden death in subarachnoid hemorrhage. *Stroke, 6:* 382–386, 1975.

119. Doshi, R., and Neil-Dwyer, G: A clinicopathological study of patients following a subarachnoid hemorrhage. *J Neurosurg, 52:* 295–301, 1980.

120. Andrews, R.J., and Spiegel, P. K.: Intracranial aneurysms: Age, sex, blood pressure, and multiplicity

in an unselected series of patients. *J Neurosurg, 51:* 27–32, 1979.

121. Cummings, T.J., Johnson, R.R., et al.: The relationship of blunt head trauma, subarachnoid hemorrhage, and rupture of pre-existing intracranial saccular aneurysms. *Neurol Res, 22:* 165–170, 2000.

122. Nanda, A., Vannemreddy, P.S., et al.: Intracranial aneurysms and cocaine abuse: Analysis of prognostic indicators. *Neurosurgery, 46:* 1063–1067, 2000.

123. Contostavlos, D.L.: Massive subarachnoid hemorrhage due to laceration of the vertebral artery associated with fracture of the transverse process of the atlas. *J Forensic Sci, 16:* 40–56, 1971.

124. Opeskin, K., and Burke, M.P.: Vertebral artery trauma. *Am J Forensic Med Pathol, 19:* 206–217, 1998.

125. Pollanen, M.S., Deck, J.H., et al.: Injury of tunica media in fatal rupture of the vertebral artery. *Am J Forensic Med Pathol, 17:* 197–201, 1996.

126. Sahjpal, R.L., Abdulhak, M.M., et al.: Fatal traumatic vertebral artery aneurysm rupture. Case report. *J Neurosurg, 89:* 822–824, 1998.

127. Ingram, M., and Hamilton, W.: Cephalohematoma in the newborn. *Radiology, 55:* 503–507, 1950.

128. Tandon, P., Banerji, A., et al.: Craniocerebral erosion (growing fracture of the skull in children). Part II. Clinical and radiologic observations. *Acta Neurochir, 88:* 1–9, 1987.

129. Kingsley, D., Till, K., et al.: Growing fractures of the skull. *J Neurol Neurosurg Psychiatry, 41:* 312–318, 1978.

130. Duhaime, A.C., Alario, A.J., et al.: Head injury in very young children: Mechanisms, injury types and ophthalmologic findings in 100 hospitalized patients younger than 2 years of age. *Pediatrics, 90:* 179–185, 1992.

131. Lindenberg, R., and Freytag, E.: Morphology of brain lesions from blunt trauma in early infancy. *Arch Pathol, 87:* 298–305, 1969.

132. Caffey, J.: On the theory and practice of shaking infants. Its potential residual effects of permanent damage and mental retardation. *Am J Dis Child, 124:* 161–169, 1972.

133. Pounder, D.J.: Shaken adult syndrome. *Am J Forensic Med Pathol, 18:* 321–324, 1997.

134. Duhaime, A.C., Gennarelli, T.A., et al.:The shaken baby syndrome: A clinical, pathologic and biomechanical study. *J Neurosurg, 66:* 409–415, 1987.

135. Johnson, D.L., Boal, D., et al.: Role of apnea in nonaccidental head injury. *Pediatr Neurosurg, 23:* 305–310, 1995.

136. Aldrich, E.F., Eisenberg, H.M., et al.: Diffuse brain swelling in severely head injured children. A report from the NIH Coma Data Bank. *J Neurosurg, 76:* 450–454, 1992.

137. Geddes, J.F., Hackshaw, A.K., et al.: Neuropathology of inflicted head injury in children. I. Patterns of brain damage. *Brain, 124:* 1290–1298, 2001.

138. Geddes, J.F., Vowles, G.H., et al.: Neuropathology of inflicted head injury in children. II. Microscopic brain injury in infants. *Brain, 124:* 1299–1306, 2001.

139. U.S. Department of Justice: Guns used in crime. 1993.

140. Sosin, D.M., Sacks, J.J., et al.: Head injury associated deaths in the United States from 1979 to 1986. *JAMA, 262:* 2251–2255, 1989.

141. Freytag, E.: Autopsy findings from firearms. Statistical evaluation of 254 cases. *Arch Pathol, 76:* 215–221, 1963.

142. Kirkpatrick, J.B., and Di Maio, V.: Civilian gunshot wound of the brain. *J Neurosurg, 49:* 185–198, 1978.

143. Cary, M.E., Sarna, G.S., et al.: Experimental missile wounds to the brain. *J Neurosurg, 71:* 754–764, 1989.

144. Kalsbeck, W.D., McLaurin, R.L., et al.: The national head and spinal cord survey: Major findings. *J Neurosurg, 53:* 19–43, 1982.

145. DeVivo, M.J., Fine, P.R., et al.: Prevalence of spinal cord injury: A reestimation employing life table techniques. *Arch Neurol, 37:* 707–708, 1980.

146. Oliver, N.J.: Annual estimates: Stroke and central nervous system trauma. Office of Scientific and Health Reports. Bethesda, MD: NINDS, 1992.

147. Lobosky, J.M.: The epidemiology of spinal cord injury. In *Neurotrauma,* Eds., Narayan, R.J., Wilberger, J.E., Jr., and Povlishock, J.T. New York: McGraw-Hill, 1996, pp. 1049–1996.

148. Case records of the Massachusetts General Hospital. Case 5-1991. *New Engl J Med, 324:* 322–332, 1991.

149. *Principles of Neural Sciences,* 4th ed. Eds., Kandel, E.R., Schwartz, J.H., and Jessell, T.M. New York: McGraw-Hill, 2000, ch. 36.

150. Kiss, Z.H.T., and Tator, C.H.: Neurogenic shock. In Geller, E.R. (ed.), *Shock and resuscitation.* New York: McGraw-Hill, 1993, pp. 421–440.

151. Schneider, R.C.: Traumatic spinal cord syndromes and their management. *Clin Neurosurg, 20:* 424–492, 1970.

152. Nathan, P.W., and Smith, M.C.: Long descending tracts in man: I. Review of present knowledge. *Brain, 78:* 248–304, 1956.

153. Eidelberg, E.: Consequences of spinal cord lesions upon motor function, with special reference to locomotor activity. *Prog Neurobiol, 17:* 185–202,1981.

154. Muller, C., Rahn, B.A., et al.: The incidence, pathogenesis, diagnosis and treatment of fat embolism. *Orthop Rev, 23:* 107–117, 1994.

155. Watson, A.J.: Genesis of fat emboli. *J Clin Pathol, 23:* 132–142, 1970.

156. Kamenar, E., and Burger, P.C.: Cerebral fat embolism: A neuropathological study of a microembolic state. *Stroke, 11:* 477–484, 1980.

157. Levy, D.: The fat embolism syndrome. A review. *Clin Orthop, 261:* 281–286, 1990.

158. McTaggart, D.M., and Neubuerger, K.T.: Cerebral fat embolism: Pathologic changes in the brain after survival of 7 years. *Acta Neuropathol, 15:* 183–187, 1970.

159. Temkin, N.R., Dikmen, S.S., et al.: A randomized, double-blind study of phenytoin for the prevention of post-traumatic seizures. *N Engl J Med, 323:* 497–502, 1990.

160. De Santis, A., Cappricci, E., et al.: Early post-traumatic seizures in adults. A study of 84 cases. *J Neurosurg Sci, 23:* 207–210, 1979.

161. Annegers, J.F., Grabow, J.D., et al.: Seizures after head trauma. A population study. *Neurology, 30:* 683–689, 1980.

162. Jennett, B.: *Epilepsy after nonmissile injuries,* 2nd ed. Chicago: Year Book, 1975.

163. Salazar, A.M., Jabbari, B., et al.: Epilepsy after penetrating head injury. I. Clinical correlates: A report of the Vietnam head Injury Study. *Neurology, 35:* 1406–1414, 1985.

164. Annegers, J.F., Shirts, S.B., et al.: Risk of recurrence after an initial unprovoked seizure. *Epilepsia, 27:* 43–50, 1986.

Part 2

BOXING INJURIES

FRIEDRICH UNTERHARNSCHEIDT[1] AND JAMES M. HENRY[2]

THERE IS GENERAL AGREEMENT among physicians that boxing can cause debilitating or fatal injuries, including the *punch-drunk* syndrome. Despite the health risks, professional and amateur boxing has become increasingly popular, continually recruiting new participants. In many countries, women are boxing professionally and in the United States boxing classes are growing in popularity, reflecting the latest fitness fad.

For the forensic pathologist, the following observations are relevant: Boxing injuries can be divided into two categories, including immediate and remote effects. Boxers who succumb to fatal incidents suffered in the ring may die minutes to hours later, whereas others may survive severe head injuries for some days or weeks. Fatal injuries associated with brief survival times include subdural hemorrhages or intracerebral hematomas, resulting in increased intracranial pressure with herniation of brain tissue and shift of midline structures. The brains of pugilists who survive a head injury for days or weeks should not be dissected in the fresh state, but first fixed in formalin, followed by selection of multiple representative tissue blocks for embedding and staining with hematoxylin-eosin.

Ex-boxers may survive their ring career for years, only to later develop clinical signs of *encephalopathia pugilistica* or *dementia pugilistica,* commonly referred to as the *punch-drunk syndrome.*

It is noteworthy that the extent of brain damage in cases of closed head injury often exceeds the anatomic findings. Even a relatively minor concussive force, sometimes without loss of consciousness, may be associated with residual clinical manifestations.

Translational and Rotational Acceleration

There are two kinds of impact to be considered in boxing, central and oblique.

In the first, the impact axis of the blow passes through the center of the head. The resulting motion is translational or linear acceleration, as exemplified by a straight blow to the face.

In the second instance, the axis of impact is not centered, and the resulting motion represents combined translational and rotational acceleration of the head. This occurs in swinging blows to the head, including uppercuts and hooks. The degree to which both forms of acceleration participate depends on the obliquity of the blow. Tangential impacts, such as hooks or uppercuts to the chin, produce virtually pure rotational acceleration. Initially, the skull begins to rotate, while the brain, by reason of its inertia, does not immediately follow. This relative displacement of the brain stretches and strains the bridging veins between the brain and superior sagittal sinus, and may cause tearing, resulting in subdural hemorrhage or hematoma.[1-4]

Facial Injuries

The intensity of injury inflicted by boxing blows to the head and brain was derived from experimental measurements of head acceleration by boxing blows.[1] Action photographs of boxers taken immediately after a hard blow to the face illustrate the intensity pictorially, confirming experimental measurements of head acceleration in boxing. The action photographs taken by press photographers were divided into two groups. The first shows the immediate effects of a single hard blow to the face. The second group

---

[1] Dedicated to the memory of Wilheim Holczabek, Wien, Austria.

[2] The opinion or assertions contained herein are those of the authors and do not necessarily reflect the view of the Department of the Army or the Department of Defense.

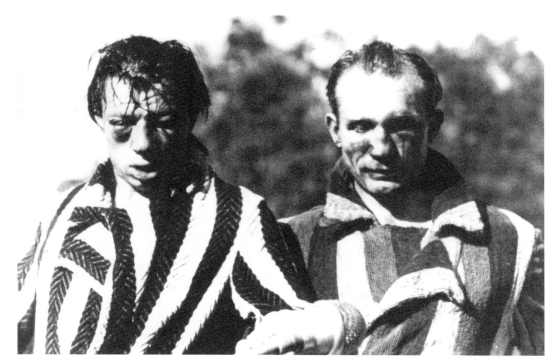

FIGURE XIX-71. Professional lightweight fight between Gerhard Hecht (left) and Herbert Kleinwachter (right). The fight ended after 10 rounds in a draw. Both eyes of Hecht are closed; the left eye of Kleinwachter is partially closed. The faces of both boxers are severely marked and swollen, *puffed,* and covered with blood. The scars and hemorrhages of the skin of the face are visible. Photo: Helmuth Rudolph.

reveals the residual sequelae of injury to the face following a knockout, a technical knockout, or at the end of a fight (Fig. XIX-71). The force of the blow deforms and distorts facial features. Inspection of action photographs of boxers' heads, taken at the moment of impact or milliseconds later, reveals that features are deformed, distorted, and displaced beyond recognition (Fig. XIX-72a–b). The human countenance literally functions as a shock absorber (Figs. XIX-73 and XIX-74), although we do not know the extent of brain injury associated with these hammer-like blows impacting the head.

The skin of the face may be diffusely swollen and puffy, or there may be focal swelling due to edema and hemorrhage. The extent of facial injuries ranges from virtually none, to severe cosmetic deformity and functional impairment. Orbital hematomas, or *black eyes,* may reach such dimensions that the eye is swollen shut.

Eye Injuries

Doggart[5,6] presented a comprehensive survey of eye injuries, including retinal detachment, one of the most devastating ocular hazards of the ring (Fig. XIX-75). The literature reveals a long list of ocular derangements, such as paralytic diplopia, iritis, cataract, glaucoma, vitreous opacity, choroidoretinal degeneration, and optic atrophy.[7,8]

Hearing Impairment

The extent of hearing loss depends mainly on two factors: The weight class of a boxer, corresponding to the intensity of head trauma and the number of fights in which he participated.[9] Heavyweights usually have more severe hearing loss than featherweights. The distribution of hearing loss after repeated blows is first noted in the low frequency range, although it later appears in

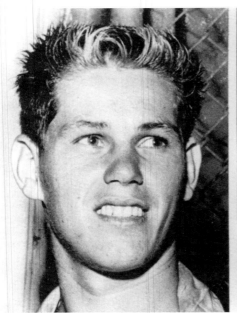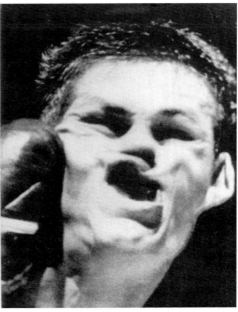

FIGURE XIX-72a–b. Professional lightweight fight between Mark Tessman (Houston) and Ronnie Williams (Fort Worth). A hard left by Tessman deforms and distorts the features of Williams, who has been hit on the right side of his face. The photo demonstrates how parts of the face and the subcutaneous tissue are displaced by the considerable kinetic energy of the blow. Both eyes are closed; the mouth is wide open. It also reveals that while the features are affected by the direct impact of the blow, the left ear is bent forward due to its inertia. The photo clearly demonstrates, the tremendous intensity of a blow by a lightweight! The picture on the left shows Williams face before the fight. Photo: AP.

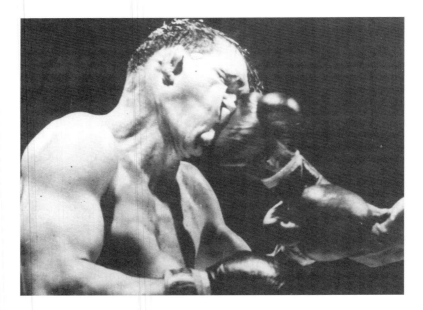

FIGURE XIX-73. Professional middleweight fight between Willie Vaughan and Ralph "Tiger" Jones. The photo shows the moment in which a hammering right of "Tiger" Jones connects with the face of Vaughan. The tremendous kinetic energy of the blow produces a grotesque displacement and flattening of the face, especially on the left side. Eyelids, nose, and upper and lower lips are completely deformed and distorted. The tremendous impact has accelerated the head, while the right ear lags behind due to its inertia. The face is acting as a shock absorber. Photo: UPI.

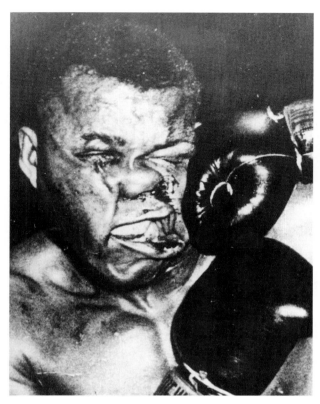

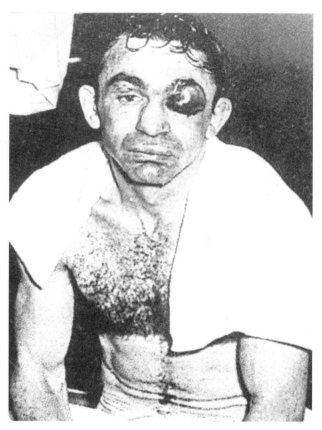

FIGURE XIX-74. Professional heavyweight fight between Rocky Marciano and Keen Simmons on January 29, 1951, in Providence, Rhode Island. The features of Simmons are completely distorted by a hard right blow of his opponent. The hammer-hard blow impacts against his left cheek, producing an immediate closure of both eyes. The nose is in a grotesque corkscrewlike bend; the tip of the nose remains behind due to inertia. There is bleeding, especially from the left nares. Left-sided parts of the mouth are completely pulled out of shape. Photo: David Lamontagne.

FIGURE XIX-75. Second professional middleweight fight between "Sugar" Ray Robinson and Carmen Basilio on March 26, 1958, in Chicago Stadium. The left eye of Basilio after the end of the fight is completely closed due to a massive hemorrhage in the upper eyelid.

the higher frequency range with extension into midrange. Usually, the left ear shows greater hearing losses than the right due to the greater incidence of boxing blows to the left side of the head, as most boxers are right-handed.

Acute and Chronic Neurological Clinical Findings

Clinically, boxing injuries can be grouped into acute and chronic types. The most notable example of the acute group is the *knockout*. One must distinguish between (1) a *knockout sui generis* and (2) a *technical knockout*.

A *knockout sui generis* occurs when a boxer is so disabled by a single blow, or series of blows, that he is incapacitated for a count of ten seconds. A *technical knockout* is declared when the fight is stopped due to an injury, or to the defenseless state of one participant.

In a *knockout sui generis,* a distinction must be made between a *cerebral knockout* and a *body knockout.* A knockout is not the result of concussion or *commotio cerebri* in every case. A boxer may be knocked down without having suffered a cerebral concussion, although he is unable to regain his footing after ten seconds. Cerebral concussion with immediate loss of consciousness and muscle tone may result from a heavy blow with acceleration of the freely movable head. The intensity of the impacting glove is sufficient to accelerate the head to an adequate threshold of unconsciousness, resulting in the concussive syndrome. Loss of consciousness and posture occur instantly, within fractions of a second after impact, and the boxer collapses on the spot. Hypoxemia due to brain swelling cannot explain this type of cerebral concussion, since this process would require at least eight to ten seconds.

The pathologist Harrison Martland[10] called attention to the fact that fight fans and promoters recognized a peculiar condition occurring among prizefighters called, in ring parlance, *punch-drunkenness*. This condition is known by several terms, such as *dementia pugilistica*,[11] *punch-drunkenness*,[10] and *chronic progressive traumatic encephalopathy* of the boxer.[12]

Martland[10] observed that many cases remained mild and did not progress beyond the initial symptoms. In others, a very distinct dragging of the legs developed, associated with a general slowing of muscular movements, a stereotyped attitude characterized by hesitancy of speech, tremors of the hands, and nodding movements of the head, necessitating withdrawal from the ring. Later, in severe cases, a peculiar head tilt developed with a staggering, propulsive gait and facial characteristics of Parkinsonism, or a backward swaying of the body with tremor, vertigo, and deafness. Eventually, marked mental deterioration led to commitment to an asylum.

Types of Traumatic Intracranial Lesions

All types of intracranial hemorrhages known to be caused by trauma to the head have been described in boxers. Epidural hemorrhages do not occur often, but one fatal case was recorded.[13] Subdural hemorrhages are a frequent type of injury, comprising approximately 75% of all acute brain injuries and taking first place as a cause of ring fatalities. Numerous observations of fatal subdural hemorrhages, involving primarily amateur boxers, have been published.[4,14] Intracerebral hemorrhages have also been reported. The cumulative effect of blows to the head may produce severe cerebral edema and other CNS lesions, leading to thrombotic occlusion (Fig. XIX-76).[15-18] Rupture of internal layers of the vessel wall with intralamellar hemorrhages and thrombosis have been described, resulting in compromised cerebral blood supply.

The effects of boxing blows against the lateral region of the neck reflect still another source of acute injury, involving compression and damage to the walls of arteries supplying the brain, particularly the carotid arteries.[19-21] Blows to the lateral side of the neck may trigger a carotid sinus syndrome, although these blows are legal in boxing and occur quite frequently in matches.

Thrombotic occlusion of the basilar artery was described by Kalges[22] in a 16-year-old male who had trained from seven years of age and with more than 60 amateur bouts. Six days after winning a championship fight, he reported minor complaints, then suddenly became unconscious. He died 11 days after the onset of sudden illness, 17 days after his last fight. The autopsy disclosed signs of increased intracranial pressure and tonsillar herniation of the cerebellum. No post-traumatic alterations of the cerebral cortex were observed. There were numerous foci of necrosis in the thalamus and substantia nigra bilaterally, as well as in both cerebellar hemispheres, resulting from a thrombus of the basilar artery at the rostral pons, which was partly organized. Although no severe blows to the neck had been reported, an isolated lesion of the intima of the basilar artery was held accountable for the thrombus, presumably of traumatic origin.

Numerous studies of brains of ex-boxers with permanent brain damage have been conducted.[16,23-30] Brandenburg,[23] described a case of a young man who began boxing at age eighteen. After 11 years of boxing, he retired from the ring. Ten years later, the first symptoms of a lingering change of personality began, with episodes of nervousness, restlessness, and anxiety. He was frequently depressed and occasionally euphoric, resulting in discharge from military service. Progressive forgetfulness became more noticeable. He became garrulous, less articulate, and clumsy. In subsequent years, his condition deteriorated to one of total disability and helplessness, with disorientation in time and space and anxiety states. The development of progressive dementia and a typical parkinsonian syndrome necessitat-

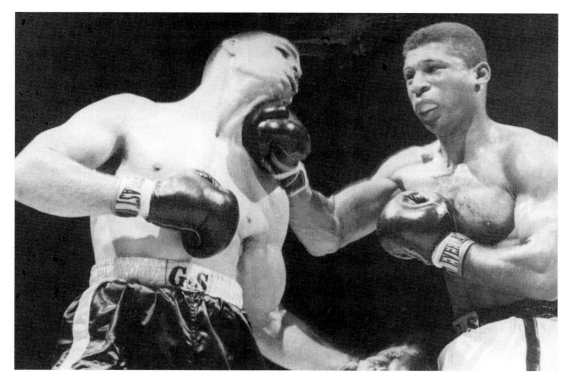

FIGURE XIX-76. Professional middleweight fight between Teddy Wright (right) and Phil Moyer (left) on May 26, 1962 in Madison Square Garden, New York. A hard right from Wright lands on the left neck region of his opponent Moyer and displaces the soft tissue of the neck. Such blows may result in a thrombotic occlusion of the carotid artery, or trigger a carotid sinus reflex. Wright won the fight after 10 rounds on points. Photo: UPI.

ed nursing care. A massive hemorrhage occurred in the rostral parts of the right cerebral hemisphere causing death.

Macroscopically, the brain was moderately atrophic with an enlarged ventricular system, in the absence of cortical contusions. Histologic examination revealed atherosclerosis of the cerebral vessels with an unusually prominent number of senile plaques throughout the entire cerebral cortex, striatum, thalamus, and, to a lesser degree, in the brain stem. Senile plaques were also present in the molecular and granular cell layers of the cerebellum. Abundant intraneuronal neurofibrillary tangles were noted in the cortex and striatum, as well as in the hypothalamus, substantia nigra, and locus coeruleus. The spinal cord showed moderate degeneration of the lateral corticospinal tracts. Brandenburg's[23] seminal description of senile plaque formation was criticized, based on the allegation that a sin-

gle case report may represent a fortuitous coincidence of a former boxer suffering from superimposed Alzheimer's disease. Moreover, it was argued that many years had elapsed between the end of the boxer's professional career and the onset of the clinical picture, suggesting that these findings were not directly attributable to boxing injury.

Grahmann and Ule[24] reported the case of a 48-year-old former boxer with similar brain findings. This ex-boxer had joined an amateur boxing club at the age of fifteen, fought in boxing exhibits for several years, and, although supposedly never knocked out, was frequently groggy. He subsequently suffered a focal seizure with clonic movements of the right arm and leg, followed by progressive mental deterioration and impaired speech. The EEG was irregular, without focal signs. The pneumoencephalogram revealed a communicating hydrocephalus, in addition to an enlarged cavum septi pellucidi. A discrete Parkinsonian syndrome later developed, characterized by slight rigor of the left arm. Microscopically the brain revealed diffuse loss of neurons in the cerebral cortex, substantia nigra, and the cerebellum. Alzheimer's neurofibrillary changes were seen in the midbrain, cerebellum, and Ammon's horns.

Neubûrger[25] reported the cases of two professional boxers who came to medical attention 15 and 20 years, respectively, after their active careers had ended.

The first, a 46-year-old ex-boxer, had fought from age fourteen to age thirty-six, as a light-heavyweight and heavyweight, including 130 professional fights and 30 knockouts. A biopsy specimen from the frontal lobe exhibited a slight reduction of neurons in the lower layers of the cerebral cortex and a striking, diffuse proliferation of astrocytes.

The second case, a 53-year-old ex-boxer, had fought from age eighteen to twenty-four. He fought as a middleweight. He stopped boxing because of left hemiparesis. Examination of the brain revealed severe atrophy of the frontal lobes, thinning of the cerebral cortex, abnormal stratification of neurons and prominent gliosis.

Spillane[26] published the neurological findings of five ex-boxers. One, who died suddenly, suffered from permanent dysarthria and ataxia. At autopsy, there were small foci of softening in the cerebral cortex of the left parietal and temporal lobes, internal capsule and the left cerebellar lobe.

Mawdsley and Ferguson[27] reported ten cases of ex-boxers who showed clinical evidence of neurological disease, of which dysarthria, ataxia, and tremors were the principal features. There was evidence of dementia in all but one. In six cases, radiographs showed symmetrical dilatation of the lateral ventricles.

Courville[31] published findings in reference to the professional lightweight boxer Denny Moore, who was involved in a boxing match with "Sugar" Ramos on March 21, 1963, in Dodger Stadium, San Francisco, California. Moore was dropped over the ropes, beaten and helpless, at the end of the 10th round. A heavy blow against Moore's head resulted in a knockdown, and he fell first on his buttocks, then backwards, hitting the lowest rope with the back of his head. The vibrating rope allegedly struck Moore's head several times, resulting in a technical knockout. About 45 minutes later, Moore complained of severe headache and became unconscious. He was admitted to a hospital in a deeply comatose state, where he died 72 hours later. The autopsy revealed a slight subdural hemorrhage over the right cerebral hemisphere. There was marked bilateral brain edema with bilateral uncal herniation. There was also hemorrhagic necrosis in the basal parts of the cerebrum, around the aqueduct, and in the left substantia nigra.

Quant and Sommer[16] published the case of a 24-year-old amateur boxer who had suffered a knockout during a match, resulting from blows to the left eyebrow and right mandible. There were several remote cortical contusions in the frontotemporal region, interpreted by the authors as injuries related to blows, although cortical contusions in boxers are usually the result of falls in the ring with occipital head impact against the canvas or, less frequently, against ring ropes. Another pattern of injury consisted of extensive, almost-symmetrical necroses in the basal parts of the cerebral hemispheres and basal ganglia with gliosis.

Payne[28] reported morphologic abnormalities in six professional ex-boxers. The main pathologic features consisted of an enlarged ventricular system, glial scars in the grey matter, foci of myelin degeneration, scattered chronic inflammatory cells and phagocytes in the perivascular spaces, and irregular areas of glial proliferation on the surface of the gyri, indicating the presence of small foci of brain damage in each of these brains.

Corsellis[29] studied the brains of 15 retired boxers. This publication is considered to be one of the most thorough and comprehensive pathomorphological reviews. A characteristic pattern of cerebral damage emerged, which appears to characterize the results of boxing injury, representing the morphologic substrate of the *punch-drunk syndrome*. Sufficient emphasis cannot be placed on the importance of pursuing the histories and observations of Corsellis and other authors, since they portray in detail the shocking and pitiful decline of the personalities of former boxers who became *punch-drunk* as a result of *encephalopathia pugilistica*, including many who suffered some form of dementia. The characteristic pattern of cerebral damage identified by Corsellis includes an enlarged *cavum septi pelluci-di*, identified in 12 of 13 brains and measuring in coronal dimensions from 1 to 8 mm, with a mean of 5.12 mm (Fig. XIX-77a–b). The striking incidence of 92% is vastly higher than that of 28% in age-matched controls. Repeated blows to the heads of boxers result in an enlargement of this structure, which is present in nearly every case *(cavum pugilisticum)*, often in association with septal fenestration *(cavum pugilisticum rupturum)*.

Mawdsley and Ferguson[27] had previously described six air encephalograms of boxers with *cavum septi pellucidi*. These authors noted in an addendum that they had examined two more boxers, in each of whom air encephalography revealed a *cavum septi pellucidi*. Isherwood[32] had an opportunity to review encephalographic studies of 16 ex-boxers, all of whom had evidence of neurological disease. A *cavum septi pellucidi* was present in nine cases.

Corsellis[29] also described a significant loss of cerebellar Purkinje cells, in addition to a Parkinsonian syndrome, cited in the hospital records of four clinical cases. In several others, the description of onset of movement disorders later in life suggests that Parkinsonism had emerged to some degree. Gross examination revealed loss of nigral pigment in the four cases diagnosed clinically (Fig. XIX-78a–b), while seven of the remaining boxers were less severely affected. There was a tendency for the medial portion of the nigra to be spared, whereas the intermediate and lateral areas were more vulnerable. According to Corsellis, the distribution of neurofibrillary tangles did not correspond to a specific topographic pattern, as they were disseminated diffusely throughout the cerebral cortex and brain stem. The most noticeable feature, however, was the intensity of neurofibrillary change in the medial temporal grey matter, where vast numbers of neurons in the uncus, amygdala, and the fusiform gyrus were involved. When these reports are considered together, Corsellis continues, "a pattern begins to emerge. First, septal anomalies have occurred suspiciously often, particularly when the evidence from air encephalographic studies is taken into account. Second, Parkinsonism, as well as neuronal degeneration

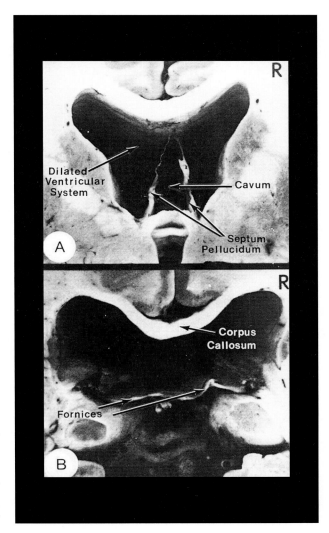

FIGURE XIX-77a–b. Case 1 (a). Coronal cut through the anterior horn of the lateral ventricles. Only a few strands of the septum pellucidum have survived, and they are widely separated by an intervening cavum. (b) coronal cut at a more posterior level, showing the flattened bodies of the fornices completely detached from the under surface of the corpus callosum. There is no septal remnant at this level. (From JAN Corsellis et al. 1973)

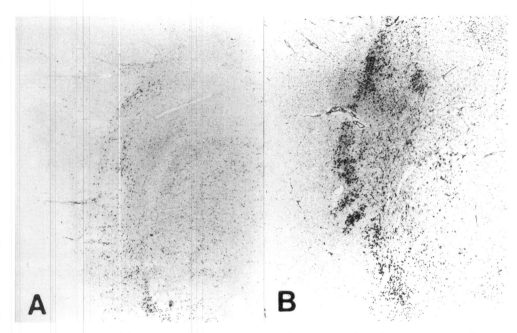

FIGURE XIX-78a–b. (a) Case 3. Depletion of pigmental neurons in the substantia nigra can be seen when compared with the normal picture in (b). a and b. Cresyl violet (Nissl) technique, 11:1. (From JAN Corsellis et al. 1973)

with loss of pigment in the substantia nigra, has been mentioned several times. Third, a diagnosis of Alzheimer's disease has sometimes been broached, although in this connection the more striking and the more anomalous feature has been the tendency for neurofibrillary tangles to occur in the absence of senile plaques."

A classic study was published by Drachman and Newell:[30] A 67-year-old, right-handed boxer was admitted to the hospital because of progressive dementia. At autopsy, the frontal and anterior temporal lobes were slightly atrophic, with a slight reduction of the white matter in the frontal lobes and a slight enlargement of the lateral ventricles. There was thickening and fenestration of the left septal leaf of the *cavum septi pellucidi.* The substantia nigra was pale. Microscopic examination revealed neuronal loss of nigral cells and many scattered neurofibrillary tangles showing immunoreactivity to a polyclonal antibody against phosphorylated tau. These tangles were most numerous in the superficial cortical layers of the inferior frontal and temporal lobes. Abundant tangles in the hippocampus were associated

with marked neuronal loss and gliosis, in addition to occasional senile plaques. The final diagnosis was "multisystem neurodegenerative disease characterized by neurofibrillary changes and a few plaques, findings consistent with *dementia pugilistica.*"

As noted in the preceding review, structural similarities link *dementia pugilistica* and Alzheimer's disease, including the presence of neurofibrillary tangles and senile plaques, as described by Brandenburg and Hallervorden.[23] Corsellis[29] emphasized the preponderance of neurofibrillary tangles associated with *dementia pugilistica,* in the relative absence of senile plaques, as a hallmark of boxing injury to the brain, although the assertion remains controversial. Stritch[33] published the initial description of diffuse loss of white matter as a sequel of severe brain injury, attributing the pathogenesis to primary shearing of axons, followed by secondary degeneration of myelin: Her concept of traumatic primary axonal injury was subsequently reinforced by the term diffuse axonal injury (DAI), based on experimental evidence in animals[34] and

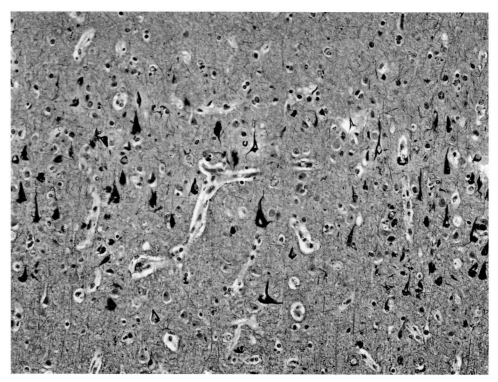

FIGURE XIX-79. Laminar distribution of cortical neurons containing neurofibrillary tangles. Bielschowsky, 150X.

on observations derived from human autopsy material.[35] Although a frequent and well-established microscopic signature associated with myriad forms of brain injury, DAI has not been adequately documented as a significant component of boxing injury to the brain. The following example illustrates the presence of neurofibrillary tangles and DAI, related to a case of dementia pugilistica.

A 52-year-old male competed in more than 75 amateur bouts and participated in the Olympic Games. His medical profile included progressive weakness and stiffness of the arms and legs, in addition to recent episodes of urinary and fecal incontinence. Shortly after admission, he suffered a convulsion and died a few days later of urinary infection complicated by sepsis.

The brain weighed 1225 grams and showed minimal atrophy of the frontal lobes. Cerebral white matter, basal ganglia, thalamus, brain stem, cerebellum, and spinal cord were grossly unremarkable.

Representative sections were stained with hematoxylin and eosin (H&E), Luxol fast blue (LFB), and Bielschowsky, in addition to immunohistochemical methods for glial fibrillary acidic protein (GFAP), neurofilament protein (NFP), and beta-amyloid. Sections of neocortex contained isolated, flame-shaped neurofibrillary tangles (NFT), contrasting markedly with random cortical areas containing densely distributed, linear foci of neurofibrillary change involving virtually each adjacent neuron for a distance of several cells. The neurofibrillary change in these linear clusters of abnormal neurons involved, predominantly, the deep cortical layers adjacent to the gyral white matter (Figs. XIX-79 and XIX-80).

Scattered NFT were noted within the neurons of the hippocampus and midbrain, although the neuronal complement in the latter structure was normal with no evidence of neuronal loss, gliosis, or Lewy bodies. Prominent displays of NFT within the basal ganglia were also noted (Fig. XIX-81).

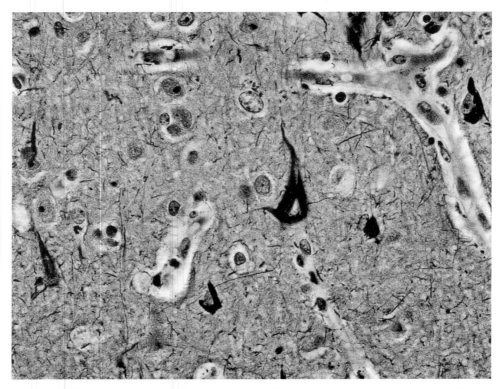

FIGURE XIX-80. Cortical neuron containing neurofibrillary tangles. Bielschowsky, 396X.

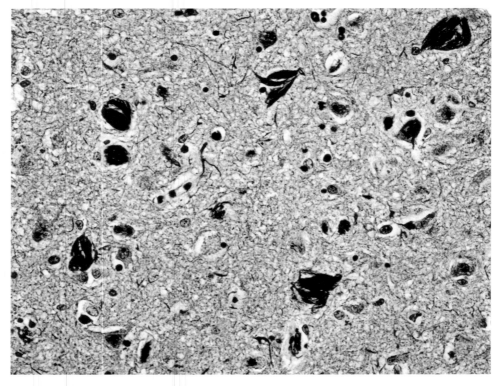

FIGURE XIX-81. Basal ganglia neurons containing neurofibrillary tangles. Bielschowsky, 300X.

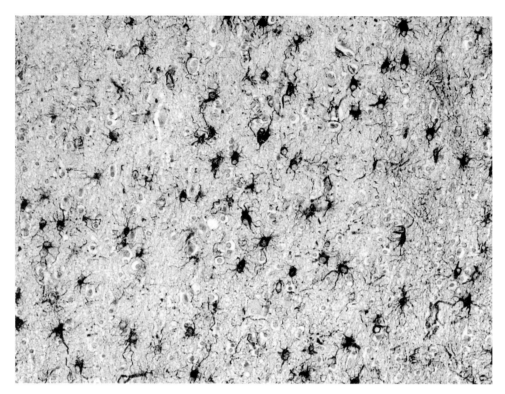

FIGURE XIX-82. Diffuse gliosis in centrum semiovale. GFAP, 135X.

Senile plaques (SP) were conspicuously absent throughout the CNS parenchyma, in marked contrast to the focal prominence of NFT. There was no evidence of granulovacuolar change, Hirano bodies, or amyloid angiopathy, frequently associated with Alzheimer's disease (AD), suggesting an alternative pathogenesis of NFT in this instance, including traumatic brain injury related to boxing. The gyral white matter showed subtle foci of rarefaction and pallor associated with varying degrees of subcortical gliosis, as readily seen with H&E and confirmed with GFAP (Fig. XIX-82). Prominent swollen axons or axonal bodies were conspicuous within the gyral white matter and centrum semiovale, which stained intensely with the Bielschowsky and NFP methods (Figs. XIX- 83 and XIX-84). A definite correlation between the presence of neocortical NFT and axonal bodies could not be ascertained with certainty, as the swollen axons were ubiquitous throughout the white matter, reflecting a variant of diffuse axonal injury. A positive correlation was noted between the intensity of gyral white matter rarefaction and associated reactive gliosis.

The striking display of sporadic, linear NFT within neurons of the lower neocortical layers, interposed between areas of normal neurons, in the absence of senile plaques (SP) and other histologic hallmarks of AD, represents a relatively unique finding. In conjunction with evidence of DAI, this change may reflect a pathognomonic aspect of boxing injury to the CNS, underpinning the clinical phenomenon of *dementia pugilistica,* or the *punch-drunk* syndrome. Although a putative relationship between trauma and AD exists, the changes noted in the brain of boxers, as exemplified by this case, contain predominantly NFT with few or no SP, in contrast to AD.

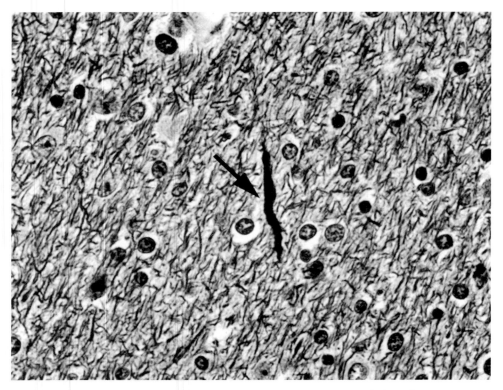

FIGURE XIX-83. Swollen, fragmented axon in centrum semiovale. Bielschowsky, 474X.

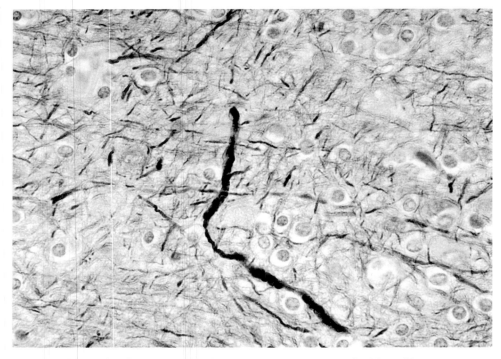

FIGURE XIX-84. Swollen, fragmented axon in centrum semiovale. Neurofilament protein, 447X.

REFERENCES

1. Sellier, K., and Unterharnscheidt, F.: Mechanik und Pathomorphologie der Hirnschäden nach stumpfer Gewalteinwirkung auf den Schädel. Hefte Unfallheilkunde, Heft 76, Springer, Berlin, 1963.

2. Unterharnscheidt, F., and Ripperger, E.A.: Mechanics and pathomorphology of impact-related closed brain injuries. In Perrone, N. (ed), *Dynamic response of biomechanical systems*. New York: The American Society of Mechanical Engineers, 1970, pp. 46–83.

3. Ripperger, E.A., and Unterharnscheidt, F.: Prototypes of head injury: Application to animal experiments. Internat Conf on Biokinetics of Impact. Amsterdam, 26–27 June, 1973, pp. 259–270.

4. Unterharnscheidt, F., and Unterharnscheidt, J.: *Boxing–Medical aspects*. Amsterdam: Elsevier, 2003.

5. Doggart, J.H.: The impact of boxing on the visual apparatus. *Arch Ophthalmol, 54:* 161–169, 1955.

6. Doggart, J.H.: Eye injuries. In Bass, A.L., Blonstein, J.L., James, R.D., and Williams, J.C.P. (eds), *Medical aspects of boxing*. Oxford London New York: Pergamon Press, 1965, pp. 3–7.

7. Maguire, J.I., and Benson, W.E.: Retinal injury and detachment in boxers. *JAMA, 255:* 2451–2453, 1986.

8. Giovinazzo, V.J., Yannuzzi, L.A., Sorensen, J.A., Delrowe, D.J., and Cambell, E.A.: The ocular complications of boxing. *Ophthalmology, 94:* 587–598, 1987.

9. Paulsen, K., and Hundhausen, T.: Hörschäden durch Boxen. *Z Laryngol Rhinol Otol, 50:* 297–324, 1971.

10. Martland, H.S.: Punch drunk. *JAMA, 91:* 1103–1107, 1928.

11. Millspaugh, J.A.: Dementia pugilistica (punch drunk). *US Naval Med Bull, 35:* 297–303, 1937.

12. Critchley, McD.: Medical aspects of boxing, particularly from a neurological standpoint. *Br Med J, I:* 357–362, 1957.

13. Krefft, F.: Uber Todesfalle beim Boxen. *Deutsch Gesundheitswes, 7:* 1559, 1952.

14. Unterharnscheidt, F.: Traumatische Schäden des Gehirns (forensische Pathologie). In Doerr, W., and Seifert, G. (eds), *Spezielle pathologische Anatomie. Pathologie des Nervensystems. Band 13/VI.B*. Berlin Heidelberg New York: Springer, 1993.

15. McAlpine, D., and Page, F.: Midbrain syndrome in a professional boxer. *Proc R Soc Med 42:* 792–793, 1949.

16. Quant, J., and Sommer, H.: Beitrag zur Pathogenese der Encephalopathia pugilistica (Boxerencephalopathie). *Psychiatr Neurol Med Psychol* (Leipzig) *17:* 448–451, 1965.

17. Colmant, H.J., and Dotzauer, G.: Analyse eines tödlich ausgegangenen Boxkampfes mit ungewöhnlich schweren cerebralen Schäden. *Z Rechtsmed, 84:* 163–278, 1980.

18. Strassmann, G., and Helpern, M.: Tödliche Hirnverletzungen im Boxkampf. *Deutsch Z Ges Gerichtl Med, 63:* 70–83, 1968.

19. Rosegay, H.: Limited value of carotid pulse in diagnosis of internal carotid thrombosis. *Neurology, 6:* 143–145, 1956.

20. Hockaday, T.D.R.: Traumatic thrombosis of the internal carotid artery. *J Neurol Neurosurg Psychiatry, 22:* 229–231, 1959.

21. Murphy, F., and Miller, J.H.: Carotid insufficiency diagnosis and surgical treatment. A report of twenty-one cases. *J Neurosurg, 16:* 1–23, 1959.

22. Kalges, U.: Thrombose der Arteria basilaris bei einem jugendlichen Boxer. *Deutsch Z Ges Gerichtl Med, 66:* 75–85, 1969.

23. Brandenburg, W., and Hallervorden, J.: Dementia pugilistica mit anatomischen Befund. *Virchows Arch, 325:* 680–709, 1954.

24. Grahmann, H., and Ule, G.: Beitrag zur Kenntnis der chronischen cerebralen Krankheitsbilder bei Boxern (Dementia pugilistica und traumatische Boxer-Encephalopathie). *Psychiatr Neurol* (Basel) *134:* 261–283, 1957.

25. Neubürger, K.T., Sinton, D.W., and Denst, J.: Cerebral atrophy associated with boxing. *Arch Neurol Psychiatr, 81:* 403–408, 1959.

26. Spillane, J.D.: Five boxers. *Br Med J, II:* 1205–1210, 1962.

27. Mawdsley, C., and Ferguson, F.R.: Neurological disease in boxers. *Lancet, II:* 795–901, 1963.

28. Payne, E.E.: Brains of boxers. *Neurochirurgica, 11:* 173–188, 1968.

29. Corsellis, J.A.N., Bruton, C.J., and Freeman-Browne, D.: The aftermath of boxing. *Psychol Med, 3:* 270–303, 1973.

30. Drachman, D.A., and Newell, K.L.: Presentation of a case (12-1999) in the weekly clinicopathological exercises of the Massachusetts General Hospital. *N Eng J Med, 340:* 1269–1277, 1999.

31. Courville, C.B.: The mechanism of boxing fatalities: Report of an unusual case with severe brain lesions incident to impact of the boxer's head against ropes. *Bull Los Angeles Neurol Soc, 29:* 58–69, 1964.

32. Isherwood, I., Mawdsley, C., and Ferguson, F.R.: Pneumencephalographic changes in boxers. *Acta Radiol, 5:* 654–661, 1966.

33. Stritch, S.J.: Diffuse degeneration of the cerebral white matter in severe dementia following head injury. *J Neurol Neurosurg Psychiat, 19:* 163–186, 1956.

34. Gennarelli, T.A., Thibault, L.E., Adams, J.H., et al.: Diffuse axonal injury and traumatic coma in the primate. *Ann Neuro, 12:* 564–574, 1982.

35. Adams, J.H., Graham, D.I., Murray, L.S., and Scott, G.: Diffuse axonal injury due to non-missile injury in humans: An analysis of 45 cases. *Ann Neurol, 12:* 557–563, 1982.

Chapter XX

MICROSCOPIC FORENSIC PATHOLOGY

JOSHUA A. PERPER

THE GROSS APPEARANCE and patterns of traumatic injuries and disease are so important to the practicing forensic pathologist that he is tempted to relegate the microscopic examination to a back seat, if not to neglect it altogether. Therefore, it is particularly important to emphasize that failure to perform a satisfactory microscopic examination may lead to important diagnostic failures and to inadequate corroboration and substantiation of crucial forensic findings. This is true not only in cases where there is an absence of demonstrable gross pathological changes and/or toxicological findings, but also when there is an abundance of gross pathology. A blunt force vehicular fatality may be triggered by a myocarditis diagnosed only on microscopic examination. Similarly, fatal myocardial infarction triggered by a prior traumatic event, may be discovered only through microscopic aging. Substantiation of a battered child case may hinge on the microscopic differentiation between alleged resuscitation trauma and earlier antemortem injury.

The major contribution of forensic microscopy is particularly evident in the following instances: investigation of sudden unexpected death, determination of premortem nature of injuries, aging of traumatic and natural processes, interpretation of gross findings of natural and unnatural diseases and injuries, diagnoses of poisoning, substantiation of occupational diseases, and identification of trace evidence. This chapter will highlight a few of the more common situations in which microscopic examination is indispensable to forensic investigation.

SUDDEN UNEXPECTED DEATH IN INFANCY AND CHILDHOOD

The value of microscopic evaluation in cases of sudden unexpected death in infancy is self-evident.

Sudden infant death syndrome (SIDS), an idiopathic condition and essentially an exclusionary diagnosis, is the most common cause of death in infants below one year of age. Absence of gross pathological findings per se is not sufficient evidence for a SIDS diagnosis, and microscopic examination is essential to exclude other causes of death. The microscopic changes in SIDS are non-specific and may include subserosal petechial hemorrhages, thymic and pulmonary intra-alveolar hemorrhages, low grade bronchiolitis and peribronchiolitis, and various degrees of alveolar septal thickening and chronic inflammatory cell infiltrate *(interstitial pneumonitis)*[1,2] (Fig. XX-1).

The non-inculpatory nature of SIDS and, in particular, the inability to predict or prevent it's occurrence make it a popular and acceptable diagnosis to treating physicians and bereaved parents alike.

It is therefore understandable why many forensic pathologists resort to SIDS as a choice diagnosis, in the presence of significant microscopic pathological findings not known to be associated with SIDS. In the presence of such non-SIDS related findings, the conscientious pathologist should feel compelled to initiate a thorough search for a clearly defined pathological process which may be the actual cause of death.

The presence of fatty change of the liver in an apparent SIDS should certainly prompt additional investigation. The fatty liver may be due to Reye's Syndrome, enzymatic carnitine deficien-

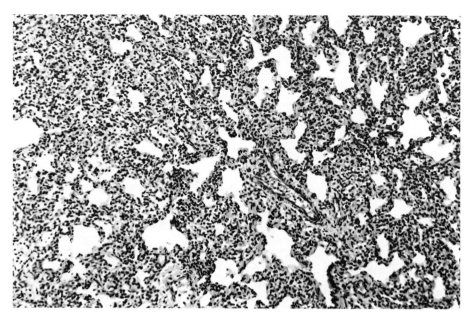

FIGURE XX-1. SIDS: (×32, H&E stain). Lung section of six-month-old victim of SIDS, showing thickening of alveolar septa and round cell infiltration.

cy, acute alcoholic intoxication, sepsis or undetermined causes.

The pattern of fatty change may assist in the differential diagnosis. In Reye's syndrome, a syndrome of fatal encephalopathy, cerebral edema and hepatic failure associated with certain strains of the influenza virus and often triggered by aspirin intake, the fatty change of hepatocytes is typically microvesicular and the nuclei remain central[3,4] (Fig. XX-2). *In alcohol-related fatty liver, on the other hand, the vacuoles tend to be macrovesicular and displace the nucleus eccentrically.* Fatty change may be also seen in the renal tubular epithelium and occasionally in the cardiac conduction system. Rarely, cases of Reye's syndrome may show periportal hepatocellular necrosis which has been related to fatty acid toxicity.[5] The brain in Reye's syndrome shows marked edema and electron microscopy has demonstrated astrocyte swelling, myelin bleb formation, and universal injury of neuron mitochondria with pleomorphism and matrix disruption.[6]

Biochemical testing for absence of medium-chain Acyl-CoA dehydrogenase (MCAD) may substantiate the diagnosis of carnitine deficiency, a condition known to be associated with fatty liver and sudden infant death[7,8] (Fig. XX-3). MCAD is an autosomal recessive inborn error of metabolism in the intramitochondrial beta-oxidation of fatty acids. It usually manifests in the first two years of life with recurrent episodes of hypoglycemia provoked by fasting. Patients have low carnitine levels in the plasma, skeletal muscle, and liver. They show, however, an increased urinary excretion of medium chain fatty acid metabolites, dicarboxylic acids (adipic, suberic, and sebacic), glycine conjugates, and carnitine esters. The liver is occasionally enlarged and microscopically marked microvesicular or macrovesicular fatty change and altered mitochondrial ultrastructure. Congenital deficiencies of other types of dehydrogenases (i.e., long chain Acyl-Co dehydrogenase, short chain Acyl-Co dehydrogenase, multiple Acyl-CoA deficiency) although much less common than MCAD, may also result in fatty change of the liver and sudden infant death.[9]

Acute alcoholic intoxication in infants may also occasionally result in fatty liver. Infants are known to be extremely sensitive to alcohol. Even when given small amounts of alcohol as a sedative–hypnotic, they may develop critical hypoglycemia and die at blood alcohol concentrations

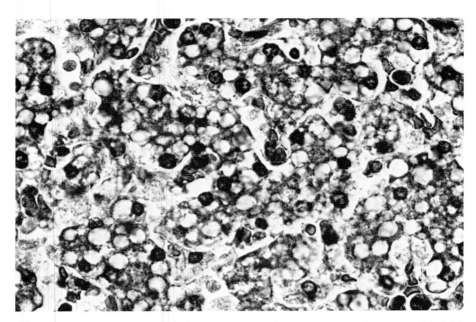

FIGURE XX-2. Reye's Syndrome (×200, H&E stain). Fatty liver in a three-year-old child with Reye's Syndrome who presented clinically with vomiting, convulsions and intractable hypoglycemia. Microvesicular pattern of fatty change with undisplaced nuclei.

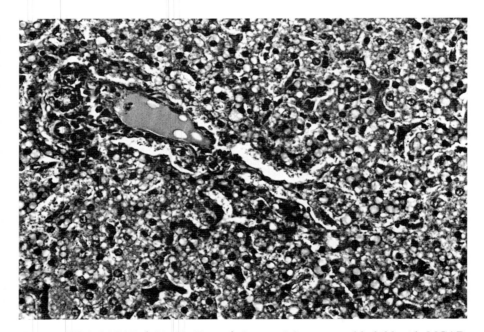

FIGURE XX-3. MCAD (×80, H&E stain). Liver of three-year-old child with MCAD (Medium Chain Acyl Dehydrogenase Deficiency). Microvesicular fatty change with undisplaced hepatic nuclei.

as low as 20 mg%.[10,11] Finally, the possibility of septicemia, a condition which also may be associated with fatty liver, should be evaluated by appropriate bacteriological cultures.

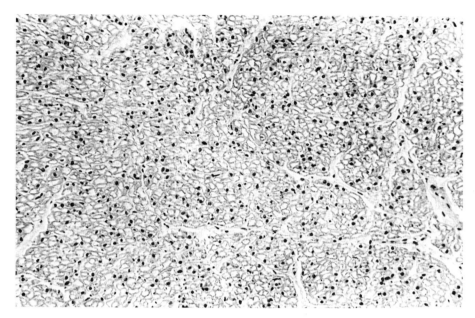

FIGURE XX-4. Pompe Disease (×40, H&E stain). Lacework-like microscopic pattern of myocardial fibers in two-month-old infant with generalized glycogenesis.

The microscopic examination may also reveal grossly undetected infectious processes such as pneumonia and myocarditis. The gross diagnosis of pneumonia in infants is difficult, if not virtually impossible.

One should also carefully screen microscopic sections for subtle diagnostic findings. For example, the presence of intra-nuclear inclusions in salivary glands and renal tubular epithelium may point to fatal cytomegalic viral disease. The presence of enlarged, foamy or vacuolated parenchymal cells in liver, spleen, or brain, raises the possibility of metabolic storage diseases, such as Tay-Sachs, Nieman-Pick, Gaucher, or Hurler's

disease. The possibility of myocardial glycogenesis or glycolipidosis (i.e., Pompe's disease, Fabry's disease) should also be considered, particularly in the presence of an enlarged or *globular* heart, and a lacework microscopic appearance of the muscle cells (Fig. XX-4).

Foamy edematous-like eosinophilic intra-alveolar pulmonary exudates should be screened by appropriate special stains (i.e., methenamine silver) in order to exclude pneumonia caused by *Pneumocystis carinii*, a parasitic protozoan, prone to attacking individuals with compromised immune function (Fig. XX-5a–b).

SUDDEN UNEXPECTED NATURAL DEATH IN ADULTS

The most common cause of sudden, unexpected, natural deaths in adults is arteriosclerotic cardiovascular disease (ASCVD) and accounts for as much as 55% of all such deaths.[12] Although most clinicians tend to label these deaths as *acute myocardial infarction* or *acute coronary thrombosis,* autopsy findings in more than 65% of these cases fail to substantiate such conditions and, in the

majority of the cases, the coronary arteries show only chronic stenotic changes with diffuse calcifications.[13]

In cases where recent occlusions or acute infarctions are present, the following questions often arise:

• What was the nature of the acute occlusion?
• Did an acute infarction occur?

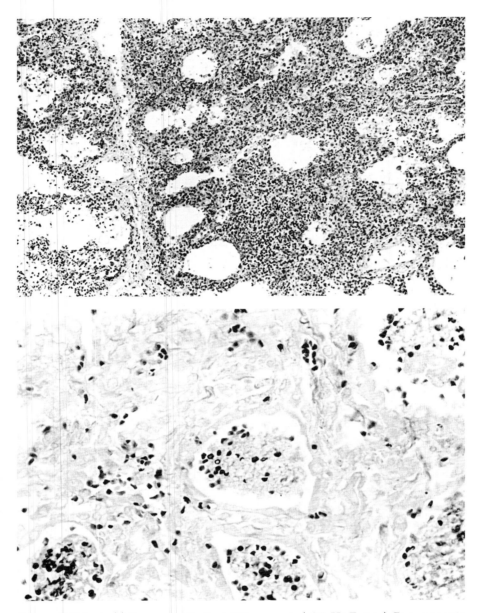

FIGURE XX-5a–b. (a) Pneumocystis Carinii Pneumonia (×25, H&E stain). Pneumocystis carinii pneumonia with heavy septal infiltrates of chronic inflammatory cells and plasmocytes. (b) (×100, H&E stain, Methenamine Silver). Circular parasites of Pneumocystis carinii within foamy alveolar exudate.

- What is the age of recent occlusion or infarction?
- Were the occlusion or infarction and death precipitated or accelerated by exogenous unnatural causes such as trauma and physical or mental stress?

Microscopic examination is crucial in answering these questions.

Recognition and Aging of Coronary Thrombosis and Myocardial Infarction

Most acute occlusions consist of a fresh thrombosis, fresh hemorrhage in a plaque, or a ruptured plaque. Embolic occlusions are rare. Recognizing a particular type of acute occlusion based on the gross diagnosis alone may be misleading. It may be difficult to differentiate between a postmortem coronary blood clot and a genuine thrombus, especially in embalmed bodies. Furthermore, fresh thrombi and hemorrhages in plaques may grossly look similar, and ruptured plaques may easily be missed. Multiple adjacent or serial sections may in some cases substantiate the co-existence of all three types of acute occlusion.

It has been suggested that the acute occlusive process may start with rupture of the roof of an arteriosclerotic plaque by the circulating blood flow.[14] As a result, the following phenomena occur simultaneously:

• spillage of atheromatous material from the plaque, with partial or total occlusion.
• blood from the lumen penetrating the plaque, with resulting hemorrhage into the plaque.
• triggering of thrombosis by highly thrombogenic atheromatous material released from the plaque.

Determination of the precise age of coronary thrombosis is particularly difficult. Initially, the thrombus is composed mainly of fibrin, platelets and entrapped red blood cells. After 12 to 24 hours, there is progressive infiltration by polymorphonuclear cells which reaches its peak about 3 to 4 days after thrombosis. At about 5 days to one week, chronic inflammatory cells can be seen within the thrombus. Endothelialization and ingrowth of young connective tissue from the periphery is evident at about 7 to 10 days. Full organization, with or without recanalization, is present after 3 to 4 weeks. Coronary thrombi are occasionally composed of several layers of various ages, indicating an episodic growth by repeated mural deposits, and may show occasional distal microembolizations and microinfarctions.[15]

The aging of myocardial infarction is more accurate. Although the area of fresh infarction may be paler than the surrounding areas, no macroscopic changes are detected within the first 6 to 12 hours. By 20 to 24 hours, the infarcted area grossly appears pale, and, after approximately 30 hours, it becomes surrounded by a crenated border of red discoloration. Between the fourth and tenth days, the infarcted area progres-

sively turns yellow. Histochemical methods may, however, demonstrate early infarcts, as early as 3 to 4 hours. Immersion of the myocardium in a solution of triphenyl tetrazolium chloride stains the normal myocardium red-brown, leaving the infarcted area as an unstained pale zone. Other histochemical stains may demonstrate similar enzymatic depletions of dehydrogenases, phosphorylases and oxidases.[16]

The disadvantage of enzymatic methods is that they require use of fresh tissue and cryostat sectioning. A number of histochemical methods, using fixed tissues and/or paraffin blocks, have also been developed. A convenient histochemical method, using paraffin embedded tissue, is hematoxylin basic fuchsin picric acid (HBPA). HBPA stains the ischemic fuchsinophilic area red, while the healthy myocardium is counterstained yellow by picric acid.

A more sensitive method recently developed by Fujiware, et al., also uses formalin fixed paraffin embedded tissue which is immunohistochemically labeled with myoglobin markers. This method can age an acute myocardial infarction at four, six, and 24 hours after a coronary occlusion.[17] Fat stains demonstrating fine droplets of lipids scattered in the cytoplasm of the myocardial fibers, (i.e., Sudan IV, osmium tetroxide) are positive in the area of infarction at between six to eight hours. Electron microscopic changes of infarction, such as mitochondrial swelling and margination of nuclear chromatin, become evident within two hours. Routine hematoxylin-eosin (H&E) histological stains do not detect coagulative necrosis within the first six to eight hours. However, a number of early and potentially reversible morphological manifestations of myocardial ischemia may be observed (Fig. XX-6). Stretched and wavy myocardial fibers may be observed at the borders of infarction as early as two hours. Another marker of early myocardial infarction, seen at the periphery of the lesion, is myocytolysis, a potentially reversible degeneration which imparts to the myocardial fibers a vegetal cell-like appearance, with large clear vacuolar spaces outlined by a peripheral rim of compressed cytoplasm and an eccentrically displaced nucleus (Fig. XX-7).[18]

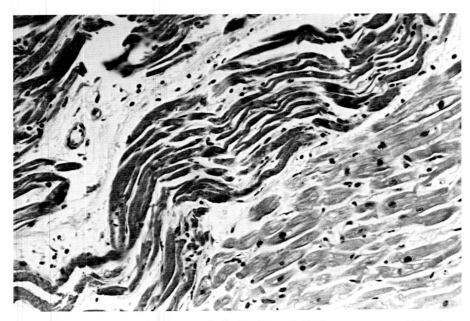

FIGURE XX-6. Myocardial Infarction (×25, H&E stain). Early acute myocardial infarction. Intense eosinophilia, indistinct or absent cross striation, thinning and marked waviness of the myocardial fibers.

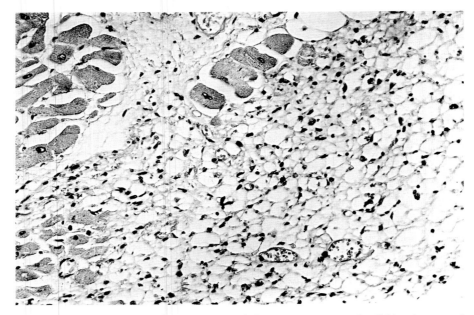

FIGURE XX-7. Myocytolysis (×50, H&E stain). Degenerative vegetal cell-like changes of myocytolysis at edge of recent myocardial infarction.

An early microscopic manifestation of acute myocardial infarction on routine H&E stained sections is the presence of intensely eosinophilic transverse contraction-band degeneration-necrosis resulting from coagulative changes of contractile proteins. Myofibrillar degeneration manifested by contraction bands is not unique to myocardial infarction, and may be seen in a vari-

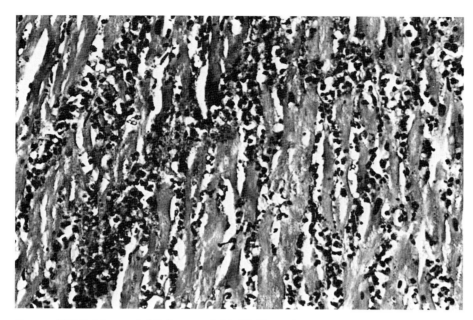

FIGURE XX-8. Myocardial Infarction (×80, H&E stain). Acute myocardial infarction at 48 hours with total disappearance of striation of muscle fibers and heavy granulocytic infiltration. Many of the granulocytes show degenerative or lytic changes.

ety of conditions associated with hypoxia and sudden release of catecholamines, such as hemorrhagic shock, carbon monoxide poisoning, drowning, drug overdose, acute brain injury and stress cardiomyopathy.[19]

Frank coagulative necrotic changes become clearly evident by light microscopy only at about eight to 12 hours. At about 24 hours, the necrotic fibers show increased eosinophilia, blurriness of cross striations and varying degrees of nuclear shrinkage and fragmentation. Polymorphonuclear infiltration is observed at about 20 to 24 hours and increases markedly by 48 hours (Fig. XX-8). By the third day, coagulative changes are markedly advanced, with dissolution of the internal structure of most affected fibers. Many of the polymorphonuclear leukocytes show fragmentation, and small numbers of mononuclear cells may be observed. By the fourth to fifth day, mononuclear cells containing hemosiderin may be demonstrated. By the seventh to tenth week, fully developed granulation tissue is present and, by the seventh week, there is complete scarring.[20–22]

However, an extensive infarction may take a considerable time to heal, and, even after 2 or more months, entrapped areas of unorganized coagulative necrosis may still be evident.

This fact is particularly important in the aging of myocardial infarction. In certain cases, the entrapped areas of yellow necrosis look very much like acute infarction and many pathologists mistakenly label the process as such. In a number of cases, the sequestrated anuclear necrotic material becomes *mummified* with only the striation preserved, and mimics, microscopically, a very recent infarction.

Pitfalls in Aging Myocardial Infarction

Histochemical stains which are positive for myocardial ischemia, such as hematoxylin and basic fuchsin picric acid (HBFP), are not specific markers of acute myocardial infarction. The myocardium may stain positive in other ischemic conditions, such as poisoning by cyanide or carbon monoxide.

A common error is the misdiagnosis of residual myocardial necrosis within an organizing infarct as an acute myocardial infarction. This is more likely to happen if the residual necrosis

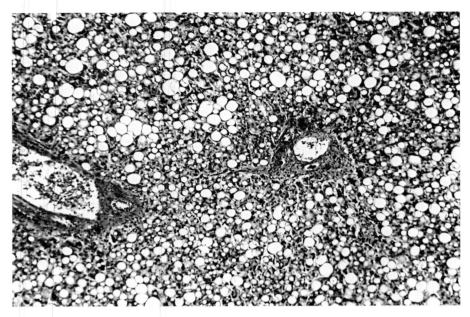

FIGURE XX-9. Alcoholic Fatty Liver (×20). Alcoholic macrovesicular fatty change of liver with relative sparing of the periportal areas.

shows mummification changes with loss of nuclei, but retention of the striation pattern. The differential diagnosis is, however, simple. In contrast to mummified myocardial necrosis, lysis of myocardial nuclei in an acute myocardial infarction is invariably associated with disappearance of striation and presence of acute inflammatory infiltrates.

Therefore, the recognition of sequestrated necrosis can be easily made if one observes the discrepancy between preservation of striation, total absence of nuclei, and lack of any acute inflammatory infiltrate.

The proper aging of thrombi and myocardial infarction is important in determining the sequential and causal relationship between precipitating agents such as physical and/or mental trauma and a coronary catastrophe.

As previously noted, in the majority of sudden deaths, acute occlusion and/or acute myocardial infarction is absent, and the death results from either mechanical or electrical cardiac failure. The increased load placed on a chronically compromised coronary circulation is often the culprit in such a sudden unexpected death.

Fatty Change of the Liver

Many physicians are not aware that fatty change of the liver associated with chronic alcoholism may be the only significant finding in sudden, unexpected death. In some regions of United States, this is the second most common cause of sudden, unexpected death of adults, following arteriosclerotic cardiovascular disease, accounting for 17% of all sudden, natural deaths.[23]

Although most of the victims are asymptomatic, some may arrive at emergency rooms with unexplained arrhythmias, hypokalemia and/or hypoglycemia.

The microscopic features of the fatty liver associated with chronic alcoholism may include all or some of the following elements (Fig. XX-9):

- Macrovesicular steatosis with eccentric displacement and compression of nuclei, and swelling of hepatocytes with compression of sinusoids and a pavement-like pattern. Only rarely is micro-vesicular steatosis the predominant pattern.
- Relatively spared periportal areas.

TABLE XX-1

MICROSCOPIC PATHOLOGY OF CHRONIC ALCOHOLISM

Organ	Process	Pattern
Liver	Fatty change	Macrovesicular steatosis, common; microvesicular steatosis, rare (see text)
	Alcoholic hepatitis	Pleomorphism of hepatocytes with focal necrosis and drop-out, neutrophilic satellitosis around degenerated hepatocytes, perinuclear clumping of cytoplasm, pericentral and mid-zonal fatty change, alcoholic hyaline (Mallory bodies), PMN and mononuclear infiltrate, Perivenular and pericellular fibrosis.
	Alcoholic cirrhosis	Early = micronodular-fat rich Late = mixed micro-macronodular-fat poor, increased cytoplasmic hemosiderin, bile stasis.
Pancreas	Acute and chronic pancreatitis	Non-specific-often chronic calcific with pseudocysts.
Brain	Cerebral atrophy	Neuronal degeneration, gliosis.
	Wernicke - Korsakoff	Focal symmetric softening and petechiae in periventricular areas of thalamus, hypothalamus, mammillary bodies, aqueduct, floor of 4th ventricle and anterior cerebellum. Hyperplasia of small blood vessels. Neuronal degeneration, necrosis and glial reaction.
	Marchiafava-Bignami Syndrome	Degeneration to necrosis of corpus callosum.
	Central pontine myelinolysis	Demyelination of central axons with preserved cell bodies, except in areas of cavitation, reactive astrocytosis, lipidization, also similar extrapontine lesions (in cerebellum, striatum, thalamus and white matter).
	Chronic cerebellar syndrome	Degeneration of Purkinje cells in cerebellar cortex, cortical atrophy.
	Peripheral neuropathy	Myelin degeneration, axonal disruption.
Heart	Cardiomyopathy	Non-specific myocardial hypertrophy, interstitial myocardial fibrosis, mitochondrial swelling with enlarged cristae.
	Peripheral myopathy	Focal necrosis of muscle fibers.
Gastrointestinal	Gastritis, Gastric ulcer	Non-specific.
Testicles	Atrophy	Non-specific, with various degrees of fibrosis and Leydig cell hyperplasia.

- Various degrees of alcoholic hepatitis with presence of Mallory bodies (P.A.S. negative intra-cytoplasmic purple hyaline-like bodies), focal intraparenchymal infiltrates of lymphoid cells, bile plugs and intracanalicular bile stasis, etc. (Table XX-1) .
- Increased hemosiderin in hepatocytes.
- Various degrees of fibrosis ranging from excessive fibrosis of periportal areas and central veins to radiating rays of fibrosis emanating from these areas, bridging of periportal areas and central veins, formation of pseudo-lobules and frank cirrhosis.

It should be emphasized that although chronic alcoholism is the most common cause of fatty change of the liver, other etiological agents should be carefully excluded.[24]

Hepatic macrovesicular steatosis, the more common pattern encountered in alcoholism, may also be seen in diabetes mellitus, obesity, starvation, malabsorption, jejunoileal bypass, and exposure to various drugs and toxins.

Microvesicular steatosis, with central nuclei and small vacuoles (as previously described in Reye's syndrome), although rarely seen in alcoholism, is frequently observed in association with acute fatty liver of pregnancy, certain types of medication (i.e., tetracyclines, salicylates, valproate) and in some metabolic disorders. The rare microvesicular steatosis seen in alcoholics is sometimes referred to as *alcoholic foamy degeneration.*[25]

It should also be noted that although Mallory bodies are characteristically present in alcoholic hepatitis, they have also been observed in primary biliary cirrhosis, hepatolenticular degeneration, jejunoileal bypass, and various toxic injuries.

The mechanism of death in fatty change of the liver has not been definitively elucidated. A number of possibilities, have been excluded, such as fat embolism from ruptured hepatic fatty microcysts, fulminant sepsis and acute alcoholic intoxication. The most likely mechanism of death is apparently an electrolyte imbalance with hypoglycemia, hypokalemia, and fatty acid hyperlipidemia as central abnormalities.

Embolism

Embolism is defined as the pathological process through which abnormal particulates, known as emboli, circulate in the blood and are eventually trapped in blood vessels smaller than their diameter. The emboli may be endogenous or exogenous. Endogenous emboli includes, thromboemboli, fat emboli, bone marrow emboli, fragmented tissue emboli, amniotic fluid emboli, septic and cholesterol emboli, etc. Exogenous emboli includes, air emboli, bullet emboli, and foreign materials infused intravenously, accidently, or by design. In most cases the diagnosis of embolism is made by microscopic examination, except in the case of large thromboemboli, bullet emboli, and air emboli, which are grossly visible.

Thromboemboli and Postmortem Blood Clots

Very fresh thromboemboli may be difficult to differentiate from postmortem clots by naked eye examination. The differentiation is much easier microscopically, through the difference in pattern between the homogenous architecture of postmortem blood and heterogenous appearance of thromboemboli.

Postmortem clots are usually microscopically characterized by masses of red blood cells with few scattered leukocytes in between. In cases of topical or generalized infections, the number of leukocytes is increased in postmortem clots, but such clots lack a fibrinous component. Acute thromboemboli show a characteristic heterogenous diffuse or layered pattern of platelets, red blood cells and leukocytes. Aging of thromboemboli is particularly difficult, because they are usually fragments detached from a distal thrombus, i.e., deep veins of calf in the case of pulmonary embolism. Acute thromboemboli can undergo processes similar to that of primary local thrombi, such as resolution, organization and recanalization. *Showers* of microscopic thromboemboli may not be recognized at all grossly and may result in sudden death.

Fat Embolism

Fat embolism is secondary to many medical conditions that release fat into the circulation, or promote the aggregation of droplets of fat in the circulation. In the majority of cases, fat embolism is a result of long bone trauma or bone joint surgery. However, soft tissue trauma as well, and a variety of conditions associated with soft tissue injuries may also result in fat embolism.

Such conditions include, burns, sickle cell disease and other hemoglobinopaties, pancreatitis osteonecrosis, rhabdomyolysis, systemic lupus erythematosus, etc. Fatty liver has been reported to be associated with fat embolism (i.e., acute fatty liver of pregnancy, fatty liver change and necrosis following Amanita mushroom poisoning).

A number of therapeutic procedures involving fat tissue manipulations may also be complicated by fat embolism. Plastic surgery procedures such as lipectomy and/or liposuction or procedures involving injection of fat to increase mass in face or breast and peri-urethral injection of autologous fat for stress incontinence, have been reported to be associated with fat embolism.

Finally, intra-venous injection, intentional or accidental of lipid solutions is associated with fat embolism.

Fat embolism may be clinically totally silent or present as a fat embolism syndrome with respiratory, neurological, hematological and cutaneous manifestations. The pathogenesis of fat embolism is still elusive, but is probably multifactorial. Both traumatic and biochemical etiologies have been proposed, including fragmentations of fat from the marrow cavity of long bones, activation of lipases by intravascular released fats, release of catecholamines and corticosteroids that cause sludging of blood with precipitation of fat particles or mobilized platelets, etc. The forensic evaluation should consider fat embolism as a possible contributory cause of death. Because fat dissolves in alcohol during routine histological procedures, fat emboli appear on H&E stained slides as empty round intravascular spaces surrounded by a peripheral line or crescent of compressed red blood cells and be easily missed. Therefore, verification of the diagnosis by special histochemical stains of lung, brain and kidney is always indicated by Sudan stain on formalin preserved tissue or frozen sections, or osmium tetraoxide stain on paraffin block sections.

It should be noted that both fat embolism and fat embolism syndrome are potentially treatable and survivable, and if survived there are usually no complications. An isolated case of fat embolism complicated by intravascular calcifications has been reported in recent years.

The determination whether the microscopic findings of fat embolism were significant enough to constitute a substantial immediate or contributory cause of death depends on a number of variables, including clinical data, the predominant affected organ (i.e., brain, lungs) and the profusion of fat emboli.

Bone Marrow Emboli

Bone marrow emboli are commonly present after bone fractures and may occasionally be fatal, if present in large numbers.

Cholesterol Emboli

Cholesterol emboli may be localized or part of a sporadic cholesterol embolic syndrome. Almost 75% of all cases occur in males with severe atherosclerotic disease and commonly

occurs days or weeks following an intravascular arterial instrumentation. Other causes include trauma and anticoagulation treatment. Spontaneous emboli occur mainly in patients with abdominal aortic aneurysms.

Cholesterol emboli are identified microscopically by the typical elongated polyhedric crevices seen in routine H&E stains.

Clear spaces or superimposed thrombi in various stages of development can be observed around the cholesterol crystals. Clinically, the cholesterol embolic syndrome is a result of end organ ischemia and may result in a rash with skin mottling, blue toes and nail bed infarction, ARSD, mesenteric ischemia, gangrene, and myocardial ischemia.

Myocarditis, Significance and Differential Diagnosis

Asymptomatic non-specific myocarditis is sometimes found to be a cause of sudden unexpected death, particularly in young people and children. In the majority of cases, the intramyocardial infiltrate is mononuclear, primarily lymphocytic, and viral cultures are often positive for Coxsackie viruses (Fig. XX-10). The adjacent myocardial fibers show varying degrees of degenerative changes, including focal necrosis. One should be prudent in making the diagnosis of fatal myocarditis, particularly if examination of multiple heart sections yields only a rare inflammatory infiltrate. It has been reported in the literature and confirmed in our experience, that such solitary infiltrates may be seen in young adults who die of unrelated causes. Furthermore, one may see severe and diffuse, asymptomatic myocarditis in otherwise healthy young adults dying of incidental traumatic causes.[26] However, in the latter situation, it may be difficult to exclude the possibility that myocarditis precipitated the unnatural event or that myocarditis may have developed after the injury.

Diabetes-Related Deaths

Recognizing diabetes mellitus as a cause of sudden unexpected death may be difficult, par-

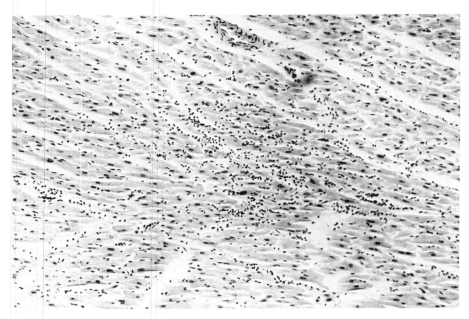

FIGURE XX-10. Myocarditis (×25, H&E stain). Non-specific myocarditis, most likely viral with, focal infiltrates of chronic inflammatory cells. Sudden death of previously healthy two-year-old.

ticularly when prior medical history is unavailable, when the patient failed to seek prior medical attention, or in the presence of an asymptomatic, atypical or unrecognized clinical course.

A number of microscopic markers may prompt suspicions of a diabetes-related death. Such markers include diabetic nephropathy, hepatic nuclear changes and distorted architecture of the pancreatic islets of Langerhans. The diabetic nephropathy often seen in neglected diabetes is Armani-Ebstein glycogen nephrosis, manifested on routine hematoxylin-eosin (HE) stains by marked vacuolization of epithelial cells of renal tubuli. This change is usually seen in the loops of Henle and in the distal tubuli. In infants, Armani-Ebstein nephropathy has been also described in certain cases of Fanconi syndrome.[27]

Severe hyperkalemia may also result in tubular changes mimicking Armani-Ebstein nephropathy, although in such cases the clear cell appearance of the renal epithelium is not due to glycogen, but to hydropic change associated with electrolyte imbalance (Fig. XX-11).

Kimmelstiel-Wilson nephropathy (intercapillary glomerulosclerosis) is a reliable indicator of long-standing diabetes mellitus, often associated with renal failure.

Another common histopathological finding in diabetes is the intranuclear vacuolization of hepatic cells, with the nuclear chromatin compressed and displaced to the periphery. Although this change is held to be non-specific, it is useful as a possible marker of diabetes (Fig. XX-12).

Other pathological changes which may point to diabetes include a reduction in the number of Langerhans cells in the usually island-rich tail of the pancreas and distortion of the architecture of the islets with interstitial sclerosis and pseudoglandular arrangements of the islets' cells.

Obviously, suspicions of a diabetes-related death should be confirmed by biochemical testing. Postmortem glucose levels in blood and cerebrospinal fluid are usually unreliable because they are affected by both hepatic glycogenolysis and bacterial decomposition. The vitreous fluid of the eyes is generally recommended for postmortem glucose and electrolyte analysis.

The presence of ketones in the urine is not per se evidence of hyperglycemic coma, because ketonuria may also be seen in starvation or as a result of acetone poisoning.

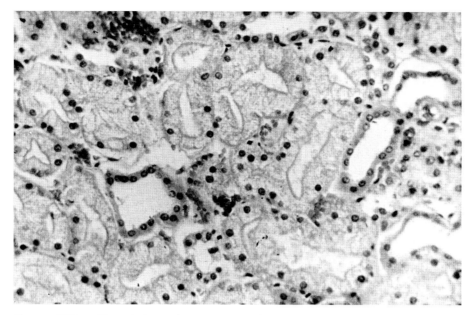

FIGURE XX-11. Hyperkalemia (×40, H&E stain). Vacuolization of renal tubuli in fatal hyperkalemia, mimicking glycogen nephrosis (Armani-Ebstein) of diabetes.

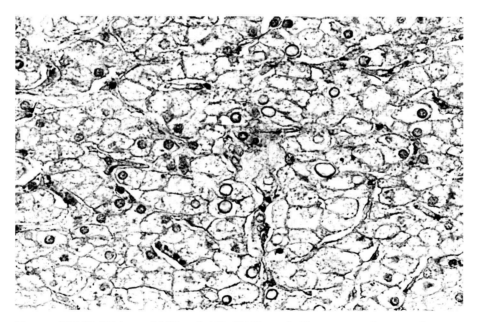

FIGURE XX-12. Diabetes Mellitus (×100, H&E stain). Hepatocytes showing glycogen vacuolization of nuclei—a non-specific marker of diabetes mellitus.

Sickle Cell Disease

Sickle cell hemoglobinopathies affect Blacks, individuals of Mediterranean extraction (Italians, Greeks), and natives of Saudi Arabia and India. Considering that 50,000 of the African Americans in the United States are homozygous for sickle cell hemoglobin and suffer from sickle cell disease and that 7–9% of all black Americans carry the sickle cell trait, it is not surprising that sickle cell crisis is occasionally encountered as a significant cause of sudden unexpected death. The entity is not always clinically recognized or known at the time of autopsy, and sudden unexpected death may well be its first diagnosed manifestation.

The autopsy may fail to reveal recognizable findings of chronic sickle cell disease, such as fatty change of heart, liver and kidneys, splenic infarcts and fibrosis, with the only diagnostic clues being microscopic in nature. It should be emphasized, however, that microscopic evidence of sickling of blood cells per se, is not necessarily an indication of sickle cell crisis.

The process of preparing histologic tissue sections may induce in vitro sickling, particularly in individuals with sickle cell disease or trait. The diagnosis of sickle cell crisis as a cause of death can be made only in the presence of characteristic microscopic changes. Such changes include marked distention and *packing* of the liver's sinusoids and central veins by large plugs of sickled cells with or without associated degenerative or destructive parenchymal changes (Fig. XX-13a–b). Similar plugs of sickled cells may also be seen in other organs such as the spleen, kidneys and brain. Phagocytosis of sickled red cells by Kupffer's cells is a common manifestation.

Fatal sickling may be precipitated by a variety of hypoxic circumstances from high altitude exposure to administration of narcotic drugs. Although fatal sickle cell crisis has been traditionally reported to occur only in patients with sickle cell disease (homozygous hemoglobin SS) and not in those with sickle cell trait (heterozygous hemoglobin SA), in recent years a number of studies have shown that particularly susceptible individuals with sickle cell trait may die when subjected to critical hypoxic conditions. Such cases have been described in anesthetized black children with sickle cell trait and in unacclimatized black military recruits subjected to rigorous training.[28,29] The pathological diagnosis of sickle cell disease at autopsy should always be confirmed by hemoglobin electrophoresis.

Primary Cardiomyopathies

Clinically undiagnosed primary cardiomyopathies are an uncommon cause of sudden death occurring primarily in young people. The microscopic picture varies considerably.[30] The myocardium of congestive (dilated) type of primary cardiomyopathy shows long strands of attenuated muscle fibers with mild vacuolization, focal hypertrophy, occasional enlarged or hyperchromatic nuclei, increased interstitial fibrosis and scattered chronic inflammatory cells.[31]

Primary hypertrophic cardiomyopathy (idiopathic hypertrophic stenosis) shows disarrayed, focally hypertrophic, or atypical interlacing myocardial fibers with an occasionally swirled or whorled pattern separated by thick strands of interstitial fibrosis.[32,33]

The obliterative type of primary cardiomyopathy (i.e., endomyocardial fibrosis, amyloidosis) is almost never seen as an asymptomatic cause of sudden unexpected death. Endomyocardial fibrosis, an obliterative type of cardiomyopathy, particularly prevalent on the African continent, also shows extensive subendocardial myocardial fibrosis and frequently, mural thrombosis.

Isolated endocardial fibroelastosis, a condition primarily affecting infants and young children, is equally exceedingly rare as a cause of sudden unexpected death. Microscopically, there is a marked thickening of the endocardium of the left ventricular wall with striking hyperplasia of elastic fibers.

Right Ventricular Dysplasia (Uhl's Disease)

In recent years, attention has been drawn to right ventricular dysplasia (Uhl's disease), a rare type of idiopathic cardiomyopathy associated with cardiac arrhythmia and sudden death.[34,35] Most patients with this condition are young adults in their twenties who are rarely symptomatic for anginal pains and/or episodes of ventricular arrhythmia. Often the sudden death occurs following recreational exercise.

The autopsy demonstrates right ventricular dilatation with severe thinning and fatty infiltration of the muscular walls, and marked reduction in the right ventricular mass, sparing the left ventricular muscle. The coronary arteries are unremarkable.

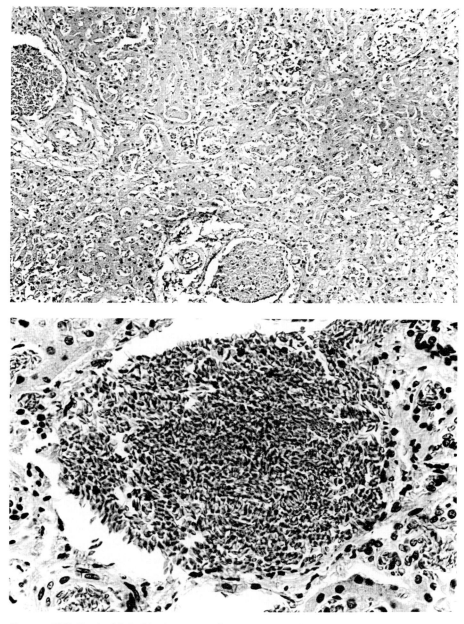

FIGURE XX-13a–b. (a) Sickle Cell Crisis (×25, H&E stain). Liver with distended central veins plugged by compact masses of sickled red blood cells, in sudden death due to sickle cell crisis precipitated by heroin use. *Note also the associated focal hepatitis and fatty change.* (b) (×100, H&E stain). Sickled red blood cells distending and plugging a central hepatic vein.

Microscopically, the right myocardium shows fatty infiltration, focal fibrosis and, occasionally prominent lymphoid infiltrates, which may at times involve the left ventricle as well.

Focal Myocardial Fibrosis

Focal myocardial fibrosis is not uncommon in sudden, unexpected death. Masson Trichrome

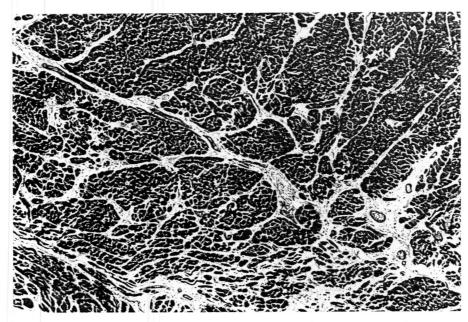

FIGURE XX-14. Focal Myocardial Fibrosis (×20, H&E stain). Myocardium with focal *spiderweb-like* pattern of interstitial fibrosis in sudden death of otherwise healthy thirty-five-year-old man.

stain for connective tissue may be helpful in substantiating a greater degree of focal myocardial fibrosis than is apparent on the routine hematoxylin-eosin stains. The etiology of the fibrosis is multifactorial and includes hypertensive cardiovascular disease, coronary heart disease, idiopathic cardiomyopathy, mitral valve prolapse, epilepsy, cocaine addiction, and bronchial asthma. A significant number of cases do not show any pathological findings other than focal myocardial fibrosis, which is most likely the result of healed myocarditis. In such cases, focal myocardial scars are often delicate and have a spidery or web-like configuration (Fig. XX-14).

A Pittsburgh-based study[36] identified a subgroup of women who died suddenly, with minimal pathologic findings at autopsy. These women had slight coronary arteriosclerosis, were usually on minor sedatives and had a psychiatric history of minor depression, marital discord or divorce. Some of the cases showed minimal focal myocardial fibrosis. The presumed mechanism of sudden death in focal myocardial fibrosis is a malignant arrhythmia.

Sarcoidosis of the Heart

Sarcoidosis of the heart is occasionally encountered as a cause of sudden unexpected death in adults, with sudden death being reported as *the most common cardiac manifestation of clinically significant sarcoidosis.*[37]

Microscopically, the pattern of the granulomatous infiltrate in the myocardium is at times different from that seen in other organs. While sarcoid infiltrates in lungs, lymph nodes, and spleen are usually in the form of distinct discrete granulomas with only occasionally coalescence, the myocardial infiltrates may present as non-discrete, diffuse, broad, granulomatous infiltrates with scattered giant cells and various degrees of fibrosis. The differential diagnosis from giant-cell myocarditis may be difficult at times.[38]

Conduction System Lesions

Another group of pathological findings which might explain sudden, unexpected death in adults involves the cardiac conduction system.[39]

Unfortunately, the conduction system is not routinely examined at autopsy because a reliable evaluation of its pathology requires a more time-consuming dissection and, often, serial sections.

Each station of the conduction system, the SA (sinoatrial) node, the atrial preferential pathway, the AV (atrioventricular) node, the approaches to the atrioventricular node, the bundles of His and the bundle branches may be affected by pathological changes and are likely to precipitate a sudden fatal arrhythmia.

Masson trichrome and silver impregnation reticulum stains are useful in demonstrating the abnormalities of the conduction system. The most common pathological changes of the conduction system include fibrosis, fatty tissue replacement, and calcifications, although many other types of lesions are also encountered, including abnormal formation of the central fibrous body, trauma, myocarditis, sarcoidosis and, rarely, tumors or hamartomas.[40] Among the latter, one should mention mesothelioma of the heart, a subendothelial hamartomatous lesion which microscopically resembles a cluster of dilated thyroid follicles or lymphatic channels.

Stress Cardiomyopathy

Most fatalities of blunt force trauma exhibit critical injuries which permit a unequivocal determination of cause, manner, and mechanism of death. However, a small subgroup of victims of homicidal assaults do not have sufficient internal injuries to explain the underlying cause or mechanism of death. In such circumstances, determination of the manner of death as a homicide is fraught with obvious difficulties.

The microscopic examination of the myocardium in such cases may reveal changes consistent with stress and the associated release of catecholamines. Microscopic changes described in such *stress cardiomyopathy* deaths include contraction bands of myocytes, granular degeneration, and non-uniform eosinophilia of subendocardial myocardial fibers (Fig. XX-15).[41] With longer survival, the myocardial lesions may exhibit focal mononuclear infiltrates and loose or compact foci of interstitial myocardial fibrosis. Experimentally stressed animals have been shown to exhibit a similar pattern of myocardial changes.[42]

A thorough microscopic examination should also include special fat stains (i.e., Sudan or Oil red O of brain, lungs and kidneys) to exclude fat embolism, a subtle complication of trauma which may be easily missed on routine examination.

It should be emphasized that potentially fatal fat embolism does not necessarily require brain involvement and that massive pulmonary fat embolism in itself can cause death (Fig. XX-16a–c).

PATTERNS OF PHYSICAL INJURIES

Gunshot Wounds

Microscopic examination may also be helpful in differentiating gunshot entrance wounds from exit wounds (Fig. XX-17). Gunshot wounds of entrance, even in the absence of powder particles, can be recognized by the presence of heat-induced denaturation of collagen at the beginning of the wound track. Gunshot wounds of exit usually lack this feature. Contaminating soil particles should not be mistaken for gunpowder particles. The presence or absence of gunpowder in *stippled* gunshot wounds may differentiate between true *stippling* caused by gunpowder which is indicative of medium range firing, and *pseudo-stippling* caused by fragmentation of frangible objects interposed between the gun and the targeted skin (i.e., a glass window, wood door).

Battered Child

Microscopic findings in child abuse are important in differentiating between agonal or post-mortem injuries associated with resuscitation and genuine premortem injuries and evaluating of the age of different traumatic injuries. Therefore, multiple samplings of injuries, including an adja-

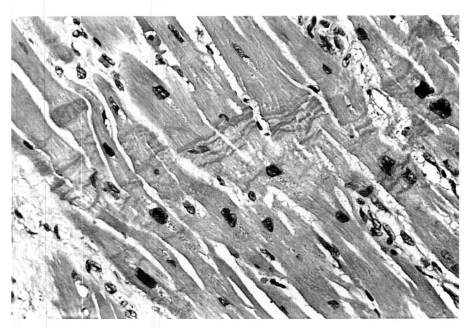

FIGURE XX-15. Stress Cardiomyopathy (×80, H&E stain). Stress cardiomyopathy with multiple transverse *contraction bands* of myocytes, granular degeneration and non-uniform staining of myocardial fibers.

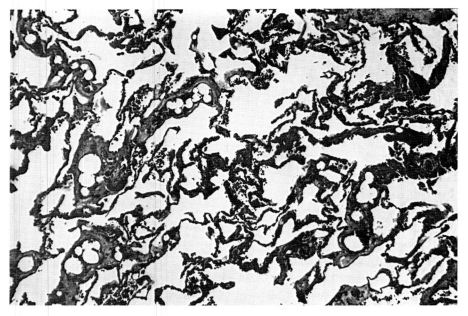

FIGURE XX-16a. Fat Embolism (×10 Lung, H&E stain). Pulmonary fat embolism. Under HE staining the emboli are invisible, and marked only by distended capillaries which are bloodless, or contain a small eccentric rim of compressed erythrocytes.

cent wedge of normal tissue, are required. Microscopic examination of the fundus of the eyes should be performed in all cases of suspected abuse. The eyes should be carefully extracted

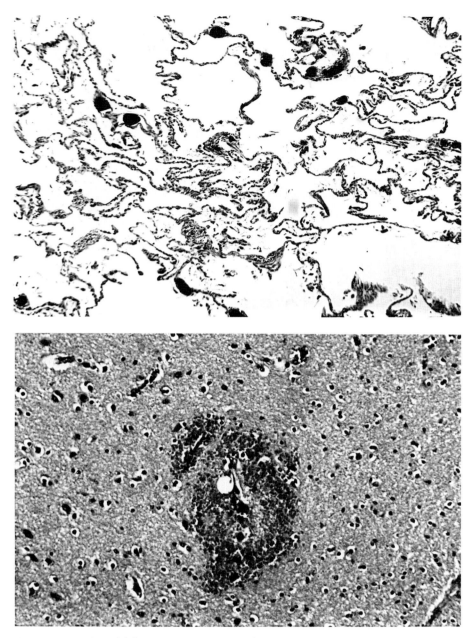

FIGURE XX-16b–c. (b) (×10 Lung, Sudan Black). Fat stains confirm the HE suspicion of fat embolism. (c) (×50, H&E stain). Fat embolus distending capillary, surrounded by large ring hemorrhage.

after removal of the viscera, in order to prevent postmortem artefactual hemorrhages. Retinal hemorrhages, as seen in *Shaken Baby Syndrome,* may be the only significant marker of possible abuse aside from the intracranial hemorrhages. It has been shown that retinal hemorrhages are often the result of abusive shaking and are not usually related to resuscitation (Fig. XX-18).[43]

Whereas, retinal hemorrhages do on occasion occur in resuscitation, they are usually much coarser and fewer in number than those incurred as a result of shaking. However, hemorrhages

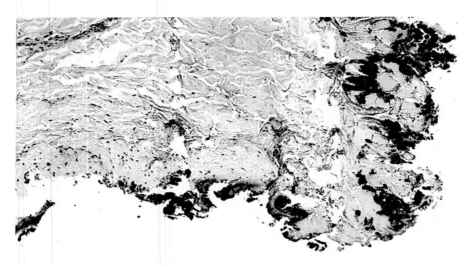

FIGURE XX-17. Near-contact gunshot wound (×32). Near-contact gunshot with heavy deposits of soot and burnt powder, destruction of the epidermis and heat denaturation changes of dermal collagen.

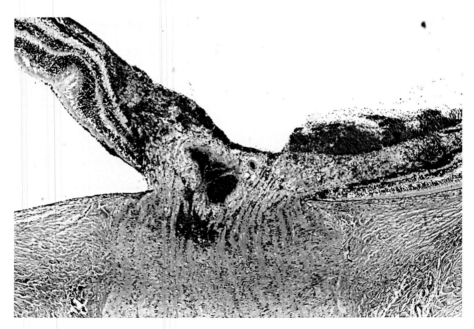

FIGURE XX-18. Shaken Baby Syndrome (×12, H&E stain). Eye section of shaken baby showing fresh hemorrhages in the retina, extending into the optic nerve.

within the optic nerve are practically indicative of shaking.

Electrical and Thermal Burns

Microscopic examination may be very helpful in the diagnosis of electrical burns.[44] Electrical burns differ from regular thermal burns by the following features (Fig. XX-19):

- Sharp borders with abrupt transition from normal to injured tissue.
- Honeycomb vacuolization of the stratum corneum (a pattern similar to that observed in electrically cauterized biopsies).

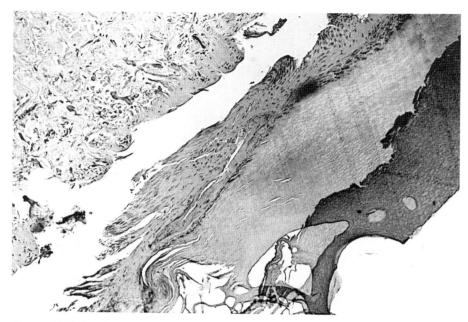

FIGURE XX-19. Electrocution Burn (×25, H&E stain). Typical electrocution burn with honeycomb vacuolization of stratum corneum, *streaking* of epithelial nuclei and intraepidermal bulla.

- Subepidermal bullae due to detachment of the epidermis from the dermis.
- Denaturation of the dermal collagen (demonstrated by the failure of subdermal collagen to stain blue and its counterstaining in red by fuchsin with Masson trichrome).
- Metallization (deposition of vaporized metal on the surface of the skin), usually seen in lightning and high voltage injuries.

Finally, the absence of electrical burns does not exclude electrocution. Electrical burns occur as a result of heat generated by the electrical resistance of the skin at the site of entrance of the electric current. If skin resistance is substantially lowered, electrical injuries may not be observed.

Diffuse Axonal Injury

Severe rotation and angular acceleration of the head may cause microscopic shearing of cerebral tissue. Such trauma may result in diffuse axonal injury (DAI), leading to coma and often death. Over 50% of victims with diffuse axonal injury expire within less than two weeks.[45] Typically the affected individuals have no lucid interval and remain unconscious until death.

DAI usually affects the corpus callosum, the rostral brain stem and white matter, and is manifested on H&E stains as oval or round eosinophilic axonal swellings ranging in size from 5 to 40 microns (retraction balls), which are scattered throughout the neuropile and are often surrounded by a clear halo (Fig. XX-20). Silver stains are used to confirm the argyrophilic axonal origin of the retraction balls. If the patient survives for weeks or months, clusters of microglia and demyelination may also be seen in the white matter.

The recognition of DAI as a cause of traumatic death is particularly important when other significant findings of impact injury are missing.[45]

Vital Reactions and Aging of Injuries

Reliable differentiation of premortem from postmortem injuries and aging of premortem injuries obviously requires histological and histochemical studies.

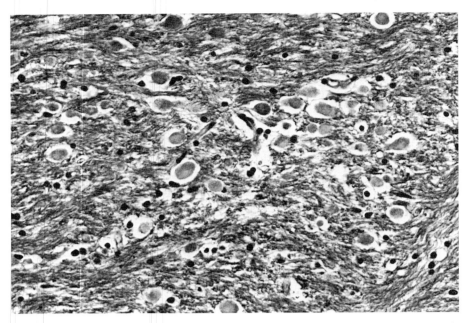

FIGURE XX-20. Diffuse Axonal Injury (×80, H&E stain). Diffuse axonal injury with numerous bulb and racquet shaped swollen axons scattered throughout the cerebral white matter.

The age of injury is the time elapsed from the infliction of tissue damage. Aging of injuries is important for medicolegal purposes in correlating the injury to an alleged precipitating event, in establishing the post-injury survival time, and in differentiating injuries inflicted at different times. Microscopic aging of injuries is based on the character, degree, and extent of cellular dissolutive changes (degeneration and necrosis) and reactive enzymatic, vascular, and cellular changes. Most of the studies reported in the forensic literature relate to aging of skin, brain, and brain-membrane injuries. Histochemical methods are particularly sensitive in the aging of early stages of injury.

Inflammatory changes cannot be detected microscopically in the first four hours following skin injury, and grossly detectable skin hemorrhage is not always reliable as a marker of vital injuries.

Polymorphonuclear cells are seen perivascularly as early as four hours after injury, increase progressively in number and form a clear peripheral front at about 12 hours and peak between at one to three days, with necrosis seen in the central area of injury. Although macrophages may appear as early as eight hours following injury, they peak at 16 to 24 hours and may even exceed the number of neutrophils in the infiltrate. Hemosiderin may be seen within macrophages as early as 72 hours from the injury. At two to four days, fibroblasts appear at the periphery of the wound and epithelization of small wounds is generally completed. At four days the first collagen fibers start to form and between four and five days there is a rich ingrowth of capillaries. At six days, the lymphocytic infiltrate reaches a peak at the periphery of the wound. After 10 to 14 days, large wounds show progressive maturation of granulation tissue.

The type and patterns of enzymes within the central and peripheral zones of skin lesions vary with the time interval following injury. The general pattern is an enzymatic depletion in the central area of the injured skin, which is paralleled, or shortly followed, by a corresponding increase in the peripheral zone. According to Rekallio,[46] after only one to two hours following the injury, adenosine triphosphatases and esterases decrease in the central area of injury and increase in the peripheral zone. Acid phosphatase decreases in the central area only after four to eight hours and increase in the peripheral zone between four to six hours.

In Europe, enzymatic histochemical staining is much more popular than in America, where few, if any forensic centers use such procedures. However, on both continents, routine hematoxylin-eosin slides and basic histochemical stains (iron stain for hemosiderin and Masson trichrome for demonstration of collagen) are commonly used for aging.

Aging of Brain Contusions

According to Loberg and Torvik,[47] aging of brain contusions is fairly accurate when based on the microscopic patterns of neuronal and glial injuries, granulocytic response, vascular changes and presence of fat and hemosiderin within macrophages. Early neuronal changes consist of diffuse cytoplasmic eosinophilia and decreased nuclear basophilia and may be seen as early as one hour after injury and may persist for weeks. Another early neuronal change seen minutes after injury is the presence of dark neurons with wavy apical dendrites. Within two to three days, many of the dark neurons evolve into eosinophilic shrunken cells. Axonal swelling (retraction balls) similar to those seen after recent infarcts and diffuse axonal injury start to be seen at the edges of the injury after two to five days and is common after five days.

Subpial glial swelling, apparently oligodendroglia, can be observed from a few minutes to four to five days after trauma. Necrotic glial cells with eosinophilic nuclei are commonly observed as early as six to 12 hours, and, in almost all cases, surviving longer. Astrocytes showing reactive changes can be seen as early as five days after injury and gemistocyte transformation is apparent by the tenth to fifteenth day. Extravascular karyorrhectic granulocytes may be seen as early as the end of the second day and thereafter. Presence of hemosiderin and fat within macrophages may be observed at the margins of the injury at three to four days. Finally, endothelial swelling is observed after 12 to 24 hours followed by sprouting of new capillaries after three to four days. It has been pointed out that this early change is in stark contrast to ischemic injury in which comparable changes are not seen until 12 to 24 hours after the hypoxic event.

Aging of Complicating Bronchopneumonia

Accurate aging of acute bronchopneumonia is difficult and evaluation should cautiously consider the following factors:
- Acute bronchopneumonia may develop within a short period of time, (within 4 to 6 hours, and the earliest we have seen is 2 hours).
- Presence of aspirated material may relate the start of bronchopneumonia to a known episode of aspiration prior to death.
- Presence of organizing pneumonia is indicative of a process in excess of 7 to 10 days.

Heat Stroke

Heat stroke occurs when persistently high environmental temperatures coupled with endogenous heat production result in failure of the body's thermoregulatory mechanisms. Microscopic changes in heat stroke can be seen in the peripheral muscles, heart, liver, and brain.[48-50] These changes are primarily due to dramatic elevations in body temperature, greater than or equal to 40 degrees Celsius, and therefore, are not dissimilar to those seen in drug induced hyperpyrexia and malignant hyperthermia.

The peripheral muscle injury ranges from rhabdomyolysis with severe degenerative changes to full necrosis of striated muscle fibers, reactive proliferation of sarcolemmal nuclei, and dystrophic calcifications. Rhabdomyolysis and necrosis are particularly evident in the muscles of locomotion (Fig. XX-21a–b). The myocardium may also show evidence of heat stroke with focal degeneration and necrosis and a peculiar *teased* or *moth eaten* appearance.

Liver injuries range from focal degeneration and necrosis in mild cases to severe and widespread centrilobular necrosis in cases of shock. The brain may show varying degrees of focal neurological damage, including focal neuronal

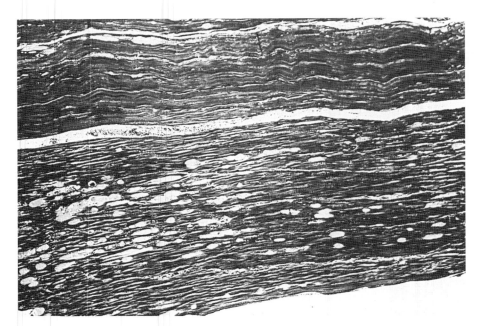

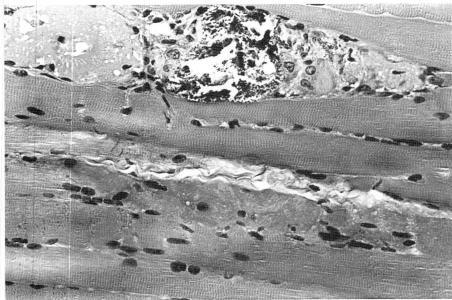

FIGURE XX-21a–b. (a) Heatstroke - Rhabdomyolysis (×5, H&E stain). Peripheral muscle with focal necrosis in twenty-two-year-old man who developed heat stroke and severe rhabdomyolysis following exercise during hot weather. (b) (×80, H&E stain). Necrosis of myocardial fibers with swelling and calcifications.

shrinkage and necrosis, especially within the Purkinje cerebellar cortical cells which show a greater selective loss. Similar changes may be seen in other conditions such as global brain ischemia, pontocerebellar degeneration, and Friedrich's ataxia. However, in global brain ischemia the process is not restricted to the cerebellum, and involves the entire brain, while in the other two conditions, the cerebellar damage is more limited. Secondary gross and microscopic changes are also common and reflect the presence of complicating hepatorenal failure and sepsis.

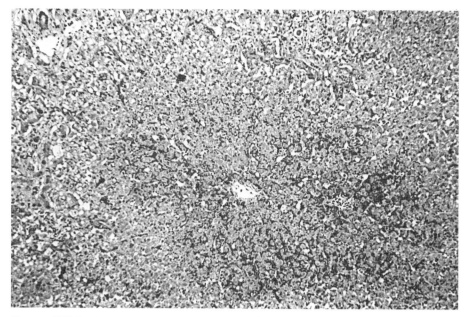

FIGURE XX-22. Aceto-Aminophen Liver Injury (×20, H&E stain). Extensive pericentral and midzonal hepatic necrosis in acetaminophen poisoning.

Cold Exposure

Gross pathological findings in cold exposure (hypothermia) are generally rare and non-specific, including cherry-red lividity, excoriation of ears, nose and hands, gastric erosions, and petechiae in peripheral muscles. Microscopic examination may reveal intra-pulmonary hemorrhages, particularly in infants, acute hemorrhagic pancreatitis or focal pancreatitis with fat necrosis and small myocardial degenerative foci.[51]

Toxic Injuries and Poisoning

Microscopic patterns of toxic injuries depend on the target-tissue specificity of the agent, intra-organ and tissue predilection, systemic and focal physiological effects, common adulterants, and related complications. Certain organs such as the liver show a monotonous reaction to different types of injury, whether ischemic or toxic. Survived liver injuries progress in uniform fashion, although hydropic degeneration, fatty change, parenchymal cell dropout and necrosis, reactive inflammatory infiltrates, fibrosis, to full blown cirrhosis. However, even with such monomorphic reactions, localization and intensity of microscopic findings may provide clues as to the etiology of the injury. Phosphorus poisoning is associated with periportal fatty change and necrosis. Dimethyl glycol toxicity, on the other hand, is associated with marked pericentral hydropic degeneration of the liver. Fatty change associated with alcohol toxicity is also predominantly pericentral and mid-zonal and, except for the most severe degree of liver steatosis, the periportal spaces are usually well preserved. Carbon tetrachloride poisoning is initially associated with pericentral fatty change and later with frank pericentral necrosis. Acetaminophen toxicity typically shows centrilobular necrosis (Fig. XX-22). However, hypoxic or ischemic injuries are also primarily centrilobular and may result in centrilobular necrosis. On the basis of the microscopic examination of the liver alone, it is often difficult, if not impossible, to differentiate between toxic and hypoxic injuries with the same hepatic localization.

On the other hand, in the cerebellum, toxic injuries can be easily differentiated from ischemic injuries. Toxic injuries affect the granular layer of

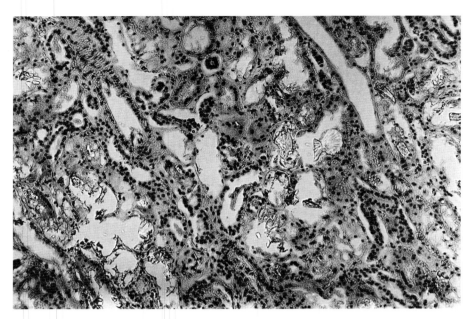

FIGURE XX-23. Ethylene-glycol Poisoning (×20 Polarized, H&E stain). Ethylene-glycol poisoning with focal necrosis of renal tubuli, many containing birefringent oxalates with typical fan-like or sheaf configuration.

the cortex which becomes focally or diffusely hypocellular with sparing of Purkinje cells. In ischemic injuries, the Purkinje cells of the cerebellar cortex show degeneration necrosis or lysis, while the granular cell layer is largely spared.

The severity of cerebral edema may also be helpful in diagnosis. Hexachlorophene poisoning has been reported to cause severe edema with a microscopic lattice-like appearance of the cerebral parenchyma, *(spongiosis)*.

Toxic by-products may manifest as cytoplasmic or intranuclear inclusion bodies, with distinct morphological characteristics, assisting in identification of the toxic agent. *(See discussion below on markers of poisoning.)*

It should be emphasized that compounds which are chemically related may show great variation in their potency, pathophysiological effects and corresponding microscopic findings. Methanol (wood alcohol), for example, is more toxic than ethanol (grain alcohol), is bio-oxidized to formic acid, and displays a specific affinity for optic nerve injury.[52] Ethylene glycol and di-ethylene glycol, two closely related compounds, display different histological patterns of injury.

Ethylene glycol causes severe kidney injury with production of large amounts of oxalates, an almost unique type of chemical meningitis secondary to presence of oxalates in the subarachnoidal vessels, indolent precipitation of oxalates in the cerebral parenchyma, and no liver damage (Fig. XX-23). Di-ethylene glycol, on the other hand, while also producing severe degeneration and necrosis of the renal tubular epithelium, generates little or no oxalates, does not cause chemical meningitis and is associated with pericentral hydropic degeneration of the liver (Fig. XX-24).[53,54]

Inorganic and organic mercury poisoning also show marked differences in pathophysiology and correspondent histological changes in spite of their chemical kinship. Inorganic mercury compounds cause hemorrhagic colitis, severe renal damage with tubular necrosis affecting primarily the terminal proximal tubuli, and non-specific neuronal injuries.[55] On the other hand, organic mercury poisoning causes severe and selective central nervous system injuries with dissolution of granular cells of the cerebellum, sparing of the Purkinje cells, and no renal injuries.[56]

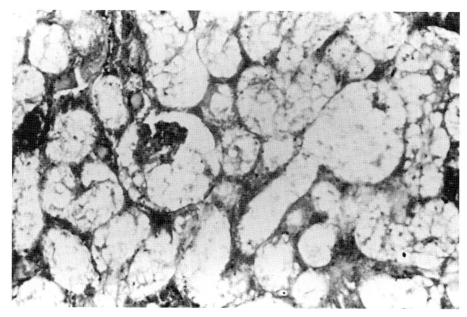

FIGURE XX-24. Diethylene Glycol Poisoning (×25, H&E stain). Renal tubuli in diethylene glycol poisoning, showing severe dilation and necrosis, but no oxalate crystals.

Drug Abuse

The microscopic patterns of drug abuse are a function of the type of drug, route of administration, various adulterants or contaminating substances, and drug-related complications. Intravenous administration of drugs is associated with:
- Topical phlebitis and periphlebitis at site of injection.
- Periportal hepatic triaditis, characterized by presence of chronic inflammatory infiltrates in hepatic periportal spaces, occasionally with presence of foreign body type multinucleated giant cells and asteroid bodies (Fig. XX-25).
- Embolization of foreign body contaminants of narcotics such as insoluble crystalline filler material and cotton or other fibers (Fig. XX-26a–b).

The foreign material triggers a foreign body reaction which varies from presence of isolated multinucleated giant cells to a florid granulomatous reaction. The latter usually occurs when an addict injects himself with a narcotic which has been primarily intended for oral consumption, such as Talwin (pentazocine) tablets or amphetamine pills, which contains large amounts of a calcium complex insoluble filler. Often, the insoluble adulterants are birefringent and can easily be demonstrated under a polarizing microscope, even if the inflammatory reaction is minimal. Most of the time, however, foreign body embolization, as marked by the birefringent crystals, is evident in lung capillaries and hepatic periportal spaces. In rare instances, emboli can break through or bypass the pulmonary circulation and reach the systemic blood vessels with embolization into coronary, renal and cerebral arteries. Other complications associated with intravascular administration of addictive drugs include sepsis, bacterial endocarditis, viral hepatitis and AIDS.

Topical reactions to the administration of a drug may result from vasoreactive changes induced by the drug. For example, intranasal administration of cocaine, which is a potent vasoconstrictor, may cause ischemic necrosis of the nasal mucosa and nasal cartilage with septal perforation. Necrosis of the nasal sinus, pharynx and soft palate have also been described in recent years.[57] This midline necrosis is often associated with a granulomatous inflammation and may be mistaken for Wegener's granulomatosis.

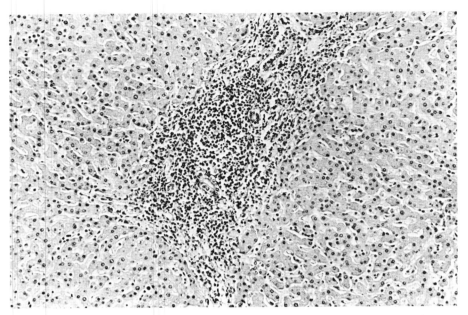

FIGURE XX-25. (×25, H&E stain). Heavy lymphocytic infiltration in a periportal space of the liver in intravenous narcotic addict.

Systemic manifestations of drug abuse may also include a variety of microscopic changes, some extensive enough to be reflected grossly, others more subtle. Cocaine intoxication, because of its associated hypertensive and vaso-constrictive effects, may result in hypertensive cerebral hemorrhage, focal myocardial necrosis, focal myocardial fibrosis, and, rarely, focal or zonal fatty change and necrosis of the liver. The liver necrosis is apparently primarily due to the specific hepatoxicity of norcocaine oxide, a metabolite which induces the formation of toxic lipid peroxides.[58]

Other drugs of addiction have also been shown to have specific toxicity for certain organs. For example, 1-methyl-4 phenylpyridium (MPP+), a toxic metabolite of a meperidine derivative, 1-methyl-4-phenyl-1,2,3,6 tetrahy-dropyridine (MPTP or new heroin), one of the designer drugs, is specifically destructive of the dopaminergic neurons of the substantia nigra in the brain, and produces irreversible Parkinson-ism and/or dopamine deficiency related cogni-tive changes.[59,60] Intravenous addiction also results in a decreased immunological status which sensitizes patients to a plethora of bacteri-al, viral, and fungal infections.

Alcohol Toxicity

The most common type of addiction is that related to ethanol consumption. Acute and chronic alcoholism and related conditions affect millions of individuals throughout the United States and the world. The chronic toxic effects of alcohol affect virtually every organ.

The associated microscopic changes are important in recognizing the various alcohol-related diseases (see Table XX-1).[61,62] Some of the changes are related to the direct toxicity of alco-hol (i.e., alcoholic hepatitis and pancreatitis) while others are related to secondary dietary or electrolyte disturbances. For example, Wer-nicke's encephalopathy is related to thiamine deficiency, while central pontine myelinolysis is ascribed to a too rapid correction of alcohol-related hyponatremia.[63-65]

Intracellular Markers of Poisoning

Recognition and diagnosis of birefringent crys-tals within human tissues may reveal the cause of death, detect the presence of intravenous addic-tion, or unmask exposure to significant toxic agents. Detection of birefractile substances does

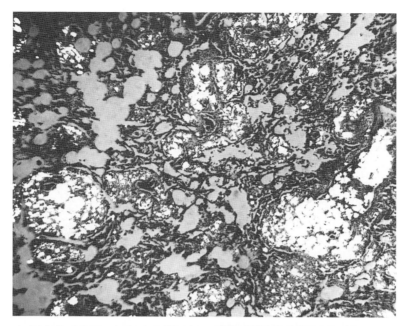

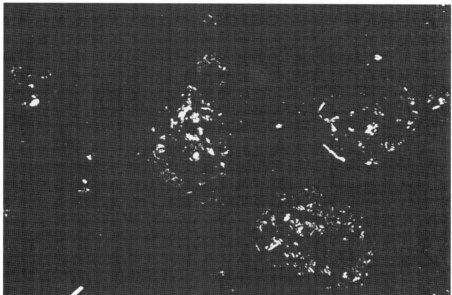

FIGURE XX-26a–b. (a) Embolic Filler Granuloma (×6 Lung, H&E stain). Pulmonary foreign-body granuloma in a thirty-five-year-old addict who injected crushed tablets of Talwin (Pentazocine). (b) (×12 Polarized, H&E stain). Under polarized light birefringent crystals are demonstrated within giant cells.

not necessarily require availability of an inbuilt polarizing microscope. Two inexpensive polarizing lenses from sunglasses may serve as a polarizer/analyzer set.

The most commonly encountered birefringent crystals in forensic practice are oxalates, talc, starch, and calcium complex fillers of drugs or medication. These crystals show different morphological and polarizing patterns which permit relatively easy identification. Oxalates may appear in tissue as a result of oxalate poisoning, ethylene glycol poisoning, or methoxyflurane (an

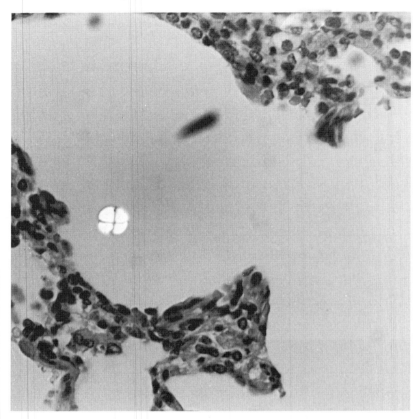

FIGURE XX-27. Starch Crystals (×100 Polarized, H&E stain). Birefringent glove powder starch (amylose) crystals showing typical Maltese Cross pattern.

anesthetic) toxicity and under polarizing light are seen as a typical laminated sheaf or fan. In ethylene glycol poisoning, deposits of oxalates with associated chemical meningitis may also be seen in subarachnoidal blood vessels and within the white matter of the brain. Oxalates may also be seen in acute and chronic renal failure. Magnesium silicate crystals (talc) are seen as birefringent, thin, prismatic crystals. Starch (amylose), a complex crystalline carbohydrate which stains faintly eosinophilic and is strongly PAS positive and birefringent, presents under polarized light a typical _Maltese cross_ pattern (Fig. XX-27). Its relative chemical inertness accounts for its widespread use as surgical glove powder although it has been reported to occasionally cause granulomatous peritonitis in sensitized patients.[66] Starch crystals are often observed in microscopic sections as artefactual contaminants from technician's gloves.

Calcium-Complex Fillers

Birefringent crystalline emboli, originating from contaminants of narcotics or from fillers of oral medications, are often seen in addicts who inject themselves with dissolved narcotic powders (i.e., heroin, cocaine) or with narcotic oral tablets such as Pentazocine (Talwin) or amphetamines.

These birefringent emboli may be seen in capillaries of the lungs and in hepatic periportal spaces. If the embolization is massive, it may result in a severe and diffuse granulomatous inflammation and fibrosis of the lungs. Occasionally, the crystalline emboli may break through the pulmonary filter into the systemic circulation. In many intravenous addicts of heroin and cocaine, the pulmonary findings are minimal and under polarized light a few birefringent crystals may be observed within or outside sparsely scattered giant cells.

Intracellular Inclusion Bodies

Intranuclear inclusion bodies may also be markers of poisoning. For example, lead poisoning is associated with eosinophilic intranuclear inclusion bodies in the epithelial cells of the renal proximal tubuli and in hepatocytes. The intranuclear inclusion bodies are composed of a lead protein complex, and may disappear following adequate chelating treatment.[67] Similarly, boric acid poisoning is associated, in about 10% of cases, with the presence of intracytoplasmic inclusions in acinar cells of the pancreas. Similar inclusions may be seen in other conditions, such as fatal gastroenteritis.[68,69]

ENVIRONMENTAL DISEASES

Environmental and occupational disease fatalities are categorized by most coroners or medical examiners as natural conditions outside the proper forensic jurisdiction, and, therefore, most autopsies of such cases are hospital based.

Unfortunately, many hospital pathologists are unaware of the full spectrum of medicolegal problems associated with the above conditions and often the forensic pathologist is called upon to act as a private consultant. When evaluating the microscopic findings of an environmental disease, the forensic reviewer must first determine whether the microscopic sections were properly sampled and whether they appear to be consistent with the locations, extent and severity of the diagnostic lesions grossly described by the initial prosector. Furthermore, a thorough clinicopathological correlation is required in order to fully appreciate the significance of the microscopic changes.

The two most common occupational diseases coming to the attention of forensic pathologists in the United States are coal-worker's pneumoconiosis (CWP) and asbestosis.[70] This is not the place to enter into a detailed description of these two pathological conditions. However, it is important to point out a few salient aspects of the forensic importance of the microscopic findings in these conditions.

Coal Worker's Pneumoconiosis

Pneumoconiosis, resulting from long-standing occupational exposure to silica and coal, has a wide spectrum of lung findings ranging from non-significant anthracosis to various degrees of simple coal worker's pneumoconiosis (CWP), and finally to the highly disabling progressive massive fibrosis (PMF).

Although the presence of positive microscopic pulmonary findings is obviously essential in establishing the diagnosis, it is not sufficient in itself and must be correlated to particular occupational exposure, clinical history and findings, radiological, respiratory and other laboratory tests, and the gross pathology at the autopsy. This will permit evaluation of the significance of the disease process.

In simple coal worker's pneumoconiosis, the major types of lesions observed are macules and nodules, with associated chronic emphysema and interstitial fibrosis (Fig. XX-28). The macules are grossly non-palpable black foci, measuring up to 5 mm, which are composed of peribronchiolar aggregates of macrophages laden with anthracotic pigment. Nodules are more advanced lesions and consist of grossly palpable black foci varying in size from a few mm to 2 cm.

Microscopically, the nodules typically show an acellular hyaline layered core or whorled hyaline center surrounded by fibrous tissue and infiltrated by macrophages containing anthracotic pigment (Fig. XX-29). Free anthracotic pigment is also seen. The periphery of the fibrous area is less compact than the lesion's core, and often exhibits radial, spidery projections. Under polarized light, small birefringent acicular crystals, indicative of silica, are seen inside nodules. Varying degrees of interstitial fibrosis, scar, and centrilobular emphysema are present around the nodules (Fig. XX-30).

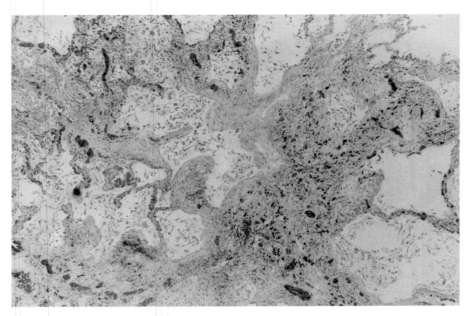

FIGURE XX-28. Interstitial type of coal workers' pneumoconiosis.

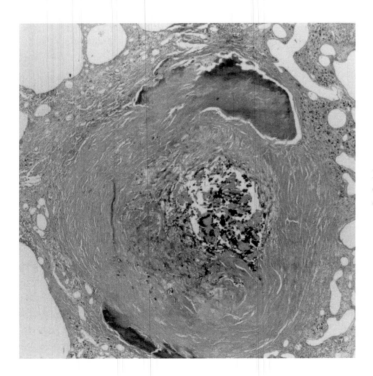

FIGURE XX-29. Hyaline (silicotic type) micronodule of coal workers' pneumoconiosis with central anthracotic pigmentation and focal calicification.

The pneumoconiotic nodules may be considered to be micronodules (0.1–0.6 cm) or macronodules (0.6 cm or more). The likelihood of the simple coal workers pneumoconiosis being a substantial cause of death, depends on the profusion and extent of pneumoconiotic lesions and consideration of symptomatology and clinical laboratory and circumstantial pertinent data.

Complicated coal worker's pneumoconiosis, or progressive massive fibrosis (PMF), is the

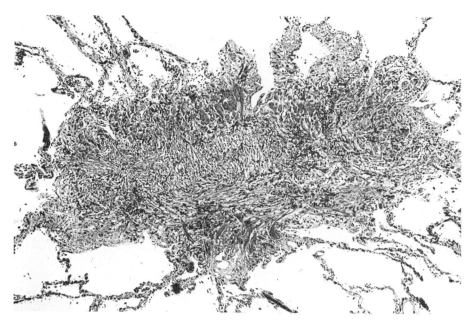

FIGURE XX-30. (×12, H&E stain). Lung of sand-blasting worker with nodule of silicosis showing adjacent scar and emphysema.

most severe stage of the disease, and present when the fibrous anthracotic scars or nodules measure in excess of 2 cm. It should be emphasized that one solitary focus is sufficient to establish the diagnosis of progressive massive fibrosis. The hilar lymph nodes may also contain pneumoconiotic nodules and often show peripheral (eggshell) calcifications. Smoking contributes to the severity of coal worker's pneumoconiosis by adding an additional component to the coal dust-related bronchiolitis. It should also be noted that recent studies have linked long-term exposure to coal and silica to the development of carcinoma of the lung and stomach.

In the past decades studies have revealed an additional pattern of coal workers pneumoconiosis characterized by interstitial pulmonary fibrosis with anthracotic pigmentation and presence of silica crystals, and few or no nodules. In recent decades it has also been amply substantiated in the medical literature that simple coal workers' pneumoconiosis is associated not only with focal (scar) emphysema around the pneumoconiotic nodules (Fig. XX-31), but also with diffuse centrilobular emphysema and chronic obstructive lung disease.

A number of studies have also alleged a causal connection between exposure to mixed coal dust containing silica and associated pneumoconiosis and the development of lung carcinoma.

Asbestos

Asbestos fibers are straight or serpentine fibrous silicates with the most common being chrysotile, crocidolite, and amosite.[71] Inhalation of asbestos fibers can result in a variety of injuries, such as pneumoconiosis (asbestosis) with severe pulmonary fibrosis, pleural adhesions, fibrocalcific plaques of the parietal pleura, pleural and peritoneal mesotheliomas, and bronchogenic carcinoma.

A significantly elevated number of cases of gastrointestinal cancer in asbestos-exposed individuals has also been described.

The typical microscopic marker of the asbestos exposure is the presence of *asbestos bodies* in the lungs. Asbestos bodies are beaded drumstick or dumbbell-like structures having an asbestos core and a coat of complex glycoproteins and hemosiderin (Fig. XX-32).[72]

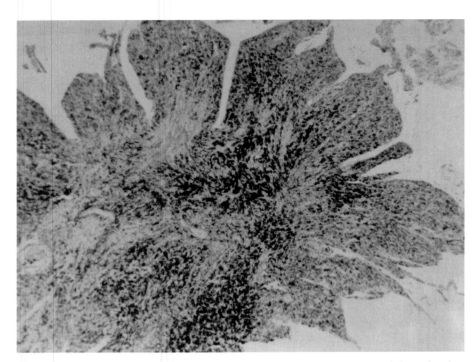

FIGURE XX-31. Stellate, mixed coal dust-type pneumoconiotic micronodule with adjacent scar (focal) emphysema.

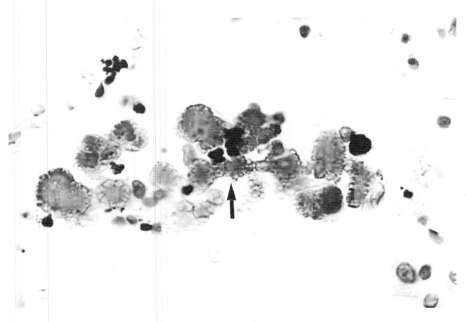

FIGURE XX-32. Asbestos Body (×100, H&E stain). Asbestos body with typical drum-stick configuration (arrow). Note additional adjacent asbestos bodies in cross section.

When evaluating the microscopic pattern of asbestos (fibrous silicates) related diseases, several facts should be kept in mind:

1. The significant pathological finding of asbestosis is the interstitial pulmonary fibrosis, caused by the fibrogenic asbestos dust. However, the

fibrosis is non-specific, and the diagnosis of asbestosis can be substantiated only by the presence of asbestos bodies.

2. Presence in the lungs of asbestos fibers per se, is not necessarily an indication of asbestosis. Isolated asbestos fibers, with typical golden drumstick configuration, may be seen in most urban dwellers' lungs. Furthermore, the diagnosis of asbestos bodies rests not just on the appearance, but also on the presence of asbestos at their core, because on rare occasions other fibers may become coated in a similar fashion, by iron-complex proteins, so called *ferruginous bodies.*[73]

3. The damaged alveolar epithelium may show eosinophilic intracytoplasmic hyaline inclusions resembling Mallory bodies. However, these inclusions are non-specific and may be seen with other types of injury such as organizing pneumonia and radiation pneumonitis.

4. Presence of parietal hyaline pleural plaques is not an indication of the severity of exposure to asbestos, because such plaques are often seen following light exposure with no pulmonary impairment.

5. Hyaline plaques as a rule, do not contain asbestos fibers.

6. All types of asbestos are fibrogenic.

7. All types of asbestos are carcinogenic, especially crocidolite.

8. The concentration, i.e., the severity of exposure to asbestos fibers may be determined by quantitative chemical analysis of lung tissue.

ABORTION

The medicolegal evaluation of abortion is particularly difficult and almost invariably requires the assistance of microscopic evaluation. The major problems which must be addressed in such instances include an adequate substantiation of the presence of abortion and the determination of the nature and actual quality of the abortion method used and its relationship to the death of the woman, if death occurred. Proper documentation and evaluation of the findings are essential, particularly in cases of criminal abortion. One should realize that criminal abortion occurs not only in countries in which abortions are by-and-large illegal, but also in countries which have legalized abortion. In the United States for example, the estimates of the annual number of illegal abortions performed between 1872–1979 varied from 5,000 to 23,000 per year, a ratio of at least 1 to 1,000 legal abortions performed during this time. Criminal abortions have a particularly high morbidity and mortality, but even therapeutic abortion carries a certain percentage of morbidity and death.

Substantiating the Presence of Abortion

The circumstances of death and findings of uterine bleeding and laceration may raise suspicion of abortion. However, these findings are not diagnostically sufficient because rape or violent voluntary sexual practices may induce similar injuries. Abortion may be substantiated by the presence of enlargement of the uterus, decidual changes and the intra- and/or extrauterine presence of trophoblastic material or fetal remains. Obviously, the presence of abortion does not indicate how it occurred, whether it occurred spontaneously or was induced, and by whom it was performed (i.e., by a physician, a non-medical person or the woman herself).

Spontaneous abortion is a common occurrence and should be properly considered and excluded before a diagnosis of induced abortion is made. In attempting to make the diagnosis of a spontaneous abortion it is suggested that the examination of the products of conception be made according to the Rushton classification.[74,75]

Rushton described the products of conception in spontaneous abortion as consisting of one of the following types:

Blighted Ova

The blighted ovum consists of an intact, delicate sac containing a slightly mucoid material, with either no embryo or deformed or vestigial embryonal and/or placental remains. The gestational age in such cases is usually between nine and 14 weeks. Microscopically, the chorionic villi show hydatiform changes, with an attenuated trophoblastic layer, and a myxomatous, avascular stroma. Occasionally, clusters of trophoblastic cells become engulfed in the villous stroma.

Macerated Embryo or Fetus and/or Macerated Placenta

Even if a fetus is absent, it is possible to recognize such cases by examination of the placenta. The histological changes in such cases include villous stromal fibrosis with collapse or obliteration of the villous vasculature, deposition of iron and calcium salts in the villous stroma, basement membrane of the blood vessels and trophoblast, and before 11 weeks gestation on degenerated, nucleated red cells. Also present are increased syncytial knotting, irregular villi and entrapped, intravillous trophoblastic islands. Increased fibrin deposition in the basal area of the placenta may be visible even grossly and is known as maternal floor infarction of the placenta.

Fresh Embryo or Fetus

In such cases, the placental findings are either normal or the placenta appears to be older than suggested by the clinical history. The presence of abnormalities of the fetus obviously increases the likelihood that the abortion was spontaneous.

In order to substantiate the above findings, one should sample for histological examination, not only the uterine wall, but also any intra- and/or extrauterine blood clots or curettage material, if available.

The presence of microscopic, fetal, or placental tissue is indicative of abortion. One should be cautious in diagnosing abortion on the basis of decidual endometrial changes alone because hormonal treatment or ectopic pregnancy may produce almost identical changes.

An autopsy of the formed fetus is mandatory in order to evaluate the presence of congenital malformations or trauma which might have precipitated the abortion. The microscopic examination may reveal manifestations of fatal intrauterine hypoxia, such as amniotic fluid aspiration (Fig. XX-33), or findings of overwhelming intrauterine infection. Cytogenetic studies should be carried out on the fetal and/or placental tissue in order to exclude the possibility of chromosomal abnormalities such as those occurring in Down's Syndrome (mongolism), trisomy 18 (Edwards' Syndrome), or Turner's Syndrome.

Spontaneous abortion may have resulted from an iatrogenic cause such as a postamniocentesis fetal hemorrhage or exposure to environmental pollutants. Occupations with exposure to anesthetic agents, laboratory work, chemical sterilization with ethylene oxide and glutaraldehyde, copper smelting, and soldering, have been shown to carry an increased risk of spontaneous abortion.

How the Abortion was Performed?

In general, the clinical history or the gross examination is more likely to answer this question. The accepted methods of therapeutic or selective legal abortion include dilatation and curettage, catheter insertion, with or without vacuum suction, the intrauterine instillation of hypertonic saline or urea, prostaglandins, or other abortifacients.

Criminal abortion, whether self-induced or performed by a non-medical person, is generally done by administering toxic abortifacients, such as quinine, or by applying intrauterine trauma using a variety of non-sterilized objects (metal rods, clothes hangers, wooden sticks, etc.). Occasionally, in cases of fatal criminal abortion, the physical object used may be retrieved or the abortifacient may be substantiated by chemical analysis. Microscopic changes in some tissues may also suggest the nature of the abortifacient used *(see below)*.

The increased incidence of alcoholism and drug abuse in pregnant women has resulted in a parallel increase in the mortality of fetuses exposed to addictive drugs. Therefore, in addition to the standard pathological examination, a

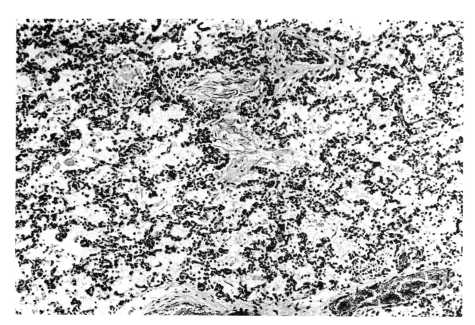

FIGURE XX-33. Amniotic Fluid Aspiration (×32, H&E stain). Lung of stillborn (40+ weeks) with alveoli flooded by amniotic fluid with proteinaceous material and multiple keratine squamae. The distended, well-developed alveoli demonstrate the difficulty in differentiating between the lung of a mature stillborn and that of an infant born alive.

thorough toxicological screening of the deceased fetuses is required to exclude the possibility of a drug-related death.

Pathological Findings in Fatal Abortions

Medical abortion is not free of complications or deaths, although criminal abortion is undoubtedly more risky. Amniotic fluid embolism, disseminated intravascular coagulation and uncontrolled infections do occur and may occasionally result in death.

The demonstration of complications as a cause of death is largely based on microscopic examination. Amniotic fluid embolism may occur in obstetric situations other than abortions, including difficult labor, traumatic deliveries and following the use of Pitocin or other uterine stimulants. Microscopically, lung capillaries may be found to transport various components of amniotic fluid, including epithelial squamae, lanugo hair, mucin, and meconium (Fig. XX-34a–b).

Disseminated intravascular coagulation may sometimes be seen in conjunction with amniotic fluid embolism, but occurs mainly as a complication in itself. Microscopically, thrombi composed of platelets and fibrin may be seen in the viscera including the brain, lungs, kidneys, heart, liver, etc. Associated with the capillary thrombi are microinfarcts of affected organs. The kidneys may show bilateral renal cortical necrosis. Disseminated intravascular coagulation (D.I.C.) is a particularly common complication of septic abortion.

Quinine induced abortion may be suspected as the cause of death when acute intravascular hemolysis and hemoglobinuria lead to fulminant anemia and renal failure, especially when the victim has previously experienced nausea, vertigo, tinnitus, deafness, and amblyopia. The pathological findings in the kidneys are typical of hemoglobinuric nephrosis, with numerous casts, degenerative and necrotic tubular changes and interstitial edema.

Fetal Pathology in Saline-Induced Abortion

A particular category of abortion in which the microscopic pathological changes in the aborted

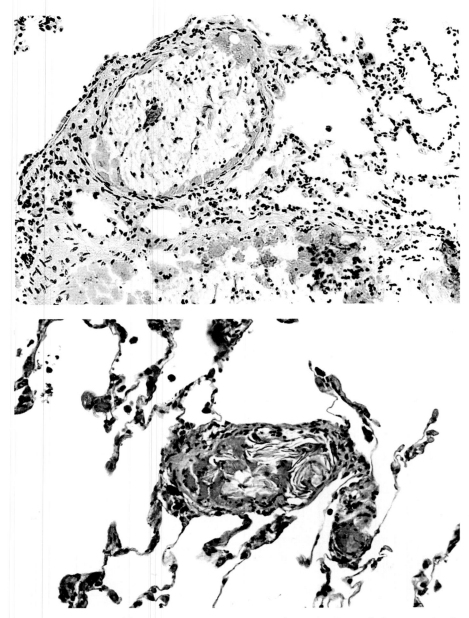

FIGURE XX-34a–b. (a) Amniotic Fluid Embolism (×32, H&E stain). Lumen of pulmonary capillary occluded by amniotic fluid embolus with wavy mucus streaks and semilunar keratin squamae. The intravascular blood is compressed peripherally by the embolus into a dark rim, overlying the intima. (b) (×50, H&E stain). Plug of keratin squamae occluding capillary.

fetus and membranes may reveal the type of procedure used is that of saline-induced abortion.[76]

Saline-induced abortion consists of amniocentesis replacement of 200 to 220 mL of amniotic fluid with a 23.5% solution of hypertonic saline. Most saline-induced abortions are administered in the second trimester of gestation, with approximately one-quarter of the fetuses weighing between 100 and 199 grams and two-thirds weighing between 200 and 299 grams. The instillation of the hypertonic solution causes placental and umbilical lesions consisting of subamniotic

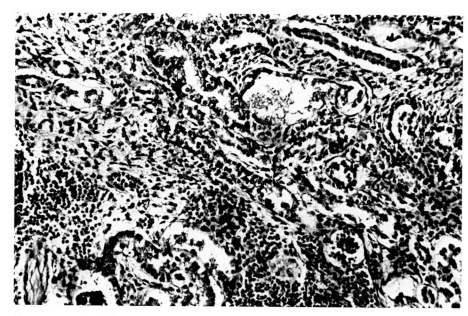

FIGURE XX-35. Kidney of Fetus Aborted by Hypertonic Urea Solution (×50, H&E stain). Changes similar to those seen in hypertonic saline abortion, with detachment of tubular epithelium from basement membrane, degeneration and necrosis of tubular epithelium and interstitial hemorrhages.

and chorionic hemorrhages, villous edema and a bloodless and collapsed cord.

Microscopically, the placenta may show focal coagulative necrosis of the chorioamnion and chorionic villi, and thrombosis and vasculitis of chorionic vessels. Microscopic changes of the cord include thrombosis and edema.

Gross findings in the fetus, in almost all cases, consist of petechial hemorrhages of the skin. In a minority of cases, extensive, purpuric hemorrhages may be observed.

Common microscopic findings are:
• Visceral congestion and hemorrhages. The most severe hemorrhages are in the lungs, in which marked pools of blood are seen around thin-walled, dilated veins and arteries. The pulmonary arteries are congested and non-hemorrhagic. Hemorrhages are also seen in other locations, including subdural and subarachnoid areas.
• Marked distention of pulmonary alveoli, with or without presence of edematous fluid or amniotic epithelial squamae (i.e., aspiration of amniotic fluid).

• In at least 50% of cases, striking detachment of tubular epithelium of proximal and distal tubuli from the basement membrane in the kidneys (Fig. XX-35).

Most pathological changes of the fetus and placenta apparently result from hyperosmolar damage caused by highly elevated concentrations of the saline solution.

The pulmonary change and, in particular, the aspiration of amniotic fluid appear to be secondary to anoxia. However, that the aborted fetus fails to show a number of microscopic features described in other types of acute salt poisoning (i.e., necrotizing arteritis).

Saline abortion is generally not associated with maternal mortality, although at least one case of related amniotic fluid embolism has been reported.[77]

An adequate medicolegal investigation of an abortion fatality requires a particularly thorough clinical history, the autopsy of both the pregnant woman and fetus, and an adequate microscopic examination, toxicology and bacteriology.

REFERENCES

1. Valdes-Dapena, M.: Sudden infant death syndrome: Morphology update for forensic pathologists. *Forensic Science Internat, 30:* 177–186, 1986.

2. Krovs, H.F.: The microscopic distribution of intrathoracic petechiae in sudden infant death syndrome. *Arch Pathol Lab Med, 108:* 77–79, 1984.

3. Maheady, D.C.: Reye's syndrome: Review and update. *J Pediatr Health Care, 3:* 246–250, 1989.

4. Svoboda, D.J., and Reddy, J.K.: Pathology of the liver in Reye's syndrome. *Lab Invest, 32:* 571–579, 1975.

5. Brown, R.E., and Ishak, K.G.: Hepatic zonal degeneration and necrosis in Reye's syndrome. *Arch Pathol Lab Med, 100:* 123–126, 1976.

6. Partin, J.C., Partin, J.S., Schubert, W.K., and McLaurin, R.C.: Brain ultrastructure in Reye's syndrome. *J Neuropath Exp Neurol, 34:* 425–444, 1975.

7. Beaudet, A.L., Sly, W.S., and Valle, D. (ed), Roe and Coates: Acyl CoA Deficiencies. In *The metabolic basis of inherited disease.* New York: McGraw-Hill, 1989, pp. 889–914.

8. Teem, W.R., Witzleben, C.A., Piccoli, D.A., Stauley, C.A., Hales, D.A., Coates, P.M., and Watkins, J.B.: Medium chain and long chain Acyl CoA dehydrogenase deficiency: Clinical, pathological, and ultrastructural differentiation from Reye's syndrome. *Hepatology, 66:* 1270–1278, 1986.

9. Harpey, J.P., Charpentier, C., Coude, M., Divry, P., and Paturneau, J.M.: Clinical and laboratory observations: Sudden death syndrome and multiple Acyl-Coenzymes dehydrogenase deficiency, Ethylmalonic-Adipic Aciduria or systemic carnitine deficiency. *J Pediatr, 110:* 881–884, 1987.

10. Cummins, L.H.: Hypoglycemia and convulsions in children following alcohol ingestion. *J Pediatr, 58:* 23–61, 1961.

11. Ricci, L.R., and Holfunon, S.A.: Ethanol induced hypoglycemia in a child. *Ann Emer Med, 11:* 202–204, 1982.

12. Kuller, L.H., Perper, J.A., and Cooper, M.: Sudden and unexpected death due to arteriosclerotic cardiovascular disease: A review of recent studies, 1968–1972. *Modern Trends in Cardiology, 3:* 292–332, 1974.

13. Perper, J.A., Kuller, L.H., and Cooper, M.D.: Arteriosclerosis of coronary arteries in sudden unexpected deaths. Supplement III to *Circulation 51* and *52:* 27–33, 1975.

14. Friedman, M.: The coronary thrombus: Its origin and fate. *Human Pathol, 2* (1): 81–128, 1971.

15. Falk, E.: Morphological features of unstable atherothrombotic plaques underlying acute coronary syndromes. *Amer J Cardiology, 63* (10): 114E–120E, 1986.

16. Fallon, J.T.: *Post mortem histochemical techniques.* The Hague: Martin Nijhoff Publisher, Wagner, G.S. (ed), 1981.

17. Fujiware, H., Fujiware, T., Tanaka, M., Onodera, T., Miyazaki, S., Wu, D.-J., Matsuda, M., Sasayama, S., and Kawai, C.: Detection of early myocardial infarction in formalin fixed paraffin embedded tissue. *Amer J Cardiovascular Pathol, 2* (1): 57–61, 1988.

18. Edwalds, G.M., Said, J.W., Bloci, M.I., Herscher, L.L., Siegel, R.J., and Fishbein, M.C.: Myocytolysis (vacuolar degeneration) of myocardium: Immunohistochemical evidence of viability. *Human Pathol, 15:* 753–756, 1984.

19. Oehmichen, M., Pedal, I.L., and Hohmann, P.: Diagnostic significance of myofibrillar degeneration of cardiocytes in forensic pathology. *Forensic Sci Internat, 48:* 163–173, 1990.

20. Mallory, G.K.: The speeding of healing of myocardial infarction: A study of the pathological anatomy in 72 cases. *Amer Heart J, 18:* 747–751, 1939.

21. Fishbein, M.C., Maclean, D., and Maroko, P.R.: The histopathologic evolution of myocardial infarction. *Chest, 73* (6): 843–849, 1978.

22. Reimer, K.A., and Ideker, R.E.: Myocardial ischemia and infarction: Anatomic and biochemical substrate for ischemic cell death and ventricular arrhythmias. *Human Pathol, 18:* 462–475, 1987.

23. Kuller, L.H., Cooper, M., and Perper, J.A.: Epidemiology of sudden death. *Arch Internal Med, 129:* 714–719, May, 1972.

24. Silverberg, S.G. (ed.): *Principles and practice of surgical pathology.* New York: Churchill-Livingston, 1990.

25. Uchida, T., Kao, H., Quispe-Sjogren, M., and Peters, R.L.: Alcoholic foamy degeneration: A pattern of acute alcohol injury of the liver. *Gastroenterology, 84* (4): 683–692, 1983.

26. Claydon, S.M.: Myocarditis as an incidental finding in young men dying from unnatural causes. *Med Sci Law, 29* (1): 55–58, 1989.

27. Bendon, R.W., and Hug, G.: Glycogen accumulation in the pars recta of the proximal tubule in Fanconi syndrome. *Pediatr Pathol, 6* (4): 411–429

28. McGory, P., and Duncan, C.: Anesthetic risks in sickle cell trait. *Pediatrics, 51:* 507–512, 1973.

29. Kark, S.A., Posey, D.M., Schumacher, H.R., and Ruehle, C.J.: Sickle cell trait as a risk factor for sudden death in physical training. *New Eng J Med, 317:* 781–787, 1987.

30. Davies, M.J.: The cardiomyopathies: A review of terminology, pathology and pathogenesis. *Histopathology, 8* (3): 363–393, 1986.

31. Johnson, R.A., and Palacios, I.: Dilated cardiomyopathies of the adult. *New Eng J Med, 307:* 1051–1058, 1982.

32. Maron, B.J., Bonow, R.O., Cannon, B.O., Leon, M.B., and Epstein, S.E.: Hypertrophic cardiomyopathy: Interrelations of clinical manifestations, pathophysiol-

ogy, and theory. *New Eng J Med, 316* (14): 844–852, 1987.

33. Rose, A.G.: Evaluation of pathological criteria for diagnosis of hypertrophic cardiomyopathy. *Histopathology, 8:* 395–406, 1987.

34. A previous undescribed congenital malformation of the heart: Almost total absence of the myocardium of the right ventricle, Uhl HSM. *Bull Johns Hopkins Hospital, 91:* 197–209, 1952.

35. Thiene, G., Naur, A., Corrado, D., Rossi, L., and Penelli, N.: Right ventricular cardiomyopathy and sudden death in young people. *New Eng J Med, 318:* 129–133, 1988.

36. Kuller, L.H., Talbott, E., and Perper, J.A.: Sudden and unexpected death among women: Possible precipitating events. *Critical Care Med, 9* (5): 411–412, 1981.

37. Roberts, W.C., McAllister, H.A., Jr., and Ferrans, V.J.: Sarcoidosis of the heart: A clinicopathologic study of 35 necropsy patients and review of 78 previously described necropsy patients. *Amer J Med, 63:* 86–108, 1977.

38. Piette, M., and Timperman, J.: Sudden death in idiopathic giant cell myocarditis. *Med Sci Law, 30:* 280–284, 1990.

39. Bharati, S., and Lev, M.: Cardiac disease in sudden death. *Arch Internal Med, 144:* 1811–1812, 1984 and Lev, M., and Bharati, S.: A method of study of the pathology of the conduction system for electrocardiograph and His' bundle electrogram correlations. *Anatomical Record, 201:* 43–49, 1981.

40. Balsaver, A.M., Morales, A.R., and Whitehouse, F.W.: Fat infiltration of myocardium as a cause of cardiac conduction defect. *Amer J Cardiology, 19:* 261–265, 1967.

41. Cebelin, M.S., and Hirsch, C.S.: Human stress cardiomyopathy: Myocardial lesions in victims of homicidal assault without internal injuries. *Human Pathol, 11:* 123–132, 1980.

42. Reichenbach, D., and Benditt, E.P.: Myofibrillar degeneration: A common form of cardiac muscle injury. *New York Acad Sci, 156:* 164, 1970.

43. Kanter, R.K.: Retinal hemorrhage after cardiopulmonary resuscitation or child abuse. *J Pediatr, 108:* 430–432, March, 1986.

44. Perper, J.A., and Wecht, C.H. (ed): *Electrical injuries in microscopic diagnosis in forensic pathology.* Springfield, IL: Charles C Thomas, 1980.

45. Parker, J.R., Parker, J.C., Jr., and Overman, J.C.: Intracranial diffuse axonal injury at autopsy. *Ann Clin Lab Sci, 20* (3): 220–224, 1990.

46. Rakallio, J.: Histochemical and biochemical estimation of the age of injuries. In Perper, J.A., and Wecht, C.H. (eds.), *Microscopic diagnosis in forensic pathologies.* Springfield, IL: Charles C Thomas, 1980.

47. Loberg, E.M., and Torvik, A.: Brain contusions: The time sequence of the histological changes. *Med Sci Law, 29* (2): 109–115, 1989.

48. Heat stroke: A clinicopathologic study of 125 fatal cases. *Military Surgeon, 99:* 397–449, 1946.

49. Rubel, L.R., and Ishak, K.G.: The liver in fatal exertional heat stroke. *Liver, 3:* 249–260, 1983.

50. Shibolet, S., Lancaster, M.C., and Danon, Y.: Heatstroke: A review. *Aviator Space Environ Med, 47* (3): 280–301, 1976.

51. Devos, C.H., and Piette, M.: Hypothermia and combined postmortem determination of amylase and isoamylase in the serum and vitreous humor. *Med Sci Law, 29* (3): 218–228, 1989.

52. Bennett, T.T., Cary, F.H., Mitchell, G.C., and Cooper, M.N.: Acute methylalcohol poisoning: A review based on experiences in an outbreak of 323 cases. *Medicine, 32:* 431–463, 1953.

53. Geiling, E.M.K., and Cannon, P.R.: Pathologic effects of elixir of sulfanilamide (diethylene glycol) poisoning, clinical and experimental correlation: Final report. *JAMA, 111:* 919–926, Sept. 3, 1938.

54. Winek, C.L., Singleton, D.P., and Shanor, S.P.: Ethylene and diethylene glycol toxicity. *Clin Toxicol, 13* (2): 297–324, 1978.

55. Gonote, C.E., Reimer, K.A., and Jennings, B.: Acute mercury poisoning: An electronic microscopic and metabolic study. *Lab Invest, 3:* 633–647, 1974.

56. Takeuchi, T.: Pathology of Minamata disease with special reference to its pathogenesis. *Acta Pathol Jpn, 32:* 73–99, 1982.

57. Deutsch, H.L., and Millard, D.R.: A new cocaine abuse complex. Involvement of nose, septum, palate, and pharynx. *Arch Otolaryngol Head Neck Surg, 115* (2): 235–237, 1989.

58. Wanless, I.R., Dore, S., Gopinath, N., Tan, J., and Cameron, R.: Histopathology of cocaine hepatotoxicity: A report of our patients. *Gastroenterology, 98:* 497–501, 1990.

59. Marsden, C.D., and Jenner, P.G.: The significance of 1-methyl-4-phenyl-1,2,3,6- tetrahydropyridine (review). *CIBA Found Symp, 126:* 239–256, 1987.

60. Stern, Y., Tetrud, J.W., Martin, W.R., and Langston, J.W.: Cognitive change following MPTP exposure. *Neurology, 40:* 261–264, 1990.

61. Charness, M.E., Simon, R. P., and Greenberg, D.A.: Ethanol and the nervous system. *New Eng J Med, 321:* 442–453, 1980.

62. Kuller, L.H., May, S.J., and Perper, J.A.: The relationship between alcohol liver disease and testicular pathology. *Amer J Epid, 108:* 192–199, 1978.

63. Nakada, T., and Knight, R.T.: Alcohol and the central nervous system. *Med Clin North Amer, 68:* 121–131, 1984.

64. Haibach, H., Ansbacher, L.E., and Dix, J. D.: Central pontine myelinolysis: A complication of hyponatremia or therapeutic intervention. *J Forensic Sci, 32:* 444–451, 1987.

65. Victor, Adams, and Collins: *The Wernicke-Korsakoff syndrome and related disorders due to alcoholism and malnutrition,* 2nd edition. Philadelphia: F.A. Davis Co., 1989.

66. Perper, J.A., Pidlaon, A., and Fisher, R.S.: Granulomatous peritonitis induced by rice starch glove powder: A clinical and experimental study. *Amer J Surg, 122:* 812–817, 1971.

67. Gover, R.A., and Wilson, M.H.: Lead induced inclusion bodies: Results of ethylenediaminetetraacetic acid treatment. *Lab Invest, 32:* 149–156, 1975.

68. Fisher, R.S.: Boric acid poisoning. *Amer J Pathol, 27:* 745–749, 1951.

69. Sanusi, I.D., Tio, F.O., and Manno, J.E.: Pancreatic inclusions and its relation to boric acid poisoning. *Forensic Sci, 6:* 165–174, 1975.

70. Spencer, H.: *The pneumoconioses and other occupational diseases in pathology of the lung,* Volume 2, IV Edition. Elmsford, NY: Pergamon Press, 1985.

71. Gazer, R.: The physical and molecular structure of asbestos. *Ann New York Acad Sci, 132:* 23–30, 1965.

72. Suzuki, Y., and Churg, S.: Structure and development of the asbestos body. *Amer J Pathol, 55:* 79–107, 1969.

73. Gaensler, E.A., and Addington, W.W.: Asbestos or ferruginous bodies. *New Engl J Med, 280:* 488–492, 1969.

74. Rushton, D.I.: Simplified classification of spontaneous abortion. *J Med Genet, 15:* 1–9, 1978.

75. Rushton, D.I.: Examination of products of conception from previable human pregnancies. *J Clin Pathol, 34:* 819–835, 1981.

76. Galen, R.S., Chavhan, P., Wietzner, H., and Navarroc: Fetal pathology and mechanism of fetal death in saline induced abortion: A study of 143 gestations and critical review of literature. *Amer J Obstet Pathol, 120:* 347–355, 1974.

77. Mirchandani, H.G., Mirchandani, I.H., and Parikh, S.R.: Hypernatremia due to amniotic fluid embolism during a saline induced abortion. *Amer J Forensic Med Pathol, 9:* 48–50, 1988.

Chapter XXI

FORENSIC ASPECTS OF RADIOLOGY

B. G. BROGDON

IN THE AUTUMN OF 1895, Dr. Wilhelm Conrad Röntgen seemed to be at the zenith of a well-established scientific career. Although only 50 years of age, he had already published 48 papers bringing him widespread recognition and admiration from his peers. He held appointments as Professor of Physics and Director of the Physical Institute at the University of Würzburg and had been elected rector. Nevertheless, he continued a busy schedule of independent research.[1]

On November 8th of that year while investigating properties of cathode ray tubes, Dr. Röntgen accidentally discovered *a new kind of ray* (eine neue Art von Strahlen). During the next 50 days of intensive research he made virtually all of the fundamental observations on this ray he called *'X'* for unknown. This led to a manuscript readily accepted for publication in the Annuals of the Würzburg Physical Medicine Society and presentation at the society's January 1896 meeting. But, as sometimes happens today, news of this exciting discovery was leaked to the press and disseminated throughout the world with the blinding speed of cable and telegraph. In the United States, the *New York Sun* scooped the country with the story on January 8, 1896.[2]

The materials required to build a primitive x-ray generator were already available throughout the civilized world, and interested parties so enabled rushed to replicate Röntgen's images. Professor Arthur Williams Wright, Director of the Sloan Physical Laboratory at Yale University, is credited with producing the first x-ray images in the United States on January 27, 1896. His test objects included scissors, a pencil and coins. More important to our purpose, a few days later Professor Wright purchased a rabbit at the market. Let the professor tell it, ". . . An exposure of one hour to the rays, left upon the plate a com-plete representation of the bony skeleton. . . . Particularly interesting in this photograph were several small round spots which appeared dark in the positive print. They were at once surmised to be shot, and from the indication of their location in the print were readily found and extracted. The mode of death of the animal was not previously known."[3]

Thus, Professor Wright became, somewhat fortuitously, the father of the application of radiology to medicolegal investigation of death. From his description we can assume that the cause of death was penetration of vital organs with shotgun pellets. The manner of death was unnatural, perhaps best labeled as *cuniculicide*. The mechanism of death remains with the ages.

Radiologic Identification of the Dead

The radiologic identification of human remains can be definitive in some cases where mutilation, decomposition, incineration, fragmentation or skeletization precludes more simple and conventional methods such as facial features, birthmarks, scars, tattoos, fingerprints, palmprints or footprints. However, radiologic identification is dependent totally and absolutely on the availability of comparable antemortem and postmortem radiologic images.

When antemortem radiographs of the presumed decedent are known to exist and are accessible, it is relatively easy to concentrate on producing similar postmortem images. When such information is lacking, prudence demands total body postmortem radiography *before autopsy* in anticipation of a potential match with whatever antemortem radiographs, often quite limited in scope, may be acquired in the course of time.

Antemortem Radiologic Studies

Due to currently prevailing medical standards in the United States, most people undergo some type of radiologic examination at some time during their lives. However, these examinations do not always lend themselves to the application of radiology to identification.

A study of the distribution of radiologic examinations of both in- and out-patients in a university medical center[4] in recent years showed about 80% to be conventional x-ray procedures. Of those, about 40% were of the chest. The upper and lower extremities each accounted for about 10%. Radiography of other body parts in diminishing frequency involved the spine, abdomen, head and neck, pelvis and hip, and *"other"* (Table XXI-1).

Mammography, although comprising eight to 10% of x-ray studies is useless for identification purposes as are nuclear medicine studies (4%) and most catheter procedures (1%).

About 10% of medical imaging is by computed tomography (CT) and some identifying matches have been made with this method[5-7] (Fig. XXI-1a–c). CT and magnetic resonance imaging (MRI) now probably constitute almost 15% of radiologic examinations, and their use is expanding rapidly. So far, these modalities have found only limited use in forensic applications because of their cost, complexity of operation and inaccessibility of such work. Increasing use of these sectional imaging systems undoubtedly will follow, but trail substantially behind increasing clinical use.

In a series of successful antemortem and postmortem comparisons, Murphy et al.[8] found the chest most commonly useful and the pelvis least useful (Table XXI-2). On the other hand, we have found more success with the spine, pelvis and chest. When only incomplete skeletonized remains are available, the odds change again. Bass and Driscoll[9] reported that individual bones most commonly retrieved in that situation were skull, femur, mandible and pelvis (Table XXI-3).

TABLE XXI-1

DISTRIBUTION OF RADIOLOGIC EXAMS
BY BODY PART AND MODALITY

Type Exam	Body Part		Percent of Total
Roentgenograms			82
(X-rays)			% of Total X-rays
	Chest	43	36
	Lower Extremity	11	9
	Upper Extremity	10	8
	Spine	8	7
	Breast (Mammogram)	8	7
	Abdomen	7	6
	Head/Neck	5	4
	Pelvis/Hip	4	3
	Other	4	2
Other Modalities			18
Nuclear Medicine			4
MRI			4
Catheter Procedures			1
CT:		% of Total CT	9
	Head/Neck	44	
	Abdomen	22	
	Pelvis	10	
	Thorax	9	
	Spine	9	
	Other	6	

From Brogdon, B.G. (ed): *Forensic radiology.* © CRC Press, Boca Raton, Florida, 1998; with permission.

Postmortem Radiologic Studies

We will limit our remarks to conventional x-ray studies, assuming that other modalities will be appropriately employed when available.

Despite frequent pressures to quickly release the body, whole-body radiography of remains should be attempted if the availability of antemortem studies is unknown and/or their extent unpredictable. Every effort should be made to replicate standard radiographic positions and projections in at least one plane (antero-posterior for most of the body with added lateral views for the skull and spine, if feasible). Standard positioning illustrations and exposure charts are available.[10] Total body radiography takes time and usually requires 12 to 15 of the largest size films (14x17 in.) for an adult.[4,11-13] Compliance with these ideal standards depends largely upon whether or not the examining facility has its own radiographic equipment and personnel to oper-

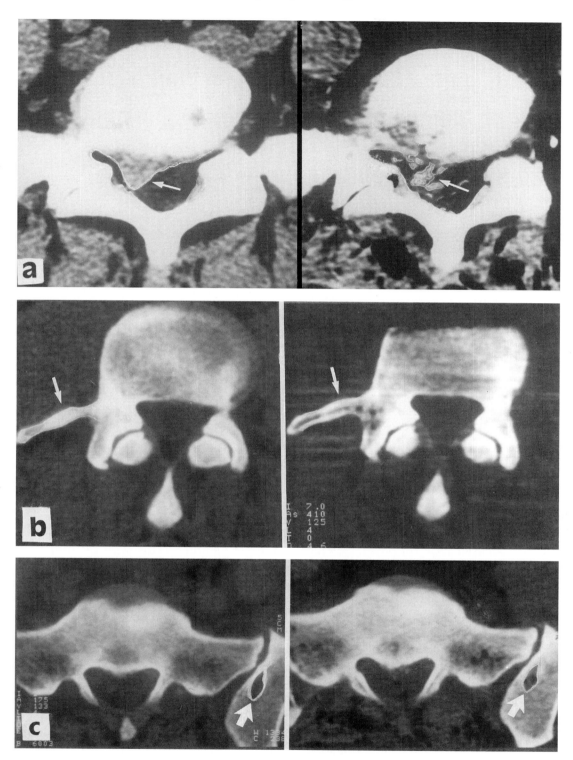

FIGURE XXI-1a–c. Identification through comparison of antemortem and postmortem computed tomography. The antemortem study is on the viewer's left in each instance. (a) Shows a posterolateral disc herniation of L5-S1. (b) Shows a peculiar thickening of the right transverse process of L4 and (c) shows identical lucencies in the left ilium at the sacroiliac joint. (Original images courtesy the authors, reproduced with permission, © ASTM.)

TABLE XXI-2

POSITIVE RADIOLOGIC IDENTIFICATION BY
ANATOMIC REGION

Region	Number*	Percent*
Chest	16 of 30	53
Skull	6 of 30	20
Extremities	6 of 30	20
Lumbar Spine	5 of 30	17
Cervical Spine	3 of 30	10
Pelvis	1 of 30	3

* Some bodies could be identified by comparison of more than one region. (© ASTM, reproduced with permission.)

TABLE XXI-3

SKELETAL ELEMENTS PRESENT IN 58 FRAGMENTED
SKELETONS

Bone	Percent
Skull or Skull Bones	66
Femur	48
Mandible	41
Innominate	40
Tibia	38
Ulna	33
Humerus	29
Fibula	28
Scapula	28
Clavicle	22
Radius	22
Sacrum	17
Patella	13
Sternum	12

(© ASTM, reproduced with permission)

ate it. The use of clinical facilities for forensic purposes is increasingly difficult, largely due to concerns of contamination by blood and other body fluids.

For example, the Oklahoma City bombing (1995) took place within 0.6 miles of a large metropolitan medical center where 173 of the survivors were received; the remainder were distributed to other area hospitals, the most distant 21 miles away from the blast. However, all 168 bodies were radiographed in the medical examiner's office.[13]

Radiologic Identification of Unknown Remains

Non-skeletal soft tissues generally are of similar (water) density on radiographs and, hence, of little value for identification purposes. Calcifications in the lungs have been helpful or specific in several of Murphy's cases.[8] Physiologic calcifications, such as falx cerebri, vascular calcifications, calcified scars or post-traumatic myositis ossificans, might be useful on occasion, as may enteric accretions, such as gallstones, kidney and bladder stones, phleboliths, thrombi, or parasitic encrustations. Increasingly, surgical sutures, stents, filters, connectors and appliances are available and useful for comparative identification[4] (Fig. XXI-2). For example, comparison of post and antemortem supine chest radiographs will show matching patterns of wire sutures in the sternum. However, there may be angulation due to shifting of deeper clips so they may not match precisely. Others may move out of posi-

tion with death and collapse of the thoracic viscera.

Skeleton

Apart from teeth, the skeleton is the most durable tissue of the body and is the basis for most radiologic identifications. Two kinds of information can be derived from the radiologic examination of skeletal remains: general and specific.

General information can be obtained from skeletal remains without comparable antemortem studies. This type of information has been called a *biological profile* and is actually the establishment of anthropological parameters: 1) are the remains human or animal; 2) one body or commingled remains of two or more individuals; 3) sex; 4) age at death; 5) population ancestry; 6) stature.[14]

The radiologic advantage is that these parameters can be evaluated in remains still totally or partially covered with soft tissue. The forensic physical anthropologist can derive equal or better information if the remains are completely skeletonized or if there are facilities and time to deflesh the bones.

The criteria are essentially the same for both disciplines, depending on size and configuration of bony parts (especially the skull and pelvis),

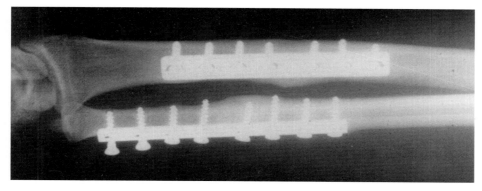

FIGURE XXI-2. Antemortem roentgenogram of the forearm of an air crash victim with a *plate and screws* fixation device in place was matched with a postmortem x-ray. (Reprinted with permission from Brogdon, B.G. (ed): *Forensic radiology,* © CRC Press, Boca Raton, Florida, 1998.)

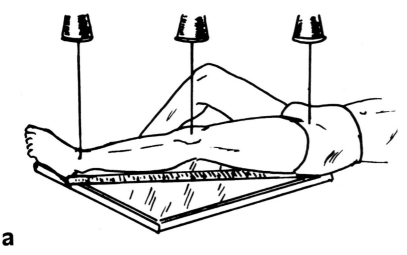

a

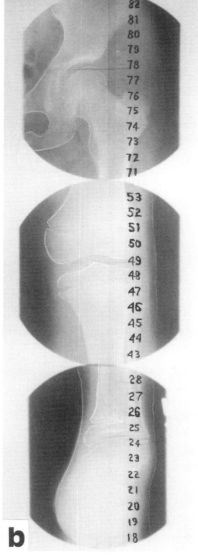

b

FIGURE XXI-3a–b. (a) Method of obtaining magnification-free measurements of long bone using collimated non-divergent x-rays over the bone ends with a partially opaque ruler in the field of exposure. (b) Example of image obtained by this method. (Reprinted with permission from Brogdon, B. G. (ed): *Forensic radiology,* © CRC Press, Boca Raton, Florida, 1998.)

degree of skeletal maturation or degeneration, measurement of certain long bones for comparison with standard tables (Fig. XXI-3a–b) and gender-predictive calcifications (Fig. XXI-4), decalcification and degeneration or disease processes (Fig. XXI-5a–d). On occasion thinning of skull bones has been observed involving the parietal or occipital areas.

Specific information derived from radiologic study of the skeleton depends on the observation of certain individual peculiarities that can be suc-

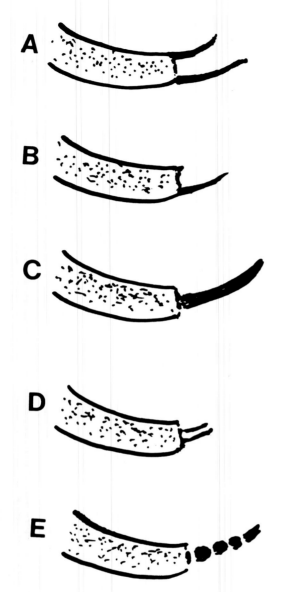

FIGURE XXI-4. Schematic drawing of patterns of costal cartilage ossification useful in determining the sex of human remains. (A) Typical male pattern. (B) Male pattern initially involving only the inferior margin of the costal cartilage. (C) Typical female pattern. (D) Uncommon pattern more often found in females than males. (E) String of rounded ossifications believed specific for elderly females. (Reprinted with permission from Brogdon, B. G. (ed): *Forensic radiology,* © CRC Press, Boca Raton, Florida, 1998.)

cessfully matched with identical findings in antemortem radiologic images. Examination of some regions of the skeleton may be more fruitful than others in bearing individualizing variation; how-ever, sometimes a single bone may suffice for positive identification. We will look at these possibilities separately.

Skull

The dental arches account for the highest percentage of success in identification of unknown bodies. This is the province of the forensic odontologist who may be quite ingenious when dealing with fragmented and fragmentary remains. In cases of charred remains it may be necessary to stabilize the areas in question to avoid disintegration. Laquer (shellac) or similar products may be used for this purpose. The parts can then be reassembled with dental wax. Sometimes this match is sufficiently simple that the odontologist's expertise is not required (Fig. XXI-6).

At the end of World War II when the Russians moved into Berlin, Hitler's driver was instructed to destroy his body after his suicide to avoid identification. He did so by dousing the body with large amounts of gasoline and igniting it.

Antemortem radiographs of Adolf Hitler showed only five of his teeth were his own, and the extensive and unusual dental work allowed the Russians to identify his remains, despite extensive charring.[15]

The paranasal sinuses and mastoid air cells allowed Culbert and Law[16] to make the first radiologic identifications of human remains in 1927. Patterns of pneumatization in these areas are distinctive; the frontal sinuses in particular are as unique to the individual as fingerprints.[17,18] Once developed, the frontal sinuses do not change with age unless substantial trauma or disease intervenes. A match is readily determined even if the projections are different. Unfortunately, the frontal sinuses may explode in high temperature fires and frequently are shattered against the dashboard or forward seat back in automobile and aircraft crashes.

The sella turcica, because of its deep central location in the skull often survives fire and trauma.[19] The configuration of the sella, the clinoid processes, and the underlying sphenoid sinuses may allow a quick positive or negative radiologic identification.[11]

Other features in the skull: The overall configuration of the skull, including salient features like

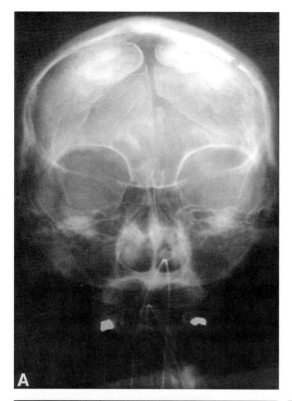

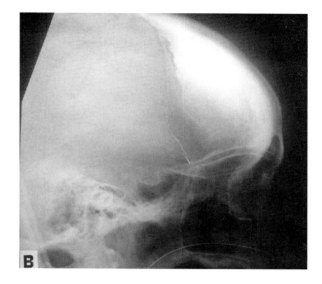

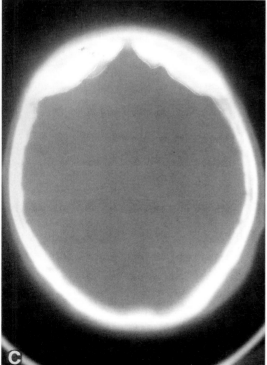

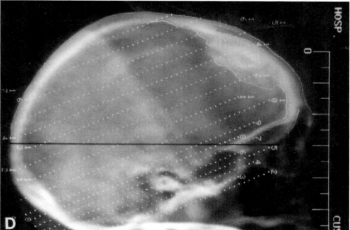

Figure XXI-5a–d. Hyperostosis interna frontalis. Dense bony thickening of the inner table of the frontal bone seen in (a) frontal and (b) lateral roentgenograms and (c) on a CT scan of the skull using *bone window*. The *topogram* preliminary to the CT scan (d) is sufficiently detailed that it could be used for purposes of identification comparison. (Reprinted with permission from Brogdon, B. G. (ed): *Forensic radiology,* © CRC Press, Boca Raton, Florida, 1998.)

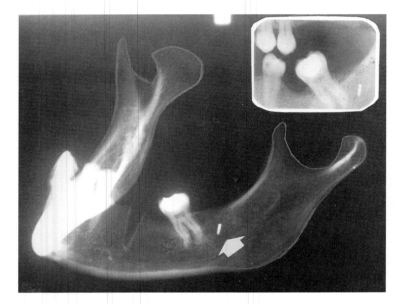

FIGURE XXI-6. Comparison of antemortem dental radiograph, with postmortem radiograph of disarticulated mandible. There is a perfect match of both the restoration in the molar and the broken-off drill bit tip (white arrow). (Reprinted with permission from Brogdon, B. G. (ed): *Forensic radiology,* © CRC Press, Boca Raton, Florida, 1998.)

the brow ridge and the inion, vascular grooves, surgical lesions, cranial sutures, trauma, and conditions secondary to disease or aging may prove useful[4] (Fig. XXI-7).

Chest

The chest is the area of the body most frequently radiographed, often can be used for comparative radiologic identification. However, the chest is relatively fragile, especially the rib cage and anterior chest wall which may be mutilated by trauma or destroyed by fire.

The cervicothoracic junction is most apt to survive calamity and the cervicothoracic vertebrae and their adjacent rib ends have considerable configurational individuality to allow comparison.

Postmortem chest radiographs were utilized to identify the mutilated, burned partial remains from a train wreck with bony structures at the cervicothoracic junction by the finding of a bony artifact at the level of T-2 on antemortem films.

The majority of clinical chest films are made with the patient erect, facing the film holder, arms akimbo and shoulders forward, with the x-ray tube behind. Most postmortem chest films are made with the body supine, the arms alongside, the shoulders back, and the x-ray tube overhead. (Fig. XXI–8) If in each instance the central ray of the x-ray beam is directed at the middle of the chest, the projection and relationships of the

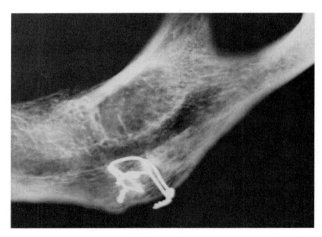

FIGURE XXI-7. Wire in the lower jaw for correction of the bite. Also, the bone pattern indicates previous surgery in the area. The body was incinerated as the result of a car fire.

bones at the cervicothoracic junction will be different. Angulation of the x-ray tube about 10–12 degrees toward the feet for the supine view will help compensate for this variation.

Costal cartilage, pleural, and *pulmonary calcification* is occasionally helpful, as are unique findings in the individual ribs.[8,20,21]

Sternal[7,22] and *scapular*[23] configuration each has proved helpful on rare occasions. The former, however, requires a lateral view for disclosure. Configurational changes in the clavicle have led to positive identification.[4,24]

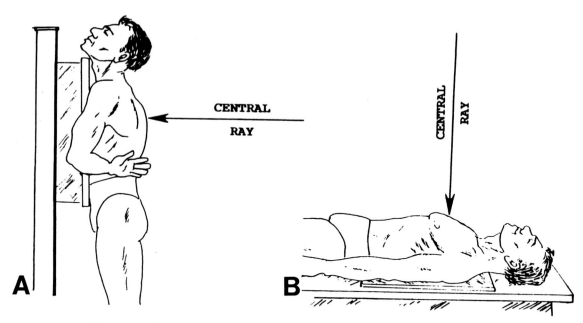

FIGURE XXI-8. (A) Positioning for a posteroanterior erect view of the chest. (B) Positioning for an anteroposterior supine view of the chest. It is obvious that the position and projection of bony structures of the pectoral girdle and at the cervicothoracic junction will be quite different from one view to the other. (Reprinted with permission from Brogdon, B. G. (ed): *Forensic radiology,* © CRC Press, Boca Raton, Florida, 1998.)

Examination of the dried skeletal remains of a young adult male yielded only one distinctive finding: an old healed fracture of the lateral third of the left clavicle. Eventually an old chest radiograph of the presumed decedent was found. With careful positioning of the dried clavicle a radiograph reproduced the fracture.

Abdomen and Pelvis

These areas of the body are most likely to survive incineration, decomposition or trauma even if the anterior abdominal wall is burned away. The heavy musculature protects the lumbar spine, pelvis and hips. Since the *lumbar spine* is most prone to anomaly and variation in development (Table XXI-4) and is susceptible to disease, trauma, tumor and degeneration, we have found it to be most useful for identification by radiologic comparison (Fig. XXI-9). Degenerative spurring and lipping of vertebral body margins, spinous processes and sometimes arteriosclerotic calcifications in iliac arteries may be matchable.

In the *pelvis* one may find evidence of old trauma, tumors or tumor metastases, disease (frequently Paget's), vascular grooves, trabecular patterns, or anomaly. One case was identified on the basis of congenital acetabular dysplasia with hip dislocation.[25] A bony excrescence on the iliac crest would fit into that category. Distinctive vascular grooves[26] and unique trabecular patterns[4] are common in the pelvis.

Other Bones

Any other part of the body may allow for radiologic identification if comparable antemortem and postmortem radiologic studies are available. Cases have been reported utilizing the elbows, assorted extremity long bones, the patella and the hands and wrists.[27-29]

Single Bone Identification

In view of the above, any single bone may hold the key to positive radiologic identification. If any antemortem studies are available simultaneously with the remains, one can concentrate on finding unique or unusual features in an antemortem image and replicate that image with the

TABLE XXI-4

THE *NORMAL* LUMBOSACRAL SPINE
(936 CASES)

Entity	Number	Percent
Spina bifida occulta	334 total	35.7
Multiple	40	4.3
Previous Scheuermann's disease	194 total	20.7
With Schmorl's nodes	96	10.3
Scoliosis greater than 1 inch	5 total	0.5
Rudimentary ribs or ununited		
transverse process	60 total	6.4
Transitional vertebrae	108 total	11.5
Sacralization	31	3.3
Bilateral	20	2.1
Unilateral	11	1.2
Lumbarization	77	8.2
Bilateral	56	6.0
Unilateral	21	2.2
Spondylolysis	71 total	7.6
Bilateral	57	6.1
Unilateral	14	1.5
Spondylolisthesis	42 total	4.5
Limbus vertebrae	9	1.0
Hemangioma	4	0.4
None of the above variations	376	40.2

Reprinted with permission from Crow, NE, and Brogdon, BG.
The "Normal" lumbosacral spine, *Radiology, 72,* 97, 1959.

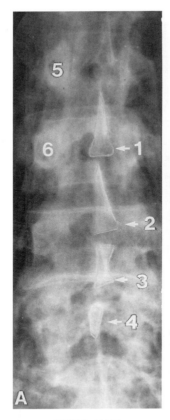
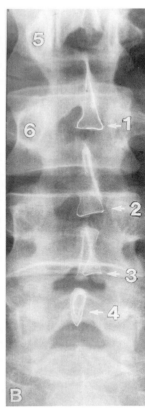

FIGURE XXI-9. (A) Postmortem and (B) antemortem frontal views of the lumbar spine. Highly individualistic configuration of the spinous processes enables positive match. Other spinal elements can also be matched. (See corresponding numbers.) (Reprinted with permission from Brogdon, B. G. (ed): *Forensic radiology,* © CRC Press, Boca Raton, Florida, 1998.)

counterpart remains. The *shadow-positioning technique* of Fitzpatrick and Macaluso[30] is ideal for this replication if the remains are skeletonized. Otherwise, trial and error positioning, and repositioning, will be required.

If antemortem radiologic studies are not immediately available, we reiterate the desirability of radiographing the total remains.

The features leading to positive identification by radiologic comparison of single bones can be categorized as follows:

1. Anomalous or unusual development (see Fig. XXI-9)
2. Disease or degeneration
3. Tumor
4. Trauma
5. Iatrogenic interference
6. Vascular grooves and trabecular patterns

MASS CASUALTIES

The principles of radiologic identification of unknown human remains are the same whether dealing with a single individual or scores of victims: comparison and detection of unique features in antemortem and postmortem images. Mass casualty situations[31] however, are unexpected, stressful, require multidisciplinary efforts and organization, depend heavily on volunteers who likely are relatively inexperienced, and usually are handled in makeshift, sometimes remote, facilities including the site of the disaster. The recovery and identification operations may be widely separated.

The radiologist will function as part of a multidisciplinary team including experts in fingerprinting, dental analysis, physical anthropology,

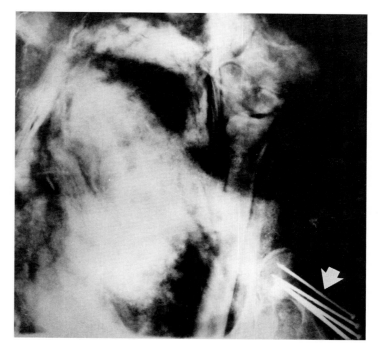

FIGURE XXI-10. Initial screening study of remains showing metallic screw fixation of a proximal femur fracture (arrow) matching an antemortem film. (Reprinted with permission from Lichtenstein, J. E., et al. *Am J Roentgen,* 150, 751, 1988.)

toxicology, blood chemistry, medical photography, investigators and forensic pathology. In the identification facility these specialists will be organized into sections resulting in an *assembly-line type* activity devoted to identification.

It may be helpful if radiology were near the front of the line. Initial screening of bodies even while in body bags may reveal helpful material not apparent on visual inspection, i.e., jewelry, surgical implants and prostheses (Fig. XXI-10), parts of a vehicle or bomb fragments. Such screening may reveal isolated skeletal or soft-tissue lesions which may be matchable with antemortem films (Fig. XXI-11).

Radiologic Equipment

Mobile x-ray units operating on standard power supply are readily available and, commonly employed. There may be temptation to take battery-operated units into the field, but their useful life is short and other inherent problems of quality control exist.

Military field units, if available, are effective. The military also has air-transportable, self-contained x-ray facilities complete with power and air-conditioning.

Mobile C-arm units have fluoroscopic capability for rapid screenings; most have filming capability, as well, for documenting screening findings.

Baggage-type scanning units with conveyor systems for transporting heavy remains, even in caskets, have been used in the military for general screening purposes and to detect live ordinance hidden inside remains.

Whatever type of x-ray equipment is employed, careful attention must be paid to radiation shielding, often with temporary lead barriers, and personnel monitoring, film badges.

Film handling and processing can be a major problem in field operations since dark room facilities and controlled-temperature water supply are essential. Fixed facilities in adjacent hospitals can be used to load and unload film cassettes and film processing but are inherently inconvenient and increase likelihood of film labeling and collation errors. Modern military self-contained units are an ideal solution. Otherwise, small table-top processors will suffice for small operations, or standard processors can be brought in and temporarily installed for large-volume activity.

Film identification must be absolutely accurate. It is best done at time of exposure with lead let-

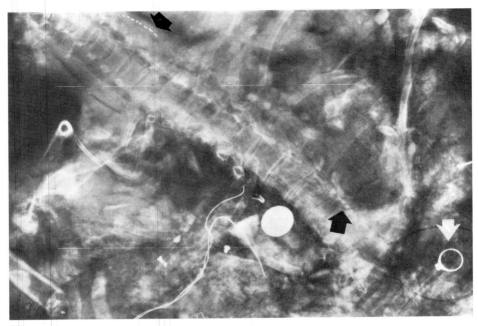

FIGURE XXI-11. Postmortem film of remains in a body bag of the Chicago DC-10 crash. The film shows a ring, later determined to belong to the victim (white arrow), other metallic foreign bodies, a severely disrupted skeleton and calcified tracheal rings (black arrows). The tracheal calcifications were matched with antemortem films. (Reprinted with permission from Lichtenstein, J. E., et al. *Am J. Roent. 150,* 751, 1998.)

ters and numbers and with all films of the same body *batched* with unique designations.

Film reporting will be abbreviated, on simple one-page forms. A multiviewer will facilitate the work.

Cause and/or Manner of Death

Radiologic examination of both the living and the dead may contribute toward determination of cause and manner of death. In an injury that results in death, however delayed, the radiologic evaluation may contribute. The radiologic contribution can be enhanced by historical information, physical examination or laboratory data (Fig. XXI-12). Radiologic training and experience with normal and abnormal findings in living patients of all ages and both sexes is the solid basis upon which forensic applications of detection, pattern recognition, interpretation, comparison and conjecture depend.[32]

The skeleton is the organ system most often targeted for this sort of evaluation, but soft tissues of the musculoskeletal system and thoracic and abdominal viscera may disclose key evidence.

Osseous Injuries

In both the living and the dead, the skeleton is best studied in standard views of two positions or projections at right angles to each other. From these two planes the experienced observer can conceptualize the third dimension of depth.

Fractures

The location and type of fracture interpreted in view of the age and level of activity of the subject may suggest whether the injury was accidental or inflicted. For instance, an undisplaced spiral fracture of the distal tibia in a 20-month-old child is a common accidental injury related to the uncertain gait at that age. Such a fracture in a six-month-old is impossible to acquire naturally in the course of infantile movement. Rather, this type of fracture would be caused by a twist-

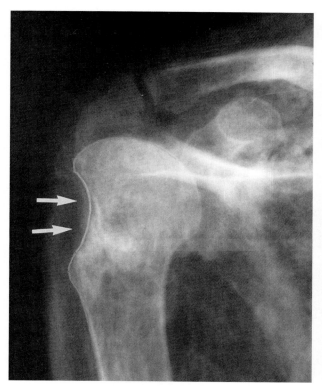

FIGURE XXI-12. A truck driver who was burned beyond recognition after a wreck had a history of dislocation of the right shoulder. Postmortem roentgenogram shows a typical Hill-Sachs deformity, an impaction fracture of the humeral head associated with anterior dislocation of the shoulder (arrows). Antemortem examination showed the dislocation and Hill-Sachs deformity, a positive identification. (Reprinted with permission from Brogdon, B. G. (ed): *Forensic Radiology,* © CRC Press, Boca Raton, Florida, 1998.)

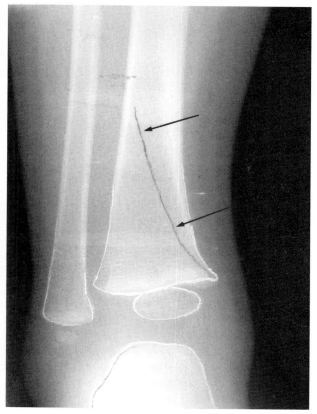

FIGURE XXI-13. This is a so-called *Toddler's Fracture,* also referred to as *torsion* or *spiral* fracture. This fracture is situated in the lower tibia and may be seen in young children in the early years as they begin to walk and run but are not yet very steady or coordinated, a *normal* fracture for this age group. (Reprinted with permission from Brogdon, B. G. (ed): *Forensic radiology,* © CRC Press, Boca Raton, Florida, 1998.)

ing force or torsion at the hands of an adult caretaker. In a six-month-old non-ambulatory infant a similar fracture would be highly suggestive of abuse (Fig. XXI-13).

In skull fractures the location, duration and sequence of blows can be determined by studying the intersection of fracture lines.[33]

A linear fracture from an earlier blow will stop propagation of a fracture from a second blow. Thus, it is possible to determine whether a fracture from a blow to the head preceded a fracture caused by the subsequent fall to the ground. A linear fracture which extends from an entrance bullet wound travels faster than the bullet causing it; a fracture from the exit wound will terminate on meeting the preexisting fracture. This

helps in deciding between entrance and exit wounds. Trajectory or direction of fire is suggested by the angle of eccentric beveling.

Some skeletal injuries clearly are defensive in origin (Fig. XXI-14a–b). Others may suggest a particular scenario.

The technician x-raying a motor vehicle accident victim noticed a bulge in the sock on one ankle and made a radiograph. The radiologist correctly predicted that this was the right foot of the driver. The talus was pushed down exerting pressure on the navicular causing it to dislodge upwards from the ankle joint by extreme dorsiflexion of the foot against the brake pedal (Fig. XXI-15).

Sometimes the neck of the talus fractures as well. In the case of a fall on the heel, the talus acts as a wedge driven into the calcaneus causing it to fracture.

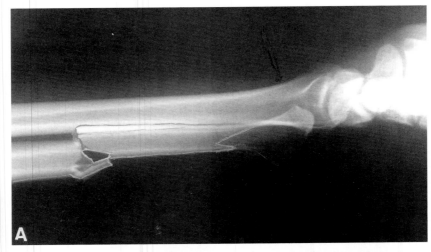

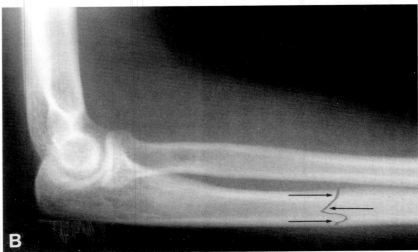

FIGURE XXI-14a–b. (A) *Fending fracture* of the ulna, the result of trying to ward off a blow by blocking it with the upraised forearm. These have also been called *night-stick* or *pool-cue* fractures. (B) A subtle, undisplaced fending fracture. (Reprinted with permission from Brogdon, B. G. (ed): *Forensic radiology,* © CRC Press, Boca Raton, Florida, 1998.)

Additional examples would include the *bumper* fracture of the pedestrian struck by an automobile (Fig. XXI-16a–b); the Y-fracture of the femur impacting a dashboard as illustrated in the chapter on the road traffic victim; the Chance fracture of the spine from hyperflexion over a lap-type belt; the tarsometatarsal fracture described as *aviator's* foot or the palmar hand fractures with thumb fracture/dislocation or avulsion from an aircraft control, whereas, flailing injuries occur on dorsal surfaces.[34,35] Certain facial fractures suggest battering, others automobile accidents, espe-

cially if related to time of presentation for medical attention.[36]

Fractures of the hyoid bone or thyroid cartilage may be associated with manual strangulation. We have seen disruption of the anterior commissure of the glottis in hanging (Fig. XXI-17).

The type of cervical spine fracture can indicate velocity at impact.[35,37]

Multiplicity of injuries at various ages may suggest different etiologies, and multiple fractures in different stages of healing in an infant or child are almost specific for child abuse.

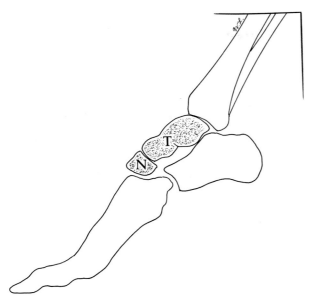

FIGURE XXI-15. During forceful dorsiflexion of the foot, the tibia will push down on the talus which in turn may dislodge the navicular. The neck of the talus may fracture to bulge under the skin at the rear of the dorsal surface of the foot.

Besides trauma, many diseases may leave a *signature* identifying the antecedent process. These are described in radiologic and anthropologic texts.

Non-Osseous Lesions

Sharp Force Injury

Stabbings and other penetrating wounds usually will not be appreciated on x-ray examination unless part of the penetrating object is left behind.

Shard of glass from a broken beer bottle was found on x-ray in the lung of a stabbing victim.

In another case a bottle was shoved into the face of an individual. The cap stayed behind, lodged in the frontal bone.

Residual bullets and pellets will be dealt with later. In rare cases, penetrating wounds with no residual inflicting instrument may have their extent and direction indicated by injection of radiopaque contrast media.

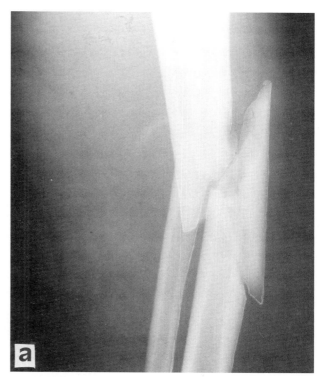

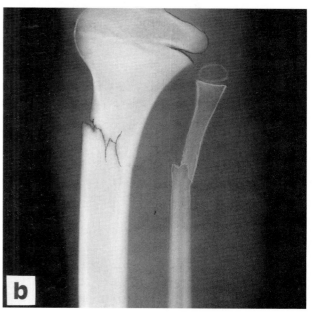

FIGURE XXI-16a–b. (a) Typical *bumper fracture* in an adult pedestrian hit from the right. (b) *Bumper fracture* in a child hit from the left is higher in the leg. Because of the increased elasticity and plasticity of young bones, the impact produced an incomplete or *green-stick* fracture. (Reprinted with permission from Brogdon, B. G. (ed): *Forensic radiology,* © CRC Press, Boca Raton, Florida, 1998.)

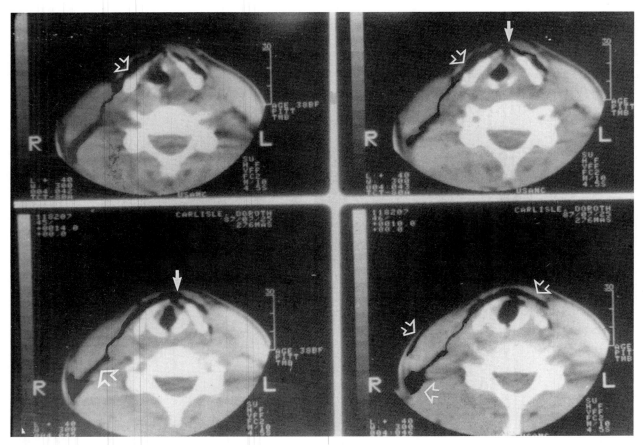

FIGURE XXI-17. CT scan of the neck shows a fracture of the anterior commisure of the larynx (arrow) with dissection of air into the soft tissues of the neck (open arrows) in this unsuccessful attempt at suicide by hanging. (Reprinted with permission from Brogdon, B. G. (ed): *Forensic radiology,* © CRC Press, Boca Raton, Florida, 1998.)

Foreign Bodies

Metallic foreign bodies are readily seen as already demonstrated. Other foreign materials also may be detected within remains and may be helpful in determining cause and manner of death.

Opaque Poisons may be seen in the stomach. Packages of narcotics can be detected in *body-bagger* smugglers, each package representing many fatal doses if broken.[38]

A man who believed he needed more lead in his system swallowed lead fishing sinkers with fatal results (Fig. XXI-18).

Chronic lead or phosphorous poisoning leaves tell-tale markers in the skeleton.

Glass commonly found in automobiles and households is radiodense with density ranging from 2.2 to 2.87 compared to 1.0 for water/soft tissue.[39,40] Whether it is detected by x-ray examination depends on the thickness and density of overlying tissues and the quality of the image. Glass in tissues may be unrecognized or misinterpreted.

Plastic as used in automobile lamp housings, is near water density and will not be revealed on x-ray examination. If embedded plastic from any source is suspected, CT or ultrasound examination will be more fruitful.

Wood is rarely detected in radiographs and should be searched for with CT or ultrasound.[40]

Animal, mineral, or vegetable matter can be aspirated, swallowed, embedded or injected and its detection by radiologic methods will depend on relative density.

Foreign bodies in inappropriate locations in the body can suggest sexual abuse, autoeroticism or psychosis (Fig. XXI-19).

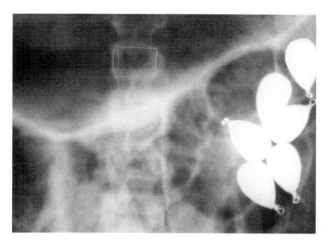

FIGURE XXI-18. Abdominal radiograph showing ingested 4-ounce lead fishing sinkers. Partially eroded or dissolved lead sinkers were removed at autopsy. (Courtesy of David R. Sipes, D.D.S.)

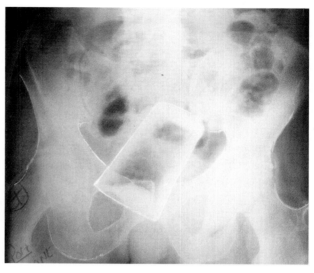

FIGURE XXI-19. Water glass in the rectum. (Reprinted with permission from Brogdon, B. G. (ed): *Forensic radiology,* © CRC Press, Boca Raton, Florida, 1998.)

Gas is a foreign substance in certain locations such as the serous cavities and spaces and in the cardiovascular system.

Infant being transported to critical care nursery, ventilated *en route* with an adult-size AMBU, was dead on arrival. Postmortem study showed air in the heart, mediastinum, hepatic and splenic veins.

Akers et al.[41] showed victims of fatal traffic accidents with craniocervical trauma had a high incidence of concomitant intravascular and intracardiac air which might be missed by the pathologist performing the autopsy unforewarned by preliminary radiography (Fig. XXI-20).

Drowning

Chest radiographs of victims of drowning will show lung density primarily due to pulmonary edema; however, there are no differentiating radiographic features between fresh water and saltwater drowning. Impacted sand in the tracheobronchial tree may be seen in a body recovered from a shoreline where there is strong surf action.[42]

Victims of scuba diving accidents may show pneumothorax, pneumomediastinum, and air embolism of varying degrees.

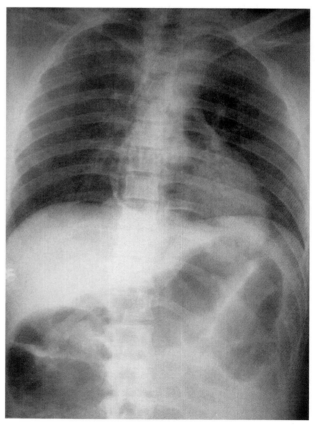

FIGURE XXI-20. Occupant of automobile in traffic collision. The victim had extensive head injuries and evidence of a massive air embolus in right chambers of the heart. (Courtesy of Daniel J. Spitz, M.D.)

Burning

Bodies that have been burned, incinerated, or cremated often are the subject of radiologic investigation. The degree of tissue destruction is a function of temperature and time. Age and size of the victim are additional factors in the equation as is whether or not the body was clothed.

Distortion of body position by shrinkage of flexor muscles produces the *pugilistic attitude* and shrinkage of extensor muscle groups will often result in wrist and ankle fractures with exposure of the respective joints. All thermal skeletal fractures complicate radiologic evaluation, however despite widespread charring of the body surface, teeth and bones may be expected to withstand an ordinary fire and the internal organs will usually be remarkably well preserved.

Bodies burned at temperatures of 800° C, such as found in ordinary house fires, will show only minimal proportional shrinkage. As temperatures increase to 1100° C, cremation temperature, so does shrinkage, up to as much as 25%, then levels off. Fleshed bones at high temperature may develop multiple fractures perpendicular to the long axis of the bone, and long bones may show some warping or bowing as they cool. Defleshed dry bones, on the other hand, tend to develop longitudinal fractures or striae.[4,43-45]

Care must be taken when trying to differentiate thermal fractures from impact fractures, as in *fuel fed* motor vehicle fires. In these cases, the critical question is whether the death of a vehicular occupant was the result of physical injuries sustained in the crash or the ensuing fire. Other times, the fire may have been intended to hide other evidence. Anytime the body surface is not amenable to detailed study, as when destroyed by fire, decomposition or other means, radiography may reveal unexpected findings not otherwise obtainable. Routine radiography of severely burned bodies may reveal other crimes.

A woman, presumably the occupant, was found burned beyond recognition after a house fire. The remains were radiographed in order to try to match with the occupant's antemortem chest film. The postmortem study was a positive match for identification but also revealed coils of wire ligature around the victim's neck.

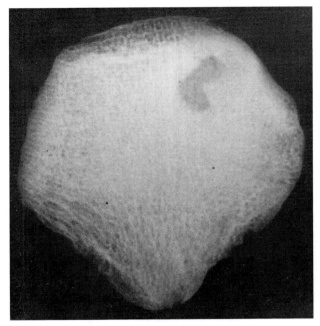

FIGURE XXI-21. A carbonized, calcined left patella was retrieved from the trunk of a burned-out automobile. When x-rayed, a rare dorsal defect of the patella (incidence = 1%) was identified in the upper outer quadrant. (Reprinted with permission from Brogdon, B. G. (ed): *Forensic radiology,* © CRC Press, Boca Raton, Florida, 1998.)

The skull may show a checkering pattern of outer table fractures from blood boiling in the diploë, or there may be complete fractures of the frontal sinuses from rapid air expansion at high temperatures, or of the calvarium from boiling blood and fluids inside the cranial vault. The bony fracture fragments will be displaced outward, whereas depression is more likely from impact injuries of blunt trauma.

For purposes of identification even calcined bones, although very delicate, will preserve enough configurational and trabecular integrity to permit radiologic comparison. Correction for shrinkage of the specimen and magnification in the fleshed antemortem study can provide superimposition of images if necessary[46] (Fig. XXI-21).

Cremains usually are purposely crushed and mixed so that there is little if any material sufficient for comparison. Individual teeth may be left, and matching of trabecular pattern in short bony segments can be attempted if bone of origin can be identified and antemortem radiographs are available. The computerized densitometric maps or densitographs of Kahana & Hiss[47] conceivably could be useful in such instances.

Gunshot Wounds

Radiologic examination in evaluation of gunfire injuries encompasses many factors of interest to the forensic pathologist.[48,49]

Location

A bullet or pellet entering the body will travel in a straight line until it loses its energy, strikes deflecting bone or exits the body. Further, the missile may be *trapped* by the cardiovascular system, gastrointestinal or urinary tract, the spinal canal or serous cavities such as the pleural or peritoneal spaces, and migrate for considerable distances from point of entry. Migration may go with or against the flow in vascular structures depending on the size of the missile and the effect of gravity. If the wound is not immediately fatal, migration may be delayed or progressive over an interval of several days.

When there is no exit wound and dissection or radiography in the area of the entry wound does not reveal the bullet, area radiography is indicated, followed by body-wide search, if necessary.

Number of Bullets

The number of bullets is important and must be correlated with entrance and exit wounds. It is unlikely that two missiles would enter through the same wound without causing a change in its appearance. Therefore, should this be suspected, consultation with a forensic pathologist may be indicated. Bullet wounds may be overlooked in the nose, mouth and body crevices. More infrequently, an entrance bullet wound may be overlooked in the eye. When this happens, the x-ray film usually shows skeletal damage of the eye socket.

Jacketed and partially jacketed bullets can lead to error since, the jacket may separate from the projectile and lead to confusion concerning the number of bullets actually present. Also, for ballistic purposes it is important to retrieve the jacket.

Caliber

Determination that bullets of different caliber are present in a body is important. Although it is generally correct that the presence of more than one caliber of bullet in the body may suggest multiple weapons have been fired and more than a single shooter, it must be remembered that a 38 caliber round can be fired from a 357 caliber pistol. Additionally, an old bullet, i.e., one from a shooting in the past, may be present in the body. Such bullet is indistinguishable from a recent shot, although on CT it may be possible to see a dense layer of surrounding scar tissue. Also, estimation of caliber from radiographs in a single plane is fraught with error since a bullet in the body is subject to some degree of magnification on the image. Elaborate methods of determining bullet caliber within the body have been suggested, but most are impractical for routine use and cannot compete for accuracy with weight and measurement of the actual bullet at autopsy.

Direction and Angle of Fire

After entering the body a bullet may fragment or shed its jacket. Fragments of the bullet may be dispersed, particularly after striking bone. These cast-off fragments clearly indicate the bullet track. If CT images are obtained, the bullet path is even more easily detected by changes in soft-tissue density due to edema and hemorrhage, whether or not bone was struck. Correlation with crime scene information often allows recreation of the relative positions of shooter and victim. Such reconstruction has been accepted in court.[50,51]

Type of Bullet

Certain types of ammunition can be identified within the body radiographically. The mush-

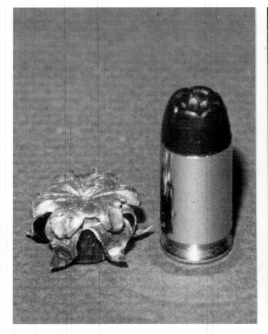
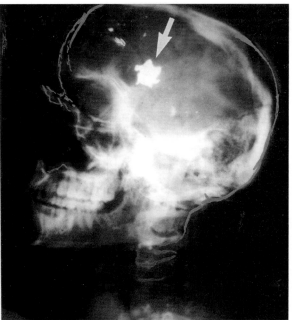

FIGURE XXI-22a–b. Fired black talon demonstrates the characteristic sharp projections that are exposed as the bullet mushrooms. The radiograph demonstrates the characteristic appearance of the black talon (arrow) and allows for a radiographic determination of the type of bullet. (Reprinted with permission from Brogdon, B. G. (ed): *Forensic radiology,* © CRC Press, Boca Raton, Florida, 1998.)

room shape of solid lead or partially jacketed bullets is characteristic. Some loads have a distinctive radiographic appearance (Fig. XXI-22a–b). High velocity hunting rifles (typically 30.06) leave a *lead snowstorm* in the body, usually after striking bone, (Fig. XXI-23) due to excessive fragmentation characteristic of unjacketed bullets. The scattering of lead fragments is usually in the shape of a funnel where the narrow end represents the entrance wound.

Range of Fire

Range of fire usually is determined by inspection of the body surface and/or its clothing. Radiology has little to offer in this area with respect to handguns and long guns. The self-contained, self-protected Faxitron® x-ray unit (Faxitron X-ray Corporation, 1670 Barclay Boulevard, Buffalo Grove, Illinois, 60089) has proved useful in examining small body fragments. It produces x-ray images of exquisite detail. It is an excellent tool for revealing gunshot residue in clothing

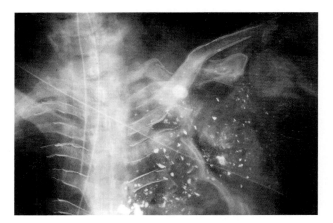

FIGURE XXI-23. A fatal high velocity rifle wound to the chest leaves a typical *lead snowstorm* of fragments. (Reprinted with permission from Brogdon, B. G. (ed): *Forensic radiology,* © CRC Press, Boca Raton, Florida, 1998.)

when visual inspection is hampered or thwarted by the presence of blood, foreign material, or dark dry patterns[52,53-55] (Fig. XXI-24).

Range of fire of shotguns can be estimated by shot patterns on the skin or clothing of the vic-

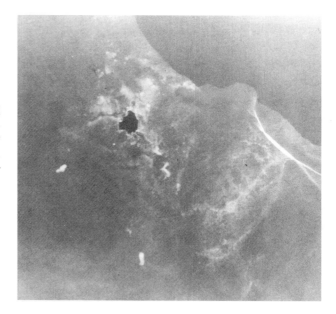

FIGURE XXI-24. A blood-soaked, dark red and black plaid flannel shirt is a difficult background for detection of gunshot residue. A low-energy radiograph with the Faxitron® unit discloses the location and distribution of residue. (Reprinted with permission from Brogdon, B. G. (ed): *Forensic radiology,* © CRC Press, Boca Raton, Florida, 1998.)

tim. Similar estimation for shot patterns within the body may be misleading because of the so-called *billiard ball effect.* The mechanism of which is described in *Chapter XII.*

Shotgun pellets, except for the steel loads mandated for waterfowl shooting, are soft and subject to deformation upon striking any firm body tissues. Large shot, 0 or 00, may resemble large caliber bullets on radiographs after deformation.[56] On the other hand, we have seen one confusing case where a decomposed body was presumed to be that of a shooting victim since it contained numerous small shotgun pellets; however, none were deformed. Actually the young decedent had died of exposure at the edge of the Sheriff's Posse Skeet Range, where spent loads had settled onto and into the decomposing body all through the winter.[57]

PHYSICAL ABUSE

Almost every application of x-ray examination to forensic matters, both criminal and civil, was predicted or initiated within two years of the announcement of Röntgen's discovery. The major exception, delayed almost half a century, was the gradual recognition and reluctant acceptance of the concept of the intentional physical abuse of infants and children by those directly responsible for their care and protection.[58]

More recently, we have come to recognize and understand that there are counterparts to the physical abuse of children to be found in two other population groups: intimate partners, and the aged and/or infirm. Each group has its patterns of injuries to be observed by direct inspection and radiologic examination.

Child Abuse

The constellation of findings leading to the radiologic diagnosis of *battered child* has not changed appreciably in 30 years; only some of those findings are more easily demonstrated with the newer radiologic modalities.

Head Trauma is the leading cause of death from child abuse and, indeed, from all trauma-related death in children.[59] Caffey's seminal paper described the association of subdural hematomas and fractures.[60] The availability of CT has greatly facilitated the diagnosis of subdural hematomas which may or may not be associated with skull fractures (*see* Figs. VIII-13 and XXI-25). Other intracranial injuries may be found as well:

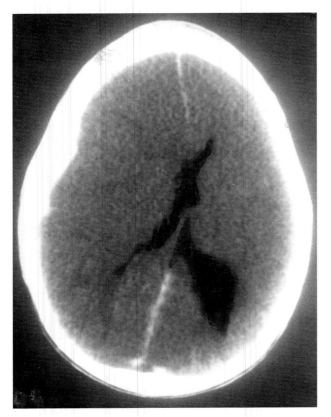

FIGURE XXI-25. Intracranial Injuries: Unenhanced CT shows blood in interhemispheric sulcus, extraapical blood on left, massive edema of left hemisphere with shift to the left, obstruction of left lateral ventricle at the forearm of Munro and cisterns. (Reprinted with permission from Brogdon, B. G. (ed): *Forensic radiology,* © CRC Press, Boca Raton, Florida, 1998.)

subarachnoid hemorrhage, intracerebral and intracerebellar hemorrhage, massive edema and, combinations of the above.

Skull Fractures: Simple linear fractures of the skull are not highly suggestive of abuse. Falls from household furniture rarely result in fractures and, usually cause only minor trauma. Complex fractures of the skull and/or serious intracranial injury, even with the history of a short fall, should raise suspicion of intentional trauma.

The head and brain oscillate asynchronously with both translational and rotational motion, shearing vessels and causing intracranial bleeding with spreading of the sutures.

Shaken baby syndrome, as described by Weston,[61] consists of massive cerebral edema and subdural hemorrhage with spread sutures but no skull fractures or soft tissue bruising.

Complete radiological examination, of any child under 3 who died under unknown, questionable, or suspicious circumstances, is warranted, if for no other reason, but to reinforce the determination that any skeletal injuries were in fact traumatic and unrelated to preexisting disease. Total body x-rays should be performed on all children whenever there is evidence suggesting abuse, even in the absence of skull fractures or intracranial injury.

Posterior Cranial Fractures

Any fracture inappropriate to the age and level of activity of the child should raise the question of intentional trauma. The frequency of posterior cranial fractures varies widely in the literature, but most occur in patients less than three years of age and half of them are found in infants.

Metaphyseal Injuries. Metaphyseal fractures are the classic injuries of physical child abuse. The fracture line crosses the extreme end of the metaphysis, creating a disc of bone between the zone of provisional calcification and the primary spongiosa of the metaphysis. The disc usually is thicker in its periphery and thinner in the center. Depending on the relationship of the fracture line to the central beam of the x-ray, the injury may appear as a transverse fracture, a *corner* fracture, a *bucket-handle* fracture, or a disc of bone (*see* Figs. VIII- 9 and XXI-26).

Diaphyseal spiral fractures are suggestive of abuse, particularly in the non-ambulatory child. Such fractures probably result from twisting or torsion forces on the extremity. Like the *toddlers* fracture, usual for activity at that age, they may be difficult to see (Figs. XXI-13 and XXI-27). Spiral fractures commonly are associated with extensive subperiosteal calcification or new bone formation if immobilization is delayed.

Periosteal new bone may occur in the absence of detectable fracture. In infants or children the periosteum is loosely attached to the underlying

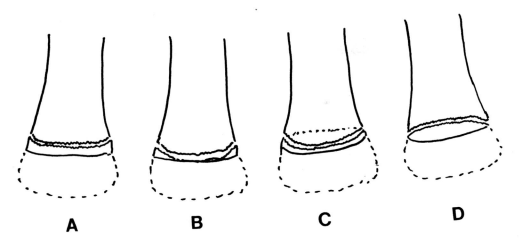

FIGURE XXI-26. Schematic drawing showing how (A) a classic transverse metaphyseal fracture can appear, by slight alteration in its relationship to the central x-ray beam, as (B) a *corner fracture,* (C) a *bucket-handle fracture* or (D) a disc of bone.

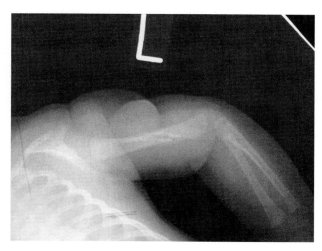

FIGURE XXI-27. Subtle spiral fracture of the distal humerus with minimal early periosteal reaction. (Courtesy of Werner U. Spitz, M.D.)

bone and is easily separated by tension and/or torsion. The resulting subperiosteal hemorrhage will calcify with time, sometimes as only a single thin line, other times as a massive collection (*see* Fig. VIII-10). Shopfner[62] has pointed out that a single thin bilateral and symmetrical, line of periosteal calcification seen in infants one to four months of age is not indicative of abuse.

Transverse fractures in long bones have a high specificity for child abuse, especially in the non-ambulant child. These relate to abusive grabbing or swinging forces which snap the bone cleanly across.

Dislocation/epiphyseal separation. True dislocations of joints are rare in the battered child. However, separation and dislocation or displacement of an epiphysis is one of the lesions first described by Caffey and is not unusual in intentional trauma.

Rib fractures are more common than fractures of the extremities, amounting to about a quarter of all skeletal fractures.[63,64] Posterior rib fractures are thought to result from grasping the chest forcefully with compression of the anterior chest. Laterally situated fractures are more likely related to direct pressure from front or back. Rib fractures are practically never seen as the result of childbirth or resuscitative effort. Fresh rib fractures are hard to see, but they heal with abundant callus and are obvious on delayed studies (Fig. XXI-28).

Fractures of the hand, excepting the uncommon fractures of the terminal phalanx of fingers caught in closing doors, are rare in infants and when found are highly suspicious of abuse.

Scapular fractures also are highly suspicious for battering. They may involve the blade, acromion, or coracoid process. Care must be taken, especially with regard to the coracoid process, not to confuse fracture with an ununited apophysis.

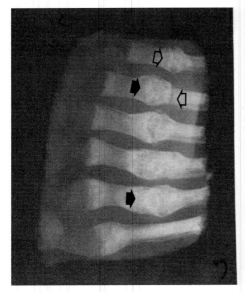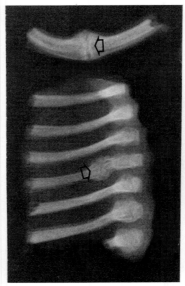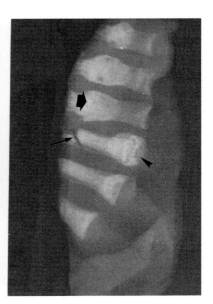

FIGURE XXI-28. Rib plate specimens removed at autopsy show evidence of repetitive trauma over time. Various fractures were estimated as (arrowhead) acute (0–7 days), (open arrow) subacute (7–14 days), (narrow arrow) healing (3–4 weeks) and (wide arrow) over (1 month or more). There are both anterior and posterior fractures suggesting squeezing and shaking. Several individual ribs show more than one fracture of different ages. Not all fractures are marked, only representative samples. (Courtesy of Werner U. Spitz, M.D.)

Clavicular fractures are the most common fractures in the newborn and typically are located in the midshaft. They are not indicative of abuse in that age group. Fractures of the lateral portion of the clavicle may result from shaking the older infant or child.

Multiple fractures and fractures of different ages. Unless there is reliable or confirmable history of major or repetitive trauma, the finding of multiple fractures in different stages of healing is the *sine qua non* in the radiologic diagnosis of child battering. The development and maturation of callus at the fracture site, or of the surrounding periosteal reaction, allows estimation of the duration of the injury. Such age estimations are not exact since the appearance, extent, proliferation and maturation of callus are related to the age of the child, the location of the fracture and the degree or absence of immobilization.

Imitative Bone Lesions: Certain diseases may produce bony changes resembling intentional trauma. They will be familiar to most radiologists, and especially those with extensive experience in pediatric radiology. These may include cases of osteogenesis imperfecta, congenital lues, rickets (vitamin D deficiency), Caffey's disease, leukemia, prostaglandin E therapy, Dilantin® therapy, Menkes' disease (kinky hair syndrome), neuroblastoma metastases, vitamin A intoxication, scurvy (vitamin C deficiency), osteomyelitis, methotrexate therapy, myelodysplasias, congenital indifference to pain, Schmid-like metaphyseal chondrodysplasia, and normal variants.

Visceral Injuries

Visceral injuries in medicolegal investigation of the dead are largely the province of the forensic pathologist. If the victim has survived long enough for medical care prior to death, there may be diagnostic studies to aid or guide the autopsy procedure. These images or their interpretation will be available in detail to the pathologist and will be dealt with only in generalities here.

Thoracic viscera are rarely involved in cases of child abuse even though the ribs are one of the most frequent sites of fracture. Minimal intrapleural blood or fluid may be demonstrated. Pulmonary contusions are occasionally seen. Cardiac and mediastinal injuries are extremely rare.

Abdominal viscera are a frequent site of abusive trauma and include duodenal hematomas, lacerations of the liver and pancreas, with or without subsequent pancreatic pseudocyst, and bowel perforation. The spleen and urinary tract are rarely injured by abusive activity.

Newer Radiologic Modalities

Increasingly, CT is used in evaluating the viscera, the head and spine.

Ultrasonography also is used extensively in head and abdominal examinations and has been utilized to demonstrate fractures and soft tissue lesions in the extremities.[65]

Nuclear medicine bone surveys are extremely sensitive to bony injury and have been strongly advocated by some for early detection of fractures[66] (Fig. XXI-29). Unfortunately, nuclear bone scans are more expensive than x-ray studies, take longer to obtain results, have a higher radiation dose, require a higher degree of technical skill, and require longer immobilization during the procedure. Also, in many areas of the country nuclear medicine studies are not immediately available at every hour of the day or night.

MRI of the brain is commonplace throughout the country. MRI is also useful in investigating the abdomen and pelvis of the traumatized child, but is used rarely in the chest or extremities. Postmortem cranial MRI has proved useful in evaluation of suspected child abuse.[67]

Abuse of Intimate Partners

Violence within marriage, cohabitation or dating mostly involves women.[36] Abuse is the most common etiology for trauma in women, exceeding motor vehicle accidents, muggings and rapes combined.[68,69] Population-based estimates indicate that battered women are more numerous than battered children.[70,71]

The head, neck and face are the principal targets of assault on women. Domestic violence and automobile accidents are the most common cause of facial injury in women and the resulting patterns are somewhat distinctive.[72] Le Fort frac-

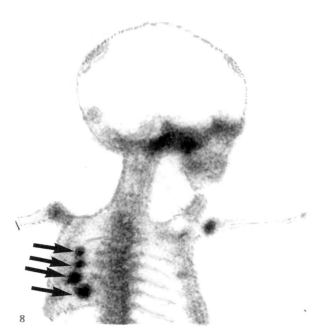

FIGURE XXI-29. Nuclear bone scan is ideal for early detection of rib fractures (arrows). Note normal high uptake at growth plate in the shoulders. Symmetrical, bilateral metaphyseal injuries would be difficult to appreciate here. The infant is slightly rotated so the proximal humeral uptake is asymmetrical. (Courtesy Dr. Damien Grattan-Smith). (Reprinted with permission from Brogdon, B. G. (ed): *Forensic radiology,* Copyright CRC Press, Boca Raton, Florida, 1998.)

ture types I and II are seen only in accident victims, while only battered women show fractures of the mandibular body/angle and the contra-lateral mandibular ramus (Figs. XXI-30a–b and XXI-31a–d). Of course, other facial fractures such as nasal, orbital, zygomaticofacial and also defensive injuries of the hand and forearm are also seen in battered women.

The chest and abdomen may be struck, but rarely produce significant injuries or rib fractures; however, common targets in the pregnant female are the breasts and abdomen. The latter has been called *prenatal child abuse.*

The majority of victims of intentional trauma delay seeking medical care for 24 hours or longer, while the vast majority of motor vehicle accident victims present for care on the day of the injury.

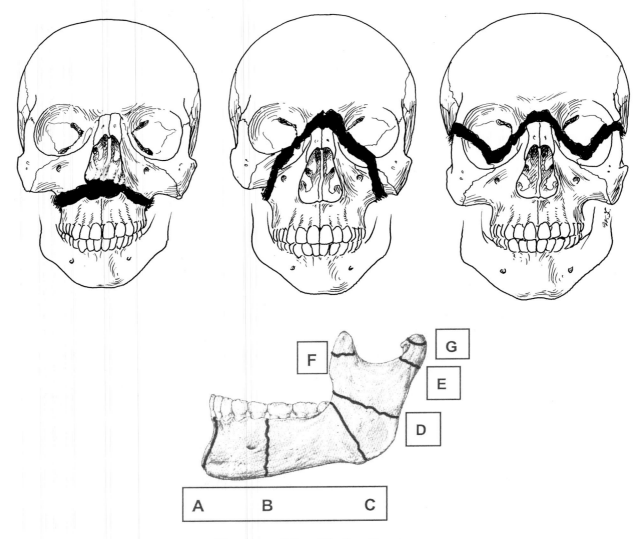

Common Mandibular Fractures

A. Symphysis   E. Condylar neck
B. Parasymphysis   F. Conoid
C. Angle   G. Intracapsular
D. Ramus

FIGURE XXI-30a–b. (a) Central fractures of the face were first classified by Le Fort in 1901 as types I, II and III. These fractures are frequently seen in drivers of automobiles following a crash, as a result of steering wheel impact. They follow the lines of least resistance and usually involve the maxillas, zygomas and the eye sockets. *Le Fort I fracture* is a horizontal fracture across the maxilla, below the nose. It is often associated with lacerations of the upper lip, malocclusion and instability of the upper jaw and its dentition. Holding the upper jaw between the index finger and the thumb, it can be moved sideways. *Le Fort II fracture* involves the midsection of the face. The fracture line runs across the cribriform plate, frequently resulting in leakage of spinal fluid through the nose. *Le Fort III fracture* involves complete separation of the central portion of the face from the base of the skull. (b) Fractures of the lower face involve the mandible and are described by the anatomical designations. Mandibular fractures are common, second only to fractures of the nose.

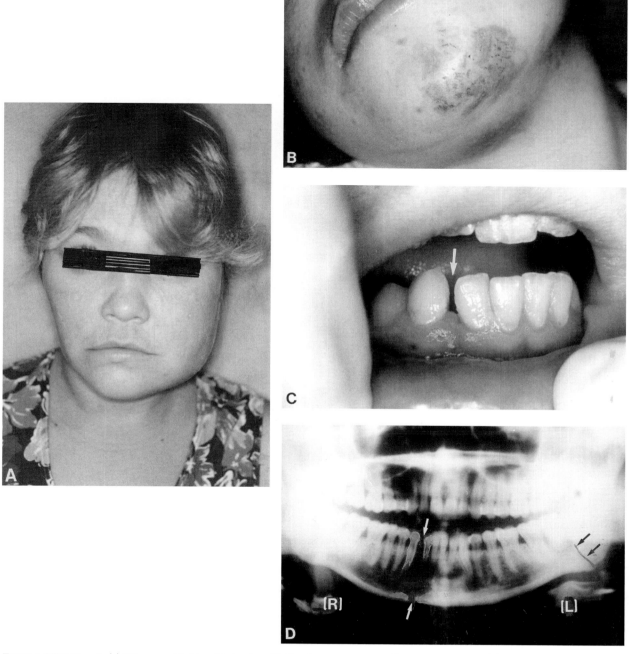

FIGURE XXI-31a–d. (a) Woman, 43, hit with husband's fist, has massive swelling over left jaw, (b) bruise and abrasions to chin, and (c) separation of teeth at fracture site. (d) Panorex study shows fractures through the left mandibular angle and right mentalis. (Reprinted with permission from Brogdon, B. G. (ed): *Forensic radiology,* © CRC Press, Boca Raton, Florida, 1998.)

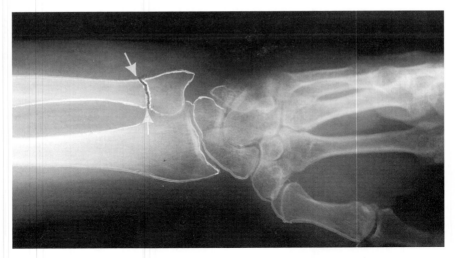

FIGURE XXI-32. This elderly female nursing home patient is profoundly osteoporotic. There is a transverse fracture of the distal ulna (arrows). Is this a defensive injury or the result of normal *handling?* The arm raised in a defensive position in front of the face will usually be palm outward, placing the ulna on top, susceptible to a blow. In a fall, on the outstretched hand, a Colles' fracture, involving the distal radius, is more likely.

Abuse of the Elderly

The first report of abuse of the elderly, *granny battering,* appeared in 1975.[36,73] Recognition of the problem has spread in the past quarter century and now all 50 states have laws on abuse of the aged. The incidence and/or recognition is increasing as is the elderly population. Diagnosis by radiologic examination is difficult. The bones of the elderly are osteopenic, often extremely fragile, sometimes broken by ordinary handling (Fig. XXI-32). Correlation with history and physical findings is important but often difficult to obtain from family caregivers or nursing home personnel (Fig. XXI-33). The victims themselves

are rarely forthcoming, fearing that compliance will result in retribution, i.e., being cast out of an abusive family situation into the more threatening care of strangers in a nursing home.

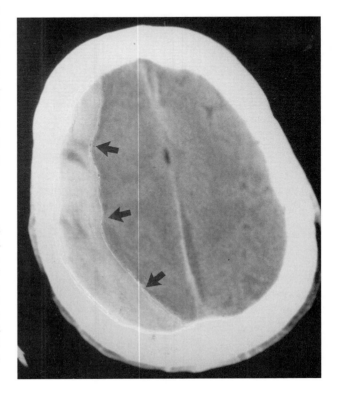

FIGURE XXI-33. This elderly male nursing home patient with dementia was taken to an Emergency Room with a split lip and bruising of the forehead and around one eye. His attendant suggested he had either fallen down or against something while walking or had fallen out of bed. He was treated and sent back to the nursing home. Two days later he was returned to the hospital with this massive fatal acute subdural hematoma (arrows). His attendant abruptly left the state that day. Review of records showed the patient to be non-ambulatory and that his mattress was already on the floor to prevent falling out of bed.

The patterns of elderly abuse are similar to those of both children and intimate partners. Maxillofacial injuries, defensive injuries and those caused by grasping, squeezing or physical restraint predominate. Thus, one looks for intra-cranial damage, facial injury, fracture of the thin, often edentulous mandible, fending fractures of the hand and forearm and twisting or turning injuries of the long bones.

REFERENCES

1. Glasser, O.: *Wilhelm Conrad Röntgen and the early history of the roentgen rays.* Springfield, IL: Charles C Thomas, 1934.
2. Eisenberg, R. L.: *Radiology: An illustrated history.* St. Louis: Mosby-Year Book, 1992, p. 63.
3. Brecher, R., and Brecher, E.: *The rays: A history of radiology in the United States and Canada.* Baltimore: Williams & Wilkins, 1969, p. 9.
4. Brogdon, B. G.: *Radiological identification of individual remains.* Chap. 8 in Brogdon, B. G. (Ed.): *Forensic radiology.* Boca Raton: CRC Press, 1998.
5. Haglund, W. D., and Fligner, C. L.: Confirmation of human identification using computerized tomography (CT). *J Forensic Sci, 38:* 708, 1993.
6. Riepert, T., Rittner, C., Ulmcke, D., Oguhuihi, S., and Scheveden, E.: Identification of an unknown corpse by means of computed tomography (CT) of the lumbar spine. *J Forensic Sci, 40:* 126, 1995.
7. Rouge, D., Telmon, N., Arrue, P., Larrouy, G., and Arbur, L.: Radiographic identification of human remains through deformities and anomalies of post-cranial bones: A report of two cases. *J Forensic Sci, 38:* 997, 1993.
8. Murphy, W. A., Spruill, F. G., and Gantner, G. E.: Radiologic identification of unknown human remains. *J Forensic Sci, 25:* 727, 1980.
9. Bass, W. M., and Driscoll, P. A.: Summary of skeletal identification in Tennessee, 1971–1981. *J Forensic Sci, 28:* 159, 1983.
10. Newell, C. W., Chucri, M. J., and Brogdon, B. G.: A primer for forensic radiology technology. Chaps. 22–24 in Brogdon, B. G. (Ed.): *Forensic radiology.* Boca Raton: CRC Press, 1998.
11. Singleton, A. C.: Roentgonological identification of victims of the "Noronic" disaster. *Am J Roentgenol, 66:* 375, 1951.
12. Mulligan, M. E., McCarthy, M. J., Wippold, F. S., et al. Radiologic evaluation of mass casulty victims: Lesions from the Gander, Newfoundland, accident. *Radiology, 168:* 229, 1988.
13. Nye, P. J., Tytle, T. L. Jarman, R. N., and Eaton, B. G.: The role of radiology in the Oklahoma City bombing. *Radiology, 200:* 541, 1996.
14. Brogdon, B. G.: Radiological identification: Anthropological parameters. Chap. 5 in Brogdon, B. G. (Ed.): *Forensic radiology.* Boca Raton: CRC Press, 1998.
15. Petrova, A., and Watson, P.: The Death of Hitler: *The full story with new evidence from secret Russian archives.* New York: Norton, 1995, p. 118.
16. Culbert, W. L., and Law, F. M. Identification by comparison of roentgenogram of nasal accessory sinuses and mastoid processes. *J Am Med Assoc, 98:* 1634, 1927.
17. Ubelaker, D. H.: Positive identification from radiograph comparison of frontal sinus patterns. Chap. 29 in Rathbun, T. A. and Buikstra, J. (Eds.): *Human identification.* Springfield, IL: Charles C Thomas, 1984.
18. Asherson, N.: *Identification by frontal sinus prints.* London: H. K. Lewis, 1965.
19. Voluter, G.: The "V" test. *Radiol Clin, 28:* 1, 1959.
20. Martel, W., Wicks, J. D., and Hendrix, R. C.: The accuracy of radiological identification of humans using skeletal landmarks: A contribution to forensic pathology. *Radiology, 124:* 681, 1977.
21. Vastine, J. H., Vastine, M. E., and Orango, O.: Genetic influence on osseous development with particular reference to the disposition of calcium in the costal cartilages. *Am J Roentgenol, 59:* 213, 1948.
22. Tsunenari, S., Uchimura, Y., Yonemitsu, K., and Oshiro, S.: Unusual personal identification with characteristic features in chest roentgenorgrams. *Am J Forensic Med Pathol, 3:* 357, 1982.
23. Ubelaker, D. H.: Positive identification of American Indian skeletal remains from radiographic comparison. *J Forensic Sci, 35:* 466, 1990.
24. Sanders, I., Woesner, M. E., Ferguson, R. A., and Noguchi, T. T.: A new application of forensic radiology: Identification of deceased from a single clavicle. *Am J Roentgenol, 115:* 619, 1972.
25. Varga, M., and Takács, P.: Radiographic personal identification with characteristic feature in the hip joint. *Am J Forensic Med Pathol, 12:* 328, 1991.
26. Moser, R. P., Jr., and Wagner, G. N.: Nutrient groove of the ilium, a subtle but important forensic marker in the identification of victims of severe trauma. *Skeletal Radiol, 19:* 15, 1990.
27. Murphy, W. A., and Gantner, G. E.: Radiologic examination of anatomic parts and skeletonized remains. *J Forensic Sci, 27:* 9, 1982.
28. Adkins, L., and Potsaid, M. S. Roentgenographic identification of human remains. *J Am Med Assoc, 240:* 2307, 1978.

29. Greulich, W. W.: Skeletal features visible on the roentgenogram of the hand and wrist which can be used for establishing individual identification. *Am J Roentgenol, 83:* 756, 1960.

30. Fitzpatrick, J. J., and Macaluso, J.: Shadow positioning technique: A method for postmortem identification. *J Forensic Sci, 30:* 1226, 1985.

31. Lichtenstein, J. E.: Radiology in mass casualty situations. Chap. 9 in Brogdon, B. G. (Ed.): *Forensic radiology*. Boca Raton: CRC Press, 1998.

32. Brogdon, B. G.: Scope of forensic radiology. Chap. 3 in Brogdon, B. G. (Ed.): *Forensic radiology*. Boca Raton: CRC Press, 1998.

33. Dixon, D. S.: Pattern of intersecting fractures and direction of fire. *J Forensic Sci, 29:* 651, 1984.

34. Kreft, S.: Who was at the aircraft's controls when the fatal accident occurred. *Aerosp Med, 41:* 785, 1970.

35. Simson, R. L., Jr.: Roentgenography in the investigation of fatal aviation accidents. *Aerosp Med, 43:* 81, 1972.

36. McDowell, J. D., and Brogdon, B. G.: Spousal abuse and abuse of the elderly–An overview. Chap. 16 in Brogdon, B. G. (Ed.): *Forensic radiology*. Boca Raton: CRC Press, 1998.

37. Jones, A. M., Bean, S. P., and Sweeney, B. G.: Injuries to cadavers resulting from experimental rear impact. *J. Forensic Sci, 23:* 730, 1978.

38. Brogdon, B. G.: Smuggling. Chap. 12 in Brogdon, B. G. (Ed.): *Forensic radiology*. Boca Raton: CRC Press, 1998.

39. deLacy, G., Evans, R., and Sandin, B.: Penetrating injuries: How easy is it to see glass (and plastic) on radiographs? *Brit J Radiol, 58:* 27, 1985.

40. Gordon, D.: Non-metallic foreign bodies: Letter to the editor. *Brit J Radiol, 58:* 574, 1985.

41. Akers, G. J., Jr., Oh, Y. S., Leslie, E. V., et al.: Postmortem radiology of head and neck injuries in fatal traffic accidents. *Radiology, 114:* 611, 1975.

42. Bonilla-Santiago, J., and Fill, W. L.: Sand aspiration in drowning and near drowning. *Radiology, 128:* 301, 1978.

43. Ubelaker, D. H.: *Human skeletal remains*. Washington, D.C.: Taraxacum, 1978, p. 33.

44. Holland, T. D.: Use of the cranial base in the identification of fire victims. *J. Forensic Sci, 34:* 458, 1989.

45. Kennedy, K. A. R.: The wrong urn: Commingling of remains in mortuary practice. *J Forensic Sci, 41:* 689, 1996.

46. Riddick, L., Brogdon, B. G., Laswell-Hoff, J., and Delmar, B.: Radiographic identification of charred human remains through use of the dorsal defect of the patella. *J Forensic Sci, 28:* 263, 1983.

47. Kahana, T., and Hiss, J.: Positive identification by means of trabecular bone pattern comparison. *J Forensic Sci, 39:* 1325, 1994.

48. Messmer, J. M.: Radiology of gunshot wounds. Chap. 10 in Brogdon, B. G. (Ed.): *Forensic radiology*. Boca Raton: CRC Press, 1998.

49. Messmer, J. M., and Brogdon, B. G.: Pitfalls in the radiology of gunshot wounds. Chap. 11 in Brogdon, B. G. (Ed.): *Forensic radiology*. Boca Raton: CRC Press, 1998.

50. Brogdon, B. G.: Two shots in the dark: Radiologic evaluation of a non-fatal shooting. *Proc Annual Mtg Am Acad Forensic Sci,* Colorado Springs, 1999, p. 119.

51. Brogdon, B. G.: Four shots in the basement: Radiologic evaluation of a non-fatal shooting. *Proc Annual Mtg Am Acad Forensic Sci,* Colorado Springs, 2001, p. 122.

52. Messmer, J. M., and Brogdon, B. G.: Pitfalls in the radiology of gunshot wounds. Chap. 11 in Brogdon, B. G. (Ed.): *Forensic radiology*. Boca Raton: CRC Press, 1998. p. 246.

53. Newell, C. W., Chucrri, M. J., and Brogdon, B. G.: Radiographic equipment, installation, and radiation protection. Chap. 22 in Brogdon, B. G. (Ed.): *Forensic radiology*. Boca Raton: CRC Press, 1998, p. 384.

54. Snell, K. S., Riddick, L., and Brogdon, B. G.: Faxitron® radiography in a forensic setting. *Proc Annual Mtg Am Acad Forensic Sci,* Colorado Springs, 1999, p. 178.

55. Snell, K. S., Carter, R. D., Riddick, L., and Goodin, J.: Identifying microscopic gunshot residue and evidence with the Faxitron®. *Proc Annual Mtg Am Acad Forensic Sci,* Colorado Springs, 2001, p. 61.

56. Froede, R. C., Pitt, M. J., and Bridgeman, R. R.: Shotgun diagnosis: "It ought to be something else." *J Forensic Sci, 27:* 428, 1982.

57. Messmer, J. M., and Brogdon, B. G.: Pitfalls in the radiology of gunshot wounds. Chap. 11 in Brogdon, B. G. (Ed.): *Forensic radiology*. Boca Raton: CRC Press, 1998, p. 239.

58. Brogdon, B. G.: Child abuse. Chap. 15 in Brogdon, B. G. (Ed.): *Forensic radiology*. Boca Raton: CRC Press, 1998.

59. Report of the U.S. Advisory Board on Child Abuse and Neglect: Fatal Child Abuse and Neglect in the United States. Washington, D.C., U.S. Department of Health and Human Services, 1995.

60. Caffey, J.: Multiple fractures in long bones of children suffering from chronic subdural hemotoma. *Am J Roentgenol, 56:* 163, 1946.

61. Weston, J. T.: The pathology of child abuse. In *The battered child,* 3rd ed., Kempe, C. H. and Helfer, R. E. (Eds.). Chicago: University of Chicago Press, 1968, p. 77.

62. Shopfner, C. F.: Periosteal bone growth in normal infants: A preliminary report. *Am J Roentgenol, 97:* 154, 1966.

63. Kleinman, P. K.: *Diagnostic imaging of child abuse*. Baltimore: Williams & Wilkins, 1987, chap. 4.

64. Kleinman, P. K., Marler, S. C., Jr., Richmond, J. M., and Blackbourne, B. D.: Inflicted skeletal injury: A postmortem radiologic-histopathologic study in 31 infants. *Am J Roentgenol, 165:* 647, 1995.

65. Nimken, K., Kleinman, P. K., Teeger, S., and Spevak, M. R.: Distal humeral physeal injuries in child abuse:

MR imaging and ultrasonography findings. *Pediatr Radiol, 25:* 562, 1995.

66. Sty, J. R., and Starsbuck, R. J.: The role of bone scintigraphy in the evaluation of the abused child. *Radiology, 146:* 369, 1983.

67. Hart, B. L.: Use of postmortem cranial CT in evaluation of suspected child abuse. Chap. 19 in Brogdon, B. G. (Ed): *Forensic radiology.* Boca Raton: CRC Press, 1998.

68. Stark, E., and Flitcraft, A.: *Spouse abuse in surgeon general's workshop on Violence and Public Health: Source book.* Leesburg, VA: Centers for Disease Control, 1985, p. SA1.

69. Drossman, D. A., Leserman, J., Nachman, G., Li, Z. M., Gluck, H., Toomey, T. C., and Mitchel, C.: Sexual and physical abuse in women with functional or organic gastrointestinal disorders. *Ann Int Med, 113:* 828, 1990.

70. Dewsbury, A. R.: Battered wives: Family violence seen in general practice. *R. R. Soc. Health, 95:* 290, 1975.

71. Collier, J.: When you suspect your patient is a battered wife. *RN, 50:* 22, 1987.

72. McDowell, J. D.: A comparison of facial fractures in women victims of motor vehicle accidents and battered women. Published thesis, University of Texas Graduate School of Biomedical Sciences, San Antonio, Texas, 1993.

73. Burston, G. R.: Granny-battering. *Br Med J, 3:* 592, 1975.

Chapter XXII

INVESTIGATION OF DEATHS FROM DRUG ABUSE

BOYD G. STEPHENS

ALCOHOL, OPIUM, AND COCAINE were probably among the first drugs abused. All three are still among the most frequently abused drugs in the world. The costs of drug abuse to society are staggering. The United States alone spends billions of dollars on drug enforcement and seizes millions of dollars worth of illegal drugs every year. Yet, the medical costs for substance abuse are in the hundreds of billions of dollars. Compare the reported 1999 budget for the Drug Enforcement Administration of $14 billion and the agency's interdiction of $24 million of the principal controlled drugs (marijuana, cocaine, heroin, and methamphetamine) in 1991 against $86 million for their 1998 interdictions[1] and the Institute of Health and Aging estimate for 1995 substance abuse medical costs of $428 billion. The estimate includes $175 billion for alcohol abuse, $114 billion for drug abuse, and $138 billion for smoking.[2] Substance abuse is part of human history and will continue to be part of our future.

Drugs of abuse are, for the most part illegal, and illegal trade carries risks. These risks must be compensated, so big profits are demanded. All these factors speak to a criminal connection and violence. For these and other reasons, drug-related death and complications are very likely to be a significant part of the medical legal investigation of death. This chapter will discuss some forensic aspects of the commonly abused drugs: cocaine, heroin, opium, amphetamines, common *designer drugs,* herbal medications, *date rape* and *club drugs,* as well as some aspects of sample collection and interpretation of analytical results.

Drug abuse is so prevalent that it should be considered as a possible cause or significant contributing factor in all death investigations, especially where death is sudden, unexpected, or where the circumstances suggest that the manner of death may not be natural. That a drug or drugs have contributed to the death may be readily apparent at the scene or be completely unsuspected. In some cases, certain features about the deceased or the scene raise suspicion that drugs may have caused or contributed to the death. Drug deaths may be readily apparent or suggested by changes noted at autopsy. As a general rule, suspicion of drug toxicity or poisoning should be entertained in most medical examiner's cases, and the appropriate samples should be routinely collected even when they are not tested initially. The collection and storage costs are low, and it is impossible to go back days later to retrieve valid specimens.

An unusual 1978 case of the political assassination of a Bulgarian defector serves as an example of the importance of proper sample collection. In addition to the investigative and medical features, which clearly indicated poisoning, the only physical evidence was the presence of a small skin puncture and the subsequent recovery of a subcutaneous particle in the soft tissue of the thigh. A small sphere of perforated plastic had been jabbed into the victim's thigh from the tip of a specially constructed umbrella. Although clearly recognized as a poisoning death, the specific poison was not confirmed until years later when new analytical techniques were developed. Ricin, the toxic alkaloid from the castor bean, was confirmed as the active agent when the stored tissue specimens were ultimately tested.

Fortunately, common drug abuse situations are less complicated and most drug analyses are much more routine. With the instrumentation and methods now available, most drugs and poisons can be detected at very low levels. Recognition of the likelihood of drug poisoning and collection and preservation of the proper samples eventually led to the diagnosis in the Ricin

1166

case. The same logic applies to routine medical examiner's cases. Collection of tissue, hair, or fluid samples for subsequent analysis by the forensic toxicologist are included in the discussion of each of the drugs discussed.

The most common types of drugs of abuse will vary from city to city and sometimes even within segments of a single jurisdiction. Ethyl alcohol is so commonly abused that collection of two or more specimens from different areas of the body should be routine. For some abusers, death comes after many years of chronic drug abuse, not from the drug itself but from chronic disease associated with that life-style, such as hepatic, cardiac, pulmonary, neurological or inflammatory disease.[3] The death may be certified as drug related or not, depending upon the investigation, policies and findings in the particular case. Chronic abuse leading to death is usually considered to be a natural manner of death, as recommended by the World Health Organization. For others, death comes because of violence and accidents. Alcohol, for example, is a common component of motor vehicle, domestic violence, and physical injuries. Because alcohol impairs judgment and increases risk taking, it is often present in trauma victims. Alcohol was commonly mentioned in combination with one or more additional drugs, and was the most frequently mentioned drug in emergency departments. While amphetamine and methamphetamine use was reported to be increasing, MDMA reports were up 58% from the level reported in 1999. There was also an increased mention of *club drugs,* which are discussed below.

In a large city, about 50% of homicides are commonly drug related. Thus, a signal issue that must be addressed by forensic medicine is the determination of the role played by drugs, if any, in a violent death. Even when there are no detectable drugs in the body of the victim, investigation may show that the motive or principal reason for the death was drug related. An example of such a case would be the shooting of a store clerk during a robbery by a person needing money to support his or her drug habit.

Following alcohol, heroin had been the leading drug of abuse for most of the past century; but sometime during 1988 that situation changed.[1] Cocaine replaced heroin as the most commonly abused drug in America primarily because of declining street costs, ready availability and the introduction of a form of cocaine called *crack*.

POSTMORTEM TOXICOLOGY

The process of collection, analysis and interpretation of postmortem toxicology can present significant difficulties. Specimens collected at autopsy are often physically and chemically, different from similar specimens collected and analyzed during life. The changes that occur with death and the biologic quality of those specimens must be considered in interpreting the significance of the toxicological laboratory findings.

When the heart stops and the blood flow ceases, the hematocrit changes locally as the cells collect by gravity, a process known as sedimentation. This same process causes livor mortis. The pH markedly decreases in some body compartments because of the build-up of acidic metabolic waste products. Drugs diffuse from higher concentrations into the surrounding tissues and organs. Native enzymes and microorganisms start the chemical degradation process, which can change or destroy pharmaceutical molecules. Protein transport mechanisms, which are pH dependent, change with the changing pH status of the body. Drugs are typically freed from carrier proteins or, in some cases, more tightly bound. This alters the form of drug that is present or the way the drug is recovered during analysis. Some drugs are present in the plasma, but not within erythrocytes. If the hematocrit is 75%, the drug concentration for a drug transported only in the plasma will be lower than if the hematocrit were 15%.

This changing nature of the blood matrix is just one example among the many factors that contribute to the alteration of drug levels within the human body following death. As a result, many drugs may not be interpretable in the same manner as the same level would be in a sample from a living person. Issues of diffusion, physiologic effect, and intoxication, as defined by a legal standard, often cannot be determined by knowing a postmortem blood level alone. Particularly over the past two decades, increasing amounts of postmortem toxicological data have been reported for many drugs and chemicals that support the existence of these changes and possible errors associated with the measurement of postmortem drug levels.

Additionally, it is often more important to compare postmortem drug levels from various fluid or tissue compartments in the process of helping eliminate the issues of contamination, redistribution and other changes that may falsely elevate or reduce the original drug level. Just the presence of a drug is often significant by itself. The ratio of the parent compound to the principal metabolites and the ratios of these compounds in various body compartments, is often the more significant argument for the interpretation of an acute versus a chronic exposure or to differentiate between the cause of death versus an incidental finding.

Generally speaking, a specific drug or chemical normally interacts with components within the body, interactions which may affect how the drug is transported, stored, or metabolized. Many of these transporter systems are pH dependent, depend upon a semi-stable complex of ions or are mechanically changed by local cellular metabolism. How drugs are stored within the body, if at all, and the metabolic pathway for their elimination also depend upon a number of variables. Ethyl alcohol, for example, is rapidly absorbed into the body and quickly distributes to equilibrium throughout all body compartments, based upon their water content. The elimination is primarily by a specific enzyme system, which is independent of concentration, except at fairly low and high ranges. There are, however, drugs that can interfere with or compete for the same metabolic pathway. The metabolism and elimi-

nation of ethyl alcohol ceases with death. The blood levels may stay stable, be affected by hematocrit and fluid changes or change if bowel or tissue diffusion occurs. Alcohol from fermentation usually takes hours to begin, depending upon the local environment.

In a similar fashion, postmortem redistribution, continued metabolism, chemical decomposition and a number of other changes make the interpretation of limited postmortem drug data the kind of information that is often misleading, even though such data are often desirable and may be important or critical to an investigation. GHB (gamma hydroxybutyrate), for example, forms *de novo* in the body after death. Thus, any postmortem data must be considered and interpreted carefully in light of all available information about the case. Some postmortem drug data, such as cocaine or morphine levels, are at best helpful guidelines, with the actual drug levels having little correlation to any physiological or psychological effect. They are examples of drugs in which the actual measured level in a deceased individual has little correlation to the clinical effect or determination of poisoning.

However, there are many important factors about postmortem toxicological data that can lead to an understanding of the cause and manner of death. Drug and chemical analysis are often the ultimate diagnostic tests that prove, refute, or make a diagnosis about the circumstances surrounding the death. Because drugs and chemicals are so often factors in deaths undergoing legal review, having a good understanding of the investigation, diagnostic findings, specimen collection and data interpretation is an important part of the forensic investigator's training. It is important to realize the need to analyze the same drug or chemical in several body compartments and, where possible, to look at the level of parent drug and the principal metabolite rather that just at the blood level alone. This is often more important in understanding the circumstances of the death than to depend upon a single blood measurement. These issues will briefly be explored in this chapter.

CALCULATING TOTAL DRUG DOSE

There is a simple formula for calculating the amount of drug necessary to produce a given blood level. This formula is most helpful in living patients. However, when blood is not flowing and mixing in a normal fashion, has changed pH so that protein binding or ionic form has changed and so forth, it should be used more as a qualitative estimation of total dose, functioning more as a guideline than an absolute.

The formula is:

Dose = wt (Kg) × blood level (mg/L) × Vd (L/Kg)

wt = weight in kilograms
blood level = reported value in mg/L
Vd = volume of distribution in L/Kg

All the units, except milligrams, cancel out so that the results are expressed in milligram of absorbed drug. Vd (volume of distribution) is readily available in many toxicological texts, pharmacological sources and drug data.[4]

This formula is helpful when contemplating how many tablets or capsules of a drug are likely to have been taken to reach a reported drug level. The calculated data are useful as long as the results are considered a guideline, not an absolute value, when working with a postmortem sample. The results can be very misleading and should always be considered along with other information from the investigation. When so indicated by the nature of the case, a forensic toxicologist who has postmortem analytical experience about the potential interpretation may be helpful.

When looking at data from the blood and another compartment, such as spinal fluid, and both are extremely high, the drug level is most likely truly high and significant in the death. Should one be high and the other low, there is postmortem redistribution, contamination or acute drug exposure without sufficient time for the drug to have moved to its usual pharmacological equilibrium. When looking at different compartments, it is necessary to know that the drug will actually go into that compartment and to what degree. For example, cocaine base freely crosses the blood brain barrier but benzoylecgonine does not. Therefore, benzoylecgonine found in the brain was formed in the brain and has to be metabolized within the brain.

ETHYL ALCOHOL

Ethyl alcohol is the most abused drug throughout the world. Determining ethyl alcohol concentration on samples from a deceased individual, especially after physical violence or injuries caused by resuscitation, is often best achieved by looking at ethyl alcohol levels in cerebral spinal fluid, urine or vitreous fluid. Allowance must be made for absorption, water content and contamination, but these compartments are frequently protected during trauma, more so than are the blood and organs within the torso. Alcohol within the gastric tract quickly diffuses into the surrounding tissues, and with mechanical injury, this effect is often magnified.[5] Therefore any sample collected from the chest or abdomen is likely to be contaminated in such cases. Peripheral blood, obtained from the proximal end of a major vessel of an extremity, is much more likely to yield a helpful sample than would a sample collected from the right heart or inferior vena cava. Without a sample from a distant and protected body compartment as a comparison basis, the central blood level may be inaccurate and misleading.

Paramedics often draw blood when they start their resuscitation procedures. This can be an important source of pretreatment peripheral blood. Blood collected in the emergency department within a tube with sodium fluoride as a preservative or the sample sent to the blood bank for cross matching may offer a chance to look at a blood sample that was taken prior to resuscitation, transfusion and the passage of time. Samples collected in serum separator tubes for drug analysis, may be faulty as some drugs are absorbed into the gel and the resulting analysis of the serum would be in error. Samples of plasma or serum that have been separated typically have a large headspace, and the alcohol concentration will continue to drop by evaporation. Opened laboratory or blood bank tubes are helpful to support the presence of ethyl alcohol, but the concentration must be considered as an approximation. Metabolism of many drugs, such as alcohol, will continue as long as there is a reasonable amount of blood flowing to the liver, even if the patient is in severe shock, on a respirator, brain dead, or being resuscitated.

Blood alcohol levels can also vary because of hematocrit changes. Alcohol is present within the water of the plasma, but typically absent or present at only low levels within erythrocytes. Replacement therapy with blood products, fluid replacement with volume expanders and other resuscitative procedures can dilute the intravascular alcohol concentration. Since alcohol quickly diffuses through all tissues, recently consumed alcohol within the stomach will not only diffuse directly into the surrounding organs and tissues (such as the inferior vena cava, liver, spleen) but can be transported to some limited extent within the vascular system by resuscitation or postmortem manipulation of the body. If there is terminal or partial aspiration of gastric contents, alcohol will rapidly be absorbed from the lungs into the pulmonary vessels or contaminate the heart by direct local diffusion.

Local diffusion into surrounding organs is also true for a number of other drugs. Thus, central vascular blood, right heart blood, bile, liver, and so forth typically are not good samples to be used alone in the determination of the blood alcohol or drug content in an autopsy case. Reliance on these sources should be considered when they are the only specimens available. In such a case, the presence of a drug or chemical should be considered as the more significant finding than any interpretation of the amount of the drug.

For ethyl alcohol, consideration must also be given to the presence of the compound secondary to the fermentation process only. In a major case, it may be necessary to look for other chemicals known to be produced during the fermentation of body sugars to discount the finding of ethyl alcohol in the absence of its presence from another body fluid compartment or investigative information supporting the ingestion of the drug. By calculation, fermentation of natural sugars within the blood and tissues could produce an ethyl alcohol of about 0.20%. Alcohol can also be used as a food source by some microorganisms or the volatile compound can be lost into the environment. Since two moles of ethyl alcohol are produced from each mole of sugar fermented, a small amount of sugar can produce a significant amount of alcohol.

The secondary products of fermentation include heat and carbon dioxide. If fermentation occurs within a rubber-stoppered tube, the resulting gas pressure is likely to blow the stopper off the tube. The presence of a preservative, such as sodium fluoride at a concentration higher than 2 mg/mL, final dilution, likely will stop bacterial or yeast metabolism. Most forensic toxicologists recommend that blood be collected with sodium fluoride at a final dilution of 10 mg/mL and the specimen stored in the refrigerator until analyzed. It is important that the blood specimen be well mixed with the preservative and that all clots are broken up so that the preservative is diluted equally throughout the specimen.

In high-energy deaths, such as explosions or aircraft crashes, the vitreous fluid should be collected as soon as possible. Each eye should be sampled and tested separately. The finding of similar levels in the two samples would be more suggestive of a true value than differing levels. Fermentation of tissues or gastric contamination can lead to high local alcohol concentrations. High concentrations and tissue exposure can lead to diffusion through the wall of the globe. If the eye is exposed to the liquid contents of the bowel, the level is more likely to increase than decrease over a short time period. The entire scene and investigative findings often have to be considered in the process of interpreting alcohol levels, especially when extreme and destructive violence to the body or extremes in the environmental conditions and decomposition are seen.

Calculating Ethyl Alcohol Levels

There is a simple formula for calculating the amount of ethyl alcohol or number of drinks represented by a given blood level or given amount or type of alcoholic beverage. For the reasons mentioned above, this is a much more reliable aid in samples from a living person than from an autopsy specimen.

Eric M.P. Widmark, a physician, investigated the absorption and metabolism of ethyl alcohol. He developed a formula that allowed calculation of the blood alcohol concentration, when the amount of consumed alcohol was known, or the amount of consumed alcohol when the blood alcohol concentration was known. The formula is:

$$C = \left[\frac{a}{P \times r} \right]$$

Where *"a"* is the weight of ethyl alcohol in grams, *"P"* is the body weight in kilograms and *"r"* is a ratio factor derived from a table based upon the person's sex and weight. *"C"* represents the blood alcohol concentration. The specific gravity of ethyl alcohol is typically reported as four significant figures, or 0.7939 grams/mL at room temperature. Usually, this is reduced to 0.79 grams/mL for calculation purposes. The value will change slightly, depending upon the temperature of the solution. The mean *"r"* factor is 0.68 for a male, 0.55 for a female.

The weight of alcohol can be determined by multiplying the reported percent concentration by the volume in milliliters. This yields the amount of ethyl alcohol in milliliters. The value has to be corrected from volume to weight by multiplying the value by the specific gravity of ethyl alcohol at a given temperature. The *"r"* factor is a relation of the distribution of alcohol within the body. This is an early statement of the volume of distribution we use today. The formula calculates the value in liters. The results have to be divided by ten to yield a result in grams/ 100 milliliters.

An easier formula to work with is attributed to C.L. Winek.[6] The formula is:

$$\frac{150 \text{ pounds}}{A} \times \frac{B}{50}\% \times \frac{C}{1} \times 0.025\% = D$$

A = weight in pounds
B = alcohol concentration in percent
C = number of ounces consumed
D = blood alcohol concentration

For example, consider a 120-pound woman who consumes beer (4% alcohol). She drinks 72 ounces. What would be her blood alcohol content? The formula becomes:

$$\frac{150 \text{ lbs}}{120 \text{ lbs}} \times \frac{4\%}{50\%} \times \frac{72 \text{ oz}}{1 \text{ oz}} \times 0.025\% = 0.180\%$$

This formula is based upon the volume of distribution of ethyl alcohol in water, and that one-ounce of 50% alcohol will elevate the blood alcohol of a 150 to 170-pound man to 0.025%. The significant advantage over the Widmark formula is that there are no conversions to calculate. The concept of the diffusion of alcohol based upon the water content within the body is something that Dr. Widmark fully understood and expressed with his *"r"* factors.

Ethyl alcohol concentration is typically reported to two significant figures in forensic toxicology, such as 0.15%, where the percent represents the weight of ethyl alcohol in a given volume of blood. This is by convention the number of grams of ethyl alcohol in 100 mL of blood. Clinical laboratory reports are more commonly in milligrams/100 mL of blood. So 100 mg/dl becomes 0.10 grams/dl or 0.10%. It is important to add the zero before the decimal so that the value is clearly indicated as being less than one.

Calculations are approximations, and a range should always be considered when giving an estimate of the results.

If the woman started drinking at a constant rate at 20:00 hours and stopped drinking at 23:00, what would her calculated blood level be if she died at midnight?

Ethyl alcohol is metabolized at the rate of 0.018% per hour for the majority, but not all, people. If you use the rate of 0.015 to 0.02% reduction per hour to cover the metabolic rate of a wide range of people, the results become:

$$0.180\% - (0.015\% \times 4 \text{ hours})$$
$$= (0.180\% - 0.060\%) = 0.120\%$$

$$0.180\% - (0.018\% \times 4 \text{ hours})$$
$$= (0.180\% - 0.072\%) = 0.108\%$$

$$0.180\% - (0.020\% \times 4 \text{ hours})$$
$$= (0.180\% - 0.080\%) = 0.100\%$$

Her blood alcohol concentration calculates to approximately 0.10 to 0.12% (see reasons for reporting a range below). Because of the variability in metabolism and the likely inaccuracies in the historical data, the calculated value is always to be considered an estimate. In this example, no allowance was made for the absorption period, which is usually short. No allowance was made for the variable rate of consumption. Again, simple calculations must be used in consideration of the known facts about the case. If the consumption data are accurate, and the calculated blood level differs greatly from the actual measured level in two compartments of the body, either the person did not die at midnight or there is another factor, such as decomposition, which alters absorption or metabolism, or the consumption statement was wrong. Comparisons with the alcohol content of the spinal fluid or vitreous will likely help determine whether the blood alcohol is correct or not.

Alcohol distribution is based upon the water content for each of the body's fluid compartments. There is more water in vitreous fluid than blood. Therefore, at exact equilibrium, the actual alcohol level will vary slightly in each body compartment, depending on which fluid source is being discussed. It is possible to calculate the blood level by correcting the alcohol level determined in another compartment by a factor reflecting the ratio of alcohol to blood at equilibrium. If the alcohol is still being absorbed and distributed into the body water, the blood alcohol level will typically be higher than in the other compartments. If alcohol absorption and diffusion have gone to completion and the patient is eliminating the drug from his or her body, the tissue and fluid compartment will be at or slightly higher than the blood alcohol level. (See Chapter XXIII on "Forensic Aspects of Alcohol" for a discussion of these ratios.)

In the case of gastric contamination, one would typically see a significant difference in the alcohol level from heart blood as compared to that of vitreous or spinal fluid, supporting that the blood level, is potentially misleading. A slightly higher blood level than seen in spinal fluid or vitreous could support that the body water deposition was going up, and there was a recent ingestion of alcohol. Spinal fluid and vitreous levels higher than the blood or equal to it could indicate that the individual was in the excretion phase, and had not recently ingested alcohol. These can be important issues in time of death considerations or in investigating given information about a case for truthfulness.

Another potential error in this example is assuming that all beer contains 4% alcohol. Most people do not realize that what is commonly called beer can range in alcohol content from 2 to 3% up to 6 to 8%. Technically, porter, ale and stouts are often at or above 6%, but some have alcohol concentrations of less than 6%, while some beers are over 6% ethyl alcohol. In reality, beer concentrations vary over a reasonably wide range of alcohol content. A number of websites monitor these data. The Bureau of Alcohol, Tobacco and Firearms (ATF), has one that lists the alcohol content for a long list of domestic and imported beers and ales. A number of popular websites also list the alcohol content of various brands of beer, and a number of papers concerning variable alcohol content have been published.[7-10] This significant issue arises in driving while intoxicated cases for court presentation where forward and backward timed calculations of consumption or blood alcohol content are often performed as part of the testimony.

Another issue is the wide variety of container sizes for beer ranging from 4 to 6 fluid ounces up to a 40 fluid ounce container and still be bottled beer. This may be an issue in an autopsy case and is sometimes an issue in cases of driving under the influence.

Alcohol is eliminated by zero order kinetics; generally speaking, the excretion of ethyl alcohol is linear in a living person after peak absorption, and tissue distribution has occurred. This statement indicates that the metabolic rate of ethyl alcohol is not affected by concentration except at high or low concentrations, and that the rate is constant. There are a number of other toxicological considerations, one would not use this information alone when evaluating a case of driving under the influence. One would need to know other facts about ethyl alcohol absorption and metabolism. Individual variability regarding the rate of metabolism of alcohol may also play a role.

For practical purposes, the metabolism of ethyl alcohol stops at death. Until fermentation, diffusion, decomposition or physical changes occur, the level tends to remain stable after death for some time. Blood, spinal fluid, urine and muscle tend to stay stable, while blood rapidly changes physically as the cellular components concentrate by the effects of gravity. Peripheral blood levels are typically stable for between 12 and 20 hours, but may be unreliable in as few as 6 hours. Vitreous, spinal fluid and typically urine levels are stable for 24 to 48 hours. These compartments may be useful beyond this time, but eventually may also become contaminated by the decomposition process.

The presence of ethyl alcohol interferes with the neurotransmitter GABA, primarily disrupting the reticular activating system, even at low concentrations. As a result, thought becomes progressively cloudy and disrupted as a function of increasing alcohol concentration. The person has increasingly impaired judgment and reduced self-criticism. Risk taking is enhanced. Higher thought processes are disrupted and short-term memory is poor. Consequently, the person is more likely to take unnecessary risks, engage in violent behavior, exhibit mood swings and be destructive.

If a person weighing 160 pounds consumed six drinks of 80 proof (40%) vodka in one hour, his or her blood alcohol concentration would increase to about 0.12%. For his or her blood alcohol level to return to zero would take about seven hours. Alcohol absorption is generally rapid, with most consumed alcohol being absorbed within 15 to 30 minutes. With large amounts of alcohol, or alcohol consumed in the presence of large amounts of food, peak absorption can be delayed to one hour or slightly longer. The neurological effect is often *felt* by the drinker more while the alcohol concentration is rising than when it is decreasing. Exercise and drinking coffee will not increase the rate of metabolism. Alcohol has a high relationship to injuries, violence and risk-taking behavior. It is therefore the most commonly detected drug in forensic cases.

Studies support that some individuals may have a genetic predisposition that makes them more susceptible to alcohol abuse. Alcohol toxicity is associated with dehydration and the accumulation of acid aldehyde, a chemical produced during the second stage of alcohol metabolism. Acid aldehyde is particularly toxic when the concentration rises to detectable levels. Alcohol poisoning generally produces respiratory depression, but alcohol toxicity can lead to death through other mechanisms such as aspiration. High levels of ethyl alcohol can be found in the alcohol tolerant. The highest level reported by our laboratory in a case of driving while intoxicated is 0.54%, and levels of over 1.0% are reported in the literature for people who survived. The lowest level reported in our office for a cause of death directly due to toxicity was 0.11% in a teenager who drank a quantity of whisky on a dare. His death was due to respiratory depression and considered accidental.

A genetic factor affects the metabolism of alcohol. Several genes express the enzyme alcohol dehydrogenase, and several express the enzyme aldehyde dehydrogenase. People who have only half or less of the genetic code for aldehyde dehydrogenase have difficulty metabolizing that compound and may become toxic or die after ingesting a moderate dose of alcohol. This fact may explain why one young person in a group dies with a blood alcohol level of less than 0.20% and another is only unconscious with a blood level of 0.45%. There are racial expressions for this genetic code. As an example, the incidence of low aldehyde dehydrogenase expression is generally higher in people of Asiatic origin than in Europeans.

ABUSE DRUGS AND LAWS

When mankind first began to use plants for medicinal purposes or first began to use them for abuse is unknown. We do know from archeological and historical data that ancient peoples were very much aware of the medicinal properties of plants and routinely used them to treat a wide variety of external and internal disorders. Similarly, modern man has often utilized the naturally occurring chemicals obtained from plants, first as extracts or isolates, then as the molecular basis for chemical analogs for the creation of new drugs. In many cases, modern chemistry simply developed synthetic sources of naturally occurring compounds or chemically altered an existing natural compound. Today, pharmaceutical compounds typically have one of two distinct origins: Those derived directly from plants and those developed synthetically.

An often-debated issue associated with the question of drug abuse is whether some drugs should be legalized in order to reduce criminality and the hazards associated with their distribution and use. The importation and distribution of illicit drugs in the United States is a multibillion dollar industry, which produces no tax revenues for the government. The enormous costs of law enforcement, medical and social complications from their use, addiction treatment and the judiciary costs are born mostly by the taxpayer.[11] However, America's and other countries' early experience with unlimited drug access was unsuccessful.

In an attempt to limit drug availability and curb drug use, laws specific to the drug abuse problem have been enacted over the years. In 1914, the Harrison Narcotic act was the first federal attempt to regulate coca and opium. This legislation was in part a response to the problem of large numbers of infant and children's deaths resulting from the over-the-counter availability of laudanum and its use for everything from controlling teething pain to infanticide. Currently, the Controlled Substance Act (Comprehensive Drug Abuse Prevention and Control Act) of 1970 is the legal foundation for government control and enforcement of drug manufacturing and use

in the United States. This act is a consolidation of numerous laws relating to the manufacture, distribution and prescription of narcotics, stimulants, depressants and hallucinogens. It extends government control of drugs from the import of raw materials or the precursor stage of manufacture to their delivery to the patient.[12] Many additional laws have been enacted on this subject since that time, many specifically pertaining to drug analogs and driving under the influence of drugs and/or alcohol.

For the drugs discussed here, a brief history of the manufacture or discovery, the importation and forms of distribution, the common method of use and the common or principal findings at autopsy are presented.

Cocaine

History

Cocaine is derived from the leaves of the coca plant *Erythroxylon coca,* which is native to the eastern half of the Andes Mountains. Although it is grown primarily in the mountains of South America, commercial cultivation has been highly successful in a number of other countries.[13] The plant is a shrub with small simple leaves that are harvested by hand. Although capable of growing to a height of 10 to 12 feet, it is usually kept pruned to a height of three to six feet to enhance harvesting. Most of the many thousands of pounds of cocaine smuggled into the United States come from the mountains of Peru, Bolivia and Columbia.

It is estimated that more than 30 million Americans have tried cocaine at least once and that five million people use the drug on a regular basis. The drug's popularity in other countries is also increasing. Every day, an estimated 5,000 people use cocaine for the first time.

According to the 2000 statistical report of the Drug Abuse Warning Network (DAWN), cocaine was the most commonly mentioned drug, other than alcohol, among reporting emergency rooms and medical examiners.[14] In the emergency room reports, cocaine was the most commonly mentioned drug in 29% of the drug-related cases reported. Cocaine mentions increased significantly in six of 21 metropolitan areas. In death reports from medical examiners, cocaine was the leading drug reported, up 13% in some areas. Even though deaths from cocaine are relatively common now, the first cocaine death was reported in 1893, more than 100 years ago.

Knowledge and use of coca leaves go back many thousands of years. The Incas used coca and it is sometimes referenced as the *Divine Drug of the Incas*. Recent excavations of Incan tombs suggest that the drug was used at least 4,000 years ago by the nobility, since classic lime pots and sticks used as spatulas for removing the lime from the pots, have been found in these burials. However, since only royalty were buried with their possessions, the level of use throughout the Incan society is unknown. Supplies of coca leaves have also been found in later burials dating from as early as 2,000 to 3,000 years B.C., again supporting that the drug was used in the region thousands of years ago. Work that is more recent has shown benzoylecgonine, the main metabolite of cocaine, in the hair of Peruvian and Chilean mummies buried more than 2,000 years ago in the arid Atacama Desert on the border of Northern Chile. Centuries later the Spanish noted its common use when they invaded Peru in the sixteenth century (Fig. XXII-1).

Today, the leaves are still chewed by Peruvian Indian men, women and even children for energy and to offset the cold and hunger associated with their lives high up in the mountains. They use the leaves by mixing them with a base, usually slaked lime, to change the pH and enhance the release of the alkaloid. The leaf is wrapped around a small amount of lime and placed between the teeth and the cheek. Alternately, lime is added to the chewed leaf from time to time in small amounts. Saliva and occasional chewing release the drug over several hours. Some suggest that the stimulant effect improves their ability to live and work at high altitude. The Spanish invaders initially refused to allow the natives to chew coca, considering it evil. However, they soon observed a significant reduction in

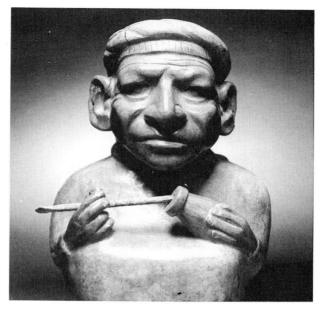

FIGURE XXII-1. A Peruvian pot depicting a man using coca. After placing coca leaves in his mouth, lime is added from the gourd. (Courtesy, *National Geographic*, Vol. 177, No. 6, June 1990. Used with permission. Photo by Nathan Benn (c). © National Geographic Society.)

the productivity of their forced laborers. Being practical, they again allowed coca chewing and the work output is reported to have increased.

In the 1800s, European travelers observed the Indians chewing coca leaves and putting saliva on wounds to reduce pain, making cocaine the first drug to be used as a local anesthetic. But centuries earlier it may have been used as a local anesthetic to allow trephination of the skull, since no source of opiates is known for South America. Skulls have been found with trephination wounds and evidence of bone healing, indicating significant survival periods. Since some of the skulls show no evidence of battle-related trauma, which might be expected to lead to loss of consciousness, the use of a drug to allow such surgery seems likely. Some skulls show multiple trephination events with healing over a period of years.

Cocaine was isolated from cocoa leaves over 100 years ago by Gaedicke (1855) and Nieman (1859). The stimulating effect of the drug made it popular in both Europe and America. Initially, cocaine was imported into the United States in small quantities, so that the numbers of recreational users was limited by its availability and cost. During this time, only the wealthy could afford the drug. Later, legal imports increased to the extent that by 1886, the price of cocaine had fallen to approximately 25 cents per gram. The public had many choices of products containing the drug, from teas and wines to salves and lotions, drops and sprays, cigarettes and patent medicines. These preparations were used for aches and pains as well as tonics. Cocaine was promoted as a safe drug, no more habit forming than was coffee or tea. Experience would show otherwise.

In the United States, William A. Hammond, a well-known neurologist, spoke and wrote favorably about the use of cocaine. In 1887, he lectured that cocaine was a safe drug. A cocaine wine he developed and sold contained two grains of cocaine per pint (one gram = 15.432 grains). He promoted it as a tonic and elixir. He claimed that it was more beneficial than the popular European elixirs, which contained only one-half grain to the pint of the drug. A wide range of cocaine-containing preparations soon became popular.

The public began to use large amounts of cocaine. Of the several tonics and soft drinks containing cocaine, probably the best-known survivor is Coca-Cola®. John Pemberton had created Coca-Cola in 1886 as a drink containing caffeine and cocaine, but without alcohol, the latter losing popularity in America with the approach of Prohibition. Lacking alcohol, Coca-Cola was considered a temperance drink and gained wide popularity. Cocaine was removed from Coca-Cola in 1900, the year before the city of Atlanta passed an ordinance, which prohibited providing cocaine to a consumer without a doctor's prescription.

In the United States, an extensive public campaign was eventually mounted to link cocaine with crime and immoral acts. Similar activities were ongoing regarding alcohol. The result was a change in public attitude about the unlimited use of cocaine, and over a period of years, laws were passed in 46 states regulating the sale and use of the drug. At that time, states, not the federal government, were responsible for health issues. It was up to the individual state to determine what was and was not a safe drug and acceptable formulation. Although products containing cocaine were still sold, its presence was often not mentioned on the label. This changed in 1906, when the Pure Food and Drug Act required that all active ingredients be listed.

Cocaine was largely introduced into medicine through the works of two Viennese physicians, Sigmund Freud and Karl Koller. Freud made a detailed study of cocaine, noting its physiologic and central nervous system effects. He published the first comprehensive paper on cocaine, *Über Coca,* in 1884.[15] Freud gave a detailed account of his studies, including the psychopharmacological effects of the drug in humans, and suggested a number of medicinal uses. He strongly supported cocaine, using it to wean one of his patients from morphine addiction. Unfortunately, in the end, he converted the patient from morphine to a cocaine addiction, from which the patient eventually died. Freud reportedly became addicted to the drug himself, but eventually was able to be cured.

Koller used cocaine as a local anesthetic for eye surgery, a practice that rapidly became popular and gained wide medical acceptance. By 1884, Hall and others had used the drug for infiltration anesthesia, and dentistry began using it as a local anesthetic. A year later, it was used as a local nerve block for surgery. Chemical research on the drug continued. Einhorn developed the first of many synthetic substitutes in 1892, resulting in the introduction to medicine in 1905 of procaine. A series of *caine drugs,* such as lidocaine became popular for medical use. The synthetic compounds lacked many of the unfavorable aspects of the parent drug, such as ulceration of the cornea and addiction.[16,17]

Karch, in his interesting book *A Brief History of Cocaine,* noted that much of the important work on the medical problems associated with cocaine use had been published in German before the turn of the twentieth century. He concludes that many of the pathologic problems associated with cocaine abuse had been described and solved by these early researchers, but their work is now largely ignored because it was published a long time ago in another language.[13]

When it was first being investigated, cocaine was used primarily for surgery of the eye, the nose and the throat. Because of its vasoconstrictor properties, which decrease bleeding, this is still its primary use in medicine today. Occasionally, however, cocaine is currently being used during some emergency intubations, a fact that must be considered when interpreting drug levels in resuscitated patients with no investigative history of drug use or exposure.

Coca is now grown on large plantations, and the mature leaves are usually harvested by manually picking each leaf, somewhat like the process for gathering tea. Women and children often perform this work. To process the crop, the leaves are placed in shallow plastic-lined or concrete pits. The mat of leaves is made alkaline, sometimes with lime or lye, and a solvent such as gasoline or alcohol is poured over them. Workers then pulverize the leaves with wooden pestles or trod upon the leaves and solution, sometimes in their bare feet, to macerate and speed up the extraction of the alkaloid into the solvent. The liquid is removed, the solvent evaporated, and the resulting material is called paste. Cocaine paste is the alkaloid form of the drug. It is chemically stable and can be smoked or taken orally. Paste is seldom seen in the United States or Canada, though it is popular elsewhere.

The typical produce for illegal import into North America is cocaine hydrochloride. Paste is transferred from the plantation to a laboratory where it is re-extracted and acidified to make the hydrochloride salt. After the secondary processing step, cocaine is present in concentrations of 60 to 89%. Depending upon the method and technique of preparation, cocaine hydrochloride may appear as solid chunks, flakes, or powder. Although the pure crystal form is white, high quality cocaine hydrochloride may sometimes have a slight color due to impurities left over from the processing. It is chemically stable and can be snorted or injected. It cannot be readily smoked.

The product is often put up as one kilogram bricks (Fig. XXII-2) by wrapping it in plastic and sometimes aluminum foil. The outside is usually waterproofed, frequently by using medical cast-

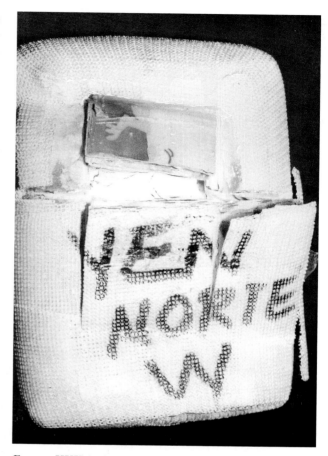

FIGURE XXII-2. A 1 Kg cocaine *brick* is wrapped in orthopedic casting material. Markings on the package identify the producer and shipper.

ing material that is set by ultraviolet light. The multiple layers are intended to insure water resistance and reduce any odor that a drug dog might detect. Each brick is currently worth approximately $36,000, and tons of cocaine in these brick forms are seized by law enforcement each year (Fig. XXII-3).

Enormous amounts of cocaine are produced each year. The DEA's year 2000 report on Columbia production indicated that the country could potentially produce up to 580 tons of the drug per year. This estimate is more than twice that indicated for 1996. The United Nations report suggests that the total potential production for Columbia could be at or more than 800 tons per year. One agency, the U.S. Coast Guard seized a total of 63 tons of cocaine in the year

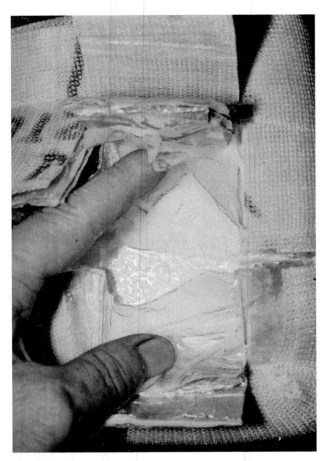

FIGURE XXII-3. Multiple layers of wrapping material are used to waterproof and reduce odors which a drug dog might detect.

2000. One ship seized in February 2001 by the Coast Guard contained 8.8 tons of cocaine.

Cocaine, a naturally occurring alkaloid, is present in the coca leaves at levels up to 7%. More commonly, the concentration is between one-half to 2%. Plants can be selectively cultivated for high concentration. Other alkaloids that are in the leaves include ecgonine, cinnamyl cocaine, and hygrine. The ratio of components in the paste can sometimes be used to identify the source of the leaves, since there is some uniqueness for drug contents by growing region. This information is useful to not only those who try to intercept the drugs coming into the country, but also for toxicologists who frequently see the other alkaloid compounds when analyzing samples with mass spectroscopy.

Most processors do not recrystallize and filter the product to increase the purity, but cocaine with purities of better than 90% is commonly seen on the street. For street sale, cocaine is often cut by five to 40%, but the drug is currently so easily obtainable in the drug trade that uncut cocaine is readily available. Physiologically active cutting agents that are used include procaine, lidocaine, Methedrine and pemoline; common inert cutting agents are lactose, mannite and corn starch.

In the early 1970s, the organized production of cocaine both lowered its street cost and increased its availability just as a wave of increased popular drug acceptance spread across the United States. Availability, coupled with social acceptance of drug use in general, led to a resurgence of cocaine use.[12] As acid or hydrochloride salt, the drug could be snorted or injected, but not smoked. From the user's point of view, cocaine was still expensive compared to heroin.

Crack cocaine, on the other hand, can be smoked. Rather than chemically decomposing or pyrolyzing as cocaine hydrochloride does when heated, crack cocaine melts at 98o C and vaporizes. The vapor, which is fat soluble, is absorbed by all mucous membranes and enters the blood stream rapidly through the lungs. Since in this form the drug can easily cross the blood-brain barrier in one minute or less, it quickly produces an intense euphoric sensation, which may last as long as 30 minutes. For many people, this effect is so overwhelmingly pleasurable that they would sell or do anything to get more of the drug.

The euphoric effect of the drug depends on the interference of dopamine reuptake, resulting in an overload of the neurotransmitter. Drug abusers report that the drug induces a feeling of power, self-esteem, sensual well being, heightened sensations perception and sexual prowess. In some circumstances, sex is exchanged for cocaine. Higher levels or prolonged use is reported to have an adverse effect upon sexuality.

Although cocaine hydrochloride had been snorted or injected for years, it was now recognized that the drug could be changed into a hydrolyzed or basic form by mixing it with an alkali solution such as ammonium hydroxide and then extracting the hydrolyzed cocaine with a water immiscible solvent such as ethyl ether. This form of the drug was fat soluble, would cross the cell membrane, and could be smoked. Smoking imparted a faster, more powerful, much more intense and long-lasting high than could be achieved by snorting or injecting the drug. This process was termed *freebasing,* from the chemical term *freebase* form of the drug. It became popular despite the danger of working with an open flame and a flammable solvent. Inexperienced or intoxicated persons handling the highly flammable solvents as they heated the extracted crystals in a pipe over a screen with a flame frequently suffered severe burns or experienced explosions of the solvent-drug mixture. Burns of the fingers, face and absent eyelashes were typical findings specific to free basing cocaine. The intense high was so desirable, the risk was considered acceptable by the users.

As the amount of available cocaine increased, street prices dropped. A safer way to manufacture base cocaine using common household chemicals was developed. Mixing the alkaline solution of cocaine with sodium bicarbonate, and then heating the mixture resulted in an off-white opaque mass. This is broken into small chunks called *rocks* (Fig. XXII-4). The *rocks* are sometimes crushed into smaller fragments or smoked whole. As they are heated, they produce a cracking and popping sound, giving birth to the name *crack cocaine.* The household stove was used to drive off the water from the mixture and fix the base to the cocaine molecule, but microwave ovens are now commonly used for that same purpose.

Crack cocaine use spread quickly and widely around the world. Engendered by its lipid solubility, crack cocaine vapors can rapidly cross the cell membrane through the lungs, enter the bloodstream and enter the brain within seconds.

Pharmacology

Definitions

Freebase: This is a term for cocaine that has been chemically converted from its acid radical.

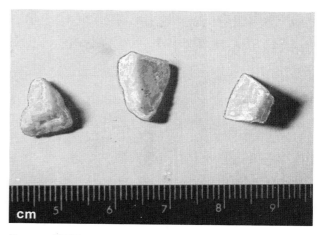

FIGURE XXII-4. Crack cocaine as sold in the street. The slightly larger center rock would be called *fat,* and sell for a slightly higher price.

The most common chemical form of newly produced illegal cocaine is cocaine hydrochloride (salt) with a melting point of 187 to 197° C. The wide melting point range reflects the variable purity of the available non-commercial compound. The salt form is water soluble and has a pH of 4 to 4.5. The base form, however, has a much lower melting range of 94 to 98° C, is water insoluble, and has a pH of approximately 7.0. It tends to form a vapor by sublimating at the lower melting point temperature rather than chemically decomposing, as does the HCl salt when heated. The freebase form tends to be unstable after preparation, and can be stored for only a short time in the freezer, whereas the HCl salt is stable.

Base must be smoked. Its production requires flammable solvents that are more difficult to obtain. The HCl salt, which can be snorted or injected, cannot be readily smoked because the water-soluble form of the drug does not easily cross the lipid-laden cellular membrane. The drug must *overload* the cell membranes of the nasal mucosa, be absorbed into the capillaries, then through the venous circulation to the heart, then to the lungs and back to the heart before being distributed to the brain. The base form, which is fat soluble, crosses the cell membrane, is rapidly absorbed through the airways and lung so that it quickly enters the blood stream and then circulates to the heart and then the brain,

TABLE XXII-1

COCAINE COMPARISONS

Water Solubility	Stability	Melting Point	Cost Per Gram	Method of Use
HCl – Soluble	Stable	187°–197° C	$60	Inject/Snort
Alkaloid – Insoluble	Unstable	94°–98° C	–	Smoke
"Crack" – Insoluble	Stable	98° C*	$75	Smoke

* Depending on purity.

where it is easily transported across the blood-brain barrier. From inhalation to central nervous system effect is largely a matter of circulation time from the heart to the brain, generally a matter of seconds. It thus produces a more rapid and more intense *high* than does the use of the salt.

Freebasing: This is the term that represents the technique for converting cocaine hydrochloride to the base (alkaloid) form. When the HCl component of the molecule is stripped off, the pH changes from acidic to near neutral and the water solubility changes. The production process consists of dissolving a quantity of cocaine HCl in water, adding a base, such as ammonium hydroxide to free the cocaine alkaloid as a white cloud of precipitate, then extracting the drug with a volatile immiscible solvent, such as ethyl ether. The ether extract is allowed to evaporate, leaving the fine white pure cocaine base. The base is then heated on a wire screen, usually in a pipe, using a propane torch. As the crystals melt and start to vaporize (sublimate), they are inhaled. The breath is held as long as possible to enhance absorption of the drug through the lungs (see Table XXII-1). Freebasing often results in explosions and burns when intoxicated persons use an open flame adjacent to flammable solvents. With the advent of *crack*, this process is no longer necessary.

Crack Cocaine: Alkalinizing solubilized cocaine salt and mixing the resulting product with bicarbonate produces this base form of cocaine. It is stable and is smoked. It is made relatively easily using commonly available chemical components that can be obtained at a local food market and an oven or microwave to *bake* the resulting material. The name comes from the *cracking* and *popping* sound made by the drug as it is heated. A number of computer websites give various formulas and procedures.

Crack cocaine is easy to make. In fact, school children have been known to make their own. The process requires no flammable solvents for extraction, and is stable over a wide range of temperatures. It has become the most common consumable form of cocaine throughout the United States. The use of crack cocaine does not require any of the preparations or time needed to consume freebase, nor is the smoking process difficult. The drug can be easily transported and concealed. During the production, a relatively small amount of cocaine hydrochloride converts to up to 10 to 15 times the original drug volume as *crack* thereby enhancing the profit significantly.

The plasma half-life of cocaine is 45 to 90 minutes. With the drug level dropping, the user is ready to smoke another rock. Blood levels of 0.2 to 0.7 micrograms/mL are common, but the individual user may have levels much higher or lower than this. Since the neurotransmitter effect is the primary neurological change that drives the perception of euphoria, the actual blood or plasma level has little meaning. This statement seems counter-intuitive, but only the cocaine in the brain produces euphoria. The drug is metabolized primarily in the liver with benzoylecgonine being the primary metabolite. Benzoylecgonine (BE) does not cross the blood-brain barrier to any appreciable extent, and when that metabolite is formed in the brain by esterases, it tends to stay in the brain until metabolized.

The principal area of activity is in the mesolimbic dopamine circuitry, which affects motivated behavior and emotion. In vitro autoradiography and ligand binding analysis of this area may map both the D3 dopamine and kappa opioid receptor sites, measure the neurotransmitters and yield a basis for supporting a diagnosis of cocaine poisoning or toxicity in the case.[14] This finding is considered specific in deaths during excited (agitated) delirium, where the drug level in the blood may be at or below detectable levels.

Since the drug is fat soluble, it is stored in tissue compartments and released slowly back into the blood stream. The metabolite can be detected in the urine for several days following a single dose. For frequent users, the metabolite may persist in the urine for a week or longer. The half-life of benzoylecgonine is about 90 minutes to four hours. Therefore, the concentration of the metabolite will increase in the plasma as the parent compound concentration drops, and the metabolite will stay elevated even when cocaine is no longer detectable. Thus, the presence of BE in the urine indicates that cocaine had been used, but not necessarily that day.

There is a number of other metabolites, such as ecgonine methyl ester. Some are unique to the presence of other drugs, such as when cocaine is metabolized in the presence of ethyl alcohol. Mixing alcohol and cocaine appears to increase the feeling of well-being. Cocaine metabolized in the presence of ethyl alcohol produces a compound identified as cocaethylene. Because it was thought to be physiologically active and has a much longer half-life than cocaine, cocaethylene was initially considered an important derivative. However, it is more probable that this metabolite is of little interest to the forensic scientist. It is an example of a cocaine metabolite unique to the presence of another drug, and is produced only when the two drugs are metabolized at the same time.

Like adrenalin, cocaine is a catecholamine stimulator. Most of the pathologic effects of cocaine appear to be catechol related, such as the effect on heart muscle and the conduction system. As the heart rate increases, so does the output, causing elevated blood pressure and tachycardia. The rise in blood pressure increases the chances of a hypertensive stroke. In addition, cardiac cell damage and arrhythmia may lead to sudden death. Cocaine is a sodium channel blocker, but unlike other anesthetics, it prevents the reuptake of neurotransmitters. This may be

directly related to the cardiac specific effects that lead to sudden death.[19-22] The incidence of agitated delirium appears to be increasing throughout the world as cocaine use increases. Not only can cocaine cause interference with the reuptake of dopamine by blocking the sodium channel of the pre-synaptic junction and changing the configuration of the transporter to effectively block the chloride ion binding site, but this neurotransmitter change appears to be the basis for the hyperthermia, rhabdomyolysis and the altered thought of this pathologic process. A similar mechanism is responsible for the malignant neuroleptic syndrome, sometimes referred to as malignant hyperthermia.

Cocaine is a powerful vasoconstrictor, and pathologic changes associated with this effect are unrelated to dose, drug form, or route of administration. Cocaine tends to prolong the QT interval of the heart. This means that the drug's effect on the heart is not necessarily dose related and a low blood level may be sufficient to cause death. In agitated delirium cases, the drug level is typically low or absent.

Studies show that maternal drug use in some areas of the United States can range up to 10 to 25% of live-born infants. There may be an adverse effect upon placental circulation producing placental insufficiency resulting in intrauterine death of the fetus.

Live-born infants typically have many problems. Because placental transfer of cocaine is associated with intrauterine growth retardation, these children are born small, premature, and addicted. The fetus depends upon placental clearance, since the fetal metabolism does not process this drug very well. Sixty to 90% of infants born to cocaine-addicted mothers show signs of drug withdrawal. Addicted babies often have developmental problems and may have behavioral or learning difficulties that require special training and skilled education care. How well they will be able to perform as adults is still largely unknown.[23]

All of these complications require extensive and frequently expensive medical care for the mother and infant. Because the fetal liver lacks the necessary enzymes, the newborn has a reduced ability to metabolize the drug, resulting in positive blood levels for one or more days after birth and prolonged excretion. The infant's urine often remains positive for a week after birth. Positive urine results two or more weeks following birth needs to include the possibility of an exogenous origin. Since this is a fat soluble drug, breast-feeding may be the source, since the drug is excreted in breast milk. There is also some evidence to support passive absorption of the drug through the inhalation of smoke, although the levels achieved in passive inhalation will be very low. Exposure to contaminated fingers or bottle nipples as a source of positive findings in infants has been suggested when no other reasonable source is apparent.

The infant may enter a second phase of withdrawal two to eight weeks after birth. The baby's increased irritability heightens the likelihood of child abuse. Some consider the probability of child abuse to be as high as 50% for parents or caretakers who are using drugs and alcohol.

The issue of the causal relation to infant morbidity or mortality is not totally resolved. Of pregnant women using cocaine, Chasnoff reported a 23% increase in spontaneous abortions, and in our experience, drug abusers are generally aware that cocaine may end a pregnancy. However, a large-scale controlled study reported by Behnke in 2001 reported no major congenital findings that were unique to cocaine babies. The data showed that there were significantly more premature infants with significantly lower birth weights, shorter body length and smaller head circumferences, but no other significant differences compared to infants of non-cocaine-using mothers.[24]

The reports of increased complications and death were not supported in a study reported by Andres et al. These authors concluded that their study "does not support an association between recent cocaine use and fetal hypoxemia or acidemia, depressed 5-min APGAR scores, meconium staining of the amniotic fluid, or caesarean delivery in cocaine-dependent pregnant women enrolled in prenatal care."[25] It is obvious that additional research is needed to resolve this medical issue.

As mentioned earlier, cocaine base imparts an intense craving for more drug, and individuals will go to any extreme to obtain cocaine. For women, this frequently involves trading sex for cocaine. Sexually transmitted disease and pregnancy are two obvious results. Unfortunately, the combination of disease and pregnancy produces a large number of infants born exposed to HIV. Some estimates are as high as 28 per 10,000 live births. In one study, 31% of addicts in a methadone treatment program were positive for HIV. The range in the San Francisco Bay area is 22 to 31% in African Americans, eight to 10% in other races and averages 16 to 18 per 10,000 newborns.

Additionally, other diseases associated with sharing smoking pipes are also increasing. One public health district reported a 13% increase in pulmonary tuberculosis, which workers associated with crack house smoking of cocaine. A crack house is a euphemism for a place where crack cocaine is sold and smoked. Somewhat similar to the shooting gallery term associated with heroin abuse. It is a place where people meet to *do* cocaine, as well as all the other illicit activities associated with drug abuse. Disputes and violence over territorial rights and control of drug sales are common. Especially for the young, the ability to control large amounts of money and the presence of semiautomatic weapons are frequently the fuel for violence. Drive-by shootings are associated with territorial disputes and usually involve people less than 25 years of age.

Toxic Effects

Cocaine's vasoconstrictor effect may produce coronary artery spasm. This change has been documented by angiography and is clinically related to angina as well as acute myocardial infarction. For some patients, this is the mechanism of sudden death.

Other mechanisms of death may be rapid or take days as cocaine increases both heart rate and output, resulting in increased blood pressure, which can lead to a hypertensive crisis. There is a significant increase in the incidence of intracerebral hemorrhage or rupture of an existing aneurysm.

Focal heart muscle damage with resulting cross-band necrosis is associated with cocaine use and is not dose related. This cellular damage is believed to be related to the cell physiology changes induced by cocaine on the fiber associated with contraction. The resulting hypereosinophilic cross-bands within the muscle fibers are not diagnostic of cocaine use, but are commonly associated with conditions that cause hypercontraction of the heart muscle. The bands represent no longer functional, fragmented and damaged contractile protein within the myofibril that can be seen on Hematoxylin and Eosin stain, and easily documented with a Luxol fast blue stain. Recent studies support that cocaine directly causes myofibril apoptosis when high doses are used.[26]

Damage of the myocardium results in impaired contractibility and multifocal microscopic areas of fibrosis. Cocaine also impairs effective conduction within the heart, which may elicit arrhythmias. The drug was believed to induce high levels of circulating catechols, causing direct cardiotoxicity, but the work reported by Wang et al. suggests that myofibril injury and death may be related to a direct inducement of cell death. Whether or not this is true in humans, has not yet been studied. Either through a direct action or the vasoconstrictor effect on nutrient vessels, potential lethal arrhythmias can be generated.

As with other drugs, an acute psychosis sometimes develops, leading to violent behavior in some, paranoid ideation in others or some combination of psychiatric effects. When paranoid or violent, cocaine users are a definite danger to themselves and others. Frequently, police involvement leads to trauma and may result in death. Analysis of biological samples, especially admitting samples for hospitalized patients, is important to understanding the possible cause of a psychotic event. However, there is little, if any, correlation between the blood levels and toxic effect of cocaine. Since the central nervous system effect of cocaine is to block the dopamine re-uptake at the synaptic junction, agitated deliriums tend to more commonly be associated with users who have reached the end of a period of heavy drug use and their body stores of drug are dropping. Sudden death is often a direct cardiac arrhythmia, generated at the cellular level. This, again frequently bears little relation to the measured blood levels.[27]

Toxicology Samples

Cocaine is unstable in biological samples, breaking down spontaneously to a number of compounds, principally benzoylecgonine. The chemical deterioration process is partly mediated by blood esterases and will continue both within the body, and to some extent within the test tube postmortem. Without effective preservation, analysis for cocaine may be negative or levels reduced from those that existed in life. While it is quite possible to quantitate both the parent compound and the metabolites, the original data about the levels and ratios, which can reflect drug dosage and exposure time, would be lost. For example, if an unpreserved sample is taken from a person with a recent drug exposure and kept at room temperature for hours, it might show only the benzoylecgonine, instead of the original ratio of cocaine to benzoylecgonine of two to one. The half-life of cocaine is generally between 45 and 90 minutes. These data may then be interpreted to support an older drug exposure, rather than a more recent one. In a specific investigation, this could be an important issue. These questions are often of importance in criminal court.

For these reasons, blood should be collected from a peripheral site, preferably in glass, with sodium fluoride or another enzyme inhibitor present in a concentration that will reduce or prevent chemical breakdown. With sodium fluoride at a final diluted concentration of 2.5 to 10 mg/mL, buffered to a pH of about 5.0 and refrigerated, the degradation rate will be slow and the sample will remain stable at refrigerator temperatures for months. If the serum is frozen, the sample will typically be stable in the freezer for at least a year.

Crack cocaine is not detectable as crack in biological materials. The metabolism of crack is the same as that of other forms of cocaine. The significance of the form is its fat solubility and the ability to cross cell membranes as well as the blood-brain barrier so rapidly. Once in the brain, the effect upon the neurotransmitter system is primarily within the midbrain. Benzoylecgonine formed in the brain cannot cross the blood-brain barrier and must be broken down by the body in the brain. Brain is therefore an excellent sample to evaluate either drug levels or with histochemical means, the effect upon the synaptic junction by studying the neurotransmitters. The latter may be an important issue in acute deaths associated with agitated delirium while in police custody. The sample collected is the midbrain, which should be recovered as soon as possible following death. One half of the midbrain or cerebral hemisphere is recovered, bisected in the sagittal plane through the corpus callosum, and the brain tissue quickly frozen at minus 70° C or in liquid nitrogen. Ideally, the sample should be collected within six to 12 hours of death. The tissue sample can then be forwarded frozen to a laboratory capable of measuring the brain chemical receptors and neurotransmitters.

Analysis of urine is usually performed for the primary metabolite and/or ecgonine methyl ester. While these compounds may be detectable for one or more days following a single dose, chronic abusers may excrete detectable amounts for weeks. Cocaine, taken at the same time as ethyl alcohol, produces cocaethylene which has a longer half-life than cocaine. The presence of cocaethylene may be important in a particular case, but recent data tend to support that it is not as significant in the neurochemistry as is the parent compound.

Analysis of blood, spinal fluid, brain and urine is commonly performed by a number of methods using antigen-antibody reactions, gas chromatography, mass spectroscopy or HPLC. Confirmation is usually by gas chromatography/mass spectroscopy, with detection limits of about 3 to 5 nanograms/mL. Hair can be used to detect cocaine, but not the amount nor whether it was used at or near the time of death.

Scene Investigation

Snorting involves making a line of the hydrochloride powder upon a flat surface, such as glass or a mirror. The powder is reduced by *chopping* it to a more uniform particle size, mixed and formed into the line. This is usually done with a single-edged razor blade. The thin two to four inch-long strips of cocaine powder are inhaled or *snorted* from the glass, typically through a straw with one end inserted into the nose. A rolled up piece of paper, straw, dollar bill or a *toot* are often used. The toot is a small piece of tubing, often found in a *kit*. Razor blades, straws, coke spoons and residues of fine white powder left on glass are common scene findings. The victim may have a coke spoon or small brown glass vial on or about his or her person (Figs. XXII-5 to XXII-7). Occasionally, one fingernail, usually on the little finger, is allowed to grow long and is used to measure out the cocaine (Fig. XXII-8). Snorting leaves few visible signs on the body. A rim of white powder may be seen around the nostrils. Methanol-soaked swabs can be used to recover the drug from the nasal mucosa.

The typical intravenous user now injects with an insulin syringe, leaving a pinprick-sized puncture site. The skin around the puncture site is commonly pale, and may be surrounded by a reddish ring. Since the cutting agents in cocaine are usually soluble, the skin reaction, granulomas and scarred needle tracks seen with other drugs are not common in these cases. As with snorting, injecting cocaine leaves few visible signs upon the body. With 26 to 28 gauge needles, the injection site may not be on the arms. Since there is often a sexual association with the drug's use, occasionally injection sites will be on the breast or penis. Any accessible vein however, will suffice.

If the victim was freebasing the alkaline form of the drug, the pipes, solvents, glassware, propane torches or cigarette lighters and extraction apparatus are often found at the scene. The victim may not die at the site where the drug use occurred, or the apparatus may have been removed prior to arrival of investigators. With the advent of the crack form, freebasing is now uncommon.

Crack cocaine, on the other hand, can be smoked in a number of methods that result in vaporizing the drug for inhalation. It may be mixed with tobacco in a cigarette, in a regular pipe, in a pipe with a screen to hold the tobacco

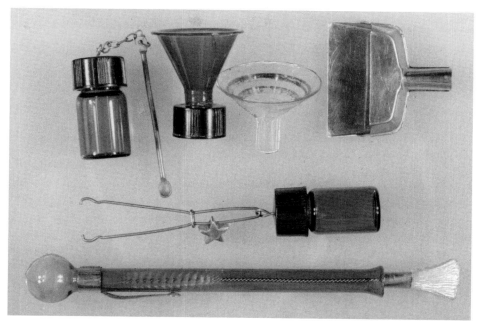

FIGURE XXII-5. Items for the packaging and use of *coke*. The pan and funnels load drug into screw top vials. The vial with the *tongs* can hold a cigarette, and the vial with the brush can be used to *snort* the powder.

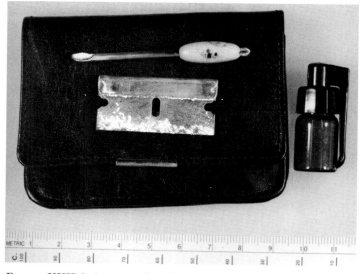

FIGURE XXII-6. A cocaine kit. Note powder on blade and spoon.

and drug mixture, or in a special crack pipe (Fig. XXII-9). Used by itself, the drug can be heated to volatility with a propane torch or butane lighter. Although both are used, propane is preferred because of the belief that other fuels impart an unpleasant taste to the vapor.

Evidence supporting drug abuse includes large numbers of used matches with few cigarette butts, propane containers, multiple butane cigarette lighters, smoking apparatus, and drug packaging material. Smoking sometimes causes burns or abrasions on fingers, and occasionally the eye-

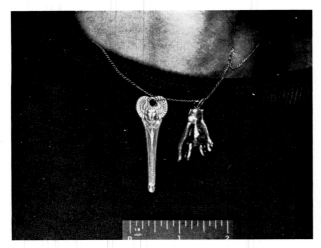

FIGURE XXII-7. *Coke spoon* worn next to a medallion around neck suggests that the deceased was a user of cocaine.

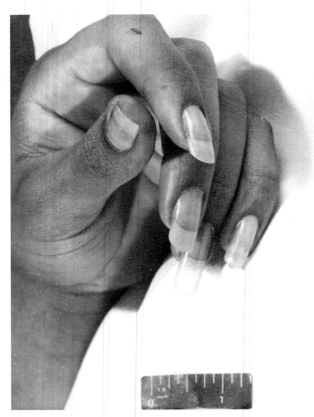

FIGURE XXII-8. Left hand of a drug dealer. Note length of fourth fingernail used as measuring device similar to spoon in Figure XXII-7.

brows or facial hair is singed. Frequent users sometimes have multiple burns on their lips and fingers from glass pipes.

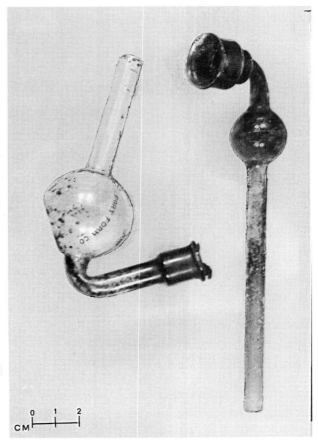

FIGURE XXII-9. Pipes used to smoke cocaine.

A drug overdose or toxic effect with a low blood level frequently results in both hyperthermia and a terminal seizure. Signs of resuscitation in the form of wet towels, wet clothing, ice (sometimes packed about the genitals) or finding the body in a bathtub or shower all support a terminal resuscitation attempt by friends. Usually, such victims do not survive long enough to develop anoxic brain changes. If the death is recent, such as in a police-related activity or citizen-involved agitated delirium case, an immediate body core temperature should be taken at the scene. In the alternate, a core temperature should be taken as soon as feasible. Other observations include whether the skin felt hot to first responders, whether the skin was dry or wet with sweat, and the respiratory rate in a pre-agonal individual are all important clues to the type of drug toxicity. Pepper sprays typically do not affect agitated delirium cases. Like other cases of drug-induced central nervous system deliriums, the use of such chemical tactics are contraindicated. Other evidence supporting drug abuse may or may not be present, but often the surroundings suggest that diagnosis. This is particularly true in the case of crack houses and shooting galleries.

Should any powder be present at a scene, it should never be tasted. Most *caine* drugs are bitter and produce a numbing effect. The differentiation of cocaine from other drugs is usually impossible by this method. There is also the real risk of tasting a poison or one of the designer drugs, either of which could be rapidly lethal. It is not unheard of for a trap to be set to intentionally harm drug investigators.

In a suspected drug-induced agitated delirium, besides the information mentioned above, the autopsy should be done as soon as feasible and specimens retained and preserved as indicated earlier. This can confirm the drug effect as the likely cause of the agitation and death. Data by Wetli supports that if the patient goes into delirium, he or she is likely to die.[28] Obviously, with police or citizen involvement, asphyxia, trauma and other factors causing or contributing to the death have to be considered prior to determining cause and manner.

Autopsy Findings

Besides the observations mentioned above, few autopsy findings are specific for cocaine poisoning or toxicity. Pulmonary congestion and edema, with the lungs weighing three to four times normal, are the most common physical findings. The right ventricle of the heart is usually distended and the pulmonary artery full, but this is a variable finding. The cardiac weight is typically increased. Resuscitation can produce a similar finding of ventricular dilation and can cause cross-band necrosis with high dose epinephrine usage. However, acute epinephrine-induced myonecrosis is not associated with the multifocal microscopic fibrosis of recurrent catechol stimulation. Rarely, individuals with a long history of heavy snorting of cocaine hydrochloride may have fenestration of the nasal septum due to necrosis as a result of the vasoconstrictor effect of cocaine. If the victim has been snorting close to the time of death, a white powder may sometimes be seen at the nares and recoverable drug from the nasal mucosa may be helpful in the investigation and support the toxicological finding of acute exposure. Other drugs are now frequently snorted, so this finding of powder in the nose is not specific to cocaine. Upper airway purging or loss of gastric content can efface this finding.

Dealers or persons who fear confrontation with someone, such as the police, often carry crack cocaine, in the form of rocks, within their mouths. The rock may be wrapped in foil or plastic, but is often just placed in the buccal sulcus. It can then be swallowed, if necessary. Sometimes the unwrapped cocaine rock is carried this way. The rocks may be found in the esophagus, mouth or stomach. A true acute drug poisoning can occur in this manner. It is uncommon, but not totally unheard of; to see the drug transported by swallowing numerous small wrapped packages (Fig. XXII-10). These are usually small rubber balloons or condoms. This method is still occasionally used to bring the drug across a border, but with the immense amounts of drug coming into the United States, the relatively small amount that could be carried this way makes this a process limited to the entrepreneur.

The diagnosis can be further supported by the microscopic examination of the heart and gross examination of the heart and lung. The lungs of a heavy crack smoker are often heavily contaminated with carbon, so that the visceral pleura and parenchyma are black with pigment. Upon microscopic examination, very large numbers of carbon particles of various sizes are seen in the tissue and within alveolar macrophages. This feature is referred to as *crack smoker's lung*. It is thought that the intense inhalation and breath holding associated with the smoking process increases the pulmonary carbon load. The increased macrophage activity is often correlated with positive toxicology or scene information supporting drug use. Increased tissue carbon deposits, with little or no polarizable foreign material, are common findings but are not spe-

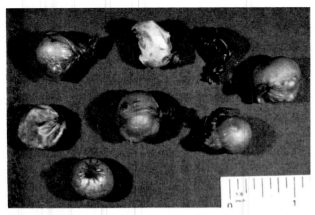

FIGURE XXII-10. Individuals smuggling drugs sometimes swallow large numbers of *bags* in an attempt to avoid detection. These are a few of the more than 100 recovered from the stomach and intestinal track during an autopsy on a *carrier* who died when several bags ruptured. Lethal levels of cocaine and benzoylecgonine were documented by toxicological analyses.

cific for cocaine abuse. The heart is typically enlarged. Often multiple cross-band necrosis is caused by the effect of cocaine upon the myofibril. Increased and multifocal fibrosis, increased perivascular fibrosis and piecemeal necrosis of the myofibril are common findings associated with cocaine's damage to the heart muscle. Spasm of the coronary vessels can be demonstrated with angiography. Cocaine produces cellular damage that leads to ischemia and arrhythmias. Either can result in sudden death.

Opium

Opium, the first known narcotic drug, is derived from the sap of the scarified seedpod of the Oriental poppy, *Papaver somniferum*. Raw opium or tincture of opium was the only known analgesic available for pain relief in early recorded history. Records from various parts of Asia Minor show a widespread industry, with trade and use of the drug in many countries.

The opium poppy will grow in a wide range of climates, but production of opium is a labor-intensive process. The unripe seedpod is lightly incised multiple times vertically along its sides. The milky fluid that collects on the surface of the

pod is raw opium. This darkens upon exposure to the air. After several hours, the collected semi-dried material is scrapped from the surface. Each seedpod produces only a small amount of fluid for each collection but can be drained several times as the pod ripens. Thousands of pods have to be incised and harvested to produce a pound of raw opium.

The word narcotic is derived from the Greek word *narkotikon,* which means to numb or be numbing. It refers to the principal effect of opium of producing analgesia and relieving pain. The term narcotic was originally used for referencing drugs derived directly from opium or for other drugs that produced analgesia or stupor, but through usage and legal definitions the term no longer refers only to drugs derived directly from opium.

In 1945, over 200 tons of opium was imported into the United States for legitimate medical needs. It was estimated that several times that amount was brought in for the illicit drug trade. Today, in spite of extensive use of synthetic analgesics, many tons of opium are imported into the United States legally, and the drug is still produced primarily in Asia where labor is still relatively cheap. Much of the illegal opium produced today is from an area referred to as the *Golden Triangle*. Some estimates are that more than 8,000 to 10,000 tons of illegal opium products, such as heroin, are brought into the country each year. Drug Enforcement Administration data for 1998 monitors four principle areas of origin. These are Mexico, Southeast Asia, Southwest Asia and South America. In 1977, 89% of the heroin seized in the U.S. came from Mexico. In 1997, only 12% came from Mexico, with 73% coming from South America. The same report indicates seizure of slightly more than 446 kilograms of heroin in 1997. On the West Coast, the most common form of heroin is the *tar* form, a viscous to solid black or brown substance, which is poorly refined, produced primarily in Mexico. Different forms are common to different areas of the world.

In 1803, the German pharmacist Serturner isolated morphine from opium. Opium contains approximately 10% morphine in addition to a number of other alkaloids. The compound was named morphine after Morpheus, the Greek god of dreams. This choice was obviously a reference to the effect in man of producing sleep. Eventually, codeine, another alkaloid occurring in opium at levels of about 0.5%, was isolated. Morphine and codeine are the principal opium derived alkaloids used in medicine today. Codeine is used as an analgesic and cough suppressant; morphine is used in several chemical forms as an analgesic; and opium is used in preparations to treat diarrhea.

There are a number of important chemical modifications of opium. In 1898, Dreser acetylated morphine with acetic acid to form heroin (3,6-diacetylmorphine). This compound was initially thought to be non-addicting. It was found to be four to five times more effective than morphine in both its analgesic effect and its direct action on the brain. Heroin has such a significant addiction quality that it is considered to offer no particular medicinal advantage over morphine and other opium derivatives. Few countries allow its medicinal use and most prohibit its manufacture or possession. Dihydrocodeine, dihydrocodeinone, dihydromorphinone and ethylmorphine are currently common medicines that are semisynthetic analog narcotics. A number of totally synthetic analgesic compounds used extensively in medicine, include meperidine, methadone and fentanyl. They are restricted and classified as narcotics.

All narcotics have shown themselves to be addicting when abused, even though several were originally introduced with the suggestion that such was not the case.

Addiction is a combination of psychological and physical dependence upon a drug. As tolerance to the drug develops, the user requires more than the usual amount to experience the same euphoric effects. The user often becomes refractory to some of the effects of the drug, so that his or her body may tolerate levels that would ordinarily be considered toxic or lethal. When tolerance and habitual use develop, a physiologic dependence also occurs, so that withdrawal of the drug progresses to clinical signs such as abdominal pain, nausea, vomiting, and restlessness. Agitation and a feeling of distress generally resolve in several days. These physical signs can be prevented by renewing the drug levels or by substitution of another drug, such as methadone. Addiction is evident when the drug user has an overpowering desire and need or compulsion to obtain and take the drug and when there is a physiologic effect when the drug is withdrawn.

Raw Opium

Although it can be absorbed by several routes, opium is most typically taken as the tincture (laudanum) or smoked. Smoking vaporizes the opium, allowing morphine and other alkaloids to be absorbed from the smoke. While the amount used initially is small, as tolerance increases, large amounts are required to achieve a similar effect. In 1822, Thomas DeQuicney wrote in his book, *Confessions of an Opium-Eater,* that "320 grains of opium may be required to stay the craving." His book, which reported favorably upon the drug's use, did much to popularize and encourage the non-medical use of opium and laudanum, which could be purchased by anyone at the time. Addiction and the attendant problems of drug abuse were not officially recognized, nor were drugs initially regulated. Opium containing compounds were common, used for such every day purposes as soothing teething infants, mild depression, and treating anxiety.

The introduction of the hypodermic syringe in the mid 1800s and the onset of the American Civil War resulted in many intravenous and subcutaneous morphine addicts. Morphine was used as a cure for opium addiction and was not, at that time, considered addicting.

At about the same time, the patent medicine industry was growing rapidly, since the means existed to distribute a product widely by the new widespread railroads. Much like cocaine, opium, morphine and even heroin enjoyed a wide over-the-counter public acceptance. By 1900, some reports estimated that there were one million addicts in the United States. Heroin, introduced in 1898, was immediately proclaimed the most effective analgesic known. Thought to be and promoted as nonaddictive, heroin was recom-

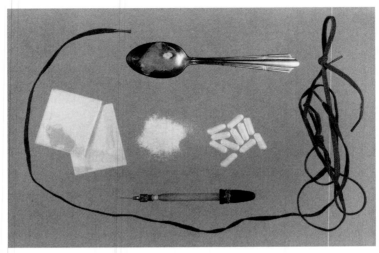

FIGURE XXII-11. The *works:* Homemade eyedropper syringe, teaspoon *cooker* with absorbent cotton intended to remove impurities, and a shoelace tourniquet. The *street* heroin mixture is usually sold in folded stamp-collector-type glassine envelopes or aluminum foil and occasionally in gelatin capsules. (In Michigan, we have not seen eyedroppers being used as syringes in many years.)

mended specifically as treatment for addiction to other opium derivatives. It was sold as an elixir and as a component in patent medicines until the early 1900s when the danger was finally recognized. The country became aware of the abuse, especially of children where it was promoted for treating such things as colic, resulting in a number of publicized infant deaths. In 1914, the Harrison Narcotic Act made such drug preparations illegal.

Heroin

Heroin became the abuse drug of choice for those who had been using the drug legally prior to passage of the law. A ready illicit market developed, with strong ties to the criminal world, which continued to manage distribution and sales (Fig. XXII-11).

In the early 1920s, Kolb studied addicted prisoners and demonstrated that the vast majority of heroin users were already involved in criminal activities prior to or in conjunction with their heroin abuse. Heroin became the major illicit drug in the United States and, until 1988, when it was replaced in some areas by cocaine, was the leading drug of addiction.

Heroin deaths peaked in the late 1970s after a five-year period of marked rise in the numbers of addicts and deaths. In 1969–70, for instance, New York City had 1000 addict deaths per year, Detroit had 450 and San Francisco had slightly less than 100. In the late 1980s and early 1990s, cocaine emerged as the principal drug of abuse, followed closely by heroin; the combined numbers of drug deaths sharply increased in most metropolitan areas of this country.

The correlation between drug use and criminal activity is demonstrated by statistics in large cities, where at least half of the homicides are often shown to be drug related. There is a high level of violence among users and dealers. Huge profits, the need to protect a drug sale territory, and the need to steal to pay for the addiction all contribute to the high level of crime associated with drug abuse. Abuse of marital partners, relatives, children and neighbors is associated with drug use. A lack of concern for care and nutrition is a common feature of child neglect cases. Occasionally, children may be given drugs to make them sleep or to cause death. Alternatively, children may ingest drugs carelessly left within their reach. Typically at such a scene, there is little food present for the child. The shelves and refrigerator contain little food, but often there are sweets in the form of candy or cookies. The living area is disheveled and drug apparatus or residue is often freely visible.

The concentration and nature of the drug varies widely from region to region, as does the form. Currently, Mexican brown or tar heroin is popular in the San Francisco area, while the powder form is more popular on the East Coast. Concentrations are typically around four to 10% for the powder and can be 40 to 70% for the tar. Physiologically active cutting agents vary from region to region, with quinine sometimes being used on the East Coast and lidocaine on the West Coast. Some other water soluble material such as mannitol may be used as an inactive agent. Cutting agents vary and may be whatever was available at the time the drug was cut. Cutting agents are used to increase bulk and increase the sale price.

Rarely is street heroin adulterated with a poison, although this has occurred. The term *hot shot* is sometimes used to indicate a particularly strong concentration or is equally used to denote an intentionally powerful dose that is given with the specific intent of causing death. The term is more commonly *street talk,* since it is often difficult to cause death by injection of heroin alone. There have been cases where injections included battery acid or some other toxic compound. These scenes or deaths were usually evident because the victim was bound or had ligature marks present on his or her extremities or there was a chemical burn evident at the injection site.

Aware of the variability of street drugs, long-term addicts prefer to buy from the same source whenever possible. The process of using the drug, however, allows some experimentation to determine the quality of the drug before injecting the full dose. Most commonly, insulin syringes are now used to inject. The small gauge needle makes finding a sclerosed vein easier. The small size of the syringe makes it easy for the user to manipulate it with one hand. The user will often inject a small amount to *gauge* the strength of the drug. It is not uncommon to have more than one person use the same batch of drugs, one dying, and the other only having the usual effect of the

high. It is also not uncommon for someone else to inject the drug. This more frequently happens at a *shooting gallery* where a person pays his or her money and the dealer prepares and injects the dose. The most common victims are the young who may not have tolerance to the drug, suffering a true respiratory depression or acute death. When such deaths occur the individual involved will be prosecuted.

The actor, John Belushi died this way. His girlfriend was charged with involuntary manslaughter and received a four-year sentence.

A similar case occurred in Macomb County, Michigan. It stands to reason that such cases are not infrequent but are not recognized.

Heroin is usually sold as a fine white powder or as a tar material. Either is wrapped in a glassine envelope, paper bindle or in a small piece of plastic or aluminum foil (Fig. XXII-12), and sometimes placed in a small balloon, which is tied into a ball (Fig. XXII-13). The contents of the container are emptied into a cooker. The cooker can be a spoon or a bottle cap, but can be anything that will hold about 5 mL of fluid and allow heating over a low flame. When water is added, most of the material is not immediately dissolved. A flame, usually in the form of a match or cigarette lighter, is used to warm the solution to increase solubility, but it is not necessary to boil it. The liquid is aspirated into an insulin or tuberculin syringe, often through a small piece of absorbent cotton or sometimes the filter of a cigarette. The filter removes the larger portions of insoluble material. The needle is inserted into a vein and a small amount of solution is injected as a test dose. The addict subjectively interprets how powerful the drug is and how much he or she will inject. This process of injecting a small amount, withdrawing some blood to keep the lumen open and insuring that the needle is within the vein is called *fooling* on the West Coast and *booting* on the East Coast. The process not only helps evaluate the concentration of the drug but also prolongs the high by introducing pulses of the drug over a period of time.

Why addicts die of overdoses is not always clear.[29,30] Blood levels are seldom helpful in supporting a drug poisoning. Although some die

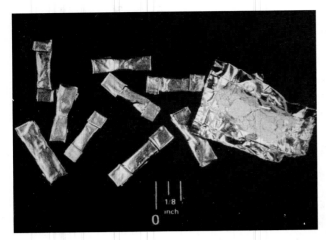

FIGURE XXII-12. Heroin packaged in aluminum foil.

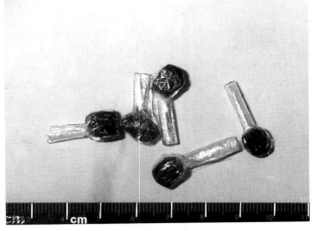

FIGURE XXII-13. *Tar* heroin in a common package form from the west coast of the United States.

with the needle still in their veins (Fig. XXII-14) and analyses of blood from several different sites show incomplete mixing of blood and heroin, undoubtedly, many of these deaths are not the result of a true drug overdose. Furthermore, situations are known in which two or more persons have injected from the same cooked solution, with one dying and the others experiencing the desired high. This tends to support that the death is either the result of a physiologic response to the drug bolus or an opioid receptor mediated reaction. Generally, testing has not supported that these are anaphylactic or endotoxin reactions. Autopsies in such cases typically show severe pulmonary congestion and edema with a dilated right ventricle (Fig. XXII-15a–b). Allergic manifestations, including mast cells, degranulation or degranulation products and eosinophils are not typically present. There does not appear to be any relation to asthmatic changes. Cultures have revealed a mixture of bacterial and fungi in the tar heroin. So far, there has not been a finding of a common factor that enhances fatal reactions to injected heroin and this consequence has been known to occur ever since the drug began to be abused by injection.

Regardless of the mechanism of death, any time more than one person is found dead or unconscious in the same location, when no injuries are evident, one should immediately suspect the cause to be either carbon monoxide or acute drug intoxication (Fig. XXII-16a–c). Often,

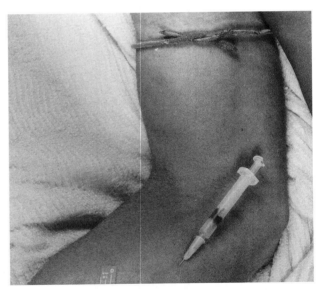

FIGURE XXII-14. Tourniquet and intravenous needle in place. Rapid injection or too potent a mixture can cause sudden respiratory arrest.

the scene will provide clues, pending autopsy and toxicological analyses.

In an unusual show of concern for the addicts' safety, quinine, which is an antimalarial drug, was first added to East Coast street heroin in the early 1940s after a series of malaria deaths. The public health director proclaimed that addicts were spreading the disease among themselves by sharing contaminated needles; mosquitoes were

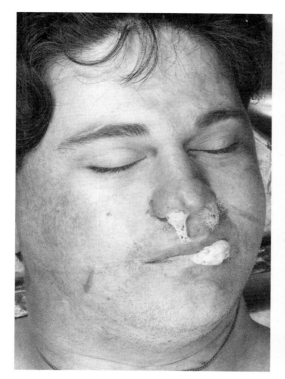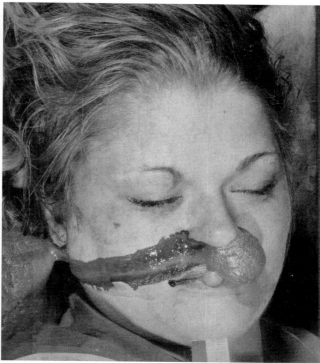

FIGURE XXII-15a–b. (a) Dense froth often exudes from the mouth and nose of addicts in mushroom fashion following death from intravenous drug use as a result of severe pulmonary edema. Initially this froth is gray-white, but it may become blood tinged as tissue autolysis progresses. In a body recovered from water, it may be difficult to determine whether the froth was due to inhalation of water, i.e. drowning or drugs. (b) Bloody foam may be due resuscitative attempts, early onset of decomposition or any one of several other causes including submersion.

not involved. Since that time, no deaths in New York from malaria have been reported to be associated with needle use. Although most alkaloids have a bitter taste, the ability to detect small amounts of quinine is far greater than the ability to taste low levels of heroin. It is thought that addicts, accustomed to gauging the presence of heroin by the taste of quinine, missed the milder taste of heroin and in some cases shot the dealer because they thought they were not getting the requested drug.

In contrast, the addition of lidocaine to heroin on the West Coast is thought to provide the characteristic bitter taste associated with the drug and/or to prolong the high and numb the injection point. Tradition aside, why quinine and lidocaine are still added at the present time is unclear, as no synergistic effect with heroin is known. This process is further enhanced by the depiction of the detective in the movies tasting the drug. With the current known presence of dangerous synthetic compounds, some that could be lethal with just a taste, such behavior is totally contraindicated at a drug scene. Further, it is evident that any type of white powder, including insoluble talc, milk sugar, flour and others can be used to cut the drug.

Generally, the local dealer does not cut tar heroin. The viscous or semisolid material represents the end product of the acetylation process. It cannot be physically manipulated like a powder. Tar heroin has been shown to contain particles of plant material, bacteria, fungi and portions of insects.

Drug addicts commonly mix drugs, including alcohol. Since there can be an additive effect, respiratory depression may occur even with experienced addicts. In cases of overdose, a mixed intoxication should always be considered. First-pass metabolism typically removes the 3-

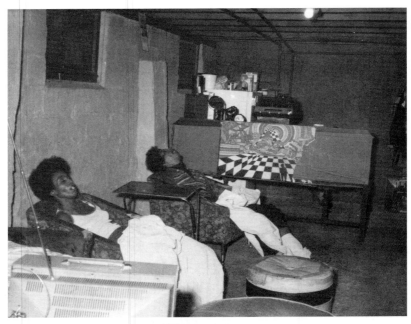

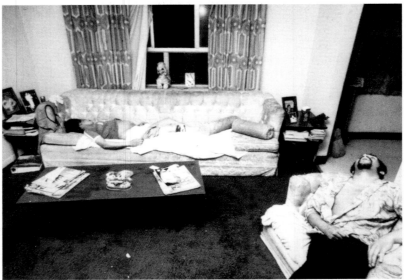

FIGURE XXII-16a–b. Non-traumatic multiple deaths are always suspicious of drug intoxication, especially if carbon monoxide is negative and the victims are young.

monoacetyl group from heroin. The 6-monoacetyl group is removed fairly quickly, primarily within the liver so that the circulating drug is morphine. The drug, effectively blocks the pain perception mechanism, thus producing analgesia, and acts upon a specific opioid receptor. Peripheral blood, urine, bile, spinal fluid and brain are the most common analyses. In an acute

death, blood levels can vary widely from an extremity and central blood specimens. Testing the contents of the syringe or tissue at the venous injection site can help make the diagnosis.

Finding the monoacetyl compound is usually considered necessary to determine that the drug used was heroin, since the compound found most commonly in the blood sample is mor-

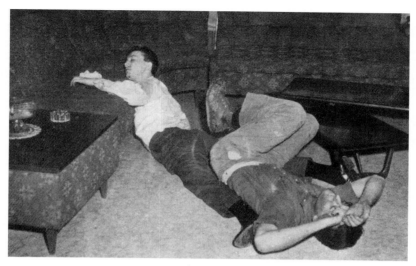

FIGURE XXII-16c. Two cousins dead of heroin intoxication. At least one of the bodies (right) has been moved after rigidity had set in.

phine. The toxicologist often simply hydrolyzes the sample and reports the results as total morphine-type alkaloids, rather than free, bound or 6-monoacetyl. Morphine is transported bound to a protein carrier, so that the analysis may report total morphine and/or free morphine. For forensic toxicology purposes, this differentiation typically does not aid in the determination of either the cause of death or the manner. To interpret the toxicology report, you need to understand how the laboratory does the analysis. This is commonly stated on the report produced by the toxicologist.

Frequently, the conclusion that a death was due to drug abuse is based upon a combination of scene investigation, physical examination of the body, the autopsy, as well as histological and toxicological findings (Fig. XXII-17). Until all data are assembled for interpretation, the final diagnosis should be withheld. Commonly, heroin addicts have many positive autopsy findings, such as old or recent myocardial or valvular disease, pulmonary fibrosis, and frequently pneumonia, malnutrition, sepsis, renal and hepatic disease.

In many jurisdictions, a drug death is listed as unclassified or drug related and the manner of death is not further classified into accident, homicide, or suicide. Death certification, which is

based upon World Health Organization (WHO) criteria, uses ICD-10 criteria and is regulated by the individual states with Center for Disease Control (CDC) guidance, does not accept such a scheme. It is not always easy to classify one of these deaths as only an accident, suicide, etc. Since death is not unexpected or reasonably unforeseen, the death is not truly accidental and is usually restricted from any insurance benefits. The addict took the drug knowing the potential for a reaction, overdose, or health risk. In the event that another person injected the drug, the differentiation of a potential homicide would not typically be evident from the autopsy alone. Similarly, if poor technique in cutting or diluting the drug resulted in high purity or an intentionally high purity was administered with the intent to cause death, the difference would not usually be apparent from the autopsy or toxicology. It is also claimed that recurrent drug abuse is a form of self-destruction, so that some would consider these deaths to be a form of suicide. For these and other reasons, it is logical not to try to classify these deaths into any one manner, but simply list them as drug related. Hopefully, attempts to get WHO to accept this logic will avoid further pseudoclassifications.

However, in many jurisdictions no such choice is available. To classify all drug deaths as

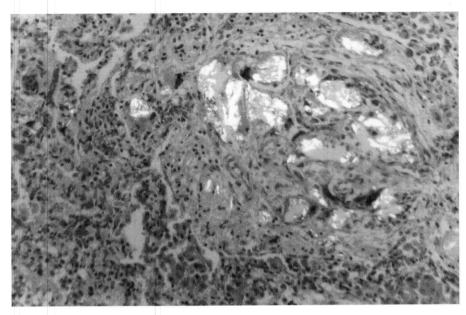

FIGURE XXII-17. Foreign body granuloma to insoluble crystals trapped in the lung of a heroin addict who had dissolved and injected methadone pills meant for oral use (×200 under polarized light).

unknown would result in an unduly large number of such deaths in the particular jurisdiction, misleading statistical results of death investigation. Death from chronic drug use complications is considered to be a natural death. Uniformity across America is needed to allow direct comparison among jurisdictions and to assemble a more accurate picture of drug use.

Scene

Heroin overdose victims are often removed from the scene of death and dumped, so that the case may first appear to be a homicide (Figs. XXII-18 to XXII-22). Property on the body is often removed, suggesting robbery or murder or both. Further, there may be a bloody oropharynx purge fluid about the face or upper clothing as a result of the pulmonary congestion. The drug injection apparatus, paraphernalia or works are typically absent, but there may be signs of resuscitation, including burns, drag marks or wet clothing (see Fig. XV-3). Sometimes ice is placed about the genitals. Any form of stimulation is used to ward off an overdose, so burns or pinch marks, often on the genitals or nipples, are some-

times noted. Generally, these are perimortem injuries with little or limited evidence of a vital response.

Because collapse and death can be rapid, many times these victims are found in obscure or unusual places where they have sought privacy to inject drugs. These factors along with a lifestyle that frequently involves abuse of alcohol and other drugs may result in bruises or injuries that can simulate an assault. As addicts sclerose their surface veins, they often turn to *skin popping,* a term which can mean subcutaneous or intramuscular injections. Rarely, they will inject directly into an internal jugular or femoral vessel. A broken needle left in the tissue can be both a source of infection and an autopsy hazard.

Skin popping has a high correlation to infections and may lead to necrotizing fasciitis. Many different bacteria have been recovered from these wounds. The ones that tend to be the most dangerous are called the *flesh eating bacteria* in the press, and often have coagulase or proteolytic enzymes. Fasciitis frequently leads to death from sepsis. Once the disease process is started these are extremely difficult cases to treat medically or surgically. The treatment often leads to massive

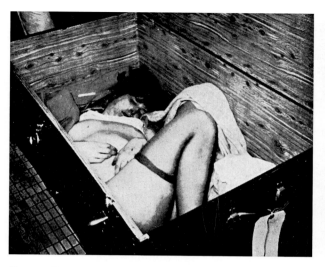

FIGURE XXII-18. Nineteen-year-old girl placed in a trunk and removed to an abandoned building following death from intravenous drug use. Note fresh injection site on the back of the left hand and the clothing disposed of with the body.

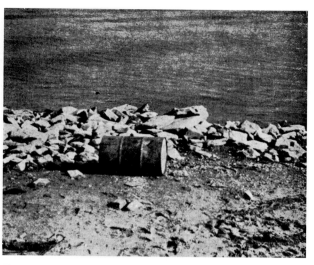

FIGURE XXII-20. Punctured oil drum found washed ashore. The drum contained the partially decomposed body of an addict who died of heroin intoxication.

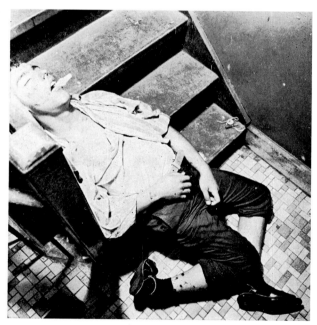

FIGURE XXII-19. Folklore remedy: Protruding paper wadding that had been forced into the mouth of an addict who lost consciousness after an intravenous injection, presumably to help him breathe, caused suffocation instead.

debridement of tissue and muscle. The organisms are often resistant to antibiotics and the dying tissue has little vascular supply to transport the treatment drugs into the necessary area.

Since addicts who are in jail or in a hospital still have the potential of getting drugs from friends or by purchase, sudden collapse in these settings should also be investigated as a potential drug-related death. In a patient with an intravenous line, injections can be given through the tubing. In a sudden unexpected death, the administration tubing should be collected for potential testing for non-prescription drugs. Such a death may be considered a homicide.

Characteristic autopsy findings depend upon the route of administration and the length of time the victim had been abusing drugs. Obviously, this ranges from one who dies after his first injection to someone with a many-year history of abuse. In San Francisco, our youngest heroin-related death was a female teenager, the oldest were men in their eighties. Since the syringe now in common use has a small-gauge needle, such as that used for insulin, the last injection site(s) may be difficult to find. However, needle tracks from previous injections can be associated with scarring and subcutaneous granulomas, which may contain polarizable foreign material (Figs. XXII-23 and XXII-24). With the small needles commonly in use today, the scars are typically much smaller than shown here. It may be necessary to incise suspicious areas along the subcutaneous veins to see perivascular hemorrhage which is

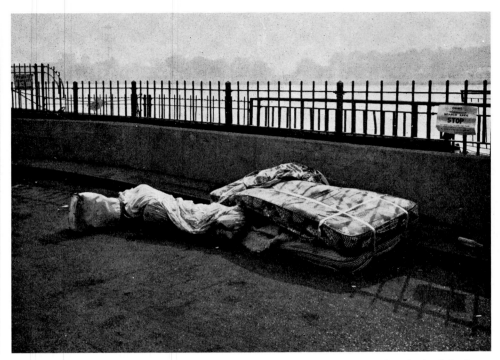

FIGURE XXII-21. The decomposing body of a twenty-four-year-old female who had died at a friend's house as a result of drug abuse was wrapped with sheets, placed between two mattresses and dropped on a highway.

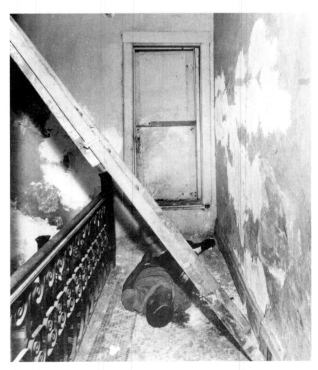

FIGURE XXII-22. Fourteen-year-old heroin addict found on a tenement roof landing used as a *shooting gallery*.

often associated with the injection site. Tissue from such areas may have both foreign materials (fibers or other substances from the filter), crystals and carbon as well as a high detectable level of monoacetyl morphine.

As indicated above, injections are not always intravenous. Skin popping or subcutaneous injections are used when entering a vein is difficult (Figs. XXII-25a–b to XXII-28). Some will resort to intramuscular injections. Because neither the drug being injected nor the technique is sterile, infections are common. Rarely, an intra-arterial injection can lead to spasm or thrombosis leading to ischemia and gangrene.

Strange and bold tattoos, sometimes homemade, are occasionally seen on the skin of narcotic addicts. Some tattoos are made with the idea of hiding needle tracks or marking a favorite injection site (Figs. XXII-29 and XXII-30). In a sudden death where drugs are suspected, these are often the areas worth incising.

Snorting heroin was uncommon. The low concentration simply did not lead to an adequate

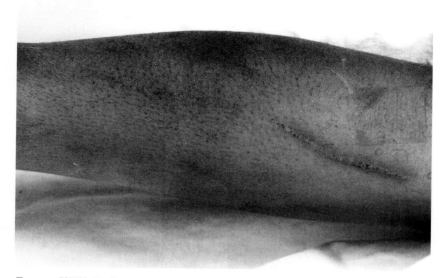

FIGURE XXII-23. Intravenous *(mainline)* track. Linear hypertrophic scars with dark spots from injections overlying veins extending from the elbow fossa to the wrist.

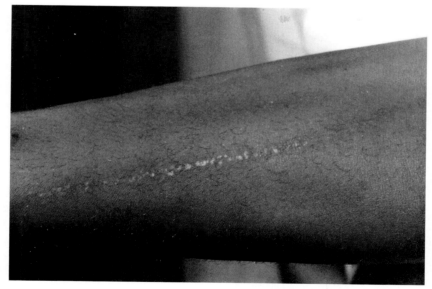

FIGURE XXII-24. Intravenous *(mainline)* track with depigmented spots from scarred injections.

blood level. That was true when the concentrations were frequently less than 10%. Now, with drug levels commonly at or over 50%, snorting, smoking or a process called *chasing the dragon* is used. In the latter, heroin is heated on a piece of aluminum foil while the user inhales the vapors with a straw or *tooter.* These methods avoid the needle, which can be a consideration for the casual user who wishes to avoid the potential of hepatitis or HIV exposure. Heroin can be recovered from the mucosa of the nose using a swab moistened with methanol (wood alcohol). Seri-

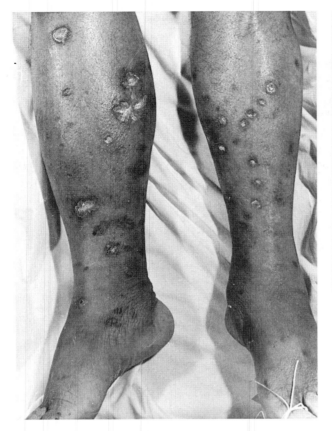

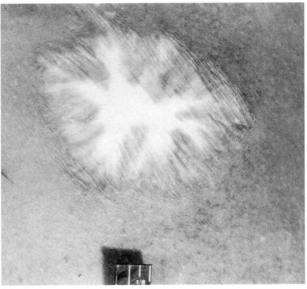

FIGURE XXII-25a–b. (a) Typical *skin-popping* scars in long-time narcotic addict. (b) Close-up of typical *skin-popping* scar.

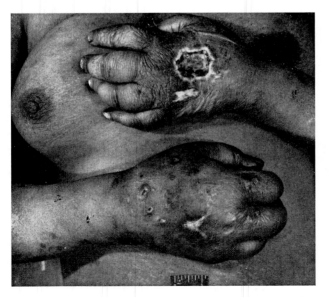

FIGURE XXII-26. Old and healing *skin-popping* ulcerations.

ous users typically inject while the recreational ones try the other methods. Heroin is typically not taken orally because of hydrolysis of the drug in the stomach and slow absorption. Occasionally, heroin is swallowed to prevent discovery of the drug during an arrest. Large amounts of swallowed heroin in a container that leaks in the bowel can lead to toxicity and death as a result of overdose.

The number of deaths related to heroin injection is probably low considering the number of addicts in the large cities. The long-term effects, however, often lead to major medical problems or trauma that adds significantly to the costs of medical care in the community.

Autopsy Findings

At autopsy, peripheral blood, urine, bile and liver should be collected. Collection of kidney tissue may be advantageous if the bladder is empty. Right heart blood can be used if peripheral blood is unavailable. It is also possible to test brain or tissue from a suspected injection site. Hair can be tested for evidence of past drug use. In the living

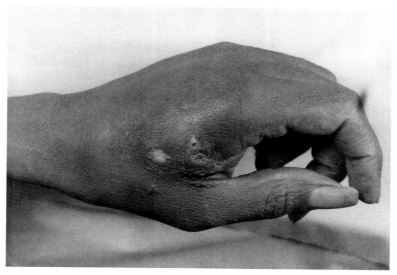

FIGURE XXII-27. Old, scarred, injection sites in the web of the thumb.

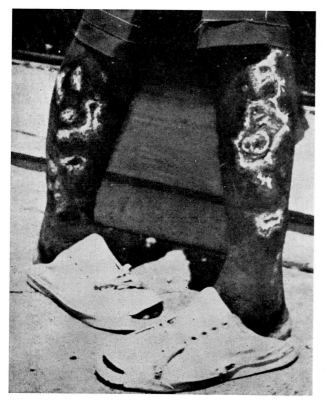

FIGURE XXII-28. Addict with extensive geographic scarring and ulcerations. (Courtesy of Baltimore City Police Department.)

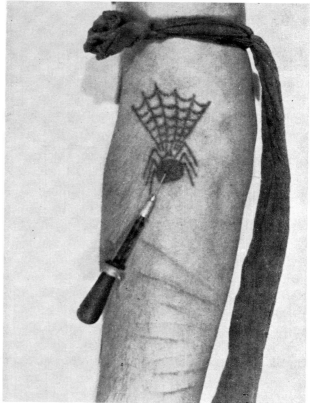

FIGURE XXII-29. Addict-type tattoo used to conceal injection sites. Note the multiple scars due to incised wounds from self-mutilation.

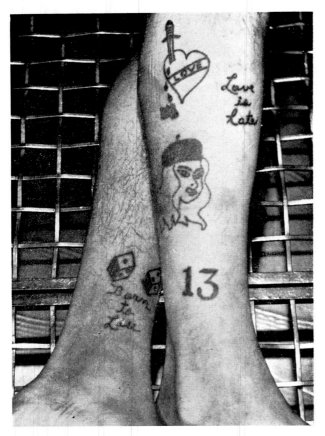

FIGURE XXII-30. Tattoos on a drug addict manifesting psychiatric significance.

patient heroin is so rapidly metabolized that even in known injection cases, no detectable drug may be found in the blood 30 to 60 minutes after administration. In the urine, however, morphine alkaloids (hydrolyzed metabolites) are detectable for hours following a single exposure. At autopsy, it is often helpful to collect blood from more than one site when the investigation supports a sudden death following injection. There can be a significant concentration difference between blood from an extremity containing the injection site and some other vascular source. Lung and brain are also good samples because of heroin's higher concentrations typically found in these organs following an acute death.

If the issue is whether the person has ever used an opioid or not, it is possible to test hair. Since it takes about two weeks for hair to grow from the root to a position above the skin sur-

face, this is not a reasonable sample in a living person for confirming acute use, but it can be a helpful sample in a decomposed case where fluids and tissues are not available and the hair can easily be removed with its roots.

Since some drugs, such as quinine, can be detected in nanogram levels and the drug is eliminated from the body more slowly than is heroin, the presence of a cutting agent could be used to suggest the presence of the opioid. This would require that quinine is routinely used as a cutting agent in the area and some other factors support a drug death. Quinine is available from a number of other sources without inferring drug use. As a medication, it is used for vascular and cardiac conditions. Some still use it to prevent malaria. It is also one of the ingredients in various common tonic waters.

If a syringe is found, it should be saved for possible analysis of the contents. Addicts often wash out their syringes following an injection, so there may not be an organic compound to detect. On the other hand, the syringe may contain a drug or drugs and, if the issue is who used the syringe, it may have fingerprints on the surface of the barrel or contain recoverable DNA. Any packets or drug containers also should be recovered, since analysis of the residue may reveal what drugs and cutting agents were used and may be a clue to the drug source. Having this material could be invaluable should it be suspected at a later time that the drugs were intentionally poisoned.

Injection sites can be incised. This should be done at the end of the autopsy when the vascular blood pressure has been relieved. By incising the skin about the vein at the end of the autopsy, local vascular bleeding will usually be reduced or eliminated. Another technique is to aspirate blood from the vein prior to making the section into the vessel. Often there is a small to moderate amount of hemorrhage surrounding the vein perforation. This area of tissue may be rich in drug and cutting agent. By eliminating vascular bleeding, the hemorrhage is easier to see and photograph.

Analysis typically starts with the urine, since it is easy to screen. If the urine is negative for morphine-type alkaloids, yet the scene or autopsy supports a drug death, analysis of blood should be performed. Although a typical drug death victim is likely to have the drug in the urine, some deaths are so rapid that the drug may be found only in the blood. Because heroin is rapidly broken down in the liver, detectable heroin from biological samples is not usually possible. The presence of monoacetyl morphine is strong support that the parent drug was heroin. In some laboratories, the extract is simply hydrolyzed so that all the metabolites, along with bound morphine, are detected and reported as morphine-type alkaloids or total morphine. The majority of forensic toxicology laboratories report morphine and monoacetyl morphine, and some report free and total. In any case, interpretation of blood levels should be related to the findings of the autopsy and the results of the investigation.

The reported blood levels have little relation to the cause of death. Some individuals will have a low level, some high. An individual with a high blood level may die from a gunshot wound, while a person with a low level may be a true drug related death. Some people die very rapidly, even prior to a complete mixing of the drug, so that the blood level detected will vary with the source of the blood. Others will survive in a coma for several hours or longer, ultimately dying from aspiration or pneumonia. The scene investigation, the autopsy findings and the exclusion of another cause of death are important factors in determining that the death is related to morphine. People in coma tend to hold the drug in the bile so that a person on a respirator following a failed resuscitation might have a negative blood and urine test, but a positive analysis of the bile. Obviously, hospital-administered medication must be ruled out as a source, since morphine is now commonly used in support of dying patients.

Because there is such variability in blood levels, some forensic scientists support that these deaths should be coded as *drug related,* rather than certifying them as accident or suicide. Deaths that follow chronic use, such as sepsis associated with endocarditis are generally considered to be of a natural manner.

Analysis has been performed on other specimens, such as fly larvae or bone marrow. In decomposed cases, skeletal tissue, clothing or hair and evidence are sometimes used to support the investigative findings that an opioid relates to the cause of death.

Analytic considerations should always include the potential action of another drug or cutting agent and should therefore encompass all common drugs. Heroin is occasionally mixed with other drugs. Cocaine and heroin used together is known as *speed-balling,* although methamphetamine, also known as *speed,* is not involved in this form of abuse. Some mixtures are reputed to take advantage of the better features of each drug, such as heroin and cocaine, while other combinations are stated to smooth out the high or potentiate it.

Concerns about a hot shot, where an intentional overdose of drugs or an intentional injection of battery acid, Drano® or some other toxic or lethal combination is given are commonly heard expressions, yet are rarely proven. Injection of a caustic or other poison usually requires restraint of the victim and often produces local change at the injection site. Sometimes the term simply means to supply an injection of high purity. With the abundance of high purity drug readily available, this is both an unlikely mechanism of murder and more street talk than fact. If a scene or investigation suggests this mode of death, injection sites should be excised and maintained frozen for potential analysis. A check of the tissue with pH paper will usually identify marked alkalinity or acidity, and in the few documented caustic injections, hemolysis or local necrosis was usually evident. In one case of injection of a liquid drain cleaner, the blood was brown, partly clotted and obviously looked abnormal. In all cases of potential drug death, abundant samples of various fluids and organs should be properly collected and held for possible analysis. This includes blood, stomach and contents, liver, kidney, bile, urine and vitreous humor. Collection of brain, lung and injection sites should be considered as appropriate to the individual case.

AMPHETAMINES

Amphetamines represented less than 2% of the 1989 National Institute of Drug Abuse cases reported by medical examiners, and the drug was nationally ranked twenty-second in all drug mentions. In 1999, that reported number had increased to closer to 6%, and with the increased use of chemical analogs, such as ecstasy, the number is likely to increase in the future. Abuse of methamphetamine has been and is common on the West Coast. Until the late 1980s, amphetamines were the second most common illicit drugs detected in San Francisco. Unlike cocaine and heroin, the amphetamine preparations are totally synthetic and do not depend upon botanical supplies or imported precursors.

The chemical class is related to ephedrine, a naturally occurring alkaloid isolated from the plant *Ephedra equisetina*. Used by the Chinese for centuries, ephedrine was first isolated by Nagai in 1887. It first became popular in the United States in 1925, following evaluation by Chen and Schmidt. Initially used for treatment of bronchial asthma and for relief of nasal congestion, Neo-Synephrine® has now largely taken its place.

MDMA (methylenedioxymethamphetamine), was synthesized in 1914, but never placed on the market. Years later, when the formula was extracted from the chemical literature, it quickly became an abuse drug. Often known on the street as ecstasy, MDMA has been associated with sudden death through cardiac arrhythmia or hyperthermia. In a recent National Institute on Drug Abuse (NIDA) survey, 11% of high school seniors indicated that they have tried ecstasy at least once. The drug has gained enormous popularity as a *rave drug,* or *club drug.* Teens and young adults participate at dance parties called *raves,* where the users take the drug, often prepared in solution and sold at booths. They may dance for long periods or to exhaustion, and sometimes place a dust mask over their faces into which a smear of menthol salve has been placed. The menthol is stated to enhance and prolong the pleasant effect of the drug. Users can become dehydrated, collapse from exhaustion or, more dangerously, suffer heat prostration or hyperthermia. Body temperature and the absence of moisture on the skin at the scene of a rave are supporting information that the drug is present and significant in the collapse or death. In a living person, muscle rigidity and changes more similar to the malignant neuroleptic syndrome are common. Body core temperature and vitreous electrolytes need to be collected as soon as possible if the body is at the scene.

Some clandestine laboratories produce a number of other drugs based upon the amphetamine structure. Some of the better known examples include MDMA (methylenedioxymethamphetamine), MDA (methylenedioxyamphetamine), DOM (2,5-dimethoxy-4-methylamphetamine) and many others. Since chemical substitution of the base compound leads to many potential products, a large number of resulting chemical compounds are possible. Although some are more powerful or more toxic than others, some will have more desirable effects. The clandestine chemist seeks out these compounds for production. They are commonly known as designer drugs and are often not illegal, even though their parent compound is restricted.

Chemically, these drugs are similar to the hallucinogen mescaline. Initially synthesized in the early 1900s, MDA did not become popular as a drug of abuse until the 1960s when it was marketed as the *love drug* because of pleasant feelings and socialization associated with drug use in the culture at the time. In moderate doses, it produced hallucinations similar to LSD.

The amphetamine analogs are known primarily for their *upper* or stimulating properties, imparting a prolonged feeling of strength and well-being in the user. Because the drugs typically increase physiologic activity, tiredness is relieved and a feeling of alertness and energy prevails. Amphetamines were used in the 1940s to increase productivity and allow prolonged activities that would normally be very tiring or tedious. Bomber pilots, for example, were given amphetamines to help them stay alert on long flights during World War II. In the 1980s, long haul truckers often used these drugs to stay awake for periods of more than 16 hours.

Because of the great propensity for abuse, the drug has now been so restricted that even medical applications are confined to conditions such as narcolepsy, limited anorexic treatment use, sleep apnea, and certain types of childhood behavioral problems. These medical uses are closely regulated.

The drug is often sold in papers, a term used for any quantity of less than one gram. A paper containing one-tenth of a gram sells for $50 to $100, one gram sells for $200 to $350, an ounce for around $4,000, and a kilogram would market for $60,000 to $100,000. Sometimes other compounds are mixed with or substituted for methamphetamine, including cocaine, phenyl-propanolamine hydrochloride, d-amphetamine, ephedrine, or pseudoephedrine. The purity of the drug ranges from a low of 30 to 40% to 99%.

The most common methods of use in order of frequency are ingestion by mouth, injection and smoking. Although typically more expensive per dose than crack cocaine, the effect of a single dose lasts for many hours, perhaps as long as ten to 16 hours. Considerable tolerance can develop in heavy users, and they may consume one or more grams of the drug per 24 hours. Because of the central nervous system stimulation, users tend to be hyperactive, go without sleep or food, or carry on other activities to excess. When used at dance parties or music events, the participants tend to be very active for long periods. Whether the drug being used is methamphetamine or an analog, such as 3,4-methylenedioxymethamphetamine (MDMA), dehydration and hyperthermia can lead to collapse and cardiac toxicity or the neurostimulation effects can lead to death.

Use of some drugs has been associated with a fulminant hepatitis. Although the most common drug associated with acute hepatic failure is acetaminophen, cocaine, solvent inhalation, phencyclidine and amphetamine-related drugs, such as MDMA, are also capable of producing severe, and sometimes fatal liver disease. MDMA is metabolized by the cytochrome CYP2D6. An estimated 5% of Caucasians and an unknown percentage of other races have a genetic deficiency that may predispose them to MDMA-related complications.[31]

The most important abuse drug is methamphetamine, and it is known by many street names such as meth, crystal, crank and speed. It is most popular on the West Coast and in the Pacific Rim countries, particularly Japan. Reports of the drug being prepared by organized gangs are widespread, but the manufacture is well within the capabilities of anyone having an understanding of practical organic chemistry. Although most of the chemical precursors are regulated, many chemical syntheses leading to these same compounds are possible, making elimination of illegal drug by precursor regulation unlikely. Since the drug depends upon a chemical synthesis, and can be prepared from a number of different routes, control of precursors is difficult. Some methods of synthesis produce almost entirely the physiologically active dextro form of the drug, while others produce a mixture of the dextro and levo forms. Chiral separation may become necessary in the analysis of some cases in order to prove the presence of the physiologically active form of the legally controlled drug.

One form of methamphetamine received excessive press coverage. Known as *ice,* it has been called *the most dangerous drug in existence,* with the suggestion that it was a *killer* drug. When volatile methamphetamine oil is allowed to crystallize slowly in a refrigerator, large crystals form. White or slightly yellow in color, they are usually the size of rock salt, about one-quarter to one-half inch long. Because of their appearance or possibly because they are formed in a refrigerator, they are called *ice.* Other street terms for this product are *crystal, batu,* and *shabu,* which are Filipino and Japanese words for rock. Because this form could be easily smoked, it was thought to be much more addicting than the powdered drug. Despite such publicity, this crystal form of methamphetamine differs from the powder only in its physical appearance. The chemical compounds are the same. Both forms can be smoked. On the East Coast, a drug known as *ice* is unrelated chemically to amphetamine, and is based upon the Demerol® molecule.

Although the powder or crystal form can be mixed with tobacco and smoked in a pipe, more often it is heated to a vapor on the screen of a pipe unmixed with tobacco, or heated in a special glass *speed* pipe and the resulting fumes inhaled. The typical effects are those of a sympathomimetic, as well as the seductive euphoric feeling and the resulting desire for more drugs. A significant problem associated with the chronic use of amphetamines is the propensity towards paranoia, violent behavior and a desire to carry weapons. Since dealers tend to be drug users, their paranoid thinking may motivate them to carry guns, money and their drugs in the belief that someone is trying to take these away. With the large amounts of money that is possible from drug sales, violence is not uncommon for the chronic user.

Given that the drug induces anxiety, and sometimes hallucinations, interactions with the police often lead to violent confrontations. Withdrawal from the drug can lead to depression and sometimes suicide.

Besides the complications described above for the *rave* drugs, prolonged use can lead to psychosis, hyperthermia, rhabdomyolysis and death. Although classed as less physiologically addicting than the narcotics, amphetamines are habituating and true withdrawal symptoms develop in long-term users.

Scene

The most significant scene findings are the types of pipes used to smoke the drug and the presence of burns about the hands, fingers, or occasionally on the lips and face. These changes are from exposure to the open flame, usually from a lighter, or the hot glass pipe being handled or placed to the lips. The pipe is usually a glass bulb with a hole in the top and a tube on one side for a mouthpiece. Shaped somewhat like a chemical retort flask, pipes come in all shapes and sizes, but tend to be about four to six inches in greatest dimension. The drug is placed in the pipe and then heated with the flame from a cigarette lighter or propane torch until a white vapor appears as the drug reaches just above its melting point. The

finger sealing the hole on the top of the pipe is removed and the user inhales from the tube as long as possible. The breath is held to increase absorption through the lungs. After inhalation, the pipe is immediately cooled with a wet cloth to condense the vapor back to a solid drug.

A single crystal can be used several times before it is consumed, and, considering the length of the *high,* it would seem to be more economical than cocaine. A used pipe will have carbon on the outside bottom and a coating of white to gray crystals on the inside walls. A source of flame and a cloth with carbon upon it are also commonly found nearby.

Scenes at meth production labs are extremely dangerous, as many of the chemicals are hazardous or explosive. Booby traps are common. Examination and the securing of the scene or removal of chemicals require specially trained people. Should a body be found in such a lab, it is advantageous to have a trained drug laboratory investigator clear the scene prior to moving the body.

Autopsy Findings

Autopsy findings are variable, as would be expected for a drug that can be smoked, snorted, injected, or absorbed from any mucous membrane. Since the drug is sometimes associated with sexual activity, it can be taken to promote sexual activity or absorbed from the rectum or vagina.

In snorting, a fine rim of powder can be seen at the nasal opening or recovered from a methanol swab of the septum. The other autopsy findings are generally non-specific.

Injections are generally made with insulin needles and the injection sites can be difficult to see. A magnifying glass can be helpful to locate the skin defect. The site may not have surrounding pallor or hemorrhage. Since the user tends to make multiple injections to maintain the high, puncture sites tend to be numerous and clustered around a favorite vein. Sometimes an elongated tattoo over the vein hides the needle marks.

If the drug is smoked or taken orally, there may be no external manifestation of use. Besides the scene information, a burn on the palmar side of the index finger that was used to apply to the opening in the heated pipe suggests drug use.

Upon internal examination, the lungs are heavy, usually 400 to 500 grams each, but weights of 1,000 grams or more per lung are not uncommon. The heart is a target organ, and is often increased in weight with concentric left ventricular hypertrophy and right dilation. On microscopic examination, there is congestion of the organs with edema. Increased amounts of carbon particles may be seen. If used intravenously, polarizable foreign material may be present in the lungs. Cross-band necrosis of myofibrils is common. Since the drug is a catecholamine stimulator and, like cocaine, is associated with increased levels of circulating catechols, the heart often has microscopic areas of ischemia and myonecrosis. There may be zone 3 hepatocytic enlargement and the cytoplasm can be vacuolated or *bubbly*. Bile plugs and *feathery degeneration* of hepatocytes can be seen on Perl's iron stain. Cases that experience hyperthermia with liver failure often have massive hepatic necrosis, microvesicular steatosis (which can also be seen in heat stroke), bile stasis and other changes of hepatocellular degeneration.[31]

The plasma half-life is such that the drug can be detected in the blood for many hours, depending upon the dose. Metabolism produces amphetamine as the primary metabolite of methamphetamine, and the ratio in blood and urine can be helpful in suggesting acute or chronic use, and may be helpful in supporting the time of administration. The urine, spinal fluid and tissues may be positive for days after a single exposure, and longer in the case of chronic users. Hair can be analyzed for the presence of the drug.

Autopsy samples should include peripheral blood without preservative, peripheral blood with sodium fluoride, urine, liver, bile, stomach contents and hair. Some laboratories use lung and brain or spinal fluid as additional samples.

An acute choreoathetoid disorder can be induced by amphetamine analog use. Hyperthermia with seizures or muscular hyperactivity with myonecrosis and rhabdomyolysis leading to acute renal failure may follow chronic or excessive use. Some people seem to be genetically more susceptible to the adverse effects of the drug. Hypertension, with complaints of chest pain is not uncommon. Like cocaine, ECG changes are absent or slight. Other complications include cerebral hemorrhage or ruptured berry aneurysm.

BARBITURATES

Under current U.S. drug regulations, many barbiturates are restricted as a class II drug because of their propensity for abuse. Some barbiturates, such as phenobarbital, which have a lesser history of abuse, are restricted as a class IV medication, while a few are listed as class III.

Among the most commonly abused forms are the short and intermediate acting barbiturates, such as secobarbital and pentobarbital. Barbiturates are the archetypical sedative-hypnotic, used as a soporific after opium and alcohol, and still filling a valuable place in the pharmacy. Replacing potassium bromide and chloral hydrate, their use in control of seizure disorders was a major medical advance.

In 1903, Fischer and Von Mering developed barbital, and over the years, many other com-

pounds have appeared with similar chemical structure. Barbiturates have been widely used because of their ability to calm, induce sleep, and reduce or prevent seizures.

Abuse is usually oral, although the drug can be injected. The sedative effect of barbiturates is by direct central nervous system action. Sleep is produced in the absence of pain, although tolerance to the drug will develop. In cases of abuse, higher-than-therapeutic doses are typically used. Stringent prescription requirements have decreased accidental and suicidal deaths. Occasional cases usually come from countries other than the United States, where barbiturates are more commonly available.

Several organizations that support suicide as a form of self-determination or euthanasia in terminal conditions recommend barbiturates as one of the preferred drugs. They may recommend a source from another country or help pool small legitimate prescriptions from other persons to constitute a lethal dose. Often no containers remain at the scene, and the source of the drug may be difficult to determine.

In other cases, there may be abundant evidence of drug use at the scene. In intentional deaths, the drugs are often mixed with alcohol and sometimes other medications. A glass with a granular, powdery residue may be near the body or a container of yogurt or a pudding mix. A will and other instructions may be displayed and a plastic bag may be tied over the head. Scene investigation and chemical analysis from the container may be as helpful in determining the manner, as are the results of the autopsy.

At autopsy, granular powder may be present on the lips or teeth or in vomitus at the scene and about the body. Medication is frequently added to the ingested medications in order to reduce vomiting and loss of drug dose from the stomach. The stomach may contain recognizable capsules or tablets. Examination of a sample of the stomach contents with polarized light may reveal crystals related to the chemical that was taken. The gastric mucosa may be eroded and there are typical signs of acute pulmonary failure, with right ventricular dilation and severe pulmonary congestion. Even individuals who do not ordinarily drink often consume alcohol to potentiate the depressive action of the drug.

In cases where the death occurs rapidly, analysis of peripheral blood, urine and liver may show high levels of alcohol and barbiturates with low levels in the urine. Stomach levels of alcohol and drug in such cases are usually very high.

LSD

Hofmann prepared lysergic acid diethylamide in 1943. While working with the compound, he noted dizziness, restlessness and slight disorientation. He ingested a small amount of the drug and confirmed its effect. LSD is the dextrorotary isomer of diethylamide or lysergic acid, an essential compound of ergot alkaloids. It probably has its central nervous system effect through a potent antiserotonin route and tends to produce a transient psychosis. Although LSD has no medicinal application, it has been available in larger metropolitan areas and sporadically appears in the drug culture (Fig. XXII-31).

Flashbacks, which are recurrent episodes of acute intoxication after days, even weeks of abstinence, are characteristic of the drug.

The scene may suggest a life-style supportive of drug abuse and may be disheveled due to prior episodes of hallucinations and/or acute psychosis. The drug can be sold as a liquid or tablet, but it is most commonly placed upon a small square of colored paper. These small squares of paper are about one-quarter to one-half inch in size and typically have a printed colored surface. Death is often the result of trauma during the psychotic phase of drug use, not the direct result of drug poisoning.

No specific autopsy findings are associated with the use of LSD. Occasionally, direct analysis of gastric material reveals the drug, but analysis by one of the specific methods is usually required for proof of exposure. Rarely, the small paper square will be found in the stomach. The part played in the death by the drug will have to be determined after full review of all the facts related to the death.

MARIJUANA

The hemp plant, *Cannabis sativa,* grows in a wide variety of habitats. Immigrants arriving in the United States to work in agriculture brought the plant with them from Mexico. The drug was specifically regulated through the *Marijuana Tax Act* of 1937, which established a special tax

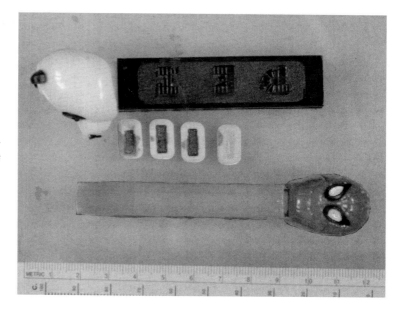

FIGURE XXII-31. LSD: Child's candy dispenser. Area of discoloration on candy is the area of drug application.

stamp, that was legally necessary to sell, possess, or transport the drug, but the stamp was never made available for public use.

During World War II, the plant was grown in large areas of the United States for the recovery of its fiber content, which is used to make rope. Partly as a result, the easily cultivated plant became even more widespread, sometimes appearing as a wild growth in uncultivated land.

Today, marijuana grows in small and large plots, indoors and out, in normal soil and hydroponically. Still illegal, this controversial drug has been a topic of discussion for years. During the 1960s, actions were taken to decriminalize possession of small amounts for medical use. In 1977, the Carter administration advocated legalizing amounts up to one ounce for personal use. However, public opinion is now changing back towards tighter regulation and control of the drug. Touted as an important appetitive and mood elevator for end stage diseases, there is currently little scientific evidence to support either side of the disagreement. A recent article in *Circulation* supported that smoking marijuana can trigger the onset of acute myocardial infarction in some rare circumstances.[32] The state of Nevada defeated legalizing marijuana at the 2002 elections.

Hashish is the resin extract of the flowering tips of the plant, which has a higher concentration of the active ingredient. Both marijuana and hashish are usually smoked, although they can be taken orally. Hashish is usually smoked in a water pipe of variable construction.

Marijuana is most commonly ingested by smoking, usually mixed with tobacco. The smoking apparatus varies, ranging from hand-rolled cigarettes to water pipes (Figs. XXII-32 to XXII-34). It can be taken orally in baked goods such as cookies and cakes. A popular form still sometimes seen is in brownies. Marijuana tea is also sometimes being used. The drug is extracted from the plant material by heating the leaves along with a fat, such as butter. The butter can then be used in baking. Fat solubility explains why the drug will elude from the body for such long periods of time following exposure. At least one study confirms impairment of smokers operating a motor vehicle.

Scene

The odor associated with the drug is herbal and somewhat specific. While detectable on the hands and fingers, lips, tongue and teeth as a green stain in recent users, determination of the principle compound and its metabolites is made from samples of peripheral blood, saliva, or urine. Deaths associated with the use of marijuana are usually the result of some activity while using the drug. Carefully controlled studies demonstrate that there is a physical and neurological impairment of safe performance of com-

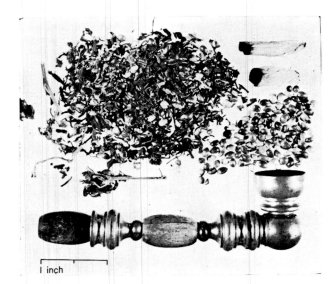

FIGURE XXII-32. *(Upper left)* Dried marijuana; stems, leaves and seeds ground together. *(Upper right)* Marijuana cigarettes that have been smoked almost to the end *(roaches)*. *(Middle right)* Characteristic marijuana seeds. *(Bottom)* Pipe for marijuana smoking.

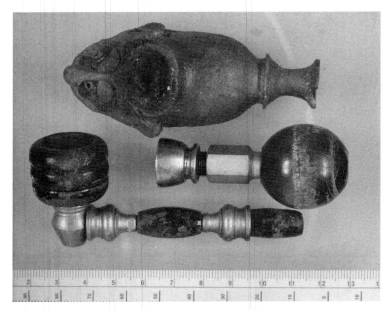

FIGURE XXII-33. Marijuana can be smoked in a number of ways. One is in a pipe, usually mixed with a small amount of tobacco.

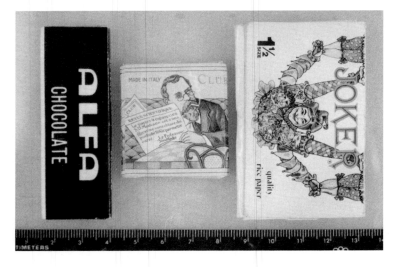

FIGURE XXII-34. Various types of tobacco paper are used to *roll* marijuana into *joints* for smoking.

plicated tasks, such as driving, while under the acute influence of the drug.

Autopsy

Autopsy examination does not reveal any specific findings. If analysis is desired from green areas on the tongue, lips or fingers, swabs are made using petroleum ether, chloroform or methanol as a solvent to recover the drug.

Interpretation of laboratory values requires caution due to the lack of a uniform and clear understanding of the relation of a value with impairment or intoxication.

PHENCYCLIDINE

Known as PCP, angel dust, the peace pill, animal tranquilizer and a number of other names, this compound was originally developed in 1958 as a short-acting anesthetic. Medical use was soon discontinued, because of the high incidence of adverse hallucinations experienced by recipients. For many, these were unpleasant events, and medical use of PCP in humans was soon abandoned. The drug is still used as an animal tranquilizer, primarily for large animals.

Its first reported illicit use was in San Francisco in 1967. It is now most commonly smoked on tobacco or taken orally, although it can be used by injection and inhalation as well. Sudden deaths have been reported following the use of the drug. PCP has a propensity for causing acute psychosis and violent behavior, which can lead to death from trauma. Confrontation with the police or citizens is common when such bizarre behavioral changes occur. Many users want to be in or near water, and some cases of drowning may be associated with the drug's use. PCP is usually easy to detect in blood, urine or other fluids.

DESIGNER DRUGS

This non-specific term is used to cover a wide range of chemical analogues to named, often regulated, or new experimental drugs. Usually, the term is reserved for illegal or unregulated compounds produced by a clandestine chemist taking advantage of a weakness in federal drug laws. Generally, federal law prevents classes of drugs from being outlawed, so by making slight or sometimes significant changes in the chemical structure of a regulated or banned chemical, the new compound becomes technically *not illegal* because it is not specifically regulated by name. In some cases, the new chemical is categorically illegal by definition, based upon existing law.

Many of these new, synthetic compounds are considered dangerous with no proven or accepted legitimate medical use. Heroin, as an example, is a potent analgesic, but has such a high likelihood of abuse that it is classed as a schedule I drug, restricted to only controlled research in the U.S. By changing the chemical structure slightly, a new drug may be legal for a time. Some drugs, like the fentanyl group, illustrate what the renegade chemist can do. Fentanyl is a synthetic, short-acting analgesic used for induction of anesthesia, brief invasive procedures and pain relief. It has over 100 identified analogues with plasma half-lives of one-tenth to 1,000 times that of the parent compound. Potency similarity ranges from slight to many times that of the original drug. Many of these known drugs have been explored and have not been introduced into medical use because of their toxicity or unduly high number of adverse reactions.

Overdoses are often difficult to prove if the syringe or drug container is not available for analysis. Blood levels may be in the nanogram or picogram range. A complete collection of samples and the help of a forensic toxicologist are often necessary to identify the specific compound. When there is a sample of the original drug, identification is frequently far easier. Assistance in a specific drug identification problem may be obtained from the local Drug Enforcement Laboratory or the police crime laboratory.

INHALANTS

Many drugs, gases, or vapors can be inhaled by accident or for abuse purposes. Some of these compounds are solvents commonly found in paint, glues, videotape head cleaner and numerous other preparations. In some cases, the solvents are a relatively pure compound, not mixed with other chemicals. In others, the solvent mixture contains a *witches brew* of chemicals. Whatever the product, it is typically placed into a container, such as a plastic or paper bag for abuse inhalation. Besides direct chemical toxicity to the physiology and neurotransmitters of the body, many of the compounds induce cardiac arrhythmia. Death can be due to asphyxiation if the container cannot be removed from the vicinity of the airway. Occasionally friends, prior to the investigator's arrival, remove the evidence from the scene. In other cases, the body may be found with the face or head still in proximity to the container. Certification of manner of the death in such situations may be problematic.

Inhalants can be used for murder or suicide. Recently, one of the self-deliverance organizations that promote the right to die has started recommending inhalation of helium to cause death. As with most of these programs, specific instructions are included in their literature. Helium is readily available in large cities, as are all the other items needed to commit this act. Death is by asphyxiation and the diagnosis is based on the investigation rather than autopsy findings.

Industrial exposures can lead to collapse and death, but these are usually evident by the circumstances. Nitrous oxide is commonly abused by inhaling the gas trapped in a balloon. A small metal cylinder about three inches long, similar to a CO_2 cylinder, is used to inflate a balloon. The contents are inhaled, producing their effect in seconds. The other most common sources are large *"B"* or *"C"* size cylinders stolen from a hospital anesthetic department, or the common *whipped cream chargers* purchased in a cooking supply store.

One case investigated by the author had a box with 51 pounds of empty discarded cylinders present at the scene. Balloons filled with the gas are sold at parties for three to five dollars each. The diagnosis is based upon investigation, the presence of the apparatus and sometimes an elevated methemoglobin level.

Scene investigation is critical in reaching the correct diagnosis. With glue and viscous compounds, material is often on the face, hands or about the nose (Fig. XXII-35a–b). However, with solvents and gases, these signs are absent. Carbon monoxide and nitrites can produce a red or pink coloration to the skin, and carbon monoxide has a tendency to blister the skin in areas of contact or pressure, i.e., the axilla or medial thighs. Solvents sometimes leave a slight odor on the clothes, in the stomach and, if the chest is compressed, the odor may be detected in the expelled air.

Special samples often need to be collected to prove the presence of a volatile gas. This includes the collection of blood in red and gray-topped vacutainer tubes by vacuum aspiration. This potentially allows for headspace analysis of the sample. A sample of bronchial air can be collected in the same manner. Some laboratories prefer a whole lung, with the bronchus tied off, submitted in a sealed container, such as an arson specimen can. This again allows the specimen to be heated and the headspace sampled for analysis. Many of the nitrate or nitrite chemicals produce methemoglobin. This can be a supportive finding in the death determination if the laboratory is not set up to do analysis of these compounds in blood.

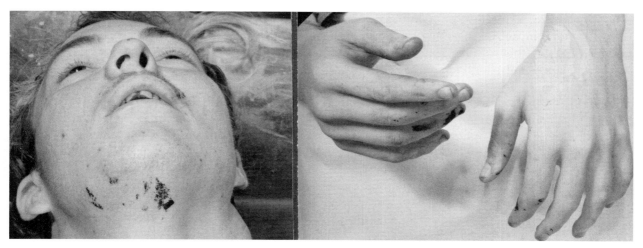

FIGURE XXII-35a–b. Dried black tarry contact cement on the fingers and below the chin was placed in a plastic bag and inhaled.

HERBAL MEDICATIONS

Herbal medications are common in most parts of the United States and other countries. Clinicians are most likely to encounter echinacea, ephedra, garlic, ginkgo, ginseng, kava, St. John's wort and valerian. These herbs are so common they can be found in many food markets or pharmacies. No prescription is needed or required for the unrestricted purchase and use of these drugs. Ephedra has been mentioned previously, and its action is primarily directly upon adrenergic receptors and indirectly by enhancing the release of endogenous norepinephrine. The adverse changes are primarily cardiac and central nervous system. Kava in larger doses acts as a sedative-hypnotic by potentiating GABA inhibitory neurotransmission. It has already been associated with several driving under the influence cases.

Other herbal medications can be more toxic or induce poisoning. Digitalis is present in a plant that grows wild or is planted as decorative foliage, the foxglove plant. *Salvia divinorum,* a member of the sage family, induces hallucinations when ingested. The same is true for a number of mushrooms, such as psilocybin. The skin of many amphibians contains chemical producing glands that can cause hallucinations, cardiac toxicity and potentially death.

Plant extracts are often powerful sources of drugs that can be abused. Their effect is often dose related. A number of deaths have been reported in the medical and toxicological literature. Some of these have been due to errors in compounding herbal prescriptions. For example, a young pregnant woman made tea of a compounded herbal medicine to ensure a strong pregnancy. She died within minutes due to an error in the amount of bufotoxin in the mixture. Unlike this case, most complications are due to abusing the herbs, and typically, from the hepatic, renal or cardiac toxicity produced by the major drug present in the mixture. Since some of these herbs are used in dieting and weight control, abuse can be excluded or included only as a *rule-out* diagnosis. Alternatively, death may result from dehydration or electrolyte imbalance with excessive diuretic use. Vitreous electrolytes provide valuable support for such a diagnosis, but are not an absolutely infallible test.

Identification of herbal medications can be difficult. A good herbalist or a school of pharmacy can be a surprisingly important source of information. A mycology program can help with fungi or spores. Spores can be recovered from uneaten food or stool. Many states have a program that can help identify physically or chemically the herb or active ingredient. The federal government has been investigating herbs, and some web sites can be a good source of information.

When the investigation suggests the potential of an herb playing a part in the death, the original container or packet may provide a lead to the source of the drug. Besides the usual toxicological samples, small and large bowel content, subcutaneous fat and hair may also be helpful.

Without a specific direction towards identification, these can be difficult cases. Any information about symptoms is important. The scene may suggest whether the patient was hallucinating or not, vomiting (which can be a sample for analysis), hyperthermic and so forth. At autopsy, evidence of disorientation based upon trauma to legs and arms, bite marks on lips or tongue, torn fingernails, and excoriations are all examples supporting a drug effect. Such case is best handled with the help of an experienced forensic toxicologist.

GHB

Gamma hydroxybutyrate, gamma butyrolactone and 1,4 butanediol are all chemicals that can convert through metabolism into one or the other. When 1,4 butanediol or gamma butyrolactone is ingested, it quickly metabolizes into GHB, which acts on the receptor sites for GABA (gamma amino benzoic acid) a naturally occurring neurotransmitter. Although not authorized as a drug for clinical use in the U.S., the drug is used as an anesthetic and to treat alcoholism in other countries. Easy to make in the home setting, it is often used at raves or club parties. It produces a sleepy, out of body experience and enhances perception of colors and sounds. Thought to enhance the sensuous nature of being touched, it is advertised as enhancing sex. At higher doses, it produces loss of muscle coordination, loss of consciousness and respiratory arrest. If resuscitated, the patient typically goes from a Glasgow coma scale of three or four to 15 within two to three hours. The drug is most likely to cause death when mixed with ethyl alcohol. Even the web sites that promote the drug caution against mixing the two.

Analysis at autopsy is associated with a major problem. The drug is produced naturally in postmortem samples unless they are collected with sodium fluoride as a preservative and refrigerated. Blood levels of less than 50 mg/L should not be considered accurate unless the drug is also proven present in the urine. Even then, any blood level of less than 75 mg/L should be considered suspect for de novo production rather than exogenous. In one study, the mean of native drug in unrefrigerated blood was 57 mg/L with a range of 9 to 433. In the presence of sodium fluoride, the same specimens had a mean of 20 mg/L and a range of 9 to 65 mg/L.[30] There are no reports of the chemical being formed in urine. Most reported studies support that the preservative should be present at a concentration of between five and ten milligrams per milliliters in the final dilution of the specimen. Storage at about 4° F should prevent chemical formation for at least one month. Again, analysis of several compartments will help demonstrate the significance of the drug. Although short-lived in the blood (detectable for up to 5 or 6 hours after ingestion), the drug can be found in the urine for 6 to 12 hours.

Sometimes used to induce unconsciousness in women for the purpose of a sexual assault, GHB is sometimes called a *date-rape* drug. It has a tendency to produce amnesia of short-term memory, as do some of the short-acting benzodiazepines. It is popular in some cities, where it is sold in bars or *clubs* for five to 10 dollars a *hit*. Analysis of other drugs is necessary to support the basis for an interpretation of the drug findings and the manner of death.[33,34]

SHORT-ACTING COMPOUNDS

Many drug users prefer compounds that have a longer effect. However, other abuse drugs produce their change for only a few minutes. Because some of these drugs have a tendency to produce amnesia and have a rapid onset, they can be used as a *knock-out* drug. The historical classic compound is chloral hydrate. Although still a commonly prescribed drug, it is rare to find the drug used for this purpose. Most commonly, drugs such as GHB, flunitrazepam (Rohypnol®), and other short-acting benzodiazepines, are removed from the blood rapidly, usually, within 6 to 12 hours. In sexual assault cases, it is important to obtain urine, bile, spinal fluid and vitreous for potential analysis. Urine can be lost from the body onto clothing or bedding. This evidence can be used to determine the presence of the drug when other specimens are absent or the patient survives on a respirator until brain death is confirmed. In living victims, blood should be taken for analysis, if less than 12 hours have passed since the assault. Ethyl alcohol is the most common drug found in sexual assault cases. Urine is the sample of choice after that time period. Although most of the short-acting drugs are absent from the urine within 24 hours, some have metabolites that survive for a longer period of time. Hair can be used for analysis to show previous exposure. In a living person, about two weeks would be necessary prior to hair collection by cutting the shaft close to the scalp. Hair should be collected from several areas of the scalp, since deposition may not be uniform. Use of a member of the drug family has to be avoided in order to give any validity to the specimen. In the deceased, other fluids, such as spinal fluid can be analyzed.

PRESCRIPTION DRUGS

Perhaps the most commonly abused *drug* in America are prescription medications. Some of these abuse patterns have other associations, both acute and chronic. Some have local, racial, historic or emotional basis for their abuse. For example, in San Francisco, carisoprodol abuse has a high correlation to Asian youth and is a frequent drug seen in driving under the influence cases. Diphenhydramine (Benadryl®) is used to *smooth-out* some of the effects of hard drug use. Regardless of the reason, prescription drugs and a number of over the counter drugs are often abused. An awareness of what is common in a particular area is important in determining both the cause and the manner of death. With abuse, circulating drug levels may be significantly higher than what would be considered toxic, and yet have little direct effect upon the death. Mixing prescription drugs with hard drugs or alcohol can lead to death. The more information available from local drug treatment programs, poison control programs, major emergency departments, or the local forensic toxicologist, the easier it is to understand and interpret laboratory results.

SUMMARY

A minister of the Irish government was quoted as stating that alcoholism was a self-inflicted plague. In a sense, all drug addictions may be so described. As with plagues, the number of cases will rise and fall over time, and the harmful agents will mutate into new analogues. We may reasonably count on the tried and true drugs of antiquity to remain as common drugs of abuse. Knowing about abused drugs and educating the population and policymakers are our best hopes for the potential control of drug abuse. There are reports supporting the value of drug education during the early elementary school years as a means of educating people of the harm, risks and social damage caused by alcohol, tobacco and drug abuse.

Investigation and analysis are our tools. We must determine what drug or drugs have been abused, how they were taken into the body, and what part they played in causing the death. Suspicion of drug involvement usually starts at the scene. When there is no scene, then the history and autopsy findings become the key. Polarization of a sample of stomach contents can support the presence of a recently ingested drug, but is a non-specific test. It is not realistic to test for all drugs in every case, nor is it necessary. Even without any investigation of background history, a negative autopsy should always evoke the need to save adequate samples for comprehensive toxicological testing.

Alcohol is a major contributor in most cases, and needs to be looked for in several body compartments. The proper collection and storage of a sample to be analyzed are critical for accurate interpretation of the results.

A single drug toxicity case is less commonly found than is the presence of multiple drugs.

Frequent exchange of information with the local poison control and/or drug abuse programs will help establish what drugs are being seen in the emergency departments and what is common on the streets. Discussions with the county, state or federal drug chemists and emergency personnel will often pick up new and emerging drugs of abuse early. Monitoring the forensic literature and a forensic toxicologist as a consultant are often necessary to know what new drugs and tests need to be considered.

It can be mutually advantageous to make arrangements, with local emergency departments or clinical laboratories, for a program to collect and hold, blood and urine specimens from major trauma victims, for an agreed-upon period of time.

REFERENCES

1. http://www.usdoj.gov/dea/stats
2. Rice, D.P.: Economic costs of substance abuse, 1995. Institute for Health and Aging, University of California-San Francisco, USA. Proc. Assoc. Am. Physicians, 1999 Mar–Apr: 111(2):119–125, 1999.
3. Fishburn, P. M.: National Survey on Drug Abuse: Main Findings: 1979, Rockville, MD., National Institute of Drug Abuse, 1980 (DHHS Publication #80-[ADM] 976.
4. Baselt, R. C.: *Distribution of toxic drugs and chemicals in man,* 5th Ed. Foster City, CA: Chemical Toxicology Institute.
5. Gifford, H., and Turkel, H. W.: Diffusion of alcohol through stomach wall after death. *JAMA, 161:* 866–868, June 30, 1956.
6. Winek, C. L.: *Forensic sciences.* Editor Cyril Wecht, Mathew Bender. New York, 1984, Vol 2, Chap. 31B.
7. http://www.brewery.org/brewery/library.html#alc.
8. http://www.theraven.com/beer.html
9. Logan, B. K., et.al.: Alcohol content of beer and malt beverages; Forensic considerations. *J Forensic Sci, 44* (6): 1292–1295, 1999.
10. Case, G. A.,Distefano, S., and Logan, B. K.: Tabulation of alcohol content of beer and malt beverages. *J Analytical Toxicology, 24:* 202–210, April 2000.
11. Rice, D. P., et al.: The economic costs of alcohol and drug abuse and mental illness: 1985. San Francisco, U.S. Department of Health and Human Services, 1990.
12. U.S. Department of Justice, Drug Enforcement Administration: The Controlled Substances Act. In *Drugs of abuse,* 1989 Edition. Washington, D.C.: U.S. Government Printing Office, 4–8.
13. Karch, S. B.: *A brief history of cocaine.* Boca Raton, FL: CRC Press, 1998.
14. http://www.samhsa.gov/oas/dawn.
15. Freud, S.: Über Coca, Wein Centralblatt fur die ges Therapie 1884, 2 (translated and reprinted in *Cocaine papers* by Sigmund Freud). New York: Stonehill Publishing Company, 1974.
16. Musto, D. F.: Opium, cocaine and marijuana in American history. *Scientific American, 265* (1): 40–47, 1991.
17. Peterson, R.: History of cocaine. *Cocaine,* 1997: Peterson, R., and Stillman, R. (eds), *National Institute on Drug Abuse Research Monograph 13,* Government Printing Office, 1977, pp. 17–34.
18. Mash, D. C, and Staley, J. K.: D3 dopamine and kappa opioid receptor alterations in human brain of cocaine-overdose victims. *Ann NY Acad Sci, 29* (877): 507–522, June 1999.

19. Karch, S. B.: Cocaine and the heart: Clinical and pathological correlations. *Advances in the Biosciences, 80:* 211–218, 1991.

20. Karch, S. B., Tazelaar, H. D., Billingham, M. E., and Stephens, B. G.: Cocaine associated sudden death syndrome. *Annals of Emergency Medicine,* Abstract *15* (5): 649, 1986.

21. Tazelaar, H.D., Karch, S.B., Stephens, B.G., and Billingham, M.E.: Cocaine and the heart, Human Pathology, 18(2):195-199, 1987.

22. Karch, S. B.: The history of cocaine toxicity. *Human Pathology, 20* (11): 1037–1039, 1989.

23. Sturner, W. Q.: Cocaine babies: The scourge of the 90s. *J Forensic Sci, 36* (1): 34–39, 1991.

24. Behnke, M., et al.: The search for congenital malformations in newborns with fetal cocaine exposure. *Pediatrics, 107* (5)e: 1–6, 2001.

25. Andres, R. L, Day, M. C., and Larrabee, K.: Recent cocaine use is not associated with fetal acidemia or other manifestations of intrapartum fetal distress. *American J Perinatology, 17* (2): 63–67, 2000.

26. Ju-Feng Wang, et al.: Differential patterns of cocaine induced organ toxicity in murine heart versus liver. *Experimental Biology and Medicine, 226:* 52–60, 2001.

27. Raval, M. P., and Wetli, C. V.: Sudden death from cocaine induced excited delirium: An analysis of 45 cases (abstract). *Am J Clinical Path, 104* (3): 329, 1995.

28. Ruttenber, A. J., Lawler-Haevener, J., Wetli, C. V., Hearn, W. L., and Mash, D. C.: Fatal excited delirium following cocaine use: Epidemiologic findings provide evidence for new mechanisms of cocaine toxicity. *J Forensic Toxicology, 42* (1): 25–31, Jan. 1997.

29. Baselt, R. C., Allison, D. J., Wright, J. A., Scannel, J. S., and Stephens, B. G.: Acute heroin fatalities in San Francisco: Demographic and toxicologic characteristics. *Western J Medicine, 122:* 455–458, 1975.

30. Hine, C. H., Wright, J. A., Allison, D. J., Stephens, B. G., and Pasi, A.: Analysis of fatalities from acute narcotism in a major urban area. *J Forensic Sci, 27:* 372–384, 1982.

31. Case records of the Massachusetts General Hospital. *New England J Medicine, 344* (8): 591–599, February 22, 2001, .

32. Mittleman, M. A., et al.: Triggering myocardial infarction by marijuana. *Circulation, 103:* 2805–2809, 2001.

33. Stephens, B. G., Coleman, D. E., and Baselt, R. C.: In vitro stability of endogenous gamma-hydroxybutyrate in postmortem blood. *J Forensic Sci, 44* (1): 231, January 1999.

34. Stephens, B. G., and Baselt, R. C.: Driving under the influence of GHB? *J Analytical Toxicology, 18:* October 1994.

Chapter XXIII

FORENSIC ASPECTS OF ALCOHOL

WERNER U. SPITZ

FROM THE STANDPOINT of the chemist, the word *alcohol* refers to a large group of chemical compounds characterized by the possession of a functional –OH group. In common usage, however, the word alcohol has been accepted as indicating a specific compound, i.e., ethyl alcohol or ethanol, having the molecular formula C_2H_5OH.

For the purpose of this chapter, the word alcohol will be used to designate the compound ethanol, present in various fermented and distilled beverages. The alcohol in such beverages is the result of fermentation of sugar by yeast. Fermentation of barley with added hops results in the production of beers and ales, while fermentation of fruits results in the formation of wines. Fermentation of grains and fruits followed by distillation results in the production of whiskey, gin, brandy and vodka. East European distilleries often use potato for vodka production. The sole purpose of distillation is to increase the concentration of alcohol in the finished product, since fermentation ceases when the alcohol concentration reaches 12% to 14% by volume.

Alcohol is the most common single substance encountered in toxicologic analyses. It is estimated that in the United States, 2/3 of all adults use alcohol occasionally and at least 12% of the users can be considered *heavy* drinkers.[1] The life expectancy of alcoholics is 10–15 years shorter than that of non-alcoholics.

Alcohol is a drug which among other manifestations, causes euphoria, dehydration and vasodilatation, hence red eyes and flushing of the face. At high concentrations, alcohol depresses the central nervous system. Respiration and circulation are predominately affected. Blood pressure falls, pulse rate rises, skin is cool and clammy, all indicative of shock.[2] Alcohol irritates the gastric lining, causing gastritis and triggers mucous secretion as a protective mechanism. Small, superficial, often bleeding gastric ulcers occur occasionally after heavy alcohol consumption. Irritation of the stomach and stimulation of certain areas in the brain contribute to nausea and vomiting. Rapid drinking enhances the irritating effect of alcohol on the gastric lining, while food protects the stomach lining and reduces irritation. At low concentration alcohol stimulates gastric secretions, increasing appetite, hence the effect of the *apéritif* or cocktail before dinner.

Chronic consumption of alcoholic beverages increases tolerance and may cause physical dependence in genetically predisposed individuals. Individual differences exist in the development of physical dependence, i.e., chronic alcoholism. Alcoholism often runs in families. By the same token great individual differences exist in those who ultimately develop liver cirrhosis as opposed to those who consume large quantities of alcohol regularly, but never develop liver complications. A genetic link to the development of cirrhosis is thought to exist.

Fatty infiltration of the liver, where the liver is enlarged, uniformly greasy, yellow and soft occurs in binge drinkers and apparently is caused by the toxic effect of alcohol on liver tissue combined with the metabolic dysfunction which results from substitution of alcohol for an ordinary balanced diet. Fatty infiltration of the liver is reversible by abstinence, however it may progress to cirrhosis if consumption of alcohol continues. Fatty infiltration of the liver is frequently found as the sole manifestation of disease in sudden deaths of alcoholics. Although the exact mechanism of such deaths is unknown, alcoholics with fatty livers occasionally have a history of seizures. Alcoholics in withdrawal, including those with a drop in their blood alcohol level below their habituated threshold, may experience delirium tremens (DTs). DTs constitutes a medical emergency usually beginning 12 to 48 hours after cessation of alcohol intake. Occasionally, tonic-clonic seizures complicate marked delirium with gross auditory and visual hallucinations, disorientation and restlessness, fast pulse and elevated temperature.

From the medicolegal standpoint, there is perhaps no chemical compound more frequently encountered than alcohol as a contributing or causative factor in violent or natural deaths. Studies in typical communities in the United States reveal that alcohol is a contributing or responsible factor in about 50% of violent deaths, and some literature indicates alcohol to be a factor in as many as 90% of motor vehicular crashes.[3,4] Each year, tens of thousands of people lose their lives in the United States in alcohol-related automobile accidents. Alcohol is also involved in many non-fatal incidents that ultimately come under the scrutiny of law enforcement agencies. Because of this ubiquity, it is advantageous to consider the various facts involved in the consumption, absorption, distribution, and elimination of alcohol by the body.

Alcohol almost invariably enters the body by ingestion of an alcoholic beverage. Alcoholic beverages are primarily a mixture of water and alcohol with small amounts of other substances, which impart the characteristic odors and tastes to the various drinks. These substances are referred to as congeners, since they are simultaneously produced during the fermentation process.[5-7] Congeners consist of organic acids and esters and, in the case of wine and brandy, include methyl alcohol. The latter is responsible for trace amounts of wood alcohol in body fluids and tissues of persons who have consumed large quantities of wine or brandy, particularly cheaper brands. Aromatic congeners are sometimes purposely added to some alcoholic beverages of inferior quality to give them an odor which the consumer associates with more expensive brands.

The so-called *odor of alcohol* frequently detected on people after consumption of alcoholic beverages is not due to alcohol, but to byproducts of alcohol manufacture or the aforementioned added congeners. Pure alcohol, i.e., 100%, is odorless. The odor of congeners may persist in tissues for several hours after all alcohol has been eliminated. Hence, the conclusion that alcohol is present based upon odor may be erroneous. Such a conclusion is valid only if founded upon a chemical analysis. We have encountered situations where a strong *odor of alcohol* was detected at autopsy, but laboratory analysis determined a negative blood alcohol concentration.

The concentration of alcohol in fermented beverages is expressed as percent by volume, while the term *proof* is used to express concentration of alcohol in distilled beverages. In the United States the term proof refers to twice the percentage of alcohol by volume. Thus, the common 80 proof whiskey sold in this country contains 40% alcohol by volume.

The alcohol content and caloric value vary in different alcoholic beverages. Most beers are 3-1/2 to 5% and contain an average of 150 calories per 12-ounce bottle or can. Light beers have lower alcohol and caloric values. The average caloric content of light beer is 90 to 120. Wines range from the light German variety at 10% alcohol and 105 calories in five ounces, to the heavier port wines of 20% alcohol and 230 calories. Most hard liquors range from 80 to 100 proof and 100 to 125 calories per 1-1/2 ounces.

Alcohol requires no preliminary digestion and, unlike foods and most drugs, is readily absorbed from the gastrointestinal tract. Almost one quarter of the total absorption occurs from the stomach. The remainder is absorbed by way of the small intestine.

The rate and relative percentage of absorption from the stomach and the intestine are affected by several factors. The amount and kind of food present are of particular significance. A large bolus of food in the stomach would act as a sponge absorbing the alcohol, trapping it for a time, delaying the metabolic process. Thus, consumption of alcohol with a meal follows different criteria than consumption of alcohol alone and *throws off* any rules of thumb usually considered in estimating blood alcohol concentration (BAC).

Alcohol is eliminated as it is absorbed. Slow alcohol absorption, such as occurs when alcoholic beverages are consumed together with a substantial meal, will account for delayed absorption with a 1–2 hour plateau, when the peak blood alcohol concentration remains unchanged, before starting the elimination phase. In such cases not all of the consumed alcohol is absorbed, and the blood alcohol concentration remains lower than expected. Whereas, the exact amount of alcohol lost to absorption is not predictable due to the multitude of intervening factors, a 30 to 60% alcohol absorption deficit, under such circumstances, is not unusual. The bolus of gastric contents traps the imbibed alcohol, releasing it for absorption and elimination at a significantly slower rate.

Carbonated beverages consumed with alcohol enhance absorption while fatty alcoholic beverages, such as kahlúa with cream are absorbed more gradually. Oily and greasy foods coat the gastric lining, and since alcohol is insoluble in fat, are particularly effective in retarding absorption of alcohol from the stomach. The amount, kind and dilution of the alcoholic beverage consumed and individual variations in the permeability of the gastric and intestinal mucosa also play a role.

While it takes only a few minutes for alcohol to pass through the intestinal wall and appear in the blood, complete absorption of alcohol from the gastrointestinal tract requires a time interval varying from 15 to 20 minutes to one hour or longer. The longer the time required for complete absorption, the lower the ultimate peak blood alcohol concentration, since some of the alcohol already in the system will be eliminated during this longer period.

An individual consuming a large number of alcohol-containing drinks over a relatively short period of time will not absorb this amount of liquid in conformity with usually accepted standards. A high concentration of alcohol in the stomach is likely to cause pylorospasm, which delays gastric emptying and alcohol absorption, thus ultimately a lower BAC. For example, someone who drinks six bottles of beer (or the same number of shots) in half an hour will reach full absorption, probably an hour or longer, after he would have, had he consumed half that amount.

Surgical removal of the stomach markedly accelerates the rate of alcohol absorption and many individuals who have undergone gastrectomy complain that they become rapidly intoxicated by amounts of alcohol which would have had little or no effect on them prior to their surgery.[8]

We have observed a case where a middle-aged man, who had a gastrectomy, performed several years earlier, parked his car between two buildings and purchased a six-pack of beer in a liquor store next door. He then consumed the beer in rapid succession sitting in his vehicle. Soon thereafter he started his car, revved the engine and drove straight ahead into the building his car was facing, killing a patron in a pizza restaurant. He blew a .20% on a police Breathalyzer a few minutes after the crash.

The rate of absorption of certain drugs from the stomach is increased by the vasodilator effect of alcohol. Alcohol consumed on an empty stomach may cause hypoglycemia and in susceptible individuals, especially diabetics, and the elderly, may induce confusion, blurred vision, weakness, altered behavior even a reduced state of consciousness, all manifestations also observed in cases of acute alcohol intoxication. Contrary to popular belief diabetes does not alter the blood alcohol concentration.

Since alcohol impairs constriction of blood vessels in the skin; high blood alcohol concentrations may aggravate hemorrhage from relatively minor wounds, increasing chances of hypovolemic shock, even death, as a result of blood loss.

Alcohol is poorly absorbed through intact skin. In years past, alcohol was used as a rubdown to reduce fever. Comparison of blood alcohol concentration using non-alcohol and alcohol-containing skin antiseptics fails to support reports whereby use of alcohol swabbing at the site of venipuncture contaminated the samples.[9] In the case of legal proceedings, however, current recommendations in the literature support a challenge to the reliability of the evidence when a blood sample obtained for the purpose of determination of alcohol content is drawn, following alcohol preparation of the skin.[10,11] Also, consideration must be given to the fact that swabbing of the skin is usually done with rubbing alcohol, i.e., isopropyl alcohol, which does not react chemically in the same way as does ethyl alcohol. On the other hand, a child with first and second-degree burns, scalded over 30% of its body treated with alcohol rubs to reduce fever was found to have a blood alcohol concentration of 0.05%. It may be presumed that alcohol absorption occurred in areas in which the upper layers of the skin had sloughed off.

Inhalation of air containing high concentrations of alcohol in the vapor state does not produce significant blood alcohol levels, even after prolonged exposure.

A truck driver for a distillery was loading 50 gallon barrels containing 80 proof whiskey when one barrel fell and ruptured spilling the contents on him and the ground. Due to severe eye irritation, the man was taken to the hospital. Because of the exposure and suspected absorption by way of the skin and inhalation, blood was drawn, which showed a negative alcohol concentration.

Alcohol is absorbed through the lining of the mouth and throat. High concentrations of alcohol (liquor) are absorbed faster than diluted forms, such as beer and wine, although the amounts absorbed from the mouth are negligible, primarily because of the relatively short duration of contact of the beverage with the oral and pharyngeal mucosa.

Negligible quantities of alcohol are also absorbed from the large bowel. Ingested alcohol is carried from the gastrointestinal tract via the portal vein to the liver. It is for this reason that, during the period of active absorption, the alcohol concentration in the blood of the portal vein exceeds that in the blood elsewhere in the body. Later the portal vein blood alcohol concentration decreases because of loss of alcohol to the liver, metabolism of alcohol by the liver and mixing with blood from the hepatic artery.

Ultimately, the blood containing alcohol reaches the right side of the heart, when it begins its circulation through the body. As the arterial blood passes through the lungs, some alcohol is lost by diffusion into the alveolar air. The concentration of alcohol in the arterial blood further diminishes as the result of passage through the capillary network.

Because alcohol is water soluble, it is lost from the blood to the tissues in proportion to the water content of the tissues with which it comes in contact. Eventually a condition of storage equilibrium is reached between blood and tissues.

However, during the period of rapid absorption, there may be some difference between the concentration of alcohol in the arterial blood and that in the venous blood.

This accounts for the difference sometimes observed in the determination of blood alcohol concentration by analysis of alveolar breath compared with direct analysis of a sample of venous blood. The former result is sometimes higher than the latter, but it more truly represents the concentration of alcohol in the blood reaching the brain and therefore accurately reveals the effect of alcohol upon the individual. The difference in the concentration of alcohol in the arterial and venous systems is at its maximum during the period of active absorption and disappears when a state of equilibrium between blood and tissues has been reached.

During the period of active absorption, the blood alcohol concentration rises quite rapidly and then continues to increase at a slower rate until the maximal concentration is reached. After the maximal blood alcohol concentration has been attained, the alcohol level in the blood decreases at a predictable, linear rate during the postabsorptive period until zero level.

In the postabsorptive phase, alcohol concentration in the different organs reaches equilibrium depending on the content of water versus fat. Alcohol, being water soluble distributes in higher concentration in watery body fluids as opposed to tissues, especially brain, due to its high fatty content. Liver tissue is the exception, in that its alcohol content is lower than that of blood, possibly due to continued alcohol breakdown by liver enzymes after death.

When equilibrium has been reached, the distribution of alcohol in the various tissues and body fluids would be of the order shown in Table XXIII-1.

The major part of alcohol that has been absorbed is eliminated from the body as the result of oxidation in the liver, which contains the enzyme alcohol dehydrogenase. More than 90% of absorbed alcohol is eliminated by this route.

In addition to oxidation, alcohol may be eliminated unchanged in the urine, by way of the kidneys, in the breath by way of the lungs, through

TABLE XXIII-1

RELATIVE CONCENTRATION OF ALCOHOL
AT EQUILIBRIUM

Sample	Relative Concentration
Whole blood	1.00
Plasma or serum	1.12–1.20
Brain	0.85
Spinal fluid	1.10–1.27
Urine (ureteral)	1.3
Alveolar air	1/2100
Liver	0.85

the skin by way of the sweat glands and through the feces by way of the colon. Of these, excretion by way of the feces is relatively insignificant. Normally, excretion by way of perspiration occurs at about one-half the rate of elimination by way of urine, and this is related to the fact that the volume of sweat is approximately one-half the urinary volume. However, in excessively hot climates, or with unusual exertion accompanied by excessive perspiration, the loss of body water by way of the skin may increase five- to tenfold. This would result in a corresponding five- to ten-fold increase in the loss of alcohol by way of the skin.

The concentration of alcohol in urine is unreliable for the purpose of estimating the amount of alcohol in the blood. Urine containing different concentrations of alcohol may be mixed in the bladder with urine devoid of alcohol which has remained in the bladder from before alcohol consumption. Urethral urine, however, i.e., urine obtained by catheterization, is known to have an alcohol content of 1.3 times that of the blood. This ratio is restricted to urine as it is being formed and does not apply to the concentration of alcohol in bladder urine.

A urine alcohol concentration that is significantly higher than that of the blood indicates that the blood alcohol concentration had been higher earlier. For example, an individual who was injured and died two hours later is likely to have a postmortem urine alcohol concentration of at least .03 to .04% higher than the level of alcohol in his blood. Obviously, during the two-hour interval some of the blood alcohol will have been metabolized. In the case of hospital admis-

sion, consideration must also be given to an artificially low blood alcohol concentration as a result of IV fluid administration, causing dilution. Due to the body's systems regulating fluid equilibrium, administration of IV fluids markedly increases urinary output carrying alcohol with it. Depending on the amounts of fluid given, the blood alcohol concentration may be reduced by as much as 50%.

The loss of alcohol by way of breath occurs at a rate approximately equal to that of urinary loss. The concentration of alcohol in alveolar breath is less than that in the blood. In accordance with Henry's law, alcohol distributes between pulmonary blood and alveolar air in a ratio of 2100 to 1. In other words, 2100 mL of alveolar air contain the same weight of alcohol as 1 mL of blood.

The question is frequently raised as to the existence of a normal alcohol content, i.e., endogenous alcohol, in human tissues and blood. The general consensus is that the normal concentration of alcohol does not exceed trace amounts.

Primary factors involved in the interpretation of postmortem results are the method of collection, preservation of the specimen and choice of sample for analysis.

In most jurisdictions, blood is the sample of choice for analysis. However, it is necessary to observe certain precautions when blood samples are collected. A blood sample should not be taken through an intact chest wall. If an autopsy has not been performed, a sample is sometimes obtained by blind puncture through the chest wall, with the needle ideally entering the heart. This method was being used frequently until it was found that erroneous results of the blood alcohol concentration occur when this procedure is used. The esophagus is situated directly behind the heart and with the relaxation of the cardiac sphincter after death, gastric contents are likely to run-up along the esophagus, contaminating the sample if the esophagus was nicked by the needle. In an average weight individual the 13 gauge, 3-1/2 inch-long autopsy needle is long enough to pass through the heart into the esophagus.

Another possible source of contamination is internal injury with rupture of the stomach and diaphragm, resulting in the presence of gastric and possibly duodenal contents in the chest cavities. If the stomach or duodenum contains alcohol, an erroneously high blood alcohol level will result. We have analyzed a blood sample, collected in the above-described way, that contained in excess of one percent ethyl alcohol. Also, pleural contents will be contaminated with aspirated gastric contents when lung tissue or bronchial branches are torn. Further, some alcohol containing stomach contents may diffuse into the interior of the heart, contaminating a blood sample, even if properly taken at autopsy.

To avoid any possibility of a subsequent argument being raised that a sample may have been contaminated, it is advisable that blood in all cases be obtained from a location removed from a potential source of contamination. The large vessels of the groin and the clavicular area best serve this purpose.

Vitreous humor may be used as an alternative to blood, when blood is unobtainable. However, vitreous alcohol concentration (VAC) lags approximately one to two hours behind the blood. Vitreous alcohol concentration (VAC) is approximately equal to that of serum less one or two hours of lag time. Consequently, vitreous alcohol concentration will vary during and following the period of alcohol consumption. In order to enable the use of VAC to estimate the BAC, it is imperative that the pattern of alcohol consumption be known. If BAC is greater than VAC, death has occurred prior to equilibrium, i.e., alcohol has not yet reached full potential in the vitreous. Theoretically, vitreous alcohol may be positive while the BAC has returned to zero.

Cerebral spinal fluid, sometimes used for analysis is equally less than optimal, since in the case of a basilar skull fracture through the sella, the CSF may be contaminated with gastric contents due to the fact that a fractured sella provides direct access to the roof of the mouth.

By the same token, it is unwise that blood which has pooled in the chest or abdomen during an autopsy be scooped up for alcohol analysis. Such practice can only give rise to a contaminated sample with an erroneous blood alcohol concentration.

However, in spite of the above caveats logic must prevail. Thus, witnessed circumstances of an event should outweigh the argument that a blood specimen is invalid solely because it was improperly collected. A urine and/or vitreous alcohol concentration, in such a case, may bolster the propriety of the blood sample.

The blood sample should be collected into a clean receptacle using a clean, dry syringe and needle. None of these items need be sterile if the sample is to be analyzed without delay.

Samples, especially blood, that are not to be analyzed immediately should be preserved by the addition of approximately five mg of sodium fluoride per mL, followed by gentle mixing without shaking. This will prevent loss or production of alcohol due to bacterial action. Samples that have been preserved in this manner will maintain their alcohol content for several weeks, even at room temperature. Refrigeration or freezing coupled with fluoride treatment will maintain the alcohol content of a sample almost indefinitely.

When blood is obtained from the heart at autopsy, it is advisable to ensure thorough mixing of the blood contained within the chambers. This is to avoid obtaining a sample with either a high or low hematocrit, which could lead to a slightly higher or lower alcohol result. Such a result would be caused by the fact that serum or plasma alcohol concentration is 12 to 20% higher than that of whole blood.

Confusion sometimes exists with regard to what specimens were analyzed in a particular case, *was the analysis performed on whole blood or on plasma or serum?* DUIL laws are based on whole blood analysis.

Hospital laboratories usually use plasma for their analyses of blood alcohol concentration. Such results will be higher than if whole blood was used. In cases where the plasma alcohol concentration mildly exceeds the level set by statute as prima facie evidence of drunken driving, such excess may make the difference between conviction and dismissal of charges.

Hospitals usually report results in mg%, thus, 100 mg per 100 mL, as opposed to results expressed as gram %, i.e., 0.10% as defined by statute. These results are synonymous. Since there are 1000 milligrams in a gram, conversion is by dividing the milligram or multiplying the gram result by 1000.

Additionally, some hospitals report the results of blood alcohol analysis in millimole (mM) instead of more conventional grams or milligram. To convert mM to milligram (mg) the following formula is applicable: mM x 4.61 = mg %

Breathalyzers are designed to measure the level of alcohol as would be found in whole blood.

Since the analysis of blood is carried out in order to obtain information concerning the concentration of alcohol in the brain, it would seem that a direct analysis of brain tissue may be more reliable. As a matter of fact, in cases where the skull is not injured, analysis of such tissue is acceptable, especially since there is less chance for contamination of the brain in the course of performing an autopsy. It is not necessary to preserve the entire brain for this purpose, since samples of tissue taken from different parts of the brain do not vary significantly in their alcohol content. When brain tissue is not available, skeletal muscle is preferable to liver, kidney or spleen. The drawback of any tissue analysis is the generally greater familiarity with the interpretation of blood/breathalyzer data. Thus, blood and breathalyzer analyses are still, the most practical, fast and easy test methods to perform in all cases where blood is available or the individual is alive.

Embalming of a body does not alter the alcohol content in the tissues, provided the fluids that are used contain no ethyl alcohol. In the United States, methanol, i.e., methyl alcohol or wood alcohol, has largely replaced ethyl alcohol in embalming solutions. The presence of methanol does not interfere with ethyl alcohol analysis. The high cost of ethyl alcohol and the fact that the laws of many states now prohibit the use of ethyl alcohol for the purpose of embalming have practically eliminated ethyl alcohol from embalming practices in this country. Nevertheless, a few foreign countries, including the U.K., still use ethyl alcohol for embalming because it is odorless and preserves the natural color of the skin.

When putrefaction has occurred, caution must be exercised in interpreting blood or tissue alcohol levels. This is due to the fact that alcohol may be lost or produced by bacterial action during the putrefactive process. Production of alcohol is by far the more serious problem, since it may lead to the conclusion that alcohol consumption was a factor in causing the death. It is, nevertheless, advantageous to do an alcohol analysis on such samples, despite the fact that it may not accurately reflect the state of intoxication of the deceased at the time of death. Also, variability of postmortem alcohol production must be considered.[12] Alcohol concentrations in skeletal muscle in excess of 0.20% and liver tissue concentrations that are three to four times as high, in a body in a state of advanced decomposition with purging of putrid fluids, bloating and discoloration and markedly foul odor indicates alcohol consumption prior to death, while levels below 0.20% may be due to possible putrefactive alcohol production. Ordinarily, in cases with mild to moderate decomposition, postmortem alcohol production in muscle does not exceed 0.10%.

The eye is relatively sheltered from bacterial contamination, thus in cases of advanced putrefaction, analysis of the vitreous humor has been found to be advantageous. Felby and Olsen[13] have shown that the alcohol concentration in vitreous humor, unlike that of blood, remains constant for a considerable length of time, and Coe and Sherman[14] report that the ratio of blood alcohol concentration to that of vitreous humor is 0.89 ± 0.02. In our experience, when putrefaction has proceeded to the stage of purging and bloating, the chances of finding vitreous humor are poor. More likely the eye has collapsed and vitreous humor has escaped. The same is true of urine and the urinary bladder.

In submerged bodies where putrefaction has progressed to the *floater stage,* alcohol produced by decomposition often reaches a level comparable to that of intoxication, even levels of 0.20 or above are not infrequent.

A hematoma found during the autopsy of a person injured shortly before death often lends itself to the determination of alcohol and drugs, and may indicate the degree of intoxication at the time the blood was shed, i.e., the time of injury. While some of these compounds in the hematoma may be lost by diffusion into surrounding tissues and the circulating blood and lymph, their concentration in the blood at the time of injury may still be approximated. Of course, this assumes an uncontaminated hematoma. With regards to subdural hematomas, it is important to recognize that brain swelling starts practically immediately following head injury. Consequently, subdural bleeding can be delayed, if the injury is severe enough to cause obliteration of the subdural space. Otherwise, alcohol or drugs will be present in a subdural hematoma, in the same way as they would in a hematoma anywhere else in the body. In fact, we have found alcohol present in subdural blood clots as long as eight days following injury.[15]

A young woman was admitted comatose to the hospital minutes after she was struck by an automobile. She had been to a bar where she consumed alcohol over a number of hours. Blood drawn on admission to the hospital indicated an alcohol concentration of 0.12%. Diagnosis was made of skull fracture and brain injury. She was treated conservatively for brain swelling until mild improvement in her condition was noted 11 hours following injury when brain swelling began to subside. Subdural bleeding which did not occur initially due to brain swelling, now began to develop, causing her condition to deteriorate gradually until she expired 21 hours after admission. Postmortem tests for alcohol in the peripheral and subdural blood were now negative.

It is evident from the toxicological results that the subdural bleeding was delayed until brain swelling was reduced, as suggested by her improved clinical condition 11 hours after injury. During this period, alcohol in the peripheral blood was metabolized, resulting in a subdural clot devoid of alcohol.

Brain swelling develops very rapidly in cases of severe brain injury, obliterating the subdural space and preventing subdural bleeding from occurring. In cases where brain injury is less severe, brain swelling is likely to be delayed, allowing for early subdural bleeding.

In older people with some degree of brain shrinkage, the subdural space is large and subdural hemorrhage occurs readily following relatively minor head trauma. In such people, brain swelling is unlikely to obliterate the subdural space allowing hemorrhage to accumulate early on with an alcohol concentration which reflects that of the peripheral blood at the time of injury. In case of survival some of the alcohol in the subdural clot will diffuse out into surrounding tissues, but a significant amount of alcohol is likely to be retained for several days. In such cases both subdural and peripheral blood should be submitted for toxicological analysis.

The most commonly utilized method by which alcohol is determined in body fluids and tissues is gas chromatography. Gas chromatography is specific, reasonably fast and inexpensive. It permits simultaneous detection and quantitation of commonly encountered interfering alcohols–methyl and isopropyl alcohol. The technique involves analysis of the head space (vapor phase) of an equilibrated blood sample and is adaptable to automation. This is most useful in situations where large numbers of samples are analyzed routinely.

The relationship of various blood alcohol concentrations to clinical signs and symptoms is shown in Table XXIII-2. It is critical, however, that certain facts be recognized in order to interpret this table properly. Among these, diabetic coma, certain drug intoxications, incipient stroke and head injuries are some examples of conditions which may mimic alcoholic intoxication. Also, in interpreting this chart it must be understood that the blood alcohol concentration shown on the left is represented by a range, where some people fall at the lower end, others at the upper.

Considerable individual variability exists to the effect of alcohol. Most people are aware of the fact that long-term use results in a greater capacity to metabolize alcohol, but Perper et al.[16] have shown that alcoholics not only develop an increased tolerance but often are functional at blood alcohol concentrations generally considered to be potentially fatal. Clinical experience, they write, contradicts the generally accepted dogma whereby, *regardless of the degree of tolerance, blood alcohol levels above 0.4% (400 mg per 100 mL) produce stupor and/or coma.* In fact, it has been found that high blood alcohol concentrations do not necessarily result in observable clinical manifestations of drunkenness in all cases. While an individual with a blood alcohol concentration of 0.08–0.10% (depending on jurisdiction) is unable to operate an automobile as required by law and

TABLE XXIII-2

PHYSIOLOGICAL EFFECTS OF ALCOHOL**

Blood Alcohol Concentration	Effects
0.00–0.04%	No significant effect to mild euphoria.
0.05–0.09%	Decreased inhibitions, increased self-confidence, decreased attention span, alteration of judgment, especially as related to time and distance.
0.10–0.14%	Singing ladies' man, happy. Some mental confusion, emotional instability, loss of critical judgment, memory impairment, sleepiness, slowed reaction time.
0.15–0.29%	Loss of muscular coordination, staggering gait, marked mental confusion, exaggeration of emotions, dizziness, decreased pain response, disorientation and thickened speech.
0.30–0.39%	Stupor, marked incoordination, marked decrease in response to stimuli, possibly coma.
0.4% and above	Anesthesia, depression of responses, deep coma, death.

** Individuals with blood alcohol concentrations below .05 have shown behavioral changes under laboratory conditions.

in accordance with road conditions, he or she may exhibit no overt evidence of intoxication and the term *visible intoxication,* as defined by dram shop statutes is in no way synonymous with *driving while under the influence of intoxicating liquor laws.*

Review of the literature on the subject of apparent sobriety in highly intoxicated people indicates publications both preceding and subsequent to Perper's article. Newman[17] quotes Jetter[18] to say that while 10.5% of examined cases were diagnosed as drunk with a BAC of 50 mg% (0.05%), 6.7% of those studied with blood alcohol concentrations of 400 mg% (0.40%) were considered sober. Paredes, et al.[19] and Lindblad[20] published similar results and Urso, et al.[21] found that some alcohol users appeared sober with a BAC as high as 0.29%.

Studies conducted to measure the effect of alcohol on individuals' behavior, in laboratory settings, indicate some degree of impairment with any departure from zero BAC. At a BAC of 0.05%, which for an individual of average weight follows consumption of three beers or the equiv-

alent of liquor within the hour, perception will be dulled and reaction time extended. Mental acuity, i.e., alertness, will be reduced. These factors coupled with a sudden emergency while driving or the added hazard of reduced lighting, as occurs at dusk, may create circumstances ideal for an accident. Reason dictates and the law supports that in a case of sudden emergency avoiding impending danger *"is best by reacting without time to consider."* Since low levels of alcohol will extend the relationship between perception and reaction time, if only by a small duration, even a low level of alcohol plays a significant role. None of the studies on low levels of alcohol drew any meaningful conclusions regarding *visible intoxication.*

Laws regarding alcohol intoxication vary worldwide. While most states in the U.S. have laws adopting a blood alcohol concentration of 0.10% as prima facie evidence of drunken driving, 18 states and the District of Columbia have imposed a level of 0.08%. Britain and Canada have adopted the same level. The U.S. House and Senate have agreed to require states to adopt the lower rate of 0.08% nationwide by 2004. States which do not abide by the new regulation will face losing federal highway funds. In the Scandinavian countries the level is 0.05%, and in Austria 0.04%. In the Czech Republic, Poland and other East European countries, it is a criminal offense to drive a motor vehicle with a blood alcohol level of 0.03%.

While the standard of 0.08% is being established for all motor vehicles, the literature is clear and unanimous regarding impairment of motorcyclists at blood alcohol concentrations as low as 0.038%,[22] and understandably so, in view of the added element of the need to maintain balance for a rider of a two-wheel vehicle. Statistical review has shown that accidents involving motorcycles occur at a substantially lower BAC than those involving cars.

Misjudgment of distances and speed occur at relatively low blood alcohol concentrations. Estimation of the speed at which we drive depends on how fast we pass stationary objects along the road, such as utility poles, trees, etc. Estimation of distances is best illustrated by the fact that an object believed to be 200 feet away, may in reality only be 20 feet away.

> Two people in a car stopped at a railroad crossing. Witnesses stated they both looked to the right and to the left, before proceeding to cross the tracks. A train 30 feet away struck their car at low speed and both men were killed. At autopsy, both had blood alcohol concentrations in excess of 0.20%.

A motor vehicle is a complicated piece of machinery, the handling of which requires skill, dexterity and mental acuity, all of which will be reduced, even eliminated by alcohol. Thus, an individual may be intoxicated to the point of being unable to operate an automobile safely, while appearing sober. Visible intoxication usually involves reduced coarse motor coordination at higher blood alcohol concentrations. Diminished fine motor coordination at levels as low as 0.05% is likely to interfere with the ability to drive.

Alcohol speeds fatigue and impairs judgment. Of course, judgment about fatigue is also impaired. Thus, drinking drivers are likely to draw the wrong conclusion about their state of intoxication and their ability to drive safely.

A point often overlooked is analysis of an individual's handwriting to establish coordination and state of sobriety. Alcohol affects motor coordination relatively early. Fine coordination is affected first. Thus, the signature on a credit receipt may be atypical, scrawled, illegible, crooked, slanted, or incomplete. Course coordination, such as exhibited by walking or picking up small objects is affected at higher blood alcohol concentrations.

In most medicolegal situations involving death, the important point at issue is the condition of the individual at the time of injury. If death was instantaneous, a postmortem blood alcohol determination will reflect the individual's state of intoxication at such time. It is generally difficult and usually unreliable to estimate a blood alcohol concentration of a person who had been drinking, from witness accounts of behavior and appearance of such an individual. No significant change in blood alcohol concentration occurs after death, until putrefaction begins. However, should some time elapse between injury and

death, the postmortem blood alcohol concentration would not necessarily reflect the condition of the individual at the time of injury. It is generally agreed that the concentration of alcohol decreases by 0.015–0.02% per hour, although it has been our experience that the rate of metabolism may be significantly higher in a large number of individuals. This is particularly true of heavy drinkers and chronic alcoholics who may eliminate alcohol from their system as much as twice as fast. The accelerated alcohol breakdown in alcoholics compensates for the loss of liver tissue in cases of cirrhosis, to the point where the rate of metabolism of alcohol in people with and without cirrhosis remains more or less unchanged.

If one can establish that a given individual was in the post-absorptive state at the time of sustaining a fatal injury, one can, based upon the above factors, estimate the probable range of alcohol concentration at the time of injury. Such estimation would be based upon the postmortem blood alcohol concentration and the time interval between injury and death.

A 24-year-old man, known to be a *social drinker,* is drinking at a neighborhood bar until closing time, at 2:00 a.m. At 5:30 a.m., he is arrested by the police as a suspect in a hit-and-run accident, which occurred at 2:30 a.m. He denies consumption of alcohol after the accident. A breathalyzer test at 6:30 a.m. indicates a blood alcohol concentration of 0.08%. Of course, the question of *driving under the influence of intoxicating liquor* is very pertinent.

Four-and-a-half hours elapsed from the time the young man left the bar until the breathalyzer test was given. During this interval, he is likely to have burned off 0.06–0.09%. Therefore, the blood alcohol concentration at the time of the collision was probably between 0.14 and 0.17%. A BAC of 0.10% currently constitutes *prima facie* evidence of drunken driving in most states.

However, should there be information indicating that alcohol consumption had occurred within the hour preceding the incident, there would remain the possibility of continued absorption of alcohol from the gastrointestinal tract after the accident. One could not, therefore, be certain when the maximal blood alcohol concentration may have been reached in relationship to the time of injury. Hence, under these circumstances, any back calculation from a given postmortem blood alcohol concentration would be speculative, subject to doubt.

In the case of an intoxicated traffic accident victim, who was injured and taken to an emergency room, consideration must be given to the quantity of intravenous fluids which may have been administered both at the hospital and during transport to the hospital. Such therapy, including blood transfusions, accounts for hemodilution and may significantly reduce the blood alcohol concentration. A 30 to 40% drop of the blood alcohol concentration have been observed under these circumstances.

Drowning in fresh water also causes hemodilution, thus reduces the blood alcohol concentration. Dilution of the blood is associated with hemolysis and electrolyte imbalance.

Innovative ideas regarding physiologic causes for an artificially high or low blood alcohol concentration are sometimes advanced by *experts* in an attempt to cast doubt on existing data. Thus, we have recently come across suggestions that menstruation may have been responsible for a drop of the BAC, and that blood loss, hypovolemic shock and dehydration were implicated in causing a false BAC in a case of a severed Achilles tendon by a shard of broken glass as a result of a fall.

The average menstrual blood loss is 60–120 mL which is an insufficient amount to cause significant blood alcohol changes. With regard to the severed Achilles tendon, the tendon is avascular and the area lacks major blood vessels to account for major bleeding. Further, loss of even large amounts of blood is not likely to change the BAC, and certainly not in the acute state, as whole blood is lost, i.e., plasma and cells, and the blood specimen which is tested expresses the BAC in percent. Of course, the situation changes once fluids are administered and dilution of the blood stream occurs.

Death due to acute alcoholic intoxication with blood alcohol concentrations below 0.40% may occur in individuals with chronic debilitating diseases, such as arteriosclerotic heart disease, chronic obstructive pulmonary disease and severe anemia. Other chronic lung diseases and conditions associated with varying degrees of hypoxia may also contribute to death in the presence of relatively low levels of alcohol. We have found that a blood alcohol concentration of 0.30% may be a contributing cause of death, especially in the elderly and individuals with chronic debilitating diseases. Prolonged coma due to acute alcoholic intoxication sometimes leads to irreversible hypoxic brain damage, which in turn may cause death. Deaths following alcoholic intoxication in cold climates, also referred to as *deaths due to exposure or hypothermia,* fall into this category. The blood alcohol level in such cases is commonly low, as would be expected after a prolonged period of coma before failure of body temperature regulatory mechanisms.

In such cases, one can frequently obtain additional information concerning the degree of intoxication at some time prior to death by analyzing both blood and urine obtained at autopsy. The urinary bladder is likely to be overly full as a result of prolonged unconsciousness, 600 mL and more is not unusual in such situations. A urine alcohol level that is significantly higher than that in the blood indicates that the blood alcohol concentration had been higher earlier.

A fact that may further complicate interpretation of alcohol findings is the simultaneous presence of another drug. Statistical review of deceased drivers found drugs in a relatively small number of instances and in low concentrations. The effect of alcohol vastly predominates.[23] Most depressants and sedative drugs will, at the very least, have an additive effect. Psychotropic drugs enhance the effect of alcohol. Perhaps the most common group of drugs in the latter category would be marijuana, cocaine and heroin. Among other drugs that are dangerous in combination with alcohol are tranquilizers, antihistamines and hypnotics. With regards to marijuana, when taken in sufficient quantity, the altered perception of time, where time seems to pass more slowly, disorientation, reduced motor coordination and cognitive ability, combines with known manifestations of alcoholic intoxication enhancing the effect of both. Further, a recent article by Bachs and Morland[24] discusses possible marijuana-related deaths caused by acute exacerbation of pre-existing cardiovascular conditions. Cannabis increases the heart rate causing greater myocardial oxygen demand. This poses a potential threat particularly to middle-aged and older individuals with coronary artery disease. The effect would be enhanced by alcohol.

Cocaine when mixed with alcohol forms cocaethylene which prolongs the effect of cocaine due to its longer half-life time.

The depressant effect of heroin and related opioids is prolonged and enhanced by alcohol and other depressants, painkillers and sedatives.

Several conditions may mimic the effect of alcohol. To name just a few, certain disorders of the central nervous system such as, an incipient stroke or a concussive head injury, with or without loss of consciousness, where balance may be lost and gait may be unsteady, speech may be slurred, double vision and dizziness may occur, hypoglycemia in a diabetic with similar manifestations, carbon monoxide and certain acute drug intoxications, specifically methamphetamine and more infrequently attention deficit disorder, with symptoms of motor incoordination and clumsiness, emotional instability and aggressiveness, may all simulate acute alcohol intoxication. An uninitiated observer may not necessarily perceive the difference between alcohol intoxication and such other conditions.

REFERENCES

1. Gilman, A., and Goodman L.: *The pharmacological basis of therapeutics,* 8th Ed. New York: Pergamon Press, 1990, p. 538.
2. *Medicolegal aspects of alcohol determination in biological specimens,* Edited by James C. Garriott, Lawyers & Judges Publishing Co., 1993, p. 37.
3. Council on Scientific Affairs: Alcohol and the Driver. *JAMA, 255* (4): 522–527, 1986.
4. Chapman, B.: Pathologists say alcohol factor greater than suspected in motor vehicle accidents. *Pathologist,* March, pp. 21–24, 1985.
5. Bonte, W., and Kuhnholz, B.: Zur Stabilitat des Begleitstoffgehalts alkoholischer Getranke. *Beitrage zur Gerichtlichen Medizin, 42:* 395–401, 1984.
6. Urban, R., Liebhardt, E., and Spann, W.: Vergleichende Untersuchungen der Konzentrationen an Begleitstoffen alkoholischer Getranke im Magen, Blut und Urin. *Beitrage zur Gerichtlichen Medizin, 41:* 223–227, 1983.
7. Bonte, W., and Russmeyer P.: Zur Frage der Normalverteilung von Begleitstoffen in alkoholischen Getranken. *Beitrage zur Gerichtlichen Medizin, 42:* 387–394, 1984.
8. Muehlberger (1958): In Goodman and Gilman's, *The pharmacological basis of therapeutics,* 6th Ed. New York: Macmillan, 1980, p. 382.
9. Goldfinger, T.: A comparison of blood alcohol concentration using non-alcohol and alcohol containing skin antiseptics. *Annals Emerg Med, 11* (12): 665–667, 1982.
10. George, J. E.: Medicolegal problems of emergency medicine. In Schwartz, G. R., Safar, P., Stone, J. H., et al. (Eds.): *Principles and practice of emergency medicine.* Philadelphia: Sanders, 1978, pp. 1495–1505.
11. Muller, F., and Hundt, H.: Ethyl alcohol: Contamination of blood specimens. *S Afr Med J, 50:* 91, 1976.
12. Zumwalt, R. E., Bost, R. O., and Sunshine, I.: Evaluation of ethanol concentrations in decomposed bodies. *J Forensic Sci, 27* (3): 549–554, 1982.
13. Felby, S., and Olson, J.: Comparative studies of postmortem ethyl alcohol in vitreous humor, blood and muscle. *J Forensic Sci, 14:* 93, 1969.
14. Coe, J. I., and Sherman, R. E.: Comparative study of postmortem vitreous humor and blood alcohol. *J Forensic Sci, 15:* 185, 1970.
15. Cassin, B. J., and Spitz, W. U.: Concentration of alcohol in delayed subdural hematoma. *J Forensic Sci, 28* (4): 1013–1015, 1983.
16. Perper, J. A., Twerski, A., and Wienand, J. W.: Tolerance at high blood alcohol concentrations: A study of 110 cases and review of the literature. *J Forensic Sci, 31* (1): 212–221, 1986.
17. Newman, H.W.: Individual variation in tolerance to alcohol. *Quart J Stud Alcohol, 2:* 453–463, 1941.
18. Jetter, W. W.: Chemical and clinical diagnosis of acute alcoholism. *New Eng J Med, 221:* 1019, 1939.
19. Paredes, A., Hood, W. R., and Seymour, H.: Sobriety as a symptom of alcohol intoxication: A clinical commentary on intoxication and drunkenness. *British Journal of Addiction, 31* (1): 233–243, 1975.
20. Lindblad, B., and Olsson, R.: Unusually high levels of blood alcohol. *J Am Med Assoc, 236:* 1600–1602, 1976.
21. Urso, T., Gavaler, J. S., and Van Thiel, D. H.: Blood ethanol levels in sober alcohol users seen in an emergency room. *Life Sciences, 28:* 1053–1056, 1981.
22. Robinson, A., Ketchum, C. H., Colburn, N., and Meyer, R.: Effect of ethyl alcohol on reaction times as measured on a motorcycle simulator. (Abst) *Clin Chem, 36:* 1170, 1990.
23. Owens, S. M., McBay, A. J., and Cook, C. E.: The use of marihuana, ethanol, and other drugs among drivers killed in single-vehicle crashes. *J Forensic Sci, 28* (2): 372–379, 1983.
24. Bachs, L., and Morland, H.: Acute cardiovascular fatalities following cannabis use. *Forensic Sci Int, 124* (2–3): 200–203, December 27, 2001.

Chapter XXIV

THE MEDICOLEGAL AUTOPSY REPORT

Werner U. Spitz

Like other medical specialties, forensic pathology has evolved into a complex field requiring not only significant textbook knowledge, but also expertise from training and daily experience. However, most medicolegal autopsies in the United States are performed by hospital pathologists with little or no medicolegal training or experience. Consequently, considerable disparity exists in the quality of these autopsies and in the documentation of postmortem findings.

Several medicolegal textbooks have been published in the United States over the years, but the space devoted to autopsy techniques and to formulation and preparation of a medicolegal autopsy report is woefully inadequate. Autopsy reports are often impressive by their length and detail, but lack the information required to enable a meaningful conclusion. A medicolegal autopsy differs from a hospital autopsy in both objective and significance. Whereas, a hospital autopsy is conducted pursuant to the wishes of the next-of-kin, an autopsy conducted by a medicolegal investigative system is pursuant to statute. Contrary to popular belief, the purpose of a medicolegal autopsy is not limited to establishing the cause of death. In fact, in a large number of cases the cause of death is already evident at the scene, and the junior police investigator has a fair idea of what it is. The *manner* and *mechanism* of death are usually not so obvious. Furthermore, a medicolegal autopsy places special emphasis on identification of the deceased, the time of death, proper handling of evidence and the recognition of any injuries or pathological conditions that may be relevant to the judicial handling of the case.

All pertinent findings have to be properly recorded and adequately described to facilitate retrieval when necessary, because legal implications of a death may arise soon after the autopsy, months, or even years later. It is, therefore, imperative that certain specific and basic information be included in every autopsy report. A case that appears to be straightforward at the time of the postmortem examination may subsequently become complicated by numerous unforeseen issues.

The basic medicolegal autopsy report, like a standard hospital autopsy report or any other medical evaluation or opinion, corresponds in essence to an established format. Yet, certain differences exist, depending upon the type of case. The following provides suggestions on how to arrange and formulate a medicolegal autopsy report. Directions are given to discern which findings need specific mention because of their presence and which are significant because of their absence. Emphasis is placed on formulation of an opinion as to cause, manner and mechanism of death. Finally, brief mention is made of special autopsy techniques to complement those in Chapter XXV. These added procedures are considered fundamental in establishing certain findings that might otherwise be overlooked.

PRELIMINARY INVESTIGATION

The individual who is charged with determining the cause and manner of death, in cases that require official investigation, must be furnished with a detailed account of the circumstances surrounding the death and of the scene where the body was found. This is usually obtained from the police. It must be understood, however, that police interest in a case usually prevails only for as long as the question of prosecution remains undecided. Once the decision is made that no criminal charges will be filed, police interest in a case rapidly wanes. This deficiency must be promptly corrected. Whereas, it would be advantageous if the medical examiner, and preferably the pathologist who will conduct the postmortem examination, were to examine every scene of death, this is neither practical nor is it essential in all cases. A phone call by him or a trained investigator to elicit pertinent information is often all that is required.

For example, in the case of an apparent nonviolent death or a suspected drug overdose, inquiry should be made into the medical background of the deceased, including old or recent surgery, recent state of mind, previous suicide attempts, alcohol consumption habits, drugs to which the individual may have had access, etc. Such information, often obtained from family physicians, hospitals, relatives, neighbors and friends, frequently eliminates unnecessary autopsies and the need for a costly, open-ended search for drugs by the toxicologist.

An individual found dead in the garage of his home may have died of carbon monoxide toxicity as a result of being overcome by exhaust fumes of the automobile he was trying to repair. In this case, the manner of death is accidental. Sometimes, however, a hose is found connected to the vehicle's exhaust pipe, leading to the interior of the car, or all openings around the doors and windows of the garage are carefully sealed with tape to prevent leakage of fumes; both are indications of a suicidal manner of death. Less than 1/4 of all suicide victims leave a note to indicate their motivations, frustrations or reasons. Of course, death may also be due to natural causes such as a heart attack or stoke. Questions as to whether the garage door was open or shut, whether the door was operated manually or electrically, evidence of work being done on the car, keys in the ignition, ignition turned on or off, amount of fuel in the gas tank and location and position of the body in relation to the automobile and the muffler should all be answered prior to autopsy. The deceased's state of health, including a history of alcohol and drug abuse, is also important.

In a traffic collision, information regarding whether the deceased was a pedestrian, driver or passenger and the year, make and model of vehicles involved in the crash are essential. Was the deceased riding a bicycle or motorcycle, snowmobile, or other type of vehicle? A sketch placing all involved parties and objects and indicating directions of travel is helpful in explaining the mechanism of certain injuries. Such a sketch also serves to corroborate anatomical findings in the victims with observations made at the scene.

Homicide scenes are frequently very informative where the medical examiner is concerned. Estimation of the time of death, using rigor, livor and temperature, is considerably more meaningful if done on location before the body is handled. Correlation of patterned injuries and other manifestations of trauma on the body surface with evidence at the scene can often be done only by viewing the place where the body was found. On the other hand, in a witnessed incident such as a barroom shooting or a family dispute, the medical examiner's presence at the scene will contribute little to the police investigation unless specific questions need to be answered.

EXTERNAL EXAMINATION

Clothing

The external examination of a body, i.e., the body surface, including the clothing, is probably the most important item in a medicolegal postmortem examination. The manner and mechanism of the death are frequently answered by this phase of the examination alone. The external examination should begin with front and back view photographs of the body in the condition in which it was received. This is followed by close-up photographs of relevant particulars. Next is a description of the clothes, with particular attention to the outer garments. In most instances of death from seemingly natural causes, a cursory statement relative to the clothes will usually suffice, but where death is caused by violence, or if foul play is suspected, meticulous examination of the clothes must be undertaken. The value of a detailed examination of the clothes sometimes exceeds that of the autopsy. For example, in an automobile collision, a minute fragment of lacquer discovered in the clothing of a hit-and-run victim may shed light on the color, make, model and year of the car involved. Tire marks imprinted on the clothing may assist the police in identifying the offending vehicle and enlighten the pathologist regarding certain findings subsequently found at autopsy (Fig. XXIV-1). In a shooting death, the frayed fibers of a coat may indicate the direction of a shot, and soot or gunpowder deposits on a garment may indicate the distance from which a weapon was fired. The pungent or fruity odor of an accelerant on the unburnt remnants of clothes of a fire victim may suggest arson. The presence of the accelerator or brake pedal imprint, on the sole of a driver's shoe, is significant in any investigation, indicating the possible motive of the crash (Fig. XXIV-2). All pockets should be checked and contents inventoried. Tears and cuts and areas of soiling, such as road dust on a particular area of the clothes, blood smears or drops, drag marks, etc. should be recorded and photographed, if possible (Fig. XXIV-3).

Clothes that are believed to be of subsequent evidentiary significance should be removed from the body with care and as little mutilation as possible. Such clothes should not be cut, except if unavoidable. Cuts are made through undamaged parts of the garments and a notation to this effect is made in the file. After the body is undressed, the clothes are handed to the police for further and more detailed examination at the crime laboratory.

Preservation of trace evidence on clothing is best accomplished by undressing the body on a clean white cotton sheet on the floor. After the nude body is placed back on the tray or autopsy table, a pouch is made of the sheet by knotting its four corners. Now the sheet with its contents is tagged for identification and handed to the police. Wet clothes, such as from a drowning vic-

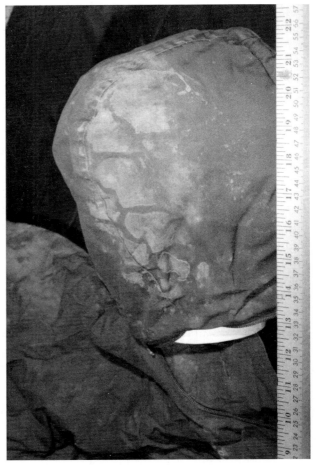

FIGURE XXIV-1. Bus tire marks on hooded jacket.

tim, or clothes soaked in blood should be thoroughly line-dried at room temperature before being folded. Drying at high temperatures may destroy evidence. Folding or packaging of wet clothes causes soiling of previously clean areas, besides promoting mildew and growth of other fungus, and renders subsequent examination more difficult or impossible.

The chain of custody of clothing, as well as the chain of custody of other retained evidence, must be maintained. A signed receipt listing each item should be obtained from the police officer who takes custody of the clothes.

Body Surface

The body surface should be carefully examined and all injuries recorded. This examination

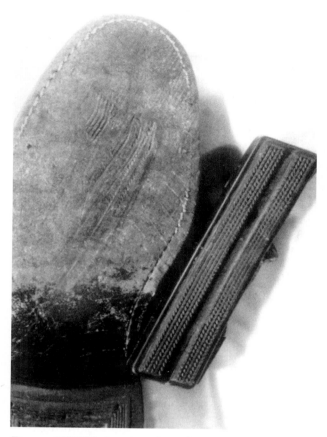

FIGURE XXIV-2. Imprint of accelerator pedal on sole of shoe.

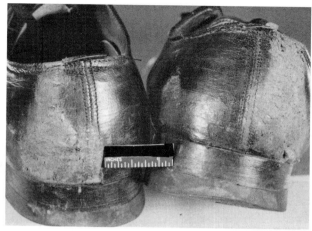

FIGURE XXIV-3. Typical scuff marks on the outer heels of the shoes occur when a body is dragged by the wrists or hands.

often will reveal the distance and sometimes the direction of fire in a gunshot case, the presence of different types of patterns on the skin which will identify a particular weapon excluding other modes of injury, the weapon involved in a stabbing case, the levels of bumper injuries on the legs of a pedestrian which will determine whether the brakes were being applied and whether the victim was walking or standing still, sometimes the very profile or contour of the bumper may be identifiable, whether the victim was the driver or passenger, and endless other examples are all the result of a thorough and accurate, albeit time-consuming, external examination.

All wounds in hairy areas should be cleaned of blood and other loose debris or dirt, shaved and photographed. A scalpel can be used for shaving. Occasionally, large areas of the hairy scalp need to be shaved to document injuries. The argument that shaving of the scalp interferes with viewing of the remains at the funeral home is invalid since, if necessary, a wig can be used or hair can be replaced with the use of special adhesives (Fig. XXIV-4).

Much of the controversy surrounding the assassination of President John Kennedy could probably have been avoided had the wound in the back of the President's head been shaved and properly documented and photographed.

Unsightly large scales and autopsy instruments, hands with bloody gloves, etc. are offensive and should not be shown in photographs.

Shaving of skin around a close-range gunshot wound does not remove gunpowder stippling embedded in the skin and only enhances evaluation of the area and estimation of the distance of fire. With adequate care, soot present around a wound may be preserved as well.

An adequate description of this part of the postmortem examination may be worded as in the following examples.

Natural Death

The body is that of a well-developed, well-nourished, fully clothed elderly white male, weighing 170 pounds and measuring 5 feet 10 inches in length. The clothes worn by the deceased are unremarkable. The deceased appears to be the stated age of 72 years.

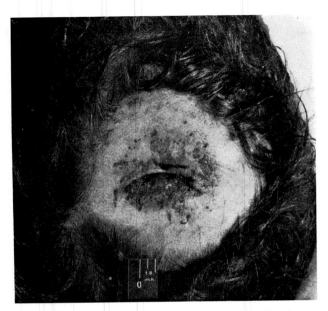

FIGURE XXIV-4. Laceration of the back of the head sustained in a fall. The edges of the injury are abraded and show the imprint of gravel. The area is shaved for the purpose of examination and photography.

Gunshot Wounds

The body is that of a . . . fully clothed white male. . . . A bullet hole measuring 1/4 inch in diameter is located in the back of the cream-colored shirt, 1 inch from the shoulder seam and 2 inches to the left of the midline. The fibers of fabric at the edges of the hole are frayed inward. Surrounding the hole are densely scattered particles of gunpowder extending over a diameter of about 1-1/2 inches. In the front of the shirt, on the right side, 6 inches below the shoulder seam, there is noted a tear apparently produced by the exiting missile. The fibers at the edges of this tear are frayed outward. The underlying T-shirt has holes in locations corresponding to those seen in the shirt. No additional bullet holes are noted in the clothing. All clothing items are listed and turned over to the police. (The signed receipt for the clothing is enclosed with the file.)

Pedestrian Struck by an Automobile

The body is that of a well-nourished, well-developed elderly white male. . . . The body is fully clothed, except for the right shoe, which is obtained separately. Examination of the clothes shows the trousers to be extensively torn, and a patterned imprint of what is believed to be a tire mark is seen in the left thigh area. A photograph is obtained of the area. The clothes are all soiled with road dirt, and the shirt is soiled with blood. (All the clothes are listed and turned over to the police).

It is advisable to mention the amount of blood present in the clothing (soaked, streaked, spotted) and describe in general terms areas that are soiled (e.g., left sleeve and back of shirt, etc.) In the case of a shooting or stabbing victim who died at the hospital, it is good practice for the police to have the clothes viewed by the pathologist before delivering them to the crime laboratory. For example, when the clothes have filtered out soot or gunpowder, and the entrance wound in the skin is devoid of evidence of close-range firing, examination of the clothes by the pathologist is invaluable to enable him to formulate an opinion regarding the manner of death. Suicidal gunshots are usually fired at contact or at very close range (Fig. XXIV-5).

To ascertain that a shooting was accidental, the circumstances of the incident must be reconstructed and correlated with the findings on the body. Examination of the clothes is essential. The presence or absence of soot and/or gunpowder will assist the pathologist in estimating the range of fire.

During a struggle for a weapon, gunpowder is often deposited on the clothes, but usually not in areas normally suggestive of suicide. Such information is important when reconstructing a case and formulating an opinion and later testimony.

A cut in an article of clothing may enlighten the examiner regarding the shape of the blade that caused a stab wound and help in identifying whether an injury was due to one or more thrusts of the weapon. Due to the relatively low elasticity of certain materials such as leather and vinyl, the shape of the blade is often better maintained in these articles than in skin or other tissues, except bone.

Clothes may be of considerable assistance when the identity of a victim is unknown. Mutilation of the face by injury or postmortem decomposition of the body may render conventional identification procedures unsuitable. The clothes should then be retained for later viewing by a potential identifier. Certain institutions, such as psychiatric hospitals, nursing homes and assisted living homes for the elderly, often mark residents' clothing.

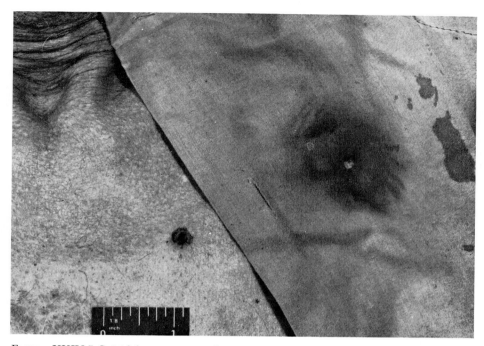

FIGURE XXIV-5. Suicidal, near-contact shot of the chest. Abundant soot is deposited around the bullet hole in the shirt. The wound in the skin is devoid of evidence of close-range firing. Without the shirt, this wound would be interpreted as a distant shot, unlikely to have been self-inflicted.

The Body

The external examination of the body documents rigor and livor mortis, postmortem decomposition, different types of injuries and patterns of injury on the skin.

Injuries on the body surface should not be listed as merely tears or lacerations, abrasions, or bruises. The findings should be descriptive, such as: brush burns, tire marks, stab wounds, bullet wounds of entrance or exit, contact shot, gunpowder stippling, etc. This provides for a concise record and enhances understanding of the report. In this way injuries produced by dragging on the ground should be described as *brush burns;* the imprint of the automobile steering column on a driver's chest should be noted, and pedestrian injuries believed to be caused by an automobile bumper may be described as *bumper injuries.* The same holds true for *dicing* produced by broken tempered glass, *dashboard injuries,* the imprint or indentation of the skin produced by the noose in a hanging victim, needle tracks in a narcotic addict, etc.

The external examination of the body lists the age, race, sex, length and weight of the deceased, as well as the state of nourishment and any congenital abnormalities. Unless the body was viewed at the scene, the presence and distribution of rigor and livor mortis as well as, body temperature, need to be recorded, although in most cases it may suffice to state whether the body is warm or cold to the touch. In cases where estimation of the time of death is important, liver or rectal temperature measurement may be of considerable value, provided the body has not been refrigerated.

The degree of corneal clouding is significant if the eyes are shut. Otherwise, corneal clouding and drying set in very rapidly. The conjunctivae may be congested or pale. Conjunctival hemorrhages, petechial or otherwise, should be noted. The presence of pinpoint hemorrhages in the eyelids must be recorded. Such hemorrhages are especially significant if strangulation is suspected. It is often necessary to slightly stretch the upper eyelids to identify these faint and very delicate reddish dots (Fig. XXIV-6). Pinpoint hemorrhag-

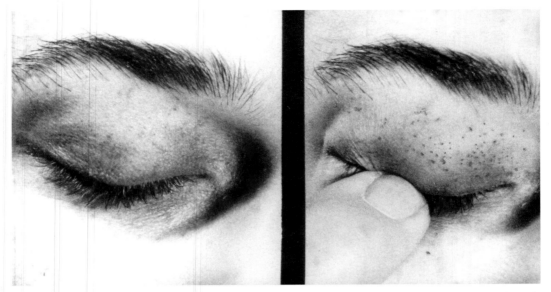

FIGURE XXIV-6. Gentle stretching of the eyelid reveals faint pinpoint hemorrhages otherwise difficult to recognize.

es are sometimes seen in the upper portions of the cheeks. The presence of cataracts or a glass eye may have special significance in the case of a traffic collision. The description should also include the oral cavity. Bruises and tears of the lining membrane and the frenulum of the upper lip caused by pressure against the teeth are sometimes noted in cases of smothering. Such injuries may be located opposite the molars. Bald spots on the head in a child and sometimes in women and the elderly may identify maltreatment.

In cases of questionable identity, all details that may be pertinent to the identity of the deceased are mentioned in the report. Thus, hair and eye color, moles, tattoos and all scars on the body are important. Identification photographs and fingerprints should be taken by police technicians. Good sets of fingerprints are often obtainable even in the presence of advanced decomposition. Postmortem dental charts and roentgenograms of both jaws, as well as other skeletal x-rays, are invaluable if antemortem data or x-ray films are available for comparison. If the face is badly mutilated or decomposition has advanced to the extent that the body is not viewable, it is often advantageous to remove the jaws from the body to facilitate a more accurate examination and possible consultation with a

dentist. The technique is discussed in Chapter XXV.

Tattoos in areas where the skin is darkened by smoke, or old tattoos that have faded and become difficult to recognize may be identified by removal of the epidermis. In a fire victim, or in the case of slippage of the skin due to decomposition, the epidermis can be removed simply by wiping the area with a moist paper towel or rag. Otherwise, a second-degree burn produced by a regular light bulb held close to the skin for a few minutes (usually less than 4 or 5), will have the same effect.

The external genitalia must be examined and described. If sexual assault is suspected, vaginal, oral and rectal specimens in females and oral and rectal specimens in males should be obtained in triplicate. One set of specimens is used for preparation of smears. These are stained with any conventional cytological stain and scanned microscopically for the presence of spermatozoa. A second set is used for determination of acid phosphatase, and a third set is typed or subjected to DNA testing. The presence of what appears to be dry semen on the thighs, abdomen, or pubic area of a body should be noted. The material may be scraped gently with a scalpel blade and placed in a test tube containing saline for later microscopic examination, blood typing, or DNA testing, if needed. Dry semen on the thigh of a man close to the genital area often results from postmortem expulsion of semen due to rigor mortis of the seminal vesicles (Fig. XXIV-7). For unknown reasons, this phenomenon is more common in asphyxial deaths.

Whereas, the postmortem expulsion of semen is the result of rigor mortis, the spillage of fecal matter and/or urine are often due to the absence of rigor, i.e., during the period where the body is flaccid and during the process of dying, when sphincter control is lost. Stools lost in this way are by gravity, therefore they are soft or semiliquid.

In every case of suspected sexual assault, pubic and scalp hair and fingernail clippings are retained, placed in separate envelopes, properly labeled and sent to the crime laboratory. The hair should be plucked rather than cut and the area from which the hair is obtained should be noted. Scalp hair and fingernail clippings or scrapings should be retained in any type of assault in which there was body contact between the parties. In such cases, the hands should be carefully inspected for foreign materials. Hairs adhering to the victim's fingers may be significant.

Gags and ligatures and bindings used to immobilize the victim should be photographed before removal from the body. Removal of any of these, or removal of a noose, is done by cutting the item, without damaging the knot, and tying the cut ends with string or wire. This prevents fraying and assures adequate preservation. It is sometimes necessary to secure the knot independently.

We have had a number of serial killings where the deaths were due to ligature strangulation. Whereas, the ligatures were different, the knots were always the same. In fact, the perpetrator was finally apprehended and convicted with this crucial evidence.

Evidence of Injury

All injuries are described, both externally and internally. Bullet wounds, stab wounds and other injuries should be precisely located on the body. For purposes of testimony, it is desirable to always use three parameters in accurately locating an injury on the body.

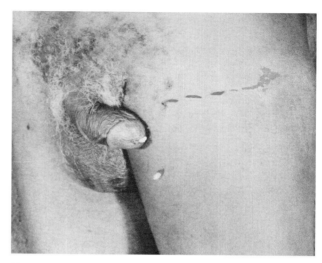

FIGURE XXIV-7. Postmortem expulsion of semen due to contraction of muscle in the wall of the seminal vesicles by rigor mortis.

1. Number of inches from the top of the head or above the sole of the foot.
2. Number of inches to the right or left of the anterior or posterior midline of the body.
3. Number of inches from a well-established landmark, such as the nipple in the male, below the collarbone, or from the navel, the groin, etc.

A wound in an extremity should be described with the limb in the anatomic position using the joints, i.e., shoulders, wrists, elbows, knees, ankles, as points of reference.

Gunshot Wounds

In the case of *gunshot wounds,* aligning a wound in a shoulder or an upper extremity with a possible re-entry wound in the trunk, neck, or head helps ascertain the total number of shots that struck the victim.

This description is not only accurate, but facilitates the demonstration of an injury on one's own body if asked to do so for the benefit of the jury at the time of a trial: "Doctor, would you please show the jury on your own body where this wound that you have just described to us, was situated?" Thus, in the case of a *gunshot wound,* the report would read:

On the front of the chest, 18 inches from the top of the head, 5 inches to the left of the midline and 2 inches below the left nipple, there is noted a gunshot wound of entrance. The wound measures 1/4 inch in diameter, and its edges are abraded. There is no evidence of soot deposit or gunpowder stippling on the skin surrounding this gunshot wound.

Note in the description of the bullet wound of entrance the mention of marginal abrasion, soot and gunpowder. As described in Chapter XII, the marginal abrasion of an entrance wound indicates the angle at which the bullet struck the body. It is therefore important that an eccentric marginal abrasion be accurately noted in the report. The *o'clock* system is best used for this purpose. Twelve o'clock is oriented superiorly. For example:

The edges of the bullet wound are abraded. The widest point of the abrasion is at three o'clock, tapering off toward one o'clock and six o'clock.

Similarly, if the gun sight or extractor rod is imprinted on the skin, the description may be worded using the same system:

A 1/4 inch diameter semicircular abrasion and bruise are situated between two and four o'clock, below the gunshot wound. . . .

If the shot was inflicted at close range, the exact diameter of the gunpowder stippling around the wound must be recorded:

Gunpowder stippling is noted scattered over a diameter of 3 inches around the entrance wound.

Or, if the vertical and horizontal distribution of the stippling is different, the dimension of each should be indicated.

After all pertinent information relative to the external appearance of the wound has been recorded, the description may proceed with an account of the wound track in anatomical order.

Regardless of the type of violence, the entire extent of the injury, beginning with the findings on the skin followed by the internal findings, should be described together in one paragraph. In this way the injury is outlined in a natural sequence, and with almost no effort one can visualize the entire wound complex. Such description significantly simplifies retrieval of this information at the time of courtroom testimony.

. . . Subsequent autopsy shows the bullet to graze the upper edge of the fifth rib and pass through the lower lobe of the left lung. A deformed small-caliber, non-jacketed lead slug is recovered from the left side of the back, 25 inches below the top of the head and 2 inches to the left of the midline, and retained. Massive bleeding (1500 cc of liquid and clotted blood) is noted within the left chest cavity. The wound path is from front to back, downward and slightly inward (medially).

The description of the slug should be noted with respect to location and type: lead, jacketed, non-jacketed, hollow point, caliber if known, otherwise described as small, medium or large caliber; and condition—intact, deformed or fragmented.

In the case of a through-and-through bullet wound of an upper extremity and re-entry into the body, the text should be worded accordingly:

Manipulation of the right upper extremity permits the through-and-through gunshot wound in the right hand to be aligned with an atypical gunshot wound in the front of the neck, suggesting that the two injuries were caused by the same missile (Fig. XXIV-8).

The bullet wound in the hand may well be a *defense-type* injury, and reference to that effect should be included in either the descriptive text of the autopsy report or, preferably, in the *opinion* at the end.

In cases of multiple gunshot wounds, it is often advisable to number each wound. The wounds may be numbered consecutively from top to bottom, regardless of whether they are entrance or exit wounds. To avoid possible misunderstanding that a wound labeled #1 was necessarily the first shot, an explanatory sentence should be added to the opinion at the end of the report: "The sequence of the shots cannot be ascertained." The description of the injuries is now complete, and there is no need to repeat this outline when detailing the individual organ systems, except for a short reference to this paragraph.

The base of a bullet recovered during autopsy should be marked for identification. If the slug is mutilated, markings may be placed in a suitable location, ensuring that rifling marks are not damaged. The markings should be recorded in the pathologist's notes, so that the slug can be identified when needed. Photographs of the bullet from different sides may be used instead of markings. Each recovered bullet is placed in a separate envelope or other secure container to

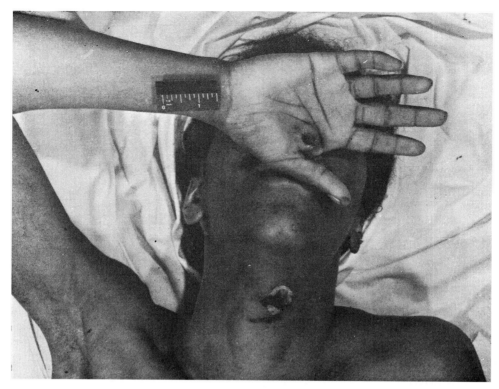

FIGURE XXIV-8. Through-and-through, close-range, entrance gunshot wound of the right hand and re-entry of the slug into the neck. The irregularity of the neck injury suggests that the wound in the hand may be a *defense-type* wound.

prevent damage to the bullet surface by scratching. The envelope states the name of the victim, the examiner's case number, date of the autopsy, name of the prosector, the part of the body where the slug was found and the name of the officer, with badge number, to whom the slug was given.

Stab Wounds

In the case of *stab wounds,* the injury in the skin should be measured and recorded in the report. Then, after adjusting the wound edges in accordance with the lines of cleavage of the skin, a second measurement of wound length and its width (representing the blunt edge of the blade) is made and recorded. Thus, a report of the external examination of a stab wound might read as follows:

On the left chest, 18 inches from the top of the head, 5 inches to the left of the midline and 2 inches below the left nipple, there is a vertical stab wound, measuring 7/8 inch in length and gapes to a width of 3/8 inch. Approximation of the sides of the wound changes its dimensions and shape. Following alignment of the wound, it becomes triangular, the upper edge representing the base of the triangle, measuring 1/8 inch in length. The sides of the triangle each measure 1 inch. The apex of the triangle points downward.

Adjacent to the upper edge of the stab wound there is a rectangular abrasion suggestive of being caused by the hilt of the blade (see Chapter XI).

Subsequent autopsy indicates the stab wound to cut through the left fifth rib cartilage and proceed into the lower lobe of the left lung to a depth of approximately 4 inches.

It is important to record the dimensions of a stab wound in any serosal surface such as the liver capsule, the pleura, or in bone. Often, these measurements more closely approximate those of the blade than the dimensions of the wound in the skin.

The entire wound track is infiltrated with a large amount of blood, and there are 1500 cc of liquid and clotted blood in the left chest cavity. The entire length of the stab wound is approximately 5-1/2 inches. The wound track passes from front to back, downward and right to left.

When there are numerous stab wounds on the body, a detailed description of each and every injury leads to a lengthy and confusing report. Instead, groups of injuries should be described and the typical wounds selected for detailed description.

Around the left nipple, over a diameter of 7 inches, there are twelve stab wounds. Most are vertical, but some are slightly slanted. They range in length from 3/4 inch to 1/8 inch.

The pathologist should then proceed to describe one typical stab wound and ascertain how many penetrate the pleural cavity and the lung, ribs involved, extent of hemorrhage, etc.

Similar grouping of injuries for the purpose of description may be done with other types of trauma. In a case of manual strangulation, for example, the following type of description may be used:

On the neck there are fingernail marks, multiple semilunar and straight linear abrasions up to 1/2 inch in length. The injuries are especially numerous on the left side of the neck.

Hammer injuries to the scalp may also be described as one entity, noting the number of wounds and their locations. Several typical wounds should be chosen for a more detailed description of their shape, diameter, underlying involvement of the skull, etc. The diameter of a hammer wound is obtained by completing the circle of the semi-circular injury on a sheet of paper. The diameter of the hammer wound determines the weight of the tool (13 oz, 16 oz etc.).

INTERNAL EXAMINATION

The description of the internal examination in a medicolegal autopsy report does not materially differ from that of any regular hospital autopsy. Findings that are described under the heading *"Evidence of Injury"* need not be repeated with the description of each organ system, except possibly for a general statement such as *the following observations are limited to findings other than injuries* described above.

Injuries that are not found on external examination, such as contusions of the scalp, are described in detail under *"Evidence of Injury."* The location and extent of such injuries may indicate the site and severity of impacts. A fracture of the skull should be described as to size and shape, depressed, comminuted, etc. A close-up photograph of the fracture, after removal of all soft tissues (including the periosteum), by scraping with the sharp edge of a scalpel, may be helpful for identification of a weapon. A subdural hematoma is best weighed or its volume determined in a graduated cylinder. Subdural blood should be analyzed for alcohol and drug content. In cases of survival, such alcohol and drug levels will reflect levels which existed at the time the blood was shed, rather than at the time of death. A traumatic clot within the brain should be handled in the same way. Alcohol, and certainly cocaine, with its short half-life time, may be eliminated from the peripheral blood during this time period.

Dissection of the cervical spine by posterior approach as outlined in Chapter XXV is necessary in certain cases. This procedure is best carried out at the end of the postmortem examination when the tissues have been drained by removal of the organs. Whiplash injuries of the upper part of the spine are not necessarily associated with fractures. In automobile drivers, they are far more frequent than is commonly acknowledged. In other cases, injury of the cervical cord may cause quadriplegia and thus immediate collapse. Injury of the medulla oblongata is likely to cause instantaneous death. Such statement in the autopsy report will immediately eliminate any chance of recovery in a later claim of pain and suffering.

A description of the degree of calcification or porosis of the skeleton provides an assessment of bone fragility. Osteoporosis is common in the elderly, in whom fractures can occur with relatively little trauma. At autopsy, after the intercostal muscles are cut, an osteoporotic rib will break from minor bending with the muffled sound of breaking cardboard. Artifactual fracture of an osteoporotic spine occurs relatively frequently above the edge of the block placed across the shoulders to facilitate removal of the organs. In severe cases, the weight of the head alone, and certainly manipulation during removal of the brain, often causes fracture of the upper thoracic spine. The hyoid bone and laryngeal cartilages, of particular significance in cases of suspected strangulation, should be evaluated for their fragility and the degree of severity noted in the autopsy description. Sectioning of the thyrohyoid ligaments between the greater cornua of the hyoid bone and the superior cornua of the thyroid cartilage permits manipulation of both structures independently and inspection for possible fractures and deep hemorrhages.

In situ examination of the larynx or removal of the neck organs is meaningful only after the brain and chest organs have been removed from the body to provide for a bloodless dissection field in the neck area. This technique practically eliminates occurrence of artifactual hemorrhages. In a fire victim, a longitudinal incision of the trachea prior to evisceration is advantageous to ascertain that soot present in the airway was inhaled rather than the result of contamination due to handling of the body.

Inspection of the organs in place is also required in gunshot and stabbing cases, where evisceration upsets normal anatomic relationships and distorts wound tracks. X-ray examination, while helpful for locating a bullet, does not outline its pathway in the body.

Injuries caused by attempted resuscitation should be described accordingly. Such injuries may include fractures of ribs and sternum, bruising and laceration of the lungs with interstitial emphysema, and tears of the heart, due to pounding on the precordial area. Periaortic and mediastinal hemorrhage occur with some regularity. Compressions may cause bruising or even tears of the heart to children or to elderly individuals. Tears of the liver are also frequent. Only a small amount of bleeding is usually associated with these injuries, but occasionally, if the heart is reactivated, a beat or two will suffice to cause extensive hemorrhage into tissues and body cavities.

Areas of aspirated blood in the lungs indicate that breathing continued for an indeterminable period of time. The origin of the inhaled blood can be anywhere in the respiratory system or the oropharynx. A possible origin of the bleeding is the base of the skull, where fracture through the sella turcica opens the pharyngeal vault, exposing the airway.

Appearance of the esophageal, gastric and intestinal mucosa is of particular significance in poisoning cases. The stomach may contain powder and undissolved partial pills. The amount, quality, color and odor of stomach contents should be described. The amount of bile in the gallbladder is significant, as is the amount of urine in the bladder. A markedly distended bladder suggests an extended period of unconsciousness preceding the death.

OPINION

Like its clinical counterpart, a medicolegal report of a postmortem examination should be concluded with a well-rounded *opinion,* tying together all salient points of the case. We have found that a properly worded explanatory note at the end of the autopsy report appreciably reduces the need for live courtroom testimony by the pathologist.

The medicolegal opinion relates the cause and manner of death, based not only on the results of the postmortem examination and laboratory analyses, but on all pertinent information that has been collected relative to the case. The scene where the body is found, circumstances surrounding the death, record of recent hospitalization and other medical history are some important considerations in formulation of a medicolegal opinion. The opinion should be concise and factual. Depending on the type of case and the manner of death, the opinion can be limited to a single short paragraph or encompass a page or two. This conclusion of the autopsy report is the only part of this document that is sure to be read by anyone with interest in the case, including law enforcement agencies, defense attorneys, judges, juries, the deceased's family and the public at large, as well as physicians. Thus, this part of the report must be worded plainly, to be understandable and leave no room for speculation. A list of technical diagnoses, in order of significance, may be included in a separate paragraph following the descriptive portion of the report or as an explanatory adjunct. In a death due to arteriosclerotic heart disease the opinion might read as follows:

This fifty-seven-year-old white male, JOHN DOE, died of a heart attack (arteriosclerotic heart disease or acute myocardial infarction with fresh thrombosis of the left anterior descending coronary artery). The manner of death is natural.

To be effective as a comprehensive summary of the report, the opinion should provide answers to certain anticipated questions, including negative statements, where appropriate, to enlighten the reader.

This twenty-eight-year-old black male, JAMES DOE, died of injuries sustained in an automobile collision. The deceased had not consumed alcoholic beverages. Or, the deceased had a blood alcohol concentration of . . .

This nineteen-year-old black male, JOHN DOE, died of what is believed to be a self-inflicted gunshot wound of the right temple. The bullet wound of entrance showed evidence of contact-range firing. A bullet wound of exit is noted in the left temple, and no fragments of metal are found along the wound track. The wrists show horizontal scars suggestive of a previous suicide attempt. The deceased had a blood alcohol level of 0.18% at the time of his death. Needle tracks on the forearms suggest chronic narcotic use.

This forty-nine-year-old black female, MARY JONES, died of gunshot wounds that involve the left hand, right forearm and the forehead. The skin around the wound of the left hand show evidence of close-range firing. The other bullet wounds show no such evidence of close-range firing. One medium caliber, non-jacketed lead slug is recovered from the back of the head and is retained. The wounds of the left hand and right forearm may not have been immediately fatal. It is conceivable that a single shot inflicted all three wound tracks, if the forearms were crossed in front of the head. Fingernail marks on the left wrist suggest an altercation. The deceased had not consumed alcoholic beverages shortly preceding her death.

This thirty-eight-year-old white male, JOHN DOE, died of an acute heart attack (acute coronary occlusion) while swimming. It cannot be excluded that he inhaled water during the attack, thus that the death was due to drowning. The manner of death is therefore, considered to be accidental.

This forty-nine-year-old white male, JOHN SMITH, died of suicidal hanging. No malignant or other tumors were found at autopsy. The deceased had a blood alcohol level of 0.05%.

This fifty-eight-year-old white male, JOHN SMITH, died of head injuries (subdural hematoma) sustained as a result of a fall. An incidental finding at autopsy is cirrhosis of the liver, as commonly found in cases of chronic alcoholism. Blood alcohol level cannot be determined due to prolonged hospitalization following the injury.

This fifty-six-year-old white female, MARY DOE, died of a heart attack (acute coronary thrombosis). The automobile crash in which she was involved is believed to have been the result of her death at the wheel. Blood alcohol level is negative.

It is not imperative that the manner of death be spelled out in each instance if it is implied. Thus, if the bullet wound of entrance shows no evidence of close-range firing, it would be highly improbable that the injury was self-inflicted. A contact shot cannot be accidental. Similarly, a stab wound in the back probably excludes suicide.

This eighteen-year-old white male, JOHN DOE, died of massive internal bleeding due to a gunshot wound of the chest involving the left lung and heart. A small caliber, non-jacketed lead slug is recovered from the spine and retained. The bullet wound of entrance shows no evidence of close-range firing on the skin. The deceased had not been consuming alcoholic beverages.

This twenty-one-year-old white male, JOHN DOE, died of a gunshot wound of the abdomen that perforated the bowel, causing spillage of bowel contents into the abdominal cavity and subsequent infection (peritonitis). . . .

Occasionally no absolute statements can be made relative to some of the postmortem findings. In such a case, the prosector should elaborate on his uncertainties and convey his impression rather than avoid the issue and leave the questions open for speculation and debate by other interested parties. The pathologist is certainly the most qualified to express an opinion relative to his findings and conclusions.

Keith Simpson, quoting Voltaire, once said, "We can none of us be certain we are right— 'Only a charlatan is certain.' But we can try to come as near the truth as the evidence allows, and we can put it in words that are understandable, not only by the lawyers, but by a jury of men and women also."

Chapter XXV

SELECTED PROCEDURES AT AUTOPSY

WERNER U. SPITZ

A MEDICOLEGAL AUTOPSY differs from a hospital autopsy in both objective and significance. Consequently, certain procedures that are of little or no use in hospital practice of pathology are applied routinely by the forensic pathologist. Several of these procedures are described in conventional autopsy manuals. The aim of this chapter is to collate selected procedures and techniques that we have found to be helpful in the routine performance of medicolegal postmortem examinations.

AIR EMBOLISM

Every autopsy in a death case involving a suspected abortion, chest trauma, or an open wound in the neck area, during childbirth, or while diving, should begin with a check for air embolism. An interrupted blood column, i.e., fragmentation of the blood line in the coronary arteries, the arteries of the meninges or elsewhere in the body, is often artifactual and must not be regarded as evidence of air embolism (Fig. XXV-1).

The following is an easy, fast and reliable method to determine the presence of air in the vascular system. A T-shaped incision is made over the heart area. Extension of the T will later constitute the usual autopsy incision through which the organs are removed. The skin and muscles are flapped back, and the precordial part of the sternum and ribs are removed. The aim at this stage is to disturb the tissues as little as possible, and care must be taken not to pull on the tissues at the time of their removal from the body. This is to avoid creating negative pressure in the tissues, which may result in suction of air into the vessels. The pericardial sac is opened anteriorly, and the edges are grasped with hemostats on each side. It is helpful to have an attendant hold the hemostats. The pericardial sac is filled with water, and the heart is submerged. The right side of the heart is then stabbed with a scalpel under the water level. The scalpel should be turned a few times when inside the heart to ensure that the wound is open. If air is present, bubbles will rise; otherwise blood will emerge from the wound.

It is recommended that the amount of air be measured. For this purpose an inverted water-filled graduated glass cylinder (preferably over 300 cc) is placed over the heart, with the open end of the cylinder in the pericardial water. When the heart is stabbed, the gas will escape into the cylinder, displacing the water. A stopper then placed on the mouth of the cylinder will ensure retention of its contents for chemical analysis if such is indicated. Aluminum foil secured with a tight rubber band will equally serve the purpose (Fig. XXV-2a–d).

PNEUMOTHORAX

Pure pneumothorax is rare. It is usually associated with injury to the lung, resulting in the presence of blood in the pleural cavity (hemopneumothorax). The pleural cavities should be checked for the presence of air in every case of chest injury. Incision of the body is as outlined in

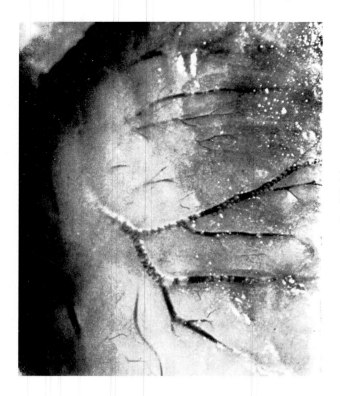

FIGURE XXV-1. Postmortem artifact. Air bubbles in coronary vessels due to removal of sternum and internal organs. This finding should not be construed as evidence of air embolism.

the section on air embolism. The skin and muscles on the injured side of the chest are reflected and dissected to form a *pocket,* which is then filled with water. A scalpel is introduced under the water level through an intercostal space into the costodiaphragmatic sinus. The scalpel should be turned a few times to ensure that the wound is open. An inverted graduated cylinder filled with water held over the pocket may be used to collect and measure the amount of air in the pleural cavity (Fig. XXV-3a–b).

DEMONSTRATION OF THROMBI IN THE CALVES

Deep vein thrombosis in the calves is a frequent complication of immobilization of the limb or prolonged bed rest and may occasionally follow direct trauma to one or both legs. Spontaneous dislodging of a deep leg vein thrombus may cause fatal pulmonary embolism. It is impossible to determine the source of an embolus in the pulmonary artery or lung by direct examination of the clot, but its origin is likely to be the calf, if other thrombi are found in that area. It is often difficult, using conventional methods of dissection, to distinguish a fresh clot in an intramuscular leg vein from a postmortem artifact. The following technique has proven to be a satisfactory alternative to other methods used to demonstrate calf vein thrombi. The calf is incised from the heel to the popliteal fossa, and the skin is reflected. The tendon of Achilles is divided. With a long knife, the calf musculature is then separated from the tibia and fibula from the heel upward. Excessive traction and handling of the muscles should be avoided, since this may liquefy and dislodge small clots.

Transverse sections about one inch apart are then placed in the calf musculature. Thrombi, if present, will *pop out* as firm, solidly structured *sausages,* which cannot be mistaken for postmortem artifacts. The major arteries of the calf

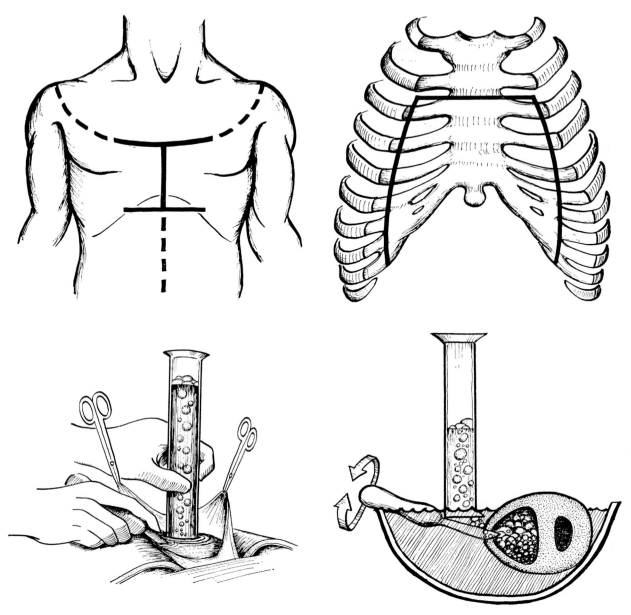

FIGURE XXV-2a–d. (a) *Step 1*–Incision of the skin for exposure of the heart. The dotted line indicates the subsequent extension of the incision for the regular autopsy. (b) *Step 2*–Indicated area represents the section of the rib cage and sternum to be removed. (c) *Step 3*–The pericardial sac is incised and filled with water. Hemostats are used to elevate the pericardium, and an inverted graduated cylinder containing water is placed over the right side of the heart, which is then punctured with a scalpel to permit the escape of gas into the cylinder. (d) Cross-sectional view, showing detail of the scalpel puncturing the heart. The escaping gas replaces the water in the cylinder. Twisting of the scalpel ensures adequate opening of the puncture.

are situated between the tibia and the fibula. They remain intact if this procedure is properly followed. Interference with subsequent injection of embalming fluids into the limb is unlikely (Fig. XXV-4a–c).

Removal of the Heart *in situ* Loses Pulmonary Embolus

Cases have occurred where a massive embolus in the pulmonary artery was lost during

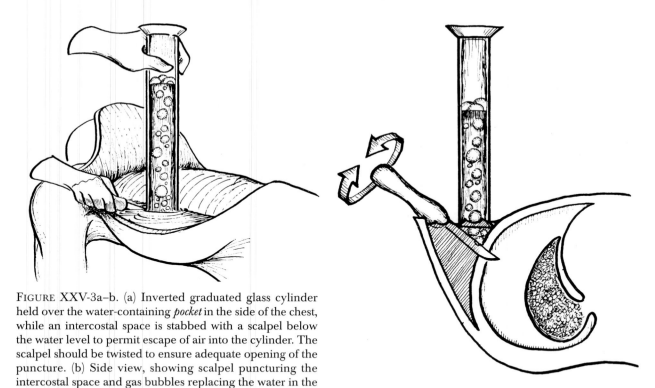

Figure XXV-3a–b. (a) Inverted graduated glass cylinder held over the water-containing *pocket* in the side of the chest, while an intercostal space is stabbed with a scalpel below the water level to permit escape of air into the cylinder. The scalpel should be twisted to ensure adequate opening of the puncture. (b) Side view, showing scalpel puncturing the intercostal space and gas bubbles replacing the water in the cylinder.

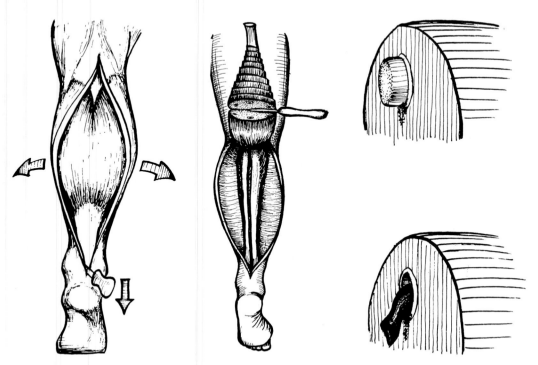

Figure XXV-4a–c. (a) *Step 1*–Skin incision for exposure of calf musculature. (b) *Step 2*–Using a long knife, the calf musculature is separated from the bones and is reflected upward. Transverse incisions of the reflected muscles will disclose the presence of thrombi. (c) Firm, solidly structured thrombi *pop out* as *sausages* from transected vein (above). The postmortem clot is flabby in comparison and does not *pop* (below).

autopsy when the heart was lifted at the apex and the major vessels were severed at the base. This allowed the embolus to fall unnoticed into the pool of blood in the pericardial sac.

In one such case, the clot was recovered at a second autopsy, 2 years later. Until then, the cause of death had been undetermined. The heart should never be removed *in situ*.

RECONSTRUCTION OF THE SKULL FOR PERSONAL IDENTIFICATION AND DETERMINATION OF TYPE OF VIOLENCE

Occasionally, the skull is fractured to the extent that facial features are not recognizable and the type of trauma responsible for the mutilation cannot be ascertained. Restoration of the contour of the skull frequently provides the answer to these questions. Replacement and fixation of the bone fragments may be done with wood glue or an electric drill and copper wire or string (Fig. XXV-5a).

The fragmented skull and extensively mutilated face of a victim of an explosion were reconstructed in this fashion.[1] Polaroid® photographs of the reconstructed face were then shown to family members who immediately identified the body. An artist's sketch and Identikit® reproductions were not recognized as being consistent with the features of the deceased (Fig. XXV-5b–c).

In another case, the body of a bound and gagged man was found in the trunk of an automobile parked alongside a road. The head was crushed, suggesting multiple blows with a blunt object, and beating was thought to be the mode of homicide. Subsequent alignment of the bone fragments and redressing of the scalp clearly indicated a circular bullet wound of entrance in the back of the head. The size of the wound and the hole in the skull, as well as the absence of shotgun pellets within the skull, suggested a single, large missile, probably a rifled slug. The secondary tears in the skin, at first thought to be blunt impacts, resulted from bone fragmentation through the scalp. A gaping exit wound was located in the right side of the forehead (Fig. XXV-6a–c).

RELEASE OF FINGERS AND EXPOSURE OF PALM DURING FULL RIGOR

Detailed viewing of the fingers, as may be necessary when searching for possible defense wounds, suspected electrical or other types of injury, obtaining finger and palm prints for identification and detection of skin and nail disease may be difficult or impossible when the fists are firmly clenched due to full rigor. A simple procedure to open the fists and extend the fingers to allow for complete exposure of the palmar aspect of the hands and fingers is to sever the flexor tendons at the wrists.

A 1/2" transverse cut of the skin at the anterior wrist permits introduction of the scalpel blade or scissors into the wound. Access to each tendon may require some rotation and twisting of the instrument under the skin, in the direction of the radial side, to reach the tendon controlling the thumb (flex. poll. long.). The entire procedure should not take longer than five minutes and does not interfere with viewing instate (Fig. XXV-7).

REMOVAL OF THE JAWS FOR DENTAL IDENTIFICATION

Identification of human remains by comparison of antemortem and postmortem dental records is often the only alternative in cases of extensive mutilation or advanced putrefaction.

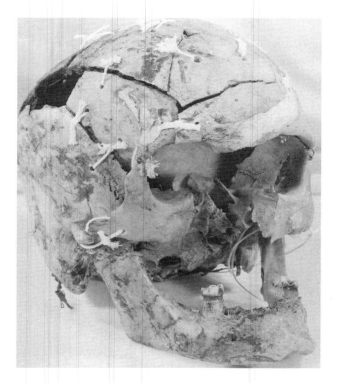

FIGURE XXV-5a. When the head is skeletonized and the skull is fragmented, identification of anthropological data and various skeletal peculiarities are best done by reassembling of the bone fragments as shown.

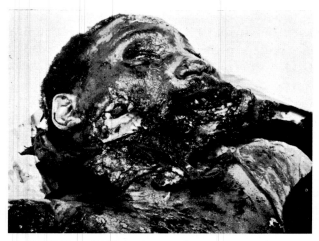 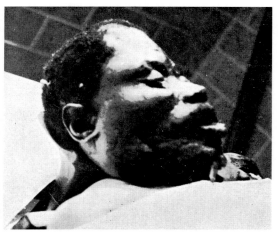

FIGURE XXV-5b–c. (b) Extensive mutilation of an explosion victim, showing vast lacerations of the lower half of the face. The entire facial skeleton was fragmented. The hands were shredded and blown off. (c) Polaroid photograph of same victim after reconstruction of the facial skeleton using copper wire and an electric drill, followed by redressing of the face with *repaired skin*. Where bone fragments were missing, wet paper towels were used to mold the contour. Finally, the lower half of the face was shaded for the purpose of this photograph. Relatives were shown this photograph and identified the victim promptly.

Disarticulation of the mandible and excision of the upper jaw may be necessary to enable adequate examination and possible preservation as evidence (Fig. XXV-8). Using an electric or manual saw, the upper jaw is excised by a horizontal cut above the hard palate. We have found this procedure useful in many instances. Due to the extent of disfigurement already present before removal of the jaws, funeral directors will usually cooperate fully when this procedure is indicated. The removed parts should be returned to the body after identification for joint burial.

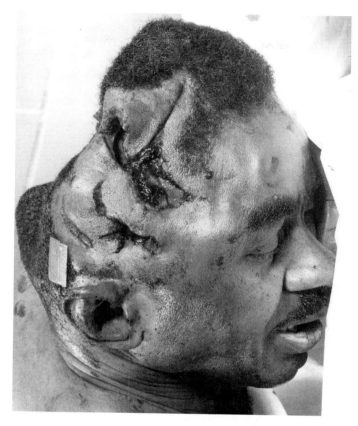

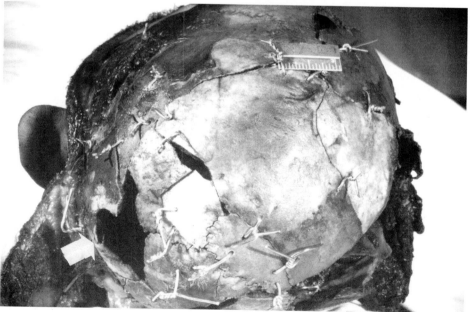

FIGURE XXV-6a–b. (a) Extensive tears of scalp and fragmentation of the skull first thought to be due to blunt impacts. (b) A circular defect behind the left ear observed after alignment (arrow) was presumed to have been caused by a missile.

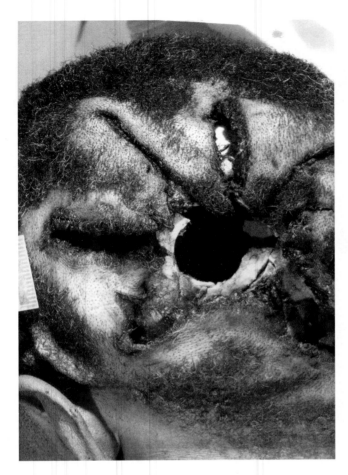

FIGURE XXV-6c. The *redressed* scalp over the circular defect in the bone shows what is now a typical shotgun wound of entrance.

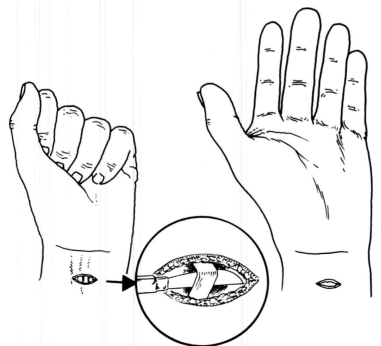

FIGURE XXV-7. Cutting wrist tendons allows a clenched fist to be opened.

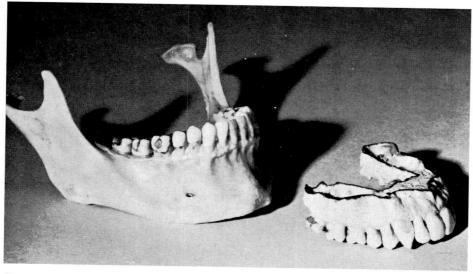

FIGURE XXV-8. Upper and lower jaws removed for comparison of antemortem and postmortem dental records for identification. The upper jaw was resected along the black (inked) line.

DOCUMENTATION OF NOSE BONE AND ADJACENT INJURIES

The term "fracture of the nose" is often a misnomer for separation of the nose bone from the septal cartilage. Exploration of this area and direct viewing may be necessary in suspected karate chops, blows to the face, falls, traffic accidents involving occupants of motor vehicles and other types of facial trauma. Sometimes, a bullet requiring retrieval may be lodged in the nasal bone or the adjacent soft tissues. Incision of the face for the purpose of exploration would interfere with the appearance of the body at the time of viewing instate.

An easy, rapid and definitive procedure is the use of the bitemporal incision of the scalp for removal of the brain extended to the level of the ear lobes. The frontal flap of the scalp is then drawn down over the lower forehead to the level of the eyebrows. Tunneling and blunt dissection enable exposure of the glabella and beyond. The use of a scalpel in the area of the glabella is discouraged to avoid cuts through the skin at the sides of the bridge of the nose.

To avoid damaging a missile requiring removal, no metal instruments should be introduced into the area, except under direct vision.

EXAMINATION OF THE CERVICAL SPINE FOR WHIPLASH INJURY

An autopsy of a traffic death, particularly one involving a rear pedestrian impact, or the victim of a fall, is incomplete without a thorough examination of the cervical spine. Other situations which require direct examination of the cervical spine include diving deaths and suspected shaken baby cases.

Meticulous examination of the cervical spine is also recommended in automobile occupants in cases of post-collision fire, when no significant injuries are found at autopsy and blood carbon monoxide saturation is low or zero. Pathologists tend to certify the cause of death in such cases as incineration or extensive body burns without exploring the cervical spine.

Clinically, so-called whiplash injuries have been described as most often located in the level of C-4 to C-6. However, a radiological study of road crash cervical injuries showed that one-half of injuries above C-3 and 22% of those below C-3 were not identified.[2] In our experience at autopsy, C-1 and C-2 are involved significantly more frequently. Injuries to this area range from severe fractures and dislocations to a few deep hemorrhages in the musculature not viewable radiographically. Most frequently encountered injuries in the level of the first two vertebrae are tears of the articular capsules and ligaments associated with intraarticular or periarticular hemorrhage.

Even in the presence of another well-documented cause of death, the significance of whiplash injury cannot be overstated. The search for whiplash injuries is greatly facilitated by the following technique. The body is placed face down. A head block is placed under the chest, and the head is bent downward. This stretches the cervical spine. Through a posterior midline incision, the musculature is dissected layerwise down to the vertebral column. The atlanto-occipital joint capsules are then incised and the articular surfaces examined. Subsequently, the atlas is disarticulated and removed. Laminectomy is now performed on the remaining cervical vertebrae, the dura mater is incised, and the spinal cord is inspected *in situ,* then removed. The underside of the base of the skull can now be inspected as far forward as the oral cavity. Replacement of the atlas and tight suture of the scalp incision permit good reconstruction with fair stability of the head.

POSTMORTEM ANGIOGRAPHY AND DISSECTION OF THE VERTEBRAL ARTERY IN SITU*

Reports in the medicolegal literature have discussed traumatic basilar subarachnoid hemorrhage, secondary to vertebral artery injuries. Variants of trauma causing this lesion include: a victim receiving a single blow to the jaw, or a victim lying on the back, ears grabbed for leverage, while the head is pummeled on the floor, or collapse after or during a boxing match, or the result of a chiropractic neck manipulation. When forces of hyperextension and rotation are applied, the head twists and impinges on the vertebral artery in the neck. The third section of the vertebral artery, as first described by Contostavlos,[3] is the most vulnerable. As the vertebral artery passes across the transverse foramen of the atlas and travels posteriorly around its lateral mass, it is most susceptible to tension trauma causing it to tear. Other areas of vulnerability are at the atlanto-axial joints. Subluxation of other cervical vertebrae can also cause fatal injury.

In a study of autopsy specimens, Johnson, et al.[4] have shown that the vertebral artery was most susceptible to stretching, as frequently occurs as a result of sudden hyperextension/flexion of the neck in victims of traffic accidents.

Laceration of a vertebral artery in its bony canal should be suspected when there is a history of trauma to the head or jaw followed by sudden collapse. Often a CT scan is available for review. When there is no subdural or epidural hemorrhage, skull fractures or contusions of the brain, but massive basal subarachnoid hemorrhage and brain edema are noted, postmortem angiography is indicated. Autopsy findings of a blow to the face or jaw, associated with massive basilar subarachnoid hemorrhage, also necessitates the use of angiography.

The autopsy should begin with a cranial examination. The brain is examined for basal subarachnoid hemorrhage before removal. If found, a small hemostat or clip is placed on the basilar artery. This may not be feasible due to the cramped space secondary to brain edema. The skullcap should then be replaced to maintain stability, proper alignment and maneuverability of the head and neck for x-ray. The vertebral arteries are located (Fig. XXV-9). They are usually the first branch of the subclavian artery, and travel posteriorly and upward into the sixth cervical vertebra. The right vertebral artery is easier to find

---

* Stanton Kessler

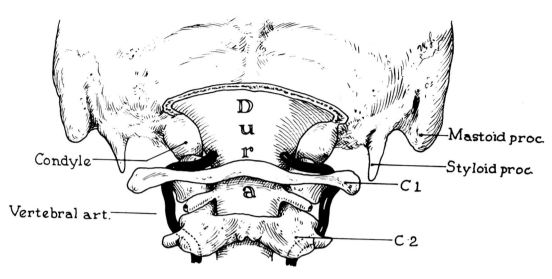

FIGURE XXV-9. Anatomical sketch showing the vertebral arteries in the upper posterior neck.

than the left, and should be found first to give the prosector familiarity with locating the other one. They are then cannulated. It is easy to obtain out-of-date angiography catheters from x-ray special procedures, along with radiopaque injection dyes. Catheters should be chosen for good fit and may range from 5 F to 10 F. An 8 F catheter is most frequently used with good results. After the extra-vertebral arterial segments are isolated and the vessels are cannulated, the catheters are secured, using an 0-silk stitch around the periarterial soft tissues. This is repeated so that there is no leakage of contrast material after injection. We have found that thinner silk sutures often break. With a head block in position under the shoulders and the neck hyperextended, an A/P baseline x-ray is taken. Each cannulated artery is injected with three to five mL of contrast medium. This process is repeated until the vessel is visible on x-ray. A transition zone, of a normal vessel going into a constricted vessel, is indicative of an intimal tear and dissection. Leakage of contrast material into soft tissues indicates a laceration. Abrupt interruption of filling suggests thrombosis.

After establishing a lesion on x-ray, a mixture of 100 mL of 60% barium sulfate and 1/4 package of Knox gelatin in water are heated together until the gelatin dissolves. As it cools the solution will gel. It is injected into the vessel while still warm. A white cast will form in the vessels, facilitating visualization of any leakage upon dissection. A cut is made around the foramen magnum and, with disarticulation of the seventh cervical vertebra, the entire neck block is removed.

After fixation in formalin for three days and, using a large magnifying glass or dissection microscope, all of the muscles of the neck are removed. An OptiVISOR magnifier worn on the head will allow free use of hands while working. The atlanto-occipital ligaments are evaluated for hemorrhage, laxity, or tearing. All of the lateral arches surrounding the vertebral arteries are removed. The arteries on both sides are then cut open and examined for signs of peri-adventitial hemorrhage, gross laceration, or traumatic aneurysm formation. The circuitous course of the vessels, as they traverse around the atlas, is usually the area of injury.

These procedures will facilitate the detection of trauma in this very protected and vital area of the body.

REMOVAL OF THE TONGUE

The tongue should be examined routinely. The presence of a fresh bite mark in the tongue lends support to the probability that a seizure preceded death. In an epileptic, a bite mark in the tongue may be the only anatomical evidence to suggest that death occurred during a seizure. As bite marks in the tongue are not usually visible on external examination, the tongue should be incised using a long blade. A single horizontal cut is recommended. *Bread-loaf-type* incisions can miss small injuries. Bite marks are mostly located along the sides of the tongue, halfway or two-thirds back, less frequently at the tip. A 3–4 mm hemorrhage under an intact mucosa is usually all that is seen.

Removal of the tongue is best done with a double-edged knife, but a regular autopsy knife will do. The use of a scalpel for this procedure is discouraged. Following the usual Y-shaped incision, the skin of the chest and neck is reflected and the knife is inserted under the chin through the floor of the mouth. The tip of the blade will emerge under the tongue. A cut is then made along the sides of the mandible to the angle of the mandible. At this point, the blade is turned inward to avoid severing the carotid artery. With the index and middle fingers, the tongue is now pushed down under the mandibular arch. The soft palate is then cut to include the uvula and tonsils with the tongue and neck organs to be removed (Fig. XXV-10a–b). Should the carotid artery be accidentally damaged during the procedure, a polyethylene tube firmly tied into the vessel will rectify the problem. This will enable subsequent injection of embalming fluids to the head.

EXAMINATION OF THE NECK

When examination of the neck organs involves a case of suspected strangulation or hanging, the European method of organ removal offers advantages not otherwise attainable. This procedure entails a straight vertical midline incision from below the chin down to the pubis. The skin of the neck is reflected laterally, followed by careful layerwise dissection of the strap muscles *in situ* and removal of the neck organs *en bloc* under direct vision, without the need of tunneling and possible creation of artefacts (Fig. XXV-11). Such artefactual hemorrhages created by massaging of blood into areas of dissection often results in misleading and confusing injuries and fractures of laryngeal cartilages caused by obscure handling, and have been known to be subject of intense subsequent debate as to whether the damage was artefactual or real. The hyoid bone and the thyroid cartilage are particularly fragile in elderly individuals and may fracture under relatively minor pressure.

Imagine the predicament of the prosector who finds a subtle hemorrhage adjacent to such fracture and is now confronted with having to explain this finding.

Such unnecessary situations can be eliminated from the start by adequate exposure, realizing the problem this procedure may create for funeral service. The ultimate question is whether this procedure is essential. A skillful embalmer should be able to conceal most, if not all of the incision.

IN-DEPTH EXAMINATION OF THE NECK FOR EVALUATION OF VIOLENCE*

The following is another practical procedure for documentation of neck trauma. Only after layer-wise examination of the tissues down to the vertebrae can it be stated that trauma was not present.

---

* Stanton Kessler

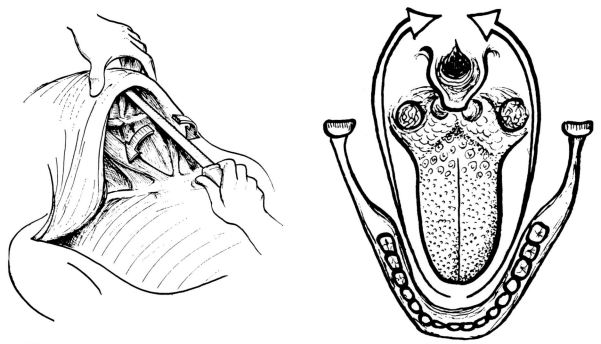

FIGURE XXV-10a–b. (a) Technique for removal of the tongue. (b) The arrows on both sides of the tongue indicate the direction of the blade to include the tonsils and the uvula, but avoid the large vessels on either side.

The usual incision from the deltoids meeting at the mid-anterior chest does not allow adequate reflection for proper examination of the lateral neck and submandibular regions. This is because of limited skin elasticity and because the platysma inserts directly into the skin. Thus, the cursory dissection of the anterior neck is limited to midline anatomy. It does not visualize the extended course of the carotid arteries and jugular veins, submandibular glands, muscles of the anterior-lateral neck, fasciae and lymph nodes.

Even in the presence of another well-documented cause of death, the importance of neck trauma cannot be ignored. Injuries to this region include contusions of lymph nodes, fasciae and submandibular glands, muscular tears and hemorrhage in the adventitia of the carotid artery at the level of the bifurcation. When this occurs, fatal arrhythmia cannot be ruled out, even in the presence of gross trauma to the larynx. Fractures of the high cervical vertebrae may be found with associated hemorrhage into the deep ligaments and soft tissues.

Examination of the neck structures is most easily performed by extending the routine intra-deltoid incisions over the crest of the shoulders to a point in the posterior neck, one-third of the distance from the midline to the lateral border of the posterior neck (Fig. XXV-12). From here the incision is extended upwards along the posterior hairline to the level of the mid-ear. The skin is then undermined from the deltoid region to the ear, while carefully positioning the blade of the scalpel down to avoid cutting the skin. The undermining should proceed to the level of the mandible on both sides. At this time all of the glands, lymph nodes, superficial muscle groups and facial planes of the anterior, lateral and posterior neck are exposed. Layerwise removal of muscles will then expose the carotid sheath, trachea, larynx and the tongue and permit detailed dissection of the posterior neck. Hemorrhage into the deep muscles of the posterior neck is often found in cases of manual strangulation.

In the rare occurrence that it becomes necessary to remove the face to retrieve subcutaneous

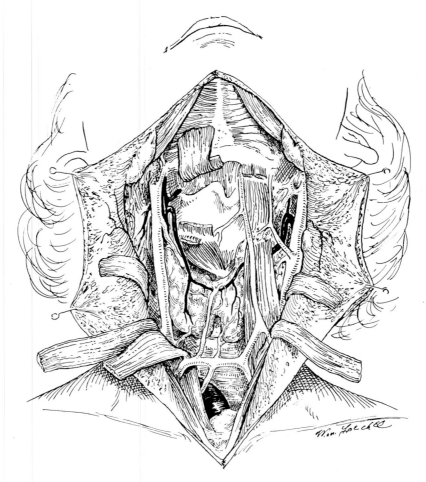

FIGURE XXV-11. Autopsy incision beginning below the chin permits a direct and
unobstructed view of the neck organs eliminating artefacts caused by tunneling.

projectiles, this dissection can be further extended by carefully undermining the facial skin, starting at the mandible. Subcutaneous cutting of the
external auditory meatus facilitates mobilization

of the skin for exposure of the facial skull, without interference with embalming procedures and
cosmetic appearance of the body.

REMOVAL OF THE SPINAL CORD BY ANTERIOR APPROACH

The spinal cord is probably the most neglected organ at autopsy. Unless a definite history
requires that it be examined, the cord usually
remains unobserved inside the body. The main
cause of this apparent lack of interest is that
removal of the cord is both laborious and time-
consuming. Yet, many years ago Kernohan, at
the Mayo Clinic, developed a method that per-

mits removal of the spinal cord without major
effort and in no more than two to three minutes.[5]
This method requires no special instruments; in
fact, a sturdy knife, Stryker saw, chisel and hammer are all the instruments that will be needed.
The cord is retrieved intact and suitable for gross
and microscopic examination. Incision of the
back is avoided, which eliminates turning the

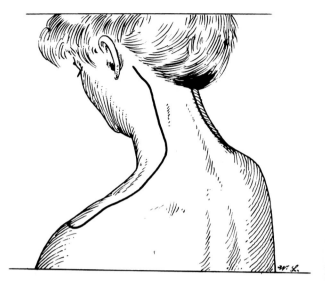

FIGURE XXV-12. Extension of the usual Y-shaped incision to encompass the posterior neck.

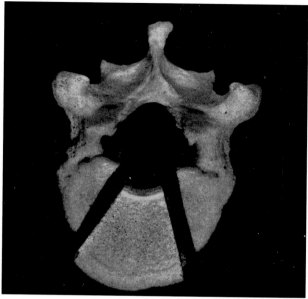

FIGURE XXV-13. Vertebra, showing wedge removed for exposure of the cord.

body and unnecessary work for the funeral director.

The autopsy is performed in the usual way. The brain is removed and the cervical nerve roots are severed through the foramen magnum. After the chest and abdominal cavities have been evacuated, removal of the spinal cord is continued, as follows: An intervertebral disc anywhere in the upper lumbar spine is transected, and another disc is cut in the lower thoracic area. A Stryker saw is then used to cut out the segment of vertebral bodies between the two separated discs (Fig. XXV-13). Prying with a chisel may be necessary to facilitate removal of the bony wedge.

This will expose 2 to 2-1/2 inches of the terminal dura, which is slit vertically and reflected sideways. The exposed portion of the cord, or the cauda equina is loosened by severing the nerves within the spinal canal. A soft moist cloth or paper towel is placed around the cord or cauda and gentle, slow downward traction (toward the feet) is applied. This permits retrieval of the cord in its entirety from within its dural encasement.

We have employed this procedure when removal of the cord was necessary and have found it to be in an excellent state of preservation, with good histologic structure and no artifactual tears.

FIXATION OF THE BRAIN

To permit a meaningful examination, the brain should be fixed in formalin for at least four to five days before being sectioned, unless fixation is accomplished by vascular injection. It is customary in many institutions to suspend the brain in a bucket of formalin, using a string under the basilar artery of the circle of Willis, to avoid flattening of the surface in contact with the bottom of the container, as a result of gravity.

Especially in cases of septicemia and in a warm environment, rapid growth of gas-forming bacteria causes bubbles throughout the brain tissue which may render it unsuitable for subsequent examination (Fig. XXV-14). This can be avoided by placing the brain into chilled formalin. A handful of kitchen salt dissolved in the formalin provides for flotation of the brain and obviates the need of tying a string through the

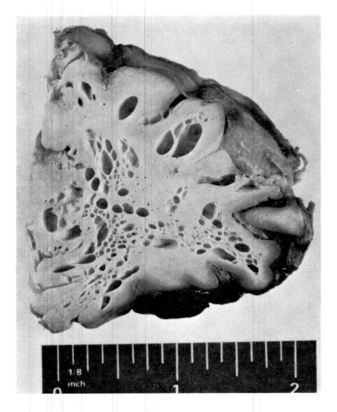

FIGURE XXV-14. Section of brain showing Swiss cheese pattern of cysts due to putrefactive gases.

basilar vessels. Drying of areas extending above the fluid level can be avoided by covering the brain with an absorbent paper towel. This will soak up the formalin and keep such areas moist. Shrinkage of tissue resulting from the added salt is minimal and causes no detectable microscopic changes. We have kept an adult human brain submerged in a saturated solution of sodium chloride for 25 years without observable changes and only minimal loss of weight.

EXPLORATION OF THE MIDDLE AND INNER EARS

Most autopsies, hospital or medicolegal, do not include exploration of the petrous portion of the temporal bones, situated at the base of the skull, containing the organs of hearing and equilibration. We have found 20% of children under 1 year, of which most end up being certified as SIDS, to have serous or purulent inflammation in one or both middle ears.

At the very least, such finding should be indicated in the autopsy report, and a swab of the exudate may be submitted for culture. Removal of the bony ridge permits decalcification and preparation of slides for microscopic examination.

After the skull has been opened, the brain removed and the dura stripped from the middle fossa, the area is thoroughly dried, preferably using an absorbent towel. Bone cutters are used for excision of the petrous ridge. The backs of the cutters' blades are pressed against the perimeter of the skull, using the fingers of the other hand. The procedure is repeated at the medial end of the ridge. The cutters are turned around and the cutters' blades are pressed against the area between the basilar portion of the occipital bone and the sella. The blades are tightened and twisted to remove the specimen. The inner surface of

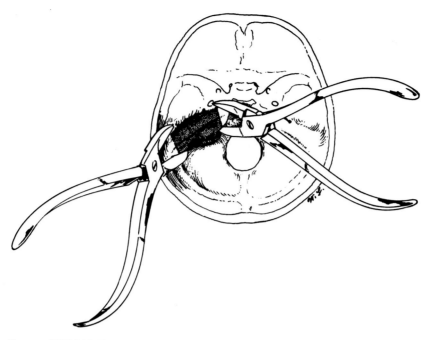

FIGURE XXV-15. Base of the skull after removal of the brain and stripping of the dura. The bone cutter is first pressed against the outer perimeter while cutting the petrous ridge, then against the area between the basilar portion of the occipital bone and the sella when cutting the medial side of the ridge. Twisting of the blades elevates and removes the ridge, exposing the tempanic membrane, the boney ridge is available for culture and microscopic examination.

the tympanic membrane can then be examined for evidence of inflammation and the presence of exudate in the middle ears. This procedure should take about five minutes (Fig. XXV-15).

WATER IN THE SPHENOID SINUS, A NON-NEGLIGIBLE FACTOR IN DIAGNOSING DROWNING

A positive autopsy diagnosis of drowning remains one of exclusion. Consequently, any item added to the list of findings places the final diagnosis on a more solid foundation. The presence of water in the sphenoid sinus, sometimes mixed with sand, even fine gravel, sea weed and diatoms is therefore significant, and has gained popularity in recent years.

A large gauge autopsy needle attached to a glass syringe is used to perforate the sphenoid bone on either side of the sella, directing the needle downward, forward and medially at a 45° angle (Fig. XXV-16). Up to 5 mL of water may be recovered (average 2–3 mL).

The same procedure may be applied to the maxillary sinus, from where a larger quantity of fluid may be withdrawn. The approach of the maxillary sinus is by raising the upper lip, through the canine fossa, with the needle directed upward and slightly backward (Fig. XXV-17).

The fluid obtained may be centrifuged and the diatom content compared to that of the water in which the suspected drowning occurred. Very few, if any, diatoms will be found in a sinus aspirate of an individual who drowned in a bathtub, due to the generally small number of diatoms in tap water. A large concentration of diatoms may be expected in swimming pool water.

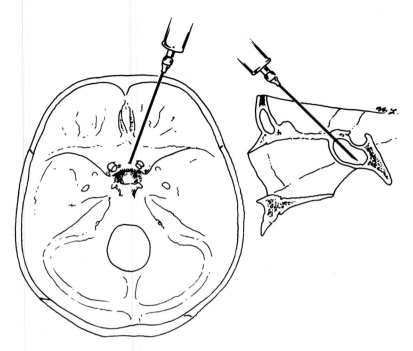

FIGURE XXV-16. Insertion of the needle into the spenoid or maxillary sinus to check for the presence of water in a case of suspected drowning.

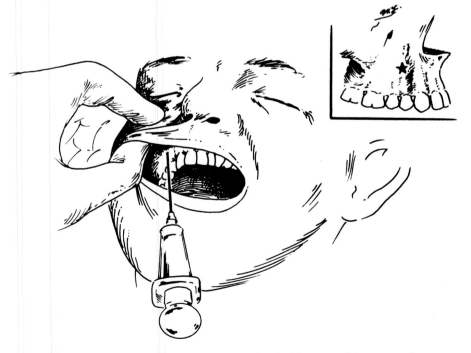

FIGURE XXV-17. The maxillary sinus is approached by way of the canine fossa.

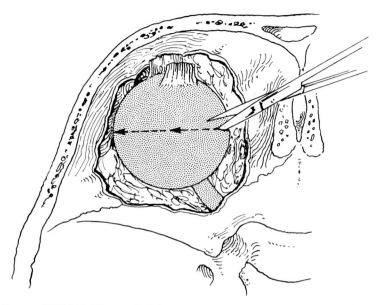

FIGURE XXV-18. The roof of the eye socket is chiseled or cut open and the eye globe is cut along the equator. The back portion of the eye and optic nerve can be removed without disturbing the front half of the globe. It is advantageous to place absorbent cotton soaked in formaldehyde to harden the posterior portion of the eye prior to removal from the socket.

DOCUMENTATION OF RETINAL HEMORRHAGES IN CHILDREN

Retinal hemorrhages play an important role in the diagnosis of *shaken baby syndrome* and other conditions. The back portion of the eye, together with the intra-orbital part of the optic nerve, can be easily removed while the front half of the eye remains intact inside the eye socket.

The roof of the eye socket is chiseled open and the eye is cut along the equator, using sharp, small, pointed scissors (Fig. XXV-18). The cavity behind the cornea is then filled with absorbent cotton soaked in formaldehyde. This procedure avoids any interference with subsequent embalming and viewing of the remains.

POSTMORTEM EXAMINATION OF A POSSIBLE VICTIM OF RAPE*

While it has been shown that physical and laboratory examination of a rape victim may be entirely negative,[6] successful prosecution in a case of suspected rape requires proof of sexual assault with penetration. It is therefore necessary that the postmortem examination of the victim include a search for such evidence whenever rape is suspected.

The examination of the victim begins with pubic combing, while carefully watching for any hair which appear foreign. Pubic and head hair samples are retained. An ultraviolet lamp is a useful tool for a preliminary search for semen on the body surface, clothes, or other suspicious areas. In a darkened room, semen stains emit a whitish-blue fluorescence under a UV light

(*Parts of this section were previously included in Chapter XIX entitled "Sex Crimes" by William F. Enos and James C. Beyer in the 2nd edition of this book.)

source. Positive stains require chemical and preferably microscopic confirmation.

The pathologist should make a detailed description of the genitalia, thighs and pubic region, including pertinent negative points, and vaginal mucus should be subjected to microscopic examination to determine the presence of spermatozoa. The use of a speculum for the examination and specimen collection is advantageous. A drop of fluid from the vaginal pool can be examined for sperm motility. The duration of sperm motility in the vagina has been variously described as ranging from 30 minutes to 60 hours, but usually sperm becomes non-motile in three to four hours.

A thorough search for spermatozoa is best conducted in a number of smears. Smears should be prepared as soon as the victim's body is available for examination by the pathologist. A cotton swab is used to prepare a smear. The material may be taken from anywhere in the vagina, but the cervical canal appears to give the best results. Smears of the oral and rectal mucosa should also be examined. In interpreting the latter, consideration must be given to contamination by vaginal contents. Therefore, collection of rectal specimens first reduces the likelihood of such contamination. The smears are stained with any of the conventional methods, but, while the Papanicolaou stain is used by most hospital cytology laboratories, hematoxylin and eosin seem to provide better differentiation of cytoplasmic and nuclear elements. This is especially important when the tail of the sperm cells is absent. Picro-indigo-carmine, which stains sperm heads red and the tails green and red is popular. The procedure is fast, easy and fairly foolproof. Methylene blue has not given very satisfactory results in that difficulties are encountered with this stain in distinguishing between sperm cells and artifacts. Whichever stain is used, preparation of a control slide will help in evaluating the results.

Decomposition of the body does not preclude the finding of identifiable spermatozoa, and embalming of the body helps preserve them. Intact spermatozoa, i.e., with tails, are rarely found in the vagina later than 72 hours after coitus. As a general rule, if the lining cells of the vaginal or oral cavity is preserved, the probability of identifying spermatozoa is reasonably good. We were able to identify spermatozoa obtained from the cervical canal in a partially frozen victim who had been dead one and one-half months. The vaginal vault was filled with ice. Wilson identified spermatozoa in a body 16 days after rape and murder.[7]

Centrifuging of vaginal aspirate creates artifacts that render identification of spermatozoa more difficult. Loss of tails occurs commonly due to centrifugation. Mucus and cell debris, especially in rectal smears as well as fungus and pollen, can also be misleading (Fig. XXV-19a–b). Identification of spermatozoa follows an all-or-none law, and reports are positive or negative. The terms *suspicious* of or *consistent with* should be avoided.

Vaginal secretions should also be obtained for acid phosphatase determination. The specimen is collected with a pipette attached to a rubber bulb using 25 to 30 cc of saline. A positive test is not necessarily proof of the presence of seminal fluid, but a high value of this enzyme is suggestive, since it does indicate the presence of prostatic secretions. The concentration of acid phosphatase gradually falls with time. Thus, in cases of alleged sexual assault, a quantitative acid phosphatase determination may indicate not only the presence of seminal fluid, but also the approximate time of coitus, even in the absence of spermatozoa.[8] The length of time acid phosphatase remains positive in the vaginal canal depends primarily on the postmortem condition of the body.[9] Values as high as 30 Bodansky units (BU) have been obtained up to 48 hours after death. Cooling of the body preserves acid phosphatase activity over an extended period. Values ranging from 10 to 30 BU suggest rape shortly before death rather than intercourse five to ten hours earlier. The determination of acid phosphatase is significant in view of the frequency of vasectomy and atrophy of the seminiferous tubules in the testicles of alcoholics with cirrhosis.

If the presence of seminal fluid is established in the vagina, oral cavity or rectum, a smear from that site should be subjected to blood type determination or preferably to DNA testing. A stain

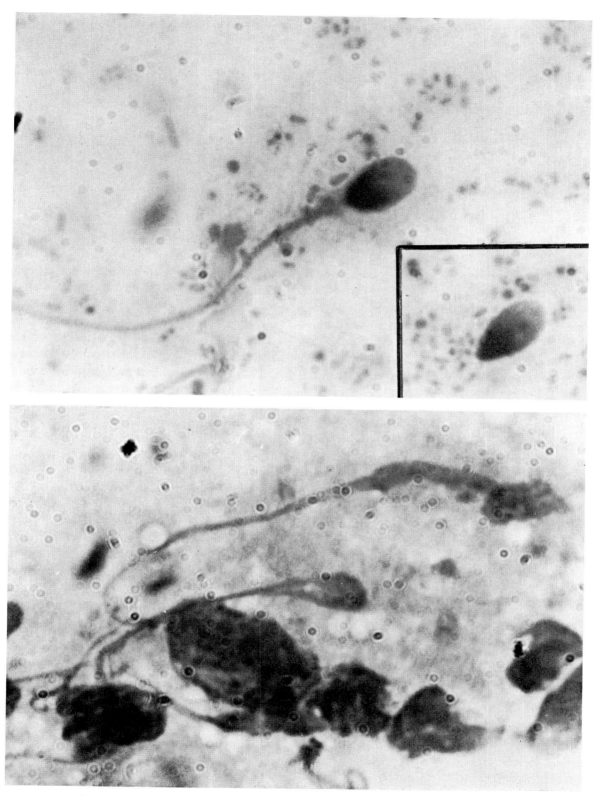

FIGURE XXV-19a–b. (a) Intact sperm cell. Insert: Tailless sperm (Both ×1500, H&E stain). (b) Mucus threads (×1500, H&E stain).

suspected of being semen on clothing or hair may be extracted with physiologic saline and the fluid from this washing treated in the same fashion. Well-preserved spermatozoa can be identified in even old and dry stains. The same is true of acid phosphatase determination. Approximately 80% of men secrete water soluble blood group substances in their seminal fluid. The identification of A, B, or H blood group substances is based on the ability of seminal fluid to at least partially neutralize the agglutinating activity of the specific antiserum. This may be used to show that the seminal fluid found in the victim is of a different blood type than that of the suspected assailant.

Pubic hair combings from the victim, may yield foreign hairs which should be properly labeled and preserved along with fingernail clippings and plucked scalp, facial and pubic hair samples. All specimens are usually examined by the police crime laboratory.

In some cases with definite sexual overtones, semen cannot be identified by any of the methods that have been described. Information gained from police investigation indicates that many of these men are impotent. Such individuals are unable to accomplish penile penetration in any of the body orifices, although premature ejaculation may occur to contaminate the skin, clothing, or surrounding environment. In such cases, swabs moistened with saline applied to such areas may be used for subsequent serologic typing and DNA testing.

Examination of Female Pelvic Organs by en bloc *Resection**

The prosector must carefully inspect the female pelvic organs when sexual assault is suspected. The vagina and rectum, however, lie deep within the pelvis, so an inspection for vaginal and rectal injuries with these organs left *in situ* is often inadequate. The dissection technique described below involves *en bloc* removal of the pelvic organs and perineum from the body. This technique not only allows a more complete inspection of the vagina and rectum under proper lighting, but also maintains the pelvic organs and perineum in their natural positions during the inspection.

Near the completion of the autopsy after the abdominal organs have been eviscerated, the prosector first incises a diamond-shaped portion of skin enclosing the vulva and anus (Fig. XXV-20a). The incisions should penetrate into the deep soft tissues bounded laterally by the ischio-pubic rami, anteriorly by the pubic symphysis, and posteriorly by the coccyx (Fig. XXV-20b). Also, an incision is made internally along the pelvic inlet, enclosing the pelvic organs (Fig. XXV-20c). The rectum and adjacent soft tissues are dissected away from the sacrum while the urinary bladder is dissected away from the pubis. Once the deep incisions made externally join the incisions made internally within the pelvis, the vulva, ureter, urinary bladder, vagina, uterus, fallopian tubes, ovaries, anus and rectum are pulled out of the body as a single tissue block. The organ block attached to the perineal skin can be pulled from the body as a single tissue block. The organ block attached to the perineal skin can be pulled from the body either superiorly through the pelvic inlet or anteriorly and inferiorly through the space bounded by the ischio-pubic rami.

Once the block is removed, the prosector opens the anus and rectum with scissors along the posterior aspect. After washing the specimen to remove feces, the muscosa is inspected for injuries or lesions. The vagina may be opened along the anterior or posterior wall, depending on how the prosector wishes to demonstrate the injuries. This opening allows inspection of the vaginal mucosa, the external os of the uterine cervix, and the junction of the vulva and vagina. The urinary bladder, uterus, fallopian tubes and ovaries are then further dissected and examined using usual techniques. All findings can be photographed easily.

At the conclusion of the autopsy, the perineal defect is closed with string prior to transport to the funeral home.

---

* Thomas W. Young

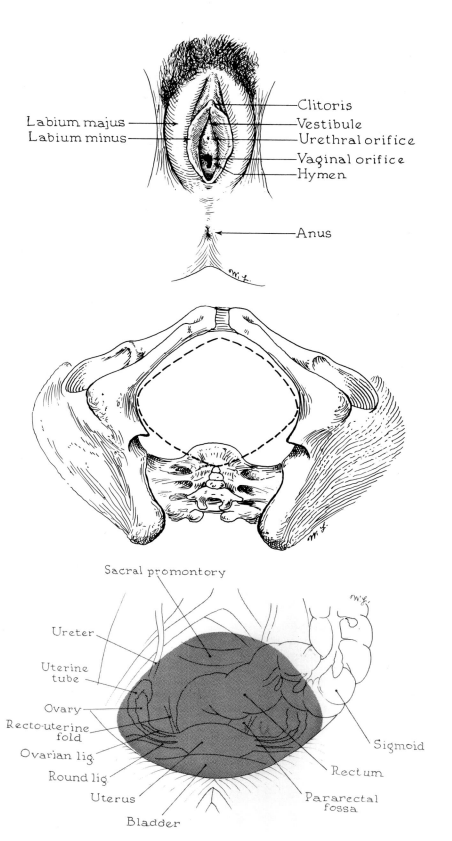

Clitoris
Labium majus
Vestibule
Labium minus
Urethral orifice
Vaginal orifice
Hymen

Anus

Sacral promontory

Ureter

Uterine
tube

Ovary

Recto-uterine
fold

Ovarian lig.

Round lig.

Uterus

Bladder

Sigmoid

Rectum

Pararectal
fossa

FIGURE XXV-20a–c. Anatomical sketches of pelvis and pelvic contents, indicating lines of dissection.

CHECK OF STOMACH CONTENTS FOR CRYSTALLINE MATERIAL

Inspection of the stomach contents is part of every autopsy and the results should be recorded. The nature of the contents indicates the type of food ingested at the last meal. The amount of stomach contents and the extent of their digestion may be helpful in estimating the time of death. It should be noted however, that slow digestion of stomach contents continues for some time after death.

By the same token, we have observed nearly undigested appearing stomach contents in autopsies of individuals who were maintained on life support for several days.

Preservation of stomach contents for subsequent chemical analyses is recommended whenever ingestion of a poison is suspected. During the autopsy, the liquid part of the stomach contents is placed in a glass funnel, the outlet of which has been sealed. Crystalline material mixed with the stomach contents will settle to the bottom of the container (Fig. XXV-21). The supernatant fluid is removed, and the crystalline material may be examined microscopically. Occasionally, the presence of crystals of familiar shape and color may direct the chemist to a specific analysis. Additional information regarding the probability of suicide versus accident may be derived from the amount of crystalline material that has settled to the bottom of the funnel. A large quantity of crystalline material tends to favor the assumption of suicidal poisoning, since it is unlikely that a large number of tablets could be ingested accidentally.

Fats in normal stomach contents sometimes convert to soaps, which settle in a manner similar to that of crystalline material. Microscopic examination of the sediment may be required to distinguish between such soaps and crystals.

COLLECTION OF BLOOD FOR TOXICOLOGICAL ANALYSIS BEFORE AUTOPSY

Collection of a postmortem blood specimen for toxicological analysis, specifically for determination of the alcohol concentration, requires special care to avoid contamination.

In the case in which a blood specimen was obtained from the heart, where no autopsy has been performed, it could be argued that the 13 gauge, 3.5" long needle went through the heart and part of the sample, however small, was actually drawn from the esophagus, situated directly behind the heart. Liquid gastric contents will run up the esophagus in a recumbent body, after muscular rigidity has passed and the gastroesophageal sphincter has relaxed.

To avoid any such allegation it is best if the specimen is obtained from a location removed from any possible source of contamination. Two such locations are suggested:

1. The groin area, where the blood is obtained from the femoral artery or vein.
2. The supraclavicular area, where the blood is obtained from the subclavian artery or vein.

Directing the needle downward and under the medial third of the clavicle will likely puncture the subclavian vein; placement of the needle at the clavicular midpoint will puncture the subclavian artery. The scalene anterior muscle, which inserts on the first rib, serves as a landmark separating the subclavian artery from the subclavian vein (Fig. XXV-22).

TOXICOLOGICAL ANALYSIS OF SKELETAL REMAINS

The biblical adage *"ashes to ashes and dust to dust"* holds true in regards to the postmortem examination of skeletal remains. When all organic matter has decomposed and been eliminated the skeleton is all that is left to examine. Such examination may reveal no evidence of the cause

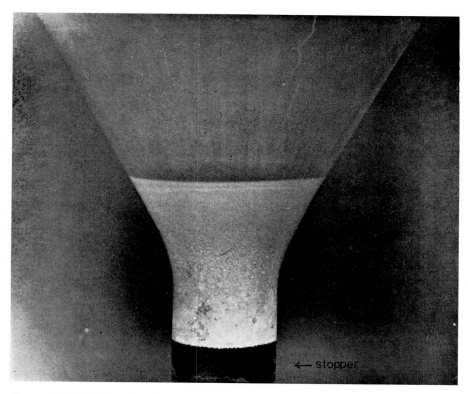

FIGURE XXV-21. Glass funnel containing stomach contents in a case of overdose of assorted pills and capsules. The large amount of crystalline material is suggestive of suicide.

of death. However, the skeleton may still contain material likely to be of toxicological significance. Non-decomposing inorganic salts would be preserved for years in skeletal remains, available for chemical analysis.

The skeleton of a 16-year-old boy who had been missing from his home in Michigan for close to four years was found buried in a shallow grave on a mountain side of Southern California. The local coroner determined that the skeleton was intact and no cause of death could be ascertained. The remains were released to the family for burial in the family's grave site in the Detroit area. Six months later at the behest of the prosecutor the body was exhumed and reexamined.

The skull was now opened and a 25-gram *cake* of dry, mud-like substance was found adherent to the petrous por- tion of one of the temporal bones. Chemical analysis of this material revealed a large amount of pentobarbital. Also, the femur and humerus were sawed open along the long axis and the marrow cavity was scraped, rinsed and analyzed with the same results.

Whereas, it would not be possible to determine a reliable blood barbiturate concentration from the results of these analyses, it is likely that a high barbiturate blood level did exist and may have been the cause of death. Because, the young man had been known to abuse various drugs, including barbiturates the court dismissed charges against a defendant at the preliminary hearing.

COLLECTION AND PRESERVATION OF TOXICOLOGIC EVIDENCE*

The pathologist who performs a medicolegal autopsy has the responsibility of collecting and preserving specimens for toxicologic testing. All too frequently, inadequate samples are obtained.

---

* Adapted in part from *Guidelines for Preservation of Toxicologic Evidence*, previously authored by Henry C. Freimuth, Ph.D.

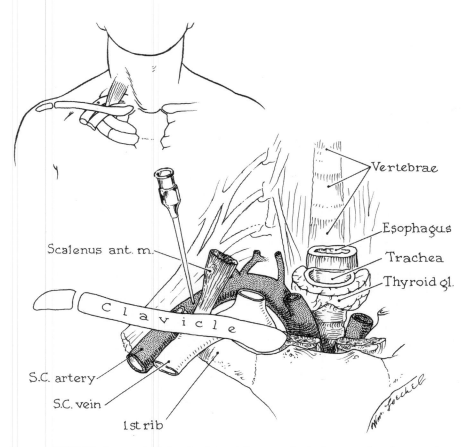

FIGURE XXV-22. Anatomical sketch of the right supraclavicular area showing puncture of the subclavian artery.

Generally, obtaining additional material after initial sample collection is impossible. It is suggested that the following samples be retained for analytical purposes: 50–100 mL of blood, 100 mL of urine or one-half a kidney if no urine is available, all of the gastric contents, all bile present in the gallbladder (many drugs are concentrated here), 50-100 grams of liver if the gallbladder is empty, 100 grams of brain, a sample of body fat, one lobe of lung (double bagged if analysis for volatiles is intended), samples of bone, finger and toe nails[10] and hair, in suspected drug abuse and chronic poisoning by metallic compounds, (segmental hair analysis provides estimates of extent and timing of drug exposure such as cocaine, heroin, methadone,[11] etc.), vitreous fluid, decomposition fluid, nasal swabs (for detection of drug snorting, such as cocaine, etc.), and maggots.[12]

Sub or epidural hematomas should be labeled as such and should also be submitted for analysis. These specimens reflect the alcohol and drug levels at the time of bleeding (not at the time of death), which is important in cases of some survival time.[13]

Each of the samples itemized should be placed in a separate container, sealed and refrigerated, or frozen without delay. Blood which is promptly analyzed needs no addition of chemical preservatives.

Certain drugs change characteristics and in some, drug levels are significantly reduced if left at room temperature. Cocaine in particular, falls into this category and although sodium fluoride retards the process, it does not prevent it from occurring. It has been reported that with storage at 4° C, blood containing 1 mg/L of cocaine lost 100% of the drug in 21 days, whereas with 0.5%

sodium fluoride 70% of the cocaine was still intact.[14]

Chemically clean plastic bags and vials make excellent containers since glass tends to break during freezing or thawing.

Each container should be labeled immediately, and the identification should bear the date and time of the autopsy, the name of the decedent, the identity of the sample and the signature of the pathologist.

When shipping specimens to a laboratory, freezing can be accomplished by packing the containers in dry ice. Samples that have been frozen and packed in this way can be transported to a laboratory even though a considerable distance or time delay might be involved. An adequate chain of custody of the specimens submitted for analysis must be maintained at all times.

The sealed containers, when they are delivered to the laboratory, should be received by the toxicologist, who then makes a record of the identities and nature of the specimens submitted, together with the date and time of their receipt and the name of the person delivering them. In the laboratory, the specimens are best stored in a locked refrigerator or freezer. In most laboratories the specimens are given an accession number when they are received, and thereafter they are handled under this number. It is important for the analyst to record the weights or volumes of any samples used in the various steps in the procedure. It is also important that the date of the analysis be recorded and that at least one-third of the original sample be preserved for possible use by another toxicologist if such is required at a later time.

In the majority of cases that involve poisoning as a cause of death, a specific substance is suspected as the causative agent and a direct analysis for such a substance can be made. The failure to find containers from which a drug or poison may have been taken suggests the need for a more thorough police investigation which may yield information leading to proof of homicide, rather than suicide or accidental overdose.

A case of homicidal poisoning with potassium cyanide developed on the basis of such an investigation. It involved the death of a woman in her seventh month of pregnancy. It was originally believed that her death had resulted from suicidal ingestion of potassium cyanide. This was supported by the finding at the scene of an unmailed letter in the handwriting of the deceased. Although this letter did not contain direct statements that the woman was going to take her own life, the general tenor of the writing suggested that the woman was in a state of agitated depression. The police were requested to search the scene for empty or partially filled containers from which the potassium cyanide may have been taken. Such a container could be expected to be present, since most persons who commit suicide with a poison, particularly with a cyanide, have neither the time nor the interest to dispose of the container. The result of this search of the scene was the finding only of some empty gelatin capsules and similar gelatin capsules that had been filled with quinine sulfate. No potassium cyanide was found in the home.

The police then began a more thorough investigation, which ultimately disclosed that the woman and her husband had been having marital difficulties, even to the point of physical violence perpetrated by the latter. A routine background check among employees of the Municipal Department of Public Works, where the husband was employed, disclosed that he had been making inquiries of a chemist in the department concerning *good poisons*. He had been told that potassium cyanide was such a substance. The police obtained the bottle of potassium cyanide reagent from the laboratory shelf and were able to develop a thumb and forefinger impression of the husband. Since the man was not employed in the laboratory, this suggested that he may have stolen some potassium cyanide from the bottle.

When confronted with this information, the man admitted the theft, although he claimed that he had done this because it was his intent to commit suicide to get away from his unhappy domestic situation. He claimed that he had filled two capsules with potassium cyanide and placed these in a dresser drawer, where there were other, similar capsules containing quinine sulfate that his wife was in the habit of taking for colds and muscle aches. His wife must have mistakenly taken the potassium cyanide capsules and thereby met her death. The man was ultimately convicted of manslaughter.

Poisoning as a possible cause of death is usually indicated by the history of the case or by gross or microscopic pathologic findings or the lack thereof. Just as the pathologist should not approach an autopsy without some preliminary background investigation, so, too, should the toxicologist not begin an analysis without having available as complete a history as possible. Toxicological analyses are quite time-consuming, and any information or aid that might shorten the procedure is most desirable. The history should generally include the following information:

1. A clinical history, obtainable either from an attending physician or from members of the family or friends of the decedent.
2. The occupation of the decedent, with a detailed description of the duties performed in this occupation.
3. Any treatment administered either for some illness, or as an antidote for a suspected poison.
4. The nature of food or drink last taken.
5. A description of gross autopsy findings.
6. Time relationships involved between the onset of symptoms, if any, and death.

Such a history will frequently suggest or rule out specific toxic agents. As an illustration, it would be futile to analyze for volatile toxic substances or for most organic drugs in a case in which an individual has been hospitalized for several weeks prior to death. During such an interval substances of this type would have been metabolized and eliminated from the body. The only toxic substances that might be detectable in such cases would be metallic poisons.

In some cases there may be no anatomic cause of death discoverable as the result of an autopsy and no information concerning the background of the deceased and the factors surrounding the death. The individual toxicologist's approach to such a problem varies and will be modified by the geographic area in which the death occurred. The availability and prevalence of use of certain substances in a particular location would make it necessary to include such substances in the general search procedure, while these same substances might not even be considered as possibilities in other areas. For example, in a highly agricultural environment organic phosphate insecticides are of major concern, whereas these same compounds are not considered a problem in most urban areas.

The most informative autopsy is one that is performed on a fresh, unembalmed body. This is especially true in cases involving possible poisoning. The embalming process will interfere with both the qualitative identification of poisons and their quantitation. Embalming, which essentially replaces most of the body's blood with a solution consisting of formaldehyde, methanol, sometime isopropyl alcohol, and small quantities of various other chemicals, materially affects the interpreta-

tion of any positive toxicological findings. As typical examples, cyanides react chemically with formaldehyde in the embalming fluid so that some are no longer identifiable, while others, are produced, albeit in trace quantities. Norpropoxyphene is converted to propoxyphene (Darvon®) in the presence of formaldehyde. Fixation of tissues by formaldehyde makes extraction procedures with organic solvents significantly less efficient. Since such extraction is involved in the separation of many organic drugs, no or low recoveries of such substances may result.

As to alcohol, embalming need not necessarily alter its concentration in body tissues. Ethyl alcohol (ethanol) is not a standard component of embalming fluids in the United States. Ethanol is a controlled substance, costly and requires permits, licenses and extensive record keeping. Caution is warranted however, since, ethanol is used in embalming fluids made in other countries; ethanol preserves the tissues and maintains the natural color of the body while it lacks the odor of formaldehyde.

In cases involving investigation of death after disinterment, where avoidance of the embalming process is not possible, it is imperative that a sample of any embalming fluids used in preparing the body for burial, be used as control, should any positive chemical findings be obtained.

The use of vitreous humor as a sample for chemical analysis in cases that involve embalming or putrefaction prior to autopsy merits some mention. It has been shown that vitreous humor may be used for analysis for a wide variety of substances of toxicological significance, including barbiturates, meprobamate, propoxyphene, pentazocine, amphetamines, digoxin and others.

As to alcohol, after consumption of alcoholic beverages on an empty stomach, it takes 15–20 minutes until absorption. It takes 45 minutes to one hour for alcohol to show up in the vitreous. Consequently, the absence of alcohol in the vitreous, must be interpreted with care, since consumption of a large quantity of alcohol over a short period of time prior to death, may result in an appreciable blood alcohol concentration, while the vitreous alcohol remains negative.

Another complicating factor in toxicological analysis is encountered when dealing with decomposed bodies. During the putrefactive process many substances that might be present in tissues undergo chemical changes, so that the parent substance may no longer be identifiable by chemical tests. Further, the putrefactive process may result in the production of substances from normal tissue components that give chemical reactions quite similar to those obtained from toxic compounds. The majority of volatile toxic substances would be lost as the result of putrefaction, while some, such as ethyl alcohol and cyanide, may be produced from normal tissue components. Although, as indicated above, the amount of cyanide so produced is in trace quantities, alcohol produced by fermentation in cases of advanced putrefaction may exceed 0.10%. Such factors may obviously lead to serious difficulties in interpretation of analytical results.

Despite the limitations placed upon the analyst by the embalming process or putrefaction, many toxic substances are still detectable. These include carbon monoxide (provided intact red blood cells are still available—the spleen may be a suitable source), fluoride, relatively stable organic compounds, such as strychnine and some barbiturates, yellow phosphorus and heavy metals, such as arsenic, lead, mercury and thallium.

Lastly, inorganic salts left behind within skeletal remains after putrefaction is complete are available for toxicological analysis. A small mass of such material may be found adherent to the interior of a previously unopened skull. Washings of the marrow cavity of long bones may also be expected to contain large quantities of the same substances (see Chapter XXV, "Toxicological Analysis of Skeletal Remains").

AUTOPSY ROOM PHOTOGRAPHY

It is unfortunate that, in spite of the popularity of amateur photography, photographic documentation of medicolegal autopsies often remains inadequate. The following are suggestions for those who wish to document pertinent findings at a postmortem examination. It would seem that these principles are to a large extent self-evident; however, experience has shown that they are practiced quite infrequently.

1. Photographs of the victim are often unsuitable because the camera is held at an incorrect angle to the body. For instance, a photograph taken from the foot end or sideways of the body on the autopsy table shows big feet and a small head and is of no real value for documentation of the upper half of the body. This is often referred to as *perspective distortion,* even though it is not a true distortion.

This fault can be readily remedied by taking the photograph from above, at right angles to the body (Fig. XXV-23). Adequate results may be obtained, by using a freestanding 6 foot ladder and a 35-mm camera. A single-lens-reflex camera is recommended.

2. Photographs of the victim must not be too gory, especially when in color. Photographs showing abundant blood on the body or the background are often considered offensive. A clean sheet of material or paper used as backdrop will be less distracting and help obtain a clearer and less gruesome picture. All extraneous objects, such as scalpels and scissors, must be rigorously excluded in case the photographs may be submitted in evidence. Many courts will object to the admission of unduly offensive photographs on the grounds that their probative value is outweighed by their prejudicial effect.

All hospital bandages and wrappings should be removed from the area to be photographed. The body must be wiped and dry blood adherent to the surface washed off to show all particulars. Care must be taken not to remove evidence of close-range gunfire when the body is prepared for photography. The case number and/or date and a scale of size suitable for the subject being photographed should be included in the picture. These should be clearly legible and positioned in the same plane as the principal points of interest. The case number is best placed in a corner or along one edge of the photograph, making it possible to cut it off should this become necessary at a later time. Suitable scales are available com-

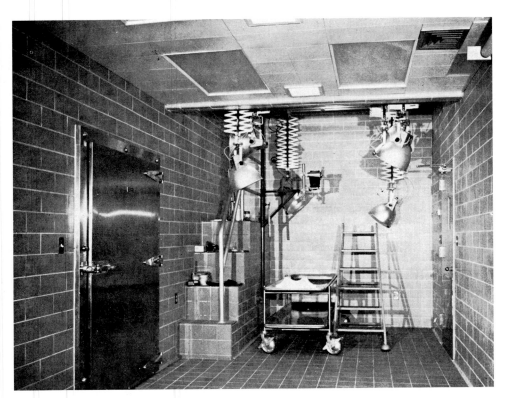

FIGURE XXV-23. Photography area of the Maryland Medical Examiner's Office. This setup has been found most advantageous.

mercially or can be made as required. A pointer, such as a narrow triangle of thin cardboard, may be used where a lesion is not readily discernible.

3. In cases of violent death, front and back of the dressed, uncleaned and nude body are recommended. It is often important to show the condition of the body when first viewed by the pathologist.

Two photographs are mandatory of the nude body: (a) distant, to indicate the location of the injuries; (b) close-up of major wounds, to show details. The close-up photograph must give the viewer a clear concept of the exact location of the injury on the body.

4. Personal identification of the victim is often made possible by a photograph of the face. Repair of facial injuries and application of make-up by a well-qualified mortician may be helpful.

Any identification photograph of a face should be taken with a lens of longer focal length than normal (e.g., 105 to 135-mm lens on 35-mm camera) to reduce distortion. Many close-up lenses

used in laboratories for specimen photography have a short focal length and cause significant distortion of features whenever the camera is moved close in order to fill the frame. Professional portrait photographers often use lenses with long focal length to cut down on such artifacts.

5. Tattoos are frequently important for identification of an unknown victim. Excessive pigmentation of the skin may obscure a tattoo. The same is true of an old tattoo which has faded. Removal of the superficial layers of the skin has proven to be advantageous in enhancing the tattooed image and enable superior documentation photographically. This is best done by producing a second-degree burn of the area, then removing by wiping the detached epidermis. Holding a hot light bulb 4–5 inches directly above the tattooed area will produce the desired effect in 2–3 minutes (Fig. XXV-24).

An incidental observation is that tattoos frequently fade with time and may even disappear

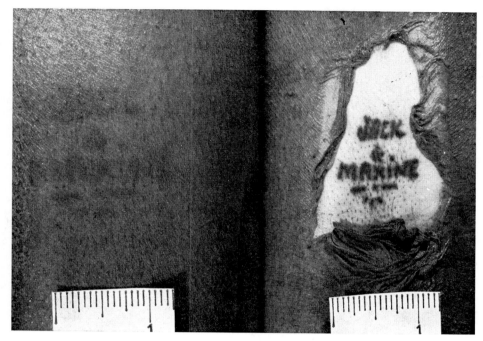

FIGURE XXV-24. Forearm of a black male. Left: Illegible tattoo. Right: Same tattoo after removal of epidermis, made possible by application of heat to the skin using a 100 watt lamp for five minutes from a distance of 6 inches.

entirely. This particularly applies to *homemade tattoos,* as are often produced in jails. In such tattoos the amount of pigment in the skin is usually much less than in tattoos made professionally. Thus, a tattoo described by relatives that is absent at the autopsy could lead to mistaken identification, unless it is realized that the pigment may have moved to the regional lymph nodes, in which it can be detected microscopically.

In a mummified body, immersion of the area believed to be tattooed in warm or hot water for as long as several hours, then scraping with a scalpel, may sometimes help remove the epidermis and significantly improve the image.

REFERENCES

1. Spitz, W. U., Sopher, I.M., and DiMaio, V. J. M.: Medicolegal investigation of a bomb explosion in an automobile. *J Forensic Sci, 15:* 537, 1970.
2. Cain, C. M. J., Simpson, M. S., Ryan, G. A., Manock, C. H., and James, R. A.: Road crash cervical injuries: A radiological study of fatalities. *Am J Forensic Med Path, 10* (3): 193–195, 1989.
3. Contostavols, D. L.: Massive subarachnoid hemorrhage due to laceration of the vertebral artery associated with fracture of the transverse process of the atlas. *J Forensic Sci, 16:* 50–56, 1971.
4. Johnson, C. P., How, T., Scraggs, M., West, C. R., and Burns, J.: A biomedical study of the human vertebral artery with implications for fatal arterial injury. *Forensic Sci International, 109:* 169–182, 2000.
5. Kernohan, J. W.: Removal of the spinal cord by the anterior route: A new postmortem method. *Am J Clin Pathol, 3:* 455, 1933.
6. Groth, A. N., and Burgess, A. W.: Sexual dysfunction during rape. *N Engl J Med, 297:* 764–766, 1977.
7. Wilson, E. T.: Sperm morphologic survival after 16 days in the vagina of a dead body. *J Forensic Sci, 19:* 561–564, 1974.
8. Findley, T. P.: Quantitation of vaginal acid phosphatase and its relationship to time of coitus. *Am J Clin Pathol, 68:* 238–242, 1977.

9. Standefer, J. C., and Street, E. W.: Postmortem stability of prostatic acid phosphatase. *J Forensic Sci, 22:* 163, 1973.

10. Garside, D., Ropero-Miller, J. D., Goldberger, B. A., Hamilton, W. F., and Maples, W. R.: Identification of cocaine analytes in fingernail and toenail specimens. *J Forensic Sci, 43* (5): 974–979, 1998.

11. Goldberger, B. A., Darraj, A. G., Caplan, Y. H., and Cone, E. J.: Detection of methadone, methadone metabolites, and other illicit drugs of abuse in hair of methadone-treatment subjects. *J Anal Tox, 22:* 526–530, 1998.

12. Levine, B., Golle, M., and Smialek, J. E.: An unusual drug death involving maggots. *Am J Forensic Med Path, 21* (1): 59–61, 2000.

13. Cassin, B., and Spitz, W. U.: Concentration of alcohol in delayed subdural hematoma. *J Forensic Sci, 28* (4): 1013–1015, 1983.

14. Baselt, R. C.: *Disposition of toxic drugs and chemicals in man,* Fifth Edition. Foster City, CA: Chemical Toxicology Institute, 2000.

INDEX